Current Veterinary Therapy

FOOD ANIMAL PRACTICE

Current Veterinary Therapy

FOOD ANIMAL PRACTICE

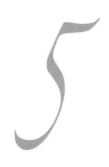

5

DAVID E. ANDERSON, DVM, MS, Diplomate ACVS
Professor and Section Head, Agricultural Practices
Department of Clinical Sciences
Kansas State University
College of Veterinary Medicine
Manhattan, Kansas

D. MICHAEL RINGS, DVM, MS, Diplomate ACVIM
Department of Veterinary Clinical Sciences
College of Veterinary Medicine
The Ohio State University
Columbus, Ohio

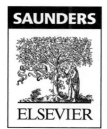

SAUNDERS

ELSEVIER

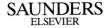

SAUNDERS
ELSEVIER

11830 Westline Industrial Drive
St. Louis, Missouri 63146

CURRENT VETERINARY THERAPY: FOOD ANIMAL PRACTICE, Fifth Volume   ISBN: 978-1-4160-3591-6
Copyright © 2009, 1999, 1993, 1986, 1981 by Saunders, an imprint of Elsevier Inc.

Notice

Knowledge and best practice in this field are constantly changing. As new research and experience broaden our knowledge, changes in practice, treatment, and drug therapy may become necessary or appropriate. Readers are advised to check the most current information provided (i) on procedures featured or (ii) by the manufacturer of each product to be administered, to verify the recommended dose or formula, the method and duration of administration, and contraindications. It is the responsibility of the practitioner, relying on their own experience and knowledge of the patient, to make diagnoses, to determine dosages and the best treatment for each individual patient, and to take all appropriate safety precautions. To the fullest extent of the law, neither the Publisher nor the Authors assume any liability for any injury and/or damage to persons or property arising out of or related to any use of the material contained in this book.

The Publisher

International Standard Serial Number: 1043-139X

Vice President and Publisher: Linda Duncan
Publisher: Penny Rudolph
Managing Editor: Teri Merchant
Publishing Services Manager: Patricia Tannian
Senior Project Manager: Anne Altepeter
Designer: Paula Catalano

Printed in the United States of America

Last digit is the print number: 9   8   7   6   5   4   3   2   1

To my wife, Lane, and sons, John and Jacob, whose understanding and support made this work possible; to the many teachers, especially Elaine Hunt and Guy St-Jean, who inspired me to accept Food Animal as a career choice; and to the many veterinary students who have continually challenged me to ask "why" or "why not"

DEA

To the many large-animal veterinarians who helped me in my academic career, especially Drs. Vernon Tharp, James C. Donham, Vaughn Larson, and Glen Hoffsis; and to my wife, Marylou, with thanks for her continued patience and love

DMR

Contributors

Eric J. Abrahamsen, DVM, Diplomate ACVA
Anesthesiologist
Ocala Equine Hospital
Ocala, Florida
Chemical Restraint in Ruminants
Inhalation Anesthesia in Ruminants
Managing Severe Pain in Ruminants
Ruminant Field Anesthesia

David E. Anderson, DVM, MS, Diplomate ACVS
Professor and Section Head, Agricultural Practices
Department of Clinical Sciences
Kansas State University
College of Veterinary Medicine
Manhattan, Kansas
Duodenal Obstruction
Fracture Management in Cattle
Intestinal Atresia
Intestinal Volvulus
Intussusception
Laparoscopic Abomasopexy for Correction of Left Displaced Abomasum
Pathophysiology of Displacement of the Abomasum in Cattle
Rectal Prolapse
Surgery of the Larynx and Trachea
Thoracic Surgery in Cattle
Trichobezoars
Umbilical Surgery in Calves
Vaginal and Uterine Prolapse

Michael D. Apley, DVM, PhD, Diplomate ACVCP
Associate Professor
Department of Clinical Sciences
Kansas State University College of Veterinary Medicine
Manhattan, Kansas
Feedlot Therapeutic Protocols

A. Catherine Barr, PhD, Diplomate ABT
Veterinary Toxicologist
Texas Veterinary Medical Diagnostic Laboratory
College Station, Texas
Hepatotoxicities of Ruminants

Ellen B. Belknap, MS, DVM, Diplomate ACVO
Metropolitan Veterinary Hospital
Akron, Ohio
Food Animal Ocular Neoplasia

Joachim F. Berchtold, Dr Med Vet, Diplomate ECBHM
Tierärztliche Gemeinschaftspraxis
Obing, Germany
Antibiotic Treatment of Diarrhea in Preweaned Calves

Joan S. Bowen, DVM
Bowen Mobile Veterinary Practice
Wellington, Colorado
Ethical Responsibilities of Small Ruminant Veterinarians in Selecting and Using Therapeutics

Carmen M.H. Colitz, DVM, PhD, Diplomate ACVO
Animal Eye Specialty Clinic
West Palm Beach, Florida
Adjunct Associate Professor
The Ohio State University
Columbus, Ohio
Food Animal Ocular Neoplasia

Michael T. Collins, DVM, PhD, Diplomate ACVM
Professor of Microbiology
Department of Pathobiological Sciences
School of Veterinary Medicine
Madison, Wisconsin
Johne's Disease (Paratuberculosis)

Anthony W. Confer, DVM, PhD, Diplomate ACVP
Regents Professor, Head, and Sitlington Endowed Chair
Department of Veterinary Pathobiology
Center for Veterinary Health Sciences
Oklahoma State University
Stillwater, Oklahoma
Mannheimia haemolytica– and Pasteurella multocida– Induced Bovine Pneumonia

Maren J. Connolly, DVM
Food Animal Intern, Department of Veterinary Clinical Sciences
Iowa State University, College of Veterinary Medicine
Ames, Iowa
Ruminal Acidosis and Rumenitis

Peter D. Constable, BVSc, MS, PhD, Diplomate ACVIM
Professor and Head
Department of Veterinary Clinical Sciences
Purdue University
West Lafayette, Indiana
Antibiotic Treatment of Diarrhea in Preweaned Calves
Function and Dysfunction of the Ruminant Forestomach

Marilyn J. Corbin, DVM, MS, PhD
Beef Cattle Technical Consultant
Elanco Animal Health
Calhan, Colorado
An Economic Risk Assessment Model for Management of Pregnant Feeder Heifers

Thomas M. Craig, DVM, PhD
Professor
Department of Veterinary Pathobiology
Texas A&M University
College Station, Texas
Helminth Parasites of the Ruminant Gastrointestinal Tract
Gastrointestinal Protozoal Infections in Ruminants

Harriet J. Davidson, MS, DVM, Diplomate ACVO
Adjunct Professor
Kansas State University
College of Veterinary Medicine
Manhattan, Kansas
Michigan Veterinary Specialists
Grand Rapids, Michigan
Ophthalmic Examination Techniques for Production
  Animals
Ophthalmic Therapeutics
Selected Eye Diseases of Cattle
Selected Eye Diseases of Sheep and Goats
Selected Eye Diseases of Swine

André Desrochers, DMV, MS, Diplomate ACVS
Professor
Départment de Science Clinique
Faculté de Médecine Vétérinaire
Université de Montréal
St-Hyacinthe, Quebec, Canada
Coxofemoral Luxation
Ligament Injuries of the Stifle

Thomas J. Doherty, MVB, MSc, Diplomate ACVA
Professor
Department of Large Animal Clinical Sciences
University of Tennessee
Knoxville, Tennessee
Pain Management in Cattle and Small Ruminants

Pascal Dubreuil, DMV, PhD
Professor
Department of Clinical Sciences
Faculty of Veterinary Medicine
Université de Montréal
St-Hyacinthe, Quebec, Canada
Small Ruminant Infectious Disease of the Foot

Misty A. Edmondson, DVM, MS, Diplomate ACT
Assistant Professor, Food Animal Section
Department of Clinical Sciences
Auburn University
Auburn, Alabama
Diagnosis and Management of Injuries to the Penis and
  Prepuce of Bulls
Pregnancy Toxemia in Sheep and Goats

Ronald J. Erskine, DVM, PhD
Professor
Department of Large Animal Clinical Sciences
Michigan State University
East Lansing, Michigan
Decision Making in Mastitis Therapy

Jennifer Ivany Ewoldt, DVM, MS, Diplomate ACVS
Scott County Animal Hospital, PC
Eldridge, Iowa
Surgery of the Urinary Tract

Virginia R. Fajt, DVM, PhD, DACVCP
Clinical Assistant Professor
Department of Veterinary Physiology and
  Pharmacology
Texas A&M University
College Station, Texas
Evidence-Based Veterinary Medicine: Therapeutic
  Considerations

Gilles Fecteau, Diplomate ACVIM
Professeur titulaire
Départment de Science Clinique
Faculté de Médecine Vétérinaire
Université de Montréal
St-Hyacinthe, Quebec, Canada
Central Nervous System Infection and Infestation
Mentation Abnormality, Depression, and Cortical
  Blindness

Marie-Eve Fecteau, DVM, Diplomate ACVIM
Assistant Professor of Food Animal Medicine and
  Surgery
University of Pennsylvania
New Bolton Center
Kennett Square, Pennsylvania
Abomasal Ulcers
Muscular Tone and Gait Abnormalities

Sherrill Fleming, DVM, Diplomate ACVIM, ABVP
  (Food Animal)
Associate Professor, Food Animal Medicine,
Department of Pathobiology and Population Medicine
College of Veterinary Medicine
Mississippi State University
Mississippi State, Mississippi
Ovine and Caprine Respiratory Disease: Infectious Agents,
  Management Factors, and Preventive Strategies

David Francoz, DMV, MSc, Diplomate ACVIM
Assistant Professor
Départment de Science Clinique
Faculté de Médecine Vétérinaire
Université de Montréal
St-Hyacinthe, Quebec, Canada
Ancillary Tests
Cranial Nerve Abnormalities
Muscular Tone and Gait Abnormalities
  (part titled Tremors)
Septic Arthritis in Cattle

Deborah S. Friedman, DVM, Diplomate ACVO
Animal Eye Care
Fremont, California
Ophthalmology of South American Camelids: Llamas,
  Alpacas, Guanacos, and Vicuñas

Robert W. Fulton, DVM, PhD, Diplomate ACVM
McCasland Foundation Endowed Chair for Food Animal
   Research
Department of Veterinary Pathobiology
Center for Veterinary Health Sciences
Oklahoma State University
Stillwater, Oklahoma
Viral Diseases of the Bovine Respiratory Tract

Franklyn B. Garry, DVM, MS, Diplomate ACVIM
Professor
Department of Clinical Sciences
College of Veterinary Medicine and Biomedical
   Sciences
Colorado State University
Fort Collins, Colorado
Rumen Indigestion and Putrefaction

Ronette Gehring, BVSc, MMedVet (Pharm)
Assistant Professor
Department of Clinical Sciences
Section of Agricultural Practices
Kansas State University
Manhattan, Kansas
*Practical Pharmacokinetics for the Food Animal
   Practitioner*

Lisle W. George, DVM, PhD, Diplomate ACVIM
Professor
University of California—Davis
School of Veterinary Medicine
Davis, California
*Central Nervous System Infection and Infestation
Mentation Abnormality, Depression, and Cortical
   Blindness*

Brian J. Gerloff, DVM, PhD
Owner, Seneca Bovine Services
Marengo, Illinois
*Fatty Liver in Dairy Cattle
Ketosis*

Juliet R. Gionfriddo, DVM, MS, Diplomate ACVO
Associate Professor
Colorado State University
Fort Collins, Colorado
*Ophthalmology of South American Camelids: Llamas,
   Alpacas, Guanacos, and Vicuñas*

Jesse P. Goff, DVM, PhD
Director of Research & Development
West Central Cooperative
Ralston, Iowa
*Milk Fever (Parturient Paresis) in Cows, Ewes, and
      Doe Goats
Phosphorus Deficiency
Ruminant Hypomagnesemic Tetanies*

Janey L. Gordon, DVM
Herrington, Kansas
Feedlot Vaccination Protocols

Dee Griffin, DVM, MS
University of Nebraska—Lincoln
Great Plains Veterinary Educational Center
Clay Center, Nebraska
*Cow-Calf Operation Beef Quality Assurance
No Loose Parts Necropsy Procedure for the Feedyard
Respiratory Disease Treatment Considerations in
   Feedyards*

**Walter Grünberg, Dr med vet, MS, Diplomate ECAR,
   and ECBHM**
Visiting Clinical Instructor
Department of Veterinary Clinical Sciences
Purdue University
West Lafayette, Indiana
Function and Dysfunction of the Ruminant Forestomach

**Thomas H. Herdt, DVM, MS, Diplomate ACVN,
   ACVIM**
Nutrition Section
Diagnostic Center for Population and Animal Health
Michigan State University
East Lansing, Michigan
*Clinical Use of Ultrasound for Subcutaneous Fat Thickness
   Measurements in Dairy Cattle
Fatty Liver in Dairy Cattle
Ketosis*

W. Mark Hilton, DVM, Diplomate ABVP (Beef)
Clinical Associate Professor, Beef Production Medicine
Purdue University, VCS—LYNN
West Lafayette, Indiana
*Marketing Beef Cow-Calf Production Medicine Programs in
   Private Practice*

Larry C. Hollis, DVM, MAg
Extension Beef Veterinarian
Kansas State University
Manhattan, Kansas
Investigating Feedlot Respiratory Disease Outbreaks

John House, BVMS, PhD, Diplomate ACVIM
Associate Professor
Livestock Veterinary Teaching and Research Unit
University of Sydney
Camden, New South Wales, Australia
Salmonellosis in Ruminants

Bruce L. Hull, DVM, MS, Diplomate ACVS
Professor Emeritus
Department of Veterinary Clinical Sciences
College of Veterinary Medicine
The Ohio State University
Columbus, Ohio
Disorders of the Upper Respiratory Tract in Food Animals

Laura L. Hungerford, PhD, DVM, MPH
Department of Epidemiology and Preventive Medicine
University of Maryland School of Medicine
Baltimore, Maryland
*An Economic Risk Assessment Model for Management of
   Pregnant Feeder Heifers*

Bradley J. Johnson, MS, PhD
Associate Professor
Animal Sciences and Industry
Kansas State University
Manhattan, Kansas
*Growth Promotants for Beef Production: Anabolic Steroids:
    Performance Responses and Mode of Action*

Meredyth L. Jones, DVM, MS, Diplomate ACVIM
Assistant Professor
Department of Clinical Sciences
Kansas State University
Manhattan, Kansas
Addressing High Dystocia Incidence in Cow-Calf Herds
Ulcerative Posthitis
Urolithiasis

Nanda P. Joshi, PhD
Assistant Professor
College of Veterinary Medicine
Michigan State University
East Lansing, Michigan
*Clinical Use of Ultrasound for Subcutaneous Fat Thickness
    Measurements in Dairy Cattle*

Ray M. Kaplan, DVM, PhD, Diplomate EVPC
Associate Professor
Department of Infectious Diseases
College of Veterinary Medicine
University of Georgia
Athens, Georgia
Anthelmintic Treatment in the Era of Resistance

Hubert J. Karreman, VMD
Affiliate Assistant Professor
Department of Animal and Nutritional Sciences
University of New Hampshire
Dairy Practitioner
Penn Dutch Cow Care, Owner
Quarryville, Pennsylvania
Therapeutic Options in Organic Livestock Medicine

**Thomas R. Kasari, DVM, MVSc, MBA, CPA, Diplomate
    ACVIM, ACVPM (Epidemiology)**
Agrivet Solutions, LLC
Fort Collins, Colorado
*Economic Analysis Techniques for the Cow-Calf
    Practitioner*

Karl W. Kersting, DVM, MS
Veterinary Diagnostic and Production Animal
    Medicine
College of Veterinary Medicine
Iowa State University
Ames, Iowa
Ruminal Acidosis and Rumenitis

Shelie Laflin, DVM
Assistant Professor, Agricultural Practices
Kansas State University College of Veterinary Medicine
Manhattan, Kansas
*Carcass Ultrasound Uses in Beef Cattle Production
    Settings*

Jeffrey Lakritz, DVM, PhD, Diplomate ACVIM
Department of Veterinary Clinical Sciences
College of Veterinary Medicine
The Ohio State University
Columbus, Ohio
Disorders of the Upper Respiratory Tract in Food Animals

**Robert L. Larson, DVM, PhD, Diplomate ACT, ACAN,
    ACVPM**
Professor, Coleman Chair Food Animal Production
    Medicine
Department of Clinical Sciences
College of Veterinary Medicine
Kansas State University
Manhattan, Kansas
Addressing High Dystocia Incidence in Cow-Calf Herds
Beef Heifer Development
Evidence-Based Veterinary Medicine: Therapeutic Considerations
Preconditioned Calves in the Feedyard
Use of Statistical Process Control in Feedlot Practice

Lynn Locatelli, DVM
Benkelman, Nebraska
Low-Stress Livestock Handling

Herris S. Maxwell, DVM, Diplomate ACT
Clinical Assistant Professor
Department of Clinical Sciences
Food Animal Section
Auburn University
Auburn, Alabama
*Diagnosis and Management of Injuries to the Penis and
    Prepuce of Bulls*

Kathryn M. Meurs, DVM, PhD
Professor, Richard L. Ott Chair of Small Animal Medicine
    and Research
Veterinary Clinical Sciences
Washington State University College of Veterinary
    Medicine
Pullman, Washington
Acquired Heart Diseases in Cattle
Congenital Heart Disease in Cattle
Examination of the Bovine Patient with Heart Disease

Matt D. Miesner, DVM, MS, Diplomate ACVIM
Assistant Professor, Clinical
Department of Clinical Sciences
Agricultural Practices Section
Kansas State University
Manhattan, Kansas
Bovine Enzootic Hematuria
Urinary Tract Infection in Food Animals
Urolithiasis
Vaginal and Uterine Prolapse

Paul E. Miller, DVM, Diplomate ACVO
Clinical Professor of Comparative Ophthalmology
Department of Surgical Sciences
School of Veterinary Medicine
University of Wisconsin—Madison
Madison, Wisconsin
Neurogenic Vision Loss

Virginia L. Mohler, BVSc (Hons)
Resident
Livestock Veterinary Teaching and Research Unit
University of Sydney
Camden, New South Wales, Australia
Salmonellosis in Ruminants

Pierre-Yves Mulon, DMV, DES, Diplomate ACVS
Clinical Instructor
Centre Hospitalier Universitaire Vétérinaire
Faculté de Médecine Vétérinaire
Université de Montréal
St-Hyacinthe, Quebec, Canada
Hygroma of the Carpus and Tarsus
Osteochondrosis in Cattle

Christine B. Navarre, DMV, MS, Diplomate ACVIM
Professor
Department of Veterinary Science
Louisiana State University Agricultural Center
Baton Rouge, Louisiana
Fluid Therapy, Transfusion, and Shock Therapy

Jonathan M. Naylor, BVSc, PhD, Diplomate ACVN, ACVIM
Professor
Department of Clinical Sciences
Ross University School of Veterinary Medicine
St Kitts, West Indies
Neonatal Calf Diarrhea

Kenneth D. Newman, BSc(Agr), DVM, MS
Locum Veterinarian
Prescott Animal Hospital
Prescott, Ontario, Canada
Bovine Cesarean Sections: Risk Factors and Outcomes
Displacement of the Abomasum in Dairy Cattle
Laparoscopic Abomasopexy for Correction of Left
  Displaced Abomasum
Laparoscopy in Large Animal Surgery
Prognostic Indicators and Comparison of Corrective
  Fixation Technique for Displacement of the
  Abomasum in Dairy Cattle

Sylvain Nichols, DMV, MS, Diplomate ACVS
Adjunct Professor
Faculté de Médecine Vétérinaire
Université de Montréal
St-Hyacinthe, Quebec, Canada
Diagnosis and Management of Teat Injury

Andrew Niehaus, DVM, MS
Assistant Professor, Food Animal Surgery
The Ohio State University
Columbus, Ohio
Displaced Abomasum in Cattle
Rumenotomy and Rumenostomy

Tom Noffsinger, DVM
Beef Production Consultant
Benkelman, Nebraska
Low-Stress Livestock Handling

Bo Norby, CMV, MPVM, PhD
Assistant Professor in Epidemiology
Department of Veterinary Integrative Bioscience
College of Veterinary Medicine and Biomedical Sciences
Texas A&M University
College Station, Texas
Antimicrobial Resistance in Human Pathogens and the Use
  of Antimicrobials in Food Animals: Challenges in Food
  Animal Veterinary Practice

Karl Nuss, Dr Med Vet, Diplomate ECVS, Diplomate ECBHM
Professor of Surgery and Orthopedics
Clinic for Ruminants
Ludwig-Maximilians-Universität München
Munich, Germany
Surgery of the Bovine Digit

Garrett R. Oetzel, DVM, MS
Associate Professor
Food Animal Production Medicine Section
School of Veterinary Medicine
University of Wisconsin—Madison
Madison, Wisconsin
Milk Fever (Parturient Paresis) in Cows, Ewes, and
  Doe Goats

Jason Osterstock, DVM
Department of Large Animal Clinical Sciences
College of Veterinary Medicine and Biomedical
  Sciences
Texas A&M University
College Station, Texas
Investigation of Lameness Outbreaks in Feedlot Cattle

Joane Parent, DMV, MVetSc, Diplomate ACVIM (Neurology)
Professor
Départment de Science Clinique
Faculté de Médecine Vétérinaire
Université de Montréal
St-Hyacinthe, Quebec, Canada
Clinical Examination

Simon F. Peek, BVSc, MRCVS, PhD, Diplomate ACVIM, ECEIM
Clinical Professor
Department of Medical Sciences
School of Veterinary Medicine
University of Wisconsin—Madison
Madison, Wisconsin
Muscular Tone and Gait Abnormalities
  (section titled *Diseases of the Peripheral Nervous System*)

J. Phillip Pickett, DVM, Diplomate ACVO
Professor
VA-MD Regional College of Veterinary Medicine
Department of Clinical Sciences
Blacksburg, Virginia
Selected Eye Diseases of Cattle
Selected Eye Diseases of Sheep and Goats

David G. Pugh, DVM, MS, Diplomate ACT, ACVN
Veterinary Consultant
Waverly, Alabama
Pregnancy Toxemia in Sheep and Goats

Richard F. Randle, DVM, MS
Technical Services Specialist
Monsanto Dairy Business
Coldwater, Michigan
Neonatal Urinary Disorders

Christopher D. Reinhardt, PhD, MS
Assistant Professor
Animal Sciences and Industry
Kansas State University
Manhattan, Kansas
*Growth Promotants for Beef Production: Anabolic Steroids:
Performance Responses and Mode of Action*

M. Gatz Riddell, Jr., DVM, MS, Diplomate ACT
Executive Vice President
American Association of Bovine Practitioners
Professor Emeritus
Auburn University
Auburn, Alabama
*Ethical Responsibilities of Bovine Veterinarians in Selecting,
Prescribing, and Using Therapeutic Drugs*

D. Michael Rings, DVM, MS, Diplomate ACVIM
Department of Veterinary Clinical Sciences
College of Veterinary Medicine
The Ohio State University
Columbus, Ohio
Abomasal Emptying Defect in Sheep
Disorders of the Upper Respiratory Tract in Food Animals
Esophageal Obstructions/Choke
*Pharyngeal Lacerations and Retropharyngeal Abscesses in
Ruminants*
Umbilical Surgery in Calves

Soren P. Rodning, DVM, MS, Diplomate ACT
Assistant Professor and Extension Veterinarian
Department of Animal Sciences
College of Agriculture
Auburn University
Auburn, Alabama
Diagnosis and Management of Inguinal Hernia in Bulls
*Diagnosis and Management of Juvenile Anomalies of the
Penis and Prepuce*
Diagnosis and Management of Penile Deviations

Ricardo F. Rosenbusch, DVM, PhD, Diplomate ACVM
Professor
Department of Veterinary Microbiology and Preventive
Medicine
College of Veterinary Medicine
Iowa State University
Ames, Iowa
Mycoplasmas in Bovine Respiratory Disease

James A. Roth, DVM, PhD, Diplomate ACVM
Distinguished Professor
Department of Veterinary Microbiology and Preventive
Medicine
College of Veterinary Medicine
Iowa State University
Ames, Iowa
*Calf Preweaning Immunity and Impact on Vaccine
Schedules*

**Allen J. Roussel, Jr., DVM, MS, Diplomate ACVIM,
ECBHM**
Professor and Associate Department Head
Large Animal Clinical Sciences
Texas A&M University
College Station, Texas
Actinomycosis and Actinobacillosis
Fluid Therapy, Transfusion, and Shock Therapy

Linda J. Saif, MS, PhD, Honorary Diplomate ACVM
Distinguished University Professor
Food Animal Health Research Program
Veterinary Preventive Medicine Department
Ohio Agricultural Research and Development Center
The Ohio State University
Wooster, Ohio
Winter Dysentery

**Michael W. Sanderson, DVM, MS, Diplomate ACVPM
(Epidemiology), ACT**
Associate Professor
Department of Clinical Sciences
College of Veterinary Medicine
Kansas State University
Manhattan, Kansas
Biosecurity for Cow-Calf Enterprises
Biosecurity for Feedlot Enterprises

Kara Schulz, DVM
Clinical Instructor, Agricultural Practices
College of Veterinary Medicine
Kansas State University
Manhattan, Kansas
Ocular Surgery: Enucleation in Cattle

Jan K. Shearer, DVM, MS
Professor and Dairy Extension Veterinarian
Department of Large Animal Clinical Sciences
College of Veterinary Medicine
University of Florida
Gainesville, Florida
Infectious Disorders of the Foot Skin

**David R. Smith, DVM, PhD, Diplomate ACVPM
(Epidemiology)**
Professor and Extension Dairy/Beef Veterinarian
Department of Veterinary and Biomedical Sciences
University of Nebraska—Lincoln
Lincoln, Nebraska
Management of Neonatal Diarrhea in Cow-Calf Herds

Geoffrey Smith, DVM, PhD, Diplomate ACVIM
Associate Professor of Ruminant Medicine
Department of Population Health and Pathobiology
North Carolina State University
Raleigh, North Carolina
FARAD and Related Drug Regulations

Joe Snyder, DVM
Owner
Myrtle Veterinary Hospital
Myrtle Point, Oregon
Ethical Responsibilities of Small Ruminant Veterinarians in Selecting and Using Therapeutics

J. Glenn Songer, PhD
Professor
Department of Veterinary Science and Microbiology
The University of Arizona
Tucson, Arizona
Clostridial Enterotoxemia *(Clostridium perfringens)*
Clostridium novyi (Myonecrosis, Black Disease, and Bacillary Hemoglobinuria) and *Clostridium septicum* (Braxy) Infections

Adrian Steiner, Prof Dr med vet, MS, Diplomate ECVS, ECBHM
Vetsuisse-Faculty of Berne, Switzerland
Head of Clinic for Ruminants
Berne, Switzerland
Fracture Management in Cattle

Douglas L. Step, DVM, Diplomate ACVIM
Department of Veterinary Clinical Sciences
Veterinary Medical Teaching Hospital
Center for Veterinary Health Sciences
Oklahoma State University
Stillwater, Oklahoma
Mannheimia haemolytica– *and* Pasteurella multocida–*Induced Bovine Pneumonia*

Robert N. Streeter, DVM, MS, Diplomate ACVIM
Adjunct Associate Professor
Veterinary Clinical Sciences
Oklahoma State University
Stillwater, Oklahoma
Bloat or Ruminal Tympany

Raymond W. Sweeney, VMD, Diplomate ACVIM
Professor of Large Animal Medicine
University of Pennsylvania
New Bolton Center
Kennett Square, Pennsylvania
Muscular Tone and Gait Abnormalities

James R. Thompson, DVM, MS
Associate Professor
Veterinary Diagnostic and Production Animal Medicine
College of Veterinary Medicine
Iowa State University
Ames, Iowa
Ruminal Acidosis and Rumenitis

Daniel U. Thomson, PhD, DVM
Jones Professor of Production Medicine and Epidemiology
Department of Clinical Sciences
College of Veterinary Medicine
Kansas State University
Manhattan, Kansas
Feedlot Hospital Management
Feedlot Vaccination Protocols

Alexander Valverde, DVM, DVSc, Diplomate ACVA
Associate Professor
Section of Anesthesiology
Department of Clinical Studies
Ontario Veterinary College
University of Guelph
Guelph, Ontario, Canada
Pain Management in Cattle and Small Ruminants

Sarel R. Van Amstel, BVSC, Diplomate Med Vet, M Med Vet (Med), ABVP, ACVIM
Department of Large Animal Clinical Sciences
College of Veterinary Medicine
University of Tennessee
Knoxville, Tennessee
Noninfectious Disorders of the Foot

David C. Van Metre, DVM, Diplomate ACVIM
Associate Professor
Department of Clinical Sciences
Colorado State University
Fort Collins, Colorado
Hemorrhagic Bowel Syndrome

Robert J. Van Saun, DVM, MS, PhD, Diplomate ACT, ACVN
Professor and Extension Veterinarian
Department of Veterinary and Biomedical Sciences
College of Agricultural Sciences
Pennsylvania State University
University Park, Pennsylvania
Metabolic Profiling

Sarah A. Wagner, DVM, PhD, Diplomate ACVCP
Assistant Professor of Veterinary Technology
Department of Animal Sciences
North Dakota State University
Fargo, North Dakota
Decision Making in Mastitis Therapy

Paul H. Walz, DVM, PhD, Diplomate ACVIM
Associate Professor
Departments of Clinical Sciences and Pathobiology
College of Veterinary Medicine
Auburn University
Auburn, Alabama
Bovine Viral Diarrhea Virus

Kevin E. Washburn, DVM, Diplomate ACVIM, ABVP
Assistant Professor
Department of Large Animal Clinical Sciences
Texas A&M University
College Station, Texas
Vesicular Diseases of Ruminants

Brad J. White, DVM, MS
Assistant Professor
Department of Clinical Sciences
Kansas State University
Manhattan, Kansas
Preconditioned Calves in the Feedyard
Use of Statistical Process Control in Feedlot Practice

Brian K. Whitlock, DVM, MS, Diplomate ACT
Auburn University
Auburn, Alabama
Preparation of Teaser Bulls, Rams, and Bucks

Robert H. Whitlock, DVM, PhD, Diplomate ACVIM
Associate Professor of Medicine
University of Pennsylvania
New Bolton Center
Kennett Square, Pennsylvania
Abomasal Ulcers
Preparation of Teaser Bulls, Rams, and Bucks

William Dee Whittier, DVM, MS
Professor, Department of Large Animal Clinical Sciences
Virginia-Maryland Regional College of Veterinary Medicine
Virginia Polytechnic Institute and State University
Blacksburg, Virginia
Investigation of Abortions and Fetal Loss in the Beef Herd

Robyn Wilborn, DVM, Diplomate ACT
Department of Clinical Sciences
College of Veterinary Medicine
Auburn University
Auburn, Alabama
Diagnosis and Management of Conditions of the Scrotum and Testes

Dwight Wolfe, DVM, MS, Diplomate ACT
Professor, Food Animal Section
Department of Clinical Sciences
College of Veterinary Medicine
Auburn University
Auburn, Alabama
Diagnosis and Management of Conditions of the Scrotum and Testes
Diagnosis and Management of Inguinal Hernia in Bulls
Diagnosis and Management of Juvenile Anomalies of the Penis and Prepuce
Diagnosis and Management of Penile Deviations
Preparation of Teaser Bulls, Rams, and Bucks

Preface

We are proud to offer this book, the fifth volume of *Current Veterinary Therapy: Food Animal Practice*. Although the veterinary textbook market has expanded tremendously in recent years, *Current Veterinary Therapy* has long been a favorite of practitioners because it offers current, concise information for busy veterinarians who need answers fast. This tradition of excellent service from *Current Veterinary Therapy: Food Animal Practice* was developed by Dr. Jimmy Howard. Although this volume is structured slightly differently from previous volumes, we are confident that the tradition of concise, state-of-the-art information continues.

The fifth volume in the *Current Veterinary Therapy* series represents a new start with a new editorial team. In continuing from previous volumes, readers will find that topics merely needing an update are brief and areas that justified expansion are afforded more space. New information has been added; for example, this volume contains considerably more surgery topics compared with previous volumes. A striking difference from previous volumes is the absence of swine information, except in Section X, Ophthalmic Examination Techniques. We believe that swine medicine has become a highly focused and specialized area of veterinary medicine and does not easily meld into a textbook oriented toward ruminants. Therefore, topics in this volume emphasize beef and dairy cattle diseases and boast new, cutting-edge information regarding cow-calf and stocker/feedlot topics.

Another expansion of content in this fifth edition is a focus on pain management and clinical pharmacology.

The food animal industries face mounting societal pressure to address animal well being, pain, and food safety. We hope that the sections dedicated to pharmacology and anesthesia will assist practitioners in serving the interests of their clients.

Veterinary medicine for ruminants is rapidly changing. Colleges of veterinary medicine increasingly are strained to offer sufficient breadth and depth of ruminant education to prepare veterinary students to enter practice in a rural setting. Food animal industries—technology, management, pharmaceutical use, economics, and epidemiology—are rapidly evolving. Veterinary colleges have not kept pace with these trends. As the veterinary profession has turned toward companion animal emphasis, food animal industries have turned to other professionals for support. Failure to train veterinarians for rural practice has led to a deficiency of food animal practitioners. One beneficial effect of this increased demand/limited supply of food animal veterinarians has been the steady increase in salaries, benefits, and quality-of-life adjustments for rural practitioners, as evidenced by organizations such as the Academy of Veterinary Consultants and the Academy of Rural Veterinarians. We hope that this text is equally helpful to the many veterinarians whose emphasis is food animal practice as well as to the multitude of mixed-practitioner veterinarians.

David E. Anderson
D. Michael Rings

Contents

Section III
Respiratory System

Jeffrey Lakritz and *David E. Anderson*

Section IV
Cardiovascular Diseases

Kathryn M. Meurs

Section V
Musculoskeletal System Medicine

André Desrochers

Section VI
Neurologic Diseases of Cattle, Sheep, and Goats

Gilles Fecteau and *Lisle W. George*

Section VII
Urinary System

Matt D. Miesner

Digestive System

Allen J. Roussel, Jr., **and** *David E. Anderson*

CHAPTER 1

Pharyngeal Lacerations and Retropharyngeal Abscesses in Ruminants

D. MICHAEL RINGS

Pharyngeal lacerations and retropharyngeal abscesses are almost always the result of injurious oral treatments using balling guns, boluses, Frick speculums, orogastric tubes, or drenching instruments. Acute downward deviation of the head during the use of any of these instruments can result in the positioning of the instrument against the dorsal pharyngeal wall rather than lining up with the esophagus. This predisposes the area to injury. Although pharyngeal trauma likely occurs frequently during the oral treatment of ruminants, most animals recover quickly with a minimum of clinical signs.

Clinical signs can range from the subtle (mild inappetence) to obvious distress (massive swelling, inspiratory distress) and death. With mild lacerations without abscessation, the animal may show some degree of dysphagia and ptyalism (hypersalivation). A necrotic odor to the animal's breath exists. Larger lacerations are more likely to become impacted with feed and cause swelling behind the ramus of the mandible. With most of the cervical musculature running down the neck, infections gaining access to fascial planes can extend to the thoracic inlet and even into the mediastinal area. Head and neck extension and inspiratory stridor can be seen when the retropharyngeal swelling deviates the larynx.

Diagnosis of pharyngeal trauma can often be made solely on the basis of the history and physical findings. Digital examination of the pharyngeal area in mature cattle can be accomplished with the use of a mouth speculum. Endoscopy of the pharynx and proximal esophagus and trachea permits visualization of the lesion and allows the veterinarian to more accurately predict the outcome. Ultrasonography is valuable in examining swellings posterior to the mandible and is helpful in differentiating between cellulitis and abscess formation. Radiography has also been used to help locate abscesses and foreign bodies in the retropharyngeal area.

Mild cases of pharyngeal trauma (irritation and localized inflammation) often resolve on their own within a few days. Lacerations with impacting of feed into the retropharyngeal area will either end up as retropharyngeal abscesses or dissecting cervical tracts. Larger lacerations may actually be easier to treat because they are easier to empty digitally even if they also are more likely to refill. Lavage of the retropharyngeal area should be done carefully so that any infection is not flushed farther down the neck. Withholding feed while the wound contracts is advisable. Many animals will continue to drink, but for those in too much pain to swallow the passage of a nasogastric tube or creation of a temporary rumen fistula will permit fluid administration during healing.

With the formation of retropharyngeal abscesses the only effective treatment is drainage. Ultrasound-guided opening of the abscess is a nice touch in that it permits the veterinarian to avoid the important vascular structures in this area. A ventral approach immediately lateral to the trachea is the safest surgical approach and provides the best long-term drainage. Lavage of the abscess with a tamed iodine or other antiseptic solution should be continued for several days to prevent premature closure of the wound that would allow the abscess to refill. Broad-spectrum antibiotics are often given to help limit spread of the infection.

The prognosis for retropharyngeal lacerations and abscesses is always guarded during the initial examination. Animals that respond to therapy within the first few days and return to eating and drinking will likely recover without incident. Animals that develop cervical swelling descending toward the thoracic inlet have a poor prognosis and will likely require extensive treatment to have any chance of recovery.

CHAPTER 2

Vesicular Diseases of Ruminants

KEVIN E. WASHBURN

Diseases that create vesicular lesions are of particular importance in ruminants due to their ability to cause high morbidity in susceptible populations. Although mortality of such diseases is relatively low, the dramatic reduction in productivity of diseased animals leads to long-lasting, widespread effects. Of the four recognized vesicular diseases, foot-and-mouth disease (FMD) and vesicular stomatitis (VS) are the only ones that affect ruminants. FMD is of particular significance due to its worldwide recognition as an economically crippling disease of livestock in endemic regions and a potentially devastating threat to FMD-free areas. Because VS is clinically indistinguishable from FMD, it is important to consider both as formidable rule outs for the appearance of vesicular lesions.

Microscopically, vesicles begin as intracellular edema that results in ballooning and degeneration of the stratum spinosum. Grossly, vesicles appear as small, clear, fluid-filled lesions that enlarge or coalesce with others to form bullae. These bullae subsequently rupture and ulcerate, leaving irregular areas of denuded, red submucosa. Therefore clinically, vesicular disease lesions progress from raised, fluid-filled blisters to reddened ulcers and may appear in any stage of development depending on time of examination. This complicates the clinical picture by forcing one to expand the list of differential diagnoses of such lesions to include diseases that produce erosions, bullae, detached areas of epithelium, and ulcers. Vesicles can occur anywhere in the integumentary system; however, locations of vesicles caused by FMD and VS include the oral cavity, coronary band, interdigital skin, and teats.

Differentials for cattle and small ruminants with one or any combination of oral, coronary band, interdigital skin and teat ulcers, erosions, and vesicles are listed in Box 2-1. Although VS is reported in small ruminants, it is important to realize that they are relatively less susceptible to the virus than cattle.

Sorting through the potential etiologies of lesions consistent with vesicular disease requires careful collection of historical data, in particular, information concerning the other animals on the premises, recent travel by owners or others in contact with the herd, and the biosecurity measures in place. Based on these data, the veterinarian can eliminate some diseases and lower others on a differential diagnosis list ranked by likelihood. For example, vesicular lesions in a horse in contact with ruminants displaying similar signs would reduce the likelihood of a diagnosis of FMD.

In today's world where bioterrorism is an increasingly more significant threat, it is paramount that private practitioners familiarize themselves with diseases considered "exotic" for their region. Therefore diseases once considered "improbable" should begin to appear on differential lists and not be discounted. If a potentially devastating disease such as FMD is introduced, private practitioners very well may be the front line of defense in recognition of disease and implementation of control and eradication procedures.

VESICULAR STOMATITIS

Etiology

Vesicular stomatitis is caused by a bullet-shaped virus of the Rhabdoviridae family. This enveloped, single-stranded RNA virus is easily inactivated by iodine, quaternary ammonium compounds, lipid solvents, phenolic compounds, and chlorine. Two serotypes, New Jersey and Indiana 1, have resulted in numerous outbreaks in the United States. These two serotypes are also present in Mexico and Central and South America. Many more serotypes have been identified in other parts of the world.

Box 2-1

Differential Diagnoses for Cattle and Small Ruminants with Signs of Any Combination of Ulcers, Erosions, and Vesicles in the Oral Cavity, Interdigital Skin, Coronary Band, or Teats

Cattle
Vesicular stomatitis
Foot-and-mouth disease
Bovine viral diarrhea
Infectious bovine rhinotracheitis
Bluetongue virus
Malignant catarrhal fever
Footrot
Pseudocowpox
Bovine herpes mammillitis
Cowpox
Pseudolumpyskin disease
Rinderpest
Ingestion of caustic agents

Small Ruminants
Vesicular stomatitis
Foot-and-mouth disease
Bluetongue virus
Footrot
Contagious ecthyma
Ingestion of caustic agents

Epidemiology

Vesicular stomatitis virus infects cattle, horses, swine, wild ruminants, and llamas resulting in clinical disease with vesicular lesions. Other species experimentally infected include opossum, rabbits, ferrets, hamsters, and other laboratory animals. The most recent outbreaks of vesicular stomatitis in the United States occurred in 1997 and 1998. Investigation into the strains responsible for these outbreaks revealed that they were not related to strains identified in past outbreaks. This suggested that the 1997 and 1998 outbreaks were due to strains newly introduced into the United States. Economic losses in dairy cattle and cow-calf operations can be substantial due to decreased productivity in the form of lower milk production, poor growth, reduced reproductive performance, and death loss. Humans can also be infected with vesicular stomatitis, usually manifesting as flulike symptoms, so appropriate precautions should be taken when handling suspected cases.

Transmission

Vesicular stomatitis is thought to be transmitted horizontally, with the aid of vectors, or by direct contact. Insects have long been thought to play a significant role in the transmission of the virus acting primarily as mechanical vectors transporting virus draining from ruptured lesions from one animal to the next. Vesicular stomatitis virus has been isolated from both blood- and non–blood-feeding insects including midges *(Culicoides),* black flies *(Simulidae),* and sand flies *(Lutzomyia).* Most recently, experimental transmission of vesicular stomatitis to cattle by *Culicoides sonorensis* has been documented. Contact transmission is also thought to occur through the presence of mucosal abrasions in uninfected animals and the sharing of fomites (water/feed troughs) with infected animals shedding virus through active lesions. The highest levels of virus are at the edges of lesions and within the vesicular fluid. The virus is incapable of invading intact epithelium.

Clinical Signs

After a relatively short incubation period (3-14 days), the animal is febrile and vesicle formation begins. Vesicles develop on the tongue, lips, and muzzle and may also be noted on the interdigital skin and teats. Vesicles may not be apparent because they rapidly rupture, leaving areas of ulceration beneath. Large portions of the tongue may be involved as multiple small vesicles coalesce into bullae. Oral lesions manifest as excessive salivation and feed refusal, whereas interdigital skin lesions may result in lameness. Cracked, dry skin on the teats may provide opportunity for development of teat lesions that could subsequently lead to secondary bacterial mastitis. Recovery may take as long as 3 weeks, and actual healing of the lesions may require as long as 2 months. Because of reduced feed intake and dysphagia, marked weight loss occurs. Deaths from vesicular stomatitis are rare but are most commonly due to secondary bacterial invasion that penetrates deeper, more vital structures.

Vesicular lesions in sheep are rare due to VS virus; nonetheless, this disease should be considered a differential, especially when sheep are present in areas experiencing outbreaks in other species. Affected animals develop antibodies that may persist for years, but there is no evidence of a carrier state of persistent infection in cattle, horses, or swine. Despite the prolonged period of the presence of neutralizing antibodies, reinfection can occur.

Diagnosis

Because VS and FMD are clinically indistinguishable, state or federal authorities should be notified if vesicular disease is suspected. Appropriate specimens to submit for diagnostics include vesicular fluid if possible, epithelium from a ruptured vesicle, serum, and swabs of the lesions. These specimens can be subjected to a number of tests for either the presence of the virus or antibodies. Virus isolation, polymerase chain reaction, and antigen capture ELISA can detect the presence of virus, whereas complement fixation, virus neutralization, IgM-capture ELISA, and competitive ELISA techniques are available to detect antibody. Contacting the laboratory before sending samples is important to determine availability and instructions on preservation during shipping.

Treatment

Animals affected with vesicular stomatitis should be isolated from unaffected individuals, allowed to rest, and offered soft feed and water. Separate feeders and waterers should be provided to these animals. All fomites contaminated with saliva should be destroyed or disinfected. Affected dairy cattle should be milked last, followed by a thorough disinfection of the milking equipment. Because flying insects have been implicated as potential means of transmitting the virus, unaffected animals should be penned in barns or stables if possible to reduce feeding of these insects.

Prevention and Control

Quarantine of affected premises, isolation of affected animals, and prevention of movement of susceptible species from these premises are steps required to gain control of a potential outbreak of VS. Unless animals are going to slaughter, movement of susceptible species from affected premises is prohibited for 30 days after the last clinical signs are noted. Any animals brought into the premises should be quarantined from the rest of the herd as well. Establishing effective fly control programs is also beneficial in controlling the spread of disease. Both live and killed vaccines have been developed against VS; however, both state and federal regulatory veterinarians should be contacted before considering vaccination.

FOOT-AND-MOUTH DISEASE

Etiology

FMD is caused by a picornavirus of the *Aphthovirus* genus, family Picornaviridae. Currently, seven different serologically distinct types of this nonenveloped RNA virus have been identified, and within these types at least

60 subtypes are recognized. The seven specific serotypes are A; O; C; SAT (Southern African Territory) 1, 2, 3; and Asia 1. The virus is very resistant to drying and environmental conditions and can survive outside of the host in body fluids, animal products, and contaminated materials for considerable periods of time; however, sunlight, high temperature, and high or low pH rapidly inactivates it. Effective disinfectants include sodium hydroxide, iodophors, sodium carbonate, chlorine dioxide, and acetic acid. Many more common disinfectants are ineffective.

Epidemiology

Natural hosts of FMD virus include cattle, swine, sheep, goats, buffalo, deer, antelope, and camelids, which are all in the mammal order Artiodactyla. The horse is resistant to infection. Cattle and swine are most susceptible, whereas sheep and goats display mild clinical symptoms. The disease is endemic in Asia, Africa, most of South America, and parts of Europe. However, within each country or region, the tendency is for the disease to be in zones rather than to be widespread. The disease has moderate spread from these zones when host susceptibilities and epidemiologic conditions are favorable. Humans are not considered susceptible to infection, although rare reports of laboratory infection exist.

Transmission

Transmission of the virus is primarily by aerosol, contact, or contaminated fomites. Ingestion, insemination with contaminated semen, and inoculation with contaminated vaccines have also been reported means of transmission. In cattle the respiratory tract is the most common route of infection, whereas in swine oral ingestion is a common portal of entry. Cattle that recover from the disease may carry and shed the virus for up to 2 years and may therefore serve as a source of infection. Some experts believe that buffalo may harbor the virus for life. Swine shed tremendous amounts of virus via the respiratory tract during the first week of infection. Sheep and goats can incubate the virus while being clinically unaffected and, thereby, serve as a maintenance host. Fomites commonly implicated in the transmission include shoes and hands of humans, bedding, feed, waterers, troughs, and equipment. The virus is also present in milk and may survive pasteurization. FMD virus does not survive in muscle tissue following postmortem autolysis; however, in areas in which the pH does not change dramatically after death such as the bone marrow, lymph nodes, and visceral organs it may persist. Therefore importation of commodities such as partially cooked or smoke-cured meat products pose a high risk to FMD-free countries.

Clinical Signs

Clinical signs of fever, depression, anorexia, and marked drop in milk production begin after a short incubation period of 2 to 4 days. Cattle usually experience excessive salivation and smacking of the lips before the development of vesicles. Vesicles may be observed on the buccal mucosa, gingival mucosa, tongue, palate, teats, and nares. Cattle are often lame as a result of development of lesions on the interdigital skin and coronary band. On rupture of the vesicles, eroded to ulcerated denuded areas remain. On the tongue specifically, large portions of the epithelium may be sloughed. Clinically, the lesions are indistinguishable from those of vesicular stomatitis. Death loss in adults is generally low; however, mortality rates may be quite high in young cattle due to the potential development of myocarditis. Morbidity, on the other hand, is high as the disease rapidly spreads to susceptible animals. Cattle that recover are nonproductive for extended periods of time. The disease can also be mild or subclinical in cattle with partial immunity resulting from vaccination or prior disease. Sheep and goats are usually subclinically affected; however, FMD should still be considered with the appearance of suspicious lesions, especially in regions experiencing an outbreak.

Diagnosis

As is the case with VS, after careful evaluation and examination of the animal and consideration of potential differentials, if a vesicular disease is suspected, the appropriate governmental authorities should be contacted. Appropriate samples for collection include vesicular fluid, epithelium from ruptured vesicles, serum, and whole blood. Governmental officials will guide submission of these samples to an official vesicular disease diagnostic laboratory for testing. Various tests including virus isolation, serology, and detection of viral antigens or nucleic acid are available.

Treatment

The treatment of FMD is primarily only a consideration for endemic areas. Considerations in these endemic regions include quarantine, local eradication, virus typing, and revaccination of at-risk and contact animals. Appropriate supportive care should include soft feeds and antimicrobials to prevent secondary bacterial infection. Although most adults survive, weight loss, loss of milk production, and abortion may eventually lead to culling.

Prevention and Control

Vaccination and quarantine form the basis of prevention and control in endemic areas, whereas in regions free of disease, cases are rapidly identified, quarantined, and slaughtered along with all other affected and contact animals. Because of short-lived immunity, vaccination should be repeated two or three times a year. In addition, the vaccines must be type specific; therefore autogenous vaccines are most effective. Protection from vaccination is partial and usually causes mild or subclinical disease.

Recommended Readings

Comer JA, Tesh RB, Govind BM et al: Vesicular stomatitis virus, New Jersey serotype: replication in and transmission by *Lutzomyia shannoi (Diptera: Psychodidae), Am J Trop Med Hyg* 42:483-490, 1990.

Cottral GE, Callis JJ: Foot-and-mouth disease. In Commission on Foreign Animal Disease, editor: *Foreign animal disease, their diagnosis and control,* Richmond, Va, 1975, US Animal Health Association.

Francy DB: Entomological investigations of a 1982 vesicular stomatitis virus epizootic in Colorado, USA. In *Proceedings of International Conference on Vesicular Stomatitis,* Mexico City, 1984, 1:208-212.

Fraser CM: Foot-and-mouth disease. In Fraser CM, editor: *The Merck veterinary manual,* ed 6, Rahway, NJ, 1986, Merck.

Goodger WJ, Thurmond M, Nehay J, et al: Economic impact of an epizootic of bovine vesicular stomatitis in California, *J Am Vet Med Assoc* 186:370-373, 1985.

Graves JH: Foot-and-mouth disease: a constant threat to US livestock, *J Am Vet Med Assoc* 174:174-176, 1979.

Hurd HS, McCluskey BJ, Mumford EL: Management factors affecting the risk for vesicular stomatitis in livestock operations in the western United States, *J Am Vet Med Assoc* 215:1263-1268, 1999.

Kahrs RF: *Viral diseases of cattle,* Ames, Iowa, 1981, Iowa State University Press.

Lubroth J: Foot-and-mouth disease: a review for the practitioner, *Vet Clin Food Anim* 18:475-499, 2002.

Mead DG, Ramberg FB, Mare CJ: Laboratory vector competence of black flies *(Diptera: Simuliidae)* for the Indiana serotype of vesicular stomatitis virus, *Ann N Y Acad Sci* 916:437-443, 2000.

Perez De Leon AA, Tabachnick WJ: Transmission of vesicular stomatitis New Jersey virus to cattle by the biting midge *Culicoides sonorensis (Diptera: Ceratopogonidae), J Med Ent* 43:323-329, 2006.

Schmitt B: Vesicular stomatitis, *Vet Clin Food Anim* 18:453-459, 2002.

Thurmond MC: Vesicular stomatitis. In *Third Annual Dairy Research Report, Department of Animal Science,* University of California, Davis, 46-54, 1984.

Webb PA, Monath TP, Reif JS et al: Epizootic vesicular stomatitis in Colorado, 1982: Epidemiologic studies along the northern Colorado front range, *Am J Trop Med Hyg* 36:183-188, 1987.

Westbury HA, Doughty WJ, Forman AJ et al: A comparison of enzyme-linked immunosorbent assay, complement fixation and virus isolation for foot-and-mouth disease diagnosis, *Vet Microbiol* 17:21-28, 1988.

Wright HS: Inactivation of vesicular stomatitis virus by disinfectants, *Appl Environ Microbiol* 19:96-99, 1970.

CHAPTER 3

Actinomycosis and Actinobacillosis

ALLEN J. ROUSSEL, JR.

ACTINOMYCOSIS

Etiology and Epidemiology

Actinomycosis is a localized bacterial infection caused by *Actinomyces bovis,* a gram-positive filamentous anaerobic bacterium. *A. bovis* is part of the normal oral and respiratory flora, a commensal organism of cattle and other ruminants. It can only invade deeper tissues when there has been a break in the epithelial or mucosal surface. Breaks in the mucosa can be caused by stemmy, sharp, or scabrous forage or by eruption of the cheek teeth. Lesions tend to be locally proliferative, but the organism is not highly invasive. Any part of the bone could be affected, but the alveoli around the roots of the cheek teeth are frequently involved. Typically the infection is polymicrobial, involving several pyogenic aerobic and anaerobic species. Therefore, when multiple cases occur in a herd, it is usually not a contagion but rather the widespread exposure to a common risk factor.

Clinical Disease

The most common clinical presentation of actinomycosis in cattle is osteomyelitis of the mandible or maxilla. This clinical presentation has led to the use of the common name "lumpy jaw." The lesion is a slow-growing, firm, nonpainful mass that is attached to or, in fact, part of the mandible and consists primarily of proliferative bone with osteolytic cavitation throughout. The osteomyelitis is often accompanied by granulomatous soft tissue reaction that increases the physical size of the lesion. In some but not all cases, ulceration with or without fistula forms over the granulation tissue. Although discrete pus-filled abscesses are uncommon, drainage of purulent exudate sometimes occurs. This exudate often has tiny yellow-white particles about 1 mm in diameter. These are the so-called sulfur granules, which are actually clusters of bacteria.

Diagnosis

A presumptive diagnosis is usually made based on history and physical examination findings. The diagnosis can be confirmed by one of several means. Although culture of the organism is the ideal and definitive diagnostic test, it is difficult to accomplish in the field situation because *A. bovis* is an obligate anaerobic bacterium and requires special culture technique. The characteristic organisms may be identified in a smear of exudate by adding 10% sodium hydroxide to the purulent material, allowing it to dissolve and soften, and then crushing the sulfur granules under a coverslip. A Gram stain of the resulting preparation will reveal gram-positive, club-shaped rods and filaments. Alternatively, a biopsy using a Michel's trephine may be obtained, fixed in formalin and stained for microscopic examination. The identification of Splendore-Hoeppli bodies is suggestive of actinomycosis but may also be seen with actinobacillosis.

Differential diagnoses for actinomycosis include abscess, mandibular fracture, actinobacillosis, and tumors. Actinobacillary pyogranulomas and common pyogenic abscesses are typically not attached to the bone. Abscesses tend to be more fluctuant and nonulcerated, and they yield plus when aspirated with a large-gauge needle. A healing mandibular fracture or neoplasia of the mandible may present with similar clinical signs to actinomycosis. History and radiograph examination will usually differentiate these conditions from actinomycosis.

Treatment and Prevention

The best treatment option, as well as the prognosis for success, depends on the chronicity and extent of the lesion. The goal of treatment is usually to arrest the spread of the lesion and reduce the active inflammation associated with it. Seldom does the lesion itself completely disappear, and frequently the disease recrudesces after a period of dormancy following treatment. Early lesions that do not involve the cheek teeth can usually be successfully treated or at least put into an extended period of dormancy. Treatment consists of intravenous administration of 20% sodium iodide solution administered several times, 5 to 10 days apart. The recommended dose is 70 mg/kg, but higher dosages have been reported.[1] In my experience, failure to administer repeated treatments is the most frequent cause of treatment failure. Sodium iodide was once thought to cause abortion in cattle, and the label still warns against this complication. However, it has been shown to be safe for use in pregnant cows and presents little risk of abortion.[2] Discussing with the owner the risks associated with treatment, as well as the risks associated with not treating the condition, allows for an informed decision to be made regarding treatment of pregnant cattle. Isoniazid (10 mg/kg/day orally for 1 month) is reported to be an effective treatment for actinomycosis.[3] However, this drug, which is not approved for use in cattle in the United States, can cause abortion and should not be used in pregnant cattle.

Concurrent administration of antimicrobial drugs is recommended. Most papers describing treatment protocols for this condition were written before many of the antimicrobials currently available were marketed. In general the organism is not highly resistant, so many microbial agents are potentially useful. Penicillin, streptomycin, and oxytetracycline are generally considered to be effective. Long-acting oxytetracycline products provide a convenient dose form for weekly or semiweekly treatment that coincides with sodium iodide administration. Some of the other long-acting antimicrobials are potentially effective as well. When fistulous tracts are present, débridement of the soft tissue lesion is recommended as an adjunct to medical therapy. When the tooth roots are affected, or when cheek teeth are loose, the cheek teeth must be removed. This can only be done safely and effectively with the animal restrained and sedated or anesthetized. Oral organic iodide such as ethylene ethylenediamine dihydriodide (EDDI) has been used as a follow-up to intravenous sodium iodide, but there is no published evidence of its effectiveness as a sole therapy.

Because *A. bovis* is a normal inhabitant of the mouth of ruminants, prevention is restricted to reducing the risk of mucosal penetration. Therefore if multiple cases occur in a herd, the forages or pasture should be examined for course, fibrous, or sharp components, and they should be eliminated from the diet. The successful use of orally administered organic iodides as a preventive has not been reported.

ACTINOBACILLOSIS

Etiology and Epidemiology

Actinobacillosis is caused by *Actinobacillus lignieresii*, a gram-negative aerobic rod that is a normal inhabitant of the gastrointestinal tract of ruminants. The disease affects primarily cattle but has also been reported in sheep and horses. The most frequent clinical presentation is a granulomatous or pyogranulomatous lesion of the tongue or subcutaneous tissues in the head and neck region. Presumably the infection can occur in any location where the epithelium has been broken and the organism has gained access to subcutaneous tissues. The disease is typically sporadic and is associated with the feeding of course or sharp feedstuffs. However, outbreaks affecting up to 73% of exposed cattle have been reported when there is common exposure to a risk factor such as stemmy forage.[4]

Clinical Disease

The classical form of actinobacillosis is a granulomatous glossitis, characterized by a firm swelling of the tongue, dysphagia, drooling and, occasionally, protrusion of the tongue. This form of the disease is also called "wooden tongue." Granulomas, and even abscesses of the neck and head region, are also common. Although the lesion may be a typical pus-filled abscess, pyogranulomas that are ulcerated and exude small amounts of pus are more frequently observed. Atypical manifestations of the disease have been reported associated with lacerations, nose rings, dehorning, and intravenous injections, and lymphadenitis with disseminated infection can also occur.[1,5]

Diagnosis

Differential diagnoses include actinomycosis, pyogenic abscesses, granulation tissue, and neoplasia. Actinobacillosis should be suspected whenever a wound heals with excessive granulation that is painful and exudative. Gross and histologic examination of biopsy specimens from masses suspected to be neoplasia or granuloma may be strongly suggestive of actinobacillosis. "Sulfur granules" like those seen in actinomycosis are commonly present in infected tissues. In cases where more typical pus filled abscesses form, the pus may contain sulfur granules. Histologic lesions are characteristic, consisting of small granulomas with clumps of bacteria. Confirmation of the disease requires isolation of the organism which is easily grown in the laboratory.

Treatment and Prevention

Treatment of actinobacillosis is similar to that of actinomycosis, but the prognosis for complete recovery is much better. Intravenous sodium iodide and parenteral antimicrobial agents such as penicillin or oxytetracycline are frequently recommended. The clinical response is usually rapid and dramatic, but several weeks of therapy may be necessary to completely eliminate the organism. When treatment is abbreviated, recurrence of the lesion is common. Debulking of large lesions may improve the prognosis for a rapid recovery. Pus-filled abscesses should be lanced and treated as other abscesses. Prevention is limited to removing the offending risk factors.

References

1. Rebhun WC, King JM, Hillman RB: Atypical actinobacillosis granulomas in cattle, *Cornell Vet* 78:123, 1988.
2. Miller HV, Drost M: Failure to cause abortion and cows with intravenous sodium iodide treatment, *J Am Vet Med Assoc* 172:466, 1978.
3. Watts TC, Olson SM, Rhodes CS: Treatment of bovine actinomycosis with isoniazid, *Can Vet J* 14:223, 1973.
4. Bottenscøn J: The occurrence of lesions in the tongue of adult cattle and their implications for the development of actinobacillosis, *J Vet Med A* 36:393, 1989.
5. Franco DA: Generalized actinobacillosis and a Holstein cow (postmortem lesions), *VM/SAC* 65:562, 1970.

CHAPTER **4**

Esophageal Obstructions/Choke

D. MICHAEL RINGS

Esophageal obstructions in ruminants are most commonly related to feedstuffs ingested by the animal. Cattle are more prone to eat objects such as apples, turnips, beets, and hedge apples without sufficient mastication and may swallow the object whole. Sheep and goats, being more delicate eaters, frequently choke on grain diet when put into a competitive feeding situation. Obstruction of the esophagus can also occur from compression of the esophagus externally from abscesses along the neck, especially at the thoracic inlet, or neoplasms such as lymphosarcoma (thymic and mediastinal lymph node). The parasite *Hypoderma lineatum* migrates around the esophagus as part of its life cycle, and poorly timed killing of the parasite has been reported to cause esophageal blockage.

Esophageal obstruction may be partial or complete, and the urgency to correct the problem will depend on this assessment. Fermentation gases become a problem with complete obstruction because of pressure applied to the diaphragm, adversely affecting respiration. Early signs of esophageal obstruction include an anxious expression on the animal accompanying retching motions, usually with the neck held extended and the head down. Ropey salivation is frequently seen flowing from the mouth, and waves of esophageal muscle contraction can be seen as the animal attempts to either swallow or regurgitate the obstruction. Rumen tympany and respiratory distress may develop quickly with complete obstruction and may, in fact, be the primary reasons for presentation. Death in most animals with complete obstruction is due to respiratory distress/arrest.

Partial obstructions that permit gas to be regurgitated may result in the persistence of clinical signs for several days. Pressure changes to the esophageal mucosa resulting from the obstruction may cause necrosis and the formation of esophageal fistulas and strictures.

TREATMENT OF ESOPHAGEAL OBSTRUCTIONS

Passage of a large-bore orogastric tube should be attempted to move the obstruction into the rumen. A large-bore, semistiff tube is more helpful than a small flexible tube in pushing the obstruction along because it engages the object over a broader surface and is less easily doubled over. The stiffer tube should be used judiciously because it can more easily traumatize or puncture the esophagus. Most of the obstructions are sufficiently far away from the pharyngeal opening that removal through the oral cavity (digitally) is not possible and passing the tube will help define the area of obstruction. Sedation may be useful in both easing the animal's anxiety and allowing for muscle relaxation along the esophagus, facilitating passage of the obstruction. It is important to address any respiratory distress by placement of a bloat trochar or creation of a rumen fistula to relieve the pressure on the diaphragm.

Obstructions caused by concentrates and forages may be of sufficient size and length that pressure applied aborally may not move the mass. Pumping small volumes of water against the mass can serve to lubricate and dilate the esophagus so that the obstruction can pass into the rumen. The use of a two-tube system as previously outlined in the third edition has been used in anesthetized cattle to successfully relieve the choke by breaking up and floating out the obstructing material. Surgical correction of cervical obstructions is not often recommended due to complications with wound healing of the esophagus.

Esophageal obstructions relating to competitive consumption of concentrates by sheep or goats usually self-correct within a few minutes, but persistence of signs beyond 30 minutes should result in some type of intervention.

Incomplete esophageal obstructions may result in chronic damage to the esophagus and the formation of strictures, which may lead to recurring choking problems. Fistula formation is rare in ruminants because sufficient pressure to cause necrosis is only encountered with complete obstructions of significant duration. Ruminants are usually dead from bloat long before rupture of the esophagus takes place.

DIFFERENTIAL DIAGNOSES

Adult ruminants showing clinical signs of esophageal obstruction should be viewed as possible rabies cases, and appropriate precautions taken to minimize the risk of human exposure. Animals with stomatitis (bovine viral diarrhea, calf diphtheria, vesicular stomatitis, pharyngeal trauma) will often have profuse, ropey saliva and have problems swallowing. Cattle with frothy bloat may show respiratory distress but can be observed to swallow water without regurgitation. Conditions such as megaesophagus are rarely encountered in ruminants.

CHAPTER 5

Bloat or Ruminal Tympany

ROBERT N. STREETER

DEFINITION

Bloat is an excessive accumulation of fermentation gases within the reticulorumen. This disorder can develop rapidly and become life threatening. The complete absence of eructation in intensively fed ruminants is a medical emergency. Bloat may occur in an individual or in numerous animals in a herd or flock. Economic losses caused by bloat can represent a significant burden to producers in the form of deaths, reduced gains, cost of preventive strategies, and inability to maximally utilize certain forages.

ETIOLOGY AND PATHOGENESIS

The capacity for eructation in a healthy ruminant exceeds the maximal rate of gas production, even at the highest rates of microbial fermentation.[1] Therefore bloat is not a consequence of excessive gas production but rather a failure of eructation. This failure may be due to a mechanical or functional disturbance anywhere along the path of the eructation mechanism (reticulorumen, esophagus, pharynx, nervous system) and result in free gas bloat. Alternatively, the failure may be in the form of the gas (foam mixed with digesta), wherein relaxation of the cardia will not occur due to reflex inhibition, resulting in frothy bloat. A complete description of ruminal motility and eructation is presented in Chapter 6.

Free gas bloat is not a disease in itself but rather a manifestation of an underlying primary disorder. Free gas bloat occurs sporadically, usually affecting a single animal without an associated change in the diet. Numerous conditions and disturbances can lead to free gas bloat as summarized in Box 5-1 and discussed elsewhere in this volume.

Box 5-1

Conditions Leading to Free Gas Bloat

Esophageal Dysfunction
Intraluminal: foreign body (choke)
Intramural: papilloma, granuloma, tetanus
Extramural: mediastinal lymphadenopathy
Positional: lateral recumbency, hypocalcemia, surgery

Ruminal Motility Dysfunction
Muscular inactivity: hypocalcemia, xylazine, atropine
Reticular adhesions: hardware, abomasal ulcers
Vagal nerve injury: many
Abnormal rumen environment:
   Grain engorgement (lactic acidosis)
   Rumen impaction with microbial inactivity
   Rumen putrifaction
Severe abomasal distention:
   Left displaced abomasum (particularly in calves)
   Milk engorgement/overeating

Box 5-2

Bloat Potential of Forages

High Risk
Alfalfa
Sweet clover
Red clover
Winter wheat

Moderate Risk
Arrowleaf clover
Spring wheat
Oats
Perennial ryegrass

Low Risk
Lespedeza
Birdsfoot trefoil
Sainfoin
Most perennial grasses

Frothy bloat is a primary disease wherein the ruminal gases are trapped in small bubbles within abnormally viscous digesta. The development of stable foam in the rumen fluid is known to be dependent on interactions among the diet, ruminal microflora, and animal. Frothy bloat occurs in animals consuming a variety of different feedstuffs. Offending diets include many legumes, lush wheat or rye grass, and high-concentrate rations. The bloat that develops is referred to as *legume bloat, wheat pasture bloat,* and *grain* or *feedlot bloat,* respectively. Several factors contribute to the pathogenesis of all causes of primary frothy bloat, the most important of which are (1) small particles in the rumen content, (2) rapidly digested feedstuffs, (3) rumen microorganisms, (4) foam-promoting compounds, and (5) foam-retarding compounds.[2]

Ruminal bacteria adhere to small feed particles (fine kernel elements or plant membrane fragments) in the digesta. The small particle size allows for a large population of adherent bacteria for subsequent fermentation. Rapid digestibility then provides adequate nutrients for explosive microbial proliferation. The multiplying bacteria release large amounts of a mucopolysaccharide, termed *slime* or *biofilm,* which is highly viscous. Small gas bubbles released during fermentation become trapped in a particle-biofilm-gas complex and make up the froth or foam.[2] The stability of the foam is enhanced by factors such as low ruminal pH and surface-active foaming agents in certain plants. Salivary mucoproteins have foam-retardant properties, so reduced saliva production enhances foam stability.

Box 5-2 summarizes significant differences in the bloat-inducing potential of pasture forages. An important forage characteristic promoting the development of frothy bloat is a high rate of digestion, which is influenced by a plant's leaf structure, mesophyll cell wall characteristics, and maturity.[2] Other factors include the concentration of foaming agents (soluble leaf proteins, pectins) and soluble nitrogen. High levels of condensed tannin in the plant afford bloat resistance to a forage, possibly by binding with soluble plant proteins.

Environmental factors can influence the bloat potential of forages. This interaction is complex but may be related to the digestibility of the forage, grazing patterns of the animals, and saliva production.

The foam-producing compounds in grain bloat are derived from the ruminal microflora. The regulation and modulation of bacterial biofilm production is an incompletely understood process. Biofilm production varies among rumen microbes but appears to be promoted with conditions of low pH and readily available energy sources in the digesta.[3] Variation in the rate and extent of ruminal digestion of cereal grains exists, but the processing of grain to produce small particle size and rapid fermentation appears to be the primary feed-related factor controlling the development of feedlot bloat. Poor feed management in terms of inadequate adaptation periods, component feeding, and inconsistent feeding can precipitate bloat attacks.

Individual cattle vary in their susceptibility to frothy bloat.[4] Bloat-susceptible cattle have slower clearance of particulate matter from the rumen and larger rumen volume than bloat-resistant cattle. Differences in the rate of eructation, saliva production, and salivary composition may also affect an animal's susceptibility to bloat. Some degree of the susceptibility to bloat appears to be inherited, but information on this subject is limited.

Omasal transport failure, a type of vagal indigestion, can cause frothy bloat. This rumen outflow disturbance results in increased rumen contents, which reflexively initiates hypermotility. The excessive mixing of digesta generates a stable foam and recurrent frothy bloat.

CLINICAL SIGNS

Bloat results in an asymmetric abdominal distention, most pronounced in the left paralumbar fossa. Mild bloat is often subclinical but may be associated with reduced feed intake and production. As the condition progresses, animals display signs of abdominal discomfort manifested by restlessness, kicking at the abdomen, and rolling.

Rumen motility is increased in the early stages but later inhibited by extreme distention. As distention becomes severe, the diaphragm and lungs are compressed, interfering with ventilation and venous return to the heart. The respiratory and heart rates progressively increase. Animals may exhibit open mouth breathing with protrusion of the tongue and eventually die of asphyxia. Acute bloat is of short duration with death occurring within 30 minutes to 4 hours after onset of mild signs, depending on the specific cause and previous diet.

DIAGNOSIS

The primary diagnostic information for a case of rumen tympany is gained while passing an orogastric tube; see Fig. 5-1. Diagnosis of the cause of free gas bloat not associated with esophageal obstruction can be challenging. Close inspection of the rumen and its motility patterns is warranted. Helpful ancillary diagnostic techniques include rumen fluid examination, esophageal endoscopy, reticular ultrasonography, and exploratory laparotomy/rumenotomy.[5]

Differential diagnoses for abdominal distention that could be confused with bloat include ruptured bladder, hydroallantois, left displaced abomasum in calves, abomasal volvulus, and mesenteric volvulus. Careful physical examination including evaluation of the abdominal contour and rectal palpation should allow differentiation.

Postmortem diagnosis of bloat is complicated by the fact that some gas accumulates in the rumen after death from any cause. In primary bloat the rumen may be markedly distended with foamy contents, but the viscosity of the digesta will decline with increasing postmortem interval. Other findings include congestion of the head, neck, and forelimbs contrasted with compression and pallor of the abdominal viscera and pelvic limbs. A line of demarcation (bloat-line) between the congested extrathoracic esophagus and the blanched thoracic esophagus is strong evidence for antemortem bloat.[6]

TREATMENT

Bloated animals that are dyspneic and recumbent require emergency ruminal decompression via trocarization (free gas) or emergency rumenotomy (frothy). For less severely affected animals, an orogastric tube is passed to facilitate gas removal. Highly frothy digesta will not escape through a tube, and antifoaming agents should be administered. Available compounds include poloxalene (2 oz/1000 lb), mineral or vegetable oils (1 to 2 pints/1000 lb), and dioctyl sodium sulfosuccinate (2 oz/1000 lb). The antifoaming agent should be deposited near the cardia and be provided in enough volume or diluent to allow dissemination throughout the rumen contents. Poloxalene is more effective in cases of forage bloat than in grain bloat. Animals should be monitored closely for response to therapy over the next hour. In outbreaks of severe frothy bloat, all animals should be removed from the offending diet. Affected animals should be encouraged to walk and should be monitored for several hours to assess the need for individual treatment.

Free gas bloat requires treatment for the primary eructation disorder. Chronic cases may be symptomatically

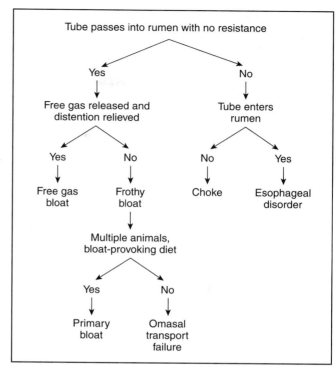

Fig 5-1   Diagnosis of bloat.

treated by a temporary rumenotomy for long-term bloat relief. Animals with recurrent bloat of any type that fails to respond to conventional measures should be considered for culling.

CONTROL AND PREVENTION

Grazing management is of paramount importance for the control of pasture bloat.[7] Cattle should not be introduced to bloat-causing forages when hungry. A full feeding of coarse roughage should precede the first exposure and may be indicated following periods of reduced feed intake (transport, processing, inclement weather). Animals should be turned onto pastures after the dew evaporates or in the afternoon. Continuous grazing should be practiced once animals are acclimated. Stocking density can be adjusted to allow for adaptation to the diet. On severely bloat-inducing pastures, the previously mentioned measures may afford incomplete protection and the provision of specific antifoaming agents is necessary.

The surfactant poloxalene is highly effective in reducing losses from wheat pasture and legume bloat if continuous intake is achieved. All at-risk animals must receive the compound daily for maximal protection and for several days before exposure. Poloxalene is available as a top dressing for grain, in molasses blocks, and in liquid supplements. Variable intake from free choice sources can limit its efficacy.

Water-soluble agents provided in the drinking water can provide more consistent intake. Formulations of alcohol ethoxylate and pluronic detergent have been widely used in Australia and New Zealand for many years, allowing grazing of legumes in pastoral dairy settings. A water-soluble pluronic detergent product was introduced in

Canada and was shown to be highly effective at reducing bloat in cattle grazing alfalfa but at the time of publication was not on the market.[8]

Cultivation of pastures with bloat-resistant legumes such as sainfoin or birdsfoot trefoil can reduce the incidence of bloat, but establishment and maintenance of these forages can be challenging. A bloat-resistant cultivar of alfalfa has been developed in Canada and was shown to reduce bloat by greater than 50% over a standard cultivar.[9]

Grain bloat is best prevented by allowing adequate adaptation to high-concentrate diets, providing adequate particle size of the ration, ensuring consistent feed intake, and providing at least 10% of the diet as course roughage. Roughage and concentrate should be fed mixed together. Other feed additives that have been used to reduce the severity of grain bloat include mineral oil, tallow, salt, and poloxalene, but their utility is reduced by constraints of cost, processing requirements, or reduced gains.

The ionophores monensin and lasalocid have been shown to reduce the incidence of legume, wheat pasture, and feedlot bloat.[10] Ionophores have the additional advantage of improving feed efficiency.

References

1. Leek BF: Clinical diseases of the rumen: a physiologist's view, *Vet Rec* 113:10-14, 1983.
2. Howarth RE, Chaplin RK, Cheng KJ et al: *Bloat in cattle. Agriculture Canada Publication 1858/E,* Ottawa, Ont, 1991, Communications Branch, Agriculture Canada, K1A 0C7, pp 6-32.
3. Cheng KJ, McAllister TA, Popp JD et al: A review of bloat in feedlot cattle, *J Anim Sci* 76(1):299-308, 1998.
4. Hegarty RS: Genotype differences and their impact on digestive tract function of ruminants: a review, *Aust J Exp Agr* 44(4-5):458-467, 2004.
5. Garry F: Managing bloat in cattle, *Vet Med* 85:643-650, 1990.
6. Mills JHL, Christian RG: Lesions of bovine ruminal tympany, *J Am Vet Med Assoc* 157:947-952, 1970.
7. Majak W, Hall JW, McCaughey WP: Pasture management strategies for reducing the risk of legume bloat in cattle, *J Anim Sci* 73:1493-1498, 1995.
8. Majak W, Lysyk TJ, Garland GJ et al: Efficacy of Alfasure (TM) for the prevention and treatment of alfalfa bloat in cattle, *Can J Anim Sci* 85(1):111-113, 2005.
9. Berg BP, Majak W, McAllister TA et al: Bloat in cattle grazing alfalfa cultivars selected for a low initial rate of digestion: a review, *Can J Plant Sci* 80:493-502, 2000.
10. Corah LR: Polyether ionophores—effect on rumen function in feedlot cattle, *Vet Clin North Am [Food Anim Pract]* 7(1):127-132, 1991.

CHAPTER 6

Function and Dysfunction of the Ruminant Forestomach

WALTER GRÜNBERG and PETER D. CONSTABLE

Ruminant digestive physiology is largely dependent on pregastric fermentation in the forestomach. Therefore in contrast to monogastric species the ruminant stomach system consists of a nonsecretory forestomach functioning as a specialized mixing and fermentation vat and an acid- and pepsinogen-secreting compartment functioning as stomach in the classical sense, the abomasum. The forestomach system anatomically consists of three primary structures: rumen, reticulum, and omasum. Because reticulum and rumen act in concert, they are functionally considered as a single unit, the reticulorumen, which is separated by a sphincter, the reticulo-omasal orifice from the omasum. Fermentation in the reticulorumen is controlled by the ruminant through forage selection, addition of buffers

contained in saliva (bicarbonate, phosphate), and constant mixing through specialized contractions of the forestomach. Reticuloruminal motility ensures a constant flow of partially digested material into the abomasum for further digestion. This constant flow of digesta into the abomasum differs markedly from the intermittent flow observed in monogastric animals.

RETICULORUMINAL MOTILITY

Four different specialized contraction patterns can be clinically identified in the reticulorumen[1-5]:

1. Primary or mixing cycle
2. Secondary or eructation cycle

3. Rumination (associated with cud chewing)
4. Esophageal groove closure (associated with suckling milk)

In addition to these extrinsic contraction patterns, the reticulorumen also exhibits some intrinsic motility that occurs autonomously even after bilateral vagal denervation. Intrinsic motility consists of low-amplitude tone variations occurring 6 to 10 times per minute. The motility pattern and function of the four specialized extrinsic contraction patterns, as well as the role of intrinsic motility, should be understood because specific disorders such as vagal indigestion, rumen bloat, lactic acidosis, and ruminal drinking produce characteristic alterations in forestomach motility.

Primary Contractions

Primary cyclic activity results in the mixing and circulation of the digesta in an organized manner. The contraction cycle begins with a biphasic reticular contraction, followed by contraction of the dorsal then ventral ruminal sac.

Ruminants are clinically categorized as having either normal forestomach motility or forestomach atony, hypomotility, or hypermotility. Forestomach *atony* is defined as the complete absence of reticuloruminal motility. Atony can result from the absence of excitatory inputs or an increase in inhibitory inputs to the gastric center of the hypothalamus; direct depression of the gastric center (associated with generalized depression, severe illness, or general anesthesia); or failure of vagal (nerve lesion) or motor pathways (e.g., hypocalcemia).

Forestomach *hypomotility* refers to a reduction in the frequency *or* strength of primary contractions and is caused by either a reduction in the excitatory drive to the gastric center, an increase in inhibitory inputs, or weakness of the motor pathway as in hypocalcemic or hypokalemic states. The distinction between primary contraction frequency and strength is clinically important, particularly in reference to therapy of reticuloruminal hypomotility. The *frequency* of primary contractions indicates the overall health of the ruminant. In the cow the primary contraction frequency averages 1 cycle/minute. The rate increases transiently during feeding and decreases during rumination and recumbency.[3] Because of this variability, auscultation should proceed for at least 2 minutes when determining the frequency of contractions. The *strength* and *duration* of each contraction is determined primarily by the nature of the forestomach contents, although alterations in serum electrolyte concentrations (particularly hypocalcemia) can also decrease contraction strength. The strength of contraction is subjectively determined by observing the movement of the left paralumbar fossa and assessing the loudness of sounds associated with rumen contraction. Hypomotility and atony of the reticulorumen have been associated with pain, fever, and endotoxemia in affected animals. This effect is presumably caused by the release of eicosanoids after activation of the inflammatory cascade because it can be reversed by administering nonsteroidal antiinflammatory drugs.[6] Pharmacologically, hypomotility or atony of the reticulorumen can be induced by a number of drugs through either a central inhibitory action,

depressing central nervous functions including the gastric centers, or a peripheral effect, or a combination of both. Xylazine and detomidine, two α_2-adrenoreceptor agonists commonly used for sedation in ruminants, decrease forestomach motility through a depression of central nervous function and through a neuromuscular transmission deficiency, likely the result of a reduced acetylcholine release. Morphine and its analogues also exert an inhibitory effect on primary cycle motility mainly through central inhibition, although at high doses peripheral inhibition is also present.[7]

Forestomach *hypermotility* refers to an increase in the frequency of primary contractions and is caused by an increase in the excitatory drive to the gastric center (typically mild reticuloruminal distention).

Secondary Contractions

Secondary contraction cycles occur independently of primary contraction cycles and at a slower frequency (usually 1 every 2 minutes). They are concerned primarily with the eructation of gas, the rate being determined by the gas or fluid pressure in the dorsal ruminal sac.[2,3] Rumen contractions are essential for eructation.[3] Tension receptors in the medial wall of the dorsal ruminal sac initiate the reflex via the dorsal vagus nerve. Contractions start in the dorsal and caudodorsal ruminal sacs and then spread forward to move the gas cap anteriorly to the cardia region, which subsequently opens.[8] The cardia remains firmly shut if foam (frothy bloat) or fluid (laterally recumbent animals) contacts the cardia. Free gas bloat is often observed in ruminants in lateral recumbency. Eructation occurs in these animals after they become sternally recumbent, when fluid moves away from the cardia. Bloat can also result when peritonitis, abscesses, or masses distort the normal forestomach anatomy, preventing active removal of fluid from the cardia region. Esophageal obstructions, associated with intraluminal, intramural, or extraluminal masses, are also a common cause of free gas bloat. Passage of a stomach tube usually identifies these abnormalities, and forestomach motility is unimpaired unless the vagal nerve is damaged. Bloat is also observed in cattle with tetanus, the bloat arising from spasm of the esophageal musculature.

A persistent mild bloat is often observed in ruminants that have ruminal atony or hypomotility secondary to systemic disease. The bloat usually requires no treatment and disappears with the return of normal motility. Although the fermentation rate is lower than normal in these cases due to reduced feed intake, the intraruminal pressure is decreased and consequently rumen contractions are not strong enough to remove all of the gas produced.[5]

Auscultation of the left paralumbar fossa (which detects rumen motility) cannot differentiate secondary contraction cycles from primary contraction cycles, unless synchronous eructation is heard. However, when palpation of the left paralumbar fossa is coupled with reticular auscultation (by placing the bell of the stethoscope at the left costochondral junction between the seventh and eighth ribs), the two contraction cycles can be distinguished.[9] Reticular contractions (indicating a primary contraction) can usually be heard a few seconds before the dorsal ruminal sac contraction is seen or palpated. The reticular contraction is not easy to identify, and this technique requires practice. The absence of a reticular contraction before dorsal ruminal sac motility indicates a secondary contraction. Reticular contractions can be more accurately identified ultrasonographically. Placement of a 3.5-5 mHz transducer immediately caudal to the xyphoid and left to the median permits easy visualization of the reticulum and reticular motility.

Rumination

Rumination is a complex process involving regurgitation, remastication, insalivation, and deglutition.[3] It is initiated by the "rumination area," located close to the gastric center in the medulla oblongata. Rumination allows further physical breakdown of food with the addition of large quantities of saliva (buffer) and is an integral part of ruminant activity. Whether hypomotility of the reticulorumen observed with increased osmolality of rumen contents is caused directly by the increase in osmolality or whether hypomotility is an indirect effect associated with the increased amount of fluid in the forestomach secondary to the osmotic drain of extracellular fluid into the rumen is currently unknown.

Esophageal Groove Closure

The esophageal groove reflex allows milk in the suckling preruminant to bypass the forestomach, directing milk from the esophagus along the reticular groove and omasal canal into the abomasum. Milk initiates the reflex by chemical stimulation of receptors in the buccal cavity, pharynx, and cranial esophagus.[10] Once the reflex is established in neonates, sensory stimuli can cause esophageal groove closure without milk contacting the chemoreceptors. Esophageal groove closure is therefore normal in calves given water in an identical manner to which the calf previously received milk or in calves abruptly changed from nipple to bucket feeding.[11] Reflex closure continues to operate during and after the development of a functional rumen, provided that the animal continues to receive milk. Esophageal groove closure has been observed in cattle up to 2 years of age and can probably be induced pharmacologically in older cattle.[12-14]

Esophageal groove closure can be induced by the oral administration of particular salt solutions. In adult dairy cows CaCl$_2$ gels administered orally appear to induce the closure of the esophageal groove, resulting in a passage of this salt directly in the abomasum. This has been associated with mucosal irritations in the reticular groove area, omasum, and entrance of the abomasum.[15] Closure of the esophageal groove in cattle younger than 2 years of age can also be induced by oral drenching with solutions of sodium bicarbonate, sodium chloride, or sugar.[12] In 93% of cattle 100-250 ml of a 10% solution of sodium bicarbonate induces esophageal groove closure.[12,16] Closure is immediate and usually lasts for 1 to 2 minutes. Oral solutions administered during this time are directed into the abomasum, avoiding dilution in the rumen. In adult sheep, 5 ml of a 10% solution of copper sulfate consistently causes esophageal groove closure. This lasts for

at least 15 seconds, during which time a second orally administered liquid will pass directly into the abomasum. Watery rumen contents favor the establishment of this reflex.[17] Repeated administration of CuSO$_4$ should be avoided because of the high risk of copper toxicity. In goats, closure is best induced by injection of vasopressin 0.5 IU/kg, whereas in cattle doses of 0.08 IU/kg have been reported to be effective.[13,14] Reflex closure can be useful in the treatment of abomasal ulcers in younger animals because magnesium hydroxide or Kaopectate can be given orally shortly after sodium bicarbonate solution. In adult cattle positive clinical results have been reported in the treatment of ketosis when administering oral carbohydrates in association with intravenous (IV) vasopressin (40 IU/animal).[13]

The esophageal groove reflex is inhibited by abomasal distension, causing milk to enter the rumen instead of the abomasum. Liquid administered to calves via an esophageal feeder will not induce groove closure; nonetheless when healthy newborn calves are tube fed, less than 10% of the administered volume is found in the reticulorumen. This volume is similar to the volume refluxing from the abomasum into the reticulorumen in suckling calves.[18]

OMASAL MOTILITY

The omasum is a compact spherical organ, comprising the omasal canal and omasal body. Motility of the omasal canal is coordinated with that of the reticulorumen, whereas omasal body contractions occur independently of and at a slower rate than reticuloruminal contractions. The function of the omasum is incompletely understood; however, the omasum plays an important role in the transport of appropriately sized feed particles from the reticulorumen to the abomasum, esophageal groove closure, fermentation of ingesta, and absorption of water, volatile fatty acids, and minerals. Sheep and goats have a relatively small omasum when compared with cattle.

Definitive evidence of an omasal disorder requires exploratory celiotomy or rumenotomy. Diseases specially affecting the omasum are rare but include omasal impaction, omasal canal obstruction, and omasal erosions. Omasal canal obstructions usually result from ingestion of baling twine or plastic and are easily diagnosed during rumenotomy. Omasal erosions may be severe enough to lead to perforation of one or more omasal leaves. These erosions are commonly seen in healthy cattle, and their etiopathogenesis is unknown, although inflammation resulting from *Fusobacterium necrophorum* infection is a likely cause.[19] Omasal lesions are also observed in cattle dying of diseases such as bovine virus diarrhea, infectious bovine rhinotracheitis, and rinderpest.

Omasal impaction is a clinical disease of controversial significance, primarily because the normal bovine omasum varies markedly in size and consistency. The disorder is characterized by anorexia, an extremely firm and enlarged omasum that may be painful on palpation, the absence of other pathologic abdominal conditions, and clinical improvement following softening of the omasum. Treatment consists of intraoperative kneading of the omasum until the contents become pliable. Four liters of mineral oil should be administered intraruminally for 3-5 days postoperatively to facilitate softening. Omasotomy is indicated in unresponsive cases. The omasum is exteriorized through a midline abdominal incision, opened along the greater curvature, and flushed with water until it becomes soft and pliable. The omasum is closed with a two-layer inverting pattern, and the abdomen is routinely closed.[20]

CLINICAL ASSESSMENT OF FORESTOMACH FUNCTION

Assessment of the primary contraction cycle should be part of the routine clinical examination of ruminant animals. Secondary contraction cycles, esophageal groove closure, and rumination need only be examined when problems associated with the gastrointestinal tract have been identified. Careful assessment of forestomach motility helps the clinician identify the nature of any dysfunction and provide a rational course for treatment.

When assessing forestomach function, the clinician must determine the following:

1. Rate and strength of rumen contractions
2. Rumen volume
3. Nature of rumen contents
4. Nature of feces

This is best approached using the following two-stage sequential technique for the cow.

Physical Examination of the Forestomach

Visual Examination
The abdominal profile is critically examined. Abnormal findings can either be a unilaterally or bilaterally distended abdomen or a sunken left paralumbar fossa and flank area. An abnormal silhouette of the left side of the abdomen is most commonly associated with abnormal rumen contents in quality or quantity but can also be caused by a left displaced abomasum. In addition, the left paralumbar fossa is inspected for periodic distension, and the frequency and strength of ruminal contractions is determined.

External Ruminal Palpation
The physical nature of ruminal contents is assessed by palpation, ballottement, and succussion of the left paralumbar fossa and flank region. Normal primary cyclic motility leads to a stratification of ruminal contents, with firmer fibrous material floating on top of a more fluid layer. A gas cap dorsal of the fibrous material moderate in size can frequently be identified. This facilitates the differentiation from the fiber mat underneath. The normal rumen therefore feels resilient in the uppermost part of the dorsal ruminal sac if a gas cap is present, doughy underneath and more fluid in the left ventral quadrant of the abdomen. Abnormal ruminal stratification, or an excessively firm or watery rumen, suggests that a forestomach disorder is present. Very watery rumen contents that splash and fluctuate on ballottement are suggestive of lactic acidosis, ileus, or prolonged anorexia. Firm rumen contents are observed with restricted water intake, after ingestion of large amounts of unchopped forages, and with some forms of vagal indigestion.

Auscultation
Identification of rumen contractions requires both auscultation and observation of the left paralumbar fossa. Sound is produced when fibrous material rubs against the rumen wall during contraction. Very little sound is audible when the rumen contains small quantities of fibrous material (i.e., watery rumen) but also when the rumen is not in its physiologic position directly apposed to the left body wall, as is the case with a left displaced abomasum. In the former case observation of the left paralumbar fossa for periodic distension is necessary to detect rumen motility. Rumen hypomotility or hypermotility is usually associated with a change in the type of sound heard during auscultation, with a distant bubbling replacing the normal close crescendo-decrescendo crackling sound. Auscultation should proceed for at least 2 minutes in two locations:

1. Left paralumbar fossa
2. Seventh to eighth intercostal space at the costochondral junction

Auscultation of the left paralumbar fossa does not differentiate primary from secondary contraction cycles unless synchronous eructation is heard, whereas auscultation at the left costochondral junction does allow differentiation of the two basic cycles. Fewer than three contractions every 2 minutes indicates hypomotility, whereas more than five contractions every 2 minutes indicates hypermotility.

Internal (Rectal) Ruminal Palpation
The caudal aspect of the rumen should be palpated during rectal examination as far as accessible, and the volume and consistency determined. The results should then be compared with those obtained during external ruminal palpation. A portion of the ventral ruminal sac may be palpated on some cows by lifting the ventral abdomen dorsally with a horizontal bar placed at the level of the umbilicus. A gradual distension of the ventral ruminal sac into the right side of the abdominal cavity giving the rumen an L shape is commonly associated with a vagal indigestion.

Examination of Fecal Material
Examination of the fecal material should encompass an estimation of the amount of feces present in the rectum, color, odor and consistency of the feces, as well as the degree of digestion. A scant amount or complete absence of feces is not necessarily consistent with a mechanical obstruction of the gastrointestinal tract but most commonly due to a functional obstruction (functional ileus) or decreased feed intake in ruminants. Color of the fecal material is not only influenced by the composition of the diet but also by the concentration of bile, as well as a possible addition of unphysiologic components like digested (melena) or undigested blood. Whereas normal feces in ruminants have a mild aromatic odor, malodorous feces are commonly the result of abnormal fermentation or putrefaction of ingesta and can be the result of an inflammatory reaction (e.g., salmonellosis). Feces with acidic odor can be the result of acute grain overload. Consistency of the feces is not only related to the type of feed but mainly to the amount of water contained in them

and the transit time of ingesta through the digestive tract. Thickening of the feces is frequently seen during stages of severe dehydration or with decreased motility of the gastrointestinal tract and of the forestomachs. Loose stool or diarrhea associated with disturbed function of the fore-stomachs is most commonly seen with rumen acidosis. The size of digested plant fragments in ruminant feces provides an indirect measure of forestomach function because solid matter normally stays in the rumen until the particle size is sufficiently small to pass through the reticulo-omasal orifice.[21] Excessively large fibers (>0.5 cm) or fine plant particles in the feces indicate rapid or prolonged rumen turnover time, respectively. The nature of the feces can also provide information about the diet; numerous corn kernels may provide evidence of excessive grain consumption.

Laboratory Examination of Rumen Fluid

Collection of Rumen Fluid

Rumen fluid can be obtained by two methods: passage of a stomach tube or rumenocentesis. Analysis is best per-formed on freshly collected samples. A detailed descrip-tion of rumen fluid analysis is available.[22]

Ororuminal collection. This involves ororuminal pas-sage of a tube to collect rumen fluid. Although this tech-nique is safe and practical, the major difficulty is avoiding saliva contamination of the rumen sample, thereby neces-sitating collection of fluid from the ventral ruminal sac. Specialized stomach tubes that minimize saliva contami-nation such as weighted stomach tubes[23] and Dirksen's guidable probe[24] have been developed, although neither tube predictably collects fluid from the ventral ruminal sac. The best method to be developed uses a magnet attached to the weighted head of the collecting tube.[25] The tube is passed ororuminally until an obstruction is felt, at which time the surface of the left ventral abdomi-nal area is scanned with a compass to confirm that the sample is being collected from the ventral ruminal sac. This technique is initially successful in 72% of attempts. If the compass indicates that the tube is not located in the ventral ruminal sac, the tube is removed and the pro-cedure repeated. Using this technique, 500 ml of ruminal fluid can be rapidly and easily removed from the ventral ruminal sac.[25] Recommendations for obtaining rumen fluid through a stomach tube for pH measurement rou-tinely include discarding the first 200 ml of fluid obtained because this initial fraction tends to have a higher pH attributable to saliva contamination.[26] Because of the poor sensitivity of orogastric probe samples for diagnos-ing subacute rumen acidosis (SARA), these samples are considered less suitable than rumenocentesis samples to rule out SARA.[26]

Rumenocentesis. This involves percutaneous aspira-tion of rumen contents from the ventral ruminal sac and is mainly indicated for the diagnosis of clinical or subclin-ical rumen acidosis. An area on the lower left ventrolat-eral abdominal quadrant, horizontal with the patella and 8 inches caudal to the costochondral junction of the last rib, is clipped and surgically scrubbed. The cow is then restrained by tail elevation and hobbling the hind feet, mild xylazine sedation (0.04 mg/kg, IV), or local lidocaine

infiltration of the puncture site. A 5-inch, 16-ga needle attached to a 10- to 20-ml syringe is thrust firmly and quickly perpendicular to the skin into the rumen. Rumen contents are then aspirated, and the pH measured imme-diately using a portable pH meter. If the needle becomes blocked with ingesta, 3 ml of air is pushed through the needle in an attempt to clear the blockage.[27,28]

Problems associated with rumenocentesis include sub-cutaneous or intraabdominal abscesses, localized peritoni-tis, hematomas, penetration of the uterus in late gestation or the abomasum in cows with left displaced abomasum, a small sample volume (<10 ml), blood contamination (affects pH through buffering capacity of blood), as well as markedly decreased feed intake and milk production in the days following the procedure.[29] The complication rates after rumenocentesis given in the literature range from 1% to 6% and are mainly classified as mild (small nod-ules at puncture site) but also as life threatening in some instances, associated with peritonitis and the formation of large abscesses.[27,29,30] To circumvent the need for rumeno-centesis, milk fat depression has been proposed as an indi-cator for the presence of SARA with a cut point of milk fat being below 3.2% in Holstein cows and below 4.2% in Jerseys.[31] Other studies report little correlation between the prevalence of SARA and milk fat concentration. This can be explained by the observation that not only do high-grain, low-fiber diets predispose the animal to SARA but that other factors such as adding unsaturated fats to the diet result in milk fat depression.[32,33] Whereas milk fat depres-sion is considered suggestive of increased risk of SARA and high milk fat percentages decrease the likelihood of SARA being present, normal milk fat percentages provide no reli-able information regarding the likelihood of SARA.[32,34]

Analysis of Rumen Fluid

Color. This is dependent on the diet; corn silage and straw diets produce yellow/brown rumen contents, con-centrates produce an olive/brown color, and pasture pro-duces a green color. A black/green color usually indicates ruminal stasis, whereas a milky gray/brown color is often observed in lactic acidosis.

Odor. Rumen fluid normally has a slightly aromatic, unobjectionable odor. Acidic/sour smells are suggestive of lactic acidosis, whereas rumen putrefaction produces a rotting odor.

Consistency. Rumen contents are normally slightly vis-cous. Excessive viscosity indicates significant saliva con-tamination, and the sample should be discarded because it is not a valid representation of rumen fluid. A watery sample with little particulate matter indicates anorexia and is usually associated with reduced protozoal and bac-terial numbers. Rumen fluid that has numerous stable bubbles that do not coalesce is indicative of frothy bloat.

pH. Rumen pH is best measured at its lowest value (i.e., 2-4 hours after feeding a concentrate meal or 4-8 hours after offering a fresh total mixed ration). Rumen pH is determined using a portable pH meter or pH papers. The normal pH of grass-fed ruminants is 6-7. A pH value of 5.5-6 is seen in cattle on high-grain diets or pasture-fed cattle with early lactic acidosis. pH values less than 5.5 are virtually pathognomonic for lactic acidosis, although feedlot cattle well adapted to high-grain diets can have rumen pH values approaching 5. A reduced feed intake of 2 or more days' duration often increases rumen pH up to 7 or 8. Rumen pH values exceeding 8 are due to (1) contamination with saliva (in which case the sample should be discarded), (2) severe putrefaction of ingested protein associated with prolonged rumen stasis, or (3) urea toxicity. For diagnosing SARA, the most commonly recommended cut points are a pH=5.5 for a diagnosis as SARA positive and a pH=5.8 for a diagnosis as SARA negative. The suitable number of samples to be analyzed for a herd or feeding group screening has been determined to be 12 animals of the specific risk group. With three or more of the 12 samples having a pH of 5.5 or lower, the prevalence of SARA should be regarded as high and thus the specific group considered as SARA affected.[27,29]

Methylene blue reduction. This test measures the reducing ability of anaerobic ruminal bacteria. Ten ml of fresh rumen fluid is added to a test tube containing 0.5 ml of a 0.03% solution of methylene blue, and the time taken for the solution to clear is measured. In cattle the clearance time is normally between 2 and 6 minutes, the faster rate being observed in cattle on high-grain diets. Clearance times greater than 10 minutes indicate inadequate anaerobic bacterial numbers, and rumen transfaunation is required. The clearance time is much faster in sheep (usually 1 to 4 minutes). This test is invalid at rumen pH less than 5.5.

Protozoa. One drop of fresh rumen contents is placed on a slide and examined under low power (×40). Normal rumen fluid contains greater than 40 protozoa per low-power field, with actively moving protozoa that can be broadly characterized into three sizes (small, medium, large). Low protozoal numbers (<8 per low-power field), nonmotile protozoa, or loss of population heterogeneity all indicate an abnormal intraruminal environment. Transfaunation is indicated if these abnormalities are identified, particularly if the methylene blue reduction time is prolonged. It is not usually necessary to identify the protozoal species present, but occasionally it is valuable to differentiate Isotrichids (formerly Holotrichs) which are usually the larger protozoa, from Oligotrichs (Entodiniomorphs), which are smaller and more resistant to pH values of less than 6. Protozoal energy stores can be assessed by adding one drop of Lugol's iodine to one drop of rumen fluid on a slide. Healthy protozoa are almost uniformly stained by iodine, whereas protozoa that have been starved have diminished starch stores, evidenced by decreasing numbers of starch granules.

Chloride concentration. The rumen fluid should be centrifuged, and the supernatant submitted for determination of the chloride concentration, which is normally 10-25 mEq/L in cattle and less than 15 mEq/L in sheep. Elevated rumen chloride concentrations result from abomasal reflux (internal vomition), ileus, or high salt intake. High Cl concentrations are most consistent with an obstruction at or distal to the pylorus. The physical examination will hopefully provide evidence as to whether this obstruction is functional or pathologic.

Rumen osmolality. The rumen osmotic pressure is actively controlled by the ruminant and closely approximates serum osmotic pressure. A constant osmotic pressure ensures homeostatic conditions for ruminal microbes,

which are susceptible to lysis or swelling if large and rapid variations in rumen osmolality occur.[35]

Gram stain. Rumen fluid normally contains a large heterogeneous population of bacteria, which are predominantly gram negative. Lactic acidosis produces a more uniform bacterial population, which is predominantly gram positive.

Other tests. A number of other laboratory tests such as sedimentation time, cellulose digestion test, and total titratable acidity have also been used in the examination of rumen fluid. These tests seldom add information than that obtained earlier, and their routine use is not recommended.

SIMPLE INDIGESTION

Definition

Simple indigestion is a common disease primarily affecting nongrazing ruminants. The disorder is relatively easy to diagnose when a large number of ruminants become inappetant immediately after a change in feeding practices. Much more difficult, however, is to diagnose simple indigestion when only one animal is affected and the diet has been unchanged. In this case simple indigestion is diagnosed by exclusion.

Pathogenesis

The cause of simple indigestion is presumed to be an altered ruminal microbial population, secondary to a rapid change in the intraruminal environment. The ruminal microbial population is normally in a continual state of flux, the population characteristics being determined by feeding frequency, nature of diet, and water intake. Diurnal variations in the rumen microbial population therefore occur. Because these variations are more pronounced in ruminants fed once or twice daily than in animals grazing pastures or fed a total mixed ration, indigestion is more likely to occur in intermittently fed ruminants.

Clinical Signs

The first indication of simple indigestion is a reduction in appetite, accompanied by a moderate decrease in milk production in lactating animals. The fecal consistency is usually altered, and typically a malodorous loose stool is voided within 12 to 24 hours of the onset of clinical signs. Reticuloruminal motility is decreased or absent, and rumination ceases. The rumen contents are more fluid on external palpation. Systemic signs of illness are not observed.

Diagnosis

Three criteria must be fulfilled before a diagnosis of simple indigestion can be made: (1) forestomach hypomotility or atony, (2) abnormal rumen contents, and (3) exclusion of all known diseases affecting the forestomach and gastrointestinal tract. Rumen fluid is required to confirm a diagnosis of simple indigestion. Strong supportive evidence for a diagnosis is a recent change in feed substrate, feeding frequency, or quantity of feed available and more than one animal being affected.

Differential diagnoses that must be strongly considered when only one animal is affected are traumatic reticulitis, left displaced abomasum, and acetonemia. Traumatic reticulitis is usually accompanied by an abrupt and marked decrease in appetite and milk production, and abdominal pain and pyrexia are often present. Forestomach motility may appear decreased in cattle with left displaced abomasum, but the characteristic "ping" of the displaced abomasum is usually identified during simultaneous auscultation and percussion. Acetonemia occurs most frequently in the first 6 weeks following parturition and is diagnosed by assessment of urine and milk aceto-acetate concentration.

Treatment

The primary goal of treatment is rapid attainment of a normal intraruminal environment. This is most easily achieved through rumen transfaunation, which provides a balanced, buffered, nutrient-dense solution that also includes essential microorganisms. At least 3 L of freshly strained rumen juice are necessary to transfaunate an adult dairy cow; 8-16 L are considered ideal. Rumen contents can be collected at the local abattoir or from cattle on the farm by passing a stomach tube and back siphoning rumen juice. The latter is a time-consuming process, and a number of cattle and special stomach tubes are required because the volume obtained varies from animal to animal. Stealing cuds from ruminating cattle has also been proposed as a means of obtaining rumen juice; however, this method is impractical for routine use and is incapable of producing adequate volumes. Probiotic agents may be of additional benefit to rumen transfaunation if imbalances in the small intestinal microbial population are suspected. Commercial probiotics consist mainly of lactate producers that are thought to create a favorable intraruminal environment that prevents accumulation of lactic acid by inducing growth of bacteria metabolizing lactic acid. The resulting enhanced ability to remove lactate from the rumen thus stabilizes the rumen pH. Further work is required to determine the optimal way to use probiotic agents. Good-quality grass hay and straw should be available to the anorexic animal because sick ruminants often prefer these feeds over alfalfa or concentrates. Oral administration of specific alkalinizing or acidifying agents should not be routinely undertaken in cases of indigestion. Magnesium oxide and magnesium hydroxide are strong alkalinizing agents able to substantially increase rumen pH and thus create a hostile environment for rumen protozoa. These compounds, when given at a label dose to dairy cattle, result in a significant decrease in rumen fermentation and a reduction in the number of rumen protozoa.[36] Therefore these compounds should only be administered to cattle with confirmed diagnosis of grain overload. Acetic acid (vinegar, 4-10 L) can be administered to cattle with putrefaction of the rumen, associated with a high rumen pH.

Ruminatorics such as nux vomica, ginger, tarter, and parasympathomimetics, although frequently used, have a limited application in modern treatment of forestomach dysfunction. Evidence for the effectiveness of these compounds to treat indigestions in ruminants is currently not available. Parasympathomimetic agents such as neostigmine or carbamylcholine should not be used when rumen atony is present. Neostigmine requires vagal activity to be effective and therefore cannot incite normal primary contractions in atonic animals. Neostigmine may be of some benefit in hypomotile states because it increases the strength of the primary contraction without upsetting rhythm or coordination. Carbamylcholine causes uncoordinated, spastic, and functionless forestomach contractions, therefore having no place in the treatment of forestomach dysfunction. The IV administration of the benzodiazepine agonist brotizolam at a dose of 0.002 mg/kg induces hyperphagia in adult cattle and goats, resulting in a transient increase in feed intake, and thus has been proposed as supportive treatment in anorectic animals with simple indigestion.[37,38]

Simple indigestion can be prevented by increasing the feeding frequency, adding buffers to the feed (e.g., crude fiber, sodium bicarbonate), and avoiding rapid changes in feeding practices and substrate.

References

1. Leek BF: Reticulo-ruminal function and dysfunction, *Vet Rec* 84:238-243, 1969.
2. Kay R: Rumen function and physiology, *Vet Rec* 113:6-9, 1983.
3. Sellers AF, Stevens CE: Motor functions of the ruminant forestomach, *Physiol Rev* 46:634-659, 1966.
4. Leek BF, Harding RH: Sensory nervous receptors in the ruminant stomach and the reflex control of reticulo-ruminal motility. In McDonald IW, Warner ACI, editors: *Digestion and metabolism in the ruminant*, Armadale, NSW, Australia, 1975, New England Publishing Unit, pp 60-76.
5. Leek BF: Clinical diseases of the rumen: a physiologist's view, *Vet Rec* 113:10-14, 1983.
6. Eades SC: Endotoxemia in dairy cattle: role of eicosanoids in reticulorumen stasis, *J Dairy Sci* 76:414-420, 1993.
7. Maas CL, Leek BF: Central and local actions of opioids upon reticulo-ruminal motility in sheep, *Vet Res Comm* 9:89-113, 1985.
8. Dougherty RW, Habel RE, Bond HE: Esophageal innervation and the eructation reflex in sheep, *Am J Vet Res* 19:115-128, 1958.
9. Williams EI: A study of reticulo-ruminal motility in adult cattle in relation to bloat and traumatic reticulitis with an account of the latter condition as seen in general practice, *Vet Rec* 67:907-911, 1955.
10. Ruckebusch Y: Pharmacology of reticulo-ruminal motor function, *J Vet Pharmacol Ther* 6:245-272, 1983.
11. Abe M, Iriki T, Kondoh K, Shibui H: Effects of nipple or bucket feeding of milk-substitute on rumen by-pass and on rate of passage in calves, *Br J Nutr* 41:175-180, 1979.
12. Riek RF: The influence of sodium salts on the closure of the esophageal groove in calves, *Aust Vet J* 30:29-37, 1954.
13. Scholz H: Utilization of the reticular groove contraction in adult cattle: a therapeutical alternative for the practitioner? *Bov Pract* 23:148-152, 1988.
14. Mikhail M, Brugere H, Le Bars H et al: Stimulated esophageal groove closure in adult goats, *Am J Vet Res* 49:1713-1715, 1988.
15. Wentink GH, Van den Ingh TSGAM: Oral administration of calcium chloride-containing products: testing for deleterious side-effects, *Vet Quart* 14:76-80, 1992.

16. Wester J: The rumination reflex in the ox, *Vet J* 86: 410-410, 1930.
17. Monnig HO, Quin JI: Studies on the alimentary tract of the merino sheep in South Africa, II. Investigations on the physiology of deglutition, II, *Onderstepoort J Vet Sci* 5:485-499, 1935.
18. Nouri M, Constable P: Comparison of two oral electrolyte solutions and route of administration on the abomasal emptying rate of Holstein-Friesian calves, *J Vet Int Med* 20:620-626, 2006.
19. Brownlee A, Elliot J: Studies on the normal and abnormal structure and function of the omasum of domestic cattle, *Br Vet J* 116:467-473, 1960.
20. McDonald JS, Witzel DA: Three cases of chronic omasal impaction in the dairy cow, *J Am Vet Med Assoc* 152:638-640, 1968.
21. Ulyatt MJ, Dellow DW, John CSW et al: Contribution of chewing during eating and rumination and the clearance of digesta from the ruminoreticulum. In Milligan LP, Grovum WL, Dobson A, editors: *Control and digestion and metabolism in ruminants*, Upper Saddle River, NJ, 1986, Prentice-Hall, pp 498-517.
22. Alonso AN: Diagnostic analysis of rumen fluid, *Vet Clin North Am Food Anim Pract* 1:363-376, 1979.
23. Geishauser T: An instrument for the collection and transfer of ruminal fluid and for administration of water soluble drugs in adult cattle, *Bov Pract* 27:38-42, 1993.
24. Dirksen G, Smith MC: Acquisition and analysis of bovine rumen fluid, *Bov Pract* 22:108-116, 1987.
25. Geishauser T: A probe for collection of ruminal fluid in juvenile cattle and cows, *Bov Pract* 28:113-116, 1994.
26. Duffield T, Plaizier JC, Fairfield A et al: Comparison of techniques for measurement of rumen pH in lactating dairy cows, *J Dairy Sci* 87:59-66.
27. Nordlund KV, Garrett EF: Rumenocentesis: a technique for collecting rumen fluid for the diagnosis of subacute rumen acidosis in dairy herds, *Bov Pract* 28:109-112, 1994.
28. Nordlund KV: Questions and answers regarding rumenocentesis and the diagnosis of herd-based subacute rumen acidosis, *Bov Proceed* 28:75-81, 1996.
29. Kleen JL, Hooijer GA, Rehage J et al: Rumenocentesis (rumen puncture): a viable instrument in herd health diagnosis, *Dtsch Tieraerztl Wschr* 111:458-462, 2004.
30. Wheeler-Aceto H, Meadows C, Ferguson J: The effects of dietary starch and nonstructural carbohydrate on production, rumen pH, and neutrophil function in Holstein cows, *J Dairy Sci* 82(suppl 1):43, 1999, abstract.
31. Pennington JA: *Factors affecting fat percent in milk of lactating cows. University of Arkansas Extension Publication No FSA4014*, Little Rock, 1999, University of Arkansas Cooperative Extension Service.
32. Garret EF: *Rumenocentesis: methodology and application in the diagnosis of subacute ruminal acidosis in dairy herds*, master's thesis, University of Wisconsin, Madison, 1996.
33. Bauman DE, Griinari JM: Regulation and nutritional manipulation of milk fat: low-fat milk syndrome, *Livest Prod Sci* 70:15-29, 2001.
34. Nortlund K, Cook NB, Oetzel GR: Investigation strategies for laminitis problem herds, *J Dairy Sci* 87(suppl):E27-E35, 2004.
35. Welch JG: Rumination, particle size, and passage from the rumen, *J Anim Sci* 54:885-894, 1982.
36. Smith GW, Correa MT: The effects of oral magnesium hydroxide administration on rumen fluid in cattle, *J Vet Intern Med* 18:109-112, 2004.
37. Van Miert AS, Koot M, Van Duin CT: Appetite modulating drugs in dwarf goats, with special emphasis on benzodiazepine-induced hyperphagia and its antagonism by flumazenil and RO 15-505, *J Vet Pharmacol Ther* 12(2):147-56, 1989.
38. Danneberg P, Bauer R, Boke-Kuhn K et al: General pharmacology of brotizolam in animals, *Arzneimittelforschung* 36(3A):540-551, 1986.

Recommended Readings

Constable PD, Hoffsis GF, Rings DM: The reticulorumen: normal and abnormal motor function. Part I. Primary contraction cycle, and Part II. Secondary contraction cycles, rumination, and esophageal groove closure, *Compend Contin Ed Pract Vet* 12:1008-1015 and 1169-1174, 1990.

Ruckebusch Y: Gastrointestinal motor functions in ruminants, In Wood J, editor: *Handbook of physiology, the gastrointestinal system*, Bethesda, MD, 1990, American Physiologic Society, pp 1225-1282.

CHAPTER 7

Rumen Indigestion and Putrefaction

FRANKLYN B. GARRY

SIMPLE AND SECONDARY INDIGESTION

DEFINITION

The term *indigestion* describes a disruption of normal reticulorumen function. By this definition, indigestion is a group of problems that involve abnormal forestomach motility or abnormal fermentative activity, which in turn lead to abnormal reticulorumen contents. The various aberrations in motility and fermentation define the type of indigestion such as rumen acidosis, vagal indigestion, and frothy bloat. The subjects of this section are probably the most common types of indigestion but are also the least dramatic and least clearly definable.

Simple indigestion is a disease with acute onset. It is associated with an abrupt dietary change that results in a self-limiting but rapid decline in rumen fermentation. If the dietary or rumen fluid change cannot be assigned to one of the more well-characterized indigestions such as acidosis, alkalosis, or rumen putrefaction, it may be characterized as simple indigestion. It can occur in an individual animal or in several members of a group.

Secondary indigestion is a disruption of normal reticulorumen function as the sequela of other disease such as endotoxemic infection, abomasal disease, and metabolic disease. It is similar to simple indigestion but typically more chronic in onset because it follows the establishment of another disease entity. The main importance of this condition is that it can confound accurate identification of the primary disease, and it can delay return to normal health as the primary disease resolves.

PATHOGENESIS

Simple indigestion results from rapid change in feedstuff or introduction of substances that rapidly change the rumen fluid environment or inhibit the present fermentation pattern. Moldy or overheated feeds, frosted forages, and partially fermented, spoiled, and soured silages are typically implicated causes. Components of the feed or fermentation products acutely, but temporarily, cause a decline in rumen fermentation and motility. Specific toxins may be involved but have not been identified. Some plants can produce indigestion as a primary sign of toxicity (e.g., azalea and rhododendron in small ruminants), but these problems are addressed elsewhere in this text.

Secondary indigestion can result when another disease reduces feed intake or specifically reduces rumen motility (e.g., endotoxemia, febrile disease). Abomasal/intestinal disease can both reduce rumen activity and reflux abomasal content into the reticulorumen. Reduced intake, depressed motility, and abnormal reflux fluid entry all result in declining fermentation, in some cases leading to complete cessation of rumen activity.

CLINICAL SIGNS

Cattle affected by simple indigestion typically demonstrate acute anorexia without overt systemic signs of disease. Heart rate is usually normal to low, and hydration status is unremarkable. Rumen motility is reduced to absent, and abdominal fill is not remarkably altered, although mild free gas bloat may occur. Malodorous diarrhea is usually observed in about 24 hours. The disease is self-limiting, and affected cattle usually return to feed within 1 to 2 days. Multiple cattle may be affected, but often the problem occurs in only one or several animals, even though the entire herd is on the same feed.

Clinical signs of secondary indigestion are concurrent with signs of the primary disease, but rumen inactivity may continue as the primary disease is resolving. Identification of this problem relies on assessing rumen function as part of the evaluation and treatment of anorexic cows affected by any of a variety of diseases. Rumen function is decreased, rumination absent, and with chronicity the rumen is underfilled. Fecal production is usually depressed, and diarrhea is common.

DIAGNOSIS

Diagnosis may be empirically based on clinical signs, history, and exclusion of other primary forestomach diseases. For secondary indigestion, diagnosis of another primary disease will have been made and the affected animal may be presumptively treated to combat depressed forestomach function. Thorough forestomach evaluation may show overtly depressed function. Rumen fluid analysis can help characterize poor fermentative activity and monitor response to treatment. Rumen fluid pH is typically normal to mildly elevated (6.5->7.5), and the odor is usually stale or sour. Rumen microbial activity is reduced, as evidenced by low protozoal numbers and activity and prolonged methylene blue reduction time. Rumen fluid is watery rather than slightly viscous, and sedimentation of feed particles occurs rapidly. Elevated rumen fluid chloride concentration helps characterize abomasal reflux as a contributor to poor forestomach activity.

TREATMENT

Careful assessment of forestomach function and rumen fluid characteristics directs the appropriate treatment. The primary goal is restoration of a normal forestomach environment. Mild cases of simple or secondary indigestion are self-correcting, and many clinicians may elect no treatment. Alternatively, some simple treatments will usually benefit the mild cases and provide greatly improved recovery rates in more severe cases.

Rumen transfaunation is the single best means of inoculating an inactive rumen. Fluid should come from a healthy individual, preferably one that is adapted to the patient's expected ration. The fluid can be obtained from a fistulated animal, siphoned via stomach tube, or from a local abattoir. Large particulate matter can be strained from the fluid using cheesecloth, and the transfaunate administered via stomach tube. The inoculum is optimal if administered immediately but remains viable for up to 9 hours at room temperature or 24 hours under refrigeration. A minimum of 3 L should be administered to an adult cow, and 8 to 16 L is preferable. Transfaunating several days in a row is desirable in severely affected cattle, but the need for multiple transfaunations can be assessed based on the animal's response. Probiotic preparations (direct-fed microbial preparations) are not a substitute for rumen fluid administration because they contain only one or several microbial species, but they may be beneficial if rumen fluid for transfaunation cannot be obtained.

For cattle with notably decreased rumen fill, additional oral fluid administration is usually beneficial. Mild rumen distention is one of the primary stimuli for active rumen motor activity. Twenty to 30 L of fluid may be required to accomplish the desired effect. Fluid should be warmed to body temperature. The oral fluid also provides a vehicle for administering other treatments that may be beneficial in most cases of indigestion. Sodium and potassium salts (table salt, Lite Salt) can be added to produce an isotonic solution ($\approx$2 teaspoons/L) for animals with prolonged anorexia or presumed electrolyte deficiency. Propylene glycol and niacin are beneficial for cattle with ketosis. Alfalfa pellets added to provide a gruel are useful for prolonged anorexia. Complete or partial resolution of the primary disease problem is usually required before cattle with secondary indigestion will respond favorably to forestomach therapy.

Historically, many other agents have been advocated for oral administration to cattle with simple indigestion. Our current understanding suggests these treatments are unwarranted or detrimental. Unless rumen fluid pH is grossly abnormal, rumen alkalinizing agents (magnesium oxide or magnesium hydroxide) and acidifying agents (acetic acid, vinegar) will not be beneficial and may result in additional disturbances. Ruminatorics (ginger, tartar emetic, nux vomica) and parasympathomimetic agents (neostigmine, carbamylcholine) can alter rumen contraction but do not induce return to normal rumen activity. Restoration of physiologic normalcy appears to be the best means of stimulating fermentative digestion and productive rumen function.

Additional treatments include provision of good-quality grass hay or other coarse feed such as dry oats. These feeds are often more acceptable to cattle recovering from indigestions than are more energy-dense rations. Parenteral administration of B vitamins may be helpful until normal rumen function is reestablished.

RUMEN PUTREFACTION (ESOPHAGEAL GROOVE DYSFUNCTION, RUMEN DRINKERS)

DEFINITION

In this indigestive disturbance a putrefactive decomposition of forestomach contents replaces the normal fermentation processes of rumen microbial digestion. The disease can occur in calves or adult cattle, but it is uncommon in adults fed typical ruminant rations. It is more frequently seen in calves before weaning, before conversion to a ruminant diet and the attainment of full rumen digestive function. The existence of an established, active, forestomach microbial population is usually effective at inhibiting the abnormal decomposition of ingesta that causes this disease. The disease has a chronic course and typically occurs in individual animals, although herdmates are exposed to similar management and a similar diet.

Putrefactive indigestion is associated with abnormal feeds or with continued deposition of milk in the rumen of the preweaned calf. The disease in calves has been associated with poor function of the esophageal groove. In milk-fed calves, this results in ongoing exposure of milk to bacterial degradation in the forestomach, with consequent abnormal fermentation and disease development. Affected calves have been called "rumen drinkers" and are characterized by chronic poor growth, a potbellied appearance, free gas bloat, poor hair coat or hair loss, abnormal feces, and sometimes a depraved appetite and licking of the hair coat.

PATHOGENESIS

Properties of ingested feed and the forestomach microbial population are primary determinants of the type of digestive processes that occur in the forestomach. High-protein diets favor a proliferation of proteolytic organisms. The resulting high rumen fluid pH, paired with repeated inoculation of abnormal bacteria, can promote the development of putrefactive decomposition. In adult cattle, spoiled fermented forages or concentrates and fecal contamination of feed or water can provide the abnormal microbial inoculum. These conditions are not common, and a well-established rumen microflora inhibits the development of such aberrant digestive patterns, so the disease is uncommon.

The young calf without well-developed rumen fermentation is apparently more susceptible to this form of indigestion. Repeated deposition of milk in the developing rumen stimulates abnormal digestion. Milk can gain access to the rumen by several means. These include failure of esophageal groove closure, prolonged maintenance of calves as preruminants (>3-4 months), and abomasal reflux. The latter can result from fluid feeding beyond the capacity of the abomasum ($\approx$5% of body weight), fluids that delay abomasal emptying or inhibit curd formation, and abomasal inflammation. The high fat and protein content and relatively low carbohydrate content of milk predispose to a microflora in the rumen that decomposes these constituents, producing spoiled and rancid rumen ingesta. Problem development is further encouraged by feeding contaminated or spoiled fluids.

CLINICAL SIGNS

Cattle affected by rumen putrefaction have reduced appetite and productivity, decreased rumen activity, recurrent bloat, and intermittent diarrhea. Occasionally, frothy rumen contents are found. Overt systemic signs of disease are usually absent.

Calves with this type of indigestion typically display poor growth and evidence of malnutrition. These signs likely result from abnormal digestive end products, and herdmates on a similar feeding regimen may be performing adequately. Affected calves typically develop a poor hair coat and sometimes a depraved appetite with excessive licking of the hair coat. The abdomen is mildly distended (potbellied) and flaccid, and the rumen is distended with fluid. Ballottement during auscultation reveals tinkling fluid sounds and/or pings of rumen origin. Rumen motility is poor, and recurrent bloat is common. Feces are commonly pasty or fluid in consistency. The disease develops gradually, so the animal's poor condition may be well advanced before it is noticed.

This disease can occur in association with neonatal enteritis in calves 1 to 2 weeks old. In these cases the evaluation of the calf is usually focused on the intestinal tract and body fluid balance, whereas the rumen is overlooked and not evaluated. Calves with esophageal groove dysfunction may have prolonged diarrhea and poor response to usual therapeutic procedures. Although the rumen is not well developed, auscultation with ballottement and percussion of the left flank usually reveals splashing and tinkling fluid sounds and pings. Auscultation during drinking can be especially revealing. Other clinical signs include prolonged mild depression and poor appetite compared with calves that have diarrhea without esophageal groove dysfunction.

DIAGNOSIS

Diagnosis requires evaluation of rumen fluid characteristics. Typically, the history is unrevealing until after the diagnosis is achieved because the animal is maintained similarly to other normal herdmates. After diagnosing the condition, a further investigation may reveal predisposing factors.

In adult cattle the rumen fluid color is typically dark green to black, solid and liquid components are mixed and sometimes frothy, the odor is foul, pH typically ranges between 7.5 and 8.5, and the number of protozoa is greatly reduced.

Milk-fed calves with this problem are also identified based on rumen fluid analysis. Rumen fluid pH in older calves (2-4 months) may be alkaline as a result of the proteolytic formation of ammonia. The rumen fluid pH is usually acidic (<pH 6) in young calves (1-2 weeks) with esophageal groove failure and neonatal enteritis,

apparently resulting from lactic acid or butyric acid generation. These pH findings contrast with normal rumen fluid pH between 6.0 and 7.0 in young calves. Color is typically milky to beige, and milk clots and curdling may be apparent. The odor is rancid to sour to stale. These findings, combined with the physical findings described earlier, define the disease but usually fail to define the cause in an individual, and further workup may be required to evaluate abomasal health and possible causal involvement. Rumen fluid chloride concentration is high in normal milk fed calves (40-95 mEq/L), and its measurement is therefore not particularly helpful in achieving this diagnosis, nor in identifying abomasal disease as the cause. Typically a specific cause is not determined, and further diagnostic efforts may be unwarranted unless response to treatment including dietary changes fails to produce satisfactory improvement.

TREATMENT

The primary goal, as for other fermentative indigestions, is restoration of a normal forestomach environment and microbial digestion pattern. Three general steps are taken to accomplish this goal: (1) correct the current fluid abnormalities, (2) reinoculate the rumen with microbes appropriate for normal carbohydrate fermentation, and (3) change the feeding pattern and the rumen ingesta available for fermentation.

Rumen fluid pH abnormality can be corrected by administration of alkalinizing (magnesium hydroxide at 1 g/kg) or acidifying (acetic acid/vinegar at 2 mL/kg) agents via stomach tube. Intraruminal administration of antibiotics such as oxytetracycline has been used to decrease undesirable populations of rumen microbes.

In my view, the best approach is removal of the accumulated ingesta. Especially in young calves that have little dry matter content in the rumen, the fluid can be drained off by siphoning via stomach tube. Emptying the contents via rumenotomy may be more expedient and more effective than siphoning when the ingesta has a significant fiber component. The rumen may be lavaged with warm fluids to enhance thorough emptying.

Following the correction of rumen fluid abnormality, rumen transfaunation is used to inoculate the rumen. This procedure is described earlier in the section on simple indigestion. Transfaunating several days in a row is desirable and has the additional benefit of providing a nutrient-dense supplement to the affected animal. Probiotic preparations (direct-fed microbial preparations) are not a substitute for rumen fluid administration, but they may be beneficial if rumen fluid for transfaunation cannot be obtained. Administration of alfalfa pellets mixed into a gruel provides substrate for fermentative activity and can be especially helpful in younger animals that have limited experience consuming solid feed.

The final treatment objective, changing the feed pattern, can include provision of good-quality grass hay or other coarse feed such as dry oats or calf starter pellets. Pasture grazing of fresh green grass remains an ideal means of stimulating normal forestomach digestion. If the calf is more than 1 month old, it is preferable to wean it and encourage conversion to full rumen function. Very young calves will require continued milk feeding, but establishing an active forestomach flora and intake of solid feed will enhance a better plane of nutrition, reduce the need for full milk feeding, and be effective in preventing recurrence of the abnormal rumen digestion.

Both the animal and the rumen microflora have trace mineral requirements that will not have been met during the period of abnormal rumen activity. Oral supplementation of minerals and parenteral administration of B vitamins may be helpful until normal rumen function is reestablished.

Recommended Readings

Breukink HJ, Wensing T, Weeren-Keverling-Buisman A: Consequences of failure of the reticular groove reflex in veal calves fed milk replacer, *Vet Q* 10:126-35, 1988.

Coverdale JA, Tyler HD, Quigley JD III, Brumm JA: Effect of various levels of forage and form of diet on rumen development and growth in calves, *J Dairy Sci* 87:2554-62, 2003.

Dirksen G: The digestive system. In Rosenberger G, editor: *Clinical examination of cattle*, Berlin, 1979, Verlag Paul Parey, pp 184-242.

Dirksen G: *Indigestions in cattle*, Konstanz, Germany, 1983, Schnetztor Verlag.

Dirksen G, Dirr L: Oesophageal groove dysfunction as a complication of neonatal diarrhea in the calf, *Bov Practitioner* 24:53-60, 1989.

Dirksen G, Garry F: Diseases of the forestomachs of calves. Part I and Part II, *Comp Cont Ed Pract Vet* 9:F140-F147, F173-F179, 1987.

Garry FB: Indigestion in ruminants. In Smith BP, editor: *Large animal internal medicine,* ed 3, St Louis, 2002, Mosby, pp 722-746.

Rademacher G, Korn N, Friedrich A: The ruminal drinker as patient in practice/Der Pansentrinker als Patient in der Praxis, *Tierarztliche Umschau* 58:115, 2003.

Rager KD, George LW, House JK et al: Evaluation of rumen transfaunation after surgical correction of left-sided displacement of the abomasum in cows, *J Am Vet Med Assoc* 225:915-920, 2004.

Ruckebusch Y: Pharmacology of reticulo-ruminal motor function, *J Vet Pharmacol Therap* 6:245-272, 1983.

van Bruinesses-Kapsenberg EG, Wensing T, Breukink HJ: Indigestionen der Mastkaelber infolge fehlenden Schlundrinnenreflexes, *Tierarztliche Umschau* 7:515-517, 1982.

CHAPTER 8

Ruminal Acidosis and Rumenitis

KARL W. KERSTING, JAMES R. THOMPSON, and MAREN J. CONNOLLY

RUMINAL ACIDOSIS

Definition

Several distinct syndromes that result in D-lactic acidosis are recognized, the most dramatic of which is the ingestion of excessive highly fermentable carbohydrate feed leading to systemic dehydration and severe depression. Ration ingredients involved include the common feed grains fed in quantities larger than those to which the animal has been accustomed. Finely ground grains present a greater surface area for fermentation and are more likely to cause severe problems, but grinding is by no means a prerequisite. Other feed sources known to cause lactic acidosis in cattle include brewers' grains and distillery byproducts such as corn gluten. Green corn, sweet corn, bakery bread, and apples and similar fruits have also been involved.

The propensity of a given feed to induce lactic acidosis is dependent on its content of lactic acid precursors. Carbohydrates that can lead to accumulation of lactic acid include starch, maltose, sucrose, lactose, cellobiose, fructose, and glucose.[1]

A syndrome of chronic rumen acidosis in which lactic acidosis may not be a prominent feature has been described. The disorder occurs in beef or dairy cattle fed for high production and results from feeding high proportions of concentrate at the expense of appropriate quantities of fibrous roughage or from too-rapid introduction to such high-energy rations. Associated findings in affected animals include low milk fat, reduced rate of gain, liver abscesses, chronic laminitis, ketosis, rumenitis or rumen parakeratosis, bloat, and obesity.

Acidosis has been associated with a diet of high-quality vegetative pasture. Short, fast-growing pasture may be sufficiently low in fiber that rapid degradation of relatively modest sugar content leads to increased ruminal production of volatile fatty acids. The increased VFA production and inadequate fiber can contribute to a decrease in rumen pH.[2]

Pathogenesis

The normal ruminant forestomachs can be thought of as a continuous culture fermentation receptacle. The normal microflora constitutes the culture; the ration being fed constitutes the medium or substrate on which the culture grows. The fermentation end-products are normally acetic, propionic, and butyric acid, short-chain volatile fatty acids that are absorbed from the rumen as the animal's primary energy source. Bacterial cell protein is also produced and is digested farther down the tract as an amino acid source. Water-soluble vitamins are produced as an additional byproduct of fermentation.

When the quantity of highly fermentable carbohydrate in the ration is increased abruptly, normal fermentation patterns change. Gram-positive streptococcus and lactobacillus organisms become predominant, and lactic acid (both D- and L-isomers) becomes a principal fermentation end product. Lactic acid production increases osmotic pressure within the rumen so that fluid is drawn into the rumen from the circulatory system and thus from other tissues as well. The rumen pH drops, resulting in rumen stasis, and a large percentage of the normal rumen microflora is destroyed. Most of the gram-negative microorganisms and protozoa disappear. Symptoms become severe when the pH reaches 4 to 5.

The D- and L-lactic acid isomers in the rumen contribute to hyperosmolality and acidity. They are absorbed into the circulation (mainly D-lactate because it is the form produced by bacteria) and contribute to a depression of the blood pH and depression of the animal. Additional lactate is absorbed from the omasum, abomasum, and intestine as a result of continuing fermentation of carbohydrate passing from the rumen. An osmotic gradient is also established within the intestine, drawing additional fluid into the lumen and contributing to the profuse diarrhea.

Chemical damage to the surface epithelium of the rumen mucosa occurs and later results in adherence of debris and facilitates penetration by particulate matter from the rumen ingesta such as hair and sharp pieces of plant material. Bacterial and mycotic organisms begin to invade the rumen wall, and absorption patterns are changed.

Acute acidosis is often followed by bacterial or mycotic rumenitis. Other possible sequelae are liver abscesses and peritonitis. Bloat may result from the decreased rumen motility and altered fermentation patterns. The development of acute, and later chronic, laminitis observed in some animals is thought to relate to the relative levels of histamine produced during the acute phases of the process. Thiaminase production by acidophilic microflora may lead to an increased incidence of polioencephalomalacia.

The entire disease process is complex and variable, and a suggested additional component is likely endotoxic shock from toxins released from the destruction of large numbers of gram-negative microorganisms from the rumen ingesta.[3,4]

Clinical Signs

The rapidity of onset of clinical signs varies and depends on the nature and quantity of the feed consumed and the adaptation of the animal to that feed. Unadapted animals may die from quantities of feed that are routinely consumed without ill effects by animals conditioned to the feed. Conversely, even animals on "full feed" can overeat and develop acute lactic acidosis under some circumstances.

Usually, clinical signs will become apparent in 12 to 36 hours after engorgement on grain or similar material. Incoordination and ataxia are first noticed, followed by profound weakness and depression. Anorexia will be apparent, and affected animals appear blind. Rumen stasis is complete, with abdominal pain evidenced by occasional grunting and grinding of the teeth. Abdominal fullness and fluid distention of the rumen are observed.

Significant dehydration will become apparent within 24 to 48 hours. Fetid diarrhea develops but may not be observed in animals that die acutely. Profuse diarrhea may be considered a sign of improvement if the animals are not seriously depressed.

In severe cases the animals may become recumbent in 24 to 48 hours because of weakness and toxemia. The respiratory rate will most likely be increased because of acidosis. Body temperature may be subnormal by the time other signs are observed. The pulse is usually weak and thready in character.

Recumbent animals will lie quietly, often with the head tucked to the side, as in parturient paresis. Crusty mucus will be present on the muzzle because the animal fails to clean its nostrils.

When a herd problem is observed, it is common to see several animals with profound depression and acute lactic acidosis. Animals with less severe cases will also be present and are likely to show only mild depression and diarrhea. Some animals may develop acute laminitis with a "walking on egg shells" lameness.

Most deaths associated with acute D-lactic acidosis occur in the first 24 to 48 hours. Many animals that appear to recover may later deteriorate and die as a result of secondary complications. It is not unusual for losses to continue for 3 to 4 weeks in severely affected herds. Secondary rumenitis may cause an increased incidence of bloat and is thought to be a major cause of unexplained deaths in feedlots, commonly diagnosed as "sudden death syndrome."

Some animals will partially recover but perform poorly in the feedlot because of chronic rumenitis, liver damage, or laminitis. Pregnant animals frequently abort some days or weeks after the acute phases of illness.

Clinical Pathology and Necropsy

Affected animals have hemoconcentration and acidic rumen content. The pH of ingesta aspirated from the rumen may be 4 or lower, and the urine pH may be as low as 5. Commercial pH paper is sufficiently accurate to determine rumen pH's < 5.0 acidemia and metabolic acidosis or usual findings. Blood samples should be collected anaerobically in heparinized tubes or syringes and refrigerated (4° C) until measured. Accurate assessment of the blood pH requires that bicarbonate or total carbon dioxide be measured also. Values below 7.2 generally indicate severe acidosis and a poor prognosis. Hypocalcemia may be superimposed on the metabolic acidosis. The urine volume will usually be greatly decreased as a result of the dehydration, and secreted urine will be high in D-lactate and acidic.

Necropsy findings of acute cases include a distended rumen filled with fluid content that smells like sour feed. The offending material is likely to be evident, but postmortem measurements of rumen pH may not be valid because of rapid changes in the dead animal.

Rumen engorgement of slightly longer duration is characterized by rumenitis. However, postmortem autolysis occurs rapidly in the rumen, so observations on the rumen mucosa must be interpreted carefully.

Diagnosis

Diagnosis is usually based on history and clinical examination. The history alone is often sufficient, but it may be misleading if the pattern of feed consumption is not known or not suspected. Laboratory evaluations, especially of rumen ingesta, as well as whole blood and urine pH, are particularly helpful.

The condition must be differentiated from polioencephalomalacia, urolithiasis, fulminating peritonitis, parturient hypocalcemia, and other diseases that cause profound depression. Most of these conditions are likely to affect individual animals within a group, whereas feed-related problems are more likely to affect multiple animals at a time, owing to mass exposure.

Treatment

Animals with mild cases may recover without treatment, but in more severe forms the damage to the animal may be so extensive that even with intensive therapy only limited success is achieved. Emptying of the rumen by oral lavage or rumenotomy is indicated if circumstances permit.

The oral administration of rumen buffers such as magnesium carbonate or magnesium hydroxide is indicated, but they should be mixed in 2 to 3 gallons (8 to 12 L) of warm water and given by stomach tube to ensure dispersion throughout the rumen. Initial doses of up to 1 g/kg body weight (454 g for an adult bovine) should be followed by smaller doses repeated at 6- to 12-hour intervals. If the rumen has been evacuated, the initial dose should not exceed 0.5 lb (225 g).

Oral sodium bicarbonate (baking soda) should be avoided as a buffer in the static rumen because of the likelihood of creating tympany (bloat) through the release of carbon dioxide.

Importantly, dehydration and acidosis must be corrected as well. Balanced electrolyte and sodium bicarbonate solutions should be given intravenously. A 450-kg animal with 10% dehydration may require as much as 50 L of fluid over a 24-hour period. For severe cases sodium bicarbonate should be given at the rate of 0.5 g/kg body weight initially and repeated in 24 hours if necessary (1 g of sodium bicarbonate supplies 12 mEq of bicarbonate ion). Correction of blood pH to within the normal range is vital for survival of the animal even if the offending rumen ingesta is removed.

Oral administration of activated charcoal at the rate 2 g/kg body weight is said to enhance clinical recovery from acute lactic acidosis. This effect may be achieved by inactivating endotoxin thought to be released by the destruction of gram-negative rumen microorganisms.[5]

Administration of antihistamines is considered to be of value by some.

In Asia, acupuncture has been used as an adjunctive therapy in cases of rumen acidosis.[6]

Prevention

Avoiding sudden and drastic changes in the ration is paramount in preventing rumen acidosis. Bunk-fed cattle need consistent quantities of ration at consistent intervals, and adequate bunk space must be available so that all animals have an equal opportunity to eat normally. The ration must include adequate roughage (generally not <10%).

Animals on self-feeder programs are particularly vulnerable to excessive consumption, especially early in the feeding program. Every precaution must be taken to ensure that roughage is available (mixed in the feed if possible) and that animals are brought onto full feed slowly. Feeders must be checked regularly and not permitted to run low or stand empty so that excessive intake by hungry animals is avoided after the feeders have been refilled. Managers must be particularly astute following sudden adverse weather conditions that may temporarily force cattle away from feed to ensure that overconsumption does not occur when the weather returns to normal.

Progress has been made in the prevention of rumen lactic acidosis by pharmacologic means. The ionophore antibiotics including monensin, lasalocid, and salinomycin appear to be particularly useful in maintaining higher rumen pH and lower rumen lactate concentrations, as well as in improving feed efficiency in treated as compared with control animals.[7]

RUMENITIS

Definition

The term *rumenitis* refers to a series of inflammatory changes that develop in the rumen mucosa and underlying tissues in cattle fed high-energy rations with inadequate roughage. Clinically, the syndrome includes the associated lesions of liver abscess and laminitis. The incidence may be as high as 100% in cattle fed all-concentrate rations for prolonged periods or those that have not been carefully adapted to such rations. Rumenitis also occurs as a secondary stage of acute rumen engorgement with acidosis.

Pathogenesis

The association between liver abscess formation and ruminal lesions was first reported by Smith[8] and later by Jensen and colleagues.[9] A definite relationship between rumen adaptation to high-energy rations and the development of rumen lesions is now generally understood. The exact pathogenesis of the rumen lesions has not been elucidated, but it is commonly accepted that the end products of rumen fermentation accumulate, causing an increase in hydrogen ion concentration and leading to inflammation of the rumen mucosa.

Fusobacterium necrophorum has been detected as the predominant organism in cases of rumenitis. Injury to the rumen mucosal allows for penetration of the vascular system and spread to abdominal organs. *F. necrophorum* has been shown to adhere to inflamed rumen tissue with increased efficacy when compared with normal rumen tissue.[10]

Lactic acidosis is often not a prominent feature of this disorder, and affected animals may not go through an acute phase of illness. Some animals may perform very well, showing acceptable weight gains or producing high volumes of milk in the case of dairy cows. The rumen fluid may be moderately acidic (<6.0), but any lactic acid produced is probably metabolized by other microorganisms, so the effects are mostly chronic and insidious.[11]

The sequence of events would appear to be (1) inflammation of the rumen mucosa, (2) adherence of debris to the mucosa, (3) ulceration and infection of deeper layers in the rumen wall, and (4) focal abscess formation in the rumen wall. Suppurative rumenitis may initiate liver abscesses via portal vein emboli. Similarly, liver abscesses may lead to caudal vena cava phlebitis, endocarditis, and pulmonary abscesses and hemorrhage.

Chronic laminitis is a later sequela, but its relationship is uncertain and appears less well correlated with the preceding events. Other independent factors may be involved in the development of chronic laminitis. It is frequently observed in cattle fed high-energy rations for 60 to 90 days, but the incidence appears to be higher among females, and laminitis sometimes occurs in the absence of rumen and liver lesions. Likewise, there is nothing specific about the lesions in the rumen or the liver; the lesions in either could arise from other causes.

Clinical Signs

Cattle do not necessarily become clinically ill during the early stages of rumenitis and liver abscess formation. Feed consumption is usually good, and weight gains on all-concentrate rations for periods more than 100 days are acceptable. However, the addition of good-quality hay or silage (at least 10% to 20% of the ration) often results in increased feed consumption and average daily gain. Dairy cattle may suffer losses in milk production related to undulating or diminished dry matter intake. Butterfat content of milk is often negatively affected.

Animals with advanced rumen and liver lesions may show reduced appetite and weight gains, usually late in the feeding period. Affected individuals show an apparent lack of fill, as evidenced by gauntness of the abdomen. Other clinical signs, possibly from developing peritonitis or septicemia, may be seen. Elongation and flatness of the hooves with a very apparent alteration in gait occurs if chronic laminitis exists.

Necropsy

Lesions are usually observed only at slaughter and result in the condemnations of livers and rumens. The rumen mucosa has edema and clumping papillae in mild cases. More advanced causes demonstrate matting and necrosis of papillae with diffuse ulcerations. Hair and debris adhere to the mucosa. Extensive thickening of the rumen wall with abscessation is also observed.

Increased thickness of the cornified portion of the rumen epithelium and increased numbers of vacuoles on histologic examination occur. The lesion is characteristic of an acid burn.

Abscesses are observed on cut sections of the liver and are apparent as light-colored spots on the uncut surface in severe cases.

Diagnosis

Chronic laminitis may be the first visible sign, but in many instances its appearance accompanies or precedes a noticeable reduction in feed consumption and rate of gain. Negative changes in herd milk production and increased culling rates of mature cattle may be observed.

The condition can be suspected in any group of cattle being fed for maximal gains on high-energy or all-concentrate rations or in dairy animals consuming a total ration containing inadequate amounts of coarse fiber.

A diagnosis of chronic acidosis may be achieved despite vague clinical signs. Documentation of the condition requires rumen fluid evaluation. Numerous methods of rumen liquor assay and collection have been described.[12] The critical determination for diagnosis of acidosis is pH. Percutaneous aspiration of rumen fluid from the lower left flank has been cited as the preferred collection method for sampling a number of animals for a herd investigation.[13] This method also avoids salivary contamination associated with oral probe sampling, which may artificially raise the pH. The fluid must be tested with a pH meter because pH paper is not precise enough to distinguish between acceptable and unacceptable rumen pH.

Treatment

Correction and prevention of this condition is accomplished by reducing the total acid production in the rumen and decreasing the fluctuation in pH during the day. This is achieved by modifying the amount and proportions of roughage fed, as well as adjusting feeding intervals and practices. As these changes could potentially alter the animal's performance, they should be made by a professional who has expertise in nutrition and familiarity with the producer's operation.

Several antibiotics are approved as feed additives for the reduction of liver abscess incidence; however, tylosin appears to be the most effective.[14] *Fusobacterium necrophorum* vaccines may offer an additional measure of control.[15]

References

1. Cullen AJ, Harmon DL, Nagoraja TG: In vitro fermentation of sugars, grains and by-product feeds in relation to initiation of ruminal lactate production, *J Dairy Sci* 69:2616-2621, 1986.
2. Westwood CT, Bramley E, Lean IJ: Review of the relationship between nutrition and lameness in pasture-fed dairy cattle, *N Z Vet J* 51(5)208-218, 2003.
3. Dougherty RW, Coburn KS, Cook HM, Allison MJ: Preliminary study of appearance of endotoxin in circulatory system of sheep and cattle after induced grain engorgement, *Am J Vet Res* 36:6, 1975.
4. Mullenox CH, Keller RR, Allison MJ: Physiologic responses of ruminants to toxic factors extracted from rumen bacteria and rumen fluid, *Am J Vet Res* 5:16, 1944.
5. Buck WB: *Proceedings, XVIII Conference Rumen Function*, Chicago, 1985, p 1.
6. Habacher G, Pittler MH, Ernst E: Effectiveness of acupuncture in veterinary medicine: systemic review, *J Vet Intern Med* 20:480-488, 2006.
7. Nogaraja TG, Avery TB, Galitzer SJ, Dayton AO: Prevention of lactic acidosis in cattle by lasalocid or monensin, *J Anim Sci* 53:206-216, 1981.
8. Smith H: Ulcerative lesions of bovine rumen and their possible relation to hepatic abscesses, *Am J Vet Res* 5:16, 1944.
9. Jensen R, Deane HM, Cooper LF et al: The rumenitis-liver abscess complex in beef cattle, *Am J Vet Res* 15:55, 1954.
10. Takayama Y, Kanoe M, Maeda K et al: Adherence of *Fusobacterium necrophorum subsp. Necrophorum* to ruminal cells derived from bovine rumenitis, *Lett Appl Microbiol* 30:308-311, 2000.
11. Garry FB: Diagnosing and treating indigestion caused by fermentative disorders, *Vet Med* 85:660-670, 1990.
12. Rings DM, Rings MB: Rumen fluid analysis, *Agri-Practice* 14:26-29, 1993.
13. Nordlund KV, Garrett EF: Rumenocentesis: a technique for collecting rumen fluid for the diagnosis of subacute rumen acidosis in dairy herds, *Bovine Pract* 28:109-112, 1994.
14. Nagaraja TG, Laudert SB, Parrott JC: Liver abscesses in feedlot cattle II. Incidence, economic importance and prevention, *Compendium* 18:S264-273, 1996.
15. Saginala S, Nagaraja TG, Tan Z et al: Serum neutralizing antibody response and protection against experimentally induced liver abscesses in steers vaccinated with *Fusobacterium necrophorum*, *Am J Vet Res*:483-488, 1996.

CHAPTER 9

Rumenotomy and Rumenostomy

ANDREW NIEHAUS

The proximal part of the ruminant digestive system is complex, consisting of four compartments between the esophagus and the duodenum. The abomasum is the "true stomach" of the ruminant and contains glandular mucosa for production and secretion of digestive juices. The abomasum is the most distal of the four aforementioned compartments and lies in the right hemi-abdomen extending from the xyphoid between the rumen and omasum caudally to the ninth or tenth intercostal space.[1] The three forestomach compartments are the reticulum, omasum, and rumen. These compartments comprise nonglandular mucosa and serve as chambers for microbial digestion and fluid absorption.

Referred to as the "hardware stomach," the reticulum is an outpouching of the cranioventral rumen. It lies against the diaphragm opposite the sixth to eighth ribs on midline with equal parts lying on either side.[1,2] It is below the cardia, and rumen contractions serve to move dense objects into this compartment. The function of the omasum is mechanical processing of food particles and fluid absorption prior to entering the abomasum. Its normal anatomic location is the ventral aspect of the seventh to eleventh ribs lying to the right of the rumen and abomasum.[1]

The rumen in the adult cow comprises approximately 80% of the abdominal cavity,[1] with a capacity around 80 L (roughly 16% of body weight).[3] Some sources report capacities varying from 102-148 L for mature cattle.[2] The rumen lies primarily on the left side of the abdomen, and its length extends from the seventh or eighth rib to the pelvis.[1] It is typically described as a "fermentation vat." Through the process of fermentation, microbes within the rumen convert complex carbohydrates, which are useless to the host animal, into volatile fatty acids, microbial protein, and B vitamins, which are useful products. Byproducts of fermentation include methane, carbon dioxide, ammonia, and nitrate, which need to be cleared.[3] The neonate has a small rumen and relatively large abomasum. The relative size of the rumen increases with the age of the animal. Ingestion of forage and fermentation products is stimulus for rumen enlargement. The ratio of abomasal volume to rumen volume is 0.5:1 at 4 weeks of age and eventually reaches 10:1 in adult cattle.[1]

The apposition of the rumen against the left body wall makes it an easy portal through which to access other proximal gastrointestinal structures including the reticulum, the reticulo-omasal orifice, and the rumen itself. Both rumenotomy and rumenostomy are performed commonly in our practice. Indications for rumenotomy include traumatic reticuloperitonitis (hardware disease) or merely retrieval of ruminal and reticular foreign bodies not associated with hardware disease. Another indication is removal of ruminal contents in cases of frothy bloat, grain overload, and toxin ingestion. Indications for performing a rumenostomy include relief of bloat and to provide enteric nutrition in cases of vagal indigestion, chronic reoccurring bloat, and creation of a permanent rumen fistula.[4-6]

An exploratory rumenotomy is commonly performed to retrieve an ingested foreign body. Using the rumen as access, the reticulum can be explored and foreign bodies penetrating the wall of the reticulum causing traumatic reticuloperitonitis can be removed. Perireticular abscesses that frequently develop secondarily to penetrating reticular foreign bodies can be surgically drained into the reticulum via a rumenotomy. In our practice, the indication for performing approximately half of the rumen surgeries is for retrieval of a foreign body in cases of hardware disease. Other indications for performing a rumenotomy include removal of rumen contents in cases of acute toxin ingestion, grain overload, or frothy bloat. A rumenostomy can be a therapeutic option for an animal with chronic bloat, to provide enteric nutrition, or to place a rumen canula.

Hardware disease is caused by foreign body ingestion with subsequent trauma to the digestive tract, specifically the reticulum and the associated adjoining structures. The disease is a continuum. In its most benign form, it merely causes irritation of the reticulum (traumatic reticulitis). If the foreign body penetrates the reticulum and enters the peritoneal cavity, the penetrating foreign body causes septic peritonitis and is termed *traumatic reticuloperitonitis.* If further migration of the foreign body occurs, the diaphragm and cardiac sac can be penetrated, causing traumatic reticulopericarditis.

Multiple techniques have been described for performing laparorumenotomy in cattle. All techniques involve making an approach in the left paralumbar fossa to gain access to the rumen, exteriorization of the rumen, securing the rumen to the body wall or skin, and limiting contamination. The techniques differ by the method in which the rumen is secured to the body wall or skin. The technique in its simplest form involves making a standard laparotomy incision in the left paralumbar fossa through the skin, external, internal, and transverse abdominal muscles followed by the peritoneum. It has been suggested to always perform an abdominal exploration before performing the rumenotomy.[4,5] Although a thorough abdominal exploration is limited from the left flank because of the overwhelming size of the rumen, the cranioventral abdomen can be palpated for the presence of reticular adhesions, a common sequela to reticuloperitonitis. Diffuse, generalized peritonitis can also be

diagnosed from the left paralumbar fossa approach. Both findings are indications for continuing with the rumenotomy to search for penetrating foreign bodies.[4] The dorsal sac of the rumen is then exteriorized and secured before creation of the rumenotomy incision. One technique described securing the rumen to the peritoneum.[7] The disadvantage with this technique is that the peritoneum can be weak and allow for retraction of the rumen into the abdomen. Contamination of the muscle layers also results because the body wall muscle layers are exposed. Most techniques describe securing of the rumen to the skin. This protects both the muscle layers and the peritoneal cavity. Another fixation technique is the skin suture fixation technique in which the rumen is sutured to the skin using a continuous inverting suture pattern such as a Connell or a Cushing.[6] The stay suture technique has also been described. This technique uses four stay sutures to anchor the rumen to the skin at the dorsal, ventral, cranial, and caudal parts of the incision.[6] Although similar to the skin suture fixation, the stay suture technique has areas where rumen contents can pass between the rumen and the body wall and allow contamination of the peritoneal cavity.

Several devices have been developed to anchor the rumen following exteriorization and speed up the rumenotomy procedure. In 1954 a report on a rumenotomy ring was published. This consisted of an aluminum ring with a rubber ring attached to its inner circumference.[8] It was designed so that the rumen could be hooked to this rubber ring. The idea was that it would keep the rumen exteriorized and prevent abdominal contamination. The hook placement is faster than suturing the rumen to the skin and thus decreases time of the rumenotomy. Weingarth's ring was based on this previous ring with some modifications for securing the hooks and lacked the inner rubber ring. The Gabel rumen retractor (rumen board) is another similar instrument used to keep the rumen exteriorized. This device has a hole in the center through which the rumen is pulled. A series of bolts around the circumference of the hole allow hooks to attach the rumen to the board. The board helps to decrease abdominal contamination but limits the accessibility of the rumen. Another method, the skin clamp technique, uses towel clamps to secure the rumen to the skin in an overlapping fashion. Dehghani compared the skin suture fixation, stay suture fixation, Weingarth's ring, and the skin clamp technique in 20 cattle. He found that the stay suture fixation was inferior to the other techniques with increased incidence of infection.[6] The rumen shroud is another device that has been developed to help limit abdominal contamination with rumen contents. This rubber device has a large, flat surface similar to a rumen board on one side and an inner flange that secures it to the inside of the temporary rumen fistula.[9]

At best, rumen surgery is considered a clean, contaminated surgery because a hollow viscus is penetrated. Antibiotics are recommended in any surgery that is considered less than clean.[10] Haven and colleagues[10] showed that prophylactic use of penicillin significantly decreased the incidence of abscess formation following rumenotomy. He also demonstrated that an initial antibiotic dose at the time of surgery was all that was necessary and continuing the therapy for several postoperative days had no significant decrease on the incidence of abscess and infection rate.[10]

Overall in our practice, the apparent complication rate associated with rumen surgery is low (<10%). The prognosis and outcome largely depends on the presenting complaint and preoperative condition of the animal rather than operative factors.

References

1. Ducharme NG: Surgery of the bovine forestomach compartments, *Vet Clin North Am Food Anim Pract* 6:371-397, 1990.
2. Oehme FW: *Textbook of large animal surgery*, ed 2, Baltimore, 1988, Williams & Wilkins, pp 399-449.
3. Church DC: *The ruminant animal: digestive physiology and nutrition*, Englewood Cliffs, NJ, 1988, Prentice-Hall.
4. Donawick W: Abdominal surgery. In Amstutz HE, editor: *Bovine medicine and surgery*, ed 2, Santa Barbara, Calif, 1980, American Veterinary Publications, pp 1207-1220.
5. Noordsy JL: Rumenotomy in cattle. In Noordsy JL, editor: *Food animal surgery*, ed 2, Lenexa, Kan, 1989, Veterinary Medicine pp 105-109.
6. Dehghani SN, Ghadrdani AM: Bovine rumenotomy: comparison of four surgical techniques, *Can Vet J* 36:693-697, 1995.
7. Hofmeyr CFB: The digestive system. In Oehme FW, editor: *Textbook of large animal surgery*, ed 2, Baltimore, 1988, Williams & Wilkins, pp 364-449.
8. Michael SJ, Mc KR: Rumenotomy simplified, *J Am Vet Med Assoc* 124:26-27, 1954.
9. Turner AS, McIlwraith CW, Hull BL: *Techniques in large animal surgery*, Philadelphia, 1989, Lea & Febiger.
10. Haven ML, Wichtel JJ, Bristol DG et al: Effects of antibiotic prophylaxis on postoperative complications after rumenotomy in cattle, *J Am Vet Med Assoc* 200:1332-1335, 1992.

CHAPTER 10

Abomasal Ulcers

MARIE-EVE FECTEAU and ROBERT H. WHITLOCK

DEFINITION AND CLASSIFICATION

Abomasal ulcers are lesions that penetrate the basement membrane of the abomasal mucosa. They can occur in cattle of all breeds and ages, but rarely in small ruminants. For the purpose of consistency with most literature on abomasal ulcers in cattle, we describe four ulcer types. Historically, abomasal ulcers have been classified among five groups, with lymphosarcoma-associated bleeding ulcers as a separate type (type III). Here, lymphosarcoma-associated bleeding ulcers are described in the section on type II ulcers. Abomasal ulcers may be classified into nonperforating and perforating ulcers. The nonperforating ulcers can further be divided into nonbleeding ulcers (type I) and ulcers with major bleeding (type II), and the perforating ulcers can similarly be subdivided between perforating with local peritonitis (type III) and perforating with diffuse peritonitis (type IV). The clinical signs resulting from an abomasal ulcer are highly variable and depend on the type and location of the ulcer. The initial erosion or early ulcer lesion may not elicit any clinical signs, yet such lesions are commonly detected in abattoir surveys.[1] Ulceration that progresses to hemorrhage or perforation of the abomasal wall results in quite different signs: anemia or peritonitis.

EPIDEMIOLOGY

Abomasal ulceration occurs in cattle of all ages, but periparturient dairy cows, dairy calves, and preweaned beef calves tend to be most frequently affected. Surveys report the prevalence of abomasal ulceration in cattle to be approximately 1% in asymptomatic dairy cows at slaughter, 3% in feedlot cattle, 9% in cows sent to emergency slaughter, 34% in preweaned beef calves, and as high as 97% in veal calves at slaughter.[1-4] Nearly all reports indicated the lesions occur most frequently in the pyloric region, yet duodenal ulceration is rare. Abomasal ulcers in feedlot cattle occur more commonly during the winter when the cattle are first placed on feed.[2] Clinically important abomasal ulcers were detected in 69 of 6385 cattle admitted to a referral hospital. Of those 69 cases, 24 were bleeding ulcers, 12 benign, and 12 associated with lymphosarcoma.[5] The prevalence of abomasal ulcers in beef calves has been increasing with reports of up 50% of calves being affected in some calf crops.[6]

ETIOLOGY AND PATHOPHYSIOLOGY

As with gastric ulcers in other animals and humans, abomasal ulcers are multifactorial in origin. They occur as a result of an imbalance of defensive factors to protect the gastric mucosa, which include local blood flow, mucus cover, mucosal cell resistance, and duodenal influence on gastric acid secretion. Aggressive factors that promote ulceration include excess pepsin, trauma, hyperacidity, hormonal factors, and stress.

The precise mechanisms that comprise mucosal resistance to the corrosive effects of acid-pepsin have not been fully defined. Gastric mucus, secreted by mucous cells of gastric glands, is a gelatinous material that coats the mucosal surface of the stomach. The mucus coating serves as an unstirred layer through which the diffusion of acid-pepsin is reduced. Normally the gastric luminal epithelial cell surfaces and intercellular tight junctions provide a nearly impermeable barrier to back-diffusion of hydrogen ions from the lumen. Such back-diffusion to intracellular and intercellular sites may result in cellular injury, release of histamine from mast cells, further stimulation of acid secretion, damage to small blood vessels, mucosal hemorrhage, and superficial ulceration. Group E prostaglandins (PGE) are of foremost importance in the preservation of mucosal integrity. PGE functions include increasing mucus secretion and microcirculation and reducing the secretion of hydrochloric acid.[7] Decreased mucosal blood flow, accompanied by back-diffusion of hydrogen ions, also appears to contribute to damage to the gastric mucosa. Both short chain fatty acids, which have a detergent action, and bile acids, which may reach the abomasum by duodenal reflux, may destroy the mucous coating.[8] Drugs such as salicylic acid, which inhibit PGE, predispose to ulcers.[6]

The so-called "stress factors" may play a role in ulcerogenesis of cattle. A higher stocking rate of dairy cattle per acre was associated with a significantly higher prevalence of ulcers.[3] This Dutch study reported bleeding ulcers to be most common during the summer (May to October) and to be highly associated with heavy nitrogen fertilization of pastures, especially new pastures. They occurred more commonly in higher-producing cows but were not associated with recent parturition. North American studies report a higher prevalence during the stabling period (January to April) with a close association with recent parturition.[5,9] Clearly, different predisposing factors must exist. Other stress factors occurring when the peak occurrence of abomasal ulceration is diagnosed include parturition; other concurrent, early postpartum diseases such as retained placenta, mastitis, metritis, and hypocalcemia; and attainment of peak lactation. Perhaps increased abomasal volatile fatty acids (VFAs) following feeding of high-concentrate diets may induce hyperacidity within the abomasum, predisposing to ulceration when compounded by the presence of concurrent disease. In a herd of 40 Jersey cattle, 5 cases of perforated fatal ulcers occurred in a 1-month period. The rapid change from pasture to a high-moisture corn and silage ration was thought to predispose to the unusual number of cases.[10] In dairy calves a study found a high prevalence of severe ulcers in loosed-housed calves with access to straw and fed free-choice milk replacer.[1] Another study in dairy calves found an increased incidence in abomasal erosions when solid feed, particularly straw, was provided along with a milk diet.[11] In beef calves, copper deficiency has been suspected as a predisposing factor for abomasal ulceration.[12]

Although abomasal hairballs have long been suspected to be a risk factor for abomasal ulcerations, this has not been proven.[4] For a comprehensive review on abomasal ulcers in calves, see Dirksen.[13]

For years similar stresses were believed to be the major factors associated with human gastric ulcers until *Helicobacter pylori* was successfully cultured from human gastric ulcers.[14] In subsequent reports of therapeutic trials, epidemiologic studies, and animal models, *H. pylori* was shown to be an important agent for human gastritis, gastroduodenal ulceration, and gastric carcinoma.[15-18] At least two reports suggest that campylobacter-like organisms observed in histologic sections of normal and ulcerated bovine abomasums may be *H. pylori*.[19,20] The results of one study indicated that spiral-shaped bacteria may be found frequently in the bovine abomasum but failed to determine whether these bacteria are associated with the inflammatory lesions observed and whether they play a role in the pathogenesis of abomasal ulcers in cattle.[20] A prospective study of beef calves failed to provide any histologic or microbiologic evidence that *H. pylori* was associated with perforating or bleeding abomasal ulcers.[21] This report is compatible with reports in humans in which perforated duodenal ulcers were not associated with *H. pylori* but were commonly associated with chronic gastric and duodenal ulceration.[22]

Other microorganisms including clostridium, campylobacter, streptococci, and fungi have been associated with abomasal ulceration in ruminants.[21,23,24] Most investigators believe mycotic or fungal agents invade the ulcer after its formation and are not causal. Only *Clostridium perfringens* continues to be considered a risk factor for abomasitis and possibly abomasal ulcers in young cattle. Earlier reports have suggested an association between acute abomasal ulcers and *C. perfringens*, especially in beef cattle.[23-25] Experimental intraruminal inoculation of *C. perfringens* type A caused depression, diarrhea, abdominal bloat, abomasitis, and abomasal ulceration in calves.[26] The ulcers produced were frequently multiple, never perforating, and associated with petechial and ecchymotic hemorrhages. By contrast, naturally occurring ulcers are typically singular, frequently perforating, rarely hemorrhagic, and often localized in the fundic portion of the abomasum. *Sarcina*-like bacteria, *Clostridium fallax*, and *Clostridium sordellii* have also been associated with abomasitis and abomasal ulcers in lambs and goat kids.[27,28]

NONPERFORATING ABOMASAL ULCERS

Clinical Presentation and Diagnosis of Type I Abomasal Ulcers

Most cases of type I abomasal erosions and ulceration in cows occur in the peripartum period and are typically associated with concurrent diseases such as left displacement of the abomasum (LDA), coliform mastitis, or septic metritis.[5,9] Type I ulcers may not cause severe disease in affected cows and may manifest solely as a reduced feed intake and reduced milk production. The clinical signs are more often attributable to the primary disease and not the abomasal ulcers. However, a number of cows with type I ulcers show characteristic clinical signs of darkened, soft to fluid feces, with minimal anemia. Clinical diagnosis of type I abomasal ulcers may be difficult and is most often a clinical suspicion or a diagnosis of exclusion. A final diagnosis of type I ulcers can only be done at necropsy or during abomasotomy. When erosions progress to ulcers, they produce a local inflammatory response with peripheral thickening of the abomasal wall, which can sometimes be detected on transabdominal ultrasound examination. Feces may be positive for occult blood, and some cows exhibit a painful response to xiphoid pressure.[29] If present, the abnormal dark feces usually resolve as the primary disease responds to therapy.

Most type I ulcers are detected at slaughter or necropsy and typically multiple and superficial. Type I abomasal ulcers were found in 20.5% of 912 abomasums examined at slaughter.[30] Other ulcer types were not found in any of these cattle; however, 32% were anemic with a packed cell volume (PCV) less than 28% and 11% of the cattle were hyperfibrinogenemic (>700 mg/dl).[30]

Clinical Presentation and Diagnosis of Type II Abomasal Ulcers

The hallmarks for bleeding abomasal ulceration are black, tarry feces and anemia.[5,9,31] Rarely, the affected cow may die peracutely from exsanguination into the abomasal lumen. This type of ulceration typically involves one large ulcer that erodes through the wall of major gastric blood vessels. Typically, cattle with this type ulcer have clinical signs referable to anemia. The history often includes a sharp drop in milk production, depression, and a capricious appetite. Concurrent disease problems such as displaced abomasum, ketosis, metritis, mastitis, and retained placenta are often present.[5] Rumen motility is usually decreased both in strength and rate of contraction. Anemia is clinically manifested by pale mucous membranes, tachycardia, muscle weakness, and melena, although occasionally an affected cow may die before melena becomes evident. Laboratory findings usually support the presence of profound anemia (PCV<15%). With loss of whole blood, total plasma protein is also lowered, usually less than 6.0 g/dl. The guaiac test for fecal occult blood can detect as little as 75 ml of blood loss per day.[32]

In a retrospective study of 296 cattle with signs of gastrointestinal dysfunction, including 26 animals with confirmed abomasal ulcers, fecal occult blood, abdominal pain, and packed cell volume were evaluated for sensitivity, specificity, and positive or negative predictive value for abomasal ulcers.[29] The fecal occult blood test had a sensitivity of 77% for all types of abomasal ulcers, whereas if all three tests were negative or normal, there was only an 11.5% chance that ulcer disease was present. Of note was that 6 of 17 cows with bleeding ulcers had evidence of abdominal pain, and 7 of 9 cows with perforating ulcers had a positive fecal occult blood test. False-positive tests occurred most commonly in cattle with traumatic reticulitis, abomasal displacement, liver disease, cecal volvulus, and pneumonia or pleuritis.[29] The usefulness of plasma gastrin determinations as a diagnostic aid in cattle with bleeding abomasal ulcers has recently been evaluated.[33]

Type II ulcers may be associated with infiltration of the abomasum with lymphosarcoma. This type of ulceration has previously been referred to as type III ulcers when abomasal ulcers were classified on a scale of I through V. These ulcers occur most often in cattle 5 years and older and in cattle at any stage of gestation and lactation.[5] Type II ulcers not associated with lymphosarcoma occur more frequently in cows younger than 5 years of age often with concurrent diseases such as metritis or mastitis and are more common in the early postpartum period.[5] Conversely, lymphosarcoma-associated bleeding ulcers tend to have more gradual blood loss with other clinical signs of lymphosarcoma such as detectable tumor masses and weight loss. The rate of progression of clinical signs in cattle with type II ulcers associated with lymphosarcoma tend to be more gradual than in cows with bleeding ulcers not associated with lymphosarcoma. Approximately 50% of cattle with bleeding ulcers associated with lymphosarcoma have enlarged peripheral lymph nodes and/or masses detectable on rectal examination.[5] A negative bovine leukemia virus (BLV) titer in an adult cow with type II abomasal ulceration would rule out lymphosarcoma as the cause because nearly all cows with the adult form of lymphosarcoma have a BLV titer. On the other hand, the presence of a BLV titer would only indicate the cow was exposed to the virus, not that clinical lymphosarcoma was present, because less than 5% of BLV-positive cows go on to develop lymphosarcoma in their lifetime.[34] Neoplastic lymphocytes may be found on abdominocentesis because some abomasal lymphosarcomas may exfoliate neoplastic cells. The prognosis for recovery is grave for lymphosarcoma-associated ulcers, so it is important for the clinician to be able to differentiate bleeding ulcers not associated with lymphosarcoma from lymphosarcoma-associated ulcers. Approximately 75% of cattle with type II (nonlymphosarcoma) bleeding ulcers survive with supportive treatment.[5]

Other causes of melena include blood loss from the duodenum and/or other parts of the small intestine[35] and hemoptysis secondary to embolic pneumonia associated with caudal vena caval thrombosis. Cows with salmonellosis, coccidiosis, winter dysentery, and rectal lacerations often have bright red blood in the feces and are thus easily differentiated from cows with abomasal ulceration. Hemorrhagic bowel syndrome usually manifests as a mixture of fresh and digested blood in the manure, with the presence of large blood clots. The hemorrhagic form of bovine viral diarrhea also manifests as fresh blood in the feces, as well as increased tendency to bleed from other sites.

Treatment of Nonperforating Abomasal Ulcers (Types I and II)

Treatment is aimed at correcting concurrent diseases, reducing stress, and correcting dietary problems. In most cases type I abomasal ulcers resolve as the primary disease process is corrected. Although the ulcers may heal with a superficial mucosal scar, secondary complications are rare. Management of a cow with type II abomasal ulceration is directed at restoring blood volume with intravenous fluids (1-2 L of hypertonic saline is often used in field situations) and whole blood, if anemia becomes severe (PCV<15%). The most reliable indication for blood transfusion is assessment of the general condition of the patient. Marked weakness with dyspnea and tachycardia (>100/minute) with pale membranes is evidence for blood transfusion. If whole blood is to be given, a minimum of 5 L is recommended. Crossmatching the donor's red cells with the recipient's plasma is not necessary because cattle have so many different blood groups.[36] Most healthy adult cows can donate up to 8 L at one time. Prudent use of analgesics such as flunixin meglumine (0.5-1.1 mg/kg) may be indicated for the alleviation of discomfort. Other supportive measures include dietary change to a more fibrous diet including high-quality hay.

Although type II histamine receptors are present in the abomasum, in one study to alter abomasal acidity, type II antagonists (cimetidine, famotidine, and ranitidine) were only partially successful.[37] In this study, ranitidine (6.6 mg/kg) has been shown to increase abomasal pH.[37] In a more recent study, in which the effect of orally administered cimetidine and ranitidine on abomasal luminal pH in clinically normal milk-fed calves was investigated, it appeared that both cimetidine and ranitidine were efficacious in raising abomasal pH in those calves, but the doses required were much greater than those used in monogastrics.[38] Doses of 50 to 100 mg/kg of cimetidine and 10 to 50 mg/kg of ranitidine were required for clinically important changes in abomasal pH to be achieved. Antacid agents containing aluminum hydroxide and magnesium hydroxide have also been investigated in their usefulness at modifying abomasal pH in clinically normal calves.[39] Results suggested that clinically normal milk-fed calves given a commercially available antacid orally have a transient increase in abomasal luminal pH. In adult ruminants, most orally administrated drugs are inactivated in the rumen and therefore have a questionable efficacy. Stimulation of the esophageal groove closure by use of copper sulfate solution or vasopressin (0.25 IU/kg IV) may help increasing efficacy of orally administered antiacids.[40] Administration of ranitidine (1.5 mg/kg TID) intravenously has successfully been used by one of the authors in the treatment of valuable cows with suspicion of abomasal ulcers. Surgical intervention is not generally recommended as the primary approach for treatment of bleeding ulcers. However, ligation of affected vessels with resection of the ulcer may be performed in rare cases.

PERFORATING ABOMASAL ULCERS: Types III and IV

History and Clinical Presentation

Abomasal ulcers may perforate the abomasal wall without involving large vessels and cause either localized (type III) or diffuse (type IV) peritonitis. In dairy cows, most cases of type III and IV ulcers occur in the early postpartum period.[9] Occasionally, cows with LDA may have concurrent abomasal ulceration with localized peritonitis. An investigation of 209 cases of fatal abomasal ulceration in Canadian beef calves showed that more than 93% were perforating with 85% occurring in calves younger than 2 months of age and a range of 5 days to 6 months of age.[41,42] Abomasal hairballs were thought to be related to the occurrence of ulcers in beef calves, but in an investigation of 56 calves with perforated ulcers, the affected group had a similar frequency of hairball (>60%), as did control

calves.[4] Cattle affected with type III ulcers resemble cattle with traumatic reticuloperitonitis (TRP). These animals may be moderately febrile and partly or totally anorectic, and milk production may decrease acutely. Abdominal pain, usually localized to the right ventral quadrant, is evident. Rumen motility may be decreased to absent, and mild bloat may be present. These signs may abate over the course of a few days if the infection is contained.

Cows with type IV ulcers often present as medical emergencies with abruptly decreased milk production, rumen stasis, and evidence of abdominal pain. These cows have more severe clinical signs including prominent tachycardia (>120/minute), complete rumen stasis, profound depression, progressive severe dehydration, and, in advanced stages, recumbency and cold extremities suggestive of shock. The rectal temperature may be normal or decreased. Many affected cows have low-volume diarrhea, but in rare instances a cow will be constipated.[9] As a rule of thumb, cattle with perforating ulcers rarely bleed and cows with bleeding ulcers rarely perforate.[5] Statistically, these events were found to be nearly mutually exclusive.[5]

Diagnosis of Perforated Abomasal Ulcers (Types III and IV)

The diagnosis of abomasal ulcers with perforation requires a comprehensive examination by an astute clinician. Local or diffuse peritonitis may be confirmed by intracellular bacteria and toxic changes in the cells on cytologic examination of fluid obtained by abdominocentesis. Cows with type III ulcers will typically show a neutrophilic leukocytosis and hyperproteinemia associated with hyperglobulinemia and hyperfibrinogenemia. Cows with type IV ulcers typically show a severe neutropenia and severe hemoconcentration (PCV > 40%) with hypoproteinemia (total plasma protein < 5.0 g/dl). The disparate values of elevated PCV and low total plasma protein concentrations signal the possibility of diffuse peritonitis, one cause of which is a perforating abomasal ulcer.[43]

Occasionally, perforating ulcers are first detected during the process of surgical correction of displaced abomasum. Depending on the surgical approach used, the ulcers may be oversewn or surgically resected and then the displacement corrected or a second approach can be made. When the surgical findings include an early perforating ulcer or a complete thickness ulcer, such cows have a fair to good prognosis for survival. Some abomasal perforations are confined to the omental bursa along the lesser curvature of the abomasum and result in local peritonitis.

Treatment of Perforating Abomasal Ulcers

The objectives for treatment of a perforating abomasal ulcer with circumscribed peritonitis are similar to TRP (i.e., broad-spectrum antimicrobials to control the infection), restricted exercise to allow a firm adhesion to develop and, perhaps, elevation of the front quarters. For cows with concurrent abomasal displacement, a paramedian celiotomy to locate and oversew the ulcerated lesion is recommended.[44] When the abomasum is displaced and adhered to the left side of the abdomen, a left-flank approach may also be used to free up the abomasum from the flank.

PROGNOSIS AND COMPLICATIONS

Type I abomasal ulcers heal as the affected animal recovers from the primary disease. In animals that die of the primary disease, multiple abomasal ulcers will be found in the abomasal mucosa. Only rarely will the blood loss associated with these ulcers ever cause clinical anemia. Prognosis for type II bleeding abomasal ulcers is often good, even with those cows requiring a blood transfusion with greater than 75% survival.[5] Cattle with lymphosarcoma-associated ulcers have a grave prognosis. Cattle with type III ulcers generally have a fair to good prognosis for survival.[9] Occasionally, adhesions develop and interfere with forestomach motility, which may lead to vagal indigestion syndrome. Type IV ulcers resultant in diffuse contamination of the peritoneal cavity carry a uniformly grave prognosis.

References

1. Welchman D, Baust GN: A survey of abomasal ulceration in veal calves, *Vet Record* 121:586, 1987.
2. Jensen R, Pierson RE, Braddy PM et al: Fatal abomasal ulcers in yearling feedlot cattle, *J Am Vet Med Assoc* 169:524, 1976.
3. Aukema JJ, Breukink HJ: Abomasal ulcers in cattle with fatal hemorrhage, *Cornell Vet* 64:303, 1974.
4. Jelinski MD, Ribble CS, Campbell JT, Janzen ED: Investigating the relationship between abomasal hairballs and perforating abomasal ulcers in unweaned beef calves, *Can Vet J* 37:23-6, 1996.
5. Palmer JE, Whitlock RH: Bleeding abomasal ulcers in adult dairy cattle, *J Am Vet Med Assoc* 183:448, 1983.
6. Jelinski MD, Jansen ED, Hoar B et al: A field investigation of fatal abomasal ulcers in western Canadian beef calves, *J Agri-Practice* 16:16, 1995.
7. Highland RL, Upson DW: Simplified role of prostaglandins in the gastrointestinal tract, *Comp Cont Educ Pract Vet* 8:188, 1986.
8. Braun U, Hausmann K, Forrer R: Reflux of bile acids from the duodenum into the rumen of cows with reduced intestinal passage, *Vet Record* 124:373, 1989.
9. Smith DF, Munson L, Erb HN: Abomasal ulcer disease in adult dairy cattle, *Cornell Vet* 73:213, 1983.
10. Sanford SE, Josephson GK: Perforated abomasal ulcers in post-parturient Jersey cows, *Can Vet J* 29:392, 1988.
11. Mattiello S, Canali E, Ferrante V et al: The provision of solid feeds to veal calves: II. Behavior physiology and abomasal damage, *J Anim Sci* 80(2):367-375, 2002.
12. Johnson JL, Schneider NR, Slanker MR: Trace element concentrations in perinatal beef calves from West Central Nebraska, *Vet Hum Toxicol* 31:521, 1989.
13. Dirksen GU: Ulceration, dilatation and incarceration of the abomasum in calves: clinical investigations and experiences, *Bov Pract* 28:127, 1994.
14. Marshall BJ: Unidentified curved bacilli on gastric epithelium in active chronic gastritis, *Lancet* 1:1273, 1983.
15. Mantzaris GJ, Hatzis A, Tamvakologos G et al: Prospective randomized, investigator-blind trial of *Helicobacter pylori* infection treatment in patients with refractory duodenal ulcers, *Dig Dis Sci* 38:1132, 1993.
16. Blaser M: Epidemiology and pathophysiology of *Campylobacter pylori* infections, *Rev Infect Dis Suppl* 1:99, 1990.
17. Lee A, Fox JG, Murphy J: A small animal model of human *Helicobacter pylori* active chronic gastritis, *Gastroenterology* 99:1315, 1990.
18. Graham DY, Go MF: *Helicobacter pylori*: Current status, *Gastroenterology* 105:279, 1993.
19. Haringsma PC, Mouwen JM: Mogelijke betekenis van spirilvormige bacterien bij het ontstaan van lebmaagzweren bij het volwassen rund. [Possible role of spiral-shaped bacteria in the pathogenesis of abomasal ulcers in adult cattle], *Tijdschr Diergeneeskd* 117:485, 1992.
20. Braun U, Anliker H, Corboz L, Ossent P: The occurrence of spiral-shaped bacteria in the abomasum of cattle, *Schweiz Arch Tierheilkd* 139(11):507-516, 1997.
21. Jelinski MD, Ribble CS, Chirino-Trejo M et al: The relationship between the presence of *Helicobacter pylori*, *Clostridium perfringens* type A, *Campylobacter* spp, or fungi and fatal abomasal ulcers in unweaned beef calves, *Can Vet J* 36:379, 1995.
22. Reinbach DH, Cruickshank G, McColl KE: Acute perforated duodenal ulcer is not associated with *Helicobacter pylori* infection, *Gut* 34:1344, 1993.
23. Mills KW, Johnson JL, Jensen RL et al: Laboratory findings associated with abomasal ulcers/tympany in range calves, *J Vet Diagn Invest* 2:208, 1990.
24. Berkhoff GA, Braun RK, Buergelt CD et al: *Clostridium perfringens* type A associated with sudden death of replacement and feeder calves, *Am Assn Vet Lab Diag 23rd Ann Proc* 45, 1980.
25. Johnson JL, Hudson DB, Bohlender RE: Perforating abomasal ulcers and abomasal tympany in range calves, *Am Assn Vet Lab Diag 24th Ann Proc* 203, 1981.
26. Roeder BL, Chengappa MM, Nagaraja TG et al: Experimental induction of abdominal tympany, abomasitis, and abomasal ulceration by intraruminal inoculation of *Clostridium perfringens* type A in neonatal calves, *Am J Vet Res* 49:201, 1988.
27. Vatn S, Tranulis MA, Hofshagen M: *Sarcina*-like bacteria, *Clostridium fallax* and *Clostridium sordelli* in lambs with abomasal bloat, haemorrhage and ulcers, *J Comp Pathol* 122(2-3):193-200, 2000.
28. DeBey BM, Blanchard PC, Durfee PT: Abomasal bloat associated with *Sarcina*-like bacteria in goat kids, *J Am Vet Med Assoc* 209(8):1468-1469, 1996.
29. Smith DF, Munson L, Erb HN: Predictive values for clinical signs of abomasal ulcer disease in adult dairy cattle, *Prev Vet Med* 3:573, 1986.
30. Braun U, Eicher R, Ehrensperger F: Type 1 abomasal ulcers in dairy cattle, *J Vet Med A* 38:357, 1991.
31. Braun U, Bretscher R, Gerber D: Bleeding abomasal ulcers in dairy cows, *Vet Record* 129:279, 1991.
32. Payton AJ, Glickman LT: Fecal occult blood tests in cattle, *Am J Vet Res* 41:918, 1980.
33. Ok M, Sen I, Turgut K et al: Plasma gastrin activity and the diagnosis of bleeding abomasal ulcers in cattle, *J Vet Med A Physiol Pathol Clin Med* 48(9):563-568, 2001.
34. Thurmond MC, Holmberg CA, Picanso JP: Antibodies to bovine leukemia virus and presence of malignant lymphoma in slaughtered California dairy cattle, *J Natl Cancer Inst* 74:711-714, 1985.
35. Ruggles AJ, Sweeney RW, Freeman DE et al: Intraluminal hemorrhage from small intestinal ulceration in two cows, *Cornell Vet* 82:181, 1992.
36. Kallfelz FA, Whitlock RH: Survival of ^{59}Fe-labeled erythrocytes in cross-transfused bovine blood, *Am J Vet Res* 34:1041, 1973.
37. Wallace LLM, Reecy J, Williams JE: The effect of ranitidine hydrochloride on abomasal fluid pH in young steers, *J Agri-Practice* 15:34, 1994.
38. Ahmed AF, Constable PD, Miks NA: Effect of orally administered cimetidine and ranitidine on abomasal luminal pH in clinically normal milk-fed calves, *Am J Vet Res* 62(10):1531-1538, 2001.
39. Ahmed AE, Constable PD, Misk NA: Effect of an orally administered antacid agent containing aluminum hydroxide and magnesium hydroxide on abomasal luminal pH in clinically normal milk-fed calves, *J Am Vet Med Assoc* 220(1):74-79, 2002.

40. Mikhail M, Brugère H, Le Bars H, Colvin HW Jr: Stimulated esophageal groove closure in adult goats, *Am J Vet Res* 49:1713-5, 1988.

41. Jelinski MD, Ribble CS, Campbell JR, Janzen ED: Descriptive epidemiology of fatal abomasal ulcers in Canadian beef calves, *Prev Vet Med* 26:9, 1996.

42. Katchuik R: Abomasal disease in young beef calves: surgical findings and management factors, *Can Vet J* 33:459, 1992.

43. Palmer JE, Whitlock RH: Perforated abomasal ulcers in adult dairy cows, *J Am Vet Med Assoc* 184:171, 1984.

44. Tulleners EP, Hamilton GF: Surgical resection of perforated abomasal ulcers in calves, *Can Vet J* 21:262, 1980.

CHAPTER 11

Abomasal Emptying Defect in Sheep

D. MICHAEL RINGS

Abomasal emptying defect (AED) presents most commonly as a syndrome of chronic, progressive weight loss in adult black-faced sheep. This syndrome is unique from abomasal impaction in that feces continue to be passed. The duration of the problem appears variable based on owner's ability to detect weight loss. Affected sheep in heavy fleece often go undiagnosed until shearing. Owners often report weight loss despite the animal continuing to eat; however, this is a misconception in that although the animal may be observed to eat one or two mouthfuls when feed is first presented, it quickly loses interest but may remain at the feeding area with other animals.

Physical examination of affected sheep will show normal to slight elevations in heart rate (70->90 bpm) with a normal body temperature and respirations. Hypermotile rumen activity and hypomotile rumen activity have been seen. Abdominal distention of the lower right quadrant is found in roughly 50% of affected sheep. Careful ballottement of this region often reveals a firm viscus extending from the xiphoid distally to an area just in front of the pelvis. As previously stated, normal pelleted feces can be found in the rectum. Varying degrees of weight loss and emaciation can be found depending on duration. A gender predisposition does not appear to exist.

Diagnosis of this condition can be made using measurement of rumen chloride values combined with abdominal ultrasound examination. Because the abomasum is slow to clear abomasal hydrochloric acid, some HCl is refluxed into the rumen, causing a slight rise in rumen chloride (normal 8-20 mEq/L). Values greater than 50 mEq/L have been found in several affected sheep. Ultrasonography of the right paramedian area shows a large viscus extending behind the liver and lying against the ventral abdominal wall. Interestingly, the serum electrolyte values for sodium, potassium, and chloride remain within the normal range, opposite of what would be expected with an abomasal outflow problem.

The etiology of AED has not been determined, but it appears that some genetic predisposition must have been present in Suffolk and Hampshire sheep. Since AED's first recognition in the 1980s, the incidence seems to have been dramatically reduced through recognition and elimination of sires known to produce an affected individual. A similar syndrome of abomasal outflow problems has been recognized in Great Britain in scrapie-affected sheep. Postmortem examination, as well as codon testing on affected sheep, has not shown any association between AED and scrapie in U.S. sheep.

No treatment or combination of therapies has shown any consistent improvement. Promotility drugs with or without surgical emptying of the abomasum have not improved survivability in affected sheep. Despite studies suggesting that metoclopramide has little effect on the abomasum, some sheep respond to twice- or three-times-daily doses of 0.1 to 0.3 mg/kg given subcutaneously. Even when response is seen, it appears to be only temporary with most, if not all, relapsing in fewer than 6 months.

The gross pathology findings in AED are cachexia (loss of body fat and muscle wasting) accompanied by distension of the abomasum. The interesting feature of AED that differentiates it from abomasal impaction is that the pyloric and antral portions of the abomasum are relatively normal (free of impacting material). Almost all distention of the abomasum is in the body. Histologic examination of the vagus nerve and abomasal musculature on a limited number of cases failed to show any consistent abnormal finding.

CHAPTER 12

Pathophysiology of Displacement of the Abomasum in Cattle

DAVID E. ANDERSON

Displacement of the abomasum (DA) in cattle is a gastrointestinal disease that was not widely recognized until the mid-twentieth century. Research initially focused on treatment and prognosis of the disease. Recently, research has focused more on risk factors, prevention, and prediction of this disease. This chapter reviews progress that has been made regarding risk factors, prediction variables, and prevention of abomasal displacement in cattle.

HISTORICAL PERSPECTIVE

Veterinarians treating dairy cattle commonly diagnose displacement of the abomasum. However, DA is a relatively recent phenomenon with respect to the development of the veterinary profession. To my knowledge the earliest reported cases of DA were by Carougeau and Prestat in 1898 and Fincher in 1927, but this disease did not become commonly reported until after the 1940s.[1-7] Before then, DAs either did not occur, were not diagnosed, or were not described as such. Begg reported three cases of left-sided displacement of the abomasum (LDA) of which one cow died because of peritonitis following surgical reduction of the abomasum and two cows returned to normal after withholding all food for 48 hours.[3] Jones described manual correction of LDA without stabilization of the abomasum in two cows.[4] The incidence of diagnosis of DA increased greatly after the mid-1960s and is an internationally recognized problem of dairy cows as we enter the twenty-first century.

DA is commonly referred to as a "disease of high milk production." This statement may be justified in that as dairy cows have been selected for genetic improvement primarily based on milk production, these same cows may have been selected into a high-risk group for development of DA. Presumably, DA has existed for many centuries and was simply not recognized. The justification for this supposition is based on the fact that DA is observed in calves, young stock, adult bulls, and beef cows. Only recently has research been directed more toward identification of risk factors and institution of prevention strategies rather than comparisons of specific treatment techniques. This chapter focuses on the clinical syndrome of DA and summarizes available information regarding risk factors and prediction variables associated with development of DA.

CLINICAL SYNDROME

Displacement of the abomasum may occur to the left (LDA ≈ 90%); right (right displaced abomasum [RDA] or right abomasal volvulus [RAV] ≈ 10%); or, rarely, medially displacing the omental sling. In 1971 Wallace reported that LDA occurs most commonly in 4- to 6-year-old Holstein cows during the first 6 weeks postpartum.[8] Historical factors, as reported by the owner, found to be common among cows with LDA were hypocalcemia (12.4%), ketosis (42%), metritis (41.2%), retained fetal membranes (30.1%), and stressors (11.7%). Also, LDA appeared to be more common among cows having twins. At the time of veterinary examination, physical examination findings common among cows with LDA included metritis (43.5%), mastitis (19%), enteritis (7.3%), and retained fetal membranes (4.8%) (Table 12-1). Research documented since this study generally has concurred with these findings.

LDA causes a 180-degree torsion of the abomasum without volvulus. The torsion is caused by rotation of the abomasum along its long axis ventral and to the left of the

Table 12-1

Concurrent Diseases in Cattle with Abomasal Displacement

Disease	% Cattle*	% Cattle† (RR)
Ketosis	42	7.7 (33.04)
Metritis	43.5	1.8 (4.26)
Retained placenta	30.1	4.7 (6.62)
Mastitis	19	
Hypocalcemia	12.4	1.8 (0.65)

*Modified from Wallace CE: *Bov Pract* 10:50-58, 1975.
†Modified from Markusfeld O: *Prev Vet Med* 4:173-183, 1986.
RR, Relative risk.

rumen. Little or no outflow obstruction of the abomasum occurs, and life-threatening abomasal obstruction is rare with LDA. LDA does result in decreased appetite and milk production possibly resulting from pain, increased forestomach transit time, and stress. Left displacement rarely causes ischemia to the abomasum, but abomasal ulcers are not uncommon among cows having LDA.[9,10]

RDA causes a similar clinical syndrome as LDA but is potentially life threatening because the 180-degree right displacement (torsion) may also rotate about the mesenteric axis and cause abomasal volvulus. Abomasal volvulus causes an outflow obstruction of the abomasum, and ischemia ensues if the gastric arteries or veins become obstructed (abomasal arterial blood is supplied by the right and left gastric arteries along the lesser curvature and the right and left gastroepiploic arteries along the greater curvature; venous drainage occurs via veins of the same name). Abomasal outflow obstruction causes progressive forestomach dilation (e.g., fluid bloat), which causes eventual respiratory and cardiovascular embarrassment. Rumen distention is most severe if the omasum becomes involved as a result of the volvulus of the abomasum (e.g., failure of eructation causing fluid and free gas bloat). Abomasal-omasal torsion and volvulus have greater risks for development of ischemia to the forestomachs because occlusion of the venous drainage and arterial supply is more likely. In my experience, less than 10% of cattle with right abomasal volvulus have concurrent omasal torsion.

Medial displacement of the abomasum is rare and causes identical clinical signs as LDA. In this type of displacement, the greater curvature of the abomasum rotates (torsion) medially and dorsally along the medial wall of the rumen (does not pass under the rumen). This results in the abomasum displacing the omentum dorsally so that it protrudes into the supraomental recess. In 10 years of bovine surgery, I have treated three cows with this type of abomasal displacement.

Definitive diagnosis of abomasal displacement is based on surgical findings or necropsy. However, clinical diagnosis based on simultaneous auscultation and percussion of the abdomen has been shown to be a reliable tool for diagnosis of DA. Smith and colleagues[11] performed a retrospective study of 366 cows with right-sided abdominal resonance ("ping"). Of 366 cattle, 137 had DA, 157 had intestinal gas involving the cecum, spiral colon, or small intestine, and 2 cattle had peritoneal gas. A definitive diagnosis was available for 151 cattle and yielded a positive predictive value of 96% for abomasal displacement and a positive predictive value of 87% for cecum or ascending colon distention.

FACTORS AFFECTING ABOMASAL MOTILITY

The prerequisite for displacement of the abomasum is abomasal atony resulting in the accumulation of gas and fluid in the abomasum. Abomasal motility may be altered under a variety of circumstances. Geishauser and Seeh[12] (1996) found that reflux of duodenal content, as defined by presence of bile acids within the abomasum, is a normal phenomenon in healthy cattle but that cattle with DA had significantly greater abomasum bile acid concentration, suggesting an abnormal duodeno-abomasal reflux. Malbert

and Ruckebusch[13] (1991) described abomasal emptying in adult ruminants including rhythm linked to duodenal motility and circadian rhythms of unknown origin. Transpyloric flow seemed to be controlled by duodenal reflexes. Geishauser and colleagues[14] studied abomasal muscle responses to electrical field stimulation in vitro and found that contractions were decreased in abomasal muscle preparations from cows with LDA (47% less), RDA (66% less), and RAV (45% less).[14] Also, sensitivity to acetylcholine was decreased in these specimens. However, this research does not establish whether the motility disturbance occurs before the displacement or is a result of it. The data are important in that therapy of cattle having DA should be aimed at encouraging return to normal abomasal motility (e.g., electrolyte therapy, prokinetic drugs if severe abomasal atony is anticipated).

Svendsen[15] (1969) studied factors affecting forestomach motility and fluid and gas production in dairy cows. In that experiment, cows fed 15 lb of concentrate feed had fewer rumen and reticulum contractions per minute during the period from 1 to 6 hours after feeding compared with cows fed 5 lb of concentrate feed. Similarly, abomasal motility was decreased, especially of the proximal abomasum, during this period. In a second trial, rumen fluid was collected from cows fed 5 or 15 lb of concentrate feed and injected directly into the abomasum of cows on roughage diets. Rumen and reticulum motility were not changed, but abomasal motility decreased similarly to cows in the previous experiment, indicating that byproducts of concentrate fermentation acted to decrease abomasal motility. In a third experiment, a solution of volatile fatty acids was injected directly in the abomasum. In this study, abomasal motility was decreased but for a shorter period of time. Also, Svendsen studied abomasal gas accumulation during these experiments. Gas production increased markedly with concentrate feeding at time intervals similar to those reported for decreased motility. In cows fed 15 lb of concentrate feed, abomasal gas increased from 0.5 L/hr to a peak of 2 L/hr 5 hours after feed consumption. Thus abomasal gas production is highest during the same time interval that abomasal motility is the least frequent. Lester and Bolton[16] (1994) studied the effect of concentrate feeding on abomasal motility in sheep. Sheep fed a ration consisting of 50% concentrates and those fed 100% concentrates had significantly less frequent abomasal slow waves and duodenal spike bursts compared with sheep fed 100% forages. Interestingly, the velocity of propagation of the slow waves and duodenal spike bursts was not affected. These data are important to establish a link between nutrition and abomasal atony—the prerequisite for DA.

FEEDING PRACTICES AS RISK FACTORS FOR DISPLACEMENT OF THE ABOMASUM

Robertson[17] (1968) found that DA was most common among herds being fed grain starting in the last month of gestation. Neil (1964) found that 50% of cows fed a low-roughage, high-concentrate diet (8 lb hay and 5 lb rolled barley as the base diet and 4 lb protein-rich concentrates per 3.87 L of milk produced) suffered displacement of the abomasum.[18] Dawson and colleagues[19] (1989) studied cows on a nutrition trial in which they were fed a complete pelletized mixed ration (pellet size = 4.8 mm) containing 15% to 20% crude protein and 30% alfalfa. Cows fed the pelletized ration were 10.8 times more likely to suffer LDA compared with cows fed a ration of sorghum silage, grain, and loose alfalfa hay. Dawson theorized that the pelletized ration was more quickly passed from the rumen to the abomasum, causing increased abomasal volatile fatty acids, gas, and fluid accumulation (e.g., abomasal fermentation). Presumably, this would cause abomasal atony and predisposition to displacement. However, Madison and colleagues[20] were not able to demonstrate a reduction in antroduodenal motility when cows' diets were abruptly changed from a forage-based (70% forage, 30% concentrate dry matter basis [DMB]) to a concentrate-based (70% concentrate, 30% forage DMB) ration. Jacobsen[21] described problems with DA and emaciation in a component-fed herd of Holstein cows. Nonesterified fatty acid (NEFA) analysis indicated negative energy balance (NEFA > 1 mEq/L), many cows were thin (BCS < 3.5 at calving or dry-off), and the incidence of DA was approximately 19%. The original ration (DM 71.5%, NE-L 0.78, CP 17.9%, ADF 26.6%, and NDF 45.5%) was changed to increase energy and decrease both acid detergent fiber and neutral detergent fiber (DM 61.2%, NE-L 0.80, CP 17.2%, ADF 22.6%, and NDF 37.1%). Feeding management was altered to improve roughage (effective fiber) intake, and no additional cases of DA occurred. In a survey of data collected on pasture-grazed dairy cattle in Australia, the incidence of DA was only 0.06%.[22] Markusfeld[23] (1989) found hypovitaminosis A in a group of dairy heifers, of which 18.5% had LDA. These heifers were confined within a barn and fed a ration consisting of orange peels, cotton peels, broiler manure, barley, and corn straw (vitamin A estimate 4750 IU total daily intake; NRC recommendation 75 IU/kg body weight/day or ≈45,000 IU for a 600-kg (1320-lb) cow[24]). Other problems encountered included anasarca, ataxia, and abortion. These studies are important to emphasize that concentrate feeding, alone, is not the cause of DA. Poor effective fiber content; low energy density; and possibly vitamin, mineral, or electrolyte imbalances are important contributors.

MECHANISMS FOR DISPLACEMENT OF THE ABOMASUM

Byproducts of fermentation seem important to the development of DA, but the management and animal factors, which culminate in DA, are not clear. Petty and colleagues[25] suggested that altered exercise and feeding patterns caused by management practices might contribute to development of LDA. The reason for displacement to the left side rather than to the right side is elusive. Contrary to popular descriptions, Mulville and Curran[26] (1993) described the abomasum as being positioned along the ventral midline medial and ventral to the omasum. Presumably, displacement of the abomasum to the left side is caused by pressure from the omasum located dorsal, lateral, and to the ride side of the abomasum. This theory is supported by an anatomy text in which the abomasum is shown lying medial and ventral to the ruminoreticular grove with the omasum located dorsal to it.[27] This orientation would cause an anatomic predisposition to left-sided displacement through the space created by the confluence of the ruminoreticular groove and the cranial grove of the rumen.

RISK FACTORS FOR DISPLACEMENT OF THE ABOMASUM

Terms commonly used to evaluate risk factors include relative risk (RR), odds ratio (OR), and likelihood ratio. Relative risk and odds ratios are measures of the odds of an animal with a given factor having the disease compared with the odds of an animal without that factor having the disease. Likelihood ratios are a means to express the odds that a certain value of a diagnostic test would be expected in a subject with the disease compared with a subject without the disease. Harman and colleagues[28] evaluated the effects of season, parity, and concurrent disease on parturition-to-conception interval in 44,450 Finnish Ayrshires. In this study 148 multiparous cows were diagnosed with abomasal disorders (0.5% lactation incidence) at a median of 29 days-in-milk, and 30 primiparous cows (0.2% lactation incidence) had abomasal disorders a median of 41 days-in-milk. Constable and colleagues[29] (1992) found that age, breed, gender, and season were risk factors for abomasal volvulus and LDA (Table 12-2). Cattle at the greatest risk of developing LDA or RAV were 4- to 7-year-old dairy cows in January (for RAV) or March (for LDA) and during the first 2 weeks of lactation. Among dairy breeds, Guernsey cattle had greater odds of LDA and Brown Swiss cattle had lower odds of RAV compared with Holstein cattle. Markusfeld[30] reported that cows in their fifth or higher lactation had the highest risk of developing DA (RR 2.41).

Periparturient diseases are common among cattle with DA (see Table 12-1).[8,29,30] Oikawa and colleagues[31] (1997) reported that ketosis and LDA were linked to fatty liver disease (Table 12-3). Interestingly, cows in Oikawa's study with LDA alone had higher NEFAs but similar β-hydroxybutyrate (BHB) concentration compared with

Table 12-2

Risk Factors for Displacement of the Abomasum in Cattle

Variable	Category	Crude Odds Ratio
Age	<2 mo	1
	2-6 mo	1.9
	6 mo-1 yr	1.4
	1-2 yr	5.2
	2-4 yr	51.4
	4-7 yr	114.0
	>7 yr	54.6
Breed category	Beef	1
	Dairy	170.1
Dairy breeds (>2 yr old)	Holstein	1
	Jersey	1.53
	Brown Swiss	1.29
	Guernsey	2.76
	Ayrshire	1.21
Gender	Male	1
	Female	98.4

Modified from Constable PD, Miller GY, Hoffsis GF et al: *Am J Vet Res* 53:1184-1191, 1992.

Table 12-3

Expected Ranges for Various Metabolic Variables in Healthy Cattle and Cattle with Fatty Liver Disease, Ketosis, and/or Displaced Abomasum

Variable	Early Lactation	Midlactation	Ketosis	LDA	Ketosis + LDA
NEFA (mEq/L)	0.336±0.15	0.208±0.07	1.43±0.63	0.957±0.31	1.65±0.55
BHB (mM)	0.852±0.32	0.595±0.12	3.24±2.27	0.657±0.24	3.65±1.75

Prediction factor	Control Cows First Week PP (mean)	Cows LDA First Week PP (mean)	Control Second Week PP (mean)	Cows LDA Second Week PP (mean)	Cutoff Value (Likelihood Ratio)
AST (U/L)	91	112	86	140	>140 wk 1 (3)
BHB (μmol/L)	868	1182	785	1554	>1400 wk 1 (2.8)

Modified from Oikawa S, Katoh N, Kawawa F et al: *Am J Vet Res* 58:121-125, 1997.
AST, Aspartate transaminase; *BHB*, β-hydroxybutyrate; *LDA*, left-sided displacement of the abomasum; *NEFA*, nonesterified fatty acids; *PP*, postpartum.

cows in midlactation. Cows with LDA and ketosis had BHB concentrations similar to cows with ketosis alone. Rehage and colleagues[32] (1996) reported that the severity of fatty liver disease, determined histologically, in cows having a DA was severe in 32%, moderate in 40%, and mild or absent in 28%.[32] Of these cattle with DA, 55% had mastitis, endometritis, or lameness. Ito and colleagues[33] (1997) found that cows with ketosis, DA, and fatty liver disease had decreased concentrations of apolipoprotein B-100 (normal for mature cows, 259±63 μg/ml).[33] Geishauser and colleagues[34,35] (1997 and 1998) found that cows having an AST greater than or equal to 180 U/L and those having a BHB of greater than or equal to 1600 μmol/L had greater odds ratio for subsequent diagnosis of LDA (Table 12-4).

Time of year, animal factors, and feed factors are important to the development of DA, but these effects are difficult to quantitate (Table 12-5, Fig. 12-1). Of 15 management factors entered into a risk factor model for LDA by Correa and colleagues,[36] only lead feeding was preserved in the model after statistical analysis.[36] Cows that had lead feeding had an odds ratio of 4.4 for development of LDA. In that study, cows having metritis had an odds ratio of 43.7. Markusfeld[30] (1986) reported the relative risk for abomasal displacement associated with peripartum factors, which included twinning (RR 2.29), retained placenta (RR 6.62), metritis (RR 4.26), aciduria (RR 6.17), and ketonuria (RR 33) (see Table 12-5).

Hypocalcemia has long been recognized as a risk factor for LDA because of abomasal atony. Massey and colleagues[37] (1993) found that cows with hypocalcemia at parturition had 4.8 times greater risk of developing LDA. Oetzel[38] (1996) prophylactically administered calcium chloride gel to cows 12 hours before calving, at calving, and 12 and 24 hours after calving. Significantly fewer cases of parturient paresis, parturient hypocalcemia, and DA occurred in treated cows. Goff and Horst[39] reported that the incidence of postpartum hypocalcemia greatly increased when potassium was added to the diet at 2.1%

Table 12-4

Summary of Variables Used to Predict Which Cows Are Likely to Develop Displaced Abomasum

Variable	Cutoff Value	Likelihood Ratio
AST (U/L)	>180	4.51 wk 1 5.94 wk 2
BHB (μmol/L)	>1600	3.69 wk 1 13.89 wk 2
First milk protein–to-fat	<0.72	8.2

Modified from Geishauser T, Habil D, Leslie K et al: *Am J Vet Res* 58: 1216-1220, 1997.
AST, Aspartate transaminase; *BHB*, β-hydroxybutyrate.

or 3.1% (sodium was present at 0.12%). When a diet of 1.3% sodium and 1.5% calcium was fed, a similar effect was observed.

PREDICTION OF DISPLACEMENT OF THE ABOMASUM

Geishauser and colleagues[34,35] (1997 and 1998) found that determination of beta-hydroxybutyrate and AST concentrations within 2 weeks after parturition were useful to predict which cows would subsequently suffer LDA (see Table 12-4). Cows having an AST greater than or equal to 180 U/L had an odds ratio (OR) of 6.7 one week postpartum and OR = 6.6 two weeks postpartum, and those having a BHB of greater than or equal to 1600 μmol/L had an OR = 4.5 one week postpartum and OR = 24 two weeks postpartum for subsequent diagnosis of LDA. Nielen and colleagues[40] (1994) evaluated two cow-side tests for detection of subclinical ketosis as defined by serum concentration of beta-hydroxybutyrate greater

Table 12-5

Summary of Risk Factors for and Prediction Factors of Displacement of the Abomasum in Cattle

VARIABLE	FACTOR	
Seasonal effects	Season	% Cases
	September-November	9.7
	December-February	23.2
	March-May	42.5
	June-August	24.9
Animal factors	Twinning	3.25 RR
	Low milk production previous 120 days prepartum	2.71 RR
	Body condition	<30mm back fat
Feed factors	Pelletized complete ration	
	Lead feeding	4.4 OR
	Low effective fiber	

Modified from Constable PD, Miller GY, Hoffsis GF et al: *Am J Vet Res* 53:1184-1191, 1992, and Markusfeld O: *Prev Vet Med* 4:173-183, 1986. *OR*, Odds ratio; *RR*, relative risk.

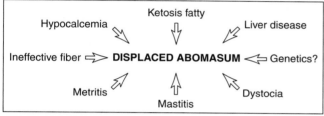

Fig 12-1 Interrelationships between various risk factors and displacement of the abomasum.

than 1.4 mmol/L. A cow-side milk ketone test (sodium nitroprusside test) had a sensitivity of 90% and a specificity of 96%. A cow-side urine ketone test (Acetest, Ames Division, Miles Laboratories, Bridgend, Glamorgan, UK) had a sensitivity of 100% and a specificity of less than 67%. Based on these studies, monitoring for ketosis may be prudent in postpartum cows and milk may be a better sample for routine monitoring for ketosis. Recent studies have shown that feeding management, diurnal variations, and lactation duration cause variation in some blood metabolites (e.g., BHB, NEFA, cholesterol).[41] These effects should be accounted for when interpreting laboratory testing results.

The milk protein–to-fat ratio was found to be useful in predicting cows that would develop DA.[42] At 19 days after calving, a protein-to-fat ratio less than 0.72 was 8.2 times more likely to be from a cow that subsequently developed a DA (sensitivity = 0.8, specificity 0.68). In a subsequent study, Geishauser and colleagues[43] (1999) found that the first milk test was useful to calculate the odds of DA. The highest odds for development of a DA were associated with lower milk yield, higher milk fat percentage, and lower milk protein percentage. Furl and

colleagues[44] (1999) reported that cows with back fat thickness greater than 30 mm, especially those suffering dystocia, were most likely to develop DA.

References

1. Carougeau, Prestat: Torsio de la caillette chez un veau, *J Med Vet* 2:340, 1898.
2. Fincher MG: Digestive disturbances of cattle, *J Am Vet Med Assoc* 71:9-20, 1927.
3. Begg H: Diseases of the stomach of the adult ruminant, *Vet Rec* 63:797, 1953.
4. Jones W: Abomasal displacement in cattle, *Cornell Vet* 42:53-55, 1952.
5. Loje K: Torsio abomasi hos kvaaget, *Mskr Dyrl* 51:85-98, 1945.
6. Loje K: Torsio abomasi beim rind mit besonderem hinblick auf die diagnose und therapie, *Medlemsbl denske Dyrlae geforen* 31:348-353, 1948.
7. Emsbo P: Lobetorsion hos kvaag, *Medlemsbl danske Dyrlaageforen* 28:182, 1945.
8. Wallace CE: Left abomasal displacement—a retrospective study of 315 cases, *Bov Pract* 10:50-58, 1975.
9. Mueller K, Merrall M, Sargison ND: Left abomasal displacement and ulceration with perforation of abdominal musculature in two calves, *Vet J* 157:95-97, 1999.
10. Cable CS, Rebhun WC, Fubini SL et al: Concurrent abomasal displacement and perforating ulceration in cattle: 21 cases, *J Am Vet Med Assoc* 212:1442-1445, 1998.
11. Smith DF, Erb HN, Kalaher KM, Rebhun WC: The identification of structures and conditions responsible for right side tympanic resonance (ping) in adult cattle, *Cornell Vet* 72:180-199, 1982.
12. Geishauser T, Seeh C: Duodeno-abomasal reflux in cows with abomasal displacement, *Zentralblatt Fur Veterinarmedzinin. Reihe A* 43:445-450, 1996.
13. Malbert CH, Ruckebusch Y: Emptying of the abomasum in adult ruminants, *Reprod Nutr Dev* 31:1-25, 1991.
14. Geishauser T, Reiche D, Schemann M: In vitro motility disorders associated with displaced abomasum in dairy cows, *Neurogastroenterol Motility* 10:395-401, 1998.
15. Svendsen PE: *Etiology and pathogenesis of abomasal displacement in cattle*. Cornell University, Ithica, NY, 1969 (master's thesis).
16. Lester GD, Bolton JR: Effect of dietary composition on abomasal and duodenal myoelectrical activity, *Res Vet Sci* 57:270-276, 1994.
17. Robertson JM: Left displacement of the abomasum: epizootiologic factors, *Am J Vet Res* 29:421-434, 1968.
18. Neil PA: Some clinical observations on the etiology of displacement of the abomasum in the dairy cow. 111th Int Meeting of the World Assoc of Buiatrics 1964, *Nord Vet Med Suppl* 1:361-366.
19. Dawson LJ, Aalseth EP, Rice LE et al: Influence of fiber form in a complete mixed ration on incidence of left displaced abomasum in postpartum dairy cows, *JAVMA* 200:1989-1992, 1989.
20. Madison JB, Merritt AM, Rice B et al: Influence of an abrupt change in diet on antroduodenal myoelectric activity in lactating cattle, *Am J Vet Res* 54:793-796, 1993.
21. Jacobsen KL: Displaced abomasa and thin cows in a component-fed dairy herd, *Compend Contin Educat* S21-27, 1995.
22. Jubb TF, Malmo J, Davis GM, Vawser AS: LDA in dairy cows at pasture, *Aust Vet J* 68:140-142, 1991.
23. Markusfeld O: Possible association of vitamin A deficiency with displacement of the abomasum in dairy heifers, *J AM Vet Med Assoc* 195:1123-1124, 1989.
24. Herdt TH, Stowe HD: Fat-soluble vitamin nutrition for dairy cattle, *Vet Clin North Am Food Anim Pract* 7:391-415, 1991.

25. Petty RD: Surgical correction of left displaced abomasum in cattle: a retrospective study of 143 cases, *JAVMA* 178:1274-1276, 1981.

26. Mulville P, Curran N: Left sided abomasal displacement in cattle: aetiology and diagnosis, *Irish Vet J* 15:21-23, 1993.

27. Ashdown RR, Done S: The abdomen. In Ashdown RR, Done S, editors: *Color atlas of veterinary anatomy. The ruminants*, Philadelphia, 1984, JB Lippincott, pp 5.1-5.45.

28. Harman JL, Grohn YT, Erb HN et al: Event-time analysis of the effect of season of parturition, parity, and concurrent disease on parturition-to-conception interval in dairy cows, *Am J Vet Res* 57:640-645, 1996.

29. Constable PD, Miller GY, Hoffsis GF et al: Risk factors for abomasal volvulus and left abomasal displacement in cattle, *Am J Vet Res* 53:1184-1191, 1992.

30. Markusfeld O: The association of displaced abomasum with various periparturient factors in dairy cows. A retrospective study, *Prev Vet Med* 4:173-183, 1986.

31. Oikawa S, Katoh N, Kawawa F et al: Decreased serum apolipoprotein B-100 and A-I concentrations in cows with ketosis and left displacement of the abomasum, *Am J Vet Res* 58:121-125, 1997.

32. Rehage J, Qualmann K, Meier C et al: Post-surgical convalescence of dairy cows with left abomasal displacement in relation to fatty liver, *Schweizer Archiv Fur Tierheilkunde* 138:361-368, 1996.

33. Ito H, Tamura K, Motoi Y, Kawawa F: Serum apolipoprotein B-100 concentrations in healthy and diseased cattle, *J Vet Med Sci* 59:587-591, 1997.

34. Geishauser T, Habil D, Leslie K et al: Evaluation of aspartate transaminase activity and β-hydroxybutyrate concentration in blood as tests for prediction of left displaced abomasum in dairy cows, *Am J Vet Res* 58:1216-1220, 1997.

35. Geishauser T, Leslie K, Duffield T et al: The association between selected metabolic parameters and left abomasal displacement in dairy cows, *Zentralblatt Fur Veterinarmedizin Reihe A* 45:499-511, 1998.

36. Correa MT, Curtis CR, Erb HN et al: An ecological analysis of risk factors for postpartum disorders of Holstein-Friesian cows from 32 New York farms, *J Dairy Sci* 73:1515-1524, 1990.

37. Massey CD, Wang C, Donovan GA et al: Hypocalcemia at parturition as a risk factor for left displacement of the abomasum in dairy cows, *J Am Vet Med Assoc* 203:852-853, 1993.

38. Oetzel GR: Effect of calcium chloride gel treatment in dairy cows on incidence of periparturient diseases, *J Am Vet Med Assoc* 209:958-961, 1996.

39. Goff JP, Horst RL: *Potassium, not calcium induces milk fever: addition of potassium or sodium, but not calcium, to prepartum rations induces milk fever in dairy cows.* 29th Annual Convention Proceedings American Association of Bovine Practitioners, 1996:170.

40. Nielen M, Aarts MG, Jonkers AG et al: Evaluation of two cowside tests for the detection of subclinical ketosis in dairy cows, *Can Vet J* 35:229-232, 1994.

41. Eicher R, Liesegang A, Bouchard E, Tremblay A: Effect of cow-specific factors and feeding frequency of concentrate on diurnal variations of blood metabolites in dairy cows, *Am J Vet Res* 60:1493-1499, 1999.

42. Geishauser TD, Leslie KE, Duffield TF, Edge VL: An evaluation of protein/fat ratio in first DHI test milk for prediction of subsequent displaced abomasum in dairy cows, *Can J Vet Res* 62:144-147, 1998.

43. Geishauser T, Leslie K, Duffield T, Edge V: The association between first DHI milk-test parameters and subsequent displaced abomasum diagnosis in dairy cows, *Berliner Und munchener Tierarztliche Wochenschrift* 112:1-4, 1999.

44. Furl M, Dabbagh MN, Jakel L: Body condition and dislocated abomasum: comparative investigations into back fat thickness and additional criteria in cattle, *Deutsche Tierarztliche Wochenschrift* 106:5-9, 1999.

CHAPTER 13

Displaced Abomasum in Cattle

ANDREW NIEHAUS

An abomasal displacement (DA) is an abnormal positioning of the abomasum within the abdominal cavity. In the truest sense of the term a DA is divided into three categories consisting of left abomasal displacement (LDA), right abomasal displacement (RDA), or right abomasal volvulus (RAV).

In the adult bovid the rumen occupies most of the abdomen. The rumen normally lies along the left body wall, and the ventral sac of the rumen extends to the right of midline. The omasum lies to the right of the cranial rumen. It lies just above the cranial aspect of the abomasum. The abomasum also lies to the right of the rumen against the ventral abdominal wall. The craniodorsal aspect of the abomasum normally lies between the rumen and the omasum.

An LDA occurs when the abomasum becomes displaced to the left of the rumen and floats up between the rumen and the left body wall. Because of the buoyancy of the gas-filled abomasum within the abdominal cavity, the abomasum cannot replace itself into its normal position to the right of the rumen. An RDA occurs when the abomasum becomes gas distended and floats dorsally but remains along the right side of the rumen. The RDA slides along the right body wall. If the RDA flips along its long axis, then an RAV is created. The abomasal volvulus may include the omasum within the twist, becoming a right abomasal omasal volvulus (RAOV).

An LDA and RDA create a partial outflow obstruction to abomasal contents. The abomasum is usually only mildly to moderately distended, and the affected animal is typically not colicky. The animal usually is depressed in feed intake. A lactating dairy cow generally drops in milk production over the course of the disease. The signs of an RAV are generally more severe. The onset of clinical signs is more acute with a RAV. The abomasum is typically severely distended, and the luminal pressures can reach upwards of 30 mm Hg.[1] Signs of colic are common with an elevated heart rate and respiratory rate. As the lumen pressure increases, the abomasal perfusion decreases.[2] The abomasal tissue may be totally devitalized, resulting in necrosis of the abomasal wall. Signs of shock and endotoxemia may result. RAV is an emergency condition. If the omasum is involved within the twist, then the condition is worsened. One study found that cattle with omasal involvement had significantly worse prognosis than cattle without omasal involvement.[3]

DIAGNOSIS

Diagnosis of abomasal displacements is usually made based on clinical signs and auscultation and percussion of the abdomen. Auscultation and percussion over the displaced abomasum typically reveal a characteristic hyper-resonant "ping." A left-sided ping will be auscaulted in cases of LDA; a right-sided ping will be auscaulted in cases of RDA and RAV. A common differential for a left-sided abdominal ping is gas within the rumen. Right-sided pings also can occur commonly in a normal animal and include gas within the spiral colon, or gas within the cecum (cecal dilatation or volvulus). Gas within the uterus (physometra) from metritis and free peritoneal gas (pneumoperitoneum) from peritonitis can cause pings on either side of the abdomen. Other ancillary tests to help support the diagnosis of a displaced abomasum include a pH analysis of fluid aspirated from the viscous in question (liptack test) and abdominal ultrasound. Passing a stomach tube into the rumen and ausculting over the left paralumbar fossa for air bubbles while an assistant blows on the tube can help to differentiate between ruminal tympany and an LDA. Usually the diagnosis can be based on location and size of the ping. An LDA will auscult lower than free ruminal gas, which usually auscults along the left transverse processes of the lumbar vertebra. Depending on the size of the LDA, it will commonly extend back into the left paralumbar fossa. In these cases a small bulge may be evident within the fossa, which can frequently be palpated, as well as percussed. The thirteenth rib may be elevated (referred to as "sprung," meaning that the rib is laterally or outwardly projected because the distended abomasum is displacing the rib), which is another sign indicative of an LDA. RDAs and RAVs can be auscaulted on the right abdominal wall anywhere from the eighth to thirteen ribs. RAVs are usually larger and frequently extend back into the paralumbar fossa. Cecal gas and spiral colon gas will typically be found higher and more caudal in the paralumbar fossa than abomasal gas. Spiral colon gas will be moving through the colon,

and therefore the ping that can be auscaulted will be transient in nature. The displaced abomasum is usually under greater pressure than other structures within the abdomen, and therefore the quality of the ping will be better than other structures within the abdomen that may also give a ping.

Rectal palpation should always be performed as part of the routine physical examination. The rectal palpation should be performed in a systematic manner. A normal rectal examination is typically found in cases of right and left abomasal displacement. The abomasum can sometimes be felt in the right paralumbar fossa with large RDAs or RAVs and in the left paralumbar fossa with distended LDAs. An LDA frequently pushes the rumen away from the left body wall. The right displacement of the rumen from an LDA may be felt on rectal palpation. Cecal dilatation or volvulus can be felt on rectal palpation, which may be a differential for a right-sided ping. It may also be useful to determine the ruminal consistency for diagnosis or treatment of gastrointestinal (GI) disorders in cattle.

A definitive diagnosis can be made with an abdominal exploratory. In normal animals the rumen contacts the left and cranioventral abdominal wall. The abomasum can typically be palpated along the right cranioventral abdomen. If the abomasum becomes trapped between the rumen and the left body wall, a left displaced abomasum has occurred. Animals that have an RDA are found to have a distended abomasum that remains on the right side of the abdomen. The greater curvature becomes displaced dorsally. Animals that have an RAV have an abomasum located on the right side of the abdominal cavity in the cranial abdominal quadrant; the abomasum is distended, causing medial displacement of the liver such that the diaphragmatic surface of the liver no longer contacts the right abdominal wall; and a firm twist is palpated at the omasal-abomasal junction. Occasionally the diagnosis of RAOV is made. The degree of abomasal distension and liver displacement for an RAOV is like that for an RAV, and palpation of the reticulo-omasal junction reveals a firm twist.

ETIOLOGY

The etiology of abomasal displacements is multifactorial. Experts believe that the genesis of all abomasal displacements is abomasal atony. Abomasal atony leads to gas accumulating within the abomasum, creating a gas-filled viscus. This gas-filled viscous is buoyant within the abdomen and floats dorsally. If it floats up on the left side of the rumen, an LDA is formed; if it remains on the right side, an RDA is formed. An RDA can twist again, creating an RAV or RAOV. The direction of the twist is described as counterclockwise as viewed from the hind (RDA) and counterclockwise as viewed from the top (RAV). All cases of abomasal volvulus likely begin as RDAs.

Any concurrent diseases or conditions that cause GI atony can lead to formation of a displaced abomasum. Infectious diseases such as mastitis, metritis, enteritis, and peritonitis, as well as noninfectious causes such as hypocalcemia, hypokalemia, and ketosis, can lead to stasis of the GI tract and subsequent GI and abomasal atony. Abrupt changes in diet can also cause upsets that can cause GI atony. Cattle that recently calve are at a much higher risk for developing a DA. Experts believe that the void created within the abdominal cavity after parturition can allow the abomasum to move more freely. Also, cows in the early postparturient period are at a much higher risk for development of other conditions such as metritis, mastitis, hypocalcemia, and ketosis.

MEDICAL THERAPY

Medical therapy is seldom used alone for treatment of abomasal displacements. Usually medial therapy is combined with surgical correction of the displacement. Medical therapy involves correction of the underlying cause and promotion of GI motility. The restoration of abomasal motility should expel gas and allow it to return to its normal anatomic position.[4] Oral or systemic calcium to correct hypomotility caused by hypocalcemia may be useful. Promotility agents such as parasympathomimetic agents can help to stimulate GI motility. Dehydrated animals or animals that suffer from severe electrolyte imbalances may benefit from oral or systemic fluid therapy.

Many animals with DAs are in a state of negative energy balance and have concurrent ketosis. A cause and effect relationship may not be able to be established. The negative energy balance can be the result of decreased intake from the DA. Or the ketosis can cause appetite suppression, as well as hypomotility, and be the cause of GI atony. The ketosis may resolve following correction of the DA and eventual increase in energy intake; however, it is the author's opinion that severe cases of ketosis should be primarily treated. Intravenous dextrose, insulin therapy, oral niacin, and oral propylene glycol are commonly used in the author's practice to decrease the negative energy balance.

SURGICAL CORRECTION

Surgical correction of DAs is one of the most commonly performed surgery on cattle by food animal surgeons.[5-7] Several surgical techniques are available for correction of abomasal displacements. The chosen technique depends largely on surgeon preference. Other factors for choosing to use one method of correction over another include direction of displacement (left flank abomasopexy can only be used for correction of an LDA), presence of adhesions, and prior displacement with surgical correction. The techniques of correction that are most widely employed at the author's practice are in order of decreasing frequency: right flank omentopexy, right flank omentoabomasopexy, and left flank abomasopexy. Other techniques of correction and fixation include right paramedian abomasopexy, "roll and tack," "roll and toggle," or laparoscopic abomasopexy.

Right flank techniques are advocated because of their versatility in working with different abdominal structures and permit a more thorough abdominal exploratory. Because of blockage by the rumen, left flank techniques do not allow for a complete exploratory of the peritoneal cavity. Right flank techniques are also preferred because they allow the surgeon to work alone.[5] The right flank omentopexy is a procedure by which the greater omentum

attaching to the greater curvature of the abomasum is fixed to the right body wall holding the abomasum in near anatomic position. The pylorus usually serves as a landmark and is brought to the level of the flank incision to assure correct positioning of the abomasum.[5] With this technique, no suture is placed in the abomasal wall. Placing suture directly in the abomasum has been associated with leakage of abomasal contents, which can result in peritonitis or fistula formation.

Disadvantages of the right flank approach include inability to visualize and work with adhesions of the abomasum to the left body wall. The right flank approach is therefore not the preferred method of correction if we have had previous bouts of peritonitis or suspect adhesions of the abomasum to the left body wall. Also, in cases of late-stage pregnancy, when the uterus is taking up a lot of abdominal space, the abomasum can be difficult to replace from a right flank approach. In these cases a left flank would be the preferred method of correction.[5] It is critical that the correct abomasal positioning be achieved and that sutures are placed through the omentum in close proximity to the pylorus. If this is not achieved, the omentum can stretch and the abomasum can redisplace.

Because the omentum can stretch or break down, allowing for redisplacement of the abomasum, many surgeons advocate adding a pyloropexy to the omentopexy to increase the strength of the pexy. With a true pyloropexy, suture is passed through the pyloric tissue at the pyloric junction.[7,8] At this teaching institution, because of possible complications of pyloric stricture and secondary abomasal outflow problems, we prefer to pexy through the pyloric antrum of the abomasum, approximately 3 to 5 cm proximal to the pylorus. It can be used as a stand-alone procedure, or it can be combined with an omentopexy to increase the security of the omentopexy. Although providing added security to the pexy, there is greater risk of abomasal perforation and fistula formation. Indications for performing a pyloricantropexy are those situations in which the surgeon believes that an omentopexy may not be secure enough to hold the abomasum in place. In overconditioned cattle the fatty omentum is friable and tears easily. In cases in which the omentum tears as the abomasum is being replaced, recurrence of displacement of the abomasum is more likely with omentopexy because the attachment of the omentum to the abomasum is compromised.[8] Studies have found that recurrence rates of LDAs are approximately equivocal[9,10] for correction via omentopexy (4%[10]) versus paramedian abomasopexy (2.4%,[11] 3.6%,[12] and 4.3%[13]).

The left flank abomasopexy technique is performed by laparotomy incision in the left paralumbar fossa. The abomasum is visualized, and multiple continuous bites of a nonabsorbable suture are placed in the greater curvature of the abomasum and passed though the ventral body wall, creating a pexy. Although methods for preventing left displaced abomasum via left flank approach have been described,[14] in general the left flank approach can only be used for the correction of left displaced abomasum, which is a clear disadvantage if the veterinarian is unsure of a diagnosis. Another disadvantage of performing a left flank abomasopexy as compared with the right flank approaches is that the left flank abomasopexy requires an assistant to guide the needle through the ventral abdominal wall so as to achieve correct positioning of the pexy and to avoid vascular structures.[15] The main indication for performing a left flank abomasopexy is the case of an LDA in which adhesions are present between the abomasum and the left body wall. These adhesions can be visualized and subsequently broken down through a left flank approach. Other forms of abomasal pathology like gastric ulcers or perforations can be oversewn from the left flank approach.[5] Surgical correction of LDAs during late-stage pregnancy may be difficult to perform from the right flank because of the large gravid uterus preventing replacement of the abomasum. These cattle may be good candidates for a left flank abomasopexy.[5]

An abomasopexy can also be performed from a right paramedian approach. With this approach, the cow is placed in dorsal recumbency. An incision is created parallel to and 3 to 4 cm to the right of midline, extending caudally from a point 4 to 5 cm caudal to the xyphoid. The incision should be approximately 15 to 20 cm in length.[4] Following reposition of the abomasum, the seromuscular layer of the abomasum is sutured to the peritoneum and the internal rectus fascia. Advantages of this approach include achievement of a stronger pexy, as well as the ability to work with adhesions. Complications with this technique include complications with maintaining the cow in dorsal recumbency during surgery, abomasal fistula formation, and herniation of abomasal leaves.

Less invasive techniques have been developed for correction and fixation of abomasal displacements. These include the roll-and-tack, toggle pin fixation, and laparoscopic techniques. These techniques are only recommended for correction of LDAs because of the possibility of creating an RAV from an RDA. The cow with an LDA is placed on her right side and then through dorsal recumbency and slightly onto her left side. The buoyant abomasum should float to the most nondependent (right ventral) part of the abdomen. Auscultation and percussion is used to verify the positioning of the gas-filled abomasum. A large needle is used to penetrate the body wall and abomasum and tie the suture to secure the abomasum (abomasopexy) to the right cranioventral abdomen. Alternatively, two cannulas placed through the right cranioventral abdomen and into the abomasum can be used to insert two toggle sutures. After placement of the toggle sutures, the abomasal gas can be evacuated via the cannula. After removal of the cannula, the toggle sutures are tied together, securing the abomasum to the body wall. These techniques are quick and relatively easy to perform.

No laparotomy incision is made, eliminating the risk of incisional complications. The major complication of these techniques is the penetration of other abdominal organs because the sutures are placed blindly. Modifications of these techniques involve using laparoscopy to verify the correct positioning of the abomasum and hence decrease the risk of inadvertent penetration of other abdominal structures.

References

1. Constable PD, St-Jean G, Koenig GR et al: Abomasal luminal pressure in cattle with abomasal volvulus or left displaced abomasum, *J Am Vet Med Assoc* 201:1564-1568, 1992.
2. Wittek T, Constable PD, Furll M: Comparison of abomasal luminal gas pressure and volume and perfusion of the abomasum in dairy cows with left displaced abomasum or abomasal volvulus, *Am J Vet Res* 65:597-603, 2004.
3. Constable PD, St Jean G, Hull BL et al: Prognostic value of surgical and postoperative findings in cattle with abomasal volvulus, *J Am Vet Med Assoc* 199:892-898, 1991.
4. Trent AM: Surgery of the abomasum. In Fubini SL, Ducharme NG, editors: *Farm animal surgery,* St Louis, 2004, Saunders, pp 196-240.
5. St-Jean GD, Hull BL, Hoffsis GF et al: Comparison of the different surgical techniques for correction of abomasal problems, *Compend Contin Educ Pract Vet* 9:F377-F382, 1987.
6. Trent AM: Surgery of the abomasum, *Agri-Practice* 13:12-14, 1992.
7. Baird AN, Harrison S: Surgical treatment of left displaced abomasum, *Compend Contin Educ Pract Vet* 23:S102-S108, 2001.
8. Wren G: In-clinic displaced abomasum surgery, *Bov Vet* 4-8, 1993.
9. Fubini SL, Ducharme NG, Erb HN: A comparison in 101 dairy cows of right paralumbar fossa omentopexy and right paramedian abomasopexy for treatment of left displacement of the abomasum, *Can Vet J* 33:318-324, 1992.
10. Wallace CE: Left abomasal displacement: a retrospective study of 315 cases, *Bov Pract* 10:50-58, 1975.
11. Mather MF, Dedrick RS: Displacement of the abomasum, *Cornell Vet* 56:323-344, 1966.
12. Kelton DF, Garcia J, Guard CL et al: Bar suture (toggle pin) vs open surgical abomasopexy for treatment of left displaced abomasum in dairy cattle, *J Am Vet Med Assoc* 193:557-559, 1988.
13. Robertson JM, Boucher WB: Treatment of left displacement of the bovine abomasum, *J Am Vet Med Assoc* 149:1423-1429, 1966.
14. Pearson H: The treatment of surgical disorders of the bovine abdomen, *Vet Rec* 92:245-254, 1973.
15. Gabel AA, Heath RB: Correction and right-sided omentopexy in treatment of left-sided displacement of the abomasum in dairy cattle, *J Am Vet Med Assoc* 155:632-641, 1969.

Prognostic Indicators and Comparison of Corrective Fixation Techniques for Displacement of the Abomasum in Dairy Cattle

KENNETH D. NEWMAN

Displacement of the abomasum is the most common bovine gastrointestinal disease encountered by dairy practitioners.[1] A displacement occurs when the abomasum fills with gas and deviates from its normal anatomic position. Correction of this disorder is accomplished by surgical intervention. This chapter discusses (1) the risk factors and clinical signs associated with abomasal displacement, (2) the advantages and disadvantages of the four most commonly used surgical techniques to correct displaced abomasums, and (3) preoperative, intraoperative, and postoperative prognostic indicators.

REVIEW—RISK FACTORS AND CLINICAL SIGNS

The etiology of this disease is multifactorial[2]; however, on a fundamental level it is considered a preventable disease that is the result of poor management. Primary causes include both insufficient effective fiber length and hypocalcemia, which predisposes for abomasal atony.[3] Contributing factors for abomasal displacement arise from the body's endotoxic or febrile reactions to disease (i.e., mastitis, retained fetal membranes, metritis). These conditions can adversely affect surgical outcome.

Abomasal displacement can be subdivided into three distinct presentations of differing prevalence and severity.[3] Left displaced abomasum (LDA) is the most common (85.3%) and least severe. Right displaced abomasum (RDA) is less common (8.8%) and potentially more severe. And abomasal volvulus (AV) is the least common (5.9%) and typically the most severe.

A number of significant ($p < 0.05$) risk factors for LDA and AV have been identified: age, breed, gender, and season.[2] The relative risk of LDA and AV increases with age, especially between 4 and 7 years. Compared with beef cattle, dairy cattle are more likely to develop either an LDA (95.2 odds ratio) or an AV (36.4 odds ratio). Brown Swiss have a lower risk ($p < 0.0001$), and Guernsey have a higher risk ($p < 0.0001$) compared with Holsteins. Female cattle are more at risk of developing either an LDA (29.1 odds ratio) or AV (3.3 odds ratio). Significantly more cases of LDA (57%) versus AV (28.3%) developed during the first 2 weeks postcalving. The prevalence of concurrent disease was significantly higher ($p < 0.0001$) in cows with LDA (53.6%) versus those with AV (28.3%). A significant seasonal difference occurred ($p < 0.0001$) between the odd ratios for LDA (March) and AV (January).

The clinical signs of an LDA can sometimes be vague.[3] These signs include, but are not limited to, moderate to total anorexia, decreased feces, decreased ruminal contractions and ruminations, and decreased milk production. Occasionally the last rib on the left is sprung out, and the heart rate is elevated. Often secondary ketosis is also present. The classic test to diagnose a displacement is auscultating a "ping." The criteria to auscultate a "ping" is a viscus with a gas/fluid interface that is under pressure and adjacent to the body wall. A "ping" can be identified by simultaneous auscultation and percussion on the left side between the eighth and twelfth ribs along a line from the tuber coxa to the olecranon. The differential diagnoses for a left-sided ping include ruminal tympany, peritonitis, pneumorectum, and physometra.

Other physical findings include a rectal examination that may reveal a medially displaced rumen. A Liptak test (percutaneous aspiration of abdominal viscera) can be done "cowside" and is expected to have a pH of less than 4.5 when the abomasum is aspirated. This would confirm the presence of an LDA. In addition, laboratory biochemistry typically reveals a hypochloremic, hypokalemic, metabolic alkalosis.

The clinical signs of RDA and AV tend to be more severe.[3] These include, but are not limited to, complete anorexia, little to no scant feces, absent ruminal contractions and ruminations, and decreased milk production. Dehydration and tachycardia usually increase with severity of the disorder. An AV often evokes higher heart rates and dehydration compared with either an RDA or LDA. The characteristic "ping" can be heard over the right side along a line from the tuber coax to the olecranon. An

RDA tends to be a smaller ping between the eighth and twelfth ribs, whereas an AV spans a larger area between the seventh and thirteenth ribs and creates a dramatic fluid wave that can be auscultated during succussion. The differential diagnoses for a right-sided ping include pneumorectum, physometra, peritonitis, cecal dilatation and volvulus, and spiral colon. With an RDA, a tight viscus can sometimes be palpated in the lower abdominal quadrant during a rectal examination. In comparison, a large, tight viscus encompassing the majority of the right abdomen would be palpated with AV.

COMPARISON OF SURGICAL TECHNIQUES

The basic principles of correction are to place the abomasum in its correct anatomic position and avoid recurrence of the displacement.[4] Numerous techniques for correction of displacement of the abomasum are listed in the literature.[5-7] These include rolling the cow, closed suture, toggle suture, left-flank abomasopexy, right paramedian abomasopexy, and right-flank omentopexy and/or pyloropexy. This section concentrates on comparing the most commonly used techniques in practice (i.e., left-flank abomasopexy, right paramedian abomasopexy, right-flank omentopexy and/or pyloropexy, and the toggle suture).

Left-Flank Abomasopexy

This procedure involves suturing the abomasums to the right ventral abdominal wall and can only be used for the fixation of LDA. This has been considered by some as the preferred method for fixation in heavily pregnant cows.[8] And its success has been reported as high as 100%.[9] The main advantage of this approach is the ability of the cow to remain standing, therefore minimizing stress on the cow and requiring less manual assistance to perform this procedure.

This approach also has a few disadvantages. Suturing can be difficult if the abomasum lies ventral to the flank incision; thus a large abomasums is preferred for easier access. On large, deep-chested cows, it may be difficult to physically reach the right paramedian area—a full rumen can compound this problem. Small intestine can become incarcerated as the suture is pulled through the body wall, which can be a serious complication. An abomasal fistulation is a postoperative complication that can occur if either the abomasal lumen is penetrated or the sutures are not removed within 2 weeks.[4] Additionally, in cases of a misdiagnosis, this approach permits limited abdominal exploratory and the inability to perform a prophylactic abomasopexy.

Right Paramedian Abomasopexy

The advantage of this technique is that the abomasum is easily positioned. Spontaneous repositioning of the abomasum to its correct anatomic position can occur while in dorsal recumbency. Therefore in the event of a misdiagnosis, the abomasum can still be pexied. This approach permits the best exposure to the cranial abdomen: The abomasum can be examined visually for ulcers and pyloric impactions. LDA, RDA, and AV can be corrected by this approach. Long arms are not required as with other approaches.[4] The adhesions formed by this technique are accepted as being the strongest and longest lasting with the fewest complications. The external scar is minimal, which is a desirable characteristic in show cattle.

This approach has some disadvantages, though. The casting procedure usually requires space, help, and sedation. Regurgitation can be a problem while in dorsal recumbency. Cows with large, full rumens are more prone to regurgitation. Xylazine is the most common sedative used in bovine practice. In addition to sedation, xylazine also desensitizes the larynx and adducts the pharyngeal anatomy, therefore restricting the cow's ability to protect its airway.[10] Preparation of the surgical site may require more time because of fecal contamination.[4] After the surgery, this site can be more difficult to keep clean and dry. In cases of periparturient edema, this approach should be avoided. Advanced pregnancy or pneumonia will further restrict lung capacity while in dorsal recumbency. Abomasal fistulation, albeit rare, can occur if the abomasum lumen is penetrated.[4,11,12] Fistulas can develop between 2 weeks and 12 months.[12] Unfortunately, the incidence rate of this complication is not known but is presumed to be low. This approach can be most physically demanding from the surgeon's point of view.[4]

This technique reportedly has a high success rate, ranging from 83.5% to 94%.[13-15] The reported prevalence of recurrence for ventral paramedian abomasopexy is 2.4% to 4.3%.[16] A retrospective study of 143 cases of LDA fixation by right paramedian abomasopexy in the Chino Valley of southern California reported a postsurgical cull rate of 9.1%.[17] Mastitis, poor postsurgical production, and infertility were the determinants for culling. Furthermore, it was observed that a higher percentage of cows that had not undergone surgery (59.6%) were pregnant versus those that had surgery (42%).

Right-Flank Omentopexy/Pyloropexy

This approach shares similar advantages with the left-flank approach. The cow remains standing, and not much help is required. This approach permits the most thorough exploratory compared with the other techniques. In the event of a misdiagnosis, a prophylactic pexy can still be done. LDA, RDA, and AV can all be corrected by this approach. There are a few disadvantages of this approach, however. This fixation method requires the most technical skill to master.[4] It can be difficult to reach around a large distended rumen, especially in deep-chested cows. Therefore it can be difficult to access adhesions between the abomasum and the left body wall.[4] The abomasum almost always requires deflating, using a 14-ga needle and tubing. However, this process does increase the potential of postoperative peritonitis, though the low pH of the abomasum reduces the likelihood of bacterial contamination.[4] The omentopexy is an indirect fixation method, unlike the previously mentioned techniques. The omental-peritoneal adhesions may not be as strong or as long lasting, especially in heifers and thin cows. Experts believe this problem can be reduced by doing a concurrent pyloropexy. This procedure secures a portion of the greater curvature of the abomasum, 10 cm craniolateral from the pylorus to the body wall. This modification, if done too closely to the pylorus, can cause abomasal outflow problems (type III vagal syndrome).

The annual postsurgical death rates were reported as 13%, 5.5%, and 12.2% for 3 consecutive years.[19] In comparison, the hospital fatality rate at Ohio State University was determined to be 5.6%.[2] A recurrence rate was calculated (minus cows that had died) to be 3.6% and 4.2% for 2 consecutive years.[19] This figure is relatively consistent with the reported prevalence by other investigators.[14,18,19]

In a more recent study comparing two techniques (right flank omentopexy versus right paramedian abomasopexy), there were no statistical significant differences reported concerning complication, death, and cull rates—the 1-year follow-up combining dead and cull rates was 38%.[20] This higher proportion was consistent with an earlier study that found cows with LDA were more likely (odds ratio 43) to be culled for miscellaneous reasons compared with cows without LDA.[21]

Toggle Suture

This approach shares some of the advantages and disadvantages of the previous techniques. The advantages are that the cow remains briefly in dorsal recumbency and the abdomen is not opened up.[7] These advantages may reduce the complications seen with open techniques and possibly reduce the amounts of antibiotic usage and discarded milk. This technique still requires space and help. The most significant disadvantage of this approach is that it is a blind procedure.[4] The abomasum is neither visualized nor palpated; therefore other abdominal viscera could be pexied by accident. Though toggle placement can be verified by checking the pH and odor, this technique does not ensure correct anatomic placement. Furthermore, the opportunity to explore the abdomen is not possible. This technique can only correct LDA, not RDA, and certainly not RAV.[4] Unlike most other techniques, this method requires a large abomasum. Although other techniques require a certain degree of surgeon skill, the success of this method is highly operator dependent. Abomasal fistulation is also a potential complication.

The initial study[7] for toggle fixation reported a success rate of 73.3%. All the cows in this study had concurrent disease processes: ketosis (63.3%), metritis (26.6%), mastitis (13.3%), and retained placenta (13.3%). The mortality rate was 13.3% but was not attributed to the procedure itself (pneumonia, perforating reticular ulcer, hemorrhagic enteritis). In a later study by the same authors,[22] an 88% success rate was reported. Of 100 cows in this study, 96 had toggle fixation. Six cases were deemed to have failed: In four cases the procedure was cancelled (failure to auscultate the abomasum with the cow in dorsal recumbency), and in two cases the sutures pulled out and were reoperated via the left-flank abomasopexy procedure. Of 96 cattle having toggle fixation, 6 died. Of these six, four had concurrent disease.

Pyloric obstruction has been reported after toggle fixation[16]—one (and three suspected) cows in 3 years. Signs of suspected outflow problems secondary to toggle

fixation can occur within 72 hours after fixation. The authors recommend close observation of cows postfixation and cutting the external knot holding the toggles if necessary. The decision then is whether to repeat the procedure or to perform a traditional laparotomy.

A third study compared the toggle versus right paramedian techniques.[23] No significant differences occurred between groups up to 60 days after fixation in return to normal milk production, return to normal feed intake, mortality, culling rate, tissue reaction at the surgical site, or redisplacement rates. Although the toggle fixation technique was developed for use in older commercial cows, or cows with concurrent disease, the authors of this study suggest that the toggle fixation is a good alternative to right paramedian technique.

A further study looked at 1-year survival of cows that had left displaced abomasums corrected using the toggle fixation technique.[24] No significant difference occurred between the cull rates of these cows and herd averages.

It takes longer to reach the first service interval with the toggle technique (92 days) compared with controls (73 days).[25] Furthermore, milk production during the first 3 months after calving was lower compared with controls. But after the third month, milk production in cows with toggle fixation surpassed controls. This phenomenon has been referred to as "super-normal milk production" and was observed in the ventral paramedian abomasopexy correction of LDA.[26]

When no metritis or little metritis was present, the toggle fixation method demonstrated a $100 advantage over pyloro-omentopexy techniques.[25] An even greater monetary advantage was realized in cases of severe metritis. Although limited to a single herd, 72 cows with LDA were enrolled in this study. The authors state that it is unlikely that a single fixation technique would be best for all cows on all farms. They also challenge the dogma that valuable cows should be treated by open surgical techniques. The results from other studies demonstrate that toggle fixation may be a reasonable alternative to open surgical fixation methods.[23,25] Furthermore, it is suggested that the toggle suture method is appropriate for use in routine LDA cases.

PROGNOSTIC INDICATORS

A retrospective study reported that 65.4% of LDA cases corrected by right flank omentopexy had concurrent disease; mastitis (43.5%) and metritis (19%) were present at the time of surgery.[18] The majority of postsurgery complications have been associated with the presence of concurrent disease.

Using retrospective analysis, a classification of severity and evaluation of outcome for AV was developed.[27] A heart rate above 100/min and chloride concentrations below 79 mEq/L were significantly ($p < 0.001$) associated with poor outcomes. Cows with omasal-abomasal volvulus had a significantly ($p < 0.005$) worse prognosis (55% survival) compared with cows with abomasal volvulus alone (87% survival).[28] In a retrospective study of 458 cows with either RDA or AV, a preoperative heart rate of 107.5 ± 18.4/min was observed in salvaged or terminal cows compared with 80.9 ± 18.6/min in productive cows

($p < 0.0001$).[29] In a prospective study that looked at cows with AV, heart rate, hydration status, and period of inappetence were found to be more useful prognostic indicators compared with laboratory tests.[30] Productive cattle had high positive predictive values: heart rate = 80/min (0.88), normal hydration (0.96), and duration of inappetence (59 hours) (0.88). The positive predictive values were much lower in the nonproductive cattle: heart rate = 120/min (0.67) or = 100/min (0.56), dehydration (0.52), and inappetence (0.39).

A retrospective study found that abomasal adhesions present at the time of surgery prevented correction of the LDA and were responsible for 30% of the 9.1% postsurgical cull rate.[17] Abomasal ulcers and fat necrosis are complications observed at the time of surgery. Fatty liver, a multifactorial syndrome, if present at the time of surgery, is a well-known complication with potentially high mortality.[31]

The degree of abomasal distention with gas and fluid has been used to classify severity and outcome of AV.[27] This retrospective classified the volume of fluid and whether this fluid had to be drained to allow correction. A positive outcome was significantly ($p < 0.001$) associated if either gas was mainly present or the AV could be corrected without draining the fluid contents. Conversely, draining was significantly ($p < 0.001$) associated with poor outcomes. Abomasal luminal pressures taken intraoperatively have been determined to be a good prognostic indicator in cases of AV.[32] Based on calculated values, a cutoff of 16 mm Hg divided the cattle into productive and nonproductive groups. Luminal pressures below 16 mm Hg had calculated values for sensitivity (0.83), specificity (0.75), positive predictive value (0.95), and negative predictive value (0.43). Luminal pressure above 16 mm Hg had calculated values for sensitivity (0.75), specificity (0.98), positive predictive value (0.55), and negative predictive value (0.95). Higher intraluminal pressures are thought to incite vascular damage to the abomasal mucosa. Poor outcomes were recorded when visual evidence (color ± edema) of abomasal vascular compromise was observed during surgery.[29] This vascular damage was positively correlated to preoperative tachycardia.

New cases of mastitis accounted for 7% of complications.[18] A prospective AV study observed that appetite was the best postoperative prognostic indicator.[28] All cows with good appetites by the third day postsurgery were productive (positive predictive value 1). Postoperative tachycardia was a poor indicator of outcome due to low sensitivity (range 0.36-0.47). The absence of diarrhea postsurgery could only be interpreted as a poor prognosis if a large, fluid-filled abomasum was identified at the time of surgery.

OVERVIEW

Displacement of the abomasum is the most common bovine abdominal surgery. Mature, older, female cattle (especially Guernseys and Holsteins) are most at risk. In descending order of prevalence but increasing order of severity, manifestations of this disorder are the LDA, RDA, and AV. Concurrent disease is more often present with LDA compared with RDA.

All four techniques have their strengths and weaknesses. The three open techniques have similar success and recurrence rates. The closed method can achieve comparable rates; however, close attention to details and aggressive follow-up is required. In an ideal world the dairy practitioner would select the technique on a case-by-case basis. In reality the technique chosen is usually based on the practitioner's preference and comfort level.

Preoperative prognostic indicators include the type of displacement, heart rate, hydration, and concurrent disease(s). Productive cows postsurgery had high preoperative positive predictive values for heart rate less than 80/min (0.88), normal hydration (0.96), and duration of inappetence (0.88). Intraoperative prognostic indicators include the presence of abomasal ulcers and adhesions, fat necrosis, fatty liver, visual evidence of abomasal vascular occlusion, and intraluminal abomasal pressure. Large, discolored abomasums that required draining to allow correction and intraluminal pressures greater than 16 mm Hg were significantly associated with poor outcomes. A good appetite by the third day postsurgery was associated as the most reliable postoperative prognostic indicator.

References

1. Trent AM: Surgery of the abomasum, *Agri-Practice* 9:12-14, 1992.
2. Constable PD, Miller GY, Hoffis GF et al: Risk factors for abomasal volvulus and left abomasal displacement in cattle, *Am J Vet Res* 53:1184-1192, 1992.
3. Guard C: Diseases of the alimentary tract. In Smith BP, editor: *Large animal internal medicine*, ed 2, St Louis, 1996, Mosby, pp 868-884.
4. St-Jean GD, Hull BL, Hoffis GF et al: Comparison of the different surgical techniques for correction of abomasal problems, *Comp Contin Edu* 9:F377-F382, 1987.
5. Turner AS, McIlwraith CW: *Techniques in large animal surgery*, Philadelphia, 1989, Lea & Febiger, pp 274-288.
6. Hull BL: Closed suturing technique for correction of left abomasal displacement, *Iowa State Univ Vet* 34:142-144, 1972.
7. Grymer J, Sterner K: Percutaneous fixation of left displaced abomasums using a bar suture, *J Am Vet Med Assoc* 180:1458-1461, 1982.
8. Baker JS: Displacement of the abomasum in dairy cows. Part 2, *Pract Vet* 45:16-22, 1973.
9. Ames S: Repositioning the displaced abomasum in the cow, *J Am Vet Med Assoc* 153:1470-1471, 1968.
10. Anderson DE, Gaughan EM, DeBowes RM et al: Effects of chemical restraint on the endoscopic appearance of laryngeal and pharyngeal anatomy and sensation in adult cattle, *Am Vet J Res* 55:1196-1200, 1994.
11. Sams AE, Fubini SL: Primary repair of abomasal fistulae resulting from right paramedian abomasopexy in eight adult dairy cattle, *Vet Surg* 22:190-193, 1993.
12. Parker JE, Fubini SL: Abomasal fistulas in dairy cows, *Cornell Vet* 77:303-309, 1987.
13. Menard L, St Pierre H, Lamothe P: Les affections de la caillete chez la vache laitiere au Quebec II Etude retrospective to 1000 cas, *Can Vet J* 19:143-149, 1978.
14. Robertson JM, Boucher WB: Treatment of left displacement of the bovine abomasums, *J Am Vet Med Assoc* 149:1423-1429, 1966.
15. Lowe JE, Loomis WK, Kramer LL: Abomasopexy for repair of left displacement in dairy cattle, *J Am Vet Med Assoc* 147:389-393, 1965.

16. Kelton DF, Fubini SL: Pyloric obstruction after toggle-pin fixation of left displaced abomasums in a cow, *J Am Vet Med Assoc* 194:677-678, 1989.
17. Petty RD: Surgical correction of left displaced abomasums in cattle: a retrospective study of 143 cases, *J Am Vet Med Assoc* 178:1274-1276, 1981.
18. Mather MF, Dedrick RS: Displacement of the abomasum, *Cornell Vet* 56:323-344, 1966.
19. Wallace CE: Left abomasal displacement—a retrospective study of 315 cases, *Bov Pract* 10:50-58, 1975.
20. Fubini SL, Ducharme NG, Erb HN, Sheils RL: A comparison in 101 dairy cows of right paralumbar fossa omentopexy and right paramedian abomasopexy for treatment of left displacement of the abomasum, *Can Vet J* 33:318-324, 1992.
21. Milian-Suazo F, Erb HN, Smith RD: Risk factors for reason specific culling of dairy cows, *Prev Vet Med* 7:19-29, 1989.
22. Sterner KF, Grymer J: Closed suturing techniques using a bar-suture correction of left displaced abomasum: a review of 100 cases, *Bov Pract* 17:80-84, 1982.
23. Kelton DF, Garcia J, Guard CL et al: Bar suture (toggle pin) vs open surgical abomasopexy for treatment of left displaced abomasum in dairy cattle, *J Am Vet Med Assoc* 193:557-559, 1988.
24. Grymer J, Bartlett PC, Houe H et al: One-year survival of cows with left displacement of the abomasum corrected with the role-and-toggle procedure, *Bov Pract* 31:80-82, 1997.
25. Bartlett PC, Kopcha M, Coe PH et al: Economic comparison of the pyloro-omentopexy vs the roll-and-toggle procedure for treatment of left displacement of the abomasum in dairy cattle, *J Am Vet Med Assoc* 206:1156-1162, 1995.
26. Ehrlich J: Super-normal milk production subsequent to ventral paramedian abomasopexy, *Bov Pract* 29:83-85, 1995.
27. Smith D: Right-side torsion of the abomasum in dairy cows: classification of severity and evaluation of outcome, *J Am Vet Med Assoc* 173:108-111, 1978.
28. Constable PD, St Jean G, Hull BL et al: Prognostic value of surgical and postoperative findings in catle with abomasal volvulus, *J Am Vet Med Assoc* 7:892-898, 1991.
29. Fubini SL, Grohn YT, Smith DF: Right displacement of the abomasum and abomasal volvulus in dairy cows: 458 cases (1980-1987), *J Am Vet Med Assoc* 3:460-464, 1991.
30. Constable PD, St-Jean G, Hull BL et al: Preoperative prognostic indicators in cattle with abomasal volvulus, *J Am Vet Med Assoc* 12:2077-2085, 1991.
31. Pearson EW, Mass J: Hepatic lipidosis. In Smith BP, editor: *Large animal internal medicine*, ed 2, St Louis, 1996, Mosby, pp 937-938.
32. Constable PD, St-Jean G, Koenig GR et al: Abomasal luminal pressure in cattle with abomasal volvulus or left displaced abomasum, *J Am Vet Med Assoc* 10:1564-1568, 1992.

CHAPTER 15

Laparoscopic Abomasopexy for Correction of Left Displaced Abomasum

KENNETH D. NEWMAN and DAVID E. ANDERSON

A number of surgical techniques are currently in use for the correction of left displaced abomasum (LDA) in dairy cows. These techniques include left paralumbar abomasopexy, right paramedian abomasopexy, right paralumbar omentopexy with or without a "pyloropexy," blind suture, and the blind roll and tack. All these techniques have their inherent advantages and disadvantages. The drawbacks of laparotomy include recurrence, peritonitis, incisional infection, incisional dehiscence, abomasal fistulation, surgical time and cost, and antibiotic usage and milk withdrawals. The drawbacks of the blind roll and tack technique include no visual control of abomasal repositioning and fixation, high dependence on operator skill and experience, abomasal fistulation, and no opportunity to explore the abdomen.

A two-step laparoscopic abomasopexy technique has been described in the literature.[1,2] This technique is developed to reduce the incidence of complications associated with traditional laparotomy and the blind roll and tack corrective techniques. The two-step laparoscopic abomasopexy technique offers the advantages of both the laparoscopy and the blind roll and tack techniques, without the disadvantages associated with the blind roll and tack technique alone. It combines the minimal invasiveness and visual control for abomasal positioning and fixation offered by laparoscopy, and the speed and minimal invasiveness of the roll and tack techniques.[1-3] The two-step technique first involves the laparoscopic-guided toggle bar placement within the abomasal lumen through the left paralumbar area in the standing cow, followed by laparoscopic suture retrieval through the right paramedian area while the cow is in dorsal recumbency.[1-3] A one-step laparoscopic abomasopexy technique is reported and purported to simplify the use of laparoscopy to accomplish abomasal fixation.[4]

TWO-STEP TECHNIQUE

In the standing cow the left paralumbar fossa and the last three ribs are aseptically prepared. Two 5-ml local infusions of 2% lidocaine hydrochloride are used for local anesthesia. Stab incisions are made using a number 10 blade for laparoscopy portals: a viewing portal 10 cm ventral to the transverse process and 10 cm caudal to the last rib and an instrument portal 20 cm caudal to the dorsal spinous processes and the eleventh and twelfth intercostal space. After the abdomen is insufflated using carbon dioxide (maximum pressure 15 mm Hg) to permit adequate visualization of the abdomen, the abomasum is identified and trocarized. The toggle pin is inserted into the abomasal lumen using the trocar and push rod. The abomasum is deflated, and the entire suture is placed within the abdomen. The portals are sutured closed using a large, nonabsorbable, braided suture material (e.g., No. 6 Vetafil) and a simple interrupted cruciate suture pattern.

In step 2 of this technique the cow is placed in dorsal recumbency, and the right paramedian area is aseptically prepared. Two 5-ml local infusions of 2% lidocaine hydrochloride are used for local anesthesia. Stab incisions are made using a number 10 blade for laparoscopy portals: a viewing portal is made 5 cm lateral from the midline and 20 cm distal from the xyphoid, and an instrument portal is made 5 cm lateral from midline and 10 cm distal from the xyphoid. If necessary, the abdomen is reinsufflated to allow adequate visualization. The abomasum and suture material are identified. The suture material is retrieved using a 30-cm long grasping forceps. The suture is withdrawn up to the preset marked on the suture, thus positioning the abomasum adjacent to the body wall, and tied over gauze stents. The abdomen is deflated, and the portals are sutured closed using No 6 Vetafil and a simple interrupted cruciate suture pattern. Finally the cow is returned to a standing position.

ONE-STEP TECHNIQUE

This technique is done similarly to step 2 of the two-step approach. The cow is placed in dorsal recumbency, and the right paramedian area is aseptically prepared. Two 5-ml local infusions of 2% lidocaine hydrochloride are used for local anesthesia. Stab incisions are made using a number 10 blade for laparoscopy portals: A viewing portal is made 5 cm lateral from the midline and 20 cm distal from the xyphoid, and an instrument portal is made 5 cm lateral from midline and 10 cm distal from the xyphoid. The abdomen is insufflated with carbon dioxide

(maximum 15 mm Hg pressure) to permit adequate visualization. The abomasum is identified and trocarized. After the toggle bar is inserted into the abomasal lumen using the trocar and push rod, the abomasum is deflated. Unlike the two-step approach, the excess suture material is *not* fully inserted into the abdomen; therefore the 30-cm long grasping forceps are not required. The excess suture material is withdrawn up to the preset marker and tied over a gauze stent. The abdomen is then deflated, and the portals are sutured closed using No. 6 Vetafil and a simple interrupted cruciate suture pattern. Finally the cow is returned to a standing position.

CLINICAL IMPACT

Two specific advantages of the two-step technique are the opportunity to confirm LDA diagnosis and the ability to evaluate adhesions among the abomasum, left body wall, and the rumen.[1] Laparoscopic anatomy of the bovine abdomen was first described in 1993.[5] The left paralumbar fossa typically provides excellent visualization of the left cranial abdomen including the diaphragm, spleen, rumen, left kidney, and the small intestine; occasionally the pancreas, spiral colon, and bladder can be adequately visualized. In contrast, laparoscopy of the bovine abdomen from the cranioventral midline laparoscopy provides visualization of the cranioventral abdomen including the diaphragm, rumen, reticulum, abomasum, pylorus, spleen, and sometimes the left liver lobe. In the present study the right paramedian approach provided excellent visualization of the abomasum, pylorus, ventral body wall, and diaphragm. This visualization made it possible to accurately trocarize and position the abomasum adjacent to the body wall.

Laparoscopy can be performed in cows with few adverse effects.[5] Complications are not observed from the carbon dioxide insufflation or from the laparoscopic procedure itself. The placement of the ventral laparoscopy instrument portals should be done to avoid the large subcutaneous cranial epigastric vessels. Though prominent when the cow is standing, these vessels are difficult to visualize when the cow is in dorsal recumbency. In one report of a horse, these vessels were accidentally damaged during placement of the laparoscopy portals.[6] Damage to these vessels increased surgical time, subcutaneous hematoma formation, and hemoperitoneum. Most cows with LDA are within the first 4 weeks of calving; therefore damage to these vessels is undesirable with respect to maximizing milk production.

In a prospective clinical trial the outcomes of the two-step laparoscopic abomasopexy compared with traditional right paralumbar omentopexy were described.[7] Ninety-six cows, divided into equal groups, had surgery for LDA. The surgical time for the laparoscopic abomasopexy is 10.2 minutes shorter compared with the traditional laparotomy. Postoperatively, cows that had a laparoscopic abomasopexy had significantly higher feed intakes (roughage +0.61 kg, concentrates +1.24 kg), and their milk yield rose significantly higher (+1.82 kg) compared with the traditional laparotomy group. These investigators suggested that less postoperative pain was experienced by cows that had the laparoscopic abomasopexy; therefore these cows had better feed intake and consequently improved milk yield. Furthermore, this procedure was performed without routine antibiotics, unless concurrent disease (i.e., metritis) indicated otherwise. This significantly reduced treatment costs and reduced the risk of antibiotic residues compared with the cows that had had a traditional laparotomy for correction of LDA. The complications of laparoscopic abomasopexy included premature suture breakage (two cows), peritonitis (two cows), and myositis at the abomasopexy site (one cow).[7] In the same study, one cow developed an incisional infection in which a right paralumbar omentopexy had been performed to correct an LDA. These investigators did not indicate where the suture broke. Possibly, either tying the suture around the stent in such a fashion that if one suture broke the other would still hold the toggle and stent in place or placing a second toggle suture bar at the time of surgery would eliminate this complication. Peritonitis has been recorded as a surgical complication of laparoscopic abomasopexy.[3,7] However, peritonitis can also develop secondary to nonsurgical complications such as abomasal ulcers, traumatic-reticuloperitonitis, and metritis. Unfortunately, concurrent diseases were not recorded in either study.

One report from the University of Utrecht in the Netherlands suggested that the two-step laparoscopic abomasopexy technique replaced the right paralumbar omentopexy as the standard approach for correcting LDA in 1998.[3] These investigators reported on the results of 108 laparoscopic abomasopexies performed under field conditions. The data from 84 returned owner questionnaires are included in this study. The survival rate is 76%, with 57 cows starting a new lactation; 40 cows are not bred, and the fates of 11 cows are unknown. Unfortunately, these results are not compared with their previous results using the right paralumbar omentopexy technique. Perioperative conditions such as ketosis, fatty liver, retained fetal membranes, metritis, and mastitis remain a challenge to manage postoperatively and can adversely affect LDA outcomes, regardless of the LDA corrective technique performed.

The long-term anatomic assessment of the laparoscopic abomasopexy correction for LDA has been recorded.[8] Nine weeks postoperatively (6 weeks after the toggle suture had been released), the fixation site between the abomasum and the ventral body wall had stretched up to 15 cm. Therefore these cows may be at higher risk of LDA recurrence. These investigators suggest that a second toggle suture bar and maintaining the suture longer may produce more permanent adhesions and, consequently, make LDA recurrence less likely. Recently, laparoscopic

suturing of the abomasums was described to provide a broader, more secure fixation of the abomasum.[9,10] Although more technically demanding than laparoscopic toggle-pin fixation, this technique may provide for longer-term fixation in dairy cows.

An advantage of the one-step technique over the two-step technique is the ability to perform the laparoscopic abomasopexy in the event of a misdiagnosis. This then raises the possibility of performing prophylactic laparoscopic abomasopexies in breeding age heifers. Prophylactic abomasopexies on farms that have high rates of LDA might reduce any adverse events or complications associated with LDA correction in the early postpartum cow.

References

1. Janowitz H: [Laparoscopic reposition and fixation of the left displaced abomasum in cattle], *Tierarztl Prax Ausg G Grosstiere Nutztiere* 26(6):308-313, 1998.
2. van Leeuwen E, Janowitz H, Willemen MA: [Laparoscopic positioning and attachment of stomach displacement to the left in the cow], *Tijdschr Diergeneeskd* 125(12):391-392, 2000.
3. van Leeuwen E, Muller K: [Laparoscopic treatment of the left displaced abomasum in cattle and results of 108 cases treated under field conditions]. XXII World Buiatrics Congress 2002 (abstract).
4. Newman K, Anderson DE, Silviera F: One-step laparoscopic abomasopexy for correction of left-sided displacement of the abomasum in dairy cows, *J Am Vet Med Assoc* 227(7):1142-1147, 1090, 2005.
5. Anderson DE, Gaughan EM, St-Jean G: Normal laparoscopic anatomy of the bovine abdomen, *Am J Vet Res* 54(7):1170-1176, 1993.
6. Ragle CA, Southwood LL, Schneider RK: Injury to abdominal wall vessels during laparoscopy in three horses, *J Am Vet Med Assoc* 212(1):87-89, 1998.
7. Seeger T, Kumper H, Doll K: [Surgical treatment of left displaced abomasum: results of laparoscopic reposition with abomasopexy (Janowitz-method) compared to right flank laparotomy with omentopexy (Dirksen-mentod)]. XXII World Buiatrics Congress 2002, 2003 (abstract).
8. Kehler W, Stark M: [Laparoscopic repositioning and fixation of the left-displaced abomasum: anatomic assessment of the development of the fixation in the abdominal cavity in the following six months]. XXII World Buiatrics Congress 2002 (abstract).
9. Mulon PY, Babkine M, Desrochers A: Ventral laparoscopic abomasopexy in 18 cattle with displaced abomasum, *Vet Surg* 35:347-355, 2006.
10. Babkine M, Desrochers A, Boure L, Helie P: Ventral laparoscopic abomasopexy on adult cows, *Can Vet J* 47:343-348, 2006.

CHAPTER 16
Hepatotoxicities of Ruminants

A. CATHERINE BARR

RUMINANT HEPATOTOXINS

As the first organ bathed in blood containing toxins absorbed from the gastrointestinal tract, the liver is in a uniquely vulnerable and important position within the body. One of the major functions it performs is to detoxify or activate incoming compounds, some of which can damage the liver itself. Depending on the type of toxin, the hepatic damage may result in the animals dying acutely or becoming chronic poor doers. Metabolic imbalances associated with hepatic compromise, especially the excess accumulation of ammonia and other neurotoxins, may lead to neurologic signs (hepatoencephalopathy). Hepatogenous photosensitization may occur as serum phylloerythrin concentrations increase as a result of the impaired liver's inability to fully metabolize chlorophyll.

PYRROLIZIDINE ALKALOIDS

Pyrrolizidine alkaloids (PAs) are a group of more than 30 phytotoxins metabolized in the liver to generate toxic pyrroles that cross-link cellular macromolecules and inhibit division of hepatocytes causing karyomegaly, cytomegaly, and hepatocellular necrosis. The recycling chain reaction of pyrrole radicals interacting with cellular components results in progressive, irreversible periportal fibrosis. Rarely, high doses of PAs produce rapid death with liver necrosis and visceral and hepatic hemorrhage. More often, after up to several months' delay, chronic ingestion of PA-containing plants and their cumulative toxins causes ill-thrift, anorexia, depression, diarrhea, ascites, secondary photosensitization, weakness, hepatoencephalopathy, coma, and death. PA poisoning is difficult to diagnose antemortem without liver biopsy because of the nonspecific clinical presentation and the delay between consumption and onset of clinical signs. By the time clinical signs are evident, serum concentrations of gamma-glutamyl transferase (GGT) and alkaline phosphatase (ALP) are elevated. Prognosis is poor but, if fibrosis is not too advanced, a high-energy, low-protein diet may be of benefit. At necropsy the liver is typically tan, shrunken, and fibrotic with a thickened capsule. Characteristic microscopic lesions include fibrosis, bile duct proliferation, and megalocytosis.

Typically, PA-containing plants (Box 16-1) are unpalatable and are only consumed when other forage is short or when they provide the only fiber source in lush pastures. Toxicity remains intact in hay and silage, and the seeds of some of these plants (especially *Crotalaria*) have caused clinical disease in ruminants consuming contaminated feed grains. Cattle may be poisoned by consuming

---

Box 16-1

Selected Plants Containing Pyrrolizidine Alkaloids

Senecio spp.
S. jacobaea (Tansy ragwort)
S. vulgaris (Common groundsel)
S. flaccidus (Threadleaf groundsel)
S. riddellii (Riddell's groundsel)
S. triangularis (Tarweed)
S. ampullaceus (Squaw weed)
S. glabellus (Butterweed)
S. alpinus (Alpenkreutzkraut)
Amsinckia spp. (Fiddleneck)
Crotalaria spp. (Crotalaria, Rattlebox)
Echium spp. (Viper's bugloss, Salvation Jane)
Heliotropium spp. (Heliotrope)
Cynoglossum officinale (Hound's tongue)
Symphytum spp. (Comfrey)
Eupatorium maculatum (Bruner's trumpet)
Erechtites spp. (Fireweed)
Trichodesma spp.

2% to 5% of their body weight in PA-containing plant material. Sheep and goats are 20 to 30 times less sensitive, although PA exposure exacerbates sensitivity to copper toxicity, especially in sheep. Young, rapidly growing animals are more susceptible to PA toxicity than are mature animals. Low concentrations of PA can be found in the milk of affected animals and can also cross the placenta, affecting the fetus.

MYCOTOXINS

Aflatoxin

Aflatoxin is produced by several different fungi, including *Aspergillus flavus, A. parasiticus,* and various species of other genera. These fungi grow on high-energy substrates at temperatures greater than 75° F and moisture content of 17% to 20%. Drought conditions and insect damage in the field tend to compromise a seed grain's protective coat (pericarp), increasing the likelihood that mold spores will gain access to the seed's starch and initiate fungal infection. Corn, peanuts, and cottonseed are the main sources of aflatoxin in ruminant feeds, although sorghum and other small grains have occasionally been implicated. Toxin production escalates postharvest unless feeds are stored dry in clean bins. Especially with corn, avoidance of mechanical injury at harvest, removal of broken and lightweight kernels, and drying to 13% moisture or below prevent aflatoxin production. Mold distribution within a bin of feed will be irregular, and "hot spots" of high aflatoxin typically occur. An adequate sample for testing includes a combination of multiple probes from all parts of a storage container.

Ingested aflatoxin is activated by cytochrome p450 in the liver, after which it binds essential enzymes, inhibits protein synthesis, and forms DNA adducts. Because of this, the damage caused by aflatoxin occurs almost exclusively in the liver. All ruminants are affected similarly. Aflatoxin concentrations over 1000 ppb in feedstuffs have caused severe liver damage, hemorrhage, bloody diarrhea, and sudden death. Feeds containing more than 650 ppb consumed over a few weeks can produce hepatic failure with icterus, anorexia, ataxia, weakness, tremors, decreased rumen motility, abortion caused by compromised maternal health, coma, and death. On necropsy the liver may appear pale yellow and friable, microscopically exhibiting centrilobular to portal fatty degeneration and necrosis with biliary hyperplasia. Aflatoxin levels over 350 ppb fed over a month or more can cause more insidious liver failure characterized by anemia; ascites; elevated ALP, GGT, aspartate transaminase (AST), and total bilirubin; decreased albumin; and decreased immune function. Chronic, long-term exposure of mature ruminants to aflatoxin at greater than 150 ppb can result in reduced feed efficiency, increased incidence of disease, and liver damage (fibrosis with regenerative nodules). Young, rapidly growing animals are more susceptible to aflatoxin than mature animals and may exhibit decreased rate of gain, poor immunity, and liver damage at lower concentrations.

Aflatoxin B_1 is the most toxic of the four major aflatoxins (B_1, B_2, G_1, and G_2), and its metabolite M_1 is secreted into milk. About 100-fold less M_1 appears in the milk than the B_1 consumed in the feed. Because aflatoxins are carcinogenic, 0.5 ppb M_1, which can be a result of consuming feed with 50 ppb aflatoxin, is actionable in milk for human consumption. According to federal regulations, aflatoxin in sheep, goat, calf, and dairy feeds shall not exceed 20 ppb; for mature beef cattle, feeds may contain up to 100 ppb; and for finishing cattle, up to 300 ppb. Interstate transport is restricted to grain containing less than 20 ppb aflatoxin. Under emergency conditions in which a large proportion of the year's seed crop (usually corn) contains a high level of aflatoxin, some states allow mixing and dilution and/or ammoniation to reduce total aflatoxin concentration. Certain smectite clays used as feed additives are effective in decreasing bioavailability of aflatoxin B_1 (hydrated sodium calcium aluminosilica [HSCAS]). Aflatoxin has a 7-day withdrawal before slaughter.

Phomopsins

Lupinosis is a syndrome characterized by inappetence, decreased rate of gain, liver damage, and death in immature sheep grazing lupin stubble in Western Australia. The fungus *Diaporthe toxica* growing in lupin after the grain has been harvested produces phomopsins, mycotoxic cyclic hexapeptides that inhibit microtubule formation and prevent mitosis. An acute, high dose of phomopsins causes fatty uptake by hepatocytes, producing yellow-orange hepatomegaly and an enlarged gallbladder. With chronic ingestion of lower levels, serum glutamate dehydrogenase and GGT concentrations are elevated and animals appear depressed, with icterus. At necropsy the liver is small, tan, and fibrotic with a granular texture. Microscopically there is evidence of hepatic necrosis. Cattle are also affected by phomopsins, exhibiting hepatogenous photosensitization when green forage is available with the lupin stubble. Phomopsin toxicity is observed at doses as low as 10 µg/kg body weight.

Sporidesmin

Sporidesmin is produced by spores of the fungus *Pithomyces chartarum* growing in the litter at the base of ryegrass pastures in areas of Australia, New Zealand, South Africa, and parts of Europe and the United States when temperatures are 55° F to 70° F (13° C-20° C) and humidity is above 90%. Alpacas and fallow deer are very susceptible to sporidesmin toxicity, whereas sheep, cattle, red deer, and goats are more resistant. Biliary fibrosis and bile duct occlusion are precipitated by sporidesmin free radical propagation, causing liver damage and hepatogenous photosensitization called *facial eczema* in New Zealand.

Strains of *Pithomyces chartarum* are present worldwide, but not all spores are toxigenic. Studies have revealed that the spore count is closely correlated to the severity of intoxication. At 50,000 spores/g fresh grass, animals are affected after several weeks of grazing, whereas spore concentrations of 200,000 to 300,000 are only tolerated for a few days. Production losses occur because of photosensitization, decreased milk production, and resultant decreased rate of gain in calves and lambs. Sheep with genetic resistance to facial eczema are being propagated. Rumen boluses of zinc salts are protective, along with increased molybdenum and sulfur.

METALS

Copper

Ruminants with copper toxicosis present with intravascular hemolysis following one to three days of depression and inappetence. Toxicity has been demonstrated in cattle injected with copper disodium edetate as treatment for copper deficiency. More often, chronic overexposure increases the liver stores to dangerously high concentrations. Stressful conditions or events trigger release of excess copper from hepatocytes into the bloodstream, causing erythrocytolysis. Clinical signs include anorexia, depression, mild to severe icterus, and hemoglobinuria. Prognosis is poor for animals with intravascular hemolysis evidenced by severe icterus and hemoglobinuria; animals often die in renal failure. The likelihood that herdmates will succumb to copper intoxication can be reduced by individual treatment with D-penicillamine (52 mg/kg) or by placing the herd on a concentrate feed containing both 10 lb per ton of a 2% sodium molybdate premix and 5 lb per ton of gypsum to reduce liver copper stores.

Measurement of urine copper concentration is the most sensitive diagnostic tool in live animals because homeostatic mechanisms tightly control serum copper concentration. Necropsy findings may include icterus; a friable, golden liver; and dark red to almost black kidneys. Microscopically, the liver exhibits centrilobular necrosis, fibrosis, and bile duct hyperplasia and hemoglobinuric casts are present in the renal tubules.

Sheep are sensitive to copper toxicosis, and dietary copper concentrations should not exceed 10 ppm (≈9 g/ton) unless balanced by the presence of molybdenum (copper-to-molybdenum ratio of 10:1). Sheep may develop copper toxicity when consuming diets formulated for cattle or goats (containing 20-35 ppm [18-32 g/ton]) over the course of a few months. Potentially toxic sources of copper for cattle and goats include chicken litter or pig manure from animals treated with copper sulfate. Chicken litter has been incorporated directly into the diet, and either source used as fertilizer may allow excess copper uptake into forages.

Pyrrolizidine alkaloid intoxication can precipitate copper-induced hemolytic crisis as the volume of viable hepatic parenchyma is reduced.

Iron

Compared with copper toxicity, iron-induced liver failure is rare. Most instances have occurred in calves after receiving injectable ferrous gluconate/ferric ammonium citrate iron supplementation. Affected calves may have black, tarry stool and may tremble, grind their teeth, vocalize, and convulse. Serum GGT, ALP, bile acids, and unconjugated bilirubin are elevated. Lobular necrosis and fibrosis, periportal hepatic necrosis, and bile duct proliferation are microscopic findings.

BLUE-GREEN ALGAE AND MUSHROOMS

Hepatotoxic cyclic peptides cause disorganization of actin filaments and consequent disintegration of the hepatocellular cytoskeleton. Animals exposed to large doses may die within an hour of ingestion because of loss of hepatic blood, hypovolemic shock, or hepatocystic embolism to the lung. Lower doses lead to typical signs of liver failure including elevated serum AST, GGT, ALP, and total bilirubin, with hepatogenous photosensitization. Necropsy reveals hepatomegaly and a swollen gallbladder. Microscopic lesions include severe centrilobular hepatocyte dissociation, degeneration, and necrosis.

Microcystin and nodularin are cyclic peptides produced by blue-green algae (*Microcystis aeruginosa* and *Nodularia spumigena*, respectively) that bloom in eutrophically enriched waters with low flow rates. Mats of algae pushed against the shore by a concentrating wind provide a rich source of toxin for thirsty animals. Amanitine, produced by *Amanita* species and various other mushrooms, is another hepatotoxic cyclic peptide.

COCKLEBUR AND CYCADS

Cocklebur (*Xanthium* sp.) is lethal at 0.3% of an animal's body weight and affects all ruminants. The glycoside toxin carboxyatractyloside causes severe hypoglycemia and massive hepatic necrosis, resulting in depression, dyspnea, weakness, convulsions with opisthotonus, and sudden death. Clinical signs in goats may mimic polio encephalomalacia. Postmortem findings may include gallbladder edema and ascites caused by increased vascular permeability, as well as a swollen and friable liver. The seeds and seedlings of cocklebur contain enough carboxyatractyloside to cause toxicity, but the mature plant does not.

Cycads (*Cycas, Zamia,* and *Macrozamia* spp.) contain the glycoside cycasin, a hepato-gastrointestinal toxin metabolized to more toxic methylazoxymethanol. Ruminants ingesting cycad-derived plant material exhibit depression, anorexia, and weight loss. Larger doses over longer periods lead to liver cirrhosis, ascites and hemorrhagic gastroenteritis.

LANTANA

Lantana is an escaped ornamental plant containing triterpenoid compounds, the metabolites of which are also toxic. The lantadenes cause intrahepatic cholestasis by damage to the canaliculi (small bile ducts). Affected animals are anorectic, dehydrated, and icteric, with rumen stasis and hepatogenous photosensitization. Rumen stasis prolongs exposure to and absorption of the toxin; rumenotomy can be helpful. At necropsy the liver is enlarged, golden-yellow, and firm or friable, and the gallbladder is typically distended. Microscopically, cholestasis and bile duct proliferation are evident, often with bilirubinuric casts in the renal tubules. About 1% of an animal's body weight in green material is acutely toxic. Toxicity is not cumulative.

SAPONINS

A variety of plants (Box 16-2) contain steroidal sapogenins that generally reach their highest concentration in early and rapid growth stages of the plant. Steroidal sapogenins are metabolized to glucuronide conjugates that crystallize in the bile ducts, leading to anorexia, weight loss, icterus, hepatogenous photosensitization, sloughing of the skin, and hepatoencephalopathy. Microscopic evaluation of the liver reveals bridging and fibrosing hepatocyte necrosis, cholangitis, and occlusion of small bile ducts with birefringent crystals that may be related to sapogenin glucuronide conjugate accumulation.

Box 16-2

Saponin-Containing Plants Associated with Hepatogenous Photosensitization

Tribulus terrestris (Puncture vine) in sheep
Panicum coloratum, P. virgatum (kleingrass, switchgrass) in sheep and goats
Brachiaria decumbens (Signal grass)
Nolina texana (Sacahuista)
Agave spp. (Century plant, Agave, Lecheguilla)
Narthecium ossifragum (Narthecium, Bog asphodel)
Yucca schidigera (Yucca)
Tetradymia spp. (Horse brush) in conjunction with *Artemisia* spp. (Black sage) in sheep

Recommended Readings

Blythe LL, Craig AM: Clinical and preclinical diagnostic aids to hepatic plant toxicosis in horses, sheep and cattle. In Colgate SM, Dorling PR, editors: *Plant associated toxins*, Wallingford, United Kingdom, 1994, CABI.

Bull LB, Culvenor CCJ, Dick AT: *The pyrrolizidine alkaloids*, Amsterdam, 1968, North Holland Publishing.

Burrows GE, Stair EL: Apparent *Agave lecheguilla* intoxication in livestock and waterfowl, *Vet Human Tox* 32:259, 1990.

Burrows GE, Tyrl RJ: *Toxic plants of North America*, Ames, 2001, Iowa State University Press.

Casteel SW: Hepatotoxic plants. In Howard JL, Smith RA, editors: *Current veterinary therapy 4: food animal practice*, Philadelphia, 1999, Saunders.

Cheeke PR: *Natural toxicants in feeds, forages, and poisonous plants*, ed 2, Danville, Ill, 1998, Interstate Publishers.

Cheeke PR: The role of the liver in detoxification of poisonous plants. In Colegate SM, Dorling PR, editors: *Plant associated toxins*, Wallingford, United Kingdom, 1994, CABI.

Croker KP, Allen JG, Gittins SP et al: The development of lupinosis in weaner sheep grazed on sandplain lupins. In Garland T, Barr AC, editors: *Toxic plants and other natural toxicants*, Wallingford, United Kingdom, 1998, CABI.

Divers TJ: Treatment of liver failure. In Pearson EG, editor: *Diseases of the hepatobiliary system*. In Smith BP, editor: *Large animal internal medicine*, ed 3, St Louis, 2002, Mosby.

Flaoyen A, Wilkins AL, di Menna ME et al: The concentration of steroidal sapogenins in and the degree of fungal infection on *Narthecium ossifragum* plants in More and Romdal County, Norway. In Acomovic T, Stewart CS, Pennycott TW, editors: *Poisonous plants and related toxins*, Wallingford, United Kingdom, 2001, CABI.

Flaoyen A, Wilkins AL, Sandvik M: The metabolism of saponins from *Yucca schidigera* in sheep. In Acomovic T, Stewart CS, Pennycott TW, editors: *Poisonous plants and related toxins*, Wallingford, United Kingdom, 2001, CABI.

Fowler ME: Hepatotoxic plants. In Howard JL, editor: *Current veterinary therapy 3: food animal practice*, Philadelphia, 1993, Saunders.

Galey FD: Disorders caused by toxicants. In Smith BP, editor: *Large animal internal medicine*, ed 3, St Louis, 2002, Mosby.

Kirkpatrick JG, Helman RG, Burrows GE et al: Transient hepatotoxicity in sheep grazing *Kochia scoparia*. In Garland T, Barr AC, editors: *Toxic plants and other natural toxicants*, Wallingford, United Kingdom, 1998, CABI.

Malone FE, Kennady S, Reilly GAC et al: Bog asphodel (*Narthecium ossifragum*) poisoning in cattle. In Garland T, Barr AC, editors: *Toxic plants and other natural toxicants*, Wallingford, United Kingdom, 1998, CAB International.

Merck: *Aflatoxicosis*: http://merckvetmanual.com/mvm/index.jsp?cfile=htm/bc/212202.htm. Accessed October 18, 2007.

Merck: *Hepatotoxins*: http://merckvetmanual.com/mvm/index.jsp?cfile=htm/bc/22811.htm&word=hepatotoxins. Accessed October 18, 2007.

Molson MT: Toxic responses of the liver. In Klaasen CL, editor: *Cassarett & Doull's toxicology: the basic science of poisons*, ed 5, New York, 1996, McGraw-Hill.

Patamalai B, Hejtmancik E, Bridges CH et al: The isolation and identification of steroidal sapogenins in kleingrass, *Vet Human Tox* 32:314, 1990.

Pearson EG: Diseases of the hepatobiliary system. In Smith BP, editor: *Large animal internal medicine*, ed 3, St Louis, 2002, Mosby.

Plumlee KH: Metals and other inorganic compounds. In Galey FD: Disorders caused by toxicants. In Smith BP, editor: *Large animal internal medicine*, ed 3, St Louis, 2002, Mosby.

Schild AL, Motta AC, Riet-Correa F et al: Photosensitization in cattle in southern Brazil. In Acomovic T, Stewart CS, Pennycott TW, editors: *Poisonous plants and related toxins*, Wallingford, United Kingdom, 2001, CABI.

Smith BL, Towers NR, Munday R et al: Control of the mycotoxic hepatogenous photosensitization, facial eczema, in New Zealand. In Garland T, Barr AC, editors: *Toxic plants and other natural toxicants*, Wallingford, United Kingdom, 1998, CABI.

Texas Cooperative Extension Service, Plant Pathology Group: *Clinical Effects of Aflatoxicosis* http://plantpathology.tamu.edu/aflatoxin/effects.htm. Accessed October 18, 2007.

CHAPTER 17

Hemorrhagic Bowel Syndrome

DAVID C. VAN METRE

Hemorrhagic bowel syndrome (HBS) is a sporadic, frequently fatal enteric disease that occurs most commonly in adult dairy cattle during the first 3 to 4 months of lactation. Dairy cattle in late lactation, dry dairy cows, dairy heifers, and beef cows and bulls may be occasionally affected. A few reports of nearly identical cases of enteric disease in dairy cattle were published throughout the 1990s; however, published case series and surveys of producers and veterinarians indicate that the incidence of HBS in North America appears to have increased dramatically toward the end of that decade through the present. Other names for this disease include jejunal hemorrhage syndrome, bloody gut, and dead gut.

The defining clinical feature of HBS is peracute to acute, often massive hemorrhage into the small intestine with subsequent intraluminal formation of large clots and casts of blood that create intestinal obstruction. Blood loss into the intestine can be rapid and severe enough to cause death from exsanguination. In most cases, however, cows show signs referable to intestinal obstruction. Affected areas of intestine undergo necrosis within 1 to 2 days of the onset of clinical signs, resulting in the superimposition of peritonitis and septic shock upon signs of blood loss and intestinal obstruction. The case fatality rate for HBS is high, reportedly ranging from 80% to 100%.

HISTORY AND CLINICAL SIGNS

Historical findings in cases of HBS typically include a peracute onset of progressive weakness and abdominal distension in a cow that showed no preceding signs of illness. Depending on the rate and volume of hemorrhage into the intestine, a cow with peracute HBS may be found dead or recumbent with severe signs of hypovolemic shock. In the latter instance a rapid, weak pulse, rapid respiratory rate, pale mucous membranes, cold extremities, and normal or subnormal rectal temperature are often detected by farm personnel. Some cows with peracute HBS are mistakenly assumed to have hypocalcemia (milk fever). More careful examination typically reveals variable degrees of abdominal distension; the quantity and appearance of feces may or may not be abnormal in peracute cases.

In acute cases, similar signs of shock and hypovolemia are present but are not fulminant because most cows can be prompted to stand. However, some degree of weakness is usually evidenced by muscle tremors and a slow, unsteady gait. Progressive abdominal distension is apparent, with most distension occurring in the left and right ventral abdominal quadrants, imparting a pear shape to the abdominal contour when the cow is viewed from the rear. The cause of distension is accumulation of multiple, blood-filled loops of intestine in the ventral aspect of the abdominal cavity. Occasional cases show generalized ileus, and the superimposed ruminal gas accumulation may impart a "papple"-shaped abdominal contour (upper left and lower right quadrant distention) to the affected cow. Low-pitched, often transient "pings" may be heard over small areas of the lower right abdomen on simultaneous auscultation and ballottement of the lower right abdomen. Fluid splashing sounds are often present on succussion of the right side of the abdomen. Feces are typically scant, dark, tarry, and often contain dark red to black clots or casts of blood. Signs of mild colic may be observed, with the affected cow treading or occasionally kicking at her abdomen. Signs of more severe colic are rare.

Rectal examination may reveal ruminal or cecal gas accumulation. Small intestinal distension may be evident; however, this is an inconsistent finding, presumably because the blood-filled segments of intestine sink to the ventral abdomen, beyond the examiner's reach. Examination of rumen fluid is usually unremarkable. Occasionally, rust-colored rumen contents may be present if there is retrograde movement of hemorrhage from the upper intestine into the forestomachs.

Transabdominal ultrasonography may allow visualization of affected bowel. A 3.5- or 5-MHz, sector- or linear-array probe is placed on the abdominal wall over the ventral half of the right paralumbar fossa. Ileus is a consistent finding. Dilated loops of small intestine are frequently detected. On occasion, material consistent with the appearance of clotted blood can be seen within the distended loops of small intestine. Rarely, if the obstruction is located in the proximal jejunum or duodenum, the majority of small intestine appears empty, but the distended descending duodenum can be visualized and traced in a horizontal path across the middle to dorsal paralumbar fossa. Abdominocentesis findings have not been well characterized with HBS, but based on surgical findings, suppurative changes are likely to be found on analysis of abdominal fluid.

Within 24 to 48 hours of the onset of clinical signs, most acute cases develop terminal septic shock that results from necrosis of affected small intestine. Transabdominal ultrasonographic examination often reveals free fluid and strands of fibrin within the abdominal cavity. Death soon follows, apparently resulting from the combined effects of blood loss, intestinal obstruction, and septic shock.

DIFFERENTIAL DIAGNOSES

Differential diagnoses for HBS include intussusception, small intestinal volvulus, enteritis/pseudo-obstruction, abomasal ulceration, and vagal indigestion. Although intussusception and small intestinal volvulus are expected to elicit more severe signs of colic, antemortem differentiation of HBS from these disorders often requires exploratory surgery. Cases of enteritis with ileus (pseudo-obstruction) may show abdominal distension, scant feces, and colic, but these signs typically resolve with analgesics and fluid and electrolyte therapy, and diarrhea becomes evident soon thereafter. Unlike HBS, abomasal ulceration rarely results in abdominal distension. Vagal indigestion is often slowly progressive in nature, and unless the underlying lesion triggers sudden cardiovascular decompensation, most cows with vagal indigestion have minimal signs of hypovolemic shock.

TREATMENT

Successful treatment of HBS is difficult. Medical treatment with parenteral fluids, laxatives, antiinflammatory drugs, and antibiotics may prolong survival but is rarely ultimately successful because intestinal necrosis and subsequent peritonitis and shock still ensue in most cases. Exploratory laparotomy typically reveals one or more segments of distended jejunum, with occasional involvement of the ileum and duodenum. Gas and fluid distension of the orad intestine is frequently present. The affected segments of intestine are often located in the ventral abdomen, presumably because the large quantity of intraluminal blood makes the affected segments relatively heavy. The serosa shows patchy to diffuse, red or purple discoloration. Clotted blood within the lumen of affected intestine imparts a turgid, gelatin-like feel to the affected segments of intestine. Devitalization of affected bowel may be evident, and iatrogenic rupture may occur even with gentle manipulation.

Surgical treatment of HBS is futile if exploration reveals extensive peritonitis or devitalization of large or multiple lengths of intestine, or both. For focal lesions, the affected intestine may be gently massaged so as to break apart the obstructing clots or casts of blood within the lumen. Alternatively, the affected segment may be removed by resection and anastomosis, or an enterotomy may be performed to remove the obstruction. Even if the surgical procedure is completed successfully, recurrent intraluminal clotting and obstruction may occur at the original site of obstruction or at additional sites. Of 22 cows affected with HBS presented to a university veterinary hospital over a period of 3 years, only 5 (23%) survived; 4 of these survivors were treated surgically. Based on subsequent case reports, anecdotal information, and my experience, surgical treatment is rarely successful.

NECROPSY FINDINGS

Gross lesions are usually distributed segmentally in the jejunum, with occasional involvement of the duodenum or ileum. Purple or red, patchy or diffuse discoloration

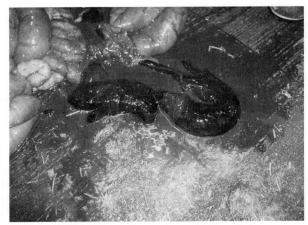

Fig 17-1   Casts of clotted blood and ingesta removed from a cow that died of hemorrhagic bowel syndrome.

of the serosa is evident. Intestinal contents are typically bloody, with unclotted blood admixed with large clots and intraluminal casts of clotted blood (Fig. 17-1). These casts may measure several inches to over a foot in length. The blood casts in affected segments are often strongly attached to the mucosa, and manual removal of the cast may result in peeling off of the adjacent mucosa. If devitalization of affected segments has occurred, fibrin may be present on the serosal surface of affected and adjacent bowel. Histologic examination reveals necrohemorrhagic enteritis, with marked, transmural accumulation of neutrophils, intraluminal and intramural hemorrhage, and ulceration and sloughing of the mucosa. A Gram stain of luminal contents or fixed tissue often reveals a dense population of gram-positive, rod-shaped bacteria within the intestinal lumen.

EPIDEMIOLOGY

In a large survey of American dairy producers, the median parity for cows affected by HBS was reported to be the third lactation, and the median number of days in milk for affected cows was 104 days. According to data from the 2002 National Animal Health Monitoring Service study, a greater percentage of producers reported seeing at least one case of HBS in the previous 5 years if they owned larger dairies, dairies with higher rolling herd average milk production, and dairies in the Western United States. In a survey of veterinary practitioners in Minnesota, there was no significant relationship among the seasons of the year and diagnosis of HBS, although producers and veterinarians have indicated that most HBS cases seem to occur during the winter and fall.

PATHOGENESIS

At present, the pathogenesis of HBS has not been described and the contributing factors for the disease have not been well characterized. Because most cases occur in dairy cows in early lactation, the physiologic stress of peak lactation and the high-concentrate, low-fiber rations typically fed to these cows have been proposed as potential risk factors.

Several studies indicate an association between HBS and *Clostridium perfringens* type A and type A with the β_2 toxin gene (type A+β_2). These bacteria can be readily isolated from the feces and intestine of affected cows. *Clostridium perfringens* is a diverse species of Gram-positive, anaerobic bacilli that can be divided into five types (designated A-E), based on the exotoxin(s) produced during rapid growth (see Chapter 19). In ruminants, this organism proliferates in the intestine under conditions of high carbohydrate or protein intake. *Clostridium perfringens* type A and type A+β_2 can be isolated from the gastrointestinal tract of healthy animals from a variety of species of livestock including cattle. The diagnostic significance of detecting *C. perfringens* type A or A+β_2 by culture of enteric contents is complicated by the tendency for type A to overgrow postmortem and by the carriage of these organisms by apparently healthy livestock. These organisms are considered more likely to be causing disease if isolation occurs from diseased bowel in the live animal or fresh cadaver, and if the corresponding exotoxins can be detected in enteric contents or blood of affected animals. The odds of isolation of *C. perfringens* type A and A+β_2 from enteric contents were shown to be significantly higher for cows with HBS relative to herd mates with left displaced abomasum (LDA); further, α and β_2 toxins were detected in the enteric contents of cows with HBS, but not in that of cows with LDA. Nonetheless, it is currently unclear what role, if any, *C. perfringens* plays in the pathogenesis of HBS. The potent exotoxins that these organisms produce could, in theory, play a central role in initiation of the disease. However, it is also possible that intraluminal enteric hemorrhage is triggered by another factor and the *C. perfringens* harbored in the intestine may proliferate as it uses blood as a substrate for growth. Efforts to experimentally induce enteric disease with *C. perfringens* type A have produced varied results, but attempts to date to induce HBS have failed.

A limited number of HBS cases have been fully investigated for enteric pathogens. Pathogens capable of inducing hemorrhagic enteritis such as *Salmonella* spp. and bovine viral diarrhea virus have been identified in a small proportion of these HBS cases. Further, the clinical, macroscopic, and histologic features of HBS do not resemble those classically attributed to these pathogens.

Aspergillus fumigatus, a toxigenic fungus that can be found in a variety of livestock feeds, has also been associated with HBS. The DNA of this organism can be detected in the blood and intestinal tissues of cattle affected with HBS, and heavy spore counts of *A. fumigatus* have been identified in the feedstuffs of dairies with a history of recent HBS. In a multicenter study the DNA of *A. fumigatus* was detected in the blood and intestine of a significantly higher proportion of cows that succumbed to HBS than cows that died from other gastrointestinal diseases. *A. fumigatus* has been postulated to contribute to the development of HBS as a primary agent that incites tissue damage. Alternatively or concurrently, the immunosuppressive mycotoxins released by this agent could reduce host resistance to yet unidentified primary pathogens or toxins. In studies of a feed supplement containing mycotoxin-binding agents (Omnigen-AF, Prince Agri Products, Inc., Quincy, Ill), neutrophils from ruminants fed the product showed enhanced activity of the genes encoding the interleukin-4 receptor and the interleukin 1-β converting enzyme, as well as increased expression of certain surface adhesion molecules relative to those of controls.

PREVENTION

At present, preventive strategies for HBS remain speculative because the etiology and pathogenesis of the disease remain largely unknown. Until further studies on these issues are published, the author recommends that all proposed agents and associated risk factors (*C. perfringens, A. fumigatus,* poor feed management, reduced host immunity) be considered when developing a preventive strategy. Given these postulated contributing factors, each dairy should be carefully scrutinized to identify ways the environment, host, and agent can be managed to minimize this disease, much as other multifactorial health problems are managed on modern dairies.

To optimize host resistance, careful analysis of the nutritional program, disease identification and control practices, and cow comfort should be performed, with particular focus paid to the transition cows and cows in early lactation. Feed formulation, mixing, and presentation should be reviewed, with particular attention paid to such parameters as the ration content of effective fiber and soluble carbohydrate to limit potential dietary influences on gut flora, mineral nutrition to maintain normal gut motility, micronutrient content to contribute to satisfactory immune function, feed bunk and pen management to maintain consistent feed intake, and feed harvest and storage practices to limit spoilage and mold formation. Carefully kept medical and feed records can be compiled to identify potential associations between the occurrence of HBS and introduction of particular feed components or batches of feedstuffs. Correlation of medical records with environmental data (e.g., rainfall, ambient temperature, stocking rate, pen location) and management events (cow movement, immunization, estrus synchronization) may also aid in identifying potential associations between HBS and certain environmental and management factors. Lastly, feed additives and vaccines directed against specific, potential contributory pathogens can be considered, with the costs of the proposed interventions and their potential efficacy weighed against the costs of the disease. According to anecdotal reports, the incidence of HBS on certain dairies has decreased following administration of an autogenous or commercially available *C. perfringens* vaccine (*C. perfringens* type A toxoid, Novartis Animal Health US, Inc., Larchwood, Iowa) to adult cows on certain dairies. Similarly, based on anecdotal evidence, the incidence of HBS has decreased on dairies following the introduction of a feed supplement (Omnigen-AF, Prince Agri Products, Inc., Quincy, Ill) into the ration. At present, data from controlled studies are not available for evaluation of the effect of these products on the incidence of or survival rate for this disease. The collateral effect that these products might have on milk production or the incidence and severity of diseases should be considered as well.

Recommended Readings

Abutarbush SM, Radostits OM: Jejunal hemorrhage syndrome in dairy and beef cattle: 11 cases (2001 to 2003), *Can Vet J* 46:711, 2005.

Berghaus RD, McCluskey BJ, Callan RJ: Risk factors associated with hemorrhagic bowel syndrome in dairy cattle, *J Am Vet Med Assoc* 226:1700, 2005.

Dennison AC, Van Metre DC, Dinsmore RP et al: Hemorrhagic bowel syndrome of adult dairy cattle: 22 cases (1997-2000), *J Am Vet Med Assoc* 221:686, 2002.

Godden S, Frank R, Ames T: Survey of Minnesota veterinarians on the occurrence of and potential risk factors for jejunal hemorrhage syndrome in adult dairy cows, *Bov Pract* 35:97, 2001.

Kirkpatrick MA, Kersting KW, Kinyon JM: Case report: jejunal hemorrhage syndrome of dairy cattle, *Bov Pract* 35:104, 2001.

Puntenney SB, Wang Y, Forsberg NE: *Mycotic infections in livestock: recent insights and studies on etiology, diagnostics, and prevention of hemorrhagic bowel syndrome.* Proceedings, Southwest Anim Nutr Conf, Dept. of Animal Science, University of Arizona, Tucson, Ariz, 2003, p 49.

Songer JG: Clostridium perfringens *type A infection in cattle.* Proceedings, 32nd Annual Convention, American Association of Bovine Practitioners, 32:40, 1999.

CHAPTER 18

Clostridium novyi (Myonecrosis, Black Disease, and Bacillary Hemoglobinuria) and *Clostridium septicum* (Braxy) Infections

J. GLENN SONGER

Clostridium novyi and *Clostridium septicum* are among numerous clostridia that cause myonecrosis in domestic animals (Table 18-1).[1] Common themes in infections by these organisms include endogenous and environmental sources of infection, pathogenesis facilitated by trauma, local multiplication, extensive local and systemic damage, and rapid death. The hallmark is ardent toxinogenesis, and toxoid vaccination has decreased the incidence of many such infections.[2]

CLOSTRIDIUM NOVYI

C. novyi type C is nontoxigenic (and therefore avirulent,) but types A and B, as well as D (also called *Clostridium haemolyticum*), cause disease in humans and domestic animals. Differential production of alpha and beta toxins determines toxin phenotype (Table 18-2).

Myonecrosis (*Clostridium novyi* Type A)

C. novyi type A causes massively edematous wound infections, most notably "bighead" of young rams. This rapidly progressive disease affects head, neck, and cranial thorax following clostridial invasion of subcutaneous tissues damaged by fighting. Type A has been recently recognized as a cause of septicemia in drug addicts who practice "muscle popping." Pathogenesis is mediated by alpha toxin.[3,4]

Black Disease (*Clostridium novyi* Type B)

Disease and Etiology

Infectious necrotic hepatitis is a peracute, highly fatal clostridial disease occurring worldwide in sheep, most often in well-nourished adults 2 to 4 years of age. Cattle, horses,[5] goats, and occasionally pigs may also be affected.

Table 18-1

Clostridia as Causes of Myonecrosis

Organism	Major Toxins	Diseases	Species Affected
C. perfringens type A	Alpha, theta	Gas gangrene, myonecrosis	All warm-blooded
C. septicum	Alpha	Abomasitis, malignant edema	Sheep, cattle
C. chauvoei	Alpha, beta	Blackleg	Sheep, cattle
C. novyi types A and B	Alpha, beta	Wound infections (bighead), infectious necrotic hepatitis	Sheep, goats
C. novyi type D (C. haemolyticum)	Beta	Bacillary hemoglobinuria	Cattle
C. sordellii	Hemolytic, lethal	Myonecrosis	Sheep, cattle

Table 18-2

Toxin Production and Diseases Caused by Types of *Clostridium novyi*

Type	Alpha	Beta	Diseases
A	+++		Myonecrosis; bighead in rams
B	++	+	Black disease in sheep
C			Avirulent
D		+++	Bacillary hemoglobinuria (redwater)

Type B may be involved in an emerging problem with sudden death in periparturient sows. Incidence is markedly greater in summer, and flock morbidity is usually approximately 5% but may be as high as 50%.

Peracute death is common. Animals with acute disease often stand alone and unmoving. Body temperature increases early on (40°-42° C) but may decrease to normal or subnormal levels in moribund animals. Sheep become sternally recumbent and die after a clinical course of no more than a few hours. Venous congestion darkens the underside of the skin, giving the disease its common name (black disease). Clinical signs in cattle are similar, but the course is usually 1 to 2 days.

At necropsy, fluid is found in pericardial sac and pleural and peritoneal cavity and endocardial hemorrhage is a consistent finding. Liver is engorged, and subcapsular necrotic foci in the diaphragmatic lobe are surrounded by leukocytes and large numbers of gram-positive rods.

Pathogenesis

Spores accumulating in the environment are ingested with feed, and some are deposited in Kupffer cells. Disease follows liver damage caused by migration of fluke metacercariae; *Fasciola hepatica* is the most commonly occurring fluke, but *Cysticercus tenuicollis* has also been implicated. Damaged tissue is sufficiently ischemic to stimulate germination of *C. novyi* spores. The resulting vegetative cells elaborate toxins that cause local and systemic damage.

Alpha toxin, a so-called large clostridial cytotoxin,[4] is the primary virulence factor of type B, although a small amount of beta toxin is produced. Ovine disease has been reproduced by administration of spores to animals previously infected with fluke metacercariae.

Bacillary Hemoglobinuria (*Clostridium novyi* Type D; *Clostridium haemolyticum*)

Disease and Etiology

C. novyi type D (*C. haemolyticum*) causes bacillary hemoglobinuria of cattle and other ruminants worldwide. Disease occurs sporadically and in North America is most common during summer and early fall. As with infectious necrotic hepatitis, fascioliasis frequently precipitates bacillary hemoglobinuria. Spores accumulate in the environment as a result of shedding by carrier animals and decomposition of carcasses of animals dead of bacillary hemoglobinuria. Outbreaks often follow flooding, which may bring spores into previously uninfected areas. In the United States, disease occurs most often in cattle grazed in poorly drained pastures with alkaline soil.

Bacillary hemoglobinuria is most common in well-nourished animals older than 1 year of age and is, in fact, rare in calves younger than 1 year old and in animals with poor body condition. Animals with peracute disease die without premonitory signs. Acutely affected animals stand apart from the herd and have arched backs and tucked-up abdomens. Tachycardia and tachypnea accompany inappetence, agalactia, and pale mucus membranes. Early constipation may give way to diarrhea. Animals are febrile throughout the course of the disease, but subnormal temperatures occur when animals are moribund. In late acute disease anemia is severe, with hematocrits as low as 10%, as few as 10^6 RBC/μL, and hemoglobin at 35 g/L. When hemoglobinuria (not hematuria) appears, 40% to 50% of red cells have lysed; urine takes on the color of port wine and giving the disease its common name, "redwater." Jaundice may be in evidence, and animals die in 18 to 36 hours as a consequence of anoxia. Herd mortality rates where the disease is endemic average 5%, although there are reports of 25% mortality in feedlots. The case fatality rate is approximately 95%.

Gross lesions include subcutaneous edema and petechial and ecchymotic hemorrhages throughout the body. Hemorrhagic abomasitis and enteritis may occur, and pleural and peritoneal cavities contain hemoglobin-stained transudate. Pulmonary edema is common. Hepatic infarcts are pathognomonic and may range in size from 5 to 25 cm. Necrotic and normal liver tissue are separated by a wide zone of bacteria and only a mild leukocytic infiltrate. Blood cultures may be positive.

Pathogenesis

Type D spores are ingested and deposit in Kupffer cells, where they may remain latent indefinitely. The organism can be isolated from normal livers obtained at slaughter. However, liver damage resulting from telangiectasis, liver abscessation caused by *Fusobacterium necrophorum* and *Arcanobacterium pyogenes*, or infestation with *Fasciola hepatica* or *Cysticercus tenuicollis* provides conditions that promote germination of spores. Vegetative cells proliferate and produce beta toxin, which causes extensive hepatic necrosis and, via dissemination through circulation, erythrolysis and hemorrhage. Beta toxin, a phospholipase that is related to the alpha toxin of *C. perfringens,* is the sole major toxin of type D strains. Thus pathogenesis of bacillary hemoglobinuria is similar to that of infectious necrotic hepatitis, except that the primary toxin is beta rather than alpha. Beta toxin also causes endothelial damage to arterioles, with extravasation of blood into tissues and body cavities.

CLOSTRIDIUM SEPTICUM (BRAXY)

C. septicum can be isolated from soil and feces and may enter hosts with one of the life stages of liver flukes. *C. septicum* in chickens can manifest as gangrenous dermatitis, and ovine umbilical infections are common and highly fatal. Iatrogenic infections are not uncommon in horses. *C. septicum* is a frequent postmortem invader.

Disease and Etiology

Malignant edema usually follows wound contamination, and hemorrhage, edema, and necrosis spread rapidly along fascial planes from the point of infection. The lesion, which is initially painful and warm with pitting edema, becomes crepitant and cold. Fever, anorexia, and depression terminate in death, usually in less than 24 hours.

C. septicum also causes enteric infections. It penetrates the abomasal lining of lambs and older sheep and produces a disease known as *braxy* or *bradsot*.[6] Braxy is a peracute form of hemorrhagic, necrotic abomasitis. Onset is sudden, with depression, high fever, and sometimes colic and tympany. Disease progresses to fatal toxemia and bacteremia. The case fatality rate approaches 100%. Braxy causes heavy mortality in sheep in the United Kingdom, Ireland, Norway, Iceland, and Faroe Islands and also occurs in Europe and Australia. It appears to be rare in sheep in North America. Disease is more common in beef and dairy calves.

Mucosal congestion and necrosis, gas accumulation, and ulceration are found in abomasal wall, and microscopic examination reveals acute severe transmural abomasitis. Microscopic lesions in other organs may result from toxemia. However, dissemination of *C. septicum* by the hematogenous route may give rise to secondary foci of infection, if animals survive long enough to allow this.

Pathogenesis

The pathogenetic mechanism by which *C. septicum* invades the abomasal lining is not known. However, ingestion of cold or frozen feed is frequently associated with disease in sheep and beef calves. Dairy calves given barely thawed colostrum are similarly affected. The resulting impaired mucosal function may allow entry of the organism, which is frequently present in the normal gastrointestinal tract. Local multiplication and dissemination follows, with local lesions and toxemia. As with most other clostridia, interaction of *C. septicum* with its hosts is mediated by toxins. Foremost among these is alpha toxin,[7,8] and purified toxin mimics features of the infection. A role for potential virulence attributes other than alpha toxin has not been proven, but they may, in combination, increase capillary permeability and contribute to myonecrosis and systemic toxicity.

DIAGNOSIS OF *CLOSTRIDIUM NOVYI* AND *CLOSTRIDIUM SEPTICUM* INFECTIONS

Infectious necrotic hepatitis and bacillary hemoglobinuria can be diagnosed by a combination of clinical presentation and history, gross and microscopic lesions, and detection of the infecting organism. With appropriate clinical signs, liver lesions can be pathognomonic. However, lesions may also be unremarkable and extensive fluke-mediated damage can complicate diagnosis. Acute ovine fascioliasis can have a high mortality rate, and postmortem findings are similar to those in black disease. Other causes of sudden death such as enterotoxemia, blackleg, and anthrax (depending on geographic locale) should be ruled out. Clinical diagnosis of redwater is based mainly on exclusion of other causes of hemoglobinuria such as acute leptospirosis and babesiosis (again, depending on appropriate locale) and postparturient hemoglobinuria. Hemolytic anemia caused by cruciferous plants can usually be ruled out by lack of severe febrile reactions. Hematuria caused by corynebacterial pyelonephritis and cystitis can usually be ruled out by the presence of intact red cells in urine. Chronic copper poisoning in sheep can be differentiated by absence of liver infarcts.

The often peracute nature of *C. septicum*–induced abomasitis in sheep limits opportunities for clinical diagnosis. *Clostridium perfringens* type D enterotoxemia may have similar signs but without lesions in abomasum. None of the liver lesions of infectious necrotic hepatitis exist.

Definitive diagnosis is based on demonstration of the organism in lesions. Bacteriologic culture is straightforward, and isolates can be identified by standard methods. *C. septicum* is likely to be the etiologic agent if it predominates in specimens obtained soon after death. Toxin typing of *C. novyi* isolates is useful but rarely done. Immunofluorescence is also useful (Table 18-3), and bacteria

Table 18-3

Use of Fluorescent Antibody Tests for Diagnosis of Histotoxic Clostridial Infections

Disease	Species	Test for *Clostridium*
Blackleg	Ruminants	*septicum, chauvoei, novyi, sordellii*
	Swine	*septicum, chauvoei*
Braxy	Sheep	*septicum*
Bighead		*novyi*
Black disease	Ruminants	*novyi*
Bacillary hemoglobinuria	Cattle	*novyi*
Malignant edema	Horses, ruminants, swine	*septicum*
Gangrenous dermatitis	Poultry	*septicum,* rarely *novyi, sordellii;* most likely etiology is *perfringens* (no conjugate available)

can be identified in smears of liver and other tissues. The test can also be performed on smears made from isolates.

PREVENTION AND CONTROL OF *CLOSTRIDIUM NOVYI* AND *CLOSTRIDIUM SEPTICUM* INFECTION

Treatment is rarely possible, because of the fulminant clinical course of these conditions. The course of black disease in cattle is longer than that in sheep and may allow use of antimicrobials. Cases may continue to occur for more than 2 months after elimination of the source of flukes, so antimicrobials may be useful for prophylaxis. In the case of redwater, *C. novyi* type D antitoxin can be used for treatment or prevention but always with procaine penicillin (20,000 IU/kg IM, bid) or tetracycline (10 mg/kg IV or IM sid).

Prevention is the preferred course of action. Commercial vaccines are usually multivalent and are composed of toxoids and/or bacterins. Antibody responses to somatic and toxin antigens yield solid immunity, although there may be differences in immunogenicity by vaccine, agent, and host species. Vaccine can be administered at any age but is recommended at 6 months of age and again within 3 to 4 weeks.[2] Annual boosters are often recommended in low-exposure areas, and twice-annual boosters should be used in high-exposure areas. Vaccination can reduce death losses in feedlot cattle by as much as 50%, with a cost-to-benefit ratio as high as 1:40.[9]

Control of flukes is an important management tool.

References

1. Songer JG: Clostridial enteric diseases of domestic animals: a review, *Clin Microbiol Rev* 9:216-234, 1996.
2. Hjerpe CA: Clostridial disease vaccines, *Vet Clin North Am Food Anim Pract* 6:222-234, 1990.
3. Hatheway CL: Toxigenic clostridia, *Clin Microbiol Rev* 3:66-98, 1990.
4. Busch C, Schomig K, Hofmann F et al: Characterization of the catalytic domain of *Clostridium novyi* alpha-toxin, *Infect Immun* 68:6378-6383, 2000.
5. Mullaney TP, Brown CM, Flint-Taylor R: Clostridial myositis in horses following intramuscular administration of ivermectin, *Proc Annu Meet Am Assoc Vet Lab Diagn* 27:171-177, 1984.
6. Ellis TM, Rowe JB, Lloyd JM: Acute abomasitis due to *Clostridium septicum* infection in experimental sheep, *Aust Vet J* 60:308-309, 1983.
7. Ballard J, Sokolov Y, Yuan WL et al: Activation and mechanism of *Clostridium septicum* alpha toxin, *Mol Microbiol* 10:627-634, 1993.
8. Gordon VM, Benz R, Fujii K et al: *Clostridium septicum* alpha-toxin is proteolytically activated by furin, *Infect Immun* 65:4130-134, 1997.
9. Knott GK, Erwin BG, Classick LG: Benefits of a clostridial vaccination program in feedlot cattle, *Vet Med* 80:95-97, 1985.

CHAPTER 19

Clostridial Enterotoxemia (*Clostridium perfringens*)

J. GLENN SONGER

Clostridium perfringens is ubiquitous in the environment and can be isolated from the alimentary tract of most healthy animals. Division of the species into five toxinotypes is based on production of one or more of the four so-called major toxins (Table 19-1). All toxinotypes can be etiologic agents of enterotoxemia in various species (Box 19-1); types A, C, and D are common causes of enterotoxemia in North America, whereas type E–associated disease is uncommon. Isolation of type B is rare in North America but common elsewhere. All of these organisms can be found in the intestines of normal animals, but disease results when conditions in the gut favor multiplication of *C. perfringens* and accumulation of toxins.[1]

TYPE A ENTEROTOXEMIA

Lamb enterotoxemia *(yellow lamb disease)* occurs primarily in the spring in the western United States. Icterus is the predominant feature and is accompanied by dyspnea, depression, anemia, and hemoglobinuria. Diarrhea is uncommon, and most animals experience acute hemolytic crisis and death after a clinical course of 6 to 12 hours. Kidneys are darkened, and the spleen is edematous. The liver is enlarged, pale, and friable, and fluid accumulates in pericardial and peritoneal cavities. Morbidity rates may be greater than 30%, and case fatality rates approach 100%. Large numbers of *C. perfringens* are often present in intestinal contents. Alpha toxin (*C. perfringens* A [CPA]) may be involved in pathogenesis.[2]

Disease is more common in calves than in lambs. It is perhaps most common in animals younger than 10 days of age, but another peak of onsets occurs in approximately 2-month-old calves. Incidence may be as high as 50%, especially in calves born to heifers. The infection is characterized by hemorrhagic, necrotic abomasitis and enteritis. Colic and tympany are common, and abomasal ulceration frequently leads to perforation and subsequent peritonitis. Microscopic examination reveals gram-positive bacilli on mucosa and in submucosa, and *C. perfringens* is isolated in large numbers. Disease has been reproduced experimentally.

CPA is also a cause of necrotizing enteritis in neonatal pigs. Mild villous atrophy and necrosis of superficial villous lamina propria may occur, but disease has the appearance of a secretory diarrhea. Bacteriologic cultures yield luxuriant growth of *C. perfringens*. Disease has been reproduced experimentally, but little is known of pathogenesis.[3]

TYPE B ENTEROTOXEMIA

C. perfringens type B (CPB) is the etiologic agent of dysentery in newborn lambs. Isolates of CPB are rare in North America, but disease is common in the border country between England and Scotland, Wales, South Africa, Mediterranean countries, and the Middle East. Lamb dysentery occurs most commonly during the first few days of life but may affect older lambs as well. Chronic disease (called *pine*) in older lambs manifests as chronic abdominal pain without diarrhea, and disease in calves is less severe, with a clinical

Table 19-1

Production of Major Toxins by Toxinotypes of *C. perfringens*

	Toxin			
Toxinotype	Alpha (CPA)	Beta (CPB)	Epsilon (ETX)	Iota (ITX)
A	X			
B	X	X	X	
C	X	X		
D	X		X	
E	X			X

Box 19-1

Disease Associated with Toxinotypes of *C. perfringens*

Toxinotype	Diseases
A	Porcine neonatal necrotizing enteritis, fowl necrotic enteritis, bovine/caprine/ovine neonatal hemorrhagic enteritis
B	Lamb dysentery
C	Porcine/bovine/ovine/caprine neonatal hemorrhagic necrotic enteritis
D	Ovine/bovine enterotoxemia
E	Bovine/ovine hemorrhagic enterotoxemia

course of 2 to 4 days. In typical lamb dysentery, organisms acquired from the dam or the environment proliferate in the gut, especially in lambs suckling heavily lactating ewes. Cessation of feeding, depression, abdominal pain, bloody diarrhea, recumbency, coma, and death in less than 24 hours are common. Hemorrhage and ulceration of small intestinal mucosa are likely mediated by CPB, and diffusion of epsilon toxin (ETX) into circulation leads to central nervous system effects. Peritoneal cavity often contains hemorrhagic fluid, liver is usually enlarged and friable, and mediastinal lymph nodes are generally enlarged. Incidence is often as high as 30%, with case fatality rates approaching 100%.

TYPE C ENTEROTOXEMIA

Infections by *C. perfringens* type C (CPC) have been reported in humans and most domestic animals worldwide. Among domestic animals, newborns are usually most susceptible, perhaps because of ready colonization of the gut by *C. perfringens* in the absence of well-established normal intestinal flora. Alteration of the flora by sudden dietary changes may provoke CPC infection in older animals.

In general, hemorrhagic inflammation of jejunum and ileum is the most striking feature of disease in young animals. Peritoneal cavity often contains serohemorrhagic fluid, and petechial hemorrhages are common on serosae and in spleen, thymus, heart, meninges, and brain.

Acute or peracute disease is common in piglets 1 to 2 days of age. Depression is followed by diarrhea and dysentery, with blood and necrotic debris in feces. The mucosal surface of small intestine is often dark red, with gas in tissue, hemorrhagic exudate in lumen, and hemorrhagic necrosis of mucosa, submucosa, and muscularis mucosa. Lesions in cecum and upper colon are not uncommon. CPC can usually be isolated in large numbers and pure culture from intestinal contents. Morbidity may be 30% to 50%, with case fatality rates of 50% to 100% and a clinical course of less than 24 hours. Piglets affected at 1 to 2 weeks of age usually have a longer clinical course, with nonbloody, yellowish diarrhea and necrosis of jejunal mucosa. Sows are probably a source of infection for newborn pigs.

Similar disease occurs in neonatal calves, lambs, and goats. Hemorrhagic, necrotic enteritis and enterotoxemia, often accompanied by abdominal pain, develop in vigorous, healthy calves usually younger than 10 days old. Disease in lambs resembles dysentery and is often accompanied by nervous signs such as tetany and opisthotonos. Death may be peracute, but it may also follow a clinical course of several days. Morbidity rates are 15% to 20%, with case fatality rates approaching 100%.

Adult sheep can be affected by type C enterotoxemia, colorfully named *struck* after the rapid death associated with the condition, which often leaves the impression that the animal has been struck by lightning. Damage to gastrointestinal mucosa, frequently caused by poor-quality feed, is followed by multiplication of type C in abomasum and small intestine. Subsequent mucosal necrosis usually occurs in the absence of dysentery or diarrhea. Peritoneal vessels are congested, and peritoneal hemorrhage may occur. The peritoneal cavity may contain

a large volume of serous fluid. The small intestine may contain areas of mucosal necrosis, and jejunal ulceration is common. Pleural and pericardial transudates provide additional evidence of acute toxemia.

CPB plays a central role in pathogenesis of CPC infections. In pigs CPB acts initially in jejunum under conditions of curtailed proteolytic activity. Pancreatic secretion deficiency shortly after birth and ingestion of colostral protease inhibitors compromise detoxification of CPB. Toxin-induced damage of jejunal mucosa begins before bacteria adhere. Mucosal necrosis is progressive, with epithelial cell death and desquamation followed by further bacterial invasion, multiplication, and more toxin production. Intestinal lesions can be impressive in extent and severity, but death is probably ultimately due to betatoxemia. Similarities of CPB for staphylococcal alpha and gamma toxins and leukocidin strengthen suggestions that CPB may affect the central nervous system.

TYPE D ENTEROTOXEMIA

Type D strains cause enterotoxemia (sudden death, overeating, or pulpy kidney disease) most commonly in 3- to 10-week-old lambs suckling heavily lactating ewes. However, enterotoxemia is also a significant cause of death in weaned animals up to 10 months of age, usually those fed rich grain rations in feedlots. Disease often follows upsets in gastrointestinal flora resulting from sudden dietary changes or continuous feeding of high levels of feed concentrates. Rapid multiplication of type D organisms and production of ETX is favored by the presence of excess dietary starch in the small intestine; ETX facilitates its own absorption.

Petechial and ecchymotic hemorrhages may be present on ruminal, abomasal, and duodenal serosae and in diaphragm and abdominal muscles. Excess pericardial fluid and hemorrhage of epicardium and endocardium are common. The term *pulpy kidney* is derived from postmortem autolysis that occurs rapidly in hyperemic kidney tissue damaged by ETX.

A primary target of ETX is the central nervous system, where it produces foci of liquefactive necrosis, perivascular edema, and hemorrhage, especially in the meninges.[4] The extent of neurologic signs including incoordination, convulsions, and sudden death is directly related to severity of lesions. Focal encephalomalacia is probably a chronic manifestation of enterotoxemia. Affected sheep are often blind and demonstrate head pressing and an inability to eat.

Type D enterotoxemia is also important in calves and goats and occasionally occurs in adult cattle, deer, domesticated camels, and horses. In goats, catarrhal, fibrinous, or hemorrhagic enterocolitis is a consistent lesion and the classic pulpy kidney is absent.

TYPE E ENTEROTOXEMIA

Type E may cause about 1% of all cases of enterotoxemia in calves,[5] and disease has also been reported in lambs and rabbits.[6] Supposed "vaccine breaks" among animals immunized with type C products are frequently caused by type E infection. Calves die acutely, and necropsy reveals hemorrhagic enteritis. Pathogenesis is mediated by iota toxin, a two-component toxin that ADP-ribosylates actin.[7,8]

DIAGNOSIS OF ENTEROTOXEMIA

Diagnosis of enterotoxemia is based on evaluation of clinical signs and gross and microscopic lesions, bacteriologic culture of appropriate specimens, and detection of toxins in pathologic specimens and in supernatant fluids of pure cultures. Demonstration of toxins by in vivo assays has become less common because of expense, variability of results, and undesirability, on humanitarian grounds, of the traditional mouse and guinea pig assays. Immunoassays for enterotoxemia-associated toxins are readily available for import (from BioX in Belgium). Polymerase chain reaction assays for genotyping *C. perfringens* have gained wide acceptance and can often make an important contribution to diagnosis.

TREATMENT AND PREVENTION

Prophylaxis in swine by the use of bacitracin methylene disalicylate (BMD) has been effective. In individual piglets, calves, kids, and foals, prevention via hyperimmune antiserum may be of value for up to 3 weeks.

The course of enterotoxemia is usually rapid, often precluding treatment. However, antimicrobial drugs effective against anaerobic bacteria might be beneficial, at least in theory. Penicillins and macrolides would be reasonable choices, and *C. perfringens* is susceptible in vitro to third-generation cephalosporins. Delivery by the IV route is indicated because time is critical and peripheral perfusion may be poor. Anecdotal reports suggest that successful treatment of clostridial myositis can be achieved by use of oral antimicrobial agents.

Immunoprophylaxis is of greatest importance. Commercial multivalent toxoids or bacterin/toxoids are typically administered to dams before parturition (two doses for single-parity animals and at least a single booster for multiparity animals). Immunization of sows during gestation is ordinarily followed by protective levels of antibodies in colostrum and can yield more than tenfold reductions in piglet mortality. Ewes may be vaccinated against infection by types A, B, C, or D, depending on the locale. Serum antibodies against ETX prevent the death of goats from toxemia but provide little protection against enterocolitis. At the time of this writing, conditional licenses are being granted in the United States for products intended to prevent enterotoxemias caused by type A.

References

1. Songer JG: Clostridial enteric diseases of domestic animals: a review, *Clin Microbiol Rev* 9:216-234, 1996.
2. Awad MM, Ellemor DM, Boyd RL et al: Synergistic effects of alpha-toxin and perfringolysin O in *Clostridium perfringens*–mediated gas gangrene, *Infect Immun* 69:7904-7910, 2001.
3. Gibert M, Jolivet-Reynaud C, Popoff MR et al: Beta$_2$ toxin, a novel toxin produced by *Clostridium perfringens*, *Gene* 203:65-73, 1997.
4. Buxton D, Morgan KT: Studies of lesions produced in the brains of colostrum deprived lambs by *Clostridium welchii* *(C. perfringens)* type D toxin, *J Comp Pathol* 86:435-447, 1976.
5. Billington SJ, Wieckowski EU, Sarker MR et al: *Clostridium perfringens* type E animal enteritis isolates with highly conserved, silent enterotoxin gene sequences, *Infect Immun* 66:4531-4536, 1998.
6. Borriello SP, Carman RJ: Association of iota-like toxin and *Clostridium spiroforme* with both spontaneous and antibiotic-associated diarrhea and colitis in rabbits, *J Clin Microbiol* 17:419-418, 1983.
7. Aktories K, Wegner A: Mechanisms of the cytopathic action of actin-ADP-ribosylating toxins, *Mol Microbiol* 6:2905-2908, 1992.
8. Daube G, Simon P, Limbourg B et al: Hybridization of 2,659 *Clostridium perfringens* isolates with gene probes for seven toxins (alpha, beta, epsilon, iota, theta, mu, and enterotoxin) and for sialidase, *Am J Vet Res* 57:496-501, 1996.

CHAPTER 20

Johne's Disease (Paratuberculosis)

MICHAEL T. COLLINS

Johne's disease, also called *paratuberculosis,* is a chronic wasting disease primarily affecting ruminants.[1] The disease is caused by infection of the small intestine with *Mycobacterium paratuberculosis;* however, some authors prefer the name *Mycobacterium avium* subspecies *paratuberculosis* because of its close genetic relationship with *Mycobacterium avium* (a cause of avian tuberculosis).[2] Unlike *M. avium, M. paratuberculosis* cannot produce the siderophore (iron-binding molecule) mycobactin, grows much slower in vitro, is much more pathogenic, and is an obligate parasite, replicating only inside macrophages of infected animals.

Johne's disease is an insidious and prevalent fatal disease of ruminants with particular economic importance for the dairy industry. U.S. Department of Agriculture herd-prevalence surveys estimated that 22% of U.S. dairy herds and 8% of U.S. beef cow-calf herds are *M. paratuberculosis* infected,[3] but experts universally acknowledge that these numbers are significant underestimates. Most agree that the dairy herd prevalence in the United States is closer to 80% and, although the infection prevalence in commercial beef cow-calf operations may be low, the prevalence among beef seed stock operations is disturbingly high based on clinical experience.

The disease occurs worldwide and also is a serious problem for ruminants other than bovids. Johne's disease in farm-raised deer and elk is an emerging disease problem. It has been reported in free-ranging wildlife and can become a significant problem in zoologic collections, particularly when diverse animal species are commingled. Johne's disease also occurs in camelids: camels, llamas, and alpacas. Sporadic infections in pigs, horses, wild rabbits, nonhuman primates, and humans also have been described.

For reasons unknown, young animals are more susceptible to infection with *M. paratuberculosis* than are adults. However, if given sufficient dose, even adult animals can become infected. Minimal infectious dose for any age animal has not been quantified. Infection occurs following ingestion of *M. paratuberculosis*–contaminated milk, water, or feed. In utero infection can also occur, particularly in pregnant animals in the latter stages of infection when the bacterium disseminates and infects multiple internal organs.[4] Offspring born to infected dams and suckled naturally until weaning have a high likelihood of becoming infected because *M. paratuberculosis* is excreted by infected animals in milk.[5,6] For animal species typically managed by hand rearing of neonates (e.g., dairy cattle),

feeding of whole milk rather than artificial milk replacer is associated with rapid dissemination of the infection in a herd.

Following ingestion, *M. paratuberculosis* is taken up by macrophages in gut-associated lymphoid tissue, particularly Peyer's patches in the terminal ileum and, occasionally, tonsils. There the bacterium multiplies intracellularly, inducing a diffuse granulomatous tissue reaction. From the primary sites of infection, *M. paratuberculosis* spreads via the lymphatics to regional lymph nodes, eventually resulting in systemic infection.[7] Infection dissemination likely occurs shortly before or at the time of onset of clinical signs because only a limited host tissue reaction is seen in tissues such as the liver, spleen, and lung and from which *M. paratuberculosis* can be isolated.

CLINICAL SIGNS

Cattle

Persistent diarrhea that is unresponsive to treatment, rapid weight loss in the face of good appetite, and the absence of fever are the constellation of signs that are typical of Johne's disease in cattle (Fig. 20-1). Most often the disease is seen in dairy cattle 3 to 5 years old. However, as the infection spreads and affects a steadily increasing percentage of cattle in the herd each year, clinical signs are often seen in animals younger than 3 years old. Presumably this is because the infection pressure (dose of bacteria to which calves are exposed) rises over time and higher doses cause more rapidly progressive infections.

Once the presence of paratuberculosis in a herd is confirmed, recognition of infected animals by clinical signs becomes easier and more subtle signs of the disease, rough lackluster hair coat and depressed milk production, are noticed by herd owners. None of the clinical signs mentioned are unique to Johne's disease, yet there is a risk of overdiagnosis (false positive) if only clinical signs are relied on. The differential diagnosis should include chronic local peritonitis, liver abscessation, helminth parasitism, pyelonephritis, and salmonellosis.

Sheep, Goats, and Other Animals

Johne's disease in ruminants other than cattle is most often recognized as a chronic wasting disease that is only sometimes accompanied by diarrhea (Fig. 20-2). For this reason, and because the progressive weight loss is often

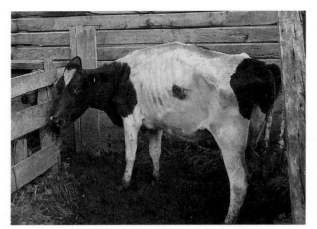

Fig 20-1   Holstein cow with clinical Johne's disease.

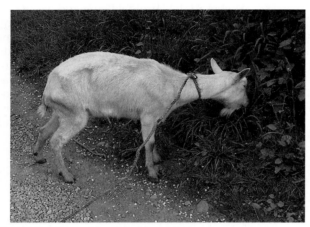

Fig 20-2   Goat with clinical Johne's disease.

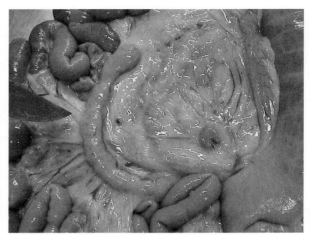

Fig 20-3   Enlarged mesenteric lymph nodes in a goat with clinical Johne's disease (the same goat as shown in Fig. 20-2).

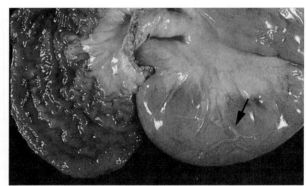

Fig 20-4   Serosal and mucosal surface of the ileum of a cow with Johne's disease. The mucosal surface is thick and corrugated, and the serosal surface has dilated lymphatic vessels *(arrow)*. (Courtesy Dr. A.J. Cooley.)

undetected because of the animal's thick hair coat, diagnosis of Johne's disease from clinical signs alone before death of the animal is not easy. Johne's disease should be included in the differential diagnosis of any ruminant or pseudo-ruminant (camelids) with poor body condition. Confirmation of the diagnosis can be made by necropsy or laboratory tests. Prominent mesenteric lymph nodes are consistent with a diagnosis of Johne's disease. Histopathology and microbiology should be performed on such lymph nodes (Fig. 20-3), as well as intestinal tissues.

DIAGNOSIS

Cattle

Consensus recommendations for testing U.S. cattle for Johne's disease were recently published. These recommendations cover both beef cattle and dairy cattle and both commercial and seedstock herds. The best tests or test regimens are recommended for each of seven different situations. Although the more common situations are covered later, interested readers should refer to these published recommendations.[8]

A fast, accurate, and inexpensive test to confirm a clinical diagnosis of Johne's disease in cattle in known infected herds is the absorbed enzyme-linked immunosorbent assay (ELISA). A positive test has a high probability of being correct. However, roughly 15% of cattle with clinical signs of Johne's disease may test negative for serum antibodies.[9] The agar-gel immunodiffusion (AGID) test is less sensitive, and the complement fixation (CF) test is less specific. Acid-fast staining of fecal sample smears is another method for rapid confirmation of a clinical diagnosis. This requires some experience, however, and is less sensitive and specific than testing by ELISA. Genetic probes for *M. paratuberculosis* are commercially available, but although faster, equally specific, and of comparable cost as fecal culture, such tests have lower sensitivity.[10] Cattle with clinical Johne's disease have a grossly thickened ileum (Fig. 20-4). Histopathology with acid-fast staining of ileum and mesenteric lymph node tissues is definitive for a diagnosis of Johne's disease (Fig. 20-5).

Diagnosis of cattle in the preclinical stages of *M. paratuberculosis* infection is challenging because of the extended period of time when animals are infected but neither shedding the bacterium in feces nor producing serum

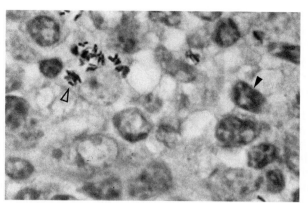

Fig 20-5 Acid-fast stained section of an ileocecal lymph node section from a cow with Johne's disease. Note the mononuclear inflammatory cells *(solid arrowhead)* and the *M. paratuberculosis* bacteria *(open arrowhead)*.

antibodies. This biologic fact presents several challenges for control programs. Repeated testing at 6- to 12-month intervals is required to ensure that an animal is unlikely to be infected. Therefore test and cull or test and segregate programs must continue for many years in infected herds. Another implication is that one-time testing of herd additions is ineffective at eliminating all infected animals. Culture of fecal samples is the most widely used reference test but has the disadvantages of being expensive and requiring 16 weeks to perform on solid culture media or 8 weeks using automated liquid culture systems. Testing for serum antibodies by absorbed ELISA is faster and less expensive and therefore more widely used, but roughly one third as sensitive as fecal culture.[9] However, ELISA sensitivity is directly correlated with fecal shedding level of *M. paratuberculosis* and ELISAs do a good job of detecting the most infectious, heavy shedding cows. Milk samples can also be used to test for antibodies to *M. paratuberculosis,* and such assays have a diagnostic accuracy (sensitivity and specificity) comparable with ELISAs performed on sera.[9-13] Economic decision analysis modeling indicates that multiple factors affect the design of the optimal Johne's disease control program for commercial dairy herds, but in general, low-cost tests such as ELISAs on milk samples are favored over more sensitive but higher-cost tests in support of herd management changes to control paratuberculosis.[14]

Detection of infected herds (herd-level diagnosis), rather than infected individual cattle, is most important to control spread of this insidious infectious disease among herds. Herd-level diagnosis can be achieved by testing a portion of the animals in the herd using serum ELISA, fecal culture, or fecal PCR. Alternatively, environmental fecal samples from six prescribed sites of animal congregation on the farm can be tested by culture. Owners of noninfected herds should keep the herd closed or, if necessary, only buy replacement cattle from test-negative herds. State and national programs are in place in the United States and other countries to classify herds based on the likelihood of being free of *M. paratuberculosis* infection, thus providing herd owners reliable, risk-based methods of animal trading.

Sheep, Goats, and Other Animals

ELISA, fecal culture, and acid-fast smears of fecal samples work as well in goats as they do in cattle for clinical diagnosis confirmation or disease management on a herd level. However, unless an ELISA kit insert does not explicitly state that the assay works on goats (or any other nonbovid species) or the testing laboratory cannot produce publications validating use of the assay in goats or any other nonbovid species, the end user should interpret ELISA results with extreme caution. When performing necropsies it should be noted that unlike in cattle, the ileum of infected goats is usually not thickened and gross pathology at necropsy is limited to slight enlargement of mesenteric lymph nodes (see Fig. 20-3).

The AGID is the preferred serologic test for use on individual sheep. Culture of *M. paratuberculosis* from sheep is more difficult than from cattle because sheep strains of the organism are more fastidious. Culture of pooled fecal samples using liquid culture media has become a preferred method for flock surveillance.[15] Like in goats, thickening of the ileum is not common and gross pathology is generally limited to extreme cachexia. Histopathology with acid-fast staining is the best method of diagnosis.[16,17]

For other animal species, serologic tests have yet to be developed and validated. Culture of fecal samples is the only antemortem diagnostic test available, and necropsy with histopathology is the most definitive diagnosis. In deer *M. paratuberculosis* can cause caseous granulomatous lesions easily confused with tuberculosis.[18]

TREATMENT

Long-term antimicrobial therapy with antituberculosis drugs results in improved body condition and somewhat prolonged life of infected animals. It does not cure the infection. Published data for recommendation of the best drugs, drug combinations, dosages, or durations for effective antimicrobial treatment of *M. paratuberculosis* infections in animals are insufficient.

PREVENTION AND CONTROL

Prevention of infection is the most effective way to manage paratuberculosis. Because *M. paratuberculosis* is an obligate pathogen, maintaining herds and flocks as closed populations, only introducing new genetic material by artificial insemination or embryo transfer will ensure that the infection remains excluded. When addition of live animals to a herd or flock is unavoidable, they should originate from herds or flocks that are at least test negative (whole herd test) and preferably at some level in a national herd certification program for paratuberculosis. Consensus biosecurity recommendations for limiting the risk of introducing *M. paratuberculosis*–infected cattle to herds have been published.[8] Many U.S. states, as well as Australia and The Netherlands, have certification programs for cattle. Similar programs for other animal species are being developed.

Control of paratuberculosis in infected herds or flocks is by (1) identifying and culling or isolating the infected animals and (2) instituting husbandry measures that limit as much as possible the opportunities for infection transmission. Both strategies must be done to achieve control in a reasonable period of time (e.g., 5 years). Vaccination of cattle herds has not proved effective at preventing infection, although it decreases the incidence of clinical disease. Economics make vaccination particularly attractive as a control measure in sheep flocks.[19]

Testing to support control programs should use quantitative interpretation of diagnostic tests to prioritize animals for culling and to identify the animals most likely to be infectious. Test-positive animals that are not culled should be visibly labeled and managed to limit opportunities to spread the *M. paratuberculosis* infection. Quantitative results for both fecal culture and ELISAs reflect the stage of infection and the level of fecal shedding of the organism. Using both types of tests on the entire adult herd or flock increases detection of infected animals and may be warranted if rapid eradication of the infection from a herd or flock is the owner's goal. To control the cost of testing, serology and culture can be done on an alternating basis at intervals of 6 to 12 months. For even faster elimination of the infection, the last offspring born to test-positive animals should also be culled. This may be less important in dairy herds where calves are immediately removed from the dam.

Dairy herd husbandry changes primarily are directed at limiting direct and indirect contact of neonates with manure from potentially infected adult animals. Prompt removal of neonates from their dam and hand rearing them using artificial milk replacer is critical for control because of the high likelihood that raw milk on the farm is contaminated with *M. paratuberculosis*. Colostrum for neonates should be obtained only from test-negative dams. Alternatively, artificial colostrum replacement products can be used. On-farm pasteurization of colostrum or milk substantially reduces the chances of *M. paratuberculosis* infection transmission. Young animals, particularly those being raised as herd or flock replacements, should remain isolated from the adult herd as long as possible. The window of susceptibility is not well defined, but for cattle it is best to ensure that calves have no contact with the adult herd for at least 6, and preferably 12, months. This includes shared feed bunks, water troughs, and pastures. Manure runoff from areas where adult animals reside also must be kept away from young herd replacements.

Options for Johne's disease control through herd management changes for beef cattle herds are more limited than for dairy herds. Strategies that generally limit fecal-oral transmission of pathogens such as decreasing the density of cows during calving season and removal of cow-calf pairs from the calving area as soon as possible are suggested. Stagnant water sources such as ponds or stock tanks are suspected to be a mode of transmission in beef cattle herds and should be fenced off with alternative, noncontaminated water provided to cattle. Because of the limited options for herd management to limit spread of Johne's disease, beef cattle herds must rely more heavily on diagnostic tests and must cull both the test-positive cow and her last calf.

Design of paratuberculosis control programs should begin with a herd risk assessment. In the United States a standardized system for doing herd risk assessments and designing herd management plans was recently implemented. Additionally, each state has a Designated Johne's Coordinator (DJC) to assist and train veterinarians to annually conduct risk assessments and write herd management plans. Contact the State Veterinarian's office for details.

ZOONOTIC CONCERNS

The zoonotic potential of *M. paratuberculosis* is a complex and controversial subject. It is beyond the scope of this chapter to thoroughly review the issue. Interested readers should consult recent reviews.[20-24] If zoonotic, the scope of state and federal programs to control paratuberculosis and ensure that *M. paratuberculosis* does not contaminate food or water will be substantial. If not zoonotic, paratuberculosis will be only one of many important animal diseases warranting control based primarily on its economic impact on herd or flock productivity. The scope and funding of federal and state control programs in the future will likely be tied to the perceived or actual zoonotic potential of *M. paratuberculosis*.

Many reasons underlie concern about the zoonotic potential of *M. paratuberculosis,* and the issue desperately needs resolution. Mounting evidence indicates that *M. paratuberculosis* may cause a chronic granulomatous bowel disease in humans known as Crohn's disease. It has been cultured from patients with Crohn's disease and detected in resected bowl samples using genetic probes for IS*900*, a genetic element unique to *M. paratuberculosis*.[25-27] Patients with Crohn's disease have antibody specific to *M. paratuberculosis*.[28] The incidence of Crohn's disease is steadily rising, and epidemiologic studies suggest that although a genetic marker for Crohn's disease has been found, called *NOD2*, the triggering factor is an infectious agent.[29-32] Crohn's disease is increasingly diagnosed in children, heightening concern about the cause of this disease.[33-35]

Foods of animal origin are potential vehicles for human exposure to *M. paratuberculosis*. It can survive pasteurization and has been recovered from retail pasteurized milk.[36,37] Animals in advanced stages of paratuberculosis (heavy fecal shedders and/or strong-positive ELISA) commonly have disseminated *M. paratuberculosis* infections.[7,38] These cattle are culled and may be used for production of ground beef. The cooking temperature required to inactivate *M. paratuberculosis* in ground beef is not known. Contamination of domestic water supplies is another potential route of human exposure to *M. paratuberculosis*.

Association of *M. paratuberculosis* with Crohn's disease does not prove causation. However, sufficient evidence exists of a potential causal association to be concerned, raising the importance of paratuberculosis control in domestic animals, particularly those used for food production.

References

1. Harris NB, Barletta RG: *Mycobacterium avium* subsp. *paratuberculosis* in veterinary medicine, *Clin Microbiol Rev* 14:489-512, 2001.
2. Thorel MF, Krichevsky M, Levy-Frebault VV: Numerical taxonomy of mycobactin-dependent mycobacteria, emended description of *Mycobacterium avium*, and description of *Mycobacterium avium* subsp. *avium* subsp. nov., *Mycobacterium*

avium subsp. *paratuberculosis* subsp. nov., and *Mycobacterium avium* subsp. *silvaticum* subsp. nov, *Int J Syst Bacteriol* 40:254-260, 1990.

3. USDA:APHIS:VS, C.N.A.H.M.S. Johne's disease on U.S. dairy operations. N245.1097, 1–52, Fort Collins, Colo, 1997, National Animal Health Monitoring System.

4. Sweeney RW, Whitlock RH, Rosenberger AE: *Mycobacterium paratuberculosis* isolated from fetuses of infected cows not manifesting signs of the disease, *Am J Vet Res* 53:477-480, 1992.

5. Sweeney RW, Whitlock RH, Rosenberger AE: *Mycobacterium paratuberculosis* cultured from milk and supramammary lymph nodes of infected asymptomatic cows, *J Clin Microbiol* 30:166-171, 1992.

6. Streeter RN, Hoffsis GF, Bech-Nielsen S: Isolation of *Mycobacterium paratuberculosis* from colostrum and milk of subclinically infected cows, *Am J Vet Res* 56:1322-1324, 1995.

7. Lombard JE, Antognolli MC, Hirst HL et al: Use of ante mortem tests to identify cattle with disseminated *Mycobacterium avium* subsp. *paratuberculosis* infection detected by post mortem culture of 15 tissues. In Manning EJB, Nielsen SS, editors: Proceedings of the 8th International Colloquium on Paratuberculosis, International Association for Paratuberculosis, Madison, Wis, 2006, p 156 (abstract).

8. Collins MT, Gardner IA, Garry FB et al: Consensus recommendations on diagnostic testing for the detection of paratuberculosis in cattle in the United States, *J Am Vet Med Assoc* 229:1912-1919, 2006.

9. Collins MT, Wells SJ, Petrini KR et al: Evaluation of five antibody detection tests for bovine paratuberculosis, *Clin Diagn Lab Immunol* 12:685-692, 2005.

10. Wells SJ, Collins MT, Faaberg KS et al: Evaluation of a rapid fecal PCR test for detection of *Mycobacterium avium* subsp. *paratuberculosis* in dairy cattle, *Clin Vaccine Immunol* 13:1125-1130, 2006.

11. Nielsen SS, Grohn YT, Enevoldsen C: Variation of the milk antibody response to paratuberculosis in naturally infected dairy cows, *J Dairy Sci* 85:2795-2802, 2002.

12. Nielsen SS, Toft N: Age-specific characteristics of ELISA and fecal culture for purpose-specific testing for paratuberculosis, *J Dairy Sci* 89:569-579, 2006.

13. Hendrick SH, Duffield TF, Kelton DF et al: Evaluation of enzyme-linked immunosorbent assays performed on milk and serum samples for detection of paratuberculosis in lactating dairy cows, *J Am Vet Med Assoc* 226:424-428, 2005.

14. Dorshorst NC, Collins MT, Lombard JE: Decision analysis model for paratuberculosis control in commercial dairy herds, *Prev Vet Med* 75:92-122, 2006.

15. Sergeant ES, Whittington RJ, More SJ: Sensitivity and specificity of pooled faecal culture and serology as flock-screening tests for detection of ovine paratuberculosis in Australia, *Prev Vet Med* 52:199-211, 2002.

16. Clarke CJ, Little D: The pathology of ovine paratuberculosis: gross and histological changes in the intestine and other tissues, *J Comp Path* 114:419-437, 1996.

17. Pérez V, Marín JFG, Badiola JJ: Description and classification of different types of lesion associated with natural paratuberculosis infection in sheep, *J Comp Path* 114:107-122, 1996.

18. O'Brien R, Mackintosh CG, Bakker D et al: Immunological and molecular characterization of susceptibility in relationship to bacterial strain differences in *Mycobacterium avium* subsp. *paratuberculosis* infection in the Red Deer *(Cervus elaphus)*, *Infect Immun* 74:3530-3537, 2006.

19. Reddacliff L, Eppleston J, Windsor P et al: Efficacy of a killed vaccine for the control of paratuberculosis in Australian sheep flocks, *Vet Microbiol* 115:77-90, 2006.

20. Hermon-Taylor J, Bull TJ: Crohn's disease caused by *Mycobacterium avium* subspecies *paratuberculosis*: a public health tragedy whose resolution is long overdue, *J Med Microbiol* 51:3-6, 2002.

21. Biet F, Boschiroli ML, Thorel MF et al: Zoonotic aspects of *Mycobacterium bovis* and *Mycobacterium avium-intracellulare* complex (MAC), *Vet Res* 36:411-436, 2005.

22. Grant IR: Zoonotic potential of *Mycobacterium avium* ssp. *paratuberculosis*: the current position, *J Appl Microbiol* 98:1282-1293, 2005.

23. Sartor RB: Does *Mycobacterium avium* subspecies *paratuberculosis* cause Crohn's disease? *Gut* 54:896-898, 2005.

24. Chamberlin WM, Naser SA: Integrating theories of the etiology of Crohn's disease on the etiology of Crohn's disease: questioning the hypotheses, *Med Sci Monit* 12:RA27-RA33, 2006.

25. Ryan P, Bennett MW, Aarons S: PCR detection of *Mycobacterium paratuberculosis* in Crohn's disease granulomas isolated by laser capture microdissection, *Gut* 51:665-670, 2002.

26. Bull TJ, McMinn EJ, Sidi-Boumedine K et al: Detection and verification of *Mycobacterium avium* subsp. *paratuberculosis* in fresh ileocolonic mucosal biopsy specimens from individuals with and without Crohn's disease, *J Clin Microbiol* 41:2920-2923, 2003.

27. Sechi LA, Scanu AM, Molicotti P et al: Detection and isolation of *Mycobacterium avium* subspecies *paratuberculosis* from intestinal mucosal biopsies of patients with and without Crohn's disease in Sardinia, *Am J Gastroenterol* 100:1529-1536, 2005.

28. Nakase H, Nishio A, Tamaki H et al: Specific antibodies against recombinant protein of insertion element 900 of *Mycobacterium avium* subspecies *paratuberculosis* in Japanese patients with Crohn's disease, *Inflamm Bowel Dis* 12:62-69, 2006.

29. Binder V, Both H, Hansen PK et al: Incidence and prevalence of ulcerative colitis and Crohn's disease in the county of Copenhagen, 1962 to 1978, *Gastroenterology* 83:583-588, 1982.

30. Fireman Z, Grossman A, Lilos P et al: Epidemiology of Crohn's disease in the Jewish population of central Israel, 1970-1980, *Am J Gastroenterol* 84:255-258, 1989.

31. Shoda R, Matsueda K, Yamato S: Epidemiologic analysis of Crohn's disease in Japan: increased dietary intake of n-6 polyunsaturated fatty acids and animal protein relates to the increased incidence of Crohn's disease in Japan, *Am J Clin Nutr* 63:741-745, 1996.

32. Loftus EVJ, Silverstein MD, Sandborn WJ et al: Crohn's disease in Olmsted County, Minnesota, 1940-1993: incidence, prevalence, and survival, *Gastroenterology* 114:1161-1168, 1998.

33. Kugathasan S, Judd RH, Hoffmann RG et al: Epidemiologic and clinical characteristics of children with newly diagnosed inflammatory bowel disease in Wisconsin: a statewide population-based study, *J Pediatr* 143:525-531, 2003.

34. Phavichitr N, Cameron DJS, Catto-Smith AG: Increasing incidence of Crohn's disease in Victorian children, *J Gastroenterol Hepatol* 18:329-332, 2003.

35. Pozler O, Malay J, Bonova O et al: Incidence of Crohn's disease in the Czech Republic in the years 1990 to 2001 and assessment of pediatric population with inflammatory bowel disease, *J Ped Gastroenterol Nutr* 42:186-189, 2006.

36. Hammer P, Kiesner C, Walte HG: Heat resistance of *Mycobacterium avium* ssp. *paratuberculolsis* in raw milk tested in a pilot plant pasteurizer, *Kieler Milchwirtschaftliche Forschungsberichte* 54:275-303, 2002.

37. Ellingson JLE, Anderson JL, Koziczkowski JJ et al: Detection of viable *Mycobacterium avium* subsp. *paratuberculosis* in retail pasteurized whole milk by two culture methods and PCR, *J Food Prot* 67:966-972, 2005.

38. Rossiter CA, Henning WR: Isolation of *Mycobacterium paratuberculosis* from thin market cows at slaughter, *J Animal Sci* 79:113-114, 2001.

CHAPTER 21

Neonatal Calf Diarrhea

JONATHAN M. NAYLOR

Diarrhea and other digestive diseases are one of the big three causes of calf loss in beef calves and are the major cause of loss in unweaned dairy heifers born alive. Overall, beef calf mortality from diarrhea should be about 1%. In dairy calves diarrhea and other digestive diseases account for about 5% of total mortality from live birth to weaning.[1,2]

ETIOLOGY

The most commonly recognized causes of neonatal calf diarrhea are rotavirus, coronavirus, and cryptosporidia.[3-7] The major mechanism by which these and pathogens cause diarrhea is malabsorption. Enterotoxigenic *Escherichia coli* with the F5 (K99) antigen is less prevalent, probably because a highly effective vaccine has been developed.

Viral

Rotaviruses are the most commonly diagnosed cause of neonatal diarrhea. Typically they affect calves 4 to 14 days old, but infections can be seen either side of this age range. Rotaviruses invade and destroy the villus epithelial cells of the small intestine. This results in malabsorption of nutrients. Asymptomatic infections may occur in older calves and in adult cows. In cows, excretion of virus is particularly common around the time of calving. This is one method by which infection persists on a farm. Once an outbreak has started, diarrheic calves are the major source of contagion.

Coronaviruses are an important cause of diarrhea in 4- to 30-day-old calves. At least three strains of bovine coronavirus are responsible for respiratory infection, neonatal diarrhea, and winter dysentery. However, the winter dysentery and neonatal calf strains can infect both calves and adults. In calves, coronaviruses invade and destroy villous epithelial cells of the small intestine, causing villous atrophy. They also invade the epithelium of the large intestine. Because coronaviruses affect the large intestine, they may be associated with signs of colitis such as straining. Like rotavirus, excretion of coronavirus by asymptomatic adults may be an initial source of infection for calves. Clinically affected calves are the major source of virus once an outbreak is established.[3,8-14]

Bovine viral diarrhea (BVD) is an occasional cause of neonatal calf diarrhea. In outbreaks of BVD infection, diarrhea in calves has been documented as part of the clinical picture. Depending on the properties of the BVD virus and the time infection was acquired, oral lesions, thrombocytopenia and mucosal hemorrhages, blood in the feces, leukopenia, and signs of persistent infection and mucosal disease can occur.[15-19] BVD may also predispose to other enteric infections by reducing immunocompetence.

A variety of other viruses have been implicated as potential causes of calf diarrhea. These include Breda virus and Calicivirus. At present the importance of these agents is unknown.

Bacterial

A number of different groups of E. coli have been incriminated in outbreaks of calf diarrhea. Enterotoxigenic E. coli has a special fimbria, known as the K99 or F5 antigen, that allows it to attach to the surface of the small intestinal mucosa of neonatal calves. A second fimbrial attachment factor, the F41 antigen, has also been identified, but it is generally found together with F5 fimbria. Other attachment factors may exist. Enterotoxigenic E. coli produces enterotoxin (a heat stable form, ST) that stimulates secretion of sodium together with water and chloride ions by the mucosal cells. Enterotoxigenic E. coli also causes some villous atrophy.[20-25] In general, enterotoxigenic E. coli causes diarrhea in calves 1 to 4 days of age; in some cases this is profuse and watery and can rapidly result in hypovolemic shock and death. Enterotoxigenic E. coli can also secondarily infect older calves in which the mucosal cell type has been altered by prior infection with another pathogen.

Attaching and effacing E. coli (AAEC) is characterized by the possession of the eae gene, which produces the attachment protein intimin. This allows these bacteria to adhere to the mucosal surfaces of the colon and small intestine. Some strains carry Shiga's toxin (verotoxin) genes, which confer cytotoxicity in the vero cell or HeLa cell assays. E. coli, Shiga's toxin, and eae genes combined are called *enterohemorrhagic*. Other eae-carrying E. coli can be pathogenic as the result of the presence of other cytotoxic genes. In general, AAEC produce diarrhea in calves from 2 days to about 6 weeks of age. The bacteria adhere to the surface of the colon and sometimes the small intestine. Some are also internalized. The bacteria efface the surface microvilli and cause patchy mucosal stunting, erosion, and sloughing. At gross postmortem examination, changes vary from minimal to ileitis with mucohemorrhagic colitis. They produce diarrhea of variable severity that may be bloody.[26-35]

Necrotoxigenic E. coli produce a toxin that interferes with cell division and kills mucosal cells. Many strains also carry the F17 fimbrial attachment factor. Necrotoxigenic E. coli have been detected in the feces of 14% of healthy calves. However, in neonatal colostrum-restricted calves some strains are capable of causing long-lasting diarrhea and septicemia. At necropsy there may be vascular congestion of the intestinal mucosa, hypertrophy of the mesenteric lymph nodes, and congestion of the lungs. Histologically, there may be enterocolitis and lymphadenitis.[36,37]

Salmonella typhimurium, dublin, newport, and other species are important causes of calf diarrhea in operations in which there is movement and mixing of calves at an early age (see Chapter 25). These risk factors are most common in dairy and veal operations. *Salmonella* sp. penetrate the mucosa and cause intense submucosal inflammation. This inflammation stimulates a secretory diarrhea. Because the organisms penetrate the mucosa, septicemia and bacteremia are common, particularly in calves younger than 1 month of age. These organisms are potentially zoonotic.

Clostridium perfringens type C may produce a terminal diarrhea. More commonly affected calves are presented in a collapsed state and rapidly die. Signs of colic and nervous signs may also be seen. *C. perfringens* type A may produce mucoid diarrhea in calves.

Protozoal

Cryptosporidia are an important cause of diarrhea in 1- to 4-week-old calves. *Cryptosporidium parvum* and the slightly larger *Cryptosporidium muris* have both been identified in calf feces. *C. muris* is primarily an abomasal parasite and is not associated with diarrhea. *C. parvum* causes diarrhea in calves and people, although different strains may be more pathogenic in a particular species. Asymptomatic infection occurs in adult cows where fecal excretion is increased around the time of calving. The oocysts are resistant and are found in the environment associated with manure and manure contamination.

C. parvum invades the epithelium of the distal small intestine and the large intestine. It resides just beneath the cell membrane and causes loss of microvilli, villous atrophy, and villous fusion. Later in the disease process inflammatory changes develop. Oocyst secretion starts at the same time diarrhea commences and generally persists for a few days after the end of clinical signs. Because the oocysts are infectious within the intestine, autoinfection can lead to chronic disease. Clinical signs vary from mild to severe with feces of variable consistency. Tenesmus and occasionally the presence of blood in the feces may be seen.[6,38-44]

Giardia duodenalis infection is common in calves. However, its role in diarrhea is unclear. Some studies suggest that temporarily reducing the load of *Giardia* by treating with metronidazole or fenbendazole can give transient improvements in calf health, but reinfection soon occurs.[45-48]

PATHOGENESIS

Intestinal pathogens produce diarrhea via three major mechanisms. Although a certain mechanism may predominate, pathogens often cause diarrhea by a variety of mechanisms. Furthermore, it is common for more than one etiologic agent to be present in an outbreak of calf diarrhea, particularly in severe cases.

Secretory diarrhea is characterized by excess net secretion from the mucosal cells, mainly those of the small intestine. Enterotoxigenic *E. coli* is the classic example of this type of diarrhea. It produces an enterotoxin that alters the concentrations of intracellular messengers; this in turn alters the activity of the cell membrane pumps with increased net secretion of sodium, potassium, and chloride ions. The cell structure is mostly left intact. Diarrhea is typically profuse with no blood or straining. Affected calves develop signs of depression, weakness, and sometimes shock and death secondary to hypovolemia; acidemia is often mild.

Villous atrophy, malabsorption, and *osmotic diarrhea* go hand in hand. Destruction of the absorptive surface results in malabsorption of water and electrolytes. In addition, malabsorbed nutrients may have an osmotic effect that helps retain water within the gastrointestinal tract. The presence of unabsorbed nutrients in the gastrointestinal tract leads to bacterial overgrowth, particularly in the distal small intestine and large intestine. Some of these bacteria may be pathogenic, and others may cross the damaged mucosal surfaces to produce endotoxemia, bacteremia, or septicemia. Bacterial fermentation of undigested nutrients can lead to the production of D-lactic acid,[49] which is a potent neurotoxin responsible for many of the clinical signs of depressed central nervous system (CNS) function in severely affected calves.[50] Affected calves have signs of diarrhea, hypovolemia, acidemia, weakness, CNS depression, endotoxemia, and bacteremia of variable severity. Because it is difficult for a calf to tolerate both severe acidemia and hypovolemia, there is no relationship between the severity of dehydration and acidemia.[51] The profuseness of diarrhea and dehydration is poorly related to the severity of weakness and CNS depression. The three most commonly recognized enteric pathogens of calves, rotaviruses, coronaviruses, and cryptosporidia all produce villous atrophy, intestinal bacterial overgrowth, malabsorption, and osmotic diarrhea.

Inflammatory diarrhea is typical of *Salmonella* sp. These invade through the mucosa and stimulate an intense inflammation. Some of the inflammatory mediators stimulate the mucosal cells to secrete electrolytes and fluid. In addition, there is some villous atrophy. In calves, bacteremia and septicemia from the invading microorganisms are common. Systemic effects are due to some mixture of endotoxemia, hypovolemia, and acidemia.

Origin of Clinical Signs

Irrespective of the inciting infectious agent, diarrheic calves suffer from common sequelae.

Diarrhea. All agents increase the loss of water and electrolytes into the intestine, in those cases in which the compensatory ability of lower parts of the intestine to resorb water and electrolytes is exceeded, diarrhea results. *Dehydration* develops if the calf cannot compensate for this increased fluid loss by drinking and absorbing more water and electrolytes. *Hyponatremia* and whole-body potassium depletion are the result of loss of electrolytes with the diarrhea.[52-55] However, calves presented to veterinarians for treatment may be either hyponatremic or hypernatremic, presumably because oral electrolyte use by farmers is now widespread. Diarrheic calves may be hyperkalemic, normokalemic, or hypokalemic despite whole-body potassium depletion secondary to increased fecal loss. Hyperkalemia is the result of several factors; acidemia and hypoglycemia favor movement of potassium from the intracellular to the extracellular space, as does hypothermia, which slows cellular metabolism. Poor renal perfusion limits the ability of the kidneys to correct hyperkalemia.

In those calves with malabsorption and continued nutrient intake, some degree of intestinal bacterial overgrowth in response to increased nutrient availability is inevitable. This, together with damage to the mucosa, predisposes to secondary bacteremia or septicemia. Bacterial overgrowth and excess luminal nutrient availability leads to fermentation and production of organic acids including D- and L-lactic acid. Luminally produced L-lactic acid is not a major cause of systemic acidosis, probably because it can be readily removed by mammalian tissues. D-lactate, however, is poorly metabolized by mammals, and plasma concentrations correlate with ruminal and fecal D-lactate.[49] Chronic malabsorption leads to weight loss, particularly if malaise or therapeutic feed restriction limit caloric intake.

Acidemia is common in the more severely sick diarrheic calves. Of the documented causes, D-lactic acid is the major component. L-lactic acid can be important, particularly in severely hypovolemic calves in which tissue anoxia increases production of L-lactic acid from glucose and hepatic removal is reduced.[49,56,57] Fecal bicarbonate loss is another cause of acidemia, but its importance and whether this is due to decreased absorption of bicarbonate or to the trapping or bicarbonate by luminal acids has not been quantified.

Causes of Weakness and Central Nervous System Depression

Signs of weakness are usually the result of some mixture of hypovolemia, D-lactatemia, hypothermia, and endotoxemia.

The most important factors affecting CNS function are hypovolemia, D-lactatemia, hypothermia, profound hypoglycemia (rare), and to some extent endotoxemia. D-lactate is a potent neurotoxin that penetrates the blood-brain barrier and produces signs of ataxia, decreased mentation, recumbency, and coma.[49,50,58,59] In calves with acidosis without dehydration syndrome, D-lactate concentrations correlate highly with weakness and loss of CNS function, suggesting it is the major neurotoxic agent.[60-62] D-lactate concentrations also correlate with the degree of weakness and CNS in diarrheic calves.[63] Acidemia alone has small effects on mentation or ambulation but may be responsible for loss of the suck reflex.[50]

Origin of Cardiac Arrhythmia

Bradycardia with a regular rhythm can be the result of hypothermia or profound hypoglycemia. Bradycardia complicated by an irregular rhythm (e.g., because of premature ventricular contractions) is caused by hyperkalemia. Cardiac arrhythmia is one cause of death.[64,65]

APPROACH TO THERAPY

The initial assessment of a diarrheic calf involves a general physical examination; assessment should include whether an arrhythmia is present, dehydration status, amount of weakness and CNS depression, severity of diarrhea, condition of the navel, presence of pneumonia, and hypothermia or fever. Following this, the veterinarian may advise monitoring and oral or intravenous (IV) therapy.

Transient diarrhea is common in calves, and many self-cure. The provision of free-choice water and a salt block will make it easier for the calf to maintain homeostasis. In some cases, this is sufficient if the calves are carefully monitored.

Fluid Therapy

Correction of fluid and electrolyte abnormalities is the foundation for treatment of diarrheic calves. For a complete discussion, see Chapter 104.

Calves that are not depressed but have profuse diarrhea or are depressed and still have a good suck reflex should be treated with oral electrolyte solutions. Depending on the severity, this may take the form of an additional feeding of 2 L of oral electrolyte solution a day to the complete removal of all milk or milk replacer feeding and the substitution of three feeds of 2 L each of oral electrolyte a day. When choosing an appropriate oral electrolyte solution for more severely affected calves, look for one that, when reconstituted, contains sodium at 100 to 120 mmoles/L and 50 to 80 mmoles of acetate or propionate as the major alkalinizing agents.[66] Avoid products containing a lot of bicarbonate because these raise abomasal pH, which may make it easier for ingested pathogens to gain entry to the intestines. Bicarbonate and high levels of citrate also interfere with milk clotting in the abomasum.[67] Clotting is part of the normal digestive process for calves fed whole cow's milk.

Intravenous Fluid Therapy

Calves that have lost their suck reflex should be treated with IV fluids to correct dehydration, correct acidemia, and reduce serum D-lactate concentrations below 1 mmol/L.

Fluid Requirements

When calculating fluid requirements, it is customary to calculate the amount of fluid to correct dehydration and add amounts for ongoing losses and maintenance requirements. In diarrheic calves fed milk and oral electrolyte solutions, ongoing fecal water losses are generally between 1 and 4 L a day.[68] Maintenance water requirements for calves are not fully documented, but 70 mL/kg body weight prevented the development of dehydration and hypovolemia in one experiment.[69] Table 21-1 shows the application of these principles. The IV route allows for the administration of relatively large volumes of fluid without inefficiencies because of incomplete absorption. It also avoids problems with poor suck reflex and ileus. Ileus delays or prevents the absorption of oral fluids.

Table **21-1**

Examples of 24-Hour Fluid Requirements for a 50-kg Diarrheic Calf

Item	Dehydration 10%, Severe Diarrhea
Replacement, L	5
Ongoing losses, L	3
Maintenance (70 mL/kg), L	3.5
Total 24-hour requirement	11.5

Table **21-2**

Predicted Base Deficit, mmol/L, of Diarrheic Calves Based on Their Age and Clinical Signs

Clinical Signs	Calves ≤ 8 days	Calves > 8 days
Standing, strong suck	0	7
Standing but weak or weak suck reflex	5	11
Sternal recumbent	12	16
Lateral recumbent	13	20

(From Naylor JM: *Can Vet J,* 30:577-580, 1989.)

Diarrheic calves fed either no or small amounts of fluid orally often rapidly develop formed feces. Usually a mixture of isotonic sodium bicarbonate and isotonic saline, lactated Ringer's, or acetated Ringer's solution are used as the IV fluid.

Correction of Acidosis

Base deficit[70] is best measured using a blood gas machine or total CO_2 apparatus.[71] It can also be empirically assessed from clinical signs when this option is not available (Table 21-2). In calves with mild acidemia and base deficits less than 10 mmol/L, rehydrating the calf with lactated or acetated Ringer's solution is often sufficient to correct acidosis. More severe acidemia responds best to sodium bicarbonate solution, a fact that has been empirically proven in randomized, controlled, blinded trials in diarrheic calves.[61,72,73] Typically, correction of acidosis requires 1 to 4 L (25 to 100 mL/kg) of isotonic 1.3% sodium bicarbonate administered over about 4 to 8 hours. The remaining fluid deficits are met with isotonic saline solution.

Correction of D-Lactic Acidosis

Several important questions still need to be answered about the correction of D-lactic acidosis. One of the more important questions is whether correction of acidemia speeds the clearance of D-lactate. Conventional IV fluid therapy with saline and sodium bicarbonate given in accordance with the preceding principles has been shown to rapidly correct hyper D-lactatemia in diarrheic calves.[49] This is also associated with the excretion of D-lactate in urine.[74] In a controlled trial in calves with acidosis without dehydration syndrome, sodium bicarbonate was more effective than an equal volume of saline in correcting CNS depression,[61] suggesting that sodium bicarbonate therapy helps speed removal of D-lactate.

Antibiotics

The common indications for administering antibiotics to some diarrheic calves are for treatment of bacterial causes of diarrhea; reduction of intestinal bacterial overgrowth; and treatment of secondary bacteremia, septicemia, or intercurrent infections.[75]

The majority of cases of enteritis are the result of non-bacterial causes. Bacterial overgrowth can be managed by antibiotic administration or nutritional management.

In one study, septicemia and bacteremia were present in about 30% of diarrheic calves. Calves with low serum immunoglobulin status, recumbent calves, calves with no suck reflex, and those younger than 1 week of age are more likely to be bacteremic or septicemic, and these calves have a higher mortality rate.[76,77] In general this means that calves sick enough to require IV fluid therapy should be placed on systemic antibiotics. A wide variety of organisms can be cultured from the blood of diarrheic calves, but *E. coli* predominates. In my opinion, ceftiofur, trimethoprim sulphonamide combinations, or amoxicillin-clavulanate combinations are good choices. Pathogenic *E. coli* can be resistant to antimicrobials; therefore culture and sensitivity can be helpful in guiding therapy.

Halofuginone (Coccidiostat)

Halofuginone lactate (60-100 μg/kg body weight or 5 mg/calf in 10-ml carrier SID) fed orally by syringe into the back of the pharynx following the morning milk feed from birth for 7 days reduces the fecal shedding of cryptosporidium oocysts and the incidence of diarrhea.[78,79] This is the only known pharmacologic method of reducing the incidence of infection with cryptosporidium in calves.

Nonsteroidal Antiinflammatory Drugs

Nonsteroidal antiinflammatory drugs only appear to be beneficial in calves that have blood in their feces.[80]

Probiotics

Depending on the study, probiotics either show no or some benefit in either the prevention or treatment of diarrheic calves.[7,81-86]

PREVENTION

The main cornerstones of prevention are to boost immunity and reduce the load of infectious agents in the environment.

About 25% of dairy calves are partially or completely deficient in colostrally derived antibody. Many, but not all, studies indicate that this is a risk factor for neonatal disease including calf diarrhea.[87-93] Therefore it is important to make sure that dairy calves receive adequate colostrum. Colostrum deprivation is less of a problem in beef calves. However, farmers should monitor newborn calves carefully and assist those that have not sucked to nurse colostrum. If this is not feasible, calves suspected to be colostrum deprived can be tube fed with a commercial colostral antibody source containing at least 80 g of immunoglobulin.

Vaccinating the cows before parturition with a product against the K99 antigen of *E. coli* is a highly effective way of reducing this type of diarrhea disease. However, *E. coli* K99 is unique in that it mainly attacks calves in the first few days of life. In North America, vaccination against other diarrheal diseases does not appear to be beneficial or has only minor benefit.

In beef operations the major risk factors for outbreaks of calf diarrhea are large herd size, high stocking density, lack of a large sheltered area, poor drainage with standing water in the nursing area, failing to separate cows and heifers, poor nutrition, and a large number of heifers in the herd.[94-96] Avoid running cows or heifers through a small calving area (e.g., one particular corral or a barn). These rapidly become contaminated and a source of neonatal infection. Small herds, fewer than 40 cows, have a lower incidence of scour problems. Large herds may be best split into groups of 50 to 75 head and managed separately. Stocking density is important; cattle managed at pasture with large amounts of space have less diarrhea than those managed more intensively in corrals at calving time. However, if the weather is adverse, cattle managed at pasture will crowd together into a small space if adequate shelter is not available. There should be a minimum of 100 m² and ideally 200 m² (1000 to 2000 ft²) of area per cow. This area must be clean and sheltered from adverse weather. Damp conditions and standing water are a major risk factor for scours, particularly if more than 5% of the nursing area is affected. Contaminated water can be ingested and directly infect calves. Damp or muddy conditions favor the accumulation of dirt on the flanks, udder, and teats of the cow, where it will be ingested during nursing or grooming. The calving and nursing areas should be well drained, and any standing water should be fenced off. Drinking water should be provided from a clean source. Separating cows and heifers before calving is critically important. This allows the heifers to receive better nutrition. Calves born to heifers are much more likely to develop diarrhea; by separating these high-risk calves, spread to the rest of the herd is reduced. The diet fed to the cows should be complete and balanced. A high percentage of heifers, more than 20%, indicates herd expansion. However, it is also a risk factor for scours. When herds are being expanded it is particularly important to ensure that all other aspects of management are optimized. Another practice that may be beneficial is having an isolation area to treat diarrheic calves. This is likely to be of particular benefit for early cases, before contagion spreads throughout the facilities. Producers should be discouraged from buying in calves to replace a calf lost to dystocia or disease—this is an easy way to import disease.

In operations in which calves are hand reared, it is important to ensure that calves get adequate colostral antibody intake at an early age. This may help protect against enteric disease and definitely helps protect against secondary septicemia.[76,88,90,97,98] The next most important factor is cleanliness; at calving both cows and calving area should be clean. The calf-rearing facility must be clean, the feeding utensils must be clean at every feeding, and the feed must be clean. Cleanliness requires constant attention. A variety of factors have been implicated in increasing the risk of calf diarrhea or fecal excretion of cryptosporidia (Table 21-3). In general, calves have least

Table 21-3

Factors Associated with Risk of Diarrhea or Cryptosporidial Infection in Hand-Reared Calves

Risk Factor	Increased Risk	Decreased Risk
Calving Area	Being born in loose housing	
Many cows in maternity pen	Yes	
Floor of maternity pen	Soil	Concrete
Daily removal of soiled bedding from maternity pen and calf-raising areas	No	Yes
Ease of calving	Assistance	No assistance
Cleanliness of cows	Dirty	Clean
Feeding Method	Use of a nipple	Feeding from bucket
Number of milk feeds a day	One	Two
Feeding Concentrate	None	Yes
Solid food	High-moisture ear corn	
Building	Damp	Dry
Bedding	Damp	Dry
Ammonia smell in building	Present	None
Restraint method for calves	Tying by a collar	Loose
Quarantine Facilities for Sick Calves or Cows	Yes	No
Stocking Density	Tie stall: Less than 1.6 m² per calf	Tie stall: More than 1.6 m²
	Free stall: Less than 1 m² per calf	Free stall: More than 1 m²
Placing calf pens against a wall	Yes	No
Vaccination Against Enteric Pathogens	Yes	Vaccination against enteric disease caused by *Escherichia coli*
Calf rearer	Adult male	Women or children
Herd Size	Large	

(From data in references 98-103.)

problems if they are fed whole cow's milk or milk replacers made only from dairy products. If waste milk is fed to calves, it is best to pasteurize the milk before it is fed.

References

1. UDSA: Dairy 2002. Part I: Reference of Dairy Health and Management in the United States USDA:APHIS:VS:CEAH. NRRC Building B., M.S. 2E7, 2150 Centre Avenue, Fort Collins, CO 80526–8117, 2002.
2. USDA: Part II: Reference of 1997 Beef Cow-Calf Health & Health Management Practices. Centers for Epidemiology and Animal Health, USDA:APHIS:VS, attn. NAHMS, 555 South Howes, Fort Collins, CO 80521, 1997.
3. Bouda J, Doubek J, Medina-Cruz M et al: Pathophysiology of severe diarrhoea and suggested intravenous fluid therapy in calves of different ages under field conditions, *Acta Veterinaria Brno* 66:87, 1997.
4. McLaren IM, Wray C: Epidemiology of *Salmonella typhimurium* infection in calves: persistence of salmonellae on calf units, *Vet Rec* 129:461, 1991.
5. Radke BR, McFall M, Radostits SM: Salmonella Muenster infection in a dairy herd, *Can Vet J* 43:443, 2002.
6. Snodgrass DR, Terzolo HR, Sherwood D et al: Aetiology of diarrhoea in young calves, *Vet Rec* 119:31, 1986.
7. Waltner-Toews D, Martin SW, Meek AH: An epidemiological study of selected calf pathogens in dairy farms in southwestern Ontario, *Can J Vet Res* 50:307, 1986.
8. Athanassious R, Marsolais M, Assaff R et al: Detection of bovine coronavirus and type A rotavirus in neonatal calf diarrhea and winter dysentery of cattle in Quebec: evaluation of three diagnostic methods, *Can Vet J* 35:163, 1994.
9. Bulgin MS, Ward ACS, Barrett DP et al: Detection of rotavirus and coronavirus shedding in two beef cow herds in Idaho, *Can Vet J* 30:235, 1989.
10. Gelinas AM, Boutin M, Sasseville AMJ et al: Bovine coronaviruses associated with enteric and respiratory diseases in Canadian dairy cattle display different reactivities to anti-HE monoclonal antibodies and distinct amino acid changes in their HE, S and ns4.9 protein, *Virus Res* 76:43, 2001.
11. Hasoksuz M, Sreevatsan S, Cho-Kyoung Oh et al: Molecular analysis of the S1 subunit of the spike glycoprotein of respiratory and enteric bovine coronavirus isolates, *Virus Res* 84:101, 2002.
12. Mebus CA, Stair EL, Rhodes MB et al: Pathology of neonatal calf diarrhea induced by a coronavirus-like agent, *Vet Pathol* 10:45, 1973.
13. Traven M, Naslund K, Linde N et al: Experimental reproduction of winter dysentery in lactating cows using BCV: comparison with BCV infection in milk-fed calves, *Vet Microbiol* 81:127, 2001.
14. Tsunemitsu H, Smith DR, Saif LJ: Experimental inoculation of adult dairy cows with bovine coronavirus and detection of coronavirus in feces by RT-PCR, *Arch Virol* 144:167, 1999.
15. Bolin SR, Ridpath JF: Differences in virulence between two noncytopathic bovine viral diarrhea viruses in calves, *Am J Vet Res* 53:2157, 1992.
16. Castrucci G, Frigeri F, Osburn BI et al: A study of pathogenetic aspects of bovine viral diarrhea virus infection, *Arch Virol* 3(suppl):101, 1991.
17. Corapi WV, French TW, Dubovi EJ: Severe thrombocytopenia in young calves experimentally infected with noncytopathic bovine viral diarrhea virus, *J Virol* 63:3934, 1989.
18. Hall GA, Bridger JC, Brooker BE et al: Lesions of gnotobiotic calves experimentally infected with a calicivirus-like (Newbury) agent, *Vet Pathol* 21:208, 1984.
19. Torgerson PR, Dalgleish R, Gibbs HA: Mucosal disease in a cow and her suckled calf, *Vet Rec* 125:530-531, 1989.
20. Acres SD, Laing CJ, Saunders JR et al: Acute undifferentiated neonatal diarrhea in beef calves. I. Occurrence and distribution of infectious agents, *Can J Comp Med* 39:116, 1975.
21. Acres SD: Enterotoxigenic *Escherichia coli* infection in newborn calves, *J Dairy Sci* 68:229-256, 1985.
22. Bywater RJ: Some effects of *Escherichia coli* enterotoxin on unidirectional fluxes of water and sodium in calf Thiry-Vella loops, *Res Vet Sci* 14:35, 1973.
23. Gulati BR, Sharma VK, Taku AK: Occurrence and enterotoxigenicity of F17 fimbriae bearing *Escherichia coli* from calf diarrhoea, *Vet Rec* 131:348, 1992.
24. Mahdi-Saeed A, Bowersock T, Runnels L et al: The role of pathogenic *Escherichia coli* in the etiology of veal calf hemorrhagic enteritis, *Prevent Vet Med* 17:65-75, 1993.
25. Moon HW, Whipp SC, Skartvedt SM: Etiologic diagnosis of diarrheal disease of calves: frequency and methods for detecting enterotoxin and K99 antigen production by *Escherichia coli*, *Am J Vet Res* 37:1025, 1976.
26. Aidar L, Penteado AS, Trabulsi LR et al: Subtypes of intimin among non-toxigenic *Escherichia coli* from diarrheic calves in Brazil, *Can J Vet Res* 64:15, 2000.
27. Fischer J, Maddox C, Moxley R et al: Pathogenicity of a bovine attaching effacing *Escherichia coli* isolate lacking Shiga-like toxins, *Am J Vet Res* 55:991, 1994.
28. Janke BH, Francis DH, Collins JE et al: Attaching and effacing *Escherichia coli* infection as a cause of diarrhea in young calves, *J Am Vet Med Assoc* 196:897, 1990.
29. Levine MM: *Escherichia coli* that cause diarrhea: enterotoxigenic, enteropathogenic, enteroinvasive, enterohemorrhagic and enteroadherent, *J Infect Dis* 155:377-389, 1987.
30. Mainil JG, Duchesnes CJ, Whipp SC et al: Shiga-like toxin production and attaching effacing activity of *Escherichia coli* associated with calf diarrhea, *Am J Vet Res* 48:743, 1987.
31. Mercado EC, Gioffre A, Rodriguez SM et al: Non-O157 Shiga toxin-producing *Escherichia coli* isolated from diarrhoeic calves in Argentina, *J Vet Med B* 51:82, 2004.
32. Pearson GR, Watson CA, Hall GA et al: Natural infection with an attaching and effacing *Escherichia coli* in the small and large intestines of a calf with diarrhoea, *Vet Rec* 124:297-299, 1989.
33. Schoonderwoerd M, Clarke RC, van Dreumel AA et al: Colitis in calves: natural and experimental infection with a verotoxin-producing strain of *Escherichia coli* O111:NM, *Can J Vet Res* 52:484, 1988.
34. Stordeur P, China B, Charlier G et al: Clinical signs, reproduction of attaching/effacing lesions, and enterocyte invasion after oral inoculation of an O118 enterohaemorrhagic *Escherichia coli* in neonatal calves, *Microbes Infect* 2:17, 2000.
35. Wray C, McLaren I, Pearson GR: Occurrence of "attaching and effacing" lesions in the small intestine of calves experimentally infected with bovine isolates of verocytotoxic *E coli*, *Vet Rec* 125:365, 1989.
36. Bost S, Roels S, Mainil J: Necrotoxigenic *Escherichia coli* type-2 invade and cause diarrhoea during experimental infection in colostrum-restricted newborn calves, *Vet Microbiol* 81:315, 2001.
37. Osek J: Characterization of necrotoxigenic *Escherichia coli* (NTEC) strains isolated from healthy calves in Poland, *J Vet Med B* 48:641, 2001.
38. Anderson BC: *Cryptosporidium muris* in cattle, *Vet Rec* 129:20, 1991.
39. Anderson BC, Bulgin MS: Enteritis caused by *Cryptosporidium* in calves, *Vet Med Small Animal Clin* 76:865-868, 1981.

40. Casemore DP, Sands RL, Curry A: *Cryptosporidium* species: a "new" human pathogen, *J Clin Pathol* 38:1321, 1985.

41. Morin M, Lariviere S, Lallier R: Pathological and microbiological observations made on spontaneous cases of acute neonatal calf diarrhea, *Can J Comp Med* 40:228, 1976.

42. Peeters JE, Villacorta I, Vanopdenbosch E et al: *Cryptosporidium parvum* in calves: kinetics and immunoblot analysis of specific serum and local antibody responses (immunoglobulin A [IgA], IgG, and IgM) after natural and experimental infections, *Infect Immun* 60:2309-2316, 1992.

43. Reif JS, Wimmer L, Smith JA et al: Human cryptosporidiosis associated with an epizootic in calves, *Am J Public Health* 79:1528, 1989.

44. Tzipori S, Angus K, Campbell I et al: *Cryptosporidium*: evidence for a single-species genus, *Infect Immun* 30:884, 1980.

45. Huetink RE, van der Giessen JW, Noordhuizen JP, Ploegar HW: Epidemiology of *Cryptosporidium* spp. and *Giardia duodenalis* on a dairy farm, *Vet Parasitol* 102:53, 2001.

46. O'Handley RM, Cockwill C, Jelinski M et al: Effects of repeat fenbendazole treatment in dairy calves with giardiosis on cyst excretion, clinical signs and production, *Vet Parasitol* 89:209, 2000.

47. Olson ME, Guselle NJ, O'Handley RM et al: Giardia and cryptosporidium in dairy calves in British Columbia, *Can Vet J* 38:703, 1997.

48. Xiao LH, Herd RP, Rings DM: Concurrent infections of *Giardia* and *Cryptosporidium* on two Ohio farms with calf diarrhea, *Vet Parasitol* 51:41, 1993.

49. Ewaschuk JB, Zello GA, Naylor JM, Brocks DR: Metabolic acidosis: separation methods and biological relevance of organic acids and lactic acid enantiomers, *J Chromatogr B Analyt Technol Biomed Life Sci* 781:39, 2002.

50. Zello GA, Abeysekara AWAS, Wassef AWA et al: Evidence for D-lactic acid as a neurotoxic agent in acidotic diseases, *S African J Clin Nutr* 49:291, 2005.

51. Naylor JM, A retrospective study of the relationship between clinical signs and severity of acidosis in diarrheic calves, *Can Vet J* 30:577-580, 1989.

52. Fisher EW, de la Fuente GH: Water and electrolyte studies in newborn calves with particular reference to the effects of diarrhoea, *Res Vet Sci* 13:315, 1972.

53. Lewis LD, Phillips RW: Water and electrolyte losses in neonatal calves with acute diarrhea: a complete balance study, *Cornell Vet* 62:596, 1972.

54. Lorenz I, Rademacher G: Bedeutung und Therapie der Hyponatriamie bei alteren Kalbern mit Durchfall. (Incidence and therapy of hyponatraemia in older calves with diarrhea), *Tierarztliche Praxis Ausgabe G, Grosstiere/Nutztiere* 27:268, 1999.

55. Whitten EH, Phillips RW: In vitro intestinal exchange of Na+, K+, Cl-,3H2O in experimental bovine neonatal enteritis, *Am J Dig Dis* 16:891, 1971.

56. Ewaschuk JB, Naylor JM, Zello GA: Anion gap correlates with serum D- and DL-Lactate concentrations in diarrheic calves, *J Vet Int Med* 17:940, 2003.

57. Naylor JM: Severity and nature of acidosis in diarrheic calves over and under one week of age, *Can Vet J* 28:168, 1987.

58. Petersen C: D-lactic acidosis, *Nutr Clin Pract* 20:634, 2005.

59. Lorenz I, Gentile A, Klee W: Investigations of D-lactate metabolism and the clinical signs of D-lactataemia in calves, *Vet Rec* 156:412, 2005.

60. Abeysekara S, Naylor JM, Wassef AW et al: D-lactic acid–induced neurotoxicity in a calf model. *Am J Physiol Endocrinol Metab* 293:E558-E565, 2007.

61. Kasari TR, Naylor JM: Further studies on the clinical features and clinicopathological findings of a syndrome of metabolic acidosis with minimal dehydration in neonatal calves, *Can J Vet Res* 50:502, 1986.

62. Schelcher F, Marcillaud S, Braun JP et al: Metabolic acidosis without dehydration and no or minimal diarrhoea in suckler calves is caused by hyper D-lactatemia, *Proc of XX World Buiatrics Congress* 371, 1998.

63. Lorenz I: Investigations on the influence of serum D-lactate levels on clinical signs in calves with metabolic acidosis, *Vet J* 168:323, 2004.

64. Fisher EW: Death in neonatal calf diarrhoea, *Br Vet J* 121:132, 1965.

65. Fisher EW, McEwan AD: Death in neonatal calf diarrhoea. Part II: The role of oxygen and potassium, *Br Vet J* 123:4, 1967.

66. Naylor JM: Alkalizing abilities of calf oral electrolyte solutions, *Proc World Congress Dis Cattle* 14:326, 1986.

67. Naylor JM: Effects of oral electrolyte solutions on clotting of milk, *J Am Vet Med Assoc* 201:1026, 1992.

68. Heath SE, Naylor JM, Guedo BL et al: The effects of feeding milk to diarrheic calves supplemented with oral electrolytes, *Can J Vet Res* 53:477, 1989.

69. Gottardo FS, Mattiello S, Cozzi G et al: The provision of drinking water to veal calves for welfare purposes, *J Anim Sci* 80:2362, 2002.

70. Ganong WF: Regulation of extracellular fluid composition & volume. In *Review of medical physiology*, ed 13, Norwalk, Conn, 1987, Appleton & Lange, pp 607-614.

71. Naylor JM: Evaluation of the total carbon dioxide apparatus and pH meter for the determination of acid-base status in diarrheic and healthy calves, *Can Vet J* 28:45, 1987.

72. Booth AJ, Naylor JM: Correction of metabolic acidosis in diarrheal calves by oral administration of electrolyte solutions with or without bicarbonate, *J Am Vet Med Assoc* 191:62, 1987.

73. Kasari TR, Naylor JM: Clinical evaluation of sodium bicarbonate, sodium L-lactate and sodium acetate for the treatment of acidosis in diarrheic calves, *J Am Vet Med Assoc* 187:392, 1986.

74. Ewaschuk JB, Naylor JM, Zello GA: D-lactate production and excretion in diarrheic calves, *J Vet Int Med* 18:744, 2004.

75. Constable PD: Antimicrobial use in the treatment of calf diarrhea, *J Vet Int Med* 18:8, 2004.

76. Fecteau G, Van Metre DC, Pare J et al: Bacteriological culture of blood from critically ill neonatal calves, *Can Vet J* 38:95, 1997.

77. Lofstedt J, Dohoo JR: A model for the prediction of sepsis in diarrheic neonatal calves, *Proc Am Coll Vet Int Med* 14, pp 473-474, 1996.

78. Jarvie BD, Trotz-Williams LA, McKnight DR et al: Effect of halofuginone lactate on the occurrence of *Cryptosporidium parvum* and growth of neonatal dairy calves, *J Dairy Sci* 88:1801, 2005.

79. Villacorta I, Peeters JE, Vanopdenbosch E et al: Efficacy of halofuginone lactate against *Cryptosporidium parvum* in calves, *Antimicrob Agents Chemother* 35:283, 1991.

80. Barnett SC, Sischo WM, Moore DA et al: Evaluation of flunixin meglumine as an adjunct treatment for diarrhea in dairy calves, *J Am Vet Med Assoc* 223:1329, 2003.

81. Abdala AA, Zimmerman G, Calvinho LF et al: Evaluacion de la eficacia de un probiotico incorporado a un sustituto lacteo y a leche entera, en la crianza de terneros (Efficacy of a probiotic added to whole milk and to a milk substitute), *Revista de Medicina Veterinaria Buenos Aires* 83:196, 2002.

82. Ewaschuk JB, Zello GA, Naylor JM: *Lactobacillus GG* does not affect D-lactic acidosis in diarrheic calves, in a clinical setting, *J Vet Int Med* 20:614, 2006.

83. Ewaschuk JB, Naylor JM, Chirino-Trejo M et al: *Lactobacillus GG* is a potential probiotic for calves, *Can J Vet Res* 68:249, 2004.

84. Goncalves GD, Santos GT, Rigolon LP et al: Influencia da adicao de probioticos na dieta sobre o estado sanitario e

desempenho de bezerros da raca Holandesa. (The influence of probiotics addition in the diet on the sanitary state and the performance of calves Holstein), *Brazil J Vet Res Animal Sci* 37:74, 2000.

85. Muscato TV, Tedeschi LO, Russell JB: The effect of ruminal fluid preparations on the growth and health of newborn, milk-fed dairy calves, *J Dairy Sci* 85:648, 2002.

86. Timmerman HM, Mulder L, Everts H et al: Health and growth of veal calves fed milk replacers with or without probiotics, *J Dairy Sci* 88:2154, 2005.

87. Dardillat J, Trillat G, Larvor P: Colostrum immunoglobulin concentration in cows: relationship with their calf mortality and with the colostrum quality of their female offspring, *Ann Recherches Vet* 9:375, 1978.

88. Naylor JM, Kronfeld DS, Bech-Nielsen S et al: Plasma total protein measurement for prediction of disease and mortality in calves, *J Am Vet Med Assoc* 171:635, 1977.

89. Parreno V, Bejar C, Vagnozzi A et al: Modulation by colostrum-acquired maternal antibodies of systemic and mucosal antibody responses to rotavirus in calves experimentally challenged with bovine rotavirus, *Vet Immunol Immunopathol* 100:7, 2004.

90. Postema HJ, Mol J: Risk of disease in veal calves: relationships between colostrum-management, serum immunoglobulin levels and risk of disease, *Zentralblatt fur Veterinarmedizin A* 31:751, 1984.

91. Smith HW: Observations on the aetiology of neonatal diarrhoea (scours) in calves, *J Path Bact* 84:147, 1962.

92. Snodgrass DR, Stewart J, Taylor J et al: Diarrhoea in dairy calves reduced by feeding colostrum from cows vaccinated with rotavirus, *Res Vet Sci* 32:70, 1982.

93. Woode GN, Jones J, Bridger J: Levels of colostral antibodies against neonatal calf diarrhoea virus, *Vet Rec* 97:148, 1975.

94. Clement JC, King ME, Salman MD et al: Use of epidemiologic principles to identify risk factors associated with the development of diarrhea in calves in five beef herds, *J Am Vet Med Assoc* 207:1334, 1995.

95. Dutil L, Fecteau G, Bouchard E et al: A questionnaire on the health, management, and performance of cow-calf herds in Quebec, *Can Vet J* 40:649, 1999.

96. Schumann FJ, Townsend HG, Naylor JM: Risk factors for mortality from diarrhea in beef calves in Alberta, *Can J Vet Res* 54:366, 1990.

97. Curtis CR, Scarlett JM, Erb HN et al: Path model of individual-calf risk factors for calfhood morbidity and mortality in New York Holstein herds, *Prev Vet Med* 6:43, 1988.

98. Harp JA, Woodmansee DB, Moon HW: Effects of colostral antibody on susceptibility of calves to *Cryptosporidium parvum* infection, *Am J Vet Res* 50:2117, 1989.

99. Frank NA, Kaneene JB: Management risk factors associated with calf diarrhea in Michigan dairy herds, *J Dairy Sci* 76:1313, 1993.

100. Greene HJ, Bakheit HA: A study of the aetiology, epidemiology and control of calf diarrhoea in Ireland, *Irish Vet J* 38:63, 1984.

101. James RE, McGilliard ML, Hartman DA: Calf mortality in Virginia Dairy Herd Improvement herds, *J Dairy Sci* 67:908, 1984.

102. Kertz AF, Reutzel LF, Mahoney JH: Ad libitum water intake by neonatal calves and its relationship to calf starter intake, weight gain, feces score, and season, *J Dairy Sci* 67:2964, 1984.

103. Lorino T, Daudin JJ, Robin S et al: Factors associated with time to neonatal diarrhea in French beef calves, *Prevent Vet Med* 68:91, 2005.

104. Matoock MY, El-Bably MA, El-Bahy MM: Management practices for minimizing environmental risk factors associated with *Cryptosporidium* in dairy calves, *Vet Med J Giza* 53:565, 2005.

Recommended Readings

Abeysekara S, Naylor JM, Wassef AW et al: D-lactic acid–induced neurotoxicity in a calf model. *Am J Physiol Endocrinol Metab* 293:E558-E565, 2007.

Constable PD, Walker PG, Morin DE et al: Clinical and laboratory assessment of hydration status of neonatal calves with diarrhea, *J Am Vet Med Assoc* 212:991, 1998.

Sigaard-Andersen O: Titratable acid or base of body fluids, *Ann New York Acad Sci* 133:41, 1966.

CHAPTER 22

Helminth Parasites of the Ruminant Gastrointestinal Tract

THOMAS M. CRAIG

NEMATODE INFECTIONS OF CATTLE

The economically important nematode parasites of ruminants residing in the gastrointestinal tract all have a similar life story outside the host but vary in where they reside within the tract, what they do to the host, and in which host they are most likely found. Even though the life cycle is similar to the geographic range, seasonality of transmission varies considerably and therefore a parasite of considerable importance in one region may be of minor significance in another. Likewise, a host that evolved in the same environmental conditions that is preferable to a species of parasite is more likely to have evolved an array of mechanisms that enable it to either resist the parasite or rebound from its specific effects. The ability to quickly recover the effects of parasitism is termed *resilience.*

The disease resulting from infection by nematodes is, to a large extent, a numbers game, and individual animals with the greatest numbers of parasites are most likely to exhibit signs of disease. In any population of hosts, some individuals will be more adversely affected than others because of sex, age, prior experience with the parasite, stage in the reproductive cycle, behavior, and genetic predisposition to presence or lack of resistance or resilience factors. Because of the differences in the pathogenicity or virulence of different parasite species, or both, the number of worms required to cause disease varies immensely.

The eggs produced by most species of gastrointestinal nematodes are indistinguishable from one another so that, with few exceptions, the finding of eggs in the feces does not tell you which parasite species produced the egg. However, the host species, age, geographic region, time of year and clinical signs exhibited may enable a clinician to give a best guess as to which parasite is most likely to be encountered. The genera that produce the thin-shelled, segmented, strongyloid-type eggs are by far the most likely to be associated with disease. However, the parasites involved can only be differentiated by examination of adult worms or by culturing to the infective third larval stage. Identification of worms by DNA profiles is possible but, with thousands of eggs in the feces of some hosts, is not a practical alternative at this time.

The genera of parasites encountered in most ruminant species are the same, but the parasite species tend to be limited to a few hosts. Even if they can survive in an alternate host, they do not tend to be successful in some hosts. A successful parasite is one that successfully establishes within its host, produces eggs that are able to hatch, and has larvae that are able to develop and infect another host. If a parasite species is able to keep its DNA going, it is successful.

Killing or even severely disabling the host is not in the best interest of either host or parasite. In the best of all possible worlds, the parasite infects the host and the host is able to tolerate a level of parasitism without undue problems. The host responds to the presence of the parasite so that it is able to either withstand the parasite's deleterious effects or make the environment at the parasite level unsuitable for its continued well-being and expel the parasite. Some host responses may result in clinical disease but rid the host of its parasite load or make it unlikely that new parasites can establish in large numbers. Resistance to infection is augmented by reexposure to parasites, and equilibrium is reached when populations of both the parasite and host survive in a state in which neither wins nor loses. However, in agriculture production units where the emphasis is on the production of animals with limited resources, this equilibrium is often disrupted.

Most infections in cattle are a combination of several parasitic species, but a few stand out as being more economically important than the others. The most important parasite of cattle in temperate regions of the world is *Ostertagia ostertagi.* The parasite is pathogenic and may cause severe clinical disease. Even when encountered in comparatively low numbers, it causes anorexia and an inability to efficiently convert forage into milk or meat. The economic importance of this parasite was not fully appreciated until the availability of anthelmintics that were extremely effective against this parasite. The primary economic effects of these anthelmintics are those of increased milk production and the increased growth rate in calves. Not only do the cows produce more milk but also there is evidence that they breed back more rapidly following calving. Not all trials have replicated these findings because there is considerable variability among herds, geographic localities, and years.

The most common genus encountered in younger cattle is *Cooperia,* and from the standpoint of egg numbers it is often the dominant worm present. However, when compared with *Ostertagia, Cooperia* is of lesser clinical significance. The genus has possibly become more important in recent years because it has apparently changed from a worm that was tolerant of macrocyclic lactones to a genus that may be resistant to this class of anthelmintics. Other genera that are locally important include *Trichostrongylus, Bunostomum, Oesophagostomum, Nematodirus,* and *Haemonchus.* At this time, control programs directed toward *Ostertagia* are likely to aid in the control of other species.

Life Cycle

All of the important gastrointestinal nematodes of cattle have a direct life cycle (i.e., eggs are passed in the feces; the L1 larva hatches and feeds on bacteria in the feces; and the larva molts to the L2 stage, feeds, and then molts to the L3 stage). The exception to this is *Nematodirus,* which has a huge egg. Larval development of *Nematodirus* to the L3 stage takes place within the eggshell. *Nematodirus* is normally predominant in environments that are unfavorable for the development and survival of nematode larvae such as in arid climates or where there are long cold winters. For the genera, *Toxocara* and *Trichuris,* larvated eggs are the infective stage. The eggs require development to the infective stage outside the host, but once developed, the egg remains infective for prolonged periods of time.

The L3 is the infective stage and is encased in the cuticle of the L2, which acts as a sheath in protecting the larva from desiccation. The L3 can now leave the fecal pat and ascend vegetation in a film of water. The sheath protects the larva but also prevents its feeding, so the energy it obtained during the L1 and L2 stages will be eventually depleted. Development and survival are dependent on ambient temperature, with development being faster at high temperatures and survival longer at lower temperatures. The larva can only move out of the fecal pat in a film of moisture but may be passively carried into the soil by burrowing insects, earthworms, or other environmental influences.

Provided there is sufficient moisture to allow larvae to move from the dung pat onto the vegetation, they are ingested by grazing cattle. In the rumen the larva exsheaths under the influence of low oxygen tension, high carbon dioxide, and body temperature. The L3 then moves to the abomasum, small intestine, or large intestine, the normal abodes of the worm species. Within a short time the larva molts to the L4, which begins to feed. The larva molts to the L5 or juvenile adult or, depending on several factors, may cease development at the early L4 stage. If normal development occurs, the worms mature and begin producing eggs approximately 3 weeks after being acquired from the pasture. If not, the worm enters hypobiosis (arrested or inhibited development), a state akin to diapause in insects, which is a cessation of metabolic activity within the host. The parasite survives by evading unfavorable conditions in the host or environment. Hypobiotic larvae are not recognized by the host immune system, so even if the host has the ability to expel that species of worm it is unable to do so. The state of hypobiosis avoids the possibility that if the worm did mature it would be damaged by the hosts'

immune response or the resulting larvae would be exposed to unfavorable environmental conditions. Larvae may remain in a state of hypobiosis for prolonged periods of time and then resume development, often in synchrony, with larvae acquired over a considerable time span.

Ostertagia

O. ostertagi is the most important species of nematode throughout most of the temperate world and may even cause disease in adult cattle. The strategies directed toward the control of parasitic gastroenteritis are based on *Ostertagia,* but the timing must be different geographically. For instance, *Ostertagia* is transmitted in the northern United States and Canada during the summer and autumn and during the winter and spring in the southern United States and is absent from south Texas and Florida. The disease ostertagiosis is caused by abomasal damage from maturing worms emerging from the abomasal glands. Two disease patterns are recognized: Type I disease occurs during the grazing period, which is seasonal (i.e., summer/autumn in the North and autumn/winter in the South). The disease is caused by the emergence of immature worms from the gastric glands 10 to14 days after the ingestion of infective larvae. Type II is seen months after pasture exposure such as during the winter/spring (North) or autumn (South) and is caused by the simultaneous emergence of previously arrested larvae that were acquired over an extended period of time during the grazing season. Larvae remain hypobiotic (usually several months) within the gastric glands until some stimulus triggers the resumption of their development.

Several factors have been implicated in the emergence of immature worms: (1) anthelmintic treatment removing adult worms, (2) change of diet (rapidly growing fresh forage), or (3) change in weather conditions. The extent of the damage depends on the number of larvae emerging at a given time. Simultaneous emergence of thousands of maturing worms from the gastric glands causes marked structural and physiologic changes within the abomasum. The abomasum becomes edematous with hypertrophy of gastric mucosa. Specialized cells of the gastric glands degenerate or are replaced by cuboidal mucus-secreting cells, resulting in lowered production of HCl and pepsinogen. The normal abomasal pH is 2 to 3. As the pH rises, the conversion of pepsinogen into pepsin decreases until diarrhea occurs followed by bacterial invasion of the gastric mucosa with sloughing.

Clinical Manifestations

Type I disease is associated with overstocking, especially in young cattle; there is a failure to gain weight and a dark green diarrhea (the color of the forage consumed). The calves become dehydrated and manifest a general unthrifty look. Death losses may occur. Most of the calves in a pasture will show signs of disease, beginning a month or so after exposure to a heavily infected pasture.

Pre–type II infection is a state of potential disease. An increase in numbers of larvae occur as they accumulate within the gastric glands, but there are no changes in abomasal activity. The cattle appear normal, although there may be an increase in serum pepsinogen levels.

Type II disease is manifest as severe emaciation with brown to green diarrhea. The cattle become dehydrated and may have intermandibular edema and even anemia. Death may occur in 1 to 2 weeks in most severe cases. Although only a small percentage of the calves in a population show signs of disease, the remainder of the herd does not grow to its genetic potential.

Treatment and Control

Treating to remove hypobiotic larvae and use anthelmintics, which have residual effects so that incoming larvae are destroyed before they can establish, is the basis of *Ostertagia* control. Winter treatment in the north and summer treatment in the south may accomplish this. Beef cows and their single suckled calves are the primary thrust of the basic program. *O. ostertagi* is a common parasite of cattle. After repeated exposure to the parasite, most cattle develop resistance to clinical disease. However, the goal of modern production is optimum productivity, not just freedom from disease. In regions of the country where cattle do not get sufficient exposure to *Ostertagia* to stimulate natural immunity, clinical disease can be seen in older cattle.

Resistance (immunity) to parasite infection appears to be primarily acquired but has a strong genetic component. Therefore species or breeds that evolved with their parasites have a greater chance of responding to those specific parasites. In the case of *Ostertagia*, Zebu cattle are generally unable or delayed in mounting an effective protective immune response. The immunity expressed is protection from disease, not infection. More or less, regular exposure is necessary to maintain resistance. However, exposure in almost all geographic regions is not constant but comes in waves, and the interval between waves may allow waning of resistance. In addition, the host's hormonal state may block the effectiveness of acquired immunity. Normally, males are more susceptible to parasitic worms, except during parturition and lactation, when females are at greatest risk. Cattle must be exposed to *Ostertagia* over time to stimulate a protective immune response. The worms also appear to have the capacity to reduce the immune competence of the host. If cattle are not exposed or minimally exposed so that they remain susceptible, this may explain the high incidence of adult ostertagiosis in cattle raised in arid areas compared with those in higher rainfall areas.

When dairy calves leave a stable or dry lot and enter the pasture, parasitic gastroenteritis infection is a major impediment to production. In climates where calves are stabled or kept in dry lots or where calves are weaned at birth, introduction to pasture forage and parasites can be overwhelming. With single suckled beef calves, the transition is easier and the provision of high-quality feed (milk) assures that the suckling calf will probably not show signs of disease. The exposure is lower than when calves are run as a group, and with an adequate nutritional intake they can compensate for numbers of parasites that may otherwise cause disease. Again, the ages of dairy and beef cattle are different when they suffer disease. The first 4 months on pasture is extremely dangerous for dairy calves, whereas beef calves do not usually show signs of disease until after weaning. In both groups the more dangerous parasites encountered in most areas are *Ostertagia* and *Cooperia* spp. During the summer, *Haemonchus placei*

can affect calves in much the same fashion as *H. contortus* does sheep or goats, with severe anemia being the most striking clinical sign. Even calves that are clinically normal benefit from removal of gastrointestinal parasites while remaining on pasture or into the feedlot.

Treating cattle with an anthelmintic that is effective against arrested larvae during the winter or summer is a strategic approach that kills worms before they do damage, and the cattle do not acquire a large population of worms following treatment. In adult cattle, benzimidazoles kill 60% to 85% of the arrested larvae, which may be sufficient if they are not reexposed. However, with macrolides (avermectins/milbemycins), calves, stockers, and replacements benefit not only from the enhanced removal of the larvae residing in the abomasum at the time of treatment but also from the residual effects of the macrolides killing incoming larvae of *Ostertagia* for 2 to 4 weeks or longer. Treatment during the warm season also affects warm-season parasites and lowers subsequent larval contamination of the pastures following spring or autumn rains.

Although suckling beef calves 3 months of age or older may benefit from deworming, it is essential to deworm calves after weaning because nutritional support from the dam is withdrawn then, exposing calves to greater vulnerability. Stocker cattle imported from regions with unfavorable conditions for parasite survival into regions with greater parasite loads are particularly susceptible to disease because they lack resistance. *Ostertagia*, *Cooperia*, and *Haemonchus* are problems in stockers and dairy replacement calves. When diagnosing cattle with worms, consider *Ostertagia* first but do not discount *Cooperia* and *Haemonchus* (Table 22-1).

Trichostrongylus

Trichostrongylus axei, the stomach hairworm, occurs in ruminants, horses, and swine is the smallest abomasal nematode. *T. axei* is seldom a primary pathogen but it contributes to the parasitic gastroenteritis complex. *T. axei* may cause weight loss and anorexia that is directly related to the numbers of adult worms present. The parasite often accompanies *Ostertagia* and is controlled when *Ostertagia* is controlled. Other species of *Trichostrongylus* are occasionally reported from cattle but cannot be considered generally important with the possible exception of young calves being grazed with small ruminants.

Haemonchus

Haemonchus placei, *Haemonchus similis*, and *Haemonchus contortus* are all seen in cattle. The first two species are generally recognized as being cattle parasites, with *H. similis* being restricted to the tropics and *H. placei* in both the tropical and temperate world. The speciation of *Haemonchus* is an open question, but molecular identification may help rectify the problem. Whatever the final decision as to species name, it is a genus that can exploit opportunities by having a wide host range, tremendous fecundity, and the ability to rapidly adapt to anthelmintics. *Haemonchus* is a warm-season parasite and undergoes hypobiosis during the winter or prolonged drought. Cattle generally become immune to disease caused by *Haemonchus* much

Table 22-1

Spectrum of Anthelmintic Activity Against Selected Ruminant Parasites

Parasite	ABZ	FBZ	OFZ	LEV	MOR	IVR	EPR	DOR	MOX	CLO	TRA
Ostertagia	X	X	X	X	X	X	X	X	X	O	O
Ostertagia L4	X	X	X	O	O	X	X	X	X	O	O
Haemonchus	X	X	X	X	X	X	X	X	X	O	O
Trichostrongylus	X	X	X	X	X	X	X	X	X	O	O
Cooperia	X	X	X	X	X	L	L	L	L	O	O
Nematodirus	X	X	X	X	X	L	L	L	L	O	O
Strongyloides	O	O	O	O	O	X	X	X	X	O	O
Bunostomum	X	X	X	X	O	O	X	X	X	O	O
Moniezia	X	X	X	O	O	O	O	O	O	O	O
Oesophagostomum	X	X	X	X	X	X	X	X	O	O	O
Trichuris	O	O	O	O	O	L	O	X	O	O	O
Dictyocaulus	X	X	X	X	O	X	X	X	X	O	O
Fasciola	O	O	O	O	O	O	O	O	O	X	X
Fascioloides	O	O	O	O	O	O	O	O	O	X	X

X = Effective against most populations; L = Limited efficacy against some populations; O = Ineffective or not tested.
ABZ, Albendazole (Valbazen); *CLO*, clorsulon (Curatrem, Ivomec Plus at low dose); *DOR*, doramectin (Dectomax); *EPR*, eprinomectin (Ivomec Eprinex); *FBZ*, fenbendazole (Safegard, Panacur); *IVR*, ivermectin (Ivomec, Ivomec Plus, Phonectin, Double Impact, ProMectin, Ultramectin, Ivercide, Ivermectin, Promectin)*; *LEV*, levamisole (Totalon, Levamisole, Levasole, Prohibit); *MOR*, morantel (Rumatel); *MOX*, moxidectin (Cadetting); *OFZ*, oxfendazole (Synanthic); *TRA*, triclabendazole (Fasinex).
*The following products are labeled but have not been tested for efficacy under controlled conditions: Phonectin, Double Impact, ProMectin, Ultramectin, Ivercide, Ivermectin, and Promectin.

more readily than do goats or sheep, but calves are fully susceptible to the parasite. *Haemonchus*, the largest worm in the abomasum, is an avid bloodsucker. The females are 2.5 to 3 cm in length with a barber pole or candy cane appearance of the white, egg-filled, uterus wrapped around the blood-filled intestine. Pastures grazed by large numbers of susceptible calves have billions of infective larvae in them, become killing grounds. Anemia with packed cell volumes (PCVs) occasionally in the single digits and hypoproteinemia as seen by intermandibular edema (bottle jaw) are the primary signs of disease.

A recent report of *Haemonchus* resistant to macrolide and benzimidazole anthelmintics in stocker calves in North America is concerning. The resistance was seen in calves that originated from many farms and were held on common small pastures to complete the weaning process. The calves are vaccinated against respiratory and other viral and bacterial diseases and administered an anthelmintic at this time. If they are then placed on a warm season perennial pasture, it may be laden with larvae that survived the winter or the calves may be carrying a few worms that escaped the anthelmintic. After a period of grazing, the numbers of infective larvae in the pasture rapidly escalates because of the susceptibility of the calves and fecundity of the worms. Disease is seen later in the grazing season if weather conditions are favorable for the transmission of the parasite. However, if the calves are grazed on a cool-season annual pasture, even if a few worms survive the anthelmintic, the exposure level never becomes sufficient to cause clinical disease.

Cooperia

Cooperia spp. inhabit the small intestine and are associated with anorexia, villous atrophy, and diarrhea when large numbers of parasites are present. As a result there will be lowered weight gains. However, when *Cooperia* spp. are present, there are usually also abomasal helminths and the combination of worms is more debilitating than each species contributes in its own right. As effective treatment of *Ostertagia* has become more widely practiced, *Cooperia* has become more common and perhaps its importance should be reassessed. From the time of first release, macrolide anthelmintics have not been as effective against *Cooperia* as with other genera. This tolerance has evolved into anthelmintic resistance in several countries. As calves mature, *Cooperia* disappear, apparently because of acquired immunity, and by the time calves are 1 year of age it is unusual to find infection except in cattle never before exposed to the local species. Because macrolide anthelmintics are not as effective against this genus in light stockers or dairy calves, if *Ostertagia* is controlled, other anthelmintics may be preferable. Some evidence indicates that in the absence of other gastrointestinal nematodes, *Cooperia* may be of greater importance in causing disease than previously thought.

Nematodirus

Nematodirus helvetianus (commonly called the *twisted wireworm*) adults are 10 to 25 mm in length and coiled in a springlike fashion. The genus is characterized by large football-shaped eggs (140-180 μm × 75-90 μm) containing eight cells, which do not hatch until the L3 has developed within the egg. The parasite is seen in dry or frigid climates where other genera die because of desiccation. The apparent prevalence of *Nematodirus* is increasing in cattle as more ranchers use avermectins and milbemycins for treatment. These drugs are effective against abomasal parasites but are less effective against *Nematodirus* and *Cooperia*. Control by treating only the young to lower pasture contamination for the next year and using an anthelmintic other than a macrolide may be preferred. Strategic treatment effective for other genera may not work with this parasite.

Bunostomum

The hookworm *Bunostomum phlebotomum* is a large (3 cm), robust, white worm capable of causing anemia and black tarry feces in calves. Infection can occur both by ingestion or skin penetration and may be a problem in young calves housed in moist environments, especially in the tropics. The eggs are large, dark, and rectangular, resembling trichostrongyle-type eggs (i.e., thin shelled and segmented [100×50 μm]), but they have rough eggshells, often with clinging debris. The prepatent period is 1 to 2 months, and apparently hypobiosis is a strategy for avoiding prolonged drought conditions. *Bunostomum* can be controlled with anthelmintics, but environmental sanitation with dry bed grounds is more realistic in the long term. Calves establish rapid immunity to reinfection. In geographic areas where anthelmintics are widely used, the parasite has largely disappeared but should be considered a cause of anemia in other areas.

Strongyloides

Strongyloides papillosus is the first helminth parasite seen in calves. It is shared with other ruminant species. The parasite has alternative free-living and parasitic generations. The eggs are 50 to 60×30 μm, thin shelled, and larvated when passed in the feces. Disease is usually not associated with the infection, although occasionally loose feces are seen. *Strongyloides* may rarely cause acute death because of cardiac arrhythmias in calves bedded in contaminated sawdust. Sanitation is key to control, and many modern anthelmintics are effective against the worms in the intestine.

Toxocara (Neoascaris)

Toxocara vitulorum is a large, robust worm up to 30 cm long with three large, prominent lips. The eggs, 75 to 95 $\times$ 60 to 75 μm, are dark, subglobular, and single celled with a thick-pitted shell and are passed by calves because transmammary acquisition is the only proven method of transmission. Clinical disease is rare because most calves undergo spontaneous cure by 3 to 5 months of age. Treatment with piperazine and probably most broad-spectrum anthelmintics should be effective. The pig ascarid, *Ascaris suum*, occasionally develops to the adult stage in calves but cannot be considered an important parasite in this host.

Oesophagostomum

The adult *Oesophagostomum radiatum* lives in the large intestine, primarily the caecum of cattle. The larvae may be found from pylorus to anus in the gut mucosa. The adults are 1- to 2-cm, robust worms, the anterior ends of which are bent in a spiral, and they have inflations or vesicles. The eggs are 70 to 90 $\times$ 34 to 45 μm, thin shelled,

and segmented when passed. Before modern anthelmintics, *Oesophagostomum* was an important parasite during cool, wet seasons.

As with other intestinal nematodes, the life cycle is direct, but transmission can be through ingestion or skin penetration by infective L3 larvae. Once in the gut, larvae penetrate intestinal wall into mucosa and molt to L4, which emerge in 7 to 10 days in a susceptible host. However, nodules surrounding larvae are formed in hypersensitive hosts. The larvae may remain within the nodules for up to a year.

Broad-spectrum anthelmintics appear to be effective against this parasite, and cattle become resistant to infection. Apparently, larvae trapped in the nodules are not exposed to anthelmintics and, if some are able to emerge, they can contaminate an environment such as a feedlot with numerous larvae that are able to infect naive animals.

Trichuris

Trichuris spp. whipworms infect cattle. The adult worms are 3.5 to 8 cm with a long, threadlike anterior end and a short, thick posterior end. The eggs are approximately 75 $\times$ 35 μm, brownish, and barrel shaped, and they have bipolar plugs. They are single celled when passed. In cattle *Trichuris* are usually not pathogenic even when present in large numbers. Treatment is usually not required, but benzimidazoles should be effective, especially if administered in feed over several days.

Control Programs for Gastrointestinal Nematodes of Cattle

In recent years, with the availability of inexpensive, safe, effective dewormers, most of the control of parasitic disease has relied on the use of drugs rather than management. With high-intensity grazing systems and the selection of cattle for maximum production of meat or milk, this approach has generally served well. However, if lessons can be learned from small ruminants, the sustained use of these drugs will require some level of management in the selection of which animals to treat and when to treat them.

Without exception the disease caused by parasitic nematodes is a numbers game. When a host has a few parasites, there is no disease, but it is an opportunity to stimulate a protective immune response. With greater numbers the opportunities for disease increase as the numbers rise. Therefore young animals with immune systems that have not encountered parasites or have not matured sufficiently to limit numbers of parasites are at greatest risk of disease. To lessen the chances of disease, the most logical approach is to lessen pasture exposure to infective larvae. Pastures can become parasite safe by producing hay or cropping. An abandoned pasture is not a source of useful forage because as vegetation matures it becomes less palatable and is of lower nutritional quality. Therefore alternate species grazing or making hay/silage is preferred. The intervals of rest from grazing by a specific host species may be as short as 1 month in a warm, wet summer, but it takes months in cool, humid climates for the larval population to dissipate.

Husbandry practices to prevent disease include improved nutrition, which may lessen the amount of grazing close to the fecal pat. Because replacement dairy heifers or stocker calves are most susceptible when they are exposed to large numbers of parasites, they should not be allowed to graze pastures recently occupied by animals that are only slightly older, since these animals shed greater numbers of eggs than do mature cattle. Most hosts develop acquired resistance if not overwhelmed by parasites, and they obtain sufficient dietary protein. Management offers a substantially cheaper and more effective means for controlling or eliminating helminthiasis than drugs alone. Most clinical helminthiasis occurs in young, naive hosts or those on marginal rations. Anthelmintics will not lead to increased weight gain unless adequate rations are consumed.

Calves are at highest risk for parasitic disease, either clinical or economic. The relative risk varies with management. Intensive production of veal calves has been associated with disease associated with *Strongyloides papillosus,* but this is an unusual situation in which stable hygiene associated with sawdust bedding is the primary cause of the condition. Calves on pasture are exposed to the gamut of nematodes in the geographic area in which they are raised. When replacement dairy calves are pastured with other replacement calves using the same pastures year after year, problems will eventually occur.

Pasture Management

No system is ideal for control of parasites unless the pasture is rested 2 to 12 months, but rotational grazing is better for animal nutrition and pasture quality. The length of time that a pasture must be "rested" depends on the parasite in question as well as the temperature and moisture of the pasture of concern. It is also necessary to consider the effect that abandoning a pasture without grazing animals has on forage quality. Grazing pastures with animals that have natural immunity or have developed a level of immunity may harvest larval nematodes, resulting in safer pastures than occurs following abandonment. Pastures, especially improved pastures, must be managed. Fifty percent of the infective larvae occur within 2.5 cm of ground. The use of temporary pastures or hay meadows after harvest is a method of creating a parasite-clean pasture. Overstocking varies with the year and available forage.

Short-duration, high-density grazing systems have become extremely popular in that more livestock can be maintained on less land. Many animals are on limited areas of forage, and the livestock are moved frequently (hours to days), with pastures rested for 2 to 4 weeks (like growing and mowing a lawn). This approach is parasite heaven, but it also produces maximum production/acre with high-quality forage. The reason that this system is so favorable for parasites is that the time span required to produce high-quality forages is similar to the time required for the development of egg to infective larvae and translation of the larvae onto the forage. Also, in high-density systems the livestock do little selective grazing and consume forage they may normally avoid such as the rank grass surrounding a fecal pat. This is because they have no choice, and the forages available are a monoculture or only a limited number of plant species.

Raising replacement heifers on permanent pastures not used by similar calves the preceding year is a wise way of avoiding overwintering larvae. Older cattle can act as biologic vacuum sweepers harvesting the larvae, of which only a small percentage will become reproducing adults. Moving spring-born replacement calves at the midpoint of the grazing season is another way of avoiding heavy exposure to infective larvae. This movement at the time of anthelmintic administration not only removes the adult worms in the calves but also gives the calves a level of exposure that may stimulate the immune system.

Cattle herds in arid areas may not benefit economically from a parasite control program, but the calves from these herds are at greater risk than others. Many different management programs exist, yet some farms and ranches lack any program at all. No one parasite program works on all farms or ranches. We need to think, "How does the parasite survive?" to control it.

No single strategy of management suffices for all herds, even in a given region. A few practices can be advantageous in most, but not all, circumstances. One practice that is widely used is moving animals to clean pastures after deworming. The idea is that animals that have been freed of infection will not immediately encounter a new worm population to replace the one just removed. This is true, and when animals enter an annual pasture that is replanted each year it is a sound approach. If, however, the worms have not all been removed and the animals are to remain on the new pasture, it is a method of establishing resistant worms onto the new pasture. The reason for this is that the only worms not removed by the anthelmintic used at the time of moving produce eggs in the new environment. The subsequent larvae will have only similar worms to mate with when they enter a host. The onset of clinical resistance may not be apparent for several years in this scenario.

NEMATODE INFECTIONS OF SHEEP AND GOATS

Although sheep and goats are behaviorally and physiologically different, they share many of the same helminth parasites. The populations of worms may be different in each species but can and do cross over. Because of the way each host acquires its nutritional needs (sheep grazing and goats browsing), sheep and goats' mechanisms of either avoiding or coping with gastrointestinal nematodes evolved differently. Where sheep and goats cohabit rangelands, gastrointestinal nematodes are most often a problem in sheep because the goats have browse available. However, where goats are forced to graze they are at least as susceptible to worms as sheep and appear to be more likely to suffer from disease. The two species should not share pastures in which grasses and legumes are the primary source of nutrition. In addition, goats metabolize anthelmintics differently than do sheep, requiring 1.5 to 5 times greater doses to present lethal doses to worms within their gastrointestinal tracts. Resistance is usually first seen in goats, and then the worms are shared with sheep.

Haemonchus

The most important parasite of small ruminants in warm, humid regions worldwide is *Haemonchus contortus,* which occurs in the abomasum of ruminants. The adults are 10 to 30 mm in length, so they are grossly visible (largest of the worms found in abomasum). When fresh, worms are red because of their intestines being filled with the host's blood. The ovaries and uterus, which are white, wrap around the intestine, giving a barber pole or candy cane appearance.

Adult females produce 5000 to 6000 eggs daily. Eggs passed in the feces develop in a temperature-dependent fashion. It takes a minimum of 5 to 10 days from the eggs being passed for development to the infective L3 stage. The larvae exit the fecal pellet and ascend vegetation in a film of moisture. The sheep or goat ingests larvae while grazing. The L3 exsheaths in the rumen, moves to the abomasum, enters gastric pits, and molts to the L4. The L4 feeds on blood and molts to the adult, which mates, and produces eggs approximately 3 weeks after being acquired. Adult worms live for months in susceptible hosts. The worms produce so many offspring that at least some survive unfavorable conditions within or outside the host. During prolonged periods of drought or winter weather conditions, ensheathed larvae survive in the fecal pellet. They are inactive and do not completely use stored energy. When rains occur, they rapidly exit the fecal pellet. Following dry periods, livestock graze closer to the fecal pat than normal and their chances of becoming infected are increased. Hypobiosis, or arrested development, is common in *Haemonchus* infections and occurs within the host's abomasum during the early L4. These larvae are inactive and are not affected by the host's immune system. They remain arrested until conditions either within the host or in the environment are more favorable for the free-living stages. Development then resumes and the egg count increases, a common phenomenon in ewes or does during the periparturient period.

The primary signs of disease are those of anemia and hypoproteinemia. The onset of disease can be sudden, with apparently healthy animals becoming weak, lying down, and becoming unable to rise. In chronic cases there may be a loss of wool, decreased fiber diameter, and weight loss. The body cavities may be fluid filled. Intermandibular edema (bottle jaw) and pallor of the mucous membranes are indicative of haemonchosis. Fecal material is of variable consistency.

Diarrhea is seldom seen with haemonchosis, although the stool may be soft. Depending on the physiologic status of the host and the number of parasites with which it is infected, the disease may present differently. The peracute disease is characterized by sudden death, with few clinical signs such as lagging behind the flock. The PCV falls to less than 10. Only a few individuals in a population are affected. The anemia is responsive, and immature erythrocytes are seen in the survivors.

Acute disease is seen in more individuals in the flock. Anemia, pale mucous membranes, and hypoproteinemia (bottle jaw) are the most common clinical signs. The host may be constipated or have a normal stool. A common sequela to acute haemonchosis is wool break, in which wool sheds off a few weeks following the acute signs. A feature of the chronic disease is that the anemia becomes unresponsive. The animals show signs of ill thrift with poor-quality wool and weight loss. Erythrocyte and hemoglobin levels are depressed. At first the disease is strictly blood loss and low PCV with normal erythrocytes. Surviving animals quickly mount a response as the body attempts to replace lost erythrocytes. A macrocytic normochromic anemia is the most common finding with acute haemonchosis. Chronic haemonchosis occurs when iron, cobalt, and copper levels are depleted (microcytic, hypochromic anemia). Serum protein concentrations are low. Because protein loss occurs through the gastrointestinal tract, both albumin and globulin levels are lowered.

Fecal flotation reveals the eggs of *Haemonchus* and other nematodes. The eggs are not diagnostic because other genera of strongylids produce identical eggs. A quantitative test such as the modified McMaster method aids the veterinarian in determining if there is evidence of sufficient numbers of worms to cause disease. A more or less linear relationship between the egg count and the number of adult worms exists. Fecal egg counts of more than 4000 eggs per gram of feces are associated with haemonchosis. In humid areas during the warm portion of the year, *Haemonchus* is usually the dominant parasite, especially where it is resistant to anthelmintics.

Most modern anthelmintics were initially effective against *Haemonchus*. However, *H. contortus* has such a rich genome that individuals within populations have genes that enable them to resist the effects of anthelmintics. Together with the extreme fecundity of the worm, *Haemonchus* has rapidly adapted to tolerate anthelmintics and some populations have become resistant to every anthelmintic available. Selection by treatment (the removal of susceptible worms), not mutation, appears to be the driving force in the establishment of resistance. The molecular mechanisms of resistance may vary with different populations of worms. Tolerant or resistant worms often accompany animals being introduced to new farms. The worms accompanying their hosts are likely to be resistant to the drug(s) previously used, so clinical disease occurs more rapidly than where there are still susceptible worms. Other factors in addition to the *Haemonchus* genome contribute to the high levels of resistance in sheep and goats. These include underdosing by underestimating weight or by selecting a dose for the average size of animal in a flock, meaning that the worms are exposed to a less than lethal level of anthelmintic, especially in larger animals.

Because *Haemonchus contortus* undergoes winter or dry season arrest, control requires effective removal of larvae during hypobiosis if there is going to be any hope of control when the transmission season begins. In arid regions a single anthelmintic administered (strategic treatment) to adult animals during the winter, especially if given before, or at the time of, the periparturient relaxation of resistance (PPRR), may be the only treatment necessary because the pastures will remain parasite safe for lambs and kids until weaning. Even though this strategic treatment is an effective approach, it is also a selection mechanism for anthelmintic resistance. However, in humid areas strategic treatment may have to be repeated after the onset of grass growth not only to affect arrested larvae but also to kill the now active larvae acquired from pasture during the spring warm-up. Strategic treatment is a selection mechanism for resistance. If, however, the producer can raise young in pastures not used the preceding autumn and winter, the spring treatment can be dispensed with. After weaning, lambs or kids should be dewormed before they enter a parasite-safe pasture. The producer can move the lambs/kids, allowing the adults to remain on the contaminated pasture.

At other times of the year, tactical use of anthelmintics is beneficial. Treatment is warranted if the mean egg counts in small ruminants are greater than 1000 eggs/gram feces before the lambs are weaned or 2000 eggs/gram during the dry period. Another tactical approach is treating 2 weeks following rainfall greater than 25 mm because the larvae acquired from the pasture following the rain will not yet have matured and begun reproducing.

The most important factor to determine how and when to treat small ruminants is how they are being managed. If animals are to remain on pasture, there are alternatives such as treating after they have been exposed to large numbers of worms. For instance, treatment 2 weeks after a rain should remove many of the recently acquired worms before they begin passing eggs. Zero grazing for a period of time after a disease outbreak may enable the host to recover both in terms of reestablishing a protective immune response and in production of erythrocytes and serum protein levels. Another strategy is to identify individual animals that have a greater number of worm eggs in their feces than the remainder of the population. If they can be identified, treating them rather than the entire host population can have almost as much impact on lessening the number of larvae on pasture as treating the entire flock. Identification of wormy individuals can be made by determining egg counts or by measuring the color of the ocular mucous membranes (for instance, FAMACHA carding, which is discussed later). Treating these animals reduces the worm population and ensures the survival of susceptible worms because those in the untreated animals will not be selected. A corollary to individual treatment is the culling of those animals that are treated most often. Not only are they not resistant to worms, but also their offspring having similar traits is likely.

Lessening exposure to susceptible hosts is paramount in control programs. In the early spring or at the onset of the rainy season, reduced pasture contamination is the most important aspect. The ewe in the periparturient relaxation of resistance, even if she has the genetic capacity for resistance, will be a source of eggs for the environment. Strategic deworming to remove arrested or recently emerged larvae before they contaminate the pasture will have a great impact on pasture contamination.

Management systems that lower the exposure of hosts to parasites have been devised. These systems may not optimize the value of forages, but they result in healthier livestock. In warm, humid climates rapid pasture rotation systems in which pastures are vacated for as few as 30 days may lower larval numbers significantly. In other climates, rapid pasture rotation ensures that infective larvae are waiting for the hosts when they return to the pasture. Using pastures that have been used for cropping,

especially in the last half of the grazing season, is an effective measure for reducing challenge.

One of the more effective ways of maintaining pastures and increasing total offtake of protein is multispecies grazing, in which a combination of cattle, sheep, and goats each exploits different plants or parts of plants. Cattle preferentially graze grasses, goats selectively browse leaves, and sheep select forbs and then grass and browse. The competition for the most palatable forage is among members of the same species, and larval nematodes are not as likely to come into contact with a preferred host. When they do find a host, the numbers are lower and unlikely to be in clinically significant numbers.

Providing sufficient protein is vital during the periparturient period. Increased protein levels lessen egg production. Pastures in which plants high in condensed tannins are grazed are safer for hosts because the incoming larvae are adversely affected. The physical structure of some plants may challenge larvae to ascend vegetation or may provide protection from adverse pasture conditions. If animals are allowed to browse, their chances of acquiring larvae diminish as the distance from the ground increases. Most infective larvae are found within 50 mm of the soil surface. Predaceous fungi have been evaluated as agents that kill larvae in pastures. One species, *Duddingtonia flagrans,* can traverse the digestive tract and is present in the fecal pat when the larvae hatch. Feeding spores or incorporating them in ruminal boluses has the potential to lower pasture contamination in specific circumstances.

The characteristics associated with resistance to, or resilience from, parasitic infections are genetic, and the selection of animals within a flock/herd for specific traits including resistance for specific parasites does not necessarily counter the selection for those traits for rapid growth, increased milk production, or fiber production. The genetic aspect of resistance to gastrointestinal parasites is not well understood. It appears that multiple genes are involved in the protective response and that different genes may be more important at different times in the course of infection. Some breeds have more individuals with resistance factors that make them more likely to survive. Even in resistant breeds, all animals are not equal and factors such as lactation, age, or nutritional status may influence the course of disease. When animals are producing at their genetic maximum, they are at greatest risk of parasitic disease because they are immunologically and nutritionally challenged. Immunity to gastrointestinal nematodes is not established in young animals until they are several months of age and have had exposure to specific parasites. In studies with different breeds of sheep exposed to *Haemonchus contortus,* the lambs in breeds with a high level of resistance show resistance earlier than those in susceptible breeds. Not only is the resistance manifested earlier, but it is also stronger in the resistant breeds as seen by lower worm egg production. When prolactin levels rise, the numbers of parasites in females increase so that the parasite progeny will be available for consumption by the offspring of the host when they begin to graze. This PPRR or spring rise in fecal egg counts leads to heavily contaminated pastures. Resistance is parasite specific; therefore resistance to the parasite species in the local environment is critical. Immunity to *Haemonchus* and *Trichostrongylus* is slow to develop, and disease may be seen in all ages but more often in the young or during the periparturient period. It may take several years, if ever, for the establishment of meaningful resistance by individual hosts. Resistance is characterized by fewer worms establishing and those worms being smaller and producing fewer eggs.

Trichostrongylus

In some geographic areas *Trichostrongylus* is the major economically important genus of parasite in small ruminants. One species, *Trichostrongylus axei,* resides in the abomasum. This is one of the few worms normally shared with cattle.

The life cycle is direct with eggs being passed in the feces. Development to the infective stage requires 5 days or longer. Infective larvae are ingested during grazing. Development of *T. axei* occurs in the stomach, with the larvae penetrating the mucosa crypts and emerging as adult worms approximately 15 days postinfection. With the intestinal species such as *Trichostrongylus colubriformis,* after ingestion larvae develop in the mucosa crypts of the small intestine and emerge as adult worms. The prepatent period is approximately 3 weeks. Hypobiosis appears to be a strategy of survival in immune hosts. When ewes or does are subject to the PPRR to nematodes, larvae resume development so that the offspring of the parasites will be in the pasture when the kids or lambs begin to graze. The most important cool season parasite of small ruminants in the southern United States, *T. colubriformis,* may undergo summer arrest, but this does not appear to be an important strategy of survival. However, *Trichostrongylus* larvae perish in summer pastures if there are rains to break up the fecal pellets.

T. axei changes the gastric mucosa, whereas *T. colubriformis, Trichostrongylus vitrinus,* and *Trichostrongylus rugatus* cause villus atrophy in the anterior small intestine. Protein loss and failure to absorb specific nutrients occur and may lead to skeletal changes in lambs. Protein is lost through the lumen of the intestine, leading to a loss of body mass. Clinical signs of anorexia, weight loss, diarrhea, dehydration, and possibly rickets in lambs are seen with the infection. The diarrhea is often dark in color—hence one of the common names, "black scours worm," is descriptive. The parasite is most likely seen in the spring and autumn when there is sufficient moisture. Lambs are at higher risk than adults. They become lethargic and appear to suffer from abdominal pain.

The diagnosis of *Trichostrongylus* spp. requires recovery of adult worms from the abomasum or small intestine. The eggs produced tend to be a bit longer and narrower than eggs of other gastrointestinal nematodes but are not diagnostic. Modern anthelmintics are the usual method of treatment. However, local resistance to one or more anthelmintics may be encountered. Therefore evaluation of anthelmintics in specific populations of hosts must be practiced.

Teladorsagia (Ostertagia)

In cool, moist climates *Teladorsagia circumcincta* is the major economic parasite of small ruminants. It is often in a mixed infection with *Trichostrongylus,* and the two genera, affecting the abomasum and small intestine, cause clinical and economic disease. The parasite produces thin-shelled, segmented eggs that are 90 × 50 μm. The life cycle is similar to other gastrointestinal nematodes. The primary damage to the host occurs when the early adult emerges from the gastric glands. The lining of the abomasum appears as a mass of umbilicated nodules, with a morocco leather appearance, and production of HCl is reduced. Edema of the abomasal folds exists, and sloughing of mucosa may occur. This results in hypoalbuminemia and elevated serum pepsinogen levels. Anorexia, diarrhea, dehydration, intermandibular edema, and weight loss are signs associated with *Teladorsagia.* A soft stool and weight loss are common, especially when there is a mixed infection with *Trichostrongylus* spp. in the small intestine. Both parasites are important to the clinical well-being of the animal, but *Teladorsagia* is more likely to be the primary cause of clinical disease. The disease appears to be more devastating in goats than sheep, possibly because of an innate failure to mount an adequate immune response.

The identification of adult worms in the abomasum is the only certain diagnosis of the worm. Adult and immature worms are generally susceptible to benzimidazole or macrolide anthelmintics. However, resistance to these compounds has developed. Evaluation of anthelmintics must be done at the local level to determine their relative value against specific parasite populations. Because the free-living stages of the parasite are susceptible to heat and desiccation, grazing lambs in pastures not occupied by weanlings the previous autumn will lower the level of exposure to pasture larvae that over wintered. Treatment of does or ewes near the time of parturition negates the effects of the periparturient relaxation of resistance, also lowering the pasture contamination present when the lambs begin to graze.

Cooperia

Cooperia curticei is a mild pathogen. Softening of the stool at the time of patency was the only sign seen in lambs. Apparently any of the modern anthelmintics are effective. The free-living stages are similar in their requirements of temperature and precipitation to that of the ostertaginae. Therefore control programs for *Teladorsagia* should be successful.

Nematodirus

Nematodirus battus is a slender, twisted worm with an anterior inflation and transverse striations. The eggs are 195 × 95 μm and brownish in color with parallel sides. The sheep is the normal host, but there are reports of the infection in cattle. The parasite is found in the ileum of hosts maintained in cool, moist, temperate areas in northern Europe and North America. The larvated eggs must undergo a period of prolonged cooling followed by warm temperatures to hatch. Levamisole, benzimidazoles, or macrolides are effective treatment. Never graze lambs on a pasture grazed by lambs the preceding year. If this is not possible, prophylactic treatment before the onset of clinical signs can be effective. However, the time of hatch varies from year to year. In the United Kingdom a predictive model based on weather conditions can provide the necessary information for sheep farmers to treat in a timely manner.

Other *Nematodirus* species are far more common and are diagnosed by the distinctly large eggs produced by this genus. If disease is seen, it is associated with poor weight gains in lambs. Most disease is associated with a combination of several parasitic species infecting a young animal simultaneously. *Nematodirus* stimulates an early protective immune response, and worms undergo hypobiosis during unfavorable conditions. Any of the modern anthelmintics should be effective in treatment, but pastures will remain contaminated from year to year.

Bunostomum

Anemia and hypoproteinemia are common signs seen with infection by *Bunostomum trigonocephalum,* especially in young animals exposed to the parasite for the first time. Foot stamping or other activities indicating local irritation may be seen when larvae are penetrating the skin. Identification of adult worms in the small intestine is the most accurate means of diagnosis. The almost rectangular, dark eggs may indicate infection with *Bunostomum,* but coproculture and larval identification are necessary for specific diagnosis. Apparently any of the modern anthelmintics are effective against *Bunostomum* because it has largely disappeared from farms where anthelmintic use is frequent.

Gaigeria

Gaigeria pachyscelis is a robust hookworm with cutting plates on the buccal cavity. The eggs are slightly larger than most strongylate eggs in the feces of small ruminants. The parasites are found in the small intestine of sheep, goats, and antelope in Southern Asia, Africa, and South America. Anemia, hypoproteinemia, emaciation, and death are the signs associated with this worm. Because of its great capacity to suck blood, as few as 24 of these hookworms can cause death in lambs.

Other Helminth Parasites

Small ruminants are infected by *Strongyloides papillosus,* which is shared with cattle, and also are infected by the small, ruminant-specific members of the genera *Oesophagostomum* and *Trichuris.* The biology of the worms and the clinical signs in their host are similar to those of cattle.

ANTHELMINTIC RESISTANCE

Largely because of the use of anthelmintics at short time intervals, anthelmintic resistance has become a problem in small ruminants. Resistance in small ruminants to *Haemonchus* in the United States and to *Ostertagia* and *Trichostrongylus* in Australia, New Zealand, Europe, and South Africa has been seen. Essentially there is a direct relationship between the number of times a worm

population is exposed to an anthelmintic and the advent of anthelmintic resistance as a clinical problem. Most anthelmintic resistance is under the control of dominant genes that are selected for. When an anthelmintic that does not kill 100% of the targeted worms is used, the survivors may be carriers of resistant genes. These survivors have no one else to mate with but another resistant worm.

Underdosing is a powerful selection mechanism. If the average animal is used for the dose for the animals in the flock or herd, then an underdose is administered to the larger animals. One practice that encourages underdosage is the subcutaneous use of cattle dewormers in small ruminants. Initially the blood levels are high, and then they drop off. In cattle this gives the long residual levels, which kills incoming worms from a week to a month or more following its use. In small ruminants, and to an extent in cattle, as the levels drop after treatment, the drug removes only the worms without any genes for resistance. This essentially turns back the "wimps" and lets the "super worms" in. Unaware of the consequences, producers and veterinarians have inadvertently selected for ivermectin resistance in small ruminants, and the opportunity for selecting resistant worms in cattle looms in the future.

Switching the families of anthelmintics used is the obvious way of preventing selection for resistance. *Unfortunately, the obvious is wrong and rotation of drugs within a grazing season selects for resistance to all of the drug families in the rotation.* This will occur with different drugs at different time intervals but will ensure that multiple resistance will occur faster than if the drug were used until no longer effective and then changed. Perhaps the most effective method to slow anthelmintic resistance is yearly rotation because the worms at the beginning of the year are the survivors of last year's treatment regimen and may be susceptible to next year's regimen, but you are not preselecting for resistance to another product. However, this approach is, in general, theoretical rather than observational over time. In many areas there is really nothing to rotate to, so the approach of using a drug until it is no longer effective is reasonable. Another problem with rotation is that some producers rotate with another drug, which affects the worms in the same way the original drug did. Side resistance to similar drugs occurs rapidly, and the worm population may already be resistant to a product the first time it is used on a specific farm. Determination of anthelmintic resistance is often made after a drug completely fails and animals die. A clinical response from an anthelmintic with only 40% to 50% efficacy will occur, but this leads to massive pasture buildup of resistant worms and numbers win. The fecal egg reduction test (FERT) is the most common method of evaluating a herd or flock. Samples are taken from 6 to 17 individual animals at the time of treatment and again in 7 to 14 days, and a comparison is made of egg counts before and after treatment. Unless there is a 95% or greater reduction in egg count, a truly effective drug against the species of adult nematodes present does not exist. But certainly a 93% or 85% reduction is better than a 20% to 50% reduction, and a different drug may have to be used even if it is not very effective.

Management Practices to Enhance the Activity of Anthelmintics

The efficacy of benzimidazoles is increased if the drug is delivered over a period of several days. That is, the total dose delivered over 3 to 5 days, or even two treatments at 12-hour intervals, is much more effective against worm populations. By incorporating the drug in palatable feed and being certain that all animals in the herd have access to and consume the drugs may accomplish this purpose. The use of blocks or minerals to administer anthelmintics has been disappointing because the consumption is too variable to ensure that a sufficient number of hosts have adequate intake. The hit or miss situation is likely to lead to low-dose selection for resistance. Fasting overnight before administering oral anthelmintics increases the effectiveness of some anthelmintics. Fenbendazole, which has low solubility, has increased efficacy when it is administered into the rumen. Rumen fluid increases the amount of the active metabolite absorbed and subsequently available to worms. However, albendazole, a more soluble compound, has greater efficacy if delivered to the abomasum. On the other hand, with a related compound, oxfendazole, it seems to make no difference if delivered to either the rumen or abomasum. As a general rule the administration of a drench over the tongue rather than into the front of the mouth is more likely to result in the drug going into the rumen rather than the abomasum.

When resistance has been documented, the simultaneous use of two or more anthelmintics that have different modes of activity is promising. Even though each anthelmintic is ineffective, combining drugs at full therapeutic levels may be clinically effective. Various combinations have been used, and it is essential that full therapeutic dosages of each anthelmintic are used concurrently. Currently this approach is used commercially in Australia in the summer rainfall *(Haemonchus)* areas, where a product used is a combination of albendazole, ivermectin, and levamisole. However, this approach is like a bandage and cannot be relied on for long-term parasite control.

In small flocks or in flocks where the owner is observing at frequent intervals, FAMACHA carding may be used to determine if members of the flock are becoming anemic and if treatment is necessary. FAMACHA, named with the acronym of the originator, is a measure of ocular mucous membrane color, which is evaluated with a color chart to determine anemia. This methodology is effective where *Haemonchus* is the predominant helminth. The idea is to first determine the individual animals with the largest numbers of worms in the abomasum and selectively treat them because 20% of the flock contains 80% of the worms. This removes most of the source of pasture contamination but puts no selective pressure on the worms in the remainder of the flock. The next step is to evaluate the flock to see how things are going before clinical signs are seen. Animals with varying levels of anemia are identified, and a score can be kept to know how the flock is doing. Even if the producer decides to treat the entire flock, the treatment will only be administered when needed (a form of tactical treatment) so that less anthelmintic is used and lower pressure is placed on the worm population. Individually identifying the treated animals is helpful because if individuals are treated multiple times, they should be removed from the flock. The greatest problem with the FAMACHA approach in summer rainfall areas is the lack of susceptible worms with which to dilute the resistant populations.

Resistant worms are purchased in a host that was treated with an anthelmintic that removed the competition with which they could mate. Therefore maintaining newly purchased animals in a barn or dry lot until they have been evaluated as parasite free, 2 weeks after treatment with a combination of anthelmintics, is an essential part of a herd health management program. This aspect is one of the most valuable contributions a veterinarian can provide to his or her clients. The veterinarian can help them remove resistant worms before the pastures become heavily laden with resistant parasites.

The most important consideration in control is to know that the anthelmintic administered actually worked. Clinical response is not sufficient. Response should be judged by a larval development assay or fecal egg reduction trial at each and every farm with small ruminants. When anthelmintic resistance is encountered, the failed drug should only be used on that farm against other parasite species if necessary because the likelihood of the resistant worms becoming susceptible again to that specific drug is low. In small ruminant flocks, anthelmintics should be evaluated yearly in high rainfall areas and every second or third year elsewhere.

Worms survive by their tremendous ability to reproduce. They avoid unfavorable environmental conditions by surviving in fecal pats or undergoing arrested development. They do best by infecting young animals in which they can more successfully reproduce. They evade host immune responses by intermittent exposure or arrested development. Nematodes produce more eggs during the periparturient period and in young hosts. They have a broad genetic base so that when environmental conditions change, there are survivors in the population that can cope with the new conditions including anthelmintics to which they have never been exposed. The offspring of tolerant worms become resistant and then dominant as the less fit individuals are removed by anthelmintics that were formerly effective against the entire population.

CESTODES AND TREMATODES IN RUMINANTS

Gastrointestinal Tract Cestodes and Trematodes in Ruminants

Adult tapeworms in the small intestine of ruminants have been blamed for a host of woes because a 2-m worm must be important. However, there is little experimental evidence that *Moniezia* spp. are economically important. Some evidence indicates that unvaccinated lambs with a *Moniezia* infection entering a feedlot are more likely to develop enterotoxemia than those without infection. Removal of the worms may stop the outbreak more rapidly than vaccination alone. As with all tapeworms,

Moniezia has an indirect life cycle, with oribatid mites serving as intermediate hosts. Infections occur in young, but by the time calves, lambs, or kids are 6 or 7 months of age the infection will disappear. Generally speaking, treating *Moniezia* is for the psychologic well-being of the owner and can be accomplished with praziquantel, where the drug is approved; albendazole; or another benzimidazole.

Thysanosoma actinoides is a fringed tapeworm. Its primary host is sheep, but other ruminants in the Western United States and South America may also be infected. The parasite is normally an inhabitant of the small intestine but is frequently found in the common bile duct. The intermediate hosts are psocids. The primary importance is the condemnation of livers. Albendazole is an effective treatment.

Rumen Flukes

The rumen reticulum is the abode of adult flukes. Larval stages are in water snails such as *Planorbis* or *Bulinus* or amphibious snails in the genus *Lymnaea*. Different primary host species and parasites are found depending on the geographic locality. Disease is more likely to occur in tropical areas. The egg hatches in water 1 to 2 weeks postexpulsion. The miracidium must quickly find a snail, which it penetrates. In the snail it reproduces asexually, developing into cercariae during a 4-week period. The cercariae exit the snail in water and attach to herbage in the water and encyst. Metacercariae, the infective stage, are ingested during grazing. They excyst in the small intestine, and the immature flukes are plug feeders in the duodenum for approximately 6 weeks. They then migrate to the rumen and attach as adults, with a prepatent period of 7 to 10 weeks.

Damage may occur during migration in the duodenum. The host becomes emaciated, with a thickened, corrugated, gelatinous, anterior small intestine and edematous, mesenteric lymph nodes. Immature flukes burrow into the intestinal wall to the muscularis mucosa, which is drawn into the oral sucker. The mucosa lifts from the muscularis in heavy infections, and there is diffuse cellular proliferation around the flukes. In most cases no clinical disease is seen, but where the number of flukes is elevated diarrhea and emaciation are associated with the development of immature flukes in the intestine.

Speciation of rumen flukes is difficult, but in a given geographic region only one or two species are likely to occur. Sedimentation or differential sieving may recover the eggs. They are similar in size and shape to those of *Fasciola* but are clear to gray, not yellow to golden. Resorantel and oxyclozanide are the drugs of choice against adult and immature rumen flukes. Neither of these drugs is available in the United States.

Liver Flukes

Fasciola hepatica, Fasciola gigantica, Fascioloides magna. Liver flukes are regionally important and within the region only on specific farms. Liver flukes are only transmitted on specific pasturelands and are of no significance elsewhere unless the infected cattle are transported. In North America two species, *Fasciola hepatica* and *Fascioloides*

magna, are important parasites of cattle. *Fasciola* is widespread, found in the Southeast and Northwest and many local places in between, whereas *F. magna* is generally found in the Great Lakes region, Northwest, and Texas Gulf Coast. Liver fluke–infested pastures tend to have clay soils and are constantly or periodically flooded but not inundated. The intermediate host snails live in shallow water with vegetation where algae, an important foodstuff, grow. The damage to cattle and the epidemiology of the two parasites are quite different, even though they both use lymnaed snails as hosts.

F. hepatica, the common liver fluke, uses a wide range of definitive hosts including humans. In tropical regions *F. gigantica* replaces *F. hepatica* as the primary liver fluke; however, the two species are similar and in general what is said about one species applies to the other. In North America cattle are the important source of infection of *F. hepatica* to snails, which is different from other countries where sheep are a major contributor. However, *Fascioloides* is unable to complete the life cycle in cattle because the eggs are trapped in thick-walled cysts within the liver. The infection of the snails all comes from cervids; white-tailed deer and wapiti are the primary hosts, and *F. magna* occurs in cattle sharing pastures with these species. Because of this difference, the results of treating cattle for liver fluke are vastly different. By treating cattle for *Fasciola,* not only is the individual animal aided but also the snails are less likely to become infected and then pass on infection to other cattle occupying the pasture. Treating cattle with *F. magna* has no effect on pasture contamination but may be of some benefit to the individual cow. Ranchers in the Texas Gulf Coast, where *Fascioloides* is a common problem, routinely administer anthelmintics to treat for this parasite. They believe that despite permanent liver damage, the cattle do better and are culled less frequently than when the drugs are not used. This perception may be false in that the drugs effective against *F. magna* are even more effective against *F. hepatica,* and the improvement may be caused by clearing this parasite. In both cases the number of flukes involved determines the level of economic loss associated with infection.

In both infections, metacercariae encysted on vegetation are ingested and larval flukes enter the liver and migrate. In the case of *F. hepatica* they eventually enter the bile ducts, where they mature and begin producing eggs 12 to 16 weeks postinfection. During acute phases of infection the mucous membranes become pale, and sheep, especially, may develop ascites. The subacute disease occurs when the flukes reach the bile ducts and there is cholangitis, as well as tracts in the liver. Anemia and hypoalbuminemia are seen, with pale mucous membranes, ascites, and bottle jaw (intermandibular edema). Chronic fascioliasis is characterized as anemia, with fibrous proliferation surrounding the bile ducts and a blockage of blood vessels in the liver causing local fibrosis. The bile ducts become hyperplastic. The liver is pale and firm, with the ventral lobe being reduced in size. In older cattle that have been repeatedly exposed to the parasite, there is a clearing of adult worms after a few months, only to be reinfected the following transmission season. There appears to be some level of resistance to reinfection. In the case of *F. magna* the flukes migrate through the liver or other tissues until they encounter another fluke when they form the cyst (each containing two or more flukes). They mature and begin producing eggs 30 to 40 weeks postinfection. However, the eggs remain within the cyst. The disease caused by *F. hepatica* is generally more severe in small ruminants, and death losses may occur during the migration because of hepatic damage and *Clostridia* disease. The number of *F. magna* required for disease in small ruminants is one. The flukes continue migration until the liver is turned into a black pâte or a large artery is severed and the animal hemorrhages into the body cavity.

During acute or subacute infections with *F. hepatica* or any time with *F. magna,* no eggs are found in the feces. Serologic tests for *F. hepatica* have been developed for use in cattle that are able to identify infections as early as 2 weeks postinfection. Serum enzyme levels of glutamate dehydrogenase (GDLH) rise during the early stages of migration, and then gamma glutamyl transpeptidase (GGT) levels rise when the flukes reach the bile ducts. During the chronic stages, finding eggs by fecal sedimentation or differential sieving is diagnostic for *F. hepatica.*

During migration through the liver parenchyma there is a failure to break down sex steroids, and if the number of parasites is high enough, there may be a delay in the onset of puberty and subsequent pregnancy in heifers exposed to *F. hepatica.* Certainly if a high number of worms is present, anemia, hypoproteinemia, and associate clinical signs are seen. There is also some evidence of lower feed efficacy in cattle with elevated *F. hepatica* infections. The condemnation of livers in cattle infected or with fibrosis and biliary hyperplasia is definitely an economic factor. Even following treatment the fibrosis may be sufficient that livers are condemned even though no flukes are present. The black tracts and thick-walled cysts in the liver and other organs associated with *F. magna* are sufficient for condemnation whether or not flukes are present.

Liver flukes are transmitted seasonally depending on the geographic location. In general transmission occurs during the latter half of the grazing season in colder climates as snails hibernate over winter. In southern climates the hot, dry summers cause snails to aestivate over summer. In both cases few infected snails are able to survive either the winters or summers while buried in the mud. Infected snails become active when conditions are suitable and rapidly reproduce. This generation of snails is ripe for infection by the hatching of eggs that are passed by parasites in the hosts' livers. The egg requires 2 to 6 weeks or longer before hatching and another month or two of development in the snail before releasing cercariae, which encyst on vegetation. The metacercariae may persist for some time in the environment if not exposed to excessively hot or cold temperatures. Based on the time necessary for development in the environment and within the host, there is only a narrow time frame in which treatment of *Fasciola* can control parasite numbers in the environment. This is especially important in North America, where the anthelmintics available are only effective after the cattle have been infected for a period of time.

Where available, triclabendazole is the most effective drug for *Fasciola* infections because it has the capacity to kill flukes as early as 1 week into migration; it is also effective against *F. magna.* Clorsulon at 7 mg/kg is effective against *F. hepatica* 8 weeks or longer after infection and has minimal effect against *F. magna.* The same drug at 3.5 mg/kg is effective against adult *F. hepatica.* The other drug available in the United States, albendazole, is approved at 10 mg/kg and has effect against adult *F. hepatica;* however, at higher doses 15 mg/kg also has an effect against *F. magna.* If available, triclabendazole is the most effective drug for *Fasciola* infections because it has the capacity to kill flukes as early as 1 week into migration. Other drugs effective in removing later migratory stages are rafoxanide, closantel, nitroxynil, and corsulon, most of which are not available in the United States. In addition to these drugs, albendazole is effective in removing adult worms. However, as with most anthelmintics, local populations of worms may be resistant to their effects.

The timing of its use against *F. magna* is not as important as for *F. hepatica* because one is not trying to protect snails from infection. Treating cattle at least 2 months after the end of the transmission season (end of grazing season in north and mid summer in the south) should effectively remove adult flukes so that when the snail activity begins, there are few fluke eggs in the environment. Of course, other hosts such as rabbits and rodents are sources of *F. hepatica* eggs but are unlikely to contribute anywhere near the level of eggs cattle do. Experimentally wild and farmed deer have been treated for *F. magna* with reasonable success. However, the use of baiting for wild populations must consider hunting season and coincide with the lack of natural feedstuff to successfully deliver the anthelmintic. This may be a less than desirable time to treat from a transmission standpoint.

Dicrocoelium dendriticum. A small (less than 1 cm) lancetlike fluke infects sheep and cattle. A number of species of land snails serve as the first intermediate host and *Formica* ants are the second intermediate host of *D. dendriticum. Dicrocoelium dendriticum* is found locally in many parts of the temperate world. Adult flukes that live in the bile ducts expel eggs that are infective to snails, which ingest the eggs. Later the cercariae are expelled from the snail in pulmonary exudates known as the "slime ball." Ants ingest the slime ball, and metacercariae are formed in the ant's brain. When the ant forages on vegetation it will grasp the forage and hang on until ingested by a grazing sheep. The immature flukes travel directly from the small intestine up the bile ducts. With hundreds of flukes present in the bile ducts, there is no change in the liver tissues. However, when thousands of flukes are present there may be fibrosis of the small bile ducts and subsequent cirrhosis. There are usually no clinical signs except with liver cirrhosis when edema and emaciation are seen. The finding of the small, brownish eggs on fecal examination or adult worms in the bile ducts is the diagnostic method. The treatment is benzimidazole given at higher rates than for other helminths or Praziquantel at double the dose for tapeworms.

The question that needs to be asked when administering an anthelmintic, for any helminth, is why? Two basic reasons to administer an anthelmintic are (1) to aid the individual by saving its life or by increasing the production of meat, milk, fiber, or possibly reproductive efficacy, and (2) to lessen the numbers of infective parasites in the environment so that someday the at-risk animals will not be exposed to the level of infection that leads to disease. With *Fasciola hepatica* and other parasites as well, treatment with the anthelmintics only effective against adult flukes is too late to really help the individual appreciably. If the drug is effective during migration, the individual may benefit. However, the use of an effective flukicide administered to livestock before the snail population has built up following aestivation or hibernation will lower the infection rate in snails. Then the snails will not pass on the infection to the next crop of calves or lambs, which has definite long-term benefit.

Liver Tapeworms

Thysanosoma actinoides, the fringed tapeworm, is normally an inhabitant of the small intestine but is frequently found in the common bile duct. The presence of the worm in the bile ducts has implicated it as causing hepatic diseases. However, there is no credible evidence of this contention. The primary importance is the condemnation of livers because of the aesthetic presence of the parasite. Albendazole is an effective treatment.

Taenia hydatigena proglottids are passed in the feces of canids. The eggs are distributed in the environment and ingested by the intermediate host ruminant or pig. The hexacanth embryo tears through the intestine and is picked up in the blood and transported to the liver. After migration through the liver, lasting approximately 1 month, the cyst of *T. hydatigena* is formed on the liver surface or in the peritoneal cavity. A dog or other canid eats the intermediate host, and the adult tapeworms mature in the small intestine. The migration of larval *T. hydatigena* through the liver may cause a condition known as "hepatitis cysticercosa," in which large tracts are seen in the liver, resembling the migration of *Fasciola hepatica.* However, the tracts appear larger. The presence of the tracts or cysticerci in the liver is a reason for condemnation. Usually no clinical disease is associated with *T. hydatigena.* However, the liver damage associated with migration of a large number of larvae through the liver may lead to anemia and hypoproteinemia. Although several anthelmintics have been used in the treatment of the cysticercus in ruminants, the lesion remains and is a cause for condemnation of the liver or carcass. Control should focus on eliminating the parasite from the dog.

CHAPTER **23**

Gastrointestinal Protozoal Infections in Ruminants

THOMAS M. CRAIG

When we think of protozoal disease and ruminants we think first of coccidiosis, which is caused by *Eimeria* spp. intracellular parasites in the digestive tract. The environmentally resistant form is the oocyst. Sporulated oocysts each contain four sporocysts, and each sporocyst contains two sporozoites. The oocyst may have a micropylar cap or residual bodies, or both. These features, plus the thickness of the oocyst wall, its size, shape, and color, aid in species identification. *Eimeria* spp. are host specific and parasitize cells of specific regions of the gastrointestinal tract and even specific locations within the host cell.

Unsporulated oocysts are passed in the feces, and sporulation occurs in the environment. The time to sporulation is temperature dependent, usually taking 2 to 7 days. The sporulated oocyst is ingested by the host.

An important difference between coccidia and helminth parasites is that coccidia do not require herbage in the environment on which to crawl. Therefore coccidiosis occurs in dry lot situations, as well as on pastures. The sporozoites enter specific cells in the gastrointestinal tract and undergo asexual reproduction, merogony. Daughter cells, merozoites, then enter other cells, and merogony is repeated. The number of generations of merogony is species specific. After two to five generations, the merozoites become either macro (female) or micro (male) gamonts. A macrogamont contains one gamete, and each microgamont contains numerous microgametes. A microgamete will exit its host cell and join with a macrogamete, forming a zygote that is incorporated in an oocyst. Most *Eimeria* species have a prepatent period of 2 to 3 weeks, and the onset of clinical signs and oocyst production usually occurs simultaneously or within a few days of each other.

Not all coccidia are pathogenic so that large numbers of oocysts may be passed in the feces of hosts without any signs of clinical disease. Even when diarrhea is observed in a potential host, it might be caused by the quality of forage consumed, gastrointestinal helminths, or other agents. Coccidiosis is seldom associated with a single *Eimeria* species, and individual animals having *Eimeria* spp. in the small intestine and the large intestine concurrently will be more adversely affected than those individuals with two species of *Eimeria* in the same organ.[1] The most virulent pathogenic species are *Eimeria bovis* and *Eimeria zuernii* in cattle,[2] *Eimeria crandallis* and *Eimeria ovoidalis* in sheep,[3] *Eimeria ninakohlyakimovae*, and *Eimeria arlongi* of goats.[4] However, most reports of coccidiosis do not indicate which species are involved, and it seems reasonable that almost any species of *Eimeria* can cause disease in susceptible hosts under crowded unsanitary conditions where large numbers of oocyst might be ingested.

Coccidiosis is a common disease in only confinement systems or where it affects stressed or naive animals. On the other hand, infection is nearly universal and most control programs are directed toward preventing the change from infection to disease. Likelihood of disease is largely a function of the magnitude of infection. When the feces of ruminants are examined, there are often *Eimeria* oocysts. However, there is a substantial and important difference between coccidiasis, an infection, and coccidiosis, a disease. The former is common and constant, the latter rare and usually confined to young animals. Once an animal has developed signs of coccidiosis, even with the best treatment, there may be some permanent effects on its future growth, resulting in runty, ill-faring young animals. Lessening exposure by reducing stocking rate lowers the magnitude of infection.[5] Keeping the environment clean, dry, and uncrowded lessens stress and the level of exposure; however, chemicals are the basis of coccidia control.

The diagnosis of coccidiosis is made by observation of clinical signs such as diarrhea with or without blood, excessive mucus in the stool, and large numbers of oocysts in the stool identified by fecal flotation techniques. Although all ruminants may pass oocysts from time to time, usually only the younger animals are at risk of disease. Older animals that have not had recent experience with the parasite or that are under stressful conditions may develop signs of disease. The finding of oocysts in the feces by flotation methods is the usual method of determining whether infection is present. Most coccidia oocysts float in a medium with a specific gravity (sp gr) of 1.10 or greater. A few species require a higher specific gravity, and centrifugal sugar flotation (sp gr 1.26) may be the most efficient in detecting oocysts. Again, it should be noted that the identification of small numbers of coccidia in the feces does not mean that coccidiosis, the disease, is present. Unless there are at least several thousand oocysts per gram of feces, the presence of oocysts alone should not be the sole basis of making a diagnosis of coccidiosis. Young ruminants may suffer from disease during the prepatent period and have signs of disease with low oocyst counts. However, this situation will be transient because most clinical cases have a large number of oocysts passed.[6]

Coccidiosis is a disease of intensive management and is seen dependent on husbandry and weather conditions before the outbreak of disease. Coccidiosis is also a disease of stress, brought on by parturition, weaning, shipping, changes of feed, or adverse weather conditions. Contaminated feed, water, or bedding leads to heavy exposure, and disease is correlated to the level of exposure and acquired immunity. The signs of coccidiosis are those of diarrhea with production of mucus or blood, or both, in the feces; rough hair coat; weakness; chronic poor doers; and death. A higher prevalence and intensity of infection occurs in young animals compared with mature animals.[7-9] Most hosts develop immunity to disease, but the immunity is not sterile, and immune hosts pass oocysts.

Very young lambs are resistant to coccidia infection and then have increased susceptibility after the first month.[10] If lambs are exposed to oocysts during the early resistant phase, they are resistant to reinfection.[11] Lambs administered a trickle infection of 2000 coccidia oocysts three times a week during the first month of life were resistant to a challenge that killed 80% of the naive controls. They also outperform lambs exposed only at birth or once a week.[12] Steer calves implanted with estradiol and progesterone and administered *Eimeria bovis* oocysts gained weight similar to noninfected controls and fared significantly better than those administered oocysts but not implanted. Apparently this difference, along with a shorter period of abnormal fecal consistency, is caused by enhanced immune function in the implanted calves.[13]

Identification of species of coccidia may be aided by examination of sporulated oocysts. Oocysts should be separated from fecal material by flotation after straining through a sieve to remove large particulate matter. Sporulation may take 1 to 2 days. The oocysts are placed in a Petri dish for adequate oxygenation and a solution of tap water with 2% potassium dichloride or 2% sulfuric acid added to limit bacterial or fungal proliferation. The identification of sporulated oocysts is aided by consulting texts.[14,15] In most instances a presumptive specific diagnosis can be made by the examination of oocysts in freshly passed feces (Figs. 23-1 to 23-4).

Coccidiostats inhibit the development of coccidia within the gut of the host. When these drugs are used prophylactically, they prevent disease. However, when an animal is already showing clinical signs of disease, most of the coccidia have developed beyond the point at which the coccidiostat is likely to exert its influence. Therefore clinical response does not occur, or if one does, it is largely because of the development of immunity. It appears desirable for a few parasites to develop in the host while on coccidiostats. This allows protective immunity to develop while the host is protected against disease. By its nature, this approach also selects for parasites resistant to the drug. Therefore specific coccidiostats may lose their effectiveness, and it becomes necessary to periodically evaluate drugs at the herd or flock level.

Coccidiostats act in different ways on the developing stages of the parasite. Amprolium, for instance, is a thiamine agonist, which is taken up by both host and parasite cells blocking the development of *Eimeria*. This drug can

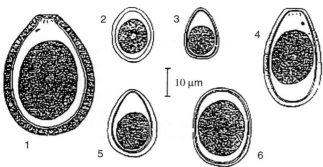

Fig 23-1 Unsporulated *Eimeria* oocysts of cattle. **1,** *Eimeria bukidnonensis* (44×32 μm); **2,** *Eimeria zuernii* (20×15 μm); **3,** *Eimeria alabamensis* (19×12 μm); **4,** *Eimeria aubernensis* (36×20 μm); **5,** *Eimeria bovis* (24×17 μm); **6,** *Eimeria ellipsoidalis* (28×20 μm).

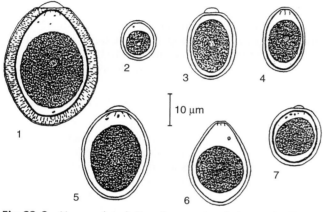

Fig 23-2 Unsporulated *Eimeria* oocysts of sheep. **1,** *Eimeria intricate* (40×29 μm); **2,** *Eimeria parva* (14×11 μm); **3,** *Eimeria ovina* (23×15 μm); **4,** *Eimeria ovinoidalis* (21×13 μm); **5,** *Eimeria ahsata* (30×21 μm); **6,** *Eimeria faurai* (27×20 μm); **7,** *Eimeria crandalis* (20×15 μm).

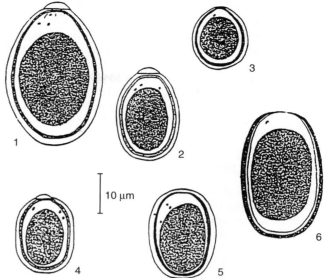

Fig 23-3 Unsporulated *Eimeria* oocysts of goats. **1,** *Eimeria christenseni* (34×24 μm); **2,** *Eimeria arlongi* (23×16 μm); **3,** *Eimeria alijevi* (16×15 μm); **4,** *Eimeria hirici* (20×14 μm); **5,** *Eimeria ninakohlyakimovae* (23×16 μm); **6,** *Eimeria caprina* (32×20 μm).

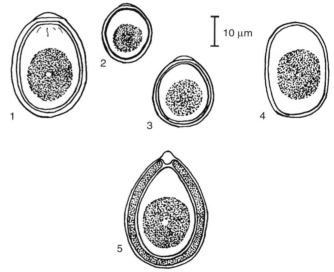

Fig 23-4 Unsporulated *Eimeria* oocysts of the *Aucheni dae.* **1,** *Eimeria lamae* (35.5×24.5 μm); **2,** *Eimeria punoensis* (20×16.5 μm); **3,** *Eimeria al pacae* (24×20 μm), **4,** *Eimeria peruviana* (32×19 μm); **5,** *Eimeria macusaniensis* (94×67 μm).

be toxic to the host if administered at an elevated dose or over a prolonged time period. Signs of toxicity mimic those of polioencephalomalacia and respond to parenteral thiamine administration. Decoquinate affects the sporozoite just as it invades the host cell by disrupting mitochondrial electron transport in the parasite but apparently not in the host, where it appears to be nontoxic at even highly elevated levels. The ionophores, lasalocid, monensin, and salinomycin, in addition to their coccidiostatic activities, also affect rumen fauna by selecting for microorganisms that produce propionic acid rather than acetic or butyric acid. Because propionic acid is used by ruminants as an energy source, animals being fed one of these substances have enhanced feed efficacy. The dose that increases feed efficacy and dose at which coccidiostatic activity occurs vary with specific hosts and may not be the same. Sulfonamides, which act on paramino benzoic acid, were the first effective coccidiostats, but they are not efficient coccidiostats because they halt maturity of the organism late in its development after most of the damage is done. However, they may be valuable in treating

clinical cases because the bacteriocidal activities may protect the host from secondary disease. Two of the more recently developed drugs, toltazuril and diclazuril, appear to have coccidiocidal, as well as coccidiostatic, properties and may be useful for treatment and protection.[2]

The practice of the use of coccidiostats year-round leads to drug resistance or susceptible hosts, or both. if the number of oocysts to which the animals are exposed becomes low, it may fall below the threshold exposure necessary to stimulate a protective response. At the same time the coccidia are becoming resistant to the coccidiostat, the host population is at risk of having low natural immunity and resistant parasites. A more rational approach is to use coccidiostats only at time of risk (i.e., parturition, inclement weather, shipping, weaning). During the rest of the time, coccidia are allowed to propagate at subclinical levels to stimulate immunity in the hosts and to develop a population of parasites that are not resistant to coccidiostats.

CRYPTOSPORIDIUM PARVUM

Cryptosporidium parvum oocysts are small (4-5 μm with four sporozoites) when they exit the microvillus border of the host enterocytes. *C. parvum* is a common parasite inhabiting the microvillus border of enterocytes and other epithelial cells in a variety of mammalian hosts. The oocyst is passed in the feces and because of the extreme small size of the oocyst, aerosol transmission is possible, although water or food is the usual transmission method. The oocyst, infective when passed, is ingested or inhaled, and the sporozoites invade the microvillus border of host cells. Merogony, gamogony, and syngamy occur in the microvillus border of enterocytes and other cells. Some of the sporozoites from oocysts are able to autoinfect the host and lead to the presence of tremendous numbers of organisms.

The host cells are not disrupted as with other coccidia, but they appear to be functionally impaired. The villi are stunted and fused and do not appear to produce membrane-bound enzymes. Young may have signs of diarrhea when infected naturally or artificially by the agent. The age of the neonate at the time of exposure largely determines the course of disease, with the younger animals being more adversely affected. *Cryptosporidium* are unaffected by most disinfectants, and the ability of the sporulated oocyst to infect immediately on being passed from the host, as well as autoinfection, leads to easy spread in the environment. In hosts with fully functional immune systems, signs will dissipate in a few days to 2 weeks but may continue indefinitely in immune-compromised hosts.

Diagnosis of *Cryptosporidium* can be made by the observation of the oocysts by acid fast or immunofluorescence staining of fecal smears or by concentration of oocysts by centrifugal sugar flotation techniques. Antigen detection detects infection in a high percentage of diarrheic stools. Previously infected individuals have specific antibody levels to the organisms. Finding organisms is not proof of disease, and in some situations nearly 100% of the population is infected from time to time and yet not show signs of disease. Large numbers of organisms and clinical signs are indicative of the disease. The ability of *C. parvum* to cause disease in humans is a concern,[16] but most outbreaks of disease in humans are caused by other species or genotypes of *Cryptosporidium*.[17]

Of the antiprotozoal agents available in North America, only decoquinate has been reported anecdotally to decrease oocyst shedding. Attempts at the use of decoquinate in preventing disease under controlled conditions did not prevent diarrhea or reduce oocyst shedding.[18]

Paromomycin has been used experimentally but is not approved for use in food-producing animals. However, halofuginone administered at the onset of clinical signs lowered the intensity of signs and oocyst production.[19] Symptomatic treatment (rehydration therapy) and providing a comfortable environment and good nursing care are usually sufficient to avoid serious clinical disease providing that the animals possess a functional immune system. Decontamination with steam or flame is usually necessary to kill the oocyst. Allowing the premises to be free of animals for weeks to months, depending on the environmental conditions, kills the oocyst by desiccation. Ammonia or formol saline are disinfectants with activity against the oocysts.

Another species of *Cryptosporidium* in cattle, *Cryptosporidium andersoni,* produces a chronic infection in the abomasum of older cattle, which has been associated with lowered weight gains in feedlot cattle and decreased milk production in dairy cattle. Clinical signs are not associated with this parasite, but there is hypertrophy of the gastric mucosa and an increased plasma pepsinogen level.[20] The prevalence of infection appears to be quite low, and differentiating the two species appears to be associated with the age of cattle infected or by postmortem examination.

GIARDIA DUODENALIS (INTESTINALIS)

Many other protozoa inhabit the intestinal tract of ruminants. The rumen is populated by a rich variety of ciliates, and there are amoeba and flagellates in the intestines. Most of these organisms are beneficial or at least harmless to the host. However, some species may occasionally cause disease. The most well known of these organisms is *Giardia duodenalis,* a flagellated organism. Its trophozoites are active when first passed in the feces. The cyst is ellipsoidal (10 × 8 μm) and has four nuclei that can be seen when the cyst is stained. The host specificity of the parasite is debatable but should be considered to be infective to most mammalian species including humans even if there are specific strains or species of the organism. However, it appears that livestock normally have strains not seen in human infections and vice versa.[21]

Giardia is a common parasite of ruminants in some geographic localities. The trophozoites attach to enterocytes lining the duodenum. They reproduce by binary fission until the host's immune system slows reproduction. Some of the organisms encyst and binary fission occurs, resulting in two trophozoites within a cyst. The cyst is the environmentally resistant stage and is ingested by the next host in food or water. The presence of the parasite adhered to the microvillus border of enterocytes causes a failure of the upper intestine to absorb nutriments, primarily fats and fat-soluble vitamins. This leads to fermentation in the bowel, resulting in steatorrhea and diarrhea. Its importance in ruminants is problematic, but it has been shown to cause clinical disease in kids, decreased production in lambs, and diarrhea in calves.[17,21,22]

Diagnosis is made by observing the activity of trophozoites in fresh feces or the recovery of cysts, flotation in zinc sulfate solution (sp gr 1.18), immune assay for coproantigens, or polymerase chain reaction (PCR) techniques that can detect low numbers of organisms in fecal material. The diagnosis of organisms may not be helpful because in some areas virtually all ruminants are infected. Because of the lack of clinical signs generally seen in most ruminants, it is doubtful that treatment is warranted under most circumstances. The benzimidazoles albendazole and fenbendazole may be effective in treating young animals, but reinfection can rapidly occur.

The cysts of *Giardia* are resistant to many disinfectants. High levels of hypochlorite solutions or quaternary ammonia compounds may kill cysts, but steam or flame of quarters previously occupied by infected animals may be the best approach. Filtration of contaminated water supplies will retain cysts.

References

1. Pout DD: Coccidiosis in sheep: a review, *Vet Rec* 98:340-341, 1976.
2. Jolley WR, Bardsley KD: Ruminant coccidiosis, *Vet Clin North Am Food Anim Pract* 22:613-621, 2006.
3. Gregory MW, Catchpole J: Ovine coccidiosis: pathology of *Eimeria ovinoidalis* infection, *Int J Parasitol* 17:1099-1111, 1989.
4. Coles GC: Control of parasites in goats, *Goat Vet Soc J* 17: 28-32, 1997.
5. O'Callaghan MG, O'Donoghue PJ, Moore E: Coccidia of sheep in South Australia, *Vet Parasitol* 24:175-183, 1987.
6. Foreyt WJ: Epidemiology and control of coccidia in sheep, *Vet Clin North Am Food Anim Pract* 2:383-388, 1986.
7. O'Callaghan MG: Coccidia in domestic and feral goats in South Australia, *Vet Parasitol* 30:267-272, 1989.
8. Alyousif MS, Kasim AA, Al-Shawa YR: Coccidia of the domestic goat *(Capra hircus)* in Saudi Arabia, *Int J Parasitol* 22:807-810, 1992.
9. Penzhorn BL, Rognile MC, Hall LL et al: Enteric coccidia of Cashmere goats in southwestern Montana, USA, *Vet Parasitol* 55:137-142, 1994.
10. Gregory MW, Catchpole J, Joyner LP et al: Epidemiology of ovine coccidiosis: effect of management at lambing, *Vet Rec* 124:561-562, 1989.
11. Gregory MW, Catchpole J: Ovine coccidiosis: heavy infection in young lambs increases resistance without causing disease, *Vet Rec* 124:458-461, 1989.
12. Catchpole J, Norton CC, Gregory MW: Immunization of lambs against coccidiosis, *Vet Rec* 132:56-59, 1993.
13. Heath HL, Blagburn BL, Elasser TH et al: Hormonal modulation of the physiologic responses of calves infected with *Eimeria bovis, Am J Vet Res* 58:891-896, 1997.
14. Anon: *Manual of veterinary parasitological laboratory techniques tech bull 18*, ed 2, Ministry of Fisheries and Food, London, 1977, Her Majesty's Stationary Office, p 129.
15. Foreyt WJ: *Veterinary parasitology: reference manual*, ed 5, Ames, Iowa, 2001, Iowa State Press, p 235.
16. Saini P, Ransom G, McNamara AM: Emerging public health concerns regarding cryptosporidiosis, *J Am Vet Med Assoc* 217:658-663, 2000.
17. Olson ME, O'Handley RM, Ralston BJ et al: Update on *Cryptosporidium* and *Giardia* infections in cattle, *Trends Parasitol* 20:185-191, 2004.
18. Moore DA, Attwell ER, Kirk JH et al: Prophylactic use of decoquinate for infections with *Cryptosporidium parvum* in experimentally challenged neonatal calves, *J Am Vet Med Assoc* 223:839-845, 2003.
19. Joachim A, Krull T, Schwartzkopf J et al: Prevalence and control of bovine cryptosporidiosis in German dairy herds, *Vet Parasitol* 112:277-288, 2003.
20. O'Handley RM, Olsen ME: Giardiasis and cryptosporidiosis in ruminants, *Vet Clin North Am Food Anim Pract* 22:623-643, 2006.
21. Olson ME, McAllister TA, Deselliers L et al: Effects of giardiasis on production in a domestic ruminant (lamb) model, *Am J Vet Res* 56:1470-1474, 1995.
22. Sutherland RJ, Clarkson AR: Giardiasis in intensively reared Saanen kids, *N Z Vet J* 32:34-35, 1984.

CHAPTER 24

Bovine Viral Diarrhea Virus

PAUL H. WALZ

Disease in cattle as a result of bovine viral diarrhea virus (BVDV) occurs worldwide and is responsible for considerable economic losses. Since the first descriptions of BVDV and its associated disease, this virus has been a source of continuous controversy in veterinary medicine and cattle production. Although the name of the virus and its associated disease implies gastrointestinal disease, BVDV is best described as a pathogen affecting multiple physiologic systems.[1] Not only has BVDV been associated with pathology involving the gastrointestinal system, but also it is responsible for considerable pathology in the reproductive, respiratory, circulatory, immunologic, integumentary, musculoskeletal, and central nervous systems. Even though initial descriptions of BVDV focused on digestive disease, it has become apparent that reproductive losses may be the most important economically, as well as the method of maintenance and transmission within and among cattle populations through the generation of persistently infected (PI) carriers.[2] Infection of pregnant cattle before day 125 of gestation may result in the birth of calves that are immunotolerant to and PI with BVDV.[3] PI calves are the most significant reservoir of BVDV.

VIRUS TAXONOMY AND CHARACTERISTICS

Bovine viral diarrhea virus is the prototypic member of the genus *Pestivirus* within the family Flaviviridae.[4] Strains of BVDV can be classified in vitro as cytopathic (CP) or noncytopathic (NCP), and this classification of the virus is referred to as the *biotype*. This differentiation is based on the effect of the virus on cultured cells, with CP strains causing vacuolation and cell death within cultured cell monolayers. Importantly, the effect of the virus in cultured cells does not correlate with virulence because strains of BVDV causing severe clinical disease are mainly NCP strains.[5] In addition, only NCP strains of BVDV have been demonstrated, both naturally and experimentally, to induce persistent infection.[6] The NCP biotype predominates in the cattle population, and distribution data from diagnostic laboratories have indicated that NCP isolates are the most common field isolate and account for approximately 65% to 90% of BVDV isolates.[7] The NCP biotype is often the source for CP strains, which arise by mutations and recombinations in the NCP strain.[8]

Because BVDV is an RNA virus, mutation and variation occurs. This variation includes antigenic, genetic, and pathogenic variation. Although there is considerable antigenic variation, all pestiviruses are antigenically cross-reactive. Therefore BVDV exists as one serotype. Genetic heterogeneity exists among BVDV isolates, and phylogenic analysis of BVDV genomic sequences has led to the conclusion that there exist two genotypes of BVDV, BVDV 1 and BVDV 2.[9] These two genotypes are now considered separate species within the *Pestivirus* genus.[4,10] Subgenotypes of both BVDV 1 and BVDV 2 are described. Specific differences in the viral nucleic acid sequences are the basis for genotyping. The classification of genotype is independent of biotype because of CP and NCP BVDV 1 and BVDV 2 strains. Several techniques are available for identifying the different genotypes of BVDV, but most genotyping procedures involve the use of molecular biology techniques that take advantage of sequence differences in specific genome segments. Differences in BVDV genotype may define antigenic differences. With respect to the distribution of genotypes within the cattle population, the BVDV 1 genotype is isolated more frequently than the BVDV 2 genotype.[7,11]

PREVALENCE AND HOST RANGE

Bovine viral diarrhea virus is distributed in cattle populations throughout the world as indicated by serologic surveys. The prevalence of seropositive cattle varies among countries and is influenced by the use of vaccines and management practices. Surveys in North America have indicated seropositive rates between 40% and 90%.[12,13] In contrast, the prevalence of PI cattle is much lower and generally believed to be less than 1% of all cattle.[14] Importantly, PI cattle may cluster within certain groups of cattle, thus elevating the prevalence within populations.[15] Although it is believed PI calves have poor survivability, the prevalence of PI calves arriving at the feedlot has been demonstrated to be between 0.1% and 0.3%,[16,17] and this PI rate in feedyards is similar to the 0.17% reported for U.S. beef cow-calf operations.[14]

Classical assignment of pestivirus isolates to BVDV 1, BVDV 2, classical swine fever virus, or border disease virus has been done according to the species from which it was isolated, with most BVDV, classical swine fever virus, and border disease virus isolates being recovered from cattle, pigs, and sheep, respectively; however, it is known that BVDV may infect other hosts in addition to cattle. Non-*Bovidae* species that have been reported susceptible to BVDV infection include pigs, sheep, goats, captive and wild cervids, and South American camelids.[18,19]

CLINICAL DISEASE SYNDROMES

Bovine viral diarrhea virus infection in cattle may result in a wide spectrum of clinical manifestations ranging from subclinical to fatal disease. Clinical manifestations depend on the interplay of host factors, environmental stress levels, and viral factors.[20] Host factors influencing the outcome of viral infection include immune status, pregnancy status, gestational age of the fetus at the time of infection, and whether the host is immunotolerant or immunocompetent. Viral factors include biotypic variation, genotypic variation, and antigenic diversity. When describing the clinical manifestations of BVDV infection in cattle, it is important to note that both BVDV 1 and BVDV 2 strains may be involved in the entire spectrum of clinical disease. The clinical manifestations of BVDV infection in cattle have been reviewed[20] and can be subdivided into three categories (Fig. 24-1): (1) BVDV infection in immunocompetent cattle; (2) reproductive consequences of BVDV (fetal infection); and (3) BVDV infection in immunotolerant cattle (mucosal disease).

BVDV INFECTION IN IMMUNOCOMPETENT CATTLE

The terms *acute* and *transient* have been used to describe BVDV infection in postnatal cattle, which possess the ability to respond immunologically to BVDV. The source of most acute infections is cattle PI with BVDV; however, acutely infected cattle can also be a source of virus to other susceptible cattle. Nose-to-nose contact between susceptible and infectious cattle is considered the most effective route of transmission.

Acute BVDV Infection

The majority of BVDV infections in immunocompetent and seronegative cattle are subclinical.[20] If observed closely, cattle undergoing a subclinical infection may exhibit a mild fever, leukopenia, and a decrease in milk production. Exposed cattle develop BVDV-specific neutralizing antibodies. Even though BVDV infection may be subclinical, if the infected animal is pregnant, deleterious effects can be manifested in the fetus.

Bovine viral diarrhea (BVD) is the term used to describe the clinical form of BVDV infection in immunocompetent cattle. Clinical signs of BVD include diarrhea, depression, oculonasal discharge, anorexia, decreased milk production, oral ulcerations, pyrexia, and leukopenia. Most commonly, the disease affects seronegative cattle between the ages of 6 and 24 months. It is generally believed that maternally derived BVDV-specific antibodies have waned and acquired immunity is not yet formed, thus making cattle older than 6 months of age susceptible; however, disease as a result of acute infection may be observed in preweaned calves.[21]

Severe Acute BVDV Infection

In 1993-1994, an atypical form of BVDV infection was recognized in Canada and the United States, and BVDV 2 strains were isolated from clinical cases.[5,22] The disease had

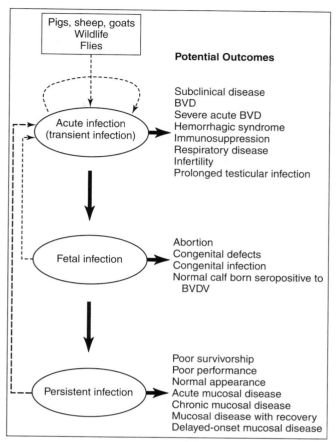

Fig 24-1 Clinical manifestations associated with bovine viral diarrhea virus infection. Routes of transmission are indicated by the dashed lines.

a peracute course, caused high morbidity, and resulted in substantial numbers of deaths in all age groups. Clinical manifestations of severe, peracute BVD include diarrhea, pyrexia, decreased milk production, and oral ulcerations in some cases. These reports of severe BVDV infections clearly demonstrate that some BVDV strains can cause severe life-threatening disease in immunocompetent cattle.

The hemorrhagic syndrome, which is characterized by thrombocytopenia, is an additional form of severe acute BVDV infection in immunocompetent cattle, and this form of infection appears to be associated with noncytopathic BVDV 2 strains.[23] Bloody diarrhea is the most common clinical sign reported, and other clinical signs include epistaxis, petechial hemorrhages, ecchymotic hemorrhages, and bleeding from injection sites or insect bites. In addition to thrombocytopenia, altered platelet function has been reported during acute BVDV infection,[24] and this may contribute to the hemorrhagic diathesis observed in infected cattle.

BVDV-Induced Immunosuppression and the Bovine Respiratory Disease Complex

Bovine viral diarrhea virus is well recognized for its ability to cause immunosuppression in cattle, leading to increased susceptibility to secondary infections. Some pathogens may induce disease alone, but in the presence of BVDV, disease is enhanced. The mechanisms responsible for BVDV-induced immunosuppression are multifactorial; however, the ability of the virus to induce quantitative and qualitative defects in leukocytes likely provides a large contribution. A transient leukopenia occurs in most cattle acutely infected with BVDV, which may be more severe with BVDV 2 than BVDV 1 strains.[25,26] In general, highly virulent strains of BVDV induce more significant depressions in the white blood cell count than less virulent strains. During acute infection, lymphoid depletion is observed in the thymus, spleen, lymph nodes, and gut-associated lymphoid tissues (Peyer's patches).[27] Decreased functional responses in immune system cells have also been described during acute BVDV infection, and affected cells include lymphocytes, neutrophils, and monocytes and macrophages.[28,29]

Substantial data exist demonstrating that BVDV infection is important in polymicrobial disease, and the bovine respiratory disease complex in feedlot animals and intensively housed calves is the best example of this type of disease process. In North American feedyards, bovine respiratory disease is the most frequently reported cause of morbidity and mortality. The role of BVDV in the bovine respiratory disease complex is debatable as to whether BVDV-induced immunosuppression or primary infection of the respiratory tract plays the major role, but BVDV is isolated from pneumonic cattle more frequently than other viruses.[30] Certain BVDV strains may be pneumotrophic, as evidenced by some BVDV strains causing interstitial pneumonia in experimentally inoculated calves.[31] BVDV may play a secondary role in bovine respiratory disease complex through immunosuppression. Although BVDV is frequently isolated from cattle with pneumonia, it is often isolated with the other infectious agents typically associated with bovine respiratory disease complex.[32] Reports from disease outbreaks and experimental studies have supported a synergistic role of BVDV with BHV-1 and BRSV.[33,34] Calves experimentally inoculated with BVDV 7 days before inoculation with BHV-1 developed more severe clinical disease, with dissemination of BHV-1 into nonrespiratory tissues including intestinal and ocular tissues, as compared with calves inoculated with BHV-1 alone.[33] Initial BVDV infection may impair the ability of calves to clear BHV-1 from the lungs and contain BHV-1 at the local infection site.

Prolonged Testicular Infections

Bulls acutely and persistently infected with BVDV are capable of shedding virus in semen.[35,36] Bulls persistently infected with BVDV shed large quantities of virus in the seminal fluid, and BVDV may survive cryopreservation and processing of semen for artificial insemination and thus infect susceptible female cattle.[36] In contrast, acutely infected bulls shed lower concentrations of BVDV in semen; however, infection of artificially inseminated heifers may result from using semen from acutely infected bulls before seroconversion.[37] Acceptable or unacceptable semen quality may be observed in bulls acutely infected with BVDV. Although acute BVDV infections generally result in a transient viremia with subsequent clearance

of the virus by the host immune system, a localized, prolonged infection of testicular tissue with NCP BVDV has been described under both natural and experimental conditions.[35,38] The original description of prolonged testicular infection with BVDV was identified in the testes of a seropositive, nonviremic bull at an artificial insemination center.[38] Despite absence of viremia, the bull continuously shed infectious BVDV in semen throughout his life, and the semen of this bull resulted in infection and subsequent seroconversion of an inseminated seronegative heifer.[39] Protection from a systemic immune response because of a blood-testes barrier is believed to be the mechanism for the localized, prolonged testicular infection. Uncertainty currently exists regarding whether bulls with a prolonged testicular infection may become viremic and infectious to other animals.

REPRODUCTIVE CONSEQUENCES OF BVDV INFECTION (FETAL INFECTION)

Well established is the fact that infection of pregnant, susceptible cattle with BVDV results in transplacental infection. Transplacental infection is a common event in pregnant cattle exposed to BVDV, and in experimental studies, transplacental infection occurs with almost 100% efficiency.[40] Most acute, postnatal infections are subclinical, yet infection in pregnant cattle may result in significant disease. The economic damage caused by BVDV in susceptible herds is mainly associated with the outcomes of intrauterine infections. The outcome of fetal infection with BVDV depends on three main factors: (1) time of infection (i.e., gestational age of the fetus at the time of infection); (2) organ system involved in the infection; and (3) properties of the virus (i.e., biotype, virulence, and target cell range). Importantly, BVDV 1 and BVDV 2, as well as CP and NCP strains, can result in reproductive disease, although only NCP strains are capable of inducing PI cattle.

Infertility and Early Embryonic Death

Infection of cattle before insemination results in impaired conception rates.[41] This may be due in part to ovarian infection and dysfunction as a result of BVDV viremia. Viral antigen in macrophage-like cells and ovarian stromal cella and oophoritis have been described in cattle acutely infected with BVDV.[42] Conception and pregnancy rates are lower if the animals are viremic at the time of insemination. Further field studies have supported this theory that BVDV is involved in early embryonic death and repeat breeding syndrome.[2]

Abortion

Abortion may be observed at any time during gestation as a result of BVDV infection. Depending on the gestational age of the fetus at the time of infection, fetal resorption, mummification, or expulsion can occur following fetal death.[2] Although fetal death and abortion are most common during the first trimester, mid- and late-term abortions and stillbirths should be examined for BVDV. Diagnostic laboratory surveys indicate that BVDV isolation prevalence from aborted fetuses in the United States is quite variable, with BVDV being isolated from 0.1% to 27.2% of submitted fetuses.[43,44] Following BVDV infection, expulsion of the fetus may occur shortly or may be delayed for several months after infection. As a result of delayed expulsion following fetal death, isolation of BVDV from aborted fetuses may not be successful. This has also been demonstrated experimentally, with abortion being observed 30 to 50 days after experimental infection at approximately days 100 to 120 of gestation.[45]

Persistent Infection

The period of fetal development from gestation day 45 to gestation day 125 begins with the end of the embryonic stage and ends with the development of fetal immunocompetence. The most outstanding outcome of infection during this period is the development of persistent infection. By definition, cattle that are PI with BVDV are immunotolerant to BVDV. Biotype is important when discussing infection during this period of gestation. Infection with either biotype is capable of causing fetal death; however, only the NCP biotype is capable of causing persistent infection.[6] The PI animal cannot recognize the infecting NCP BVDV as foreign. Immunotolerance is specific to the infecting NCP strain of BVDV, and postnatal, PI animals can respond immunologically to heterologous strains of BVDV. For this reason, PI animals may be seropositive to BVDV and seropositive status cannot be utilized diagnostically to rule out PI.

Cattle PI with BVDV are characterized by a wide distribution of BVDV throughout their organs as a result of lacking an immune response to the persisting BVDV strain. In PI animals, the virus is present throughout all organs and tissues; therefore BVDV is shed from multiple sites including nasal discharges, urine, semen, colostrum/milk, and feces. Some PI calves are born without any observable abnormalities; thus these animals are an important source for horizontal and vertical transmissions. Vertical transmission is 100% because PI cows give birth to PI offspring. Some PI calves are born weak and stunted and die shortly after birth.[20] PI cattle have decreased survival rates, as evidenced by reports documenting a greater than 50% mortality rate in the first year of life.[46] This mortality may be due in part to the fact that PI animals may have an impaired immune response, which makes them more susceptible to opportunistic pathogens.

Congenital Defects

Congenital malformations may be produced by BVDV infection during the gestational period of organogenesis, which occurs approximately between days 100 and 150 of gestation.[40] Congenital malformations that have been reported in association with BVDV infection include cerebellar hypoplasia, hypomyelinogenesis, hydranencephaly, alopecia, cataracts, optic neuritis, brachygnathism, hydrocephalus, microencephaly, thymic aplasia, hypotrichosis, pulmonary hypoplasia, and growth retardation. Congenital malformations may be due to the direct result of viral infection on developing cells or the host immune response in destroying virally infected cells.

BVDV Infection during Later Stages of Pregnancy

Beyond day 125 of gestation, the fetus is generally considered immunocompetent. Congenital infection during this period usually results in the birth of a calf that is seropositive on a precolostral blood sample. Detrimental effects of BVDV infection in late gestation seem to be less common; however, weak calves and abortions have been reported.[40] It has generally been accepted that infection in late gestation results in the birth of calves that are clinically normal; however, calves congenitally infected with BVDV may be at greater risk for increased morbidity and mortality postnatally.[47] Calves born with neutralizing antibody titers to BVDV were twice as likely to experience a severe illness during the first 10 months of life as compared with calves born free of BVDV antibody titers.[47]

INFECTION IN PERSISTENTLY INFECTED CATTLE (MUCOSAL DISEASE)

PI cattle are at risk of developing mucosal disease. Mucosal disease is the most dramatic of BVDV-associated clinical disease because of the severity and characteristics of lesions. Mucosal disease occurs when cattle that are immunotolerant and PI with NCP BVDV become infected with a CP BVDV.[48] Because mucosal disease only occurs in PI cattle and PI cattle comprise less than 1% of the cattle population, it is characterized as a disease of low morbidity and high mortality. Although the origin of the CP BVDV can be external, such as following the use of modified-live-virus vaccines, current theory holds that in the majority of cases of mucosal disease, the CP BVDV represents a mutation of the NCP BVDV (the PI biotype).[48]

Multiple clinical forms of mucosal disease exist, with variations due to the antigenic relationship between the PI NCP strain and the superinfecting CP strain.[48] At one end of the spectrum is acute, fatal mucosal disease, in which the superinfecting CP strain is homologous to the persistently infecting NCP strain. The other end of the spectrum is mucosal disease with recovery, in which the superinfecting CP strain is heterologous to the persistently infecting NCP strain. The animal mounts an immune response to the heterologous superinfecting CP strain and recovers. The multiple clinical forms of mucosal disease can be divided into acute fatal mucosal disease; chronic mucosal disease; chronic mucosal disease with recovery; and delayed-onset mucosal disease.[48]

Acute Mucosal Disease

Acute mucosal disease occurs when the superinfecting CP strain shares close antigenic homology to the persistently infecting NCP strain. The CP strain may arise de novo by a mutational event from the NCP strain in the PI animal.[49] The mutational event affects the viral biotype but does not affect the viral antigenicity.[49] The clinical findings associated with acute mucosal disease include pyrexia, depression, anorexia, decreased milk production, profuse diarrhea, ptyalism, mucopurulent oculonasal discharge, and oral erosions.[20] Oral erosions are present on the lips, gingival margins, tongue, dental pad, and hard palate (Fig. 24-2). Experimental reproduction of acute mucosal disease indicates an incubation period of 7 to 14 days.[48] Acute mucosal disease is considered to be 100% fatal. On postmortem examination, lesions appear to be confined primarily to the gastrointestinal tract, where erosions are also present in the esophagus, on the ruminal pillars, in the reticulum, and in the omasum.[50] Peyer's patches in the intestinal tract may appear hemorrhagic and necrotic.

Chronic Mucosal Disease

Chronic mucosal disease and mucosal disease with recovery are forms of mucosal disease in which the superinfecting CP strain is heterologous to the PI NCP strain. The likely source of the superinfecting CP strain is external, rather than a mutational event in the PI NCP strain. The clinical manifestations of chronic mucosal disease are anorexia, weight loss, diarrhea, chronic bloat, alopecia, erosive lesions on the mouth and skin, and lameness.[20] The lameness may develop as a result of laminitis, interdigital necrosis secondary to erosive lesions, and hoof deformities. Rarely, a PI animal may mount an immune response to the superinfecting, heterologous CP strain, and clear the superinfection. This phenomenon has been referred to as mucosal disease with recovery.[48] Importantly, the animal remains PI with the NCP strain.

DIAGNOSIS

Numerous methods are available for detecting BVDV infection. The choice of test depends on the clinical problem, the availability of tests by different diagnostic laboratories, and financial considerations. Because the clinical manifestations of BVDV are diverse, accurate diagnosis of BVDV infection relies on laboratory testing. Once a positive diagnosis is made, rational management decisions and control procedures may be implemented to prevent further disease losses.

Virus Isolation

Virus isolation is a basic, reliable, and widely used method for diagnosis of BVDV infection and remains the gold standard for BVDV diagnostics. The BVDV may be cultured and isolated from many samples including serum, whole blood, semen, nasal swabs, and various types of tissues.[51] Mononuclear cells in the buffy coat from whole blood are the ideal sample for individual virus isolation because BVDV is highly cell associated, and the virus isolation is not interfered with neutralizing antibodies to BVDV in serum.[51] The ideal tissue samples for virus isolation from deceased animals at postmortem examination include lymphoid organ–related tissues such as spleen, the gut-associated lymphoid tissue of the distal small intestine (Peyer's patches), mesenteric lymph nodes, and thymus.[51] In addition, pooled tissues from the same animal can be applied to virus isolation. Detection of NCP BVDV strains and confirmation of CP strains as BVDV are

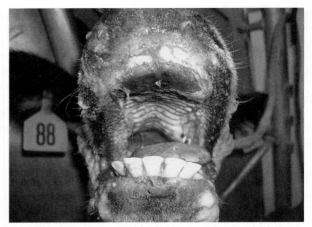

Fig 24-2   Oral erosions present in a cow with mucosal disease.

performed using immunofluorescence or immunoperoxidase staining techniques or RT-PCR.

A microtiter virus isolation that has been referred to as the *immunoperoxidase monolayer assay* (IMPA) has been developed, but the test is not ideal for detecting acute infections, nor is it advisable to use this assay for testing calves younger than 3 months of age because these calves likely have colostral antibodies that would interfere with the test.[52]

BVDV Antigen Detection

Direct antigen detection methods have been described for BVDV using blood and a variety of fresh, frozen, or fixed tissues. These methods include immunohistochemistry (IHC), antigen capture enzyme-lined immunosorbent assay (ELISA) (ACE), and immunofluorescence. Viral antigens can be detected from BVDV infected tissue, whole blood, serum, milk, or nasal swab samples.[51] These tests are advantageous in that they allow rapid and inexpensive detection as compared with virus isolation. In addition, there is no amplification of antigen, so these tests are ideally suited for the detection of animals with considerable amounts of antigen, namely the PI carrier.

Detection of BVDV antigen through IHC or ACE methods on skin samples has become widely used and applied for the detection of cattle PI with BVDV.[53,54] Skin biopsies may be obtained easily and inexpensively. A major advantage of testing by IHC or ACE on skin samples is that sampling can be performed on young PI calves, which may test negative by virus isolation, microplate virus isolation, and ACE testing on serum because of inhibition by acquired colostral antibodies.[55] Both the IHC and ACE tests are ideally suited for the detection of PI animals, and reports indicate these tests do not detect acutely infected cattle.[56,57] However, a recent report indicates positive results may be observed for acutely infected cattle with IHC and ACE tests.[58] With IHC testing, PI animals can be differentiated from acutely infected cattle based on the location of viral antigen in the skin.[53] Cattle vaccinated with modified live viral vaccines do not cause a positive result when tested by IHC or ACE methods.[59,60]

Reverse Transcription—Polymerase Chain Reaction

Since sequences of BVDV isolates became available, molecular techniques have been developed for diagnosis of BVDV and this method of BVDV diagnosis has gained widespread use as a routine diagnostic method.[54] Development of commercial kits, with rapid and simple viral RNA extraction techniques, has made molecular techniques ideal for detection of viral genomic nucleic acids from many types of samples including serum, whole blood, tissues, and bulk tank milk. The RT-PCR assay is a molecular diagnostic method that is a specific and sensitive technique for diagnosis of BVDV infection. The RT-PCR is more sensitive than virus isolation.[61] The high sensitivity of RT-PCR makes it useful for pooled testing, and pooling of whole blood, serum, milk, or skin samples is an economical way to detect BVDV infection in herd screening assays.

Serology

Detection of antibodies to BVDV is another method to demonstrate virus infection; however, it is often difficult to distinguish antibodies produced in response to a natural infection, following vaccination, or as a result of transfer of maternal antibodies from dam to offspring. Interpretation of serology results is difficult without knowing important information of the herd being tested (e.g., vaccination history). Serologic testing may be used to assess vaccine efficacy and vaccine protocol compliance, as well as determine if BVDV exposure has occurred in the herd.[51]

The BVDV-specific antibodies can be divided into two groups, neutralizing and non-neutralizing antibodies. Although there are several applicable methods, the virus neutralization (VN) test and ELISA have been most commonly used for serologic diagnosis of BVDV. The VN is considered the gold standard for serologic assays and is the most frequently utilized test for BVDV antibodies.[62] The VN test quantifies the level of inhibition of specific antibodies on virus replication in cell cultures, and the results are reported as a titer. Simultaneous testing of paired samples, acute and convalescent, are strongly recommended because of variation from antigenic diversity of BVDV isolates and variations of laboratory techniques.[62] As an alternative method to the VN test, the antibody capture ELISA is sensitive, specific, and rapid and can detect antibodies to both BVDV structural and nonstructural antigens.

PREVENTION AND CONTROL

Control of any infectious disease relies on eliminating the reservoirs of the pathogen and limiting transmission from infected individuals to susceptible animals. The goal of BVDV control is to ultimately reduce production losses associated with BVDV infection. Development and implementation of herd health programs that involve vaccination and biosecurity to limit exposure of pregnant cattle to PI cattle are important for success of control. Therefore when applying prevention and control to BVDV, three major areas should be instituted: (1) identification and elimination of PI animals, (2) enhancing immunity through vaccination, and (3) implementing strict biosecurity measures to prevent introduction of PI carrier animals into a population of susceptible cattle. Each principle has been applied to BVDV control[63]; however, BVDV continues to be a major problem to the cattle industry worldwide. This has prompted European countries to develop and apply eradication strategies[64] and has encouraged veterinary and cattlemen's organizations in the United States to adopt control statements and strategies.

Identification and Elimination of PI Cattle

The primary source of BVDV is cattle PI with BVDV because PI animals have a high and persistent viremia and shed BVDV from nearly all secretions throughout their lifetime. Identification and removal of PI animals ideally should occur in breeding herds. In beef cow-calf operations with a controlled breeding season, PI animals should be removed before entry of the bull into the breeding herd.[65] In this situation all calves, replacement heifers, bulls, and nonpregnant dams without calves should be tested for BVDV PI status. Because PI cows always produce PI calves, a negative test result of a calf indicates a negative PI status for the dam.[66] For any calves that test positive, the dam will need to be tested for BVDV PI status. Most PI calves result from an acute infection in the dam, rather than the dam of the calf being PI. For dams that test negative, they may reenter the breeding herd and will possess high natural immunity to BVDV. In beef herds with a controlled breeding season, the BVDV status of all animals can be determined if all animals are not pregnant at the time of testing. If cattle are pregnant at the time of testing, those animals will need to be segregated and their calves will need to be tested and found negative before return to the breeding herd. In dairy herds and beef herds without a controlled breeding season, young calves should be tested and removed as soon as possible to avoid possible transmission to the breeding herd. Screening young calves for PI status is best accomplished using ACE or IHC methods on skin biopsy samples. The use of skin samples for testing young calves is advantageous over other methods in that it is relatively easy for laymen to collect the samples, samples may be taken from calves that possess circulating maternal antibodies, and a single positive test usually indicates PI status. Because the occasional, acutely infected animal may be IHC or ACE positive, valuable breeding stock should be retested 30 days later using virus isolation or RT-PCR assays on blood samples.[58]

Screening all individuals in a herd for BVDV is costly, especially considering the low prevalence of PI animals among cattle herds. Instead of whole-herd testing, monitoring strategies may be initiated including evaluation of production records, BVDV evaluation of aborted fetuses, use of sentinel animals, pooling strategies using RT-PCR testing, and BVDV testing on sick or deceased individuals within the herd.[65] Monitoring breeding records, calf morbidity and mortality rates, and weaning proportions are considered the minimal level of surveillance, and these involve the least expense, but this level of surveillance is not a sensitive method for evaluating the presence of PI BVDV within a herd.[14,65] As an example of the difficulty in using clinical suspicion as a reason to perform herd testing, BVDV was isolated from cattle in 53% of herds where there was no suspicion of the infection,[67] and BVDV PI animals were not identified in 81% of herds in which veterinarians suspected BVDV was present.[14] On the other hand, identifying BVDV in sick or dead animals or in aborted fetuses provides the justification for further whole-herd testing for BVDV PI animals.

Because of high sensitivity, RT-PCR assays using pooled samples have been developed and tested to screen populations of animals for BVDV persistent infection.[61,68] Sample types that have been used in RT-PCR assays of pooled samples include serum, whole blood, bulk tank milk, and skin biopsy samples. With pooling whole blood samples, a single PI animal is detectable in pools of up to 250 negative samples. Recently, an RT-PCR assay was developed and evaluated for testing pools of skin biopsy samples.[68] Pooled sample testing by RT-PCR is a rapid and cost-effective method for screening populations of cattle for BVDV PI animals. Subsequent testing of individuals within the positive pools may be performed using IHC, ACE, virus isolation, or RT-PCR methods depending on the class of animals being tested. When testing young beef calves, it is important to perform all testing before the breeding season to identify and eliminate BVDV PI animals that pose a risk for bred cattle.

Enhancing Immunity through Vaccination

More than 160 BVDV vaccines are available for BVDV, and the majority of these USDA licensed vaccines contain BVDV in combination with other bovine respiratory and reproductive pathogens including bovine herpesvirus-1 (BHV-1), parainfluenza type 3 (PI-3), bovine respiratory syncytial virus (BRSV), *Leptospira* spp., *Campylobacter* spp., *Mannheimia haemolytica*, *Histophilus somni*, and/or *Pasteurella multocida*. Historically, most BVDV vaccines contained only BVDV 1 strains, but because of antigenic diversity among BVDV 1 and BVDV 2, modified-live and inactivated vaccines containing both BVDV 1 and BVDV 2 strains have been developed and are now widely available (Tables 24-1 and 24-2). Advantages and disadvantages of BVDV modified-live viral vaccines and inactivated vaccines have been described.[69] One disadvantage of inactivated BVDV vaccines is that two doses are required for the initial immunization. A major problem with programs using inactivated vaccines is the widespread lack of compliance among producers who use inactivated vaccines.[70] Failure to give a booster during the primary series and failure to regularly administer annual boosters with inactivated vaccines are common.[70]

Vaccines are an important component to BVDV prevention and control, and their effectiveness has been to limit disease from BVDV infection. When discussing BVDV vaccination, it is important to discuss reasonable expectations following vaccination and to remember that disease and infection are not synonymous terms. Experimental and field data indicate that vaccination with either inactivated or modified-live BVDV vaccines is effective at reducing or obviating clinical disease.[5,71] In addition, modified-live viral vaccines containing BVDV 1 strains are effective at limiting or preventing clinical disease when vaccinated animals are subsequently challenged with a virulent BVDV 2 strain.[72,73] Protection from clinical disease is important for stocker/backgrounder and feedlot operations, and immunity to BVDV has been demonstrated to be protective against bovine respiratory disease complex.[74] Preconditioning cattle by vaccinating cattle

Table 24-1

Inactivated Vaccines Containing BVDV Available in the United States

| Manufacturer | Vaccine | BVDV 1 COMPONENT | | | BVDV 2 COMPONENT | |
		Subtype	Biotype	Strain	Biotype	Strain
Boehringer Ingelheim VetMedica	Elite	1a	CP	Singer	cp	296
AgriLabs	Master Guard	1a	CP	C24V	cp	125C
Merial	Respishield	1a	CP	Singer		
Fort Dodge Animal Health	Triangle	1a	CP	Singer		
Fort Dodge Animal Health	Triangle 4+type II	1a	CP	Singer	cp	5912
Fort Dodge Animal Health	Prism	1a	CP	Singer	cp	5912
Pfizer Animal Health	CattleMaster	1a	CP	5960		
		1	NCP	6309		
Pfizer Animal Health	CattleMaster Gold FP	1a	CP	5960	cp	—
		1	NCP	6309		
Novartis Animal Health	ViraShield	1a	CP	KY22	ncp	TN 131
		1	NCP	—		
Biocor Animal Health	Surround	1a	CP	Singer		
		1b	NCP	NY		

BVDV, Bovine viral diarrhea virus.

Table **24-2**

Modified-Live Viral Vaccines Containing BVDV Available in the United States

Manufacturer	Vaccine	BVDV 1 COMPONENT			BVDV 2 COMPONENT	
		Subtype	Biotype	Strain	Biotype	Strain
Boehringer Ingelheim VetMedica	Express	1a	CP	Singer	CP	296
Pfizer Animal Health	Bovi-Shield	1a	CP	NADL		
Pfizer Animal Health	Bovi-Shield Gold	1a	CP	NADL		
Pfizer Animal Health	PregGuard Gold FP	1a	CP	NADL	CP	53637
Fort Dodge Animal Health	Pyramid 5	1a	CP	Singer	CP	53637
Fort Dodge Animal Health	Pyramid	1a	CP	Singer	CP	5912
Merial	Reliant	1a	CP	NADL		
AgriLabs	Titanium	1a	CP	C24V	CP	296
Schering-Plough Animal Health	Jencine	1b	NCP	WRL		
Novartis Animal Health	Arsenal 4.1	1a	NCP	GL760		
Intervet	Vista	1a	CP	Singer	CP	125A
Boehringer Ingelheim VetMedica	Breed-Back FP	1a	CP	Singer	CP	296

BVDV, Bovine viral diarrhea virus.

against BVDV before an expected exposure (commingling and shipping) reduces the effects of exposure of cattle to BVDV.

Protection against viremia is the true measure of BVDV vaccine efficacy. To be truly efficacious, vaccination against BVDV should protect against viremia to prevent dissemination of virus throughout the host including preventing infection of target cells of the reproductive tract that result in fetal infection. In the past decade, the focus for vaccine efficacy has shifted from protection against clinical disease to protection against fetal disease or infection. Published studies indicate the protection against fetal infections following BVDV vaccination varies anywhere from 60% to 100%. This wide degree of variation depends on whether the vaccine is inactivated or modified-live, the timing of challenge, and the degree of homology between the vaccine strains and the challenge strains. Fetal protection studies have been performed evaluating commercial vaccines containing only BVDV 1 strains[75,76] and commercial vaccines containing BVDV 1 and BVDV 2 strains.[77,78] From published studies, it would appear that protection is superior when animals are challenged with strains from the same genotype.[79,80] An extremely important observation regarding these fetal protection studies is that although protection may not be 100% against all strains of BVDV, the level of protection is far superior to that observed when proper vaccination is not used, as evidenced by high rates of PI animals in unvaccinated cattle.

Biosecurity

Although BVDV prevention and control starts with identification and elimination of PI animals, strict biosecurity is essential to prevent reintroduction of the virus. Strict biosecurity is difficult for most cow/calf and dairy operations to achieve and is even more difficult or impossible for most stocker/backgrounder and feedlot operations to achieve. Biosecurity systems with isolation and testing of all incoming cattle are necessary to ensure that BVDV does not enter the farm. All purchased cattle should be isolated and tested for BVDV persistent infection before entry into the herd. In addition, isolation of new additions for 3 weeks before entry into the resident breeding herd should prevent transmission of BVDV from acutely infected animals. Most lapses in herd biosecurity involve purchasing cattle that are PI with BVDV or by purchasing pregnant cattle where the BVDV status of the fetus is unknown. If pregnant cattle are purchased, these animals should be isolated and their offspring should be tested to ensure that they are free of BVDV. Semen should only be used from bulls that have been tested for BVDV infection. For purebred herds marketing genetically valuable embryos and livestock, it is important to test embryo transplantation recipients to ensure that they are not PI with BVDV. Exposure of cattle to other cattle or small ruminants at exhibitions should be limited, and animals should be quarantined for 3 weeks before reentry into the breeding herd. Most biosecurity principles instituted for BVDV control have the added benefit of disease control with other pathogens of cattle.

Eradication of BVDV

Because of the negative impact that a small number of PI BVDV carriers have on cattle health and the inconsistency with which vaccines have been able to control infection, several European countries have initiated BVDV eradication programs.[64] In 2002 the Academy of Veterinary Consultants presented a position statement on BVDV for eventual eradication of the virus in North America at a USDA-sponsored meeting.[81] This position statement has since been adopted by the American Association of Bovine Practitioners, the National

Cattlemen's Beef Association, and the United States Animal Health Association. Because of the importance of BVDV infections in cattle, there is support for BVDV control in the United States and individual states are developing and implementing voluntary BVDV control programs.

References

1. Brock KV: The many faces of bovine viral diarrhea virus, *Vet Clin North Am Food Anim Pract* 20:1, 2004.
2. Grooms DL: Reproductive consequences of infection with bovine viral diarrhea virus, *Vet Clin North Am Food Anim Pract* 20:5, 2004.
3. McClurkin AW, Littledike ET, Cutlip RC et al: Production of cattle immunotolerant to bovine viral diarrhea virus, *Can J Comp Med* 48:156, 1984.
4. Thiel HJ, Collett MS, Gould EA et al: Genus pestivirus. In Fauquet CM, Mayo MA, Maniloff J et al, editors: *Virus Taxonomy Classification and Nomenclature of Viruses Eighth Report of the International Committee on Taxonomy of Viruses*, San Diego, 2005, Elsevier Academic Press.
5. Carman S, van Dreumel T, Ridpath J et al: Severe acute bovine viral diarrhea in Ontario, 1993-1995, *J Vet Diagn Invest* 10:27, 1998.
6. Harding MJ, Cao X, Shams H et al: Role of bovine viral diarrhea virus biotype in the establishment of fetal infections, *Am J Vet Res* 63:1455, 2002.
7. Fulton RW, Ridpath JF, Ore S et al: Bovine viral diarrhoea virus (BVDV) subgenotypes in diagnostic laboratory accessions: distribution of BVDV1a, 1b, and 2a subgenotypes, *Vet Microbiol* 111:35, 2005.
8. Meyers G, Thiel HJ: Molecular characterization of pestiviruses, *Adv Virus Res* 47:53, 1996.
9. Ridpath JF, Bolin SR, Dubovi EJ: Segregation of bovine viral diarrhea virus into genotypes, *Virology* 205:66, 1994.
10. Ridpath JF: Classification and molecular biology. In Goyal SM, Ridpath JF, editor: *Bovine viral diarrhea virus: diagnosis, management and control*, Ames, Iowa, 2005, Blackwell Publishing.
11. Evermann JF, Ridpath JF: Clinical and epidemiologic observations of bovine viral diarrhea virus in the northwestern United States, *Vet Microbiol* 89:129, 2002.
12. Durham PJ, Hassard LE: Prevalence of antibodies to infectious bovine rhinotracheitis, parainfluenza 3, bovine respiratory syncytial, and bovine viral diarrhea viruses in cattle in Saskatchewan and Alberta, *Can Vet J* 31:815, 1990.
13. Bolin SR, McClurkin AW, Coria MF: Frequency of persistent bovine viral diarrhea virus infection in selected cattle herds, *Am J Vet Res* 46:2385, 1985.
14. Wittum TE, Grotelueschen DM, Brock KV et al: Persistent bovine viral diarrhoea virus infection in US beef herds, *Prev Vet Med* 49:83, 2001.
15. Houe H: Age distribution of animals persistently infected with bovine virus diarrhea virus in twenty-two Danish dairy herds, *Can J Vet Res* 56:194, 1992.
16. O'Connor AM, Sorden SD, Apley MD: Association between the existence of calves persistently infected with bovine viral diarrhea virus and commingling on pen morbidity in feedlot cattle, *Am J Vet Res* 66:2130, 2005.
17. Loneragan GH, Thomson DU, Montgomery DL et al: Prevalence, outcome, and health consequences associated with persistent infection with bovine viral diarrhea virus in feedlot cattle, *J Am Vet Med Assoc* 226:595, 2005.
18. Carman S, Carr N, DeLay J et al: Bovine viral diarrhea virus in alpaca: abortion and persistent infection, *J Vet Diagn Invest* 17:589, 2005.
19. Loken T: Ruminant pestivirus infections in animals other than cattle and sheep, *Vet Clin North Am Food Anim Pract* 11:597, 1995.
20. Baker JC: The clinical manifestations of bovine viral diarrhea infection, *Vet Clin North Am Food Anim Pract* 11:425, 1995.
21. Liebler-Tenorio EM, Kenklies S, Greiser-Wilke I et al: Incidence of BVDV1 and BVDV2 infections in cattle submitted for necropsy in northern Germany, *J Vet Med B Infect Dis Vet Public Health* 53:363, 2006.
22. Ridpath JF, Neill JD, Frey M et al: Phylogenetic, antigenic and clinical characterization of type 2 BVDV from North America, *Vet Microbiol* 77:145, 2000.
23. Bolin SR, Ridpath JF: Differences in virulence between two noncytopathic bovine viral diarrhea viruses in calves, *Am J Vet Res* 53:2157, 1992.
24. Walz PH, Bell TG, Grooms DL et al: Platelet aggregation responses and virus isolation from platelets in calves experimentally infected with type I or type II bovine viral diarrhea virus, *Can J Vet Res* 65:241, 2001.
25. Walz PH, Bell TG, Wells JL et al: Relationship between degree of viremia and disease manifestation in calves with experimentally induced bovine viral diarrhea virus infection, *Am J Vet Res* 62:1095, 2001.
26. Kelling CL, Steffen DJ, Topliff CL et al: Comparative virulence of isolates of bovine viral diarrhea virus type II in experimentally inoculated six- to nine-month-old calves, *Am J Vet Res* 63:1379, 2002.
27. Liebler-Tenorio EM, Ridpath JE, Neill JD: Distribution of viral antigen and development of lesions after experimental infection with highly virulent bovine viral diarrhea virus type 2 in calves, *Am J Vet Res* 63:1575, 2002.
28. Welsh MD, Adair BM, Foster JC: Effect of BVD virus infection on alveolar macrophage functions, *Vet Immunol Immunopathol* 46:195, 1995.
29. Roth JA, Kaeberle ML: Suppression of neutrophil and lymphocyte function induced by a vaccinal strain of bovine viral diarrhea virus with and without the administration of ACTH, *Am J Vet Res* 44:2366, 1983.
30. Richer L, Marois P, Lamontagne L: Association of bovine viral diarrhea virus with multiple viral infections in bovine respiratory disease outbreaks, *Can Vet J* 29:713, 1988.
31. Potgieter LN, McCracken MD, Hopkins FM et al: Comparison of the pneumopathogenicity of two strains of bovine viral diarrhea virus, *Am J Vet Res* 46:151, 1985.
32. Campbell JR: Effect of bovine viral diarrhea virus in the feedlot, *Vet Clin North Am Food Anim Pract* 20:39, 2004.
33. Potgieter LN, McCracken MD, Hopkins FM et al: Effect of bovine viral diarrhea virus infection on the distribution of infectious bovine rhinotracheitis virus in calves, *Am J Vet Res* 45:687, 1984.
34. Brodersen BW, Kelling CL: Effect of concurrent experimentally induced bovine respiratory syncytial virus and bovine viral diarrhea virus infection on respiratory tract and enteric diseases in calves, *Am J Vet Res* 59:1423, 1998.
35. Givens MD, Heath AM, Brock KV et al: Detection of bovine viral diarrhea virus in semen obtained after inoculation of seronegative postpubertal bulls, *Am J Vet Res* 64:428, 2003.
36. Kirkland PD, Mackintosh SG, Moyle A: The outcome of widespread use of semen from a bull persistently infected with pestivirus, *Vet Rec* 135:527, 1994.
37. Kirkland PD, McGowan MR, Mackintosh SG et al: Insemination of cattle with semen from a bull transiently infected with pestivirus, *Vet Rec* 140:124, 1997.
38. Voges H, Horner GW, Rowe S et al: Persistent bovine pestivirus infection localized in the testes of an immuno-competent, non-viraemic bull, *Vet Microbiol* 61:165, 1998.
39. Niskanen R, Alenius S, Belak K et al: Insemination of susceptible heifers with semen from a non-viraemic bull with

persistent bovine virus diarrhoea virus infection localized in the testes, *Reprod Domest Anim* 37:171, 2002.

40. Dubovi EJ: Impact of bovine viral diarrhea virus on reproductive performance in cattle, *Vet Clin North Am Food Anim Pract* 10:503, 1994.

41. McGowan MR, Kirkland PD, Richards SG et al: Increased reproductive losses in cattle infected with bovine pestivirus around the time of insemination, *Vet Rec* 133:39, 1993.

42. Grooms DL, Brock KV, Ward LA: Detection of bovine viral diarrhea virus in the ovaries of cattle acutely infected with bovine viral diarrhea virus, *J Vet Diagn Invest* 10:125, 1998.

43. Kirkbride CA: Viral agents and associated lesions detected in a 10-year study of bovine abortions and stillbirths, *J Vet Diagn Invest* 4:374, 1992.

44. Woodard L: BVD virus associated with outbreaks of abortion, stillbirths, and weak calves, *Vet Med* 89:379, 1994.

45. Duffell SJ, Sharp MW, Winkler CE et al: Bovine virus diarrhoea-mucosal disease virus-induced fetopathy in cattle: efficacy of prophylactic maternal pre-exposure, *Vet Rec* 114:558, 1984.

46. Houe H: Survivorship of animals persistently infected with bovine virus diarrhoea virus (BVDV), *Prev Vet Med* 15:275, 1993.

47. Munoz-Zanzi CA, Hietala SK, Thurmond MC et al: Quantification, risk factors, and health impact of natural congenital infection with bovine viral diarrhea virus in dairy calves, *Am J Vet Res* 64:358, 2003.

48. Bolin SR: The pathogenesis of mucosal disease, *Vet Clin North Am Food Anim Pract* 11:489, 1995.

49. Tautz N, Thiel HJ, Dubovi EJ et al: Pathogenesis of mucosal disease: a cytopathogenic pestivirus generated by an internal deletion, *J Virol* 68:3289, 1994.

50. Bielefeldt-Ohmann H: The pathologies of bovine viral diarrhea virus infection. A window on the pathogenesis, *Vet Clin North Am Food Anim Pract* 11:447, 1995.

51. Saliki JT, Dubovi EJ: Laboratory diagnosis of bovine viral diarrhea virus infections, *Vet Clin North Am Food Anim Pract* 20:69, 2004.

52. Saliki JT, Fulton RW, Hull SR et al: Microtiter virus isolation and enzyme immunoassays for detection of bovine viral diarrhea virus in cattle serum, *J Clin Microbiol* 35:803, 1997.

53. Njaa BL, Clark EG, Janzen E et al: Diagnosis of persistent bovine viral diarrhea virus infection by immunohistochemical staining of formalin-fixed skin biopsy specimens, *J Vet Diagn Invest* 12:393, 2000.

54. Driskell EA, Ridpath JF: A survey of bovine viral diarrhea virus testing in diagnostic laboratories in the United States from 2004 to 2005, *J Vet Diagn Invest* 18:600, 2006.

55. Zimmer GM, Van Maanen C, De Goey I et al: The effect of maternal antibodies on the detection of bovine virus diarrhoea virus in peripheral blood samples, *Vet Microbiol* 100:145, 2004.

56. Grooms DL, Keilen ED: Screening of neonatal calves for persistent infection with bovine viral diarrhea virus by immunohistochemistry on skin biopsy samples, *Clin Diagn Lab Immunol* 9:898, 2002.

57. Fulton RW, Johnson BJ, Briggs RE et al: Challenge with bovine viral diarrhea virus by exposure to persistently infected calves: protection by vaccination and negative results of antigen testing in nonvaccinated acutely infected calves, *Can J Vet Res* 70:121, 2006.

58. Cornish TE, van Olphen AL, Cavender JL et al: Comparison of ear notch immunohistochemistry, ear notch antigen-capture ELISA, and buffy coat virus isolation for detection of calves persistently infected with bovine viral diarrhea virus, *J Vet Diagn Invest* 17:110, 2005.

59. Fulton RW, Hessman B, Johnson BJ et al: Evaluation of diagnostic tests used for detection of bovine viral diarrhea virus

and prevalence of subtypes 1a, 1b, and 2a in persistently infected cattle entering a feedlot, *J Am Vet Med Assoc* 228:578, 2006.

60. Ridpath JF, Hietala SK, Sorden S et al: Evaluation of the reverse transcription-polymerase chain reaction/probe test of serum samples and immunohistochemistry of skin sections for detection of acute bovine viral diarrhea infections, *J Vet Diagn Invest* 14:303, 2002.

61. Weinstock D, Bhudevi B, Castro AE: Single-tube single-enzyme reverse transcriptase PCR assay for detection of bovine viral diarrhea virus in pooled bovine serum, *J Clin Microbiol* 39:343, 2001.

62. Brock KV: Diagnosis of bovine viral diarrhea virus infections, *Vet Clin North Am Food Anim Pract* 11:549, 1995.

63. Brock KV: The persistence of bovine viral diarrhea virus, *Biologicals* 31:133, 2003.

64. Greiser-Wilke I, Grummer B, Moennig V: Bovine viral diarrhoea eradication and control programmes in Europe, *Biologicals* 31:113, 2003.

65. Larson RL: Management systems and control programs. In Goyal SM, Ridpath JF, editors: *Bovine viral diarrhea virus: diagnosis, management and control*, Ames, Iowa, 2005, Blackwell Publishing.

66. Smith DR, Grotelueschen DM: Biosecurity and biocontainment of bovine viral diarrhea virus, *Vet Clin North Am Food Anim Pract* 20:131, 2004.

67. Houe H, Meyling A: Prevalence of bovine virus diarrhoea (BVD) in 19 Danish dairy herds and estimation of incidence of infection in early pregnancy, *Prevent Vet Med* 11:9, 1991.

68. Kennedy JA, Mortimer RG, Powers B: Reverse transcription-polymerase chain reaction on pooled samples to detect bovine viral diarrhea virus by using fresh ear-notch-sample supernatants, *J Vet Diagn Invest* 18:89, 2006.

69. Fulton RW: Vaccines. In Goyal SM, Ridpath JF, editors: *Bovine viral diarrhea virus: diagnosis, management and control*, Ames, Iowa, 2005, Blackwell Publishing.

70. Rauff Y, Moore DA, Sischo WM: Evaluation of the results of a survey of dairy producers on dairy herd biosecurity and vaccination against bovine viral diarrhea, *J Am Vet Med Assoc* 209:1618, 1996.

71. van Oirschot JT, Bruschke CJ, van Rijn PA: Vaccination of cattle against bovine viral diarrhoea, *Vet Microbiol* 64:169, 1999.

72. Dean HJ, Leyh R: Cross-protective efficacy of a bovine viral diarrhea virus (BVDV) type 1 vaccine against BVDV type 2 challenge, *Vaccine* 17:1117, 1999.

73. Cortese VS, West KH, Hassard LE et al: Clinical and immunologic responses of vaccinated and unvaccinated calves to infection with a virulent type-II isolate of bovine viral diarrhea virus, *J Am Vet Med Assoc* 213:1312, 1998.

74. Martin SW, Bohac JG: The association between serological titers in infectious bovine rhinotracheitis virus, bovine virus diarrhea virus, parainfluenza-3 virus, respiratory syncytial virus and treatment for respiratory disease in Ontario feedlot calves, *Can J Vet Res* 50:351, 1986.

75. Brock KV, McCarty K, Chase CC et al: Protection against fetal infection with either bovine viral diarrhea virus type 1 or type 2 using a noncytopathic type 1 modified-live virus vaccine, *Vet Ther* 7:27, 2006.

76. Dean HJ, Hunsaker BD, Bailey OD et al: Prevention of persistent infection in calves by vaccination of dams with noncytopathic type-1 modified-live bovine viral diarrhea virus prior to breeding, *Am J Vet Res* 64:530, 2003.

77. Ellsworth MA, Fairbanks KK, Behan S et al: Fetal protection following exposure to calves persistently infected with bovine viral diarrhea virus type 2 sixteen months after primary vaccination of the dams, *Vet Ther* 7:295, 2006.

78. Fairbanks KK, Rinehart CL, Ohnesorge WC et al: Evaluation of fetal protection against experimental infection with type 1 and type 2 bovine viral diarrhea virus after vaccination of the dam with a bivalent modified-live virus vaccine, *J Am Vet Med Assoc* 225:1898, 2004.

79. Brock KV, Cortese VS: Experimental fetal challenge using type II bovine viral diarrhea virus in cattle vaccinated with modified-live virus vaccine, *Vet Ther* 2:354, 2001.

80. Cortese VS, Grooms DL, Ellis J et al: Protection of pregnant cattle and their fetuses against infection with bovine viral diarrhea virus type 1 by use of a modified-live virus vaccine, *Am J Vet Res* 59:1409, 1998.

81. Brock KV: Strategies for the control and prevention of bovine viral diarrhea virus, *Vet Clin North Am Food Anim Pract* 20:171, 2004.

CHAPTER 25

Salmonellosis in Ruminants

VIRGINIA L. MOHLER and JOHN HOUSE

Salmonellosis is a common disease of livestock; manifestations include diarrhea, dehydration, abortion, depressed mentation, pneumonia, septic arthritis, meningitis, gangrene of distal extremities, and sudden death. More than 2500 different *Salmonella* serotypes exist. Some serotypes such as *Salmonella dublin* are host adapted, having a propensity to cause chronic infections. Most serovars are not host adapted, infecting a broad host range, and are infrequently associated with chronic infections. *Salmonella enterica* serovars *typhimurium* and *dublin* are frequently associated with disease in cattle. *S. enterica* serovar *newport* has more recently emerged as a significant pathogen causing disease in cattle and humans.[1-5] *S. typhimurium, Salmonella arizonae, Salmonella bovismorbificans,* and *Salmonella montevideo* are serovars commonly associated with disease in sheep.

Cattle—Adult Infections

Salmonella infections are usually acquired through fecal-oral and oral-oral contamination from the environment or fomites. The number of salmonellae required to produce clinical disease depends on host immunity and a serotype's virulence. The infective dose in healthy adult cattle is about 10^9 to 10^{11} *Salmonella*.[6,7] When immunity is compromised by concurrent disease or physiologic or dietary stress, the infectious dose may decrease to only several hundred salmonellae.[8]

An estimated 5% to 20% of the feed given to dairy cows in the United States is contaminated with salmonellae.[9] Healthy adult cattle normally tolerate small numbers of salmonellae in feed and do not develop clinical disease.[9] Although the number of salmonellae in the feed may be low initially, under appropriate moisture, temperature,

and pH conditions, *Salmonella* replicated about every 30 minutes. The resultant increase in *Salmonella* numbers is exponential. *Salmonella* outbreaks often result from a large challenge dose and impaired host immunity.

Salmonellosis in adult dairy cows commonly occurs close to parturition and may be associated with concurrent disease.[10] In the periparturient period, immunity is depressed and marked dietary changes occur. Dry-matter intake may be depressed by as much as 50% four days before parturition. Dietary intake before and following ingestion of *Salmonella* influences the growth of the organism in the rumen.[11] High concentrations of volatile fatty acids and a low rumen pH (normal 5.5 to 6.5) inhibit *Salmonella* growth.[12,13] Anorexia is associated with low concentrations of volatile fatty acids and a high rumen pH (approaching a pH of 7.5). Therefore *Salmonella* disappears rapidly from the rumens of regularly fed cows but maintains or increases its numbers when feed intake is decreased for a day or more.[11] Feeding after a period of starvation leads to multiplication of *Salmonella*.[14,15] After parturition, dairy cattle are fed a high-energy production ration, and clinical and subclinical ruminal acidosis is common. The increased production of lactate (a stronger, more dissociated and thus less inhibitory acid than acetate, propionate, and butyrate) favors the less fastidious salmonellae, which multiply rapidly.[12] Dietary stress and qualitative dietary changes may predispose ruminants to *Salmonella* infection.[16,17] The incidence of clinical disease may be reduced by manipulating the ration formulation and adjusting feeding practice.[17]

The shedding of salmonellae by clinically affected animals exponentially amplifies environmental contamination. Clinically infected animals may excrete 10^8 to 10^{10} salmonellae per gram of feces.[18] Considering that cattle produce 20 to 38 kg of feces a day, clinically affected cows may shed more than 10^{14} salmonellae each day. As environmental contamination increases, the balance between challenge dose and herd immunity is tipped in favor of the pathogen. For this reason, producers should isolate clinically affected animals from the herd. However, intensive dry-lot dairies rarely have adequate facilities to isolate clinically ill animals. Postpartum cows and sick cows are commonly housed and milked together to facilitate milk management. This practice exposes cows to a large challenge dose when they are most susceptible to infection. Most *Salmonella* infections in livestock are subclinical.[19] Up to 98% of dairy cows may shed *Salmonella* during the postpartum period.[20] The host outcome following pathogen exposure will reflect the size of the challenge dose; virulence of the infecting strain; and level of host immunity, which is largely influenced by environmental influences such as nutrition and weather conditions. Several studies have established that even in the absence of disease, *Salmonella* contamination of the environment and shedding by intensively managed livestock is common.[21,22] Surveys of dairy farms in California estimate a *Salmonella* prevalence of 75%.[23]

Herd outbreaks of salmonellosis commonly last several months. Their resolution appears to be largely due to increasing herd immunity in response to *Salmonella* exposure. Despite the resolution of clinical disease, salmonellae may continue to cycle through the herd and persist in the environment. *Salmonella* can survive for up to 6 years in feces.[24] Introduction of immunologically naive stock in the form of heifer replacements raised off site may provide a susceptible population that continues to experience clinical disease. *Salmonella* contamination of dairy and beef products continues even in the absence of clinical disease.[25]

Cattle—Neonatal Infections

Immunity to *Salmonella* changes rapidly during the first 3 months of a calf's life. In animals 2 weeks old, the LD_{50} for some virulent strains is 10^5 organisms, whereas the number of organisms rises to 10^7 at 6 to 7 weeks and 10^{10} at 12 to 14 weeks.[26,27] In contrast, administering 10^{10} salmonellae to calves 24 to 28 weeks old failed to induce clinical signs of disease.[27] Different age predilections, disease manifestations, and virulence are observed among *Salmonella* serotypes and among different strains of the same serotype.

Calves on endemically infected farms are commonly exposed to salmonellae in the first few days of life.[28] *Salmonella* exposure may occur via contaminated colostrum or milk, surface contamination of teats and udders, farm personnel, equipment, or the environment. Persistence of *Salmonella* for 2 years has been reported in a disinfected calf facility.[29] Chronically infected *Salmonella* carriers may shed 2.5×10^8 salmonellae a day in milk (25 kg of milk containing 10^5 salmonellae/ml).[7] *Salmonella* contamination of colostrum and milk from periparturient and sick cows is common on *Salmonella* endemic dairy farms.[25] Pooling colostrum results in poor passive transfer and increases the risk of exposing calves

to salmonellae. Outbreaks of salmonellosis in calves are commonly associated with the feeding of unrefrigerated hospital milk.

Maternity pen management also affects the amount of environmental *Salmonella* contamination calves are exposed to at birth. Personnel and feeding utensils often play important roles in transmitting *Salmonella* to calves.[30] *Salmonella* infects the salivary glands and is shed in saliva and nasal secretions.[31] To avoid contamination, feeding utensils must be cleaned and disinfected. *Salmonella* is sensitive to most disinfectants. Removing contaminating organic debris is imperative because it reduces disinfectant activity.

Sheep Infections

Salmonellosis in sheep is most commonly observed in feeder lambs and feedlot facilities. It tends to affect lambs and sheep 5 to 7 days after entry into the feedlot. Affected animals tend to have watery diarrhea with mucus and blood. Affected stock become anorexic and may be observed standing with their abdomen tucked up and their hind legs drawn forward. Fecal staining may be observed around the anus, and the sheep may be observed to make small side-to-side steps with their back feet, suggesting abdominal pain. Septicemia is common, and some sheep may simply be found dead. Morbidity and mortality are variable, largely influenced by nutritional management, environmental conditions, prefeedlot management, and the virulence of the infecting strain. A diversity of serovars may be shed in feces and isolated from the feedlot environment. Cultures of tissue swabs collected at necropsy tend to isolate a more limited number of virulent serovars. *S. typhimurium* and *S. bovis-morbificans* are common virulent serovars isolated from sheep in feedlots in Australia. Enterotoxemia, coccidiosis, and parasitism are important differential diagnoses for enteritis in feedlot sheep.

Several serotypes of *Salmonella* can cause abortions in ewes. Animals appear unwell and bacteremic at the time of abortion with *S. dublin* and *S. typhimurium* infections, whereas *S. arizonae* and *S. montevideo* can cause abortions in animals that otherwise appear healthy. *Salmonella abortus ovis* is a host-adapted serovar that causes abortion in sheep and goats in Europe.

Salmonella infections in goats are similar to those syndromes observed in cattle. They tend to occur in neonates, nursing goat kids, and adults. The enteric form is most common, presenting with watery or hemorrhagic diarrhea. Parasitism, coccidiosis, and enterotoxemia should be considered in the differential diagnosis.

NECROPSY FINDINGS

The most common postmortem findings in ruminants with acute *Salmonella* septicemia are muco-necrotic enteritis of the jejunum, ileum cecum, and large intestine. The walls are typically thickened, and the mucosal surface can vary from normal to hemorrhagic. A diphtheritic pseudomembrane may cover large areas of the mucosal surface, and the sloughed mucosa and fibrin may form casts within the lumen. Cattle may also have pneumonia, generalized lymphadenopathy, spleno-megaly, serosal hemorrhage, and hyperemic abomasal mucosa. Pneumonia is a common finding with *S. dublin* infections in calves, and the presence of clotted bile in the gallbladder or gangrene of the distal extremities is also suggestive of *S. dublin* infection.

Isolation of *Salmonella* from the tissues of animals with typical signs and lesions confirms the diagnosis. The samples of choice in septicemic cases include lung, liver, and spleen. For enteric cases, large intestine, ileum, and mesenteric lymph node samples should be collected.

Sheep

Postmortem findings in sheep that die of salmonellosis are variable. Signs of septicemia, which include splenic enlargement, congested organs, and acute enteritis, are common. Abomasitis is frequently a feature of salmonellosis in sheep and may be severe with ulceration and hemorrhage. Enteritis manifests as thickening of the intestinal wall. Hemorrhages may be observed on the serosal surface and are frequently seen on the mucosa of the small and large intestine. Lesions are most severe in the ileum, spiral colon, and cecum. Enlargement of the mesenteric lymph nodes is frequently observed. Intestinal contents tend to be muco-hemorrhagic and malodorous, reflecting protein exudation into the lumen.

PREVENTION

Preventing fecal-oral transmission of enteric pathogens is challenging in intensive livestock production systems. Subsequently, salmonellosis tends to be observed more frequently in intensive versus extensive farming systems. Livestock manure management systems reduce but do not eliminate *Salmonella,* which is subsequently recycled. Salmonellosis in livestock usually reflects a variety of management events and environmental stressors that contribute to compromised host immunity and increased pathogen exposure. Although a diversity of *Salmonella* serovars may be endemic in a given production facility, the virulence of these serovars is variable, reflected by the disparity among *Salmonella* isolates from surveillance and clinical submissions.[19]

The diversity of *Salmonella* serovars present on farms and the potential for variable virulence between serovars and within isolates of the same serovar requires the implementation of broad prophylactic strategies that are efficacious for all salmonellae. At the farm level, producers may implement programs to promote host immunity through provision of good nutrition and a comfortable environment. When this is accomplished, livestock health and productivity is promoted. In practice, consistent day-to-day implementation of these apparently simple principles is paradoxically complex with numerous variables such as changes in weather conditions, mechanical breakdowns, variable feedstuff availability and quality, and labor compliance issues all having the potential to adversely affect management programs and, subsequently, host immunity.

Salmonella Vaccines

Calves exposed to low doses of virulent salmonellae are protected against a subsequent high-dose virulent challenge, suggesting that vaccination can prevent salmonellosis.[32] *Salmonella* vaccine studies in cattle have focused on *Salmonella* bacterins and modified live *Salmonella* vaccines.

Most *Salmonella* vaccines licensed for commercial use in the United States are formalin-inactivated products with the adjuvant of aluminum.[18,33,34] The consensus of these reports is that vaccinating cattle with *Salmonella* bacterins provides partial protection against *Salmonella* challenge. However, anaphylactic reactions are occasionally reported.

A number of naturally occurring and genetically manipulated, attenuated *Salmonella* strains have been used to immunize cattle against salmonellosis. The most widely tested modified live *Salmonella* vaccines in cattle are the genetically altered aromatic amino acid (aro) and purine (pur) auxotrophic mutants.[35,36] Comparative vaccine trails indicate that modified live *Salmonella* vaccines provide greater protection against virulent *Salmonella* than do *Salmonella* bacterins.[37,38]

With modified live *Salmonella* vaccines, immunity depends on dose (amount, number, and interval), route, and age. The frequency and magnitude of adverse reactions are also dose, route, and age dependent. Immunity can be induced in young calves with a lower inoculation dose than in older calves. And with parenteral administration, lower doses are necessary than with oral administration.[36] After oral administration of modified live vaccines to calves, the vaccine strain may be isolated from the tissues and feces for 14 to 21 days. The capacity of modified live *Salmonella* vaccines to persist in the host is important for efficacy.[39] Extensive use of antibiotics in some commercial calf-raising facilities may decrease the persistence and efficacy of modified live *Salmonella* vaccines.

Passive Protection via Colostral Transfer

Whether passive protection is achieved by feeding calves colostrum from vaccinated cows is questionable. Many reports suggest that immune colostrum provides passive protection, but others show no protective effect.[40] These different results may be partly explained by differences in study design. In one study, vaccinating pregnant cows with formalin-killed *S. typhimurium* 7 and 2 weeks before parturition protected their calves against experimental *S. typhimurium* challenge in the first week of life.[40]

Feeding calves colostrum at birth and then daily for the first 8 days of life reduced mortality more than feeding them colostrum only at birth. However, no protective effect was observed when calves were challenged at 3 weeks of age. Although the duration of immunity associated with colostral transfer may be short, calves are commonly exposed to salmonellae in the first week of life, so colostral protection may be useful. The effect of colostral transfer on the development of acquired immunity to *Salmonella* has not been evaluated.

TREATMENT AND CONTROL

Therapy for Salmonellosis

Many of the clinical signs associated with salmonellosis are mediated by the proinflammatory effects of endotoxin. Systemic signs of endotoxemia include fever, tachypnea, tachycardia, scleral injection, leucopenia or leukocytosis, weakness, and ruminal stasis. Some serotypes, particularly *S. typhimurium*, tend to induce severe inflammation of the bowel mucosa, resulting in dysentery and the passage of fibrin and mucosal casts. Feces range from mucohemorrhagic to fetid watery discharge containing frank blood. Fluid, electrolyte, and protein loss may progress rapidly and become life threatening. Dehydration, electrolyte imbalances, endotoxemia, and bacteremia are common clinical features of *Salmonella* infections. Bacteremia is common in neonates.

Treatment of salmonellosis is directed at replacing fluids and electrolyte losses, limiting inflammatory cascades through use of nonsteroidal antiinflammatory drugs (NSAIDs), and at elimination of the infecting organism through the judicious use of antimicrobials.[18,41] Additionally, good nursing care in the form of an adequate diet and provision of a clean, dry, comfortable environment can greatly improve outcome.

Fluid Therapy

Loss of mucosal epithelia cells contributes to maldigestion and malabsorption. Inflammation promotes hypersecretion; some strains of *Salmonella* also produce enterotoxins that may contribute to hypersecretion. Mucosal injury contributes to intestinal loss of proteins and fluids. In neonates, diarrhea contributes to dehydration, metabolic acidosis, cardiovascular collapse, and death.[42] Saline-based fluids with alkalizing agents such as sodium bicarbonate can be useful in correcting dehydration, replacing ongoing fluid losses, and expanding vascular volume to prevent cardiovascular failure and to improve organ perfusion. Parenteral and oral fluid therapy can increase the survival rates of calves with salmonellosis.[43] Supplemental oral or intravenous glucose, or both, can prevent hypoglycemia associated with malabsorption disorders and anorexia.

Nonsteroidal Antiinflammatory Drugs

NSAIDs have been used to attenuate endotoxin-related symptoms of inflammation in the treatment of salmonellosis. NSAIDs inhibit endotoxin-induced inflammation by blocking arachidonate cyclo-oxygenase and reducing the formation of thromboxanes and prostaglandins.[44,45] They also have analgesic and antipyretic effects and can provide prolonged therapeutic activities because of extensive tissue binding and prolonged release long after serum concentrations have dropped below detection.[46] Flunixin meglumine, meloxicam, ketoprofen, and aspirin are examples of NSAIDs used in cattle.[46-48]

The efficacy of NSAID administration in the treatment of salmonellosis in calves has not been reported in the literature. NSAID therapy has been reported to improve outcome, reduce mortality in calves with bloody diarrhea,[47] and modify the response to endotoxin.[49] Empirical treatment of salmonellosis with NSAIDs is recommended in conjunction with appropriate fluid therapy.

Precautions should be taken when administering NSAIDs to animals that are hypovolemic and hypotensive. The renal toxicity associated with NSAID administration is exacerbated by dehydration, which reduces renal perfusion. Additionally, hepatic metabolism is variable in neonates and may contribute to reduced drug clearance and prolonged half-lives. Importantly, withdrawal periods have not been established for the use of flunixin in preruminant calves and it is not recommended for use in veal calves. In the United Kingdom, meloxicam is licensed for use in the treatment of calf scours in combination with antimicrobials and oral hydration therapy.[47] In Australia, aspirin, flunixin, and ketoprofen have been approved for use in cattle with specific meat withholding periods.[50]

Antimicrobials

The propensity for *Salmonella* to cause bacteremia in calves warrants antimicrobial therapy. Prompt aggressive treatment with antimicrobials early in the infection is recommended.[43,51] Ideally antimicrobial selection at the herd level should be based on the antimicrobial susceptibility testing of *Salmonella* isolated from the tissues of an infected animal and not a fecal isolate. Empirical treatment is usually implemented pending the results of susceptibility testing.[41,43,52] *Salmonella* show variable resistance to ampicillin, amoxicillin, sulfas, trimethoprim-sulpha, ceftiofur, and tetracycline and resistance to penicillin, streptomycin, erythromycin, and tylosin.[32] Because salmonellae are facultative intracellular pathogens, selecting an antimicrobial with good tissue penetration and the ability to attain intracellular therapeutic drug concentrations within macrophages is desirable.

A number of experimental studies have evaluated the efficacy of antimicrobial agents in the treatment of salmonellosis in cattle. In a comparative trial, amoxicillin and trimethoprim sulfadiazine were shown to have equivalent efficacy in the treatment of calves with *Salmonella* infections via oral (PO), intravenous (IV), and intramuscular (IM) routes when administered at doses based on minimal inhibitory concentration (MIC) of the infecting organism and peak blood levels.[53] Extra-label use of ceftiofur has also been shown to attenuate the severity of disease and reduce fecal shedding of *Salmonella*.[41] The results of therapeutic trials suggest antimicrobial therapy is beneficial when calves are treated with an antimicrobial with a dose and frequency that maintains a drug concentration in excess of the MIC of the infecting organism.

The use of antimicrobials to treat salmonellosis in livestock raises a number of issues relating to antimicrobial resistance, antimicrobial residues in tissues, as well as the environment and human safety. Emergence of antimicrobial resistance to fluoroquinolones and third-generation cephalosporins is a public health concern. Ciprofloxacin, a fluoroquinolone and the drug of choice in the treatment of human salmonellosis, is a metabolite of enrofloxacin metabolism in cattle.[54-56] Aminoglycosides may also be used in the control of *Salmonella* infection in cattle; however, drug residues and prolonged meat withholding times make the use of these drugs prohibitive in food animal species. Prudent use of antimicrobial drugs should continue to be employed, with an emphasis on treating the bacteremic and compromised patients and using the narrowest spectrum of antimicrobial available.

PUBLIC HEALTH

The Centers for Disease Control and Prevention (CDC) reported that an estimated 1.4 million human *Salmonella* infections occurred in the United States, with only 40,000 reported at a cost of $5 billion.[57,58] In 2004 the WHO reported that more than 3 million deaths were attributed to *Salmonella* infections worldwide.[59] Most cases of human salmonellosis in developed countries are derived from contaminated foods such as eggs, milk, beef, and poultry or products that have been exposed to animal feces including fruits and vegetables. Recent statistics show that 40.3 cases of salmonellosis per 100,000 population were reported in Australia,[60] whereas 13 per 100,000 population were reported in the United States over the same period.[57] The link *Salmonella* and other enteric pathogens create between livestock production and human food safety continues to drive livestock industries to adopt management practices that address waste management, prevent disease, and minimize antimicrobial use.

References

1. CDC: Outbreak of multidrug-resistant *Salmonella newport*—United States, January-April 2002, *http://www.cdc.gov/mmwr/preview/mmwrhtml/mm5125a1.htm,MortalMorWklyRep* 51(25): 545-548, 2002.
2. Clark S: *Salmonella newport*—an emerging disease in dairy cattle, *http://www.addl.purdue.edu/newsletters/2004/summer/salmnewp. htm* In Dr. Leon Thacker AD, editor: *Animal disease diagnostic laboratory,* West Lafayette, Ind, 2004.
3. Devasia RA, Varma JK, Whichard J et al: Antimicrobial use and outcomes in patients with multidrug-resistant and pan-susceptible *Salmonella newport* infections, 2002-2003, *Microb Drug Resist Mech Epidemiol Dis* 11:371-377, 2005.
4. Varma JK, Marcus R, Stenzel SA et al: Highly resistant *Salmonella newport*-MDRAmpC transmitted through the domestic US food supply: a FoodNet case-control study of sporadic Salmonella Newport infections, 2002-2003, *J Infect Dis* 194: 222-230, 2006.
5. You Y, Rankin S, Aceto H et al: Survival of *Salmonella enterica* serovar *newport* in manure and manure-amended soils, *Appl Enviro Microbiol* 72:5777-5783, 2006.
6. Jones PW: *Salmonellosis*, Oxford, 1992, Blackwell Scientific Publications.
7. Smith BP, Oliver DG, Singh P et al: Detection of *Salmonella-dublin* mammary-gland infection in carrier cows, using an enzyme-linked immunosorbent-assay for antibody in milk or serum, *Am J Vet Res* 50:1352-1360, 1989.
8. Grau FH, Brownlie LE, Smith MG: Effects of food intake on numbers of salmonellae and *Escherichia coli* in rumen and faeces of sheep, *J Appl Bacteriol* 32:112, 1969.
9. Hancock DD, Dargatz DA: *Implementation of HACCP on the farm,* Proceedings of Hazard Analysis Critical Control Point (HACCP) Symposium 1995.
10. Morisse JP, Cotte JP: Evaluation of some risk factors in bovine salmonellosis, *Vet Res* 25:185-191, 1994.
11. Brownlie LE, Grau FH: Effect of food intake on growth and survival of salmonellas and *Escherichia coli* in bovine rumen, *J Gen Microbiol* 46:125, 1967.
12. Chambers PG, Lysons RJ: Inhibitory effect of bovine rumen fluid on *Salmonella-typhimurium, Res Vet Sci* 26:273-276, 1979.
13. Mattila T, Frost AJ, Oboyle D: The growth of *Salmonella* in rumen fluid from cattle at slaughter, *Epidemiol Infect* 101:337-345, 1988.
14. Frost AJ, Oboyle D, Samuel JL: The isolation of *Salmonella* spp from feed lot cattle managed under different conditions before slaughter, *Austral Vet J* 65:224-225, 1988.
15. Grau FH, Brownlie LE, Roberts EA: Effect of some preslaughter treatments on *Salmonella* population in bovine rumen and faeces, *J Appl Bacteriol* 31:157, 1968.
16. Kahrs RF, Lewis NF, King JM et al: Epidemiologic investigation of an outbreak of fatal enteritis and abortion associated with dietary change and *Salmonella-typhimurium* infection in a dairy-herd—case report, *Cornell Vet* 62:175, 1972.
17. Pierson RE, Poduska PJ, Cholas G et al: Relationship of management and nutrition to salmonellosis in feedlot lambs, *J Am Vet Med Assoc* 161:1217, 1972.
18. House JK, Smith BP: Current strategies for managing salmonella infections in cattle, *Vet Med* 93:756, 1998.
19. Anderson RJ, House JK, Smith BP et al: Epidemiologic and biological characteristics of salmonellosis in three dairy herds, *J Am Vet Assoc* 219:310-322, 2001.
20. House JK, Ontiveros MM, Blackmer NM et al: Evaluation of an autogenous *Salmonella* bacterin and a modified live *Salmonella* serotype Choleraesuis vaccine on a commercial dairy farm, *Am J Vet Res* 62:1897-1902, 2001.
21. Huston CL, Wittum TE, Love BC et al: Prevalence of fecal shedding of *Salmonella* spp in dairy herds, *J Am Vet Med Assoc* 220:645-649, 2002.
22. Woodward MJ, Gettinby G, Breslin MF et al: The efficacy of Salenvac, a *Salmonella enterica* subsp. enterica serotype *enteritidis* iron-restricted bacterin vaccine in laying chickens, *Avian Pathol* 31:383-385, 2002.
23. Smith BP, Da Roden L, Thurmond MC et al: Prevalence of salmonellae in cattle and in the environment on California dairies, *J Am Vet Med Assoc* 205:467-471, 1994.
24. Plym-Forshell L, Ekesbo I: Survival of salmonellas in urine and dry-faeces from cattle: an experimental study, *Acta Vet Scand* 37:127-131, 1996.
25. Gay JM, Hunsaker ME: Isolation of multiple *Salmonella*-serovars from a dairy 2 years after a clinical salmonellosis outbreak, *J Am Vet Med Assoc* 203:1314-1320, 1993.
26. Mohler VL, Heithoff DM, Mahan MJ et al: Cross-protective immunity in calves conferred by a DNA adenine methylase deficient *Salmonella enterica* serovar *typhimurium* vaccine, *Vaccine* 24:1339, 2006.
27. Segall T, Lindberg AA: Experimental oral *Salmonella-dublin* infection in calves: a bacteriological and pathological study, *J Vet Med Series B-Zentralblatt Fur Veterinarmedizin Reihe B-Infect Dis Vet Public Health* 38:169-185, 1991.
28. Robinson RA, Loken KI: Age susceptibility and excretion of *Salmonella typhimurium* in calves, *J Hygiene-Cambridge* 66:207, 1968.
29. McLaren I, Wray C: Epidemiology of *Salmonella typhimurium* infection in calves: persistence of salmonellae in calf units, *Vet Rec* 129:461-462, 1991.
30. Hardman PM, Wathes CM, Wray C: Transmission of salmonellae among calves penned individually, *Vet Rec* 129:327-329, 1991.
31. Richardson A, Fawcett AR: *Salmonella-dublin* infection in calves: value of rectal swabs in diagnosis and epidemiological studies, *Br Vet J* 129:151-156, 1973.

32. Smith BP: Diseases of the alimentary tract: salmonellosis in ruminants. In Smith BP, editor: *Large animal internal medicine*, ed 3, St Louis, 2002, Mosby, pp 775-779.

33. Aitken MM, Jones PW, Brown GTH: Protection of cattle against experimentally induced salmonellosis by intradermal injection of heat-killed *Salmonella dublin, Res Vet Sci* 32:368-373, 1982.

34. Robertsson JA, Lindberg AA, Hoiseth S et al: Salmonella typhimurium infection in calves: protection and survival of virulent challenge bacteria after immunization with live or inactivated vaccines, *Infect Immun* 41:742-750, 1983.

35. McFarland WC, Stocker BAD: Effect of different purine auxotrophic mutations on mouse-virulence of a vi-positive strain of *Salmonella dublin* and of two strains of *Salmonella typhimurium, Microb Pathogen* 3:129-141, 1987.

36. Smith BP, Reina-Guerra M, Hoiseth SK et al: Aromatic-dependent *Salmonella typhimurium* as modified live vaccines for calves, *Am J Vet Res* 45:59-66, 1984.

37. Baljer G, Hoerstke M, Dirksen G et al: Comparative studies of the effectivity of oral immunization with heat-inactivated and live, avirulent (GalE-) *S. typhimurium* bacteria against salmonellosis in calves, *Zentralblattt fur Veterinarmedizin Reihe [B]* 28:759-766, 1981.

38. Cameron CM, Fuls W: Immunization of mice and calves against *Salmonella dublin* with attenuated live and inactivated vaccines, *Onderstepoort J Vet Res* 43:31-37, 1976.

39. O'Callaghan D, Maskell D, Liew FY et al: Characterization of aromatic-dependent and purine-dependent *Salmonella-typhimurium*—attenuation, persistence, and ability to induce protective immunity in balb/c mice, *Infect Immun* 56:419-423, 1988.

40. Jones BD, Falkow S: Salmonellosis: host immune responses and bacterial virulence determinants, *Ann Rev Immunol* 14:533-561, 1996.

41. Fecteau M, House JK, Kotarski SF et al: Efficacy of ceftiofur for treatment of experimental salmonellosis in neonatal calves, *Am J Vet Res* 64:918-925, 2003.

42. Naylor JM: Manifestations of disease in the neonate: neonatal ruminant diarrhea. In Smith BP, editor: *Large animal internal medicine*, ed 3, St Louis, 2002, Mosby, pp 352-366.

43. Wray C, Davies R: *Salmonella* infections in cattle. In Wray C, Wray W, editors: *Salmonella in domestic animals*, New York, 2000, CABI Publishing, pp 169-190.

44. MacKay RJ: Diseases of the alimentary tract: endotoxemia. In Smith BP, editor: *Large animal internal medicine*, ed 3, St Louis, 2002, Mosby, pp 633-641.

45. Rang HP, Dale MM, Ritter JM: *Anti-inflammatory and immunosuppressant drugs. Pharmacology*, ed 4, London, 2001, Churchill Livingstone, pp 229-249.

46. George LW: Pain control in food animals. In Steffey EP, editor: *Recent advances in anesthetic management of large domestic animals*, Ithaca, New York, 2003, International Veterinary Information Service.

47. Barrett DC: Non-steroidal anti-inflammatory drugs in cattle: should we use them more? *Cattle Pract* 12:69-73, 2001.

48. Plumb DC: *Veterinary drug handbook*, ed 3, White Bear Lake, Minn, 1999, Pharma Vet Publishing.

49. Semrad SD: Comparative efficacy of flunixin, ketoprofen, and ketorolac for treating endotoxemic neonatal calves, *Am J Vet Res* 54:1511-1516, 1993.

50. MIMS: *2005 IVS annual*, ed 17, Singapore, 2005, Kyodo Printing Co.

51. Pasquini C, Pasquini S: Guide to bovine clinics, ed 3, Pilot Point, Texas, 1996, Sudz Publishing.

52. Bell SM, Gatus BJ, Pham JN et al: *Performance of the CDS test. Antibiotic susceptibility testing by the CDS method: a manual for medical and veterinary laboratories 2004*, ed 3, Randwick, NSW, Australia, 2004, South Eastern Area Laboratory Services, pp 12–20.

53. Groothuis DG, van Miert AS: Salmonellosis in veal calves: some therapeutic aspects, *Vet Q* 9:91-96, 1987.

54. Helmuth R: Antibiotic resistance in salmonella. In Wray C, Wray W, editors: Salmonella *in domestic animals*, New York, 2000, CABI Publishing, pp 89-106.

55. Idowu OR, Peggins JO: Simple, rapid determination of enrofloxacin and ciprofloxacin in bovine milk and plasma by high-performance liquid chromatography with fluorescence detection, *J Pharmaceut Biomed Anal* 35:143-153, 2004.

56. TerHune TN, Skogerboe TL, Shostrom VK et al: Comparison of pharmacokinetics of danofloxacin and enrofloxacin in calves challenged with *Mannheimia haemolytica, Am J Vet Res* 66:342-349, 2005.

57. CDC: Salmonellosis: Centers for Disease Control and Prevention (*http://www.cdc.gov/ncidod/dbmd/diseaseinfo/salmonellosis_g. htm*), 2005.

58. Mead P, Slutsker L, Dietz V et al: Food-related illness and death in the United State, *Emerg Infect Dis* 5:607-625, 1999.

59. WHO: Drug-resistant *Salmonella. http://www.who.int/ mediacentre/factsheets/fs139/en/print.html*, World Health Organization, Food Safety Department, 2005. Retrieved Dec 14, 2007.

60. OzFoodNet: *Foodborne disease in Australia: incidence, notification and outbreaks. Annual report of the OxFoodNet network, 2002*, Canberra, Australia, 2003, OzFoodNet Working Group, Food Safety and Surveillance, Department of Health and Aging, pp 209-243.

CHAPTER 26
Winter Dysentery

LINDA J. SAIF

Winter dysentery (WD) is an acute diarrheal disease of beef and dairy cattle and captive wild ruminants that occurs mostly during the winter (November to March in the Northern United States).[1-3] WD is one of the three clinical disease syndromes associated with bovine coronavirus (BCoV) infection, the other two being calf diarrhea and shipping fever pneumonia in feedlot cattle.[4] The BCoVs from WD outbreaks in both cattle and in captive wild ruminants (Fig. 26-1) are closely related biologically and antigenically (single serotype) to BCoVs from the other two clinical disease syndromes of cattle.[3-5] Experimentally they cross-protect calves against calf diarrhea BCoV strains.[6] The WD BCoV is pH stable (pH 3-8) and survives passage through the gut. As an enveloped virus, it is heat labile, which may explain its greater survival in a frozen state and its prevalence during winter, in addition to its sensitivity to most disinfectants and steam cleaning. Besides isolation of BCoV in cell culture from WD cases,[7] BCoV has been further implicated as a cause of WD in both epidemiologic studies[8,9] and by experimental transmission studies in calves[6] and seropositive nonlactating[10] and seronegative lactating dairy cows.[11]

EPIZOOTIOLOGY

WD occurs in cattle worldwide. The seroprevalence of BCoV among adult cattle is also high.[1,4] Although earlier reports documented outbreaks associated with BCoV mostly in dairy cattle,[1] subsequent reports have confirmed similar outbreaks and clinical signs in 6- to 9-month-old feedlot calves[2] and also in captive wild ruminants including white-tailed deer, sambar deer, and waterbuck.[3] The morbidity rate of WD outbreaks is high (50%-100%), but the mortality rate is usually low (1%-2%) unless complicated by the presence of other agents such as bovine viral diarrhea virus (BVDV) or secondary bacterial infections.[1,2] Besides BCoV fecal shedding and seroconversion to BCoV or BVDV being significant epidemiologic risk factors for WD in dairy herds, various host and environmental factors may also contribute to disease expression.[1,8,9] These include age of animal (2–6-year-olds at most risk) and larger herd size, close confinement of cattle (tie stall instead of free stalls), use of manure-handling equipment for feed, and poor barn ventilation. The latter environmental factors probably relate to the documented fecal-oral and presumed aerosol transmission routes for BCoV.

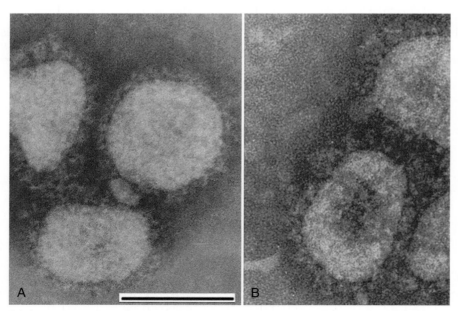

Fig 26-1   Immune electron microscopy of cell culture isolates of bovine coronavirus **(A)** and sambar deer coronavirus **(B)** from cases of winter dysentery in a dairy cow and captive sambar deer, respectively. Both samples were incubated with antiserum to bovine coronavirus. *Bar,* 100 μm.

The recent recognition of the existence of CoVs closely related to BCoVs in captive exotic (sambar deer, waterbuck) and native wild ruminants (white-tailed deer, mule deer, and elk) raises concerns of a wildlife reservoir for CoVs transmissible to cattle, as shown experimentally.[3-6] Thus the possibility exists that native wild ruminants could transmit CoV strains to cattle or vice versa, potentially serving as a reservoir for these viruses during summer with transmission initiated in winter, resulting in WD outbreaks.

CLINICAL SIGNS AND LESIONS

WD is characterized by anorexia; fever; liquid, often hemorrhagic diarrhea; frequent respiratory signs (cough, dyspnea, nasal discharge); and a marked, frequently persisting drop in milk production in dairy cattle.[1] Similar clinical signs (except decreased milk production) were evident in feedlot cattle with WD.[2] Both transient fecal and nasal shedding (1-4 days) of BCoV have been described in naturally[2] and experimentally exposed[6,10,11] cattle with WD. The fever, anorexia, bloody diarrhea, and clinical respiratory signs observed in one experimental study of BCoV seronegative lactating cows challenged with a WD BCoV[11] closely mimicked the WD clinical disease seen in feedlot outbreaks.[1,2,4] Based on the data in experimentally exposed cows or calves, the incubation period ranged from 3 to 8 days and diarrhea persisted for 1 to 6 days.[2,10,11] Intestinal lesions and distribution of BCoV-infected cells in colonic crypts of dairy and beef cattle with WD resemble those described for calf diarrhea.[2,12] The pathologic mechanism related to the profuse, dark red, bloody diarrhea and the blood within the lumen of the colon and rectum seen in some cattle is unknown, but petechial hemorrhages in the colonic mucosa are common.[2,12]

DIAGNOSIS

BCoV infections are diagnosed by the detection of virus, viral antigen, or viral RNA in intestinal tissues, feces, rectal swab fluids, intestinal contents, or nasal swab fluids and secretions of infected animals. Because WD is an acute, transient infection, definitive diagnosis requires submission of these specimens collected within 1 to 3 days of diarrhea onset. Antemortem tests are accomplished using feces or nasal or rectal swab fluids (collected in PBS or cell culture medium, pH 7-7.4) and stored frozen immediately after collection and during shipping. Bovine CoV, BCoV antigens, or BCoV RNA are detected in such samples using virus isolation techniques or immune electron microscopy (IEM), enzyme-linked immunosorbent assay (ELISA), and RT-PCR, respectively.[1-3,5-9]

Because feces contain other pleomorphic particles, IEM is useful to visualize BCoV antibody-viral aggregates and increase EM sensitivity (see Fig. 26-1), as well as to detect other enteric viruses. A commercial ELISA kit using a pool of monoclonal antibodies to BCoV has been licensed in the United States (IDEXX, Westbrook, Me). However, in one study, ELISA was less sensitive than IEM for detection of BCoV from WD cases, possibly because of interference by antibodies to BCoV that are widespread in cattle.[8] The RT-PCR assay, based on primers to the conserved BCoV N protein gene, was more sensitive than IEM for detecting WD-BCoV in feces of experimentally inoculated calves.[6]

Postmortem, BCoV antigens are detected in infected intestinal epithelial cells of the distal small intestine and colon in frozen tissue sections or acetone-fixed intestinal impression smears by immunofluorescence or immunohistochemistry.[2,12]

Seroresponses to BCoV (>two to fourfold increased titers) among cattle from WD outbreaks ranged from 59% to 100%.[1] Because most adult cattle have antibodies to BCoV, paired serum samples are necessary and should be done on a herd basis for WD affected cattle.

TREATMENT, PREVENTION, AND CONTROL

Because no antivirals for BCoV infections are available, only symptomatic treatments are possible. These include oral or IV fluids to alleviate dehydration and antibiotics if secondary bacterial infections occur. Nevertheless, in dairy cattle, anorexia and decreased milk production may persist for months after a WD outbreak.

The correlates of protective immunity associated with BCoV infections in WD outbreaks are unknown, including the role of the preexisting serum antibodies to BCoV in the affected cattle.[1] Traven and colleagues[11] reported persisting (>6 months) IgA antibodies to BCoV in milk and nasal secretions of dairy cattle recovered from experimental WD-BCoV infections. At present no BCoV vaccines are licensed to prevent WD in cattle. Whether commercially available BCoV vaccines licensed for calves would prevent WD is unknown, and they have not been tested in epidemiologic or experimental studies.

References

1. Saif LJ: A review of evidence implicating bovine coronavirus in the etiology of winter dysentery in cows: an enigma resolved? *Cornell Vet* 80:303, 1990.
2. Cho KO, Halbur PG, Bruna JD et al: Detection and isolation of coronavirus from feces of three herds of feedlot cattle during outbreaks of winter dysentery-like disease, *J Am Vet Med Assoc* 217:1191, 2000.
3. Tsunemitsu H, el-Kanawati ZR, Smith DR et al: Isolation of coronaviruses antigenically indistinguishable from bovine coronavirus from wild ruminants with diarrhea, *J Clin Microbiol* 33:3264, 1995.
4. Saif LJ: Animal coronaviruses: what can they teach us about the severe acute respiratory syndrome? *Rev Sci Tech Off Int Epiz* 23:643, 2004.
5. Tsunemitsu H, Saif LJ: Antigenic and biological comparisons of bovine coronaviruses derived from neonatal calf diarrhea and winter dysentery of adult cattle, *Arch Virol* 140:1303, 1995.
6. Cho KO, Hasoksuz M, Nielsen PR et al: Cross-protection studies between respiratory and calf diarrhea and winter dysentery coronavirus strains in calves and RT-PCR and nested PCR for their detection, *Arch Virol* 146:2401, 2001.
7. Benfield DA, Saif LJ: Cell culture propagation of a coronavirus isolated from cows with winter dysentery, *J Clin Microbiol* 28:1454, 1990.

8. Smith DR, Fedorka-Cray PJ, Mohan R et al: Evaluation of cow-level risk factors for the development of winter dysentery in dairy cattle, *Am J Vet Res* 59:986, 1998.

9. Smith DR, Fedorka-Cray PJ, Mohan R et al: Epidemiologic herd-level assessment of causative agents and risk factors for winter dysentery in dairy cattle, *Am J Vet Res* 59:994, 1998.

10. Tsunemitsu H, Smith DR, Saif LJ: Experimental inoculation of adult dairy cows with bovine coronavirus and detection of coronavirus in feces by RT-PCR, *Arch Virol* 144:167, 1999.

11. Traven M, Naslund K, Linde N et al: Experimental reproduction of winter dysentery in lactating cows using BCV—comparison with BCV infection in milk-fed calves, *Vet Microbiol* 81:127, 2001.

12. Van Kruiningen HJ, Khairallah LH, Sasseville VG et al: Calfhood coronavirus enterocolitis: a clue to the etiology of winter dysentery, *Vet Pathol* 24:564, 1987.

CHAPTER 27

Duodenal Obstruction

DAVID E. ANDERSON

Duodenal outflow problems occur as a result of obstruction or dysfunction. Duodenal dysfunction occurs as a result of peracute duodenitis, duodenal ulcers with or without perforation, clostridial duodenitis, and electrolyte abnormalities.[1-4] Duodenal obstruction occurs as a result of trichobezoars (discussed later in this chapter); foreign bodies (e.g., gravel); duodenal stricture following ulcer; obstruction by displacement of viscera (e.g., gallbladder, uterus); iatrogenic duodenal obstruction following omentopexy or pyloropexy; and extraluminal compression caused by liver abscess, omental abscess, or lyphosarcoma.[3-8]

CLINICAL SIGNS

Animals affected with duodenal obstruction may be observed to have severe bloat caused by fluid distention of all forestomachs, acute collapse and dehydration, decreased appetite, weight loss, decreased fecal production, lethargy, and apparent depression.[3] Affected animals initially show clinical signs of abdominal pain (restlessness, kicking at the abdomen, lying down and getting up frequently, arching the back, stretching out of the legs while standing) and progress to severe rumen distention, recumbency, and apparent depression. Death ensues because of dehydration and severe electrolyte disturbances.

CLINICAL PATHOLOGY

Serum biochemistry analysis reveals profound hypokalemic, hypochloremic, metabolic alkalosis, the severity of which depends on the duration of the lesion.[3] These changes are most severe with proximal intestinal obstruction and become more severe with increasing duration. Interestingly, cows with duodenal disease were reported to have severe hyperglycemia (range, 263-990 mg/dl).[9] If ischemic necrosis of the intestinal wall has occurred, an inflammatory leukogram with increased numbers of immature neutrophils may be seen. As peritonitis develops and organic acids are released into the bloodstream, the serum biochemistry changes to a metabolic acidosis with relative hyperkalemia. These changes are consistent with a poor prognosis, but death may occur before these changes occur. Perforation of the duodenum with contamination of the abdomen with ingesta carries a poor to grave prognosis.

DIAGNOSIS

In affected cattle, serum biochemistry changes are consistent with intestinal obstruction. Rumen chloride concentration may be elevated (rumen Cl > 30 mEq/l). Although not routinely done, rumen fluid bile acid concentration is helpful in differentiating duodenal and proximal jejunum obstructions from abomasal outflow obstruction. Bile acid concentrations in cattle with proximal duodenal or jejunum obstruction had significantly higher rumen bile acid concentration compared with cattle affected with reticuloperitonitis, abomasal displacement, or cecal dilation. The cause of intraluminal obstruction is rarely palpable per rectum, but small intestinal distention may be palpable. Ultrasonographic examination of the abdomen may be useful.[10] The intestinal tract appears normal, but severe distention of the duodenum and forestomachs is noted. Edema may be observed in the mesoduodenum. Duodenal obstruction should be suspected in cattle with severe rumen tympanites with marked increase in rumen chloride and classical electrolyte changes, especially if there is a history of recent surgery to correct abomasal displacement. Differential diagnoses include trichobezoars, intussusception, vagus indigestion syndrome, intestinal lymphosarcoma, fat necrosis, intestinal entrapment around anomalous fibrovascular bands, and volvulus of the jejunoileal flange.

TREATMENT

When obstruction of the duodenum is suspected, a right paralumbar fossa celiotomy and exploration of the abdomen should be performed. The obstruction is found by careful palpation and inspection of the duodenum, paying special attention to the ansa sigmoidea. If an intraluminal mass is found, this segment of intestine is exteriorized from the abdomen and isolated using moistened surgical towels, and an enterotomy performed. After removal of the foreign body, the enterotomy is closed with absorbable suture material (e.g., No 2-0 polydioxanone, polyglactin 910) using two lines of an inverting suture pattern. The enterotomy may be closed transversely to maximize the lumen of the affected segment of intestine and minimize the tension endured by the suture line during contraction of the intestinal wall. When the perceived economic value of the affected cattle is high, surgery may be performed with the patient under general anesthesia. This minimizes the risk of ingesta contamination of the abdomen during surgery. If a duodenal stricture is found, a duodeno-duodenostomy or jejuno-duodenostomy may be performed. This may be accomplished by hand-sewn anastomosis or by staple techniques. In our experience, staplers designed for use in human intestine are prone to dehiscence when used in bovine intestine. Staplers designed for use in horse intestine have a sufficient staple arm length for clinical use in bovine bowel, but these instruments are cost prohibitive in most cases. Surgical correction is best performed by side-to-side anastomosis of the cranial part of the descending duodenum to the descending duodenum. The side-to-side anastomosis should maximize the dimension of the stoma created. The most accessible segment of duodenum is placed alongside the cranial part of the descending duodenum, and seromuscular stay sutures are placed to maintain positioning without tension of the anastomotic site. Then, a 5- to 10-cm enterotomy is performed and a side-to-side anastomosis performed.

Intravenous fluid therapy is based on the clinical estimate of dehydration, severity of intestinal lesion identified at surgery, and severity of serum biochemistry changes. In general, cattle should receive 20 to 60 L of isotonic saline, intravenously, over 12 hours. We routinely add calcium (1 ml of 23% calcium gluconate/kg body weight) and dextrose (to create a 1.25% solution) to the IV fluids. Nonsteroidal antiinflammatory drugs (e.g., banamine, 1 mg/kg body weight, IV, q12h × 3 days) and antibiotics (for 3-5 days) are also administered.

PROGNOSIS

The prognosis for return to productive use is based on the animal's body condition, severity of changes in serum biochemistry variables,[11] presence of visceral perforation or peritonitis, and ability to perform surgical removal of the foreign body without contaminating the abdomen. Cattle that are less than 10% dehydrated and have mild to moderate hypochloremic (e.g., Cl >80 mEq/L) metabolic alkalosis (e.g., bicarbonate >32 mEq/L) have a fair to good prognosis for recovery. Cattle that are more than 10% dehydrated, have severe hypochloremia (e.g., Cl <80 mEq/L) and metabolic acidosis (e.g., bicarbonate <20 mEq/L), or have visceral perforation have a poor prognosis for survival. Therefore immediate surgical intervention is required for alleviation of clinical signs caused by intraluminal foreign bodies. In one study, 23 cows with duodenal ileus were reported.[3] Of these cows, 10 were slaughtered after diagnosis and 11 of 13 cows with phytobezoars survived.

PREVENTION

Duodenal obstruction occurs infrequently in cattle. The sporadic nature of the problem limits recommendations for prevention. Adequate dietary roughage should be made available to cattle at all times.

References

1. Pfeiffer CJ: A review of spontaneous ulcer disease in domestic animals: chickens, cattle, horses, and swine, *Acta Physiol Hung* 80:149-158, 1992.
2. van der Velden MA: Functional stenosis of the sigmoid curve of the duodenum in cattle, *Vet Rec* 112:452-453, 1983.
3. Braun U, Steiner A, Gotz M: Clinical signs, diagnosis, and treatment of duodenal ileus in cattle, *Schweiz Arch Tierheilkd* 135:345-355, 1993.
4. Braun U, Hausammann K, Forrer R: Reflux of bile acids from the duodenum into the rumen of cows with a reduced intestinal passage, *Vet Rec* 124:373-376, 1989.
5. Cebra CK, Cebra ML, Garry FB: Gravel obstruction of the abomasums or duodenum of two cows, *J AM Vet Med Assoc* 209:1294-1296, 1996.
6. Koller U, Lischer C, Geyer H et al: Strangulation of the duodenum by the uterus during late pregnancy in two cows, *Vet J* 162:33-37, 2001.
7. Boerboom D, Mulon PY, Desrochers A: Duodenal obstruction caused by malposition of the gallbladder in a heifer, *J Am Vet Med Assoc* 223:1475-1477, 2003.
8. Steiner A, Muller L, Pabst B: An unusual complication after the partial resection of the ascending duodenum of a cow, *Tierarztl Prax* 17:17-20, 1989.
9. Garry F, Hull BL, Ringd DM et al: Comparison of naturally occurring proximal duodenal obstruction and abomasal volvulus in dairy cattle, *Vet Surg* 17:226-233, 1988.
10. Braun U, Marmier O, Pusteria N: Ultrasonographic examination of the small intestine of cows with ileus of the duodenum, jejunum, or ileum, *Vet Rec* 137:209-215, 1995.
11. Anderson DE, Constable PD, St-Jean G et al: Small-intestinal volvulus in cattle: 35 cases (1967-1992), *J Am Vet Med Assoc* 203:1178-1183, 1993.

CHAPTER 28

Trichobezoars

DAVID E. ANDERSON

Intraluminal obstruction of the intestinal tract of cattle, sheep, and goats is most commonly caused by a trichobezoar, phytobezoar, or enterolith.[1,2] These foreign bodies form in the rumen or abomasum and may pass into the intestinal tract, where they become lodged within the small intestine or spiral colon. Hair balls (trichobezoar) are caused by frequent ingestion of hair. This is seen most commonly in cattle infested with lice or mange, or during the spring when shedding of the winter hair coat occurs. Phytobezoars and enteroliths form around undigested materials (e.g., nylon fibers, cotton fabric). In a necropsy survey of 166 dead calves younger than 90 days old in Western Canada, 56 calves died because of perforation of an abomasal ulcer.[3] Calves having an abomasal ulcer were 2.74 times more likely to have an abomasal hairball. Calves younger than 31 days old and having an abomasal ulcer were 3.81 times more likely to have an abomasal hairball. However, the authors were unable to establish a causative relationship between the presence of abomasal hairballs and a perforating ulcer. During a study of confined cattle being fed a roughage limited diet, cows began biting hair from each other's hair coat and developed multiple ruminal hair balls (range of 2-10 hairballs weighing 0.2-3.8 kg each).[4] The investigators speculated that the cows began "grazing" hair because of the lack of roughage in the diet, boredom, and high stocking density. One report describes clinical findings in 2 sheep having 107 individual hair balls.[5] The authors speculated that pruritus or some unknown dietary deficiency was the cause of excessive ingestion of the wool.

CLINICAL SIGNS

Animals affected with ruminal or abomasal bezoars may be observed to have decreased appetite, weight loss, decreased fecal production, lethargy, and apparent depression. Multiple bezoars present in the rumen or abomasum of calves, sheep, and goats may be found during transabdominal palpation or on abdominal radiographs. When an obstruction of the small intestine or spiral colon occurs, affected animals initially show clinical signs of abdominal pain (restlessness, kicking at the abdomen, lying down and getting up frequently, arching the back, stretching out of the legs while standing) and progress to recumbency and apparent depression. Progressive bloat or abdominal distention and lack of fecal production are noted.

CLINICAL PATHOLOGY

Serum biochemistry analysis reveals hypokalemic, hypochloremic, metabolic alkalosis, the severity of which depends on the duration and location of the lesion. These changes are most severe with proximal intestinal obstruction and become more severe with increasing duration. If ischemic necrosis of the intestinal wall has occurred, an inflammatory leukogram with increased numbers of immature neutrophils may be seen. As peritonitis develops and organic acids are released into the bloodstream, the serum biochemistry changes to a metabolic acidosis with relative hyperkalemia. These changes are consistent with a poor prognosis. Perforation of an abomasal ulcer or rupture of the intestine and contamination of the abdomen with ingesta carries a poor to grave prognosis.

DIAGNOSIS

In affected cattle, serum biochemistry changes are consistent with intestinal obstruction. Rumen chloride concentration may be elevated (rumen Cl > 30 mEq/L). The cause of intraluminal obstruction is rarely palpable per rectum, but small intestinal distention may be palpable. Ultrasonographic examination of the abdomen may be useful in calves and small ruminants. Intraluminal intestinal obstruction should be suspected in cattle with recurrent rumen tympanites, which is transiently responsive to decompression and is associated with minimal fecal production. Differential diagnoses include intussusception, vagus indigestion syndrome, intestinal lymphosarcoma, fat necrosis, intestinal entrapment around anomalous fibrovascular bands, and volvulus of the jejunoileal flange.

TREATMENT

Trichobezoars, phytobezoars, or enteroliths located within the rumen are unlikely to cause clinical signs unless the number and magnitude of the foreign bodies is severe (e.g., two sheep in which hair balls accounted for >10% of the animals' body weight[5]). A cow suffered esophageal obstruction after suspected attempted regurgitation of a rumen trichobezoar.[6] Ruminal foreign bodies are removed via a left paralumbar fossa celiotomy and rumenotomy (see traumatic reticuloperitonitis). We prefer to close the rumen with absorbable monofilament suture material (e.g., No 1 polydioxanone) using two layers of an inverting suture pattern (e.g., Cushing's, Lembert's patterns). Abomasal hairballs may cause pyloric obstruction, which leads to rapid onset of abdominal distention. The authors prefer to perform a right paramedian or ventral paracostal laparotomy to exteriorize the abomasum. An abomasotomy is performed along the greater curvature of the abomasum, the foreign bodies removed, and the abomasum closed with absorbable monofilament suture material (e.g., No 0 polydioxanone) using two layers of an inverting suture pattern. When obstruction of the duodenum, jejunum, or spiral colon is suspected, a right paralumbar fossa celiotomy and exploration of the abdomen should be performed. The foreign body is found by exteriorizing a segment of normal or distended intestine and tracing this segment oral, or aboral respectively, until the obstruction is found. This segment of intestine is exteriorized from the abdomen and isolated using moistened surgical towels. Then an enterotomy is performed. After removal of the foreign body, the enterotomy is closed with absorbable suture material (e.g., No 2-0 polydioxanone, polyglactin 910) using two lines of an inverting suture pattern. The enterotomy may be closed transversely to maximize the lumen of the affected segment of intestine and minimize the tension endured by the suture line during contraction of the intestinal wall. When the perceived economic value of the affected cattle is high, surgery may be performed with the patient under general anesthesia. This minimizes the risk of ingesta contamination of the abdomen during surgery.

Intravenous fluid therapy is based on the clinical estimate of dehydration, severity of intestinal lesions identified at surgery, and severity of serum biochemistry changes. In general, cattle should receive 20 to 60 L of isotonic saline, intravenously, over 12 hours. We routinely add calcium (1 ml of 23% calcium gluconate/kg body weight) and dextrose (to create a 1.25% solution) to the intravenous (IV) fluids. Nonsteroidal antiinflammatory drugs (flunixin meglumine, 1 mg/kg body weight, IV, q12h×3 days) and antibiotics (for 3-5 days) are also administered.

PROGNOSIS

The prognosis for return to productive use is based on the animal's body condition, severity of changes in serum biochemistry variables, presence of visceral perforation or peritonitis, and ability to perform surgical removal of the foreign body without contaminating the abdomen. Cattle that are less than 10% dehydrated, have mild to moderate hypochloremic (e.g., Cl >80 mEq/L), and metabolic alkalosis (e.g., bicarbonate >32 mEq/L) have a fair to good prognosis for recovery. Cattle that are more than 10% dehydrated, have severe hypochloremia (e.g., Cl <80 mEq/L) and metabolic acidosis (e.g., bicarbonate <20 mEq/L), or have visceral perforation have a poor prognosis for survival. Therefore immediate surgical intervention is required for alleviation of clinical signs caused by intraluminal foreign bodies.

PREVENTION

Intraluminal obstruction of the intestinal tract occurs infrequently in cattle. The sporadic nature of the problem limits recommendations for prevention. Adequate dietary roughage should be made available to cattle at all times. Lice control strategies, particularly during the winter, will prevent pruritus-associated ingestion of hair.

References

1. Pearson H, Pinsent PJN: Intestinal obstruction in cattle, *Vet Rec* 101:162-166, 1977.
2. Pearson H: The treatment of surgical disorders of the bovine abdomen, *Vet Rec* 92:245-254, 1973.
3. Jelinski MD, Ribble CS, Campbell JR et al: Investigating the relationship between abomasal hairballs and perforating abomasal ulcers in unweaned beef calves, *Can Vet J* 37:23-26, 1996.
4. Cockrill JM, Beasley JN, Selph RA: Trichobezoars in four Angus cows, *Vet Med Small Anim Clin* 73:1441-1442, 1978.
5. Ramadan RO: Massive formation of trichobezoars in sheep, *Agri-Practice* 16:26-28, 1995.
6. Patel JH, Brace DM: Esophageal obstruction due to a trichobezoar in a cow, *Can Vet J* 36:774-775, 1995.

CHAPTER 29

Intussusception

DAVID E. ANDERSON

Intussusception refers to the invagination of one segment of intestine into an adjacent segment of intestine. The invaginated portion of intestine is termed the *intussusceptum,* and the outer, or receiving, segment of intestine is termed the *intussuscipiens.* Intussusception occurs sporadically in cattle of all ages, breeds, and gender and may be seen at anytime during the year.[1,2] However, in a case-control epidemiologic study of 336 cattle, intussusception occurred most commonly in calves younger than 2 months old; Brown Swiss cattle appeared to be overrepresented, and Hereford cattle appeared to be underrepresented compared with Holstein cattle.[1] Although the inciting cause is rarely identified, intussusception may occur secondary to enteritis, intestinal parasitism, sudden changes in diet, mural granuloma or abscess, intestinal neoplasia (especially adenocarcinoma), mural hematoma, and administration of drugs that affect intestinal motility. Any focal disturbance of intestinal motility may facilitate the invagination of an orad segment into an aborad segment of intestine. Intussusception occurs most commonly in the distal portion of the jejunum, but intussusception has been found affecting the proximal jejunum, ileum, cecum, and spiral colon.[1-7] In a review of 336 intussusceptions in cattle, 281 affected the small intestine, 7 were ileocolic, 12 cecocolic, and 36 colocolic.[1]

CLINICAL SIGNS

Cattle affected with intussusception demonstrate clinical signs of abdominal pain (restlessness, kicking at the abdomen, lying down and getting up frequently, assuming abnormal posture) for up to 24 hours after the onset of disease. Cattle are frequently anorectic, lethargic, and reluctant to walk. After the initial signs of abdominal pain subside, affected cattle become progressively lethargic and recumbent and show apparent depression. Abdominal distention becomes apparent after 24 to 48 hours' duration. This is caused by gas and fluid distention of the forestomach and intestines, and sequestration of ingesta within the gastrointestinal tract results in progressive dehydration and electrolyte depletion. Heart rate (HR) increases proportionally to abdominal pain, intestinal necrosis, and dehydration. Fecal production may be normal for up to 12 hours after the occurrence of the intussusception, but minimal fecal production is noted after 24 hours' duration. Passage of blood and mucus from the rectum is common at this time.

CLINICAL PATHOLOGY

Hemoconcentration is usually present (increased packed cell volume and total protein), and an inflammatory leukogram may be seen if ischemic necrosis of the intussusceptum has occurred. Often, changes in the white blood cell count and differential are minimal and changes in peritoneal fluid constituents are not seen because the intussusceptum is isolated by the intussuscipiens. Hypochloremic, metabolic alkalosis is found with serum biochemistry analysis. Hyponatremia, hypokalemia, hypocalcemia, azotemia, and hyperglycemia also may be found. The magnitude of these changes is dependent on the location and duration of the lesion. Proximal jejunal intussusception causes rapid and severe dehydration, electrolyte sequestration, and metabolic alkalosis. Most lesions occur in the distal jejunum and may require more than 48 hours to develop these changes. Elevation of rumen chloride concentration (>30 mEq/L) may be found if fluid distention of the rumen is present.

DIAGNOSIS

Diagnosis of intussusception is usually made during exploratory laparotomy. Occasionally the intussusception can be felt during rectal palpation, but distention of multiple loops of small intestine is most commonly identified. In our experience, an intussusception may be present for 48 hours or more in adult cattle without being able to find intestinal distention during rectal palpation. In calves and small ruminants, percutaneous palpation and ultrasonographic examination of the abdomen may be used to identify intestinal distention and, possibly, the intussusception. It should be suspected in cattle with a history of abdominal pain and abdominal distention, scant feces consisting of blood and mucous, and palpable distention of the intestine. Differential diagnoses include primary indigestion, abomasal ulcer, functional ileus, trichobezoar, foreign bodies, intestinal incarceration or strangulation, vagal syndrome, intestinal neoplasia, fat necrosis, and jejunoileal flange volvulus.

TREATMENT

Affected cattle must be stabilized before surgical intervention is performed. Fluid therapy should be aimed to replace fluid and electrolyte deficits. Surgical correction may proceed after the patient has been assessed as a suitable candidate. Right paralumbar fossa exploratory laparotomy is the surgical approach of choice for treatment of intussusception. The majority of the small intestine of cattle has a short mesentery, preventing adequate exteriorization of the intussusception through a ventral midline incision. Also, the attachments of the greater omentum limit exposure with this approach. The presence of the rumen in the left hemi-abdomen prevents adequate exteriorization of the intussusception through a left paralumbar incision. Most often, diagnostic exploratory laparotomy is performed with the cow standing after regional anesthesia. Tension on the mesentery of the small intestine results in pain, and cattle may attempt to lie down during the procedure. Of 35 cattle having standing right paralumbar fossa laparotomy for resection of intussusception, 14% became recumbent and 26% attempted to become recumbent during the surgery.[1] Preoperative planning should include anticipation of this possibility. When intussusception is suspected and the animal is of high perceived economic value, right paralumbar fossa celiotomy may be performed with the patient under general anesthesia and in left lateral recumbency. The intussusception may be more difficult to elevate through the incision in recumbent cattle because the fluid-filled bowel gravitates away from the surgical site, but isolation and resection of the intussusception can be done without risk of the animal lying down during the procedure and with minimal risk of contamination of the abdomen.

Surgical removal by resection and anastomosis is the treatment of choice for intussusception. The intussusception is exteriorized from the abdomen and isolated using a barrier drape and moistened towels. Manual reduction of the intussusception is not recommended because of the risk for rupture of the intestine during manipulation, probable ischemic necrosis of the intestine after surgery, possible reoccurrence of the intussusception, and prolonged ileus caused by motility disturbance and swelling in the affected segment of bowel. The margins for excision are selected in healthy-appearing intestine. In general the distal margin may be 10 cm aboral to the lesion, but the proximal margin should be a minimum of 30 cm orad to the lesion. The larger proximal segment is chosen because chronic distention, inflammation, microvascular thrombosis, relative ischemia, and noxious ingesta accumulated in this segment may cause severe and prolonged postoperative ileus. Cattle have a short mesentery; therefore traction on it is painful, and the animal may go down at this moment. This short mesentery precludes adequate exteriorization of some segment of the small bowel. Only the portion to be resected should be exteriorized to avoid excessive traction and contamination during the resection-anastomosis. Infiltration of lidocaine 2% into the mesentery where it is planned to be resected may decrease the pain of traction. The mesenteric vessels (arteries and veins) are ligated using "mass ligation" with absorbable suture material (No. 3 chromic gut, No. 1 polyglactin 910), being sure not to compromise the blood supply to the intestine to be preserved. Mass ligation is required because cattle do not have an arcuate vascular anatomy as do horses, and the fatty mesentery renders vessel identification difficult and time consuming. The sutures are placed in an overlapping pattern such that double ligation of the vessels is accomplished.

This technique may be performed rapidly and efficiently. In our experience, stapling instrumentation is highly unreliable for occlusion of mesenteric vessels because of the large amount of fat normally found in the intestinal mesentery of cattle. When we have used stapling instruments, extensive manual ligation was required to control hemorrhage. After completion of mesentery ligation and transection, Doyen intestinal forceps are used to occlude the lumen of the normal and abnormal bowel. Then the intussusception and associated bowel are resected and discarded. The proximal segment of bowel is carefully exteriorized to its maximum length, and the Doyen forceps is removed. Ingesta within the intestine orad to the lesion is "milked" out through the enterectomy site, being careful not to contaminate the incision or abdomen with ingesta. This procedure will lessen the severity of postoperative ileus and shorten convalescence. The two segments of intestine are reunited by end-to-end or side-to-side anastomosis with an absorbable suture material (No. 2-0 polydioxanone or polyglactin 910) using a simple continuous suture pattern. The anastomosis is performed in three overlapping suture lines, each placed in one third of the circumference, or in four overlapping suture lines, each placed in one fourth of the circumference so that a "purse-strings" effect is not created. The initial suture line should be placed at the mesenteric attachment because this is the most likely site for leakage to occur. A second row of sutures may be placed to prevent leakage using interrupted segments of inverting suture patterns (e.g., Cushing's or Lembert's). The affected intestine is thoroughly washed with sterile isotonic fluids, checked for the presence of leakage, and replaced into the abdomen. We prefer to place a solution of antibiotic (5 million units potassium penicillin G, or 1 g of sodium ceftiofur), heparin (20 units/kg body weight), and saline (1000 ml) into the abdomen before closing the abdominal wall in routine fashion.

Postoperative management should be directed to prevent dehydration, maintain optimal blood electrolyte concentration, control for infection and inflammation, and stimulate appetite. Intravenous (IV) fluids are beneficial during the first 24 hours after surgery. We routinely perform rumen transfaunation 12 to 24 hours after surgery to stimulate forestomach motility and appetite. Withholding food after surgery should not be done. Administration of butorphanol tartrate (0.02-0.04 mg/kg, IV) may help with pain-induced ileus by providing mild visceral analgesia without direct adverse effects on intestinal motility.

PROGNOSIS

The prognosis for return to productivity after surgical correction of intussusception is variable and somewhat dependent on the duration of the lesion. In our experience, cattle respond favorably to surgery if operated within 48 hours of the onset of the disease. Cattle presenting with severe dehydration (>12%), tachycardia (HR > 120 bpm), severe decrease in serum chloride concentration (Cl < 80 mEq/L), and severe abdominal distention are considered to have a poor prognosis for survival. In our experience, calves respond more favorably to surgery than adult cattle. If viscera rupture is present at the time of surgery, the prognosis is grave. Of cattle in which surgical correction was attempted, 85 of 143 cattle with small intestinal intussusception, 0 of 4 with ileocolic, 10 of 11 with cecocolic, and 10 of 20 with colocolic were discharged from the hospital.[1]

PREVENTION

Recommendations for prevention of intussusception are difficult because the cause is seldom identified and a seasonal predilection has not been demonstrated. Changes in dietary management should be made gradually, and good hygiene and control strategies should be practiced to minimize transmission of enteric diseases or internal parasites.

References

1. Constable PD, St-Jean G, Hull BL et al: Intussusception in cattle: 336 cases (1964-1993), *J Am Vet Med Assoc* 210:531-36, 1997.
2. Pearson H: Intussusception in cattle, *Vet Rec* 89:426-437, 1971.
3. Smart ME, Fretz PB, Gudmundson J et al: Intussusception in a Charolais bull, *Can Vet J* 18:244-246, 1977.
4. Archer RM, Cooley AJ, Hinchcliff KW et al: Jejunojejunal intussusception associated with a transmural adenocarcinoma in an aged cow, *J Am Vet Med Assoc* 192:209-211, 1988.
5. Horne MM: Colonic intussusception in a Holstein calf, *Can Vet J* 32:493-495, 1991.
6. Hamilton GF, Tulleners EP: Intussusception involving the spiral colon in a calf, *Can Vet J* 21:32, 1980.
7. Strand E, Welker B, Modransky P: Spiral colon intussusception in a three-year-old bull, *J Am Vet Med Assoc* 202:971-972, 1993.

CHAPTER **30**

Intestinal Volvulus

DAVID E. ANDERSON

Volvulus refers to the rotation of viscera about its mesenteric attachment. Torsion refers to the rotation of viscera about its own (or long) axis. Although torsion of the abomasum and uterus are found in cattle, torsion of the small intestine is rare. Small intestinal volvulus may occur in different forms.[1-3] The most severe form of intestinal volvulus originates from the root of the mesentery and involves the entirety of the small intestine and mesenteries. Volvulus of the root of the mesentery causes obstruction of venous outflow and arterial blood supply to the intestines. Ischemic necrosis of the intestine occurs rapidly, causing metabolic acidosis, shock, and death. Volvulus of the jejunoileal flange refers to volvulus of the midjejunum to distal jejunum and proximal ileum where the mesentery is long. This long mesentery and associated bowel have been termed the "flange" and may rotate about its own axis without involving the remaining small intestine. Often, arterial occlusion is not found with volvulus of the jejunoileal flange, possibly because extensive fat deposits within the mesentery may prevent compression of the muscular wall of the arteries until the volvulus becomes severe. However, obstruction of outflow of venous blood may be equally detrimental because of mural edema, shunting of blood away from the mucosa, and progressive ischemia.

Cattle of any breed, age, or sex may be affected by intestinal volvulus at any time during the year. In a review of 190 cattle having intestinal volvulus, dairy breeds were at a higher risk of developing volvulus compared with beef breeds.[1] This difference was felt to be associated with differences in management. Neither lactation nor gestation were identified as risk factors, and calves were not found to be at an increased risk compared with adult cattle. In a separate study of 100 cattle having intestinal volvulus, 86 were calves between 1 week and 6 months old.[4]

CLINICAL SIGNS

Cattle having volvulus of the root of the mesentery may be found dead with severe abdominal distention. Early in the course of the disease, affected cattle demonstrate acute, severe abdominal pain (kicking at the abdomen, rolling, lying down and getting up frequently, grunting) and have marked elevation in heart rate (>120 bpm) and respiratory rate (>80 bpm). The rapid progression of the disease precludes development of significant dehydration, but cardiovascular shock is usually present.

Cattle having volvulus of the jejunoileal flange may present similarly to cattle having volvulus at the root of the mesentery. However, these cattle often demonstrate clinical signs consistent with acute intestinal obstruction rather than in cardiovascular shock. Cattle show signs of abdominal pain, are tachycardia (80-120 bpm), and pass minimal feces. Cattle may be dehydrated at the time of examination.

CLINICAL PATHOLOGY

Because of the rapid onset and progress, cattle having Intestinal volvulus may not demonstrate changes in serum biochemistry or hematology data. The changes expected with intestinal volvulus are consistent with intestinal obstruction, stress, and dehydration: azotemia, hypocalcemia, hyperglycemia, and a leukocytosis with a mild left shift.[1] In the early stages of the disease, cattle develop alkalemia with normal serum potassium concentration. As cardiovascular compromise and intestinal ischemia proceed, cattle develop metabolic acidosis and hyperkalemia. Cattle having the shift to acidosis and hyperkalemia have a poor prognosis for survival.[1]

DIAGNOSIS

Diagnosis of intestinal volvulus is by exploratory laparotomy. Rectal palpation reveals multiple loops of distended intestine filling the caudal abdomen and excessive tension on the intestinal mesentery. Simultaneous auscultation and percussion of the abdomen yields multifocal pings of variable pitch and location. Findings of scant feces, abdominal pain, sudden onset of abdominal distention, and multiple loops of distended intestine on rectal palpation in cattle are highly suggestive of intestinal volvulus. Differential diagnoses include intussusception, cecal volvulus, abomasal volvulus, intraluminal obstruction, and severe indigestion.

TREATMENT

Immediate surgical correction is the treatment of choice. Intravenous fluids should be administered to treat cardiovascular shock, but preparation for surgery should not be delayed. The volvulus must be corrected before irreversible ischemic injury or thrombosis of the mesenteric arteries has occurred. A right paralumbar fossa laparotomy with the cow standing is the approach of choice. Restoration of normal anatomic position of the intestines is more easily done with the patient standing. Cattle that are felt to be at great risk of becoming recumbent during surgery should be placed under general anesthesia, in left lateral recumbency, and the laparotomy performed through the right paralumbar fossa. The presence of the volvulus and the direction of the twist are assessed by palpating the root of the mesentery and, in the case of jejunoileal flange volvulus, following this ventrally to the location of the twist. The intestinal mass is gently derotated, being careful not to cause rupture of the viscera. This procedure may require exteriorization of various portions of the intestinal mass. After correction of the volvulus, the intestinal tract should be examined for evidence of nonviable bowel. If the intestine is compromised (arterial thrombosis, blackened serosa, friable wall of the affected segment, mural edema), then intestinal resection and anastomosis is indicated (see Chapter 29).

Also, exploration of the abdomen should be done to rule out the presence of a second lesion (e.g., abomasal displacement, fecalith, intussusception, anomalous fibrovascular bands, peritonitis).

Postoperative management is directed toward maintaining optimal hydration, electrolyte, and acid-base status. Antibiotics and antiinflammatory drugs are indicated. Ileus may be seen during the first 48 hours after surgery, but the use of prokinetic drugs should be weighed against the risk of leakage at the site of the anastomosis if intestinal resection was performed. Passage of large volumes of diarrhea within 24 hours after surgery is considered to be a favorable prognostic indicator.

PROGNOSIS

Prognosis varies with the severity and duration of the lesion. Prognosis for survival for cattle having volvulus of the root of the mesentery (44%) is less than for volvulus of the jejunoileal flange (86%).[1] Overall, dairy cattle had a better prognosis for survival (63%) than beef cattle (22%). This difference was presumed to be because dairy cattle are observed more frequently and, therefore, treatment sought earlier in the progression of the disease. Of 92 cattle in which surgical correction of intestinal volvulus was attempted, 13 were euthanatized during surgery, 25 died within 24 hours after surgery, 13 died between 2 and 7 days, and 41 (45%) survived.[4]

PREVENTION

Specific recommendations for strategies to prevent intestinal volvulus are not possible because no risk factor has been identified. Some authors have suggested that turning out to graze lush pastures is a risk factor for intestinal volvulus.[5] This has not been our experience. Feeding of concentrates, frequent dietary changes, confinement housing, and selection for high productivity may place dairy cattle at higher risk compared with beef cattle. These management techniques are also used in feedlot operations, but these cattle may not be presented for treatment to teaching hospitals because of their lower perceived economic value. Therefore recommendations should be aimed to optimize cattle health by gradual changes in diet and environment.

References

1. Anderson DE, Constable PD, St-Jean G et al: Small-intestinal volvulus in cattle: 35 cases (1967-1992), *J Am Vet Med Assoc* 203:1178-1183, 1993.
2. Fubini SL, Smith DF, Tithof PK et al: Volvulus of the distal part of the jejunoileum in four cows, *Vet Surg* 15:150-152, 1986.
3. Tulleners EP: Surgical correction of volvulus of the root of the mesentery in calves, *J Am Vet Med Assoc* 179:998-999, 1981.
4. Rademacher G: Diagnosis, therapy, and prognosis of the intestinal mesenteric torsion in cattle. Proceedings, XVII World Buiatrics Congress and XXV, *Am Assoc Bov Pract Conf, St Paul*, 1:137-142, 1992.
5. Willet MDJ: Intestinal torsion in cattle, *N Z Vet J* 18:42-43, 1970.

CHAPTER 31

Intestinal Atresia

DAVID E. ANDERSON

Atresia of various segments of the intestinal tract of calves has been described. In one study of 58 calves with intestinal atresia, 18 calves had single atretic segments, whereas 40 calves suffered multiple atretic segments (Table 31-1).[1] These congenital disorders may be obvious and diagnosed rapidly after birth, such as atresia ani, or be inapparent for several days until abdominal distension, lack of fecal output, or clinical deterioration of the calf draws attention to the abnormality. Although atresia ani is likely the most common intestinal atresia encountered, atresia coli and atresia jejuni are most represented in the scientific literature.[2-9]

Atresia coli has been most commonly reported in dairy calves, especially Holsteins. In one report, an incidence rate of 0.76% was reported in a university dairy herd of Holstein cows over a 10-year period.[7] Most calves suffering atresia coli were genetically related, but the authors also noted that pregnancy palpation before day 41 was most common among calves having atresia coli. In an epidemiologic analysis of intestinal atresia in two dairy herds in Israel, the odds of a calf being born with intestinal atresia was 119.7 times greater if rectal palpation for pregnancy had been done before day 42 of gestation.[10] I have diagnosed atresia coli in a variety of beef breeds,

including Charolais, Angus, Short Horn, and Polled Hereford. In an analysis of breed as a risk factor for atresia coli, data acquired from published literature included atresia coli calves of 10 breeds from 12 countries.[4] This analysis showed that 94% of reported cases of atresia coli were Holstein calves. The cause of atresia coli is unknown, but genetic and iatrogenic causes have been proposed. Cows having pregnancy diagnosis via transrectal palpation before 42 days' gestation seemed more likely to have calves with atresia coli, but the incidence of the anomaly is low. Also, a report of twin Holstein calves, one with and one without atresia coli, would seem to argue against a heritable trait.[11] In a breeding study designed to determine the heritability of atresia coli, early pregnancy palpation was not associated with development of atresia coli (no difference between putative carriers and general population in the same herd). However, approximately 14% of calves born to putative dams and sires had atresia coli compared with 0.15% of calves from the general population in the same herd.[8] This would seem to strongly support a heritable genetic defect as the cause of atresia coli.

CLINICAL SIGNS

Calves affected by atresia coli that have been closely monitored and evaluated from birth may be recognized by absence of fecal matter during the first 12 to 24 hours of life. Administration of cathartics or enemas has no effect, but mucous without fecal matter may be observed at the anus with increasing age. Often, atresia coli calves are not presented for evaluation until they are 3 to 5 days old. The most common client observations are decreased appetite, absence of feces, depression, and progressive abdominal distention.

DIAGNOSIS

Initially, ultrasonographic examination of the abdomen reveals the presence of normal to mildly distended intestine with normal to hypermotile activity. After several days, transabdominal palpation yields mild to moderate intestinal distension and pain is easily elicited. Careful palpation of the right paralumbar fossa reveals the presence of two to three distended intestinal loops of the spiral colon and cecum. Ultrasonographic examination of the abdomen reveals the presence of moderate to severe intestinal distention and hypermotile to nonmotile activity. Auscultation of the abdomen reveals positive "fluid and gas" sounds if intestinal motility is present. Simultaneous auscultation and percussion of the abdomen yields "pings" of variable pitch and location. Simultaneous

Table 31-1

Concurrent Findings in Calves Having Intestinal Atresia

Variable	No. Calves Affected
Intestinal Atresia	
Jejunum	5
Ileum	1
Colon	9
Rectum	3
Anus and rectum	28
Anus, rectum, distal colon	8
Rectum, colon, cecum, ileum	2
Rectum and distal colon	2
Additional Congenital Defects	
Tail absent/abnormal	4
Rectovaginal fistula	3
Rectourethral fistula	2
Rectovesical fistula	2
Horseshoe kidney	1
Hermaphrodite	1

Adapted from Martens A, Gasthuys F, Steenhaut M et al: *Vet Rec* 136:141-144, 1995.

auscultation and succession of the abdomen yields fluid waves and "sloshing" sounds as if shaking a half-filled bag of water.

Hematology variables remain normal during the first 48 hours of the disease, but dehydration ensues with fluid retention and bacterial overgrowth within the intestines. Hematocrit and total protein increase, and a degenerative left shift develops progressively as bacterial toxins are elaborated and as necrosis of the intestinal wall ensues[1] (Table 31-2). Serum biochemistry values remain normal within the first 48 hours of disease, but azotemia, hypochloremia, and hypokalemia become progressively severe with time. Failure of passive transfer of maternal antibodies is not uncommon in affected calves. However, if adequate ingestion of colostrum occurs at birth, immunoglobulin transfer is usually normal.

Definitive diagnosis is made by exploratory laparotomy. Some authors have described passage of a tube through the anus to determine the length of rectum present, performance of positive contrast rectal radiography, or rectal endoscopy for diagnosis of atresia coli or to rule out atresia recti. I prefer not to perform these procedures, but rather to make a diagnosis by exploratory laparotomy because of the high risk associated with perforation of the rectum into the abdominal cavity. Right paralumbar fossae celiotomy provides optimal access to the rectum and atretic segments. Although ventral midline celiotomy may be done, the mesenteries of the intestine, especially the terminal colons, are quite short and will prevent exteriorization or make isolation of the affected intestine difficult. Right paralumbar celiotomy should be done in the dorsal and caudal aspect of the PLF to optimize examination of the spiral colon, descending colon, and rectum. A diagnosis of atresia coli is made by examination of the spiral colon and cecum and identification of the blind-ended proximal loop. Occasionally the entire spiral colon is absent.

TREATMENT

Surgical correction may be performed by end-to-end or side-to-side anastomosis of the intestine proximal to the atretic segment to the rectum. Surgery is most easily performed with the calf under general anesthesia but may be performed using a combination of sedation, epidural anesthesia, and line blocks. A side-to-side anastomosis maximizes the dimension of the stoma created.[8] A large-bore (18-24–Fr; 6-8 mm diameter), soft rubber catheter is placed into the rectum via the anus to improve identification, handling, and anastomosis of the rectum. The rectal wall typically is underdeveloped because of absence of stimulation during gestation (e.g., absence of meconium). Thus the rectum must be handled carefully. The spiral colon is suctioned free of all gas, or a small (1-2 cm length) enterotomy can be performed to remove gas and fluid from the colon and cecum. The enterotomy is closed before conducting the anastomosis. The most accessible segment of colon is placed alongside the rectum, and seromuscular stay sutures are placed to maintain positioning without tension of the anastomotic site. Next, a 5- to 8-cm enterotomy of the rectum and colon is performed, followed by side-to-side

Table 31-2

Physical Examination, Hematology, and Serum Biochemistry Findings for Surviving and Nonsurviving Calves with Atresia Coli

Variable	Survivors (Mean)	Nonsurvivors (Mean)
Physical Examination		
Heart rate	140	156
Respiratory rate	46	60
Temperature	38.8	38.8
Age	2.5	3
Hematology		
PCV %	38	42
TP g/dl	7.4	7.5
Serum Biochemistry		
Na meq/L	140	142
K meq/L	4.6	5.1
Cl meq/L	93	91
HCO$_3$ meq/L	31	29
pH	7.4	7.36
Anion gap meq/L	20	28

Adapted from Martens A, Gasthuys F, Steenhaut M et al: *Vet Rec* 136:141-144, 1995.
PCV, Packed cell volume; *TP*, total protein.

anastomosis. The abdominal cavity is lavaged, and the abdominal wall closed in a three-layer fashion. A large Foley catheter may serve to maintain the anastomotic lumen for 48 to 72 hours after surgery because the fecal consistency is thick and prone to impaction of the anastomosis site.

Postoperatively, calves are returned to a milk diet and laxatives may be used (e.g., magnesium hydroxide) to soften the feces for 3 to 5 days after surgery. Intravenous fluids, antibiotics, antiinflammatory drugs, and pain management are integral to improving outcome of affected calves. The most common complications are peritonitis, obstruction of the anastomosis, diarrhea, dehydration, and death. Calves that survive short term are prone to prolonged diarrhea and electrolyte disturbances because of limited colon length and surface area.

PROGNOSIS

Survival of calves with atresia coli is influenced by the age at the time of surgery and the integrity of the colons. Calves having surgery before 72 hours old are more likely to survive than calves undergoing surgical correction after 5 days old. Smith and colleagues[9] found that calves having end-to-side anastomosis after resection of the blind loop/cecum had a better survival rate than calves in which side-to-side anastomosis was performed without removal of the blind loop. Overall, calves have a guarded (≈60%, Table 31-3) survival from surgery but a poor prognosis (≈40%, Table 31-4) of long-term survival for productivity.

Table 31-3

Morbidity and Mortality of Calves with Intestinal Atresia After Surgical Correction

Variable	No. Calves	Survivors/ Successful	Nonsurvivors/ Unsuccessful
Intestinal Atresia Calves			
Perineal anus	4	4	0
Laparotomy and perineal anus	7	3	4
Laparotomy and flank stoma	7	0	7
Atresia Coli			
End-to-side anastomosis	12	7	5
Side-to-side anastomosis	36	18	18
Atresia Coli			
End-to-side anastomosis	11	8	3
Side-to-side anastomosis	23	10	13

Adapted from Martens A, Gasthuys F, Steenhaut M et al: *Vet Rec* 136:141-144, 1995.

Table 31-4

Survival Rates of Calves After Surgical Repair of Atresia Coli

Outcome	Smith et al[9]	Dreyfuss et al[8]	Constable et al[5]
Survivor	27	5	24
Nonsurvivor	39	7	9
% Survivors	41	42	38
Survive to adulthood	11	NA	3
Lost to follow-up	11	NA	NA

References

1. Martens A, Gasthuys F, Steenhaut M et al: Surgical aspect of intestinal atresia in 58 calves, *Vet Rec* 136:141-144, 1995.
2. van der Gaag I, Tibboel D: Intestinal atresia and stenosis in animals: a report of 34 cases, *Vet Pathol* 17:565-574, 1980.
3. Steenhaut M, De Moor A, Verschooten F et al: Intestinal malformation in calves and their surgical correction, *Vet Rec* 98:131-133, 1976.
4. Constable PD, Shanks RD, Huhn J et al: Evaluation of breed as a risk factor for atresia coli in cattle, *Theriogenology* 48:775-790, 1997.
5. Constable PD, Rings DM, Hull BL et al: Atresia coli in calves: 26 cases (1977-1987), *J Am Vet Med Assoc* 195:118-123, 1989.
6. Syed M, Shanks RD: Incidence of atresia coli and relationships among the affected calves born in one herd of Holstein cattle, *J Dairy Sci* 75:1357-1364, 1992.
7. Syed M, Shanks RD: Atresia coli inherited in Holstein cattle, *J Dairy Sci* 75:1105-1111, 1992.
8. Dreyfuss DJ, Tulleners EP: Intestinal atresia in calves: 22 cases (1978-1988), *J Am Vet Med Assoc* 195:508-513, 1989.
9. Smith DF, Ducharme NG, Fubini SL et al: Clinical management and surgical repair of atresia coli in calves: 66 cases (1977-1988), *J Am Vet Med Assoc* 199:1185-1190, 1991.
10. Brenner J, Orgad U: Epidemiological investigations of an outbreak of intestinal atresia in two Israeli dairy herds, *J Vet Med Sci* 65:141-143, 2003.
11. Hoffsis GF, Bruner RR: Atresia coli in a twin calf, *J Am Vet Med Assoc* 171:433-434, 1977.

CHAPTER 32

Rectal Prolapse

DAVID E. ANDERSON

DEVELOPMENT

Rectal prolapse is a common occurrence in cattle and small ruminants. Prolapse of the rectal mucosa occurs following straining, which may be associated with tenesmus (as occurs with coccidiosis, colitis, etc.); dysuria (as a complication of cystitis, urolithiasis, dystocia, neoplasia, etc.); neuropathy (as a complication of being "ridden down" by other cattle during estrus, spinal lymphoma, use of epidural alcohol blocks, spinal abscess, etc.); chronic coughing (as a complication of bovine respiratory disease); or genetics.[1,2] Many other factors have been associated with the development of rectal prolapse including neoplasia, diet (e.g., clover, high estrogenic compound feedstuffs such as soybean meal), and various toxins.[3-5] Intermittent rectal prolapse has been seen in embryo transfer cows and may be caused by obesity with excessive pelvic deposition of fat and chronic administration of estrogenic hormones.

Rectal prolapse is most commonly seen in sheep as a complication of tail amputation. Typically, the tail is amputated so short that the innervation of the anal sphincter and perianal muscles are compromised. This results in chronically progressive rectal protrusion and ultimately prolapse. In a prospective study, 1227 lambs at six locations were assigned to receive (1) short tail dock at the level of the body, (2) medium tail docking at the midpoint between the body and the attachment of the caudal tail fold to the tail skin, or (3) long tail dock at the level of the attachment of the caudal tail fold to the tail skin.[6] The incidence of rectal prolapse was 7.8% of lambs with short tail dock as compared with 4% of lambs having medium tail docks and 1.8% of lambs with long tail docks. At locations with higher incidence of rectal prolapses, lambs in feedlots had rectal prolapse more often than grazing lambs. Genetic analysis of rectal prolapse using half siblings indicated a low heritability factor (0.14).

DIAGNOSIS

Diagnosis of rectal prolapse is not difficult during the physical examination, but care should be taken that the prolapse does not contain other organs and that the rectum is not further damaged during the examination. The mucosa rapidly becomes edematous and often shows bleeding lesions. Rectal prolapse may be described by the extent of involvement of various tissues as grades I to IV (Table 32-1). Grades III and IV rectal prolapse usually require surgical resection of the affected portion of the rectum (Fig. 32-1). The severity of injury to the rectum may be described by the extent of tissue damage as grades I to IV (Table 32-2).

PROCEDURES FOR CORRECTION

The simplest procedure for correction of rectal prolapse is reduction by gentle massage and retention by application of a purse-string suture pattern using umbilical tape. The suture is passed in and out through the skin around the anal opening at a distance of 2 to 4 cm from the anus. An opening should be left when tying the purse string such that defecation is possible. The suture is usually left in place for 5 to 10 days. This should be done only if the rectal mucosa is viable and no laceration is present on close inspection. Treatment of the primary cause of the prolapse must be initiated immediately to prevent subsequent prolapse. In sheep, when rectal prolapse is associated with tail amputation, pararectal injection of irritant solutions has been advocated in an attempt to create adhesions between the rectum and surrounding pelvic structures. These adhesions act to restrict the rectum within the pelvic canal and thus prevent prolapse.

When damage to the rectum is present, correction of the prolapse can be approached in different ways depending on the nature and extent of the injury. If the mucosa only is damaged, mucosal resection and anastomosis can be done. In this case the mucosa is dissected free from the submucosa, and the cut edges sutured back together, leaving the underlying submucosa and blood supply intact. This technique is uncommonly performed because of time, facility, and technical constraints of field surgery. Surgical amputation is performed most commonly when rectal prolapse is severe. For this surgery, desired instruments include hemostats, scalpel blade, scissors, thumb forceps, two 18-gauge needles (or Steinmann pins) 3 to 6 inches long, suture material, and a small-diameter rubber tube (optional) (Figs. 32-2 and 32-3). Surgery is performed after administration of epidural anesthesia. When using a tube as a stent in the rectal lumen, the tube is inserted and fixed in the rectum by inserting the two needles through the rectum at right angles to each other so that they pass through the rectum and tube and emerge from the opposite side. The dissection is started about a centimeter from the mucocutaneous border where the mucosa is still healthy, and the entire circumference of the exposed mucosa of the rectum is cut down to the serosa of the inner wall (Figs. 32-4 and 32-5). Hemorrhaging is usually minor and controlled with gauze until all the layers have been dissected and the dorsal artery of the rectum is cut. Once the dissection is completed around the prolapse,

Table **32-1**

Classification of Rectal Prolapse by Structure (Anatomic Involvement)

Classification Type	Description	Clinical Feature
I	Prolapse of rectal mucosa only. These are small and usually intermittent.	Common
II	Complete prolapse of all layers of rectal (mucosa → serosa). Length is variable. Can be intermittent.	Common
III	Type II prolapse with the addition of prolapse of the large colon (intussusception of the large colon into the rectum). These prolapses are longer and more painful, and clinical signs progress rapidly.	Uncommon
IV	Type III prolapse except that the anal sphincter is intact, causing constriction of the rectum and colon (intussusception of rectum and colon through anus).	Rare

Table **32-2**

Classification of Rectal Tears by Severity (Anatomic Extent of Injury)

Classification	Description	Clinical Feature
I	Tear of mucosa and submucosa only	Common
II	Disruption of muscular layers with mucosa and submucosa intact (causes diverticulum formation)	Uncommon
III	Tear through mucosa, submucosa, and muscular layers—serosa remains intact	Uncommon
	IIIa. Tear any location other than dorsal midline	
	IIIb. Tear dorsal midline at attachment of mesorectum	
IV	Tear through mucosa, submucosa, muscular layers, and serosa	Rare

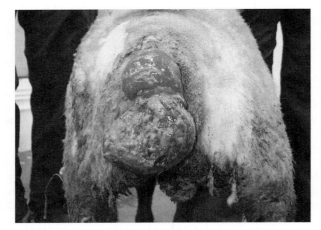

Fig 32-1   Grade III rectal prolapse in a ewe.

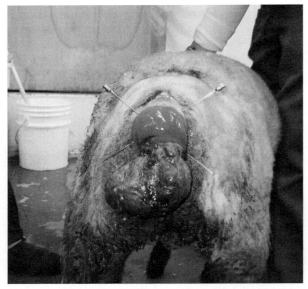

Fig 32-2   Insertion of cross-pins through the full thickness of the prolapse such that the pins transverse the lumen of the rectum.

the rectum is held in place by the needles (Fig. 32-6). The cut ends of the rectum should be sutured together using size 0 absorbable suture material in a cruciate pattern (Fig. 32-7). After the rectum has been sutured, the needles are then pulled from the tube and the tube is removed from the rectum. The rectum is allowed to retract into place (Fig. 32-8).

An alternative method of rectal amputation is to use a prolapse ring, PVC tubing, syringe case, or corrugated tube. The ring or tubing is placed in the rectum, and the halfway point on the tube needs to be inserted as far as the anal sphincter. A ligature or rubber band is then applied over the prolapse as near as possible to the anus. The ligature or rubber band must be tight enough to disrupt blood supply to the prolapse. Feces may go through the tube or may block the tube. Usually the necrotic prolapse sloughs off in 7 to 10 days with the implant in place, and then fecal production returns to normal.

Postoperative management is aimed at alleviation of the inciting cause; maintenance of soft feces (e.g., legume diet, mineral oil, cathartics such as magnesium hydroxide); and antiinflammatory and analgesic medication (e.g., flunixin meglumine). Complications seen with rectal prolapse are reoccurrence, dehiscence, constipation,

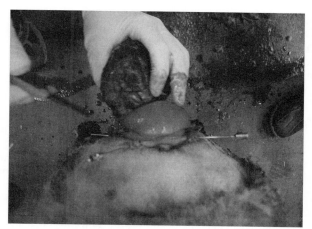

Fig 32-3   Incision site for rectal resection 1-cm proximal to healthy margin.

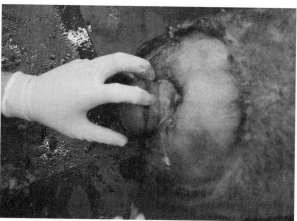

Fig 32-4   Incision into external portion of rectal prolapse (outer rectal wall = intussuscipiens).

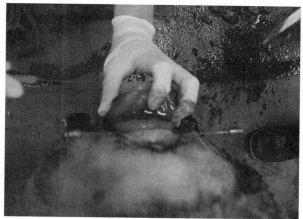

Fig 32-5   Incision through internal portion of rectal prolapse (inner rectal wall = intussusceptum).

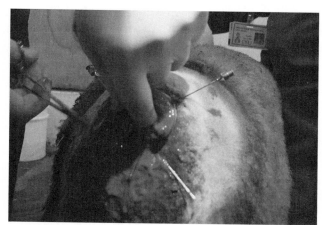

Fig 32-6   Rectal prolapse removed and end-to-end anastomosis of rectum begum using No. 0 polyglycolic acid suture.

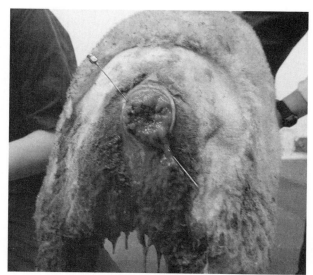

Fig 32-7   Completed anastomosis immediately before removal of final retaining pin.

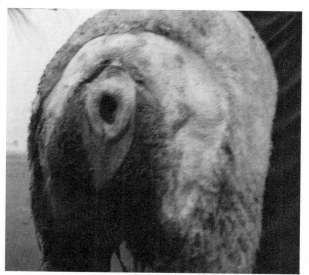

Fig 32-8   Retraction of the rectum into pelvic canal after removal of retaining pin. Note abnormal anal sphincter.

bladder retroversion, eventration of the small intestine, abscess, rectal stricture, septic peritonitis, and death. Fecal impaction of prolapse tubes is common. Significant complications such as rectal stricture, abscess, peritonitis, and death are expected to be more common with use of prolapse tubes than with surgical amputation with primary reconstruction of the rectum.

POSTOPERATIVE MANAGEMENT

In livestock with unrelenting pain and straining, epidural blocks have been used to stop nerve sensation to the rectum. Short-term epidural analgesia can be obtained using lidocaine 2% HCl (60-120 minutes), xylazine (120-180 minutes), or xylazine + lidocaine (180-240 minutes). Longer-term analgesia may be obtained using epidural morphine (12-18 hours). When analgesia is required for days to weeks, alcohol blocks (ethyl alcohol) have been used as an economical alternative. Alcohol blocks must be done cautiously and should not be done routinely. I do not support use of long-term (weeks to months) epidural nerve blocks except in extraordinary circumstances because of the potential for adverse events. Complications of alcohol blocks include fecal contamination of perineum, tail injury, death, paralysis, ataxia, and exacerbation of underlying disease.

References

1. Steiner A: Surgery of the colon. In Fubini SL, Ducharme NG, editors: *Farm animal surgery*, St Louis, 2004, Saunders, pp 257-262.
2. Haskell SR: Surgery of the sheep and goat digestive system. In Fubini SL, Ducharme NG, editors: *Farm animal surgery*, St Louis, 2004, Saunders, pp 521-526.
3. Pearson EG: Clinical manifestations of tansy ragwort poisoning, *Mod Vet Pract* 58:421-424, 1977.
4. Bertone AL: Neoplasms of the bovine gastrointestinal tract, *Vet Clin North Am Food Anim Pract* 6:515-524, 1990.
5. Van Halderen A, Green JR, Marasas WF et al: A field outbreak of chronic aflatoxicosis in dairy calves in the Western Cape Province, *J S Afr Vet Assoc* 60:210-211, 1989.
6. Thomas DL, Waldron DF, Lowe GD et al: Length of docked tail and the incidence of rectal prolapse in lambs, *J Anim Sci* 81:2725-2732, 2003.

SECTION II

Metabolic Diseases

Thomas H. Herdt

CHAPTER 33

Milk Fever (Parturient Paresis) in Cows, Ewes, and Doe Goats*

GARRETT R. OETZEL and JESSE P. GOFF

Milk fever (parturient paresis, hypocalcemia, paresis puerperalis, parturient apoplexy) is a nonfebrile disease of adult dairy cows, beef cows, ewes, and doe goats, in which acute calcium deficiency causes progressive neuromuscular dysfunction with flaccid paralysis, circulatory collapse, and depression of consciousness. Hypocalcemia in sheep and goats causes varying combinations of tetany or flaccid paralysis, or both.

OCCURRENCE

Milk fever is one of the most common metabolic diseases of dairy cattle. About 5% of U.S. dairy cattle are affected annually. Annual incidence rate of clinical milk fever within herds may vary from less than 1% to 60%.

Approximately 75% of all cases of milk fever in dairy cattle occur within 24 hours of calving. An additional 12% occur 24 to 48 hours after calving. Some cases (≈6%) occur at the time of delivery, often resulting in dystocia because hypocalcemia inhibits uterine contractility. Cases of hypocalcemia that do not occur in association with calving are termed *nonparturient hypocalcemia* rather than milk fever.

Subclinical hypocalcemia (depressed blood calcium concentrations but without clinical signs) affects about 50% of all adult dairy cattle. Subclinical hypocalcemia may lead to decreased dry matter (DM) intake after calving, increased risk of secondary disease conditions, decreased milk production, and decreased fertility later in lactation (Fig. 33-1). Therefore efforts to improve calcium metabolism in fresh cows may have payoffs even in herds without clinical milk fever problems.

Breed, age, and milk production level are important risk factors for milk fever in dairy cattle. Jerseys and Guernseys are the most susceptible to milk fever; Holsteins and Brown Swiss are moderately susceptible; and Ayrshires and Milking Shorthorns are the least susceptible.

The incidence of milk fever generally increases with parity and with higher levels of milk production, regardless of breed. First-lactation dairy cattle almost never develop milk fever.

Hypocalcemia is rare in beef cattle, probably because of their much lower milk production per unit of body weight

compared with that in dairy cattle. Milk fever incidence is also lower in sheep than in dairy cattle; however, it is possible for outbreaks of milk fever in pregnant ewes to affect up to 30% of a flock. High-producing doe goats have an incidence of milk fever similar to dairy cattle.

ETIOLOGY AND PATHOGENESIS

Milk fever is the result of severe hypocalcemia that occurs as an animal's complex mechanism for maintaining calcium homeostasis fails during a sudden and severe calcium outflow. Sudden calcium outflow occurs most commonly at the time of the initiation of lactation. The calcium demand associated with colostrum production in dairy cows (15-25 g calcium) and dairy goats (1-2 g calcium) exceeds the total prepartum calcium requirements including those associated with mineralization of the fetal skeleton (9 g and 1.2 g calcium/day).

In beef cows, ewes, and doe goats not challenged for milk production, the colostral demand for calcium is generally less than calcium demanded by the fetal skeleton. Thus these animals are at greatest risk for primary hypocalcemia in late gestation. DM intake (and thus calcium intake) decreases as parturition approaches, which

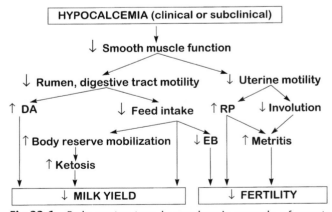

Fig 33-1 Early postpartum hypocalcemic cascade of events leading to decreased milk yield and fertility. *DA,* Displaced abomasum; *EB,* energy balance; *RP,* retained placenta. (Modified from Beede DK: *Macromineral element nutrition for the transition cow: practical implications and strategies.* Proceedings of the Tri-State Dairy Nutrition Conference, Ohio State, Michigan State, and Purdue Cooperative Extension Services, Columbus, 1995, p 185.)

---

*All material in this article is in the public domain, except for any borrowed figures and tables.

compounds the challenge to calcium homeostasis. These factors are multiplied for ewes or does carrying two or more fetuses.

An animal's ability to adapt to hypocalcemia is influenced by a number of factors. An important determinant of milk fever risk is the acid-base status of the animal at the time of parturition. Metabolic alkalosis appears to alter the physiologic activity of parathyroid hormone (PTH) so that bone resorption and production of 1,25-dihydroxycholecalciferol (1,25-[OH]$_2$D) are impaired. This reduces the animal's ability to successfully adjust to increased calcium demands.

Magnesium status is another factor influencing an animal's risk of hypocalcemia. Low blood magnesium levels can reduce PTH secretion from the parathyroid glands and can also alter the responsiveness of tissues to PTH. High dietary potassium reduces ruminal magnesium absorption. The effects of magnesium on calcium homeostasis are discussed further in this section under hypomagnesemic disorders. Excessive dietary phosphorus (>80 g/day) during late gestation is an additional risk factor for milk fever. When blood phosphorus concentration is in the range of 6 to 8 mg/dl, renal synthesis of 1,25-(OH)$_2$D is inhibited. Hypocalcemia may also be influenced by estrogen, which is a potent inhibitor of osteoclastic activity. Blood estrogen concentrations rise dramatically at the end of gestation and may blunt the effects of PTH on bone resorption.

CLINICAL PRESENTATION

The clinical effects of hypocalcemia in all species of livestock are broad because calcium serves many critical physiologic functions. Calcium is required for release of the neurotransmitter acetylcholine, which mediates transmission of nerve impulses at the myoneural junction. Lack of acetylcholine release is the likely cause of flaccid paralysis in milk fever. In addition, hypocalcemia inhibits contractility of smooth and cardiac muscle, causing a variety of additional clinical signs in affected animals.

Some hypocalcemic animals show signs of hyperesthesia and tetany, especially during the early phase of hypocalcemia. This occurs because calcium affects membrane stability in peripheral nerves and muscle fibers. Hypocalcemia may initially speed impulse conduction or even allow spontaneous impulse production in peripheral nerves and muscle fibers. Animals initially affected with hyperesthesia and tetany often later lapse into flaccid paralysis as the hypocalcemia worsens and neuromuscular junctions become blocked. Tetany is generally more pronounced in sheep and goats affected with hypocalcemia than in cattle.

Whether tetany or flaccid paralysis is seen also depends on the relative activity of magnesium and calcium. Magnesium competitively inhibits calcium at the myoneural junction. High magnesium concentration at the junction prevents calcium from stimulating acetylcholine release and promotes flaccid paralysis. Low magnesium at the junction removes the calcium inhibition and promotes tetany, so long as the hypocalcemia is not severe.

Dairy Cattle

Clinical signs of milk fever in dairy cattle may be divided for convenience into three nondiscrete stages. Stage I milk fever is characterized by mild excitement and tetany without recumbency. Dairy cattle with stage I milk fever are typically excitable, nervous, hypersensitive, anorectic, and weak. They may shift their weight frequently and shuffle their hind feet. Physical examination during stage I milk fever often reveals tachycardia and slight hyperthermia caused by increased muscular activity. Rumen contractions are weak and occur at a reduced rate.

Stage II milk fever in dairy cattle is characterized by sternal recumbency caused by flaccid paralysis. In contrast to the hypersensitivity and tetany of stage I, affected cows in stage II are depressed and paralyzed. The cow in stage II milk fever may also exhibit fine muscle tremors, particularly in the triceps muscles. Physical examination during stage II usually reveals rapid heart rate and decreased intensity of heart sounds because of reduced cardiac muscle contractility. Peripheral blood perfusion is poor, and the extremities of affected cows feel cold on palpation. Affected cows usually have lowered rectal temperature (35.6°-37.8° C or 96°-100° F), but the extent to which this occurs depends on ambient temperature. Impaired smooth muscle function caused by hypocalcemia leads to clinical signs such as gastrointestinal atony, mild bloat, constipation, and loss of the anal reflex. Pupils may be dilated and unresponsive to light owing to atony of the dilator pupillae muscle. Clinical signs of stage II generally last from 1 to 12 hours. Rumen contractions are almost undetectable.

Dairy cows in stage III milk fever are laterally recumbent and progressively lose consciousness to the point of coma. They are often severely bloated at this stage as a result of lateral recumbency combined with profound gastrointestinal atony. Cardiac output becomes severely compromised, heart sounds may be nearly inaudible, and heart rate increases to 120 bpm or more. Cows in stage III milk fever do not survive for more than a few hours without treatment.

About 7% of all cases of milk fever in dairy cattle are nonparturient. In these cases, sudden calcium outflow associated with the onset of lactation is not the stimulus for hypocalcemia. Instead, severe stress, hypomagnesemia, or feed deprivation interrupting calcium delivery to the intestine may be sufficient to cause a sudden shift in calcium balance and development of nonparturient hypocalcemia.

Beef Cattle

Milk fever in beef cattle is rare and is most likely to occur in late gestation under conditions of severe dietary mineral imbalances. If the mineral imbalances are chronic, then affected cows may present with clinical signs of osteoporosis rather than acute hypocalcemia with paresis. These problems are often corrected by simply increasing calcium or magnesium, or both, in the late-gestation diet. In recumbent beef cows suffering from general energy or protein malnutrition, or both, hypocalcemia is often observed along with hypomagnesemia and hypophosphatemia. These animals respond poorly to correction of the mineral imbalances (see Chapter 37). Occasional cases of nonparturient hypocalcemia may also occur in beef cattle.

Sheep

Milk fever in ewes is more likely to occur in late gestation rather than at the onset of lactation because ewes have a larger relative fetoplacental unit calcium drain (particularly ewes carrying multiple fetuses) and lower milk production calcium drain than do dairy cattle. Hypocalcemia in ewes may reduce feed intake and lead to concurrent pregnancy toxemia. Milk fever in ewes is primarily characterized by flaccid paralysis; however, severe muscle tremors or tetany (similar to those caused by hypomagnesemia) are frequently seen. Some affected ewes exhibit a stiff and uncoordinated gait before falling into rigid, sternal recumbency.

Goats

Milk fever may occur in doe goats either prepartum or postpartum because they have both the potential for high milk production and relatively large fetoplacental requirements associated with multiple births. The parturient form of milk fever predominates when goats are managed intensively for milk production. The prepartum form of milk fever predominates when goats are managed for multiple births or are not challenged for high milk production.

Clinical signs of milk fever in doe goats are similar to those in sheep and include both hyperesthesia with tetany and flaccid paralysis. Clinical signs in doe goats tend to be less severe than those observed in dairy cows. Goats may also be affected with nonparturient hypocalcemia.

CLINICAL PATHOLOGY

Milk fever is confirmed by low serum calcium concentrations. Clinical signs may begin as total blood calcium values fall below 7.5 mg/dl; however, more than half of all mature dairy cows will have total blood calcium concentrations below 7.5 mg/dl following calving without any evidence of clinical signs. Animals in stage I milk fever usually have mild hypocalcemia (5.5-7.5 mg/dl of calcium). Some animals are able to remain standing with total calcium concentrations as low as 5 mg/dl, but most become recumbent before this concentration is reached. Animals in stage II milk fever typically have total calcium concentrations of 3.5 to 6.5 mg/dl, and calcium levels may be as low as 1 to 2.5 mg/dl in animals with stage III milk fever.

Blood concentrations of phosphorus are typically below normal in milk fever, whereas magnesium concentrations are usually high. Phosphorus and magnesium abnormalities are further discussed elsewhere in this section.

Laboratory confirmation of the diagnosis of milk fever is often not necessary because response to treatment is a useful and commonly used diagnostic method. Most cases of milk fever respond rapidly to a single parenteral treatment with calcium salts. Collecting a blood sample before initial treatment of milk fever cases is good practice. If the animal does not respond to initial treatment, then an accurate diagnosis can be made from the pretreatment blood sample. Posttreatment samples are of limited value in diagnosing milk fever because they are temporarily influenced by the calcium administered. Ruling out other possible causes of recumbency in parturient animals before initiating calcium treatment is important.

Milk fever must be diagnosed antemortem because no gross lesions or histologic changes in affected animals are seen at necropsy. Urine obtained from the bladder will have low calcium concentration, but this alone is not sufficient evidence to make a diagnosis. Postmortem blood samples cannot be used to assess calcium status.

TREATMENT

Milk fever should always be treated as promptly as possible, particularly if the animal is already recumbent. Stage I milk fever may be treated with either oral calcium supplements or intravenous calcium salts. Animals in stage II or III require immediate treatment with intravenous calcium salts. Animals affected with milk fever do not usually recover spontaneously, and 75% of all affected animals will eventually die if left untreated.

Standard intravenous treatment for cattle affected with milk fever is 500 ml of a calcium gluconate or borogluconate solution to provide 10 to 11 g of calcium. Intravenous calcium should always be administered slowly to prevent sudden cardiac arrest caused by hypercalcemia. At least 12 minutes should be allowed for injection of intravenous calcium (8- to 12-g dose) into cattle. Adult sheep and doe goats affected with milk fever require only 50 to 100 ml of calcium solution intravenously.

The addition of magnesium or potassium to milk fever treatment solutions may be beneficial. In most cases the phosphorus provided in calcium solutions is not beneficial because it is not in the biologically relevant phosphate form. Therapeutic use of these electrolytes is discussed in other portions of this section.

Glucose added to treatment solutions may be detrimental because excretion of unneeded glucose in the urine causes increased excretion of much-needed phosphorus. More importantly it may increase risk of osmotic injury to tissues if used subcutaneously or injected outside the vein.

A precise calculation of the dose of calcium salts necessary to correct milk fever cannot be made because of the dynamic nature of calcium metabolism. The immediate total body calcium deficit in a dairy cow with milk fever is about 6 g, so a standard dose of 10 to 11 g of calcium should be adequate in most cases. Use of higher doses of intravenous calcium (e.g., two bottles instead of one) increases the risk for hypocalcemic relapses.

Approximately 60% of recumbent animals affected with uncomplicated milk fever get up within 30 minutes after a single intravenous treatment with calcium salts. Another 15% can be expected to rise within the next 2 hours. However, intravenous treatment only assists animals in getting through the temporary hypocalcemic crisis. Full restoration of normal calcium homeostasis usually requires 2 or 3 days.

Animals with unresponsive cases of milk fever should be reevaluated and retreated at about 12-hour intervals until they recover, die, or are salvaged. About 10% of dairy cows with milk fever stay recumbent for more than 24 hours but eventually recover.

Cases of stage I milk fever may be treated by administering calcium via a slowly absorbed route. For example, subcutaneously administered calcium is gradually absorbed over a period of several hours. Solutions containing glucose should be avoided or only given subcutaneously in small volumes because they often cause tissue destruction, abscess formation, or sloughing at the site of injection.

Calcium provided by oral dosing is also gradually absorbed. A variety of oral calcium salt preparations are now available. They typically contain between 25 and 100 g of calcium as either calcium chloride or calcium propionate. They work by rapidly raising calcium in the intestine to such a high concentration that a proportion of the calcium is absorbed by a passive process rather than the vitamin D dependent active transport of calcium across the intestine. For example, about 4 g of calcium will be absorbed and enter the bloodstream of a cow given an oral solution containing 50 g of calcium chloride. Calcium chloride also rapidly causes a compensated metabolic acidosis, which improves the animal's own calcium homeostatic mechanisms. However, high or repeated doses of calcium chloride can cause uncompensated metabolic acidosis, which is undesirable. Calcium chloride is irritating and may cause transient erosions in the mouth, esophagus, rumen, and abomasum of some cows. Calcium propionate is less irritating. Care must be taken during administration of any oral calcium supplement to avoid laceration of the pharyngeal region or aspiration of the solution. Typical doses of oral calcium supplements will increase blood calcium concentrations by 1 to 3 mg/dl within 30 minutes of administration. Blood calcium levels return to baseline values by 6 to 12 hours posttreatment.

About 25% to 40% of dairy cows with milk fever that respond favorably to initial intravenous calcium therapy will relapse into hypocalcemia within 12 to 48 hours. Animals with prepartum milk fever have an even greater relapse rate. Older cows are at greatest risk for a hypocalcemic relapse. Risk for relapse may be reduced by giving oral or subcutaneous calcium around the time of intravenous treatment or by giving another intravenous, oral or subcutaneous treatment 12 to 24 hours after the initial treatment.

PREVENTION

Dietary Calcium Restriction

Calcium-deficient diets (<15 g of absorbable calcium per day) fed for at least 10 days before calving greatly reduces the risk of milk fever. They work by causing a calcium deficiency in the animal. The parathyroid gland responds by releasing parathyroid hormone to stimulate bone resorption and renal production of 1,25-dihydroxyvitamin D before calving. At calving the animal is placed on a calcium adequate diet, and because intestinal calcium absorption mechanisms have been turned on by the 1,25-dihydroxyvitamin D, the animal is able to use bone and intestine to replace calcium lost to milk. Unfortunately, such diets are difficult to formulate and have proved largely impractical, especially for confined cows consuming 11 to 14 kg DM/day. Generally, the calcium in forages is only 30% to 40% available for absorption because it is tied up with plant oxalates and other organic compounds. Some types of warm-season grass pastures such as Kikuyu grass can have just 0.4% calcium. At this level the amount of available calcium from the forage may facilitate formulation of a low calcium diet to prevent milk fever. This is also aided by the reduced DM intake of cows on pasture, which may be just 7 to 10 kg DM/day.

Another approach is to add substances to the diet such as zeolite A to bind calcium in the diet so that it is unavailable for absorption. At present this approach requires about 0.5 kg zeolite A added to the diet, and some experts are concerned about whether the zeolite binds other essential minerals along with calcium.

Acidification Through Diet

The effect of diet on acid-base balance is more important in controlling milk fever than is calcium intake. Diets fed before parturition that evoke an acidic response in the animal reduce milk fever risk, whereas diets that evoke an alkaline response increase it.

The potential of a diet to cause either alkalosis or acidosis can be estimated by calculating the dietary cation-anion difference (DCAD). Dietary electrolytes can be classified as either cations (positively charged) or anions (negatively charged). Inorganic ions that are highly dissociated in aqueous solutions and absorbed across the intestine into the blood influence acid-base status. Important dietary cations are sodium (Na), potassium (K), calcium (Ca), and magnesium (Mg); important dietary anions are chloride (Cl), sulfur (S), and phosphorus (P).

Several methods of calculating DCAD have been used, including the following equations:

$$\text{DCAD (mEq)} = (Na + K + .2\,Ca + .16\,Mg) \\ - (Cl + .6\,S + .68\,P) \quad (1)$$
$$\text{DCAD (mEq)} = (Na + K) - (Cl + S) \quad (2)$$
$$\text{DCAD (mEq)} = (Na + K) - (Cl) \quad (3)$$

Note that the units are given in milliequivalents and the values are usually expressed on the basis of 100 g or 1 kg of dietary DM. The first equation takes into account the bioavailability of all of the potential strong ions. Theoretically it should be the most accurate, but it is new and has not been widely applied. The second two equations are used more commonly. The equations used to calculate DCAD and the units used to express it vary among ration evaluation software programs.

Low-DCAD diets cause metabolic acidosis and reduce the risk of milk fever. A diet can have a low DCAD because it is low in cations, high in anions, or a combination of both. Typical diets fed to dry cows have a DCAD (using equation 2 shown earlier) of about +50 to +250 mEq/kg of diet DM. Reducing DCAD by 300 mEq/kg of diet DM reduces the risk for clinical milk fever about fourfold.

In common feedstuffs, potassium is the most variable of the ions in the DCAD equation, and it is usually the most important determinant of DCAD in unsupplemented feed. A good first step in formulating a low-DCAD prepartum diet is to reduce dietary potassium to less than 1.5% of diet DM. Removing potassium from a diet can be difficult, owing to its presence in forages. Forage potassium levels depend largely on soil potassium content, which tends to be high wherever manure has been applied to soils.

Once the cation content of a prepartum diet has been reduced as much as possible by diet selection, anions can then be added to further reduce DCAD to the desired end point. Anion sources include anionic salts (any mineral salt high in chloride and sulfur relative to sodium and potassium) and mineral acids (hydrochloric or sulfuric acids). Optimal acidification generally occurs when anions are added to achieve a final DCAD (using equation 2 above) between 0 and 100 mEq/kg of DM. Lowering DCAD further may reduce the risk for milk fever but may also decrease DM intake enough to cause fatty liver or other disorders related to inadequate energy intake.

Monitoring urinary pH after feeding supplemental anions may be a direct and useful approach to establishing the optimal dose of anions within a dairy herd. An advantage of this approach (overrelying on calculated DCAD alone) is that it accounts for inaccuracies in mineral analyses and for unexpected changes in forage mineral content. Mean urinary pH can be evaluated by obtaining urine from a group of at least six animals near parturition. When acidification is optimal, mean urinary pH values will be between 6 and 7. Mean urinary pH values below 6 indicate overacidification and suggest that the DCAD could be increased. Conversely, urinary pH values greater than 7 reflect inadequate acidification and suggest that a lower DCAD is required for optimal milk fever prevention. When some cows are low (5.5 to 6) and some cows are high (7.5 to 8), overacidification may have occurred. Cows with the low urine pH ate the diet well in the past 12 to 24 hours and are now entering uncompensated metabolic acidosis. Cows with higher urine pH are recovering from uncompensated metabolic acidosis by reducing feed intake dramatically. It will be necessary to reduce anion supplementation to correct the feed intake issues.

Some uncertainty exists regarding the optimal dietary calcium concentration that should be used when low-DCAD diets are fed. Low-DCAD diets work well when they provide 90 to 140 g calcium/day.

Prophylactic Calcium Administration

Prophylactic treatment of cows with intravenous calcium gluconate immediately after calving may reduce the risk for clinical milk fever. Oral calcium supplements and subcutaneous calcium injections may reduce the risk for both clinical and subclinical milk fever. Treatment with four doses of an oral calcium supplement (providing 50 g calcium/dose, given before calving, at calving, 12 hours postcalving, and 24 hours postcalving) reduces the risk of clinical and subclinical milk fever in dairy cows by about half. This protocol works best when at least one dose of oral calcium can be administered before calving.

Recommended Readings

Charbonneau E, Pellerin D, Oetzel GR: Impact of lowering dietary cation-anion difference in nonlactating dairy cows: a meta-analysis, *J Dairy Sci* 89:537-548, 2006.

Goff JP, Horst RL: Effects of the addition of potassium or sodium, but not calcium, to prepartum rations on milk fever in dairy cows, *J Dairy Sci* 80:176-186, 1997.

Jardon PW: Using urine pH to monitor anionic salt programs, *Compend Cont Educ Practicing Vet* 17:860, 1995.

Oetzel GR: Effect of calcium chloride gel treatment in dairy cows on incidence of periparturient diseases, *J Am Vet Med Assoc* 209:958, 1996.

CHAPTER 34

Phosphorus Deficiency*

JESSE P. GOFF

Phosphorus deficiency is fairly common in grazing ruminants, especially those fed on poor-quality pastures. Except for rickets and postparturient hemoglobinuria, the clinical problems associated with phosphorus deficiency are general and nonspecific.

OCCURRENCE

The most common of the phosphorus deficiency syndromes is unthriftiness and poor growth. In arid areas of the world, where soil fertility is low, infertility and poor growth resulting from inadequate energy and protein intake goes hand in hand with phosphorus deficiency and affects nearly all animals. Because of this association, infertility has long been erroneously attributed to phosphorus deficiency. In more temperate areas, phosphorus deficiency is observed in animals subsisting on overly mature forages or on crop residues such as corn stalks. Sheep may be more resistant to phosphorus deficiency than are cattle.

ETIOLOGY AND PATHOGENESIS

Phosphorus is a component of phospholipids, phosphoproteins, nucleic acids, and energy-transferring molecules such as adenosine triphosphate (ATP). Phosphorus is an essential component of the acid-base buffer system. It is second only to calcium as the major component of bone mineral.

Plasma inorganic phosphorus concentration is normally between 4 and 8 mg/dl. Phosphorus exists in blood serum and other body fluids in organic and inorganic forms. Clinical laboratories typically measure inorganic phosphorus as phosphate. In mature ruminant animals the major phosphorus requirement is for salivary buffering, milk production, and fetal skeletal development. Salivary secretion is substantial. It is the major source of phosphorus to the rumen microbes that require phosphorus to efficiently break down cellulose and produce microbial protein. Most, but not all, of salivary phosphorus is reabsorbed and recycled.

Ruminants, unlike monogastrics, are able to use phytate phosphorus, a major source of phosphorus in plants. Plasma phosphorus concentrations are well correlated with dietary phosphorus absorption. Phosphorus absorbed in excess of needs is excreted in urine and saliva.

Rickets and Osteomalacia

Rickets is a disease of young, growing animals in which the cartilaginous matrix at the growth plate and the osteoid matrix formed during bone remodeling fail to mineralize. In adults (no active growth plates) the term *osteomalacia* is used to describe the failure of osteoid matrix to mineralize during bone remodeling. Failure to supply phosphorus in the diet results in low plasma phosphorus concentrations, which do not support bone mineralization.

Chronic Hypophosphatemia

Animals fed diets containing less phosphorus than necessary to meet physiologic needs suffer hypophosphatemia and all the physiologic consequences of failure to grow, inappetence, and unthriftiness. Milk production, but not phosphorus content of the milk, will decline.

Acute Hypophosphatemia

Beef cows fed a diet marginal in phosphorus have chronic hypophosphatemia (plasma phosphorus, 2-3.5 mg/dl). In late gestation, plasma phosphorus can decline precipitously in these animals as the growth of the fetus accelerates and removes substantial amounts of phosphorus from the maternal circulation. Affected animals often become recumbent and are unable to rise, although they appear fairly alert and may eat feed placed in front of them. Cows carrying twins are most often affected. Plasma inorganic phosphorus concentration in these recumbent animals is often less than 1 mg/dl. The disease is usually complicated by concurrent hypocalcemia; hypomagnesemia; and, in some cases, hypoglycemia.

At the onset of lactation in the dairy cow, production of colostrum and milk draw large amounts of phosphorus out of extracellular phosphorus pools, depressing blood phosphorus concentrations out of the normal range. Within a day or two of calving it is typical to find blood phosphorus concentrations between 3.2 and 4 mg/dl in normal, healthy cows. However, cows that develop milk fever have blood phosphorus concentrations that are even further depressed. Plasma inorganic phosphorus concentrations in cows with milk fever are often between 1 and 2 mg/dl. Plasma phosphorus concentrations usually increase rapidly following treatment of the hypocalcemic cow with intravenous calcium solutions. Restoring normocalcemia decreases parathyroid hormone secretion, which reduces urinary and salivary loss of phosphorus and stimulates resumption of gastrointestinal motility,

*All of the material in this article is in the public domain.

which in turn allows absorption of dietary phosphorus and reabsorption of salivary phosphorus secretions. Protracted hypophosphatemia in some cows appears to be an important factor in some nonresponsive milk fever or downer cow cases. Unlike typical cases of milk fever, plasma phosphorus levels in these cows remains low, despite successful treatment of the hypocalcemia. Why plasma phosphorus remains low is unclear, although it does not seem to be caused by low dietary phosphorus and the incidence is not reduced, and may actually be worsened by feeding more phosphorus than the close-up dry cow requires. In my experience, most cases occur in colder climates and seem to be precipitated when a cold front moves into an area. Why is unknown. Instituting a program to control hypocalcemia and milk fever generally is an effective means of preventing the low phosphorus downer cow syndrome.

CLINICAL SIGNS

Moderate, chronic hypophosphatemia, with plasma phosphorus between 2 and 4 mg/dl, causes subtle decreases in animal performance. With more severe hypophosphatemia, performance of the animals becomes poor and feed intake is depressed. The reduction in feed intake is often accompanied by pica. Recumbency and paresis when plasma calcium is normal (the hypophosphatemic downer cow) are associated with plasma phosphorus concentrations below 1 mg/dl.

Rickets and Osteomalacia

Young, growing animals with rickets exhibit joint pain and reluctance to move. Growth rate is greatly depressed. Affected animals have narrow chests, and the costochondral joints are enlarged and readily palpable. Adult animals with osteomalacia exhibit joint pain and lameness.

CLINICAL PATHOLOGY

Adult animals with plasma phosphorus concentration between 2 and 4 mg/dl are likely to perform poorly and, with time, develop osteomalacia. Plasma phosphorus concentration in young, growing animals should be between 5 and 8.5 mg/dl. Otherwise, growth impairment and rickets develop. Animals recumbent as a result of hypophosphatemia have plasma phosphorus concentrations below 1 mg/dl (often closer to 0.5 mg/dl). Hypocalcemia, hypomagnesemia, and hypoglycemia are often concurrently present in recumbent beef cows in late gestation, which is generally complicated by energy deficiency.

Bones from animals with chronic phosphorus deficiency show a reduction in bone ash content. The ratio of calcium to phosphorus in the bone is not significantly altered.

Cows with postparturient hemoglobinuria exhibit true hemoglobin in the urine. The packed cell volume of blood is reduced, and Heinz bodies are readily observed in blood smears. Many of the animals also suffer from concurrent copper or selenium deficiency, or both, casting doubt as to whether phosphorus deficiency alone is the true cause of the red blood cell fragility.

DIAGNOSIS

Clinical signs coupled with low plasma phosphorus concentration help in the diagnosis of phosphorus deficiency. Hemolysis of the blood sample causes a falsely elevated plasma phosphorus concentration. Also, if more than 12 hours have passed from sample collection until serum removal, the phosphorus can leach out of the red blood cells to the serum.

Rickets is always accompanied by hypophosphatemia. Bones of rachitic animals tend to bend without breaking. Bone lesions are the only postmortem lesion that is pathognomonic of phosphorus deficiency. Vitamin D deficiency causes hypophosphatemia and hypocalcemia, even when dietary content of these minerals is normal. The presence of more than 10 ng of 25-hydroxyvitamin D per milliliter of plasma rules out rickets caused by vitamin D deficiency.

TREATMENT

Recumbent Cows

Beef cows in late gestation and dairy cows that remain recumbent following treatment for milk fever are often hypophosphatemic. Some of these "downer cows" benefit from intravenous administration of phosphate to restore normal plasma phosphorus concentrations. Monosodium phosphate is a soluble form of phosphate that can be administered intravenously (30 g of monosodium phosphate in 300-500 ml of distilled water). Calcium salts cannot be included in these solutions because insoluble calcium phosphate salts will form. Commercial preparations containing phosphorus often use more soluble hypophosphite salts so that addition of calcium or magnesium to the solution does not cause a precipitate to form. Unfortunately, hypophosphite salts are not biologically functional and do not correct hypophosphatemia.

Intravenous phosphate treatment maintains normal plasma phosphorus concentration for only a short time (6-10 hours). In most cases these animals also require oral administration of phosphate (0.5 kg monosodium phosphate in warm water administered as a drench or via stomach tube). Dicalcium phosphate may also be used (0.5 kg), but it is poorly soluble and difficult to administer. A cocktail that includes calcium, magnesium, and an energy source, as well as phosphorus, can benefit the recumbent cow. A recipe we have used is 0.5 to 0.75 kg of calcium propionate, 0.35 kg of magnesium sulfate (Epsom salt), 0.20 kg of monosodium phosphate, and 0.5 L of propylene glycol or glycerin dissolved in 6 to 12 L of warm water administered via stomach tube as a means of supplementation for recumbent cows. Calcium chloride (0.25-0.35 kg) can be substituted for calcium propionate.

Rickets and Osteomalacia

Animals with rickets and osteomalacia will, with time, recover once dietary phosphorus is supplied to them, providing the disease has not progressed to the point of irreparable joint damage.

PREVENTION

Phosphorus deficiency is a possibility whenever animals are on pasture, especially mature pasture, that consists of less than 0.25% phosphorus. Heavily lactating dairy cows and ewes may develop phosphorus deficiency when pasture contains less than 0.32% phosphorus. Grains serve as good sources of phosphorus. In addition, mineral sources of phosphorus can be easily incorporated into the grain. Daily ingestion of 80 g of monosodium phosphate or 100 g of dicalcium phosphate prevents phosphorus deficiency in almost every case. Dicalcium phosphate is the most commonly used source of phosphate in the United States, and free choice supplementation of dicalcium phosphate can often prevent phosphorus deficiency in most of the pastured herd if it is made readily accessible. Intake of dicalcium phosphate is often enhanced if mixed 1:1 with salt. Defluoridated phosphate, along with lesser amounts of ammonium polyphosphate and phosphoric acid, are also used in grain as phosphorus supplements.

Improving pasture phosphate is an option in some areas, and it often has the added benefit of improving forage yield. However, the price of phosphate fertilizer and the size of the area to be treated often renders this approach impractical in areas where phosphorus deficiency is endemic.

Recommended Reading

Goff JP: Macromineral disorders of the transition cow, *Vet Clin North Am Food Anim Pract* 20:471-494, 2004.

CHAPTER **35**

Ruminant Hypomagnesemic Tetanies*

JESSE P. GOFF

Extracellular magnesium is vital to normal nerve conduction, muscle function, and bone mineral formation. Hypomagnesemia generally leads to hyperexcitability, tetany, convulsion, and, too often, death. Hypomagnesemia is often accompanied and complicated by hypocalcemia and hypophosphatemia.

OCCURRENCE

Hypomagnesemic tetany is most often associated with beef cows and ewes in early lactation that are grazing in spring or fall on lush pastures that are high in potassium and nitrogen and low in magnesium and sodium. This is the most common situation, and it is often referred to as *grass tetany, spring tetany, grass staggers,* or *lactation tetany.* Ewes suckling more than one lamb and higher-producing cows are at greatest risk. Magnesium is not mobilized from tissue stores to maintain plasma magnesium concentration, so it must be ingested continually. Conditions associated with hypomagnesemia as a result of feed restriction include transport (transport tetany) or sudden exposure to inclement weather. Hypomagnesemia can also develop in late gestation, often in association with and complicated by inadequate energy intake. This syndrome is sometimes referred to as *winter tetany* and is seen in animals subsisting on crop residues such as corn stalks or cereal grain stubble. Animals grazing wheat pasture (wheat pasture tetany) or other early-growth cereal forages can develop hypomagnesemia with concurrent severe hypocalcemia, resulting in a clinical picture that closely resembles milk fever. Hypomagnesemia can also occur in veal calves, especially if they are fed only milk or milk replacer beyond the first 2 months of age (milk tetany). Hypomagnesemic tetany can reach epidemic proportions on some farms, affecting nearly 20% of cows and ewes in early lactation on some pastures, although death losses of 2% to 3% are more commonly observed.

ETIOLOGY AND PATHOGENESIS

Bovine and ovine plasma magnesium concentrations are normally between 2 and 2.3 mg/dl, and 2.2 and 2.8 mg/dl, respectively. Blood and extracellular fluid

*All of the material in this article is in the public domain.

magnesium are in equilibrium with and similar to magnesium concentration in cerebrospinal fluid (CSF), although changes in CSF magnesium concentration lag behind changes in plasma magnesium concentration because the blood-brain barrier slows diffusion.

The tetany characteristic of hypomagnesemic disorders is the result of intracellular, cellular membrane, and extracellular metabolic effects of magnesium. Tetany is the result of the following factors:

1. Lower central and peripheral nervous membrane potential
2. Excessive acetylcholine release at myoneural junctions
3. Sustained myofibril contractions caused by reduced intracellular adenosine triphosphatase (ATPase) activity
4. Hypocalcemia caused by hypomagnesemic influences on parathyroid function and tissue recognition of parathyroid hormone

Despite the physiologic importance of magnesium, no hormonal mechanism is concerned principally and directly with magnesium homeostasis. Constant absorption of ingested magnesium is necessary to maintain normal plasma magnesium concentration. Dietary magnesium absorbed in excess of needs is excreted in the urine. The renal threshold for magnesium is 1.85 mg/dl in cows and 2.2 mg/dl in sheep. At plasma magnesium concentrations below these levels, little or no magnesium will be detected in urine. Maintenance of normal plasma magnesium concentration is nearly totally dependent on dietary magnesium absorption. In young ruminants, as in monogastric animals, magnesium is absorbed well from the small intestine. As the rumen develops, it becomes the main site for magnesium absorption and the intestines are a site of net secretion of magnesium.

Magnesium absorption from the rumen is dependent on the concentration of magnesium in solution in the rumen fluid and the integrity of the magnesium transport mechanisms.

The soluble concentration of magnesium in rumen fluid is dependent on the following factors:

1. *Dietary magnesium content and form of magnesium.* Magnesium oxide is the most common form of magnesium used in animal diets. Unfortunately, the bioavailability of magnesium oxide can vary tremendously. To be soluble in the rumen, the magnesium oxide must be finely ground—it should pass through a 200-μm mesh screen. High magnesium content in the magnesium oxide (>56%) may signal overheating of the magnesium ores during the calcining process. It will not be soluble in the rumen fluids. An effective magnesium oxide will be rapidly soluble in dilute acid solution (0.4 M hydrochloric acid). Magnesium sulfate and magnesium chloride are more readily absorbed, but they are not palatable.
2. *Rumen pH.* Lower pH increases magnesium solubility.
3. *Presence of nonesterified, long-chain fatty acids.* These can form insoluble magnesium salts.
4. *Presence of plant dicarboxylic acids and tricarboxylic acids.* These form insoluble magnesium complexes.

However, the role of these complexes in hypomagnesemic tetany is unclear.

Factors affecting magnesium transport across the rumen epithelium include the following:

1. *Dietary sodium-to-potassium ratio.* High dietary potassium can interfere with the sodium-linked active transport of magnesium across the rumen wall.
2. *Availability of lush, high-moisture pastures.* Such pastures increase the rate of passage of material from the rumen.
3. *Diet magnesium concentration.* If diet magnesium concentration is greater than 0.35%, the concentration of soluble magnesium in rumen fluid can be high enough to allow transport of magnesium across the rumen wall by a passive transport process.

CLINICAL SIGNS

Cattle

The clinical signs in affected cows depend on the severity of hypomagnesemia. The disease progresses more rapidly and tends to be more severe if it is accompanied by hypocalcemia, which is often the case. Both beef and dairy cows are usually affected 1 to 3 weeks into lactation, especially if they are on pasture, which tends to be low in magnesium and high in potassium. Moderate hypomagnesemia (between 1.1 and 1.8 mg/dl) is associated with reduced feed intake, nervousness, and reduced milk fat and total milk production. This can be a chronic problem in some dairy herds that often goes unnoticed. It can also predispose the animals to milk fever.

When plasma magnesium levels fall below 1.1 mg/dl, twitching is sometimes seen in the muscles of the face, shoulders, and flanks. Cows become restless and irritable, and rumen motility is reduced. Affected animals may separate themselves from herdmates and take on a spastic, stiff-legged gait. Frequent urination and bellowing are common. Some animals become aggressive. The animals are particularly sensitive to sound. Blowing a car horn and forced movement of the cows often initiates the appearance of tetany in cows with more than moderate hypomagnesemia.

As hypomagnesemia progresses, tetanic spasms of the muscles become more common and eventually cause the cow to stagger and fall. Clonic convulsions quickly follow, with chomping of the jaws and frothy salivation. Affected cows usually lie with the head arched back and the legs paddling. The heart rate can approach 150 bpm and the heartbeat is often audible without a stethoscope. Respiratory rate approaches 60 breaths/min, and the rectal temperature rises and can approach 40.5° C (105° F) as a result of the excessive muscular activity; the eyelids flutter, and marked nystagmus is present. The animal may rise after several minutes, and the convulsive episodes may be repeated several times before the cow finally dies.

Hypomagnesemic tetany in calves is clinically similar to that in adult cows, and it is often accompanied by moderate hypocalcemia.

Ewes and Goats

Affected ewes are generally hypocalcemic, as well as hypomagnesemic. They are usually in the second to fourth week of lactation and are often suckling more than one lamb. Affected ewes are generally depressed, stand with their heads down, and are reluctant to move. As hypomagnesemia and hypocalcemia progress, they suffer tetany and clonic convulsions, just as cattle do. The clinical signs in goats are similar to those observed in cattle.

CLINICAL PATHOLOGY

Plasma or serum magnesium concentrations below 1.8 mg/dl in cattle and below 2.2 mg/dl in sheep are considered to be low and indicative of inadequate magnesium absorption. Plasma magnesium concentrations below 1 mg/dl indicate the risk of developing tetany. Plasma calcium concentrations are often low as well, generally between 5 and 7.5 mg/dl. CSF magnesium concentrations less than 1 mg/dl are responsible for the clonic convulsions seen in animals with hypomagnesemic tetany. Blood samples obtained during or shortly after an episode of tetany may have near-normal levels of magnesium as a result of muscle damage and leakage of magnesium from intracellular pools. The CSF magnesium concentration remains low during tetany and also can be a reliable indicator of magnesium status for up to 12 hours after death. Vitreous humor magnesium concentrations less than 1 mg/dl are also found in animals with tetany and can be a reliable indicator for 24 to 48 hours after death, provided that environmental temperatures have not exceeded 23° C (73° F). Aqueous humor has not proved reliable as a sample. Urine magnesium concentration is nearly undetectable in animals that are hypomagnesemic.

Animals in tetany or those that have just had a tetanic episode often exhibit hyperkalemia (potassium >7 mEq/L) and elevated serum aspartate aminotransferase (AST) and creatine phosphokinase (CPK) activity as a result of muscle cell damage and leakage.

DIAGNOSIS

A diagnosis is often made after one or two animals have already died of hypomagnesemic tetany. No pathognomonic necropsy lesions are associated with hypomagnesemic tetany. A history of sudden death in early-lactation cows and ewes grazing on fast-growing, cool-season grass or green cereal crop pasture is diagnostic in many cases. The CSF and urine magnesium concentrations may be of some aid postmortem. Blood analyses will confirm low plasma magnesium concentrations in herdmates.

Dairy herds grazing pasture and having suboptimal milk fat and total milk production may have mild hypomagnesemia. A response to supplementation is the most satisfactory confirmation of diagnosis. In growing calves, 43 calcium atoms are incorporated into bone for every magnesium atom (71 mg of calcium per 1 mg of magnesium). Bone formed during chronic magnesium deficiency will have a calcium-to-magnesium ratio of greater than 100.

TREATMENT

Animals exhibiting hypomagnesemic tetany need immediate treatment. Slowly injecting 500 ml (50-100 ml for ewes) of a solution of calcium borogluconate (8-10 g of calcium) and magnesium hypophosphite, magnesium borogluconate, magnesium chloride, or magnesium gluconate (1.5-4 g of magnesium) intravenously is the safest and most effective general recommendation. Intravenous administration of solutions containing only magnesium increases the risk of respiratory failure as a result of medullary depression. The risk of cardiac failure during treatment is also reduced by addition of calcium to the intravenous solutions. In addition, most hypomagnesemic animals suffer from hypocalcemia and solutions containing magnesium with no calcium do not effect a recovery. Treatment of these animals can be challenging because insertion of the intravenous needle often initiates a tetanic episode. Some veterinarians use intramuscularly administered tranquilizers or sedatives such as acepromazine to reduce the risk of injury to the cow and to themselves from continuous clonic convulsions. Intravenous administration of tranquilizers has been associated with sudden hypotension and death. Response to therapy can be disappointing, and success is related to the interval between onset of tetany and treatment. To avoid initiation of tetany and convulsion, cows should not be stimulated to rise for at least 30 minutes after treatment. Cattle that will recover do so 1 hour after treatment, when CSF magnesium concentration returns to normal. Many of these cows suffer relapse and require further treatment within 12 hours.

The rate of relapse can be reduced with the following treatments:

1. *Subcutaneous injection of 100 to 200 ml of a 20% to 50% magnesium sulfate solution.* The stronger solutions are essentially fully saturated and hyperosmotic, and no more than 50 ml should be injected in any one site to avoid tissue damage.
2. *Magnesium enemas, 60 g of magnesium chloride or 60 g of magnesium sulfate dissolved in 200 ml of water, administered into the descending colon.* This treatment increases plasma magnesium concentration within 15 minutes. It can cause some mucosal sloughing, especially if more highly concentrated solutions are used.
3. *Magnesium salts.* Oral administration of magnesium salts can be given to provide longer maintenance of plasma magnesium concentration once the animal has regained good esophageal reflexes so that the risk of aspiration pneumonia is reduced. Drenching the cow with a slurry of 100 g of magnesium oxide in water has been reported to be effective. This provides 50 g of magnesium to the animal. Addition of 50 g of calcium carbonate, 100 g of dicalcium phosphate, and 50 g of sodium chloride may enhance the effectiveness of the slurry, especially if hypocalcemia and hypophosphatemia accompany the hypomagnesemia. The addition of sodium may enhance ruminal magnesium absorption. Alternatively, 200 to 400 ml of a 50% magnesium sulfate solution can be administered by drench. Magnesium sulfate is much more available

for absorption than is magnesium oxide. Slurries can be difficult to administer. Gel formulations containing magnesium in comparable concentrations are also available commercially.

PREVENTION

If hypomagnesemic tetany has occurred in one cow or ewe in a herd or flock, steps should be taken immediately to increase magnesium intake to prevent further losses. Getting an additional 10 to 15 g of magnesium into each pregnant cow, 20 g of magnesium into each lactating beef cow, and 30 g of magnesium into each lactating dairy cow each day usually prevents further cases of hypomagnesemic tetany. The problem with prevention is successfully getting the extra magnesium into the animal.

Individual drenching of cows at risk is effective but highly laborious. Addition of magnesium salts to grain supplements is practical in some situations. Most magnesium salts are unpalatable, making free-choice consumption ineffective. However, magnesium is readily accepted in grain concentrates. Including 60 g of magnesium oxide in just 0.5 to 1 kg of grain is effective. However, the expense of the grain and the problems associated with feeding concentrates to pastured cattle often make this option difficult to implement. Feeding mature grass or legume hay to the cows or ewes can often improve magnesium intake by increasing total dry matter intake of cattle on pasture. Hay is usually higher in magnesium content than are rapidly growing immature grasses. Hay is also lower in potassium and therefore presents less inhibition of ruminal magnesium absorption. Adding magnesium oxide (60 g/cow, mixed with water and molasses) to the hay, at the time of baling or just before feeding, can increase the effectiveness of this option. Unfortunately, cows with access to lush pasture may not eat enough hay unless they are confined for that purpose each day. Dusting of pasture foliage with magnesium oxide is also an approach that has been used to increase magnesium intake. Feeding ionophores, in situations in which they are legal, can increase dietary magnesium availability.

Adding 5 to 10 kg per 2000 L or 10 to 20 lb per 500 gal of magnesium sulfate·7H$_2$O (Epsom salts) or magnesium chloride·6H$_2$O to drinking water can be an economical means of supplementing magnesium if cows have access to no other water supply. Molasses licks and mineral blocks containing magnesium oxide and salt can help supply magnesium to animals at pasture if made readily available and if the animals learn to use the licks before parturition. A problem with many of these methods is that some cows in the herd may not voluntarily consume enough of the magnesium supplement and, on some tetanogenic pastures, cows that do not receive supplementation are often found dead.

Intraruminal magnesium-releasing boluses and bullets, which remain in the reticulum and release low levels of magnesium (1-1.5 g) daily for periods of up to 90 days, have been developed. These devices do not supply enough magnesium to raise blood magnesium levels substantially, although they may prove successful in some situations despite the low level of supplementation achieved.

Agronomic practices to increase forage magnesium content and reduce hypomagnesemic tetany are in various stages of development and show good promise.

Recommended Readings

Fontenot JP, Allen VG, Bunce GE et al: Factors influencing magnesium absorption and metabolism in ruminants, *J Anim Sci* 67:3445-3455, 1989.

Littledike ET, Goff JP: Interactions of calcium, phosphorus, magnesium and vitamin D that influence their status in domestic meat animals, *J Anim Sci* 65:1727-1743, 1987.

Martens H, Schweigel M: Pathophysiology of grass tetany and other hypomagnesemias. Implications for clinical management, *Vet Clin North Am Food Anim Pract* 16:339-368, 2000.

CHAPTER 36

Ketosis

THOMAS H. HERDT and BRIAN J. GERLOFF

OCCURRENCE

Ketosis is generally a disease of dairy cows in the period from parturition to 6 weeks postpartum. Recent reports of lactational ketosis incidence range from approximately 5% to 16%. In some herds, ketosis can affect a large proportion of at-risk cows (i.e., those in early lactation). Ketosis is occasionally seen prepartum in dairy and beef cows, in which case the condition resembles pregnancy toxemia of ewes. Cows carrying twins and receiving low-energy diets are at increased risk of prepartum ketosis.

Recent estimates of ketosis heritability range from 0.14 to 0.16 based on Norwegian Red Cattle, indicating that ketosis has low to moderate heritability.[1] The occurrence of ketosis in one lactation does not greatly increase the risk of development of the disease in a subsequent lactation. Age has little influence on ketosis risk, although in specific herds it may occur as a problem in one age group. However, the age group affected is not consistent among herds. Dry cows and pregnant heifers that are overly fat are at increased risk of developing ketosis after calving.

Clinical ketosis is frequently associated with concurrent diseases, both infectious and metabolic. In many cases, ketosis may occur secondary to another disease. In other instances, ketosis may be the initial disease or it may at least be a predisposing factor with respect to the occurrence of other diseases. This may be related, in part, to suppressed immune function associated with hyperketonemia, although other factors may also come into play.

Ketosis may be clinical or subclinical, and both forms are associated with reduced milk production and reduced reproductive efficiency. In addition, subclinical ketosis is a risk factor for the development of clinical ketosis or displaced abomasum, or both. The economic impact of ketosis is derived from treatment costs, reduced milk production, a generalized increase in morbidity, and reduced fertility. Subclinical ketosis, by one estimate, may reduce milk production by 1 to 1.5 kg/day.[2] The disease is seldom fatal, so death loss is not an important economic factor.

ETIOLOGY AND PATHOGENESIS

The initial events in the pathogenesis of all forms of ketosis are negative energy balance and the accompanying mobilization of nonesterified fatty acids (NEFAs) from adipose tissue. Negative energy balance is prevalent, perhaps universal, in dairy cows during the first 2 to 6 weeks of lactation because feed intake does not keep pace with the rapid increase in energy demands for milk production. The occurrence of ketosis is determined by the metabolic fate of NEFAs. Research indicates that distinct metabolic types of ketosis might exist, dependent on hepatic patterns of gluconeogenesis and NEFA metabolism.

Figure 36-1 illustrates two potential pathways of hepatic NEFA metabolism. With respect to metabolic disease development, ketogenesis and esterification are the most important pathways. NEFA entry into the ketogenic pathway predisposes to development of clinical ketosis, whereas entry into the esterification pathway favors fatty liver development. It is likely that glucose availability is an important factor in determining the relative activity of the two pathways of NEFA disposal. When glucose availability is low, entry of NEFA into the ketogenic pathway is favored. With somewhat higher glucose availability, esterification and fat accumulation are favored. Thus glucose availability, in addition to negative energy balance and NEFA mobilization, is an important factor in the pathogenesis of clinical ketosis.

Glucose supply is a constant metabolic challenge for ruminants because fermentative digestion destroys most of the available carbohydrates in their diets. Early lactation is a particularly challenging period because of the high glucose requirement for milk production. Two factors determine glucose availability in ruminants: (1) rate

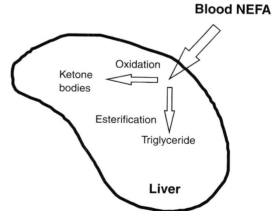

Fig 36-1 Metabolic pathways of nonesterified fatty acids (NEFAs) in the liver. After being absorbed by the liver, NEFAs can undergo esterification, resulting in triglyceride formation, or oxidation, resulting in ketone body formation. The consequence of high blood NEFA concentrations is determined by the relative activity of these two pathways: When ketogenesis predominates, ketosis is favored; when esterification predominates, fatty liver is favored. Glucose availability influences the activity of these pathways, with low glucose availability favoring oxidation.

of gluconeogenesis and (2) availability of gluconeogenetic substrate. The metabolic type of ketosis that develops is probably dependent on which of these two factors is most adversely affected.

The first factor, rate of gluconeogenesis, may be impaired in those cases of ketosis that develop within the first week of lactation. Some evidence suggests that hepatic fat accumulation before calving may reduce hepatic gluconeogenic capacity.[3,4] Thus the progression of metabolic events in this type of ketosis is proposed to be (1) prepartum adipose lysis and NEFA mobilization, (2) NEFA esterification with fatty liver development, (3) reduced gluconeogenesis, (4) reduced glucose availability, (5) a shift in NEFA metabolism from esterification to ketogenesis, and (6) ketosis development. The term *type II ketosis* has been used to describe this type of ketosis, although *periparturient,* or *early-lactation ketosis* might be more descriptive. Type II ketosis is reported to respond experimentally to glucagon administration, further suggesting that reduced gluconeogenesis plays a role in its pathophysiology.[5]

Ketosis cases that develop later during lactation, near the time of peak milk production, may be of a different metabolic type. In this case it appears that availability of gluconeogenetic substrate is simply insufficient to meet the demands of milk production. This results in high NEFA concentrations, with a large portion of NEFA being directed into ketogenesis rather than esterification. This type of ketosis has been referred to as *type I ketosis,* although *peak-lactation ketosis* might be a more suitable descriptive term. It is this manifestation of ketosis that fits the classical description of the disease, as set forth in many older textbooks of veterinary medicine. This type of ketosis is reported to be nonresponsive to experimental glucagon therapy.[5]

CLINICAL SIGNS AND SIGNALMENT

Cows that develop periparturient ketosis are frequently fat, whereas those that develop peak-lactation ketosis may be thin. The most common complaints at presentation include a sharp drop in milk production, a generally depressed attitude, and partial or complete anorexia. Slight dehydration may be evident, but vital signs are usually normal and findings on physical examination are generally unremarkable.

Occasionally, marked central nervous system signs occur with ketosis. This has been referred to as *nervous ketosis.* The signs are variable and may include excitement and hyperesthesia, depraved chewing and licking (occasionally with self-mutilation), or abnormal gait (including hypermetria or ataxia).

CLINICAL PATHOLOGY

Clinical pathologic signs include hyperketonemia, ketonuria, ketolactia, hypoglycemia, and high blood concentrations of NEFA. Values for these variables do not correspond closely with clinical signs, so exacting cutoff values are difficult to establish. Clinical cases are usually associated with plasma glucose concentrations less than 35 mg/dl and NEFA concentrations greater than 1000 μEq/L. Care must

be taken in the interpretation of blood ketone body concentrations because they may be expressed differently depending on the nature of the laboratory determination. Cases of clinical ketosis are usually associated with total ketone body (acetone, acetoacetate, and β-hydroxybutyrate) concentrations greater than 30 mg/dl. β-hydroxybutyrate concentrations alone are usually greater than 25 mg/dl. For quantitative determination of serum or plasma concentrations, β-hydroxybutyrate is preferable to acetoacetate or acetone because it is stable in the sample. It should be recognized, however, that commonly used semiquantitative methods (e.g., dipsticks) often measure only acetoacetate or acetoacetate plus acetone. The concentration of acetoacetate plus acetone usually constitutes only 10% to 20% of the total ketone body concentration, although this proportion increases in clinical ketosis. Urine ketone body concentrations are usually two to four times higher than blood concentrations, whereas milk ketone body concentrations are usually 40% to 50% of blood concentrations.

DIAGNOSIS

Diagnosis is usually based on clinical signs and the presence of detectable concentrations of ketone bodies in urine or milk. Field testing of urine and milk is done with semiquantitative methods based on visually discernible color changes. Dipsticks should be protected from moisture during storage to avoid false-negative results. The difference in ketone body concentrations between urine and milk make urine testing more sensitive but less specific than milk testing. Urine ketone body (acetoacetate) concentrations in peak-lactation ketosis are frequently high (80-160 mg/dl), whereas those for periparturient ketosis frequently are lower (20-40 mg/dl), as estimated by dipstick analysis.

The diagnosis of subclinical ketosis is important for herd management and disease prevention. Blood serum concentrations of β-hydroxybutyrate are generally taken as the gold standard for diagnosis of subclinical ketosis. The threshold concentration for classification as subclinical ketosis has been variably estimated from 10 to 14.6 mg/dl. Reported overall prevalence of subclinical ketosis ranges from 6.9% to 14.1% in the first 2 months of lactation.[6] In many well-managed, high-producing herds the prevalence is 0%, whereas a prevalence value above 30% is not unusual in problem herds. Days-in-milk is a critical factor in determining the prevalence of subclinical ketosis, and herd-level evaluations are best limited to cows in the first 3 weeks of lactation. Cow-side tests are available for estimation of subclinical ketosis. Ketostix strips (Bayer Corp., Elkhart, Indiana) detecting acetoacetate in urine samples were 78% sensitive and 96% specific using a cutoff point of "small" in the interpretation of strip color change. The KetoTest strip (SanWa Kagaku Kenkyusho Co. Ltd., Nagoya, Japan) used on milk samples had a sensitivity of 73% and specificity of 96% when a cutoff point of 100 μmol of β-hydroxybutyrate/L (10.4 mg/dl) was applied.

TREATMENT

The prognosis and response to therapy are dependent on the type of ketosis. Peak lactation ketosis (type I) usually responds quickly to therapy, but relapses are common if the diet is not corrected. Periparturient ketosis (type II) responds less rapidly to treatment. Periparturient ketosis is closely associated with fatty liver.

Treatment is aimed at reducing ketogenesis and reestablishing glucose homeostasis. Bolus administration of 500 mL of 50% glucose or dextrose solution has been a standard treatment.[7] Much of this dose is probably lost in the urine owing to the induction of serum glucose concentrations in excess of the renal glucose threshold. Nevertheless, the treatment is often effective. The high blood glucose concentrations associated with bolus intravenous (IV) infusion suppress both adipose NEFA release and hepatic ketogenesis, both favorable effects in ketosis therapy. The mechanisms by which these effects are induced are probably both insulin dependent and non–insulin dependent. The major problem with bolus IV glucose therapy is that relapses are common. In situations in which it is practical, continuous IV infusion of glucose is beneficial. Fructose and sorbitol have been used as alternatives to glucose therapy. This sugar and sugar alcohol, respectively, are expected to supply glucose directly at the hepatic level. This is in contrast to the direct administration of glucose, in which the administered glucose would be available to all tissues.

Glucocorticoid therapy is also effective. Appropriate dosages of dexamethasone (Azium, Schering Corporation, Union, NJ) and isoflupredone acetate (Predef 2X, Pharmacia-Upjohn Company, Kalamazoo, Mich.) are 1.33 mg per 45 kg of body weight. Glucocorticoids do not appear to induce gluconeogenesis in ruminants, but rather they seem to affect glucose distribution and kinetics. This may be favorable in terms of ketosis therapy because increased gluconeogenesis is usually associated with increased ketogenesis. Ketotic cows treated with glucocorticoids are less subject to relapses than are those treated with IV glucose therapy alone, although relapses can still occur. Because of the immunosuppressive nature of glucocorticoids, care should be observed in their administration to animals with infectious disease concurrent with ketosis.

Insulin, in conjunction with glucocorticoid therapy, may be more effective than glucocorticoids alone. Insulin is a powerful antiketogenic agent and also suppresses NEFA mobilization. It is important to provide a glucocorticoid or other agent, however, to counteract the hypoglycemic effects of insulin. A long-lasting form of insulin should be used. The usual dose is 200 to 300 IU per animal. Administration is repeated as needed, usually at 24- to 48-hour intervals. Insulin therapy is usually reserved for cases that have been nonresponsive to initial therapy. These are usually cases of type II, or periparturient, ketosis.

Several compounds, if administered orally, can serve as glucose precursors in ruminants. Of these, propylene glycol and salts of propionic acid have been most popular. Dosages of propylene glycol usually have been in the range of 250 to 400 g (≈8-14 oz), administered twice daily as an oral drench. Excessive dosage can result in incoordination and depression of consciousness.

PREVENTION

Prevention of peak lactation ketosis is directed toward maximizing energy intake and providing adequate glucose precursors. Feed intake is usually the most critical factor in determining energy balance of early-lactation dairy cows, so the first effort should be to maximize feed intake. This is achieved by making sure that feed is available nearly constantly and that there is not excessive competition at the feed bunk. Rations should be well balanced for all nutrients, especially for carbohydrate components. Intake of insufficient amounts of starches and other nonstructural carbohydrates results in ration-energy densities that are too low to provide maximum energy intakes. In addition, nonstructural carbohydrates promote a relatively high proportion of propionate in the ruminal volatile fatty acids. Propionate is an important glucose precursor. However, excessive dietary nonstructural carbohydrates, relative to structural carbohydrates and effective fiber, can lead to rumen acidosis and reduced feed intake, thus reducing total energy intake. Thus rations must be well formulated to provide maximum starch intake with sufficient effective fiber.

Forage quality for early lactation cows should be the best available. This promotes both energy intake and total feed intake. Fermentation characteristics of fermented forages can influence the incidence of ketosis. Hay crop forages ensiled at high moisture contents are prone to fermentation patterns that produce butyric acid. In addition to being unpalatable to cows, much of the butyric acid is converted to β-hydroxybutyric acid as it is absorbed through the rumen wall. This enhances the total ketone body load on the animal and increases the risk of ketosis.

The effect of dietary fat on the incidence of ketosis is unclear. Addition of fat to diets does increase their energy density. Dietary fat is absorbed in the form of chylomicrons and should not contribute substantially to blood NEFA concentrations. Fat, however, cannot contribute to glucose synthesis, so calories from fat do not directly improve glucose balance. Experts have speculated that provision of supplemental dietary fat may reduce the need for fatty acid synthesis in the mammary gland. This may indirectly improve glucose balance because glucose is an important energy source for fatty acid synthesis in the mammary gland. The effectiveness of supplemental dietary fat, either prepartum or postpartum, has generally been disappointing relative to ketosis prevention.

In 2004, monensin was approved as a feed additive for the improvement of milk production efficiency in dairy cows. Monensin may be fed at approved rates to both dry and lactating cows. In addition to improving milk production efficiency, monensin improves energy status and reduces the incidence of both clinical and subclinical ketosis, in some studies by as much as 40%.[6]

References

1. Heringstad B, Chang YM, Gianola D et al: Genetic analysis of clinical mastitis, milk fever, ketosis, and retained placenta in three lactations of Norwegian Red Cows, *J Dairy Sci* 88: 3273-3281, 2005.
2. Dohoo IR, Martin SW: Subclinical ketosis: prevalence and associations with production and disease, *Can J Comp Med* 48:1-5, 1984.
3. Cadorniga-Valino C, Grummer RR, Armentano LE et al: Effects of fatty acids and hormones on fatty acid metabolism and gluconeogenesis in bovine hepatocytes, *J Dairy Sci* 80: 646-656, 1997.

4. Murondoti A, Jorritsma R, Beynen A et al: Activities of the enzymes of hepatic gluconeogenesis in periparturient dairy cows with induced fatty liver, *J Dairy Res* 71:129-134, 2004.
5. Holtenius P, Holtenius K: New aspects of ketone-bodies in energy-metabolism of dairy-cows: a review, *J Vet Med* 43 (series A):579-587, 1996.
6. Duffield T, Bagg R, DesCoteaux L et al: Prepartum monensin for the reduction of energy associated disease in postpartum dairy cows, *J Dairy Sci* 85:397-405, 2002.
7. Herdt TH, Emery RS: Therapy of diseases of ruminant intermediary metabolism, *Vet Clin North Am Food Anim Pract* 8: 91-106, 1992.

Recommended Reading

Carrier J, Stewart S, Godden S et al: Evaluation and use of three cowside tests for detection of subclinical ketosis in early postpartum cows, *J Dairy Sci* 87:3725-3735, 2004.

CHAPTER 37

Pregnancy Toxemia in Sheep and Goats

MISTY A. EDMONDSON and DAVID G. PUGH

PATHOPHYSIOLOGY

Pregnancy toxemia (ketosis, hepatic lipidosis) is most commonly encountered in late-term gestation of sheep or goats carrying multiple fetuses, exacerbated by an inability to consume adequate energy to match metabolic demands.[1] Environmental conditions that increase energy requirements and decrease energy intake predispose to this condition. The causes of pregnancy toxemia can be divided into four broad categories: (1) primary pregnancy toxemia, (2) fat-ewe (doe) pregnancy toxemia, (3) starvation pregnancy toxemia, and (4) secondary pregnancy toxemia.[2] Primary pregnancy toxemia results from a decline in nutritional plane, such as occurs when ewes are switched from adequate to poor-quality feed or after a brief period of fasting. Fat-ewe (doe) pregnancy toxemia occurs when ewes or does are overconditioned in early gestation. These animals may suffer a decline in nutrition during late gestation, which may be partially caused by smaller rumen capacity associated with the expanding uterus and large intra-abdominal fat deposits. Starvation pregnancy toxemia occurs in extremely thin sheep and goats usually because of lack of feed following periods of drought, heavy snow, or flood. Secondary pregnancy toxemia occurs with concurrent disease such as lameness, dental problems, and parasites.[2]

In most instances, pregnancy toxemia can be prevented by balancing nutritional demands of the dam and increased requirements of the fetus during late gestation.[2] In late gestation, ewes carrying twins require 180% more energy than those carrying singletons and those carrying triplets require 240% more than ewes carrying singletons.[3] In addition, 80% of fetal growth occurs during the last 6 weeks of gestation. Some animals may not be capable of consuming enough feedstuffs to meet the demands required for late gestation. Environmental stresses or chronic illnesses that result in weight loss, depressed appetite, and a negative energy balance all lead to alterations in the insulin-glucagon ratio. Fatty acids (as nonesterified fatty acids, NEFAs) and glycerol are mobilized from body fat for use in energy production.[1] A large portion of the fatty acids are extracted by the liver and used in ketone body synthesis. If energy supply does not keep pace with demands, the liver may become overwhelmed with NEFAs, leading to the excessive release of ketone bodies and the development of the clinical signs of pregnancy toxemia.[3,4]

CLINICAL SIGNS AND DIAGNOSIS

Pregnancy toxemia most commonly occurs during the last 2 to 4 weeks of gestation. Early during the course of disease, clinical signs may often go unnoticed. Affected animals are anorexic and may lag behind and isolate themselves from the flock. As the disease progresses, neurologic signs manifest as progressive depression, tremors, "star-gazing," incoordination, circling, bruxism, and impaired vision, followed by recumbency and death. The diagnosis is confirmed by detecting an increase in urine and blood ketone concentrations. These animals are often acidotic and may be hypocalcemic and hypokalemic. Hypoglycemia may or may not be present. Azotemia may also be present because of dehydration and secondary renal disease. Blood concentrations of β-hydroxybutyric acid greater than 7 mmol/L are often observed in cases of pregnancy toxemia.[3]

TREATMENT

Treatment involves correcting energy, electrolyte, and acid-base imbalances, as well as stimulating appetite and treating dehydration. Females should be offered a palatable, energy-rich, highly digestible feed stuff. In the early stages of disease (animal still ambulatory), females may be treated with oral or intravenous glucose, balanced electrolyte solution with additional calcium (25 ml of a 23% calcium borogluconate per liter), potassium chloride (10-20 mEq/L), 5% dextrose, and sodium bicarbonate. Propylene glycol can be administered (15-30 ml every 12 hours) as a glucose precursor. Supplementation with vitamin B complex and transfaunation with rumen liquor may help stimulate appetite. In the later stages of disease, when the animal is recumbent, the prognosis is poor and treatment must be aggressive. The aforementioned treatments must be initiated immediately, and removal of the fetuses is crucial.[3] Treatment usually involves cesarean section or induction of parturition and is aimed at saving the life of the dam at the expense of the lambs or kids. Lambs or kids born more than 7 days premature seldom survive.[2]

PREVENTION

The single most important factor for preventing pregnancy toxemia is proper nutrition of the dam. Other management issues that may help prevent pregnancy toxemia include providing adequate bunk space, identifying those animals carrying twins or triplets (e.g., transabdominal ultrasonography) and feeding them accordingly, maintaining proper body condition throughout gestation, and decreasing the incidence of chronic disease.[3] Other strategies aimed at prevention include meeting energy, protein, mineral, and vitamin requirements; decreasing stress in late gestation (e.g., parasite control, predator control, hauling); dietary supplementation of niacin or ionophores, or both, to increase feed efficiency; and shearing of pregnant sheep in late gestation.[3,5] Measuring serum β-hydroxybutyric acid concentrations may serve as a useful method for monitoring the energy status. Values of 0.8 to 1.6 mmol/L are indicative of a negative energy balance. Managers should then take appropriate measures to correct the problem by feeding better-quality, highly digestible feedstuffs.[3]

References

1. National Academies of Science: Nutrient requirements of small ruminants, sheep, goats, cervids, and new world camelids, Washington, DC, 2007, National Academy Press.
2. Rook JS: Pregnancy toxemia of ewes. In Howard JL, editor: *Current veterinary therapy for food animal practice*, Philadelphia, 1993, Saunders.
3. Navarre CB, Pugh DG: Diseases of the gastrointestinal system. In Pugh DG, editor: *Sheep and goat medicine*, Philadelphia, 2002, Saunders, pp 97-99.
4. Marteniuk JV, Herdt TH: Pregnancy toxemia and ketosis of ewes and does, *Vet Clin North Am Food Anim Pract* 4:307, 1988.
5. Austin AR, Young NE: The effect of shearing pregnant ewes on lamb birth weights, *Vet Rec* 100:527, 1977.

Recommended Readings

Bauman DE, Durrie WB: Partitioning of nutrients during pregnancy and lactation: a review of mechanisms involving homeostasis and homeorrhesis, *J Dairy Sci* 63:1514-1529, 1980.
Lynch GP, Jackson C: A method for assessing the nutritional status of gestating ewes, *Can J Anim Sci* 63:603-611, 1983.
Sigurdsson H: Susceptibility to pregnancy disease in ewes and its relation to gestational diabetes, *Acta Vet Scand* 29:407-414, 1988.
Wastney ME, Arcus AC, Bickerstaffe R et al: Glucose tolerance in ewes and susceptibility to pregnancy toxemia, *Aust J Biol Sci* 35:381-392, 1982.

CHAPTER 38

Fatty Liver in Dairy Cattle

THOMAS H. HERDT and BRIAN J. GERLOFF

OCCURRENCE

Health problems in fat cows have been clinically associated with fatty infiltration of the liver and other organs. Clinical disease and subclinical effects of mild fatty liver have been described around the time of calving in all breeds of dairy cattle in all parts of the world. The clinical and subclinical problem usually occurs in obese dairy cattle within 1 to 2 weeks of calving. Clinical problems are usually apparent after calving, but they occasionally become evident before calving. The disease is unusual in primiparous cows, but it does occur. It is most common in mature, high-producing cattle. Mild cases of fatty liver are associated with reduced fertility and severe cases with increased culling, disease, and death.

ETIOLOGY AND PATHOGENESIS

The intrahepatic fat that accumulates in bovine fatty liver is primarily triglyceride. Cattle do not synthesize fatty acid precursors of triglyceride in the liver; thus fatty acids that accumulate as triglycerides in bovine fatty liver must be extrahepatic in origin. Fatty acids are stored as triglycerides in adipose tissue until mobilized. When they are mobilized in response to energy demand, adipose triglyceride is converted to nonesterified fatty acid (NEFA) and glycerol. The NEFAs are transported in the circulation bound to albumin. They can be extracted from the blood and used as an energy source by various tissues including the mammary gland, liver, spleen, and muscle. However, the liver extracts a large portion of circulating NEFA because of its high blood flow and high NEFA extraction efficiency.

In the liver, these fatty acids can undergo partial or complete oxidation or, alternatively, reesterification to triglyceride. Fatty acids esterified as triglyceride remain in the liver until they can be oxidized or secreted from the liver. Secretion of triglyceride from the liver is a process requiring repackaging of the triglyceride into serum lipoprotein particles. These particles have a core of triglyceride and an outer envelope of cholesterol, phospholipid, and specific proteins. Lipoprotein synthesis and secretion is, however, a naturally slow process in bovine liver, and it may be even further reduced in cows developing fatty liver. This means that once fatty acids are taken up by the liver and reesterified to triglyceride, their removal is a slow process.

Fatty liver development can occur rapidly. Within 48 hours, hepatic triglyceride concentrations can increase from less than 5% wet weight to more than 25%, under conditions of extreme adipose mobilization.[1] The pattern of hepatic lipid accumulation appears variable among herds. In many herds lipid accumulation begins to occur in the last 2 to 3 weeks of gestation,[2] whereas in other herds the primary accumulation occurs after calving. When measured quantitatively by chemical extraction methods, liver fat concentration has usually been expressed as a percentage of either total fat or triglyceride, both usually expressed on a wet tissue basis. The severity of liver fat accumulation has been typically classified into mild, moderate, and severe, corresponding to liver triglyceride concentrations of 1% to 5%, 5% to 10%, and greater than 10%, or liver total fat concentrations of 5% to 10%, 10% to 15%, and greater than 15%, respectively. Bovine liver normally contains approximately 5% fat of nontriglyceride origin, leading to the difference in concentrations between classifications based on triglyceride or total fat. The spectrum of liver fat concentrations seen in spontaneously occurring fatty liver in dairy cows is large, with extremely severe cases having hepatic total fat concentrations of nearly 50%. Liver total fat concentrations in most cases of clinically apparent fatty liver disease in cows are greater than 15% to 20%, although in cows with clinically apparent fatty liver disease the association between disease severity and liver fat concentration appears to be poor.

Hepatic lipid accumulation is triggered by increasing serum NEFA concentrations, which occur in association with negative energy balance. Negative energy balance occurs when feed and energy intake do not match energy demand. A reduction in feed intake (dry matter intake or DMI) occurs in almost all cows as they approach parturition, but it is exacerbated in obese cows and also under conditions of environmental and nutritional stress. In some cows this leads to negative energy balance before calving, and in nearly all cows energy is in negative balance in early lactation as the postpartum increase in DMI fails to keep pace with increased energy demands of milk production. The period of most severe negative energy balance is usually in the first 2 to 3 weeks of lactation.

Other factors may reduce the ability of some cows to adapt to negative energy balance, resulting in increasing serum NEFA concentrations and an increased propensity for fatty liver development. These include obesity, insulin resistance, and inflammation.

An important function of insulin is to suppress adipose mobilization and serum NEFA concentrations. As cows approach calving, the sensitivity of tissues to insulin is normally reduced, apparently in association with hormonal changes associated with impending parturition.

Obesity further suppresses insulin sensitivity. Thus obese cows in late gestation are particularly susceptible to high rates of adipose mobilization, and consequently to fatty liver.[3] Furthermore, low-level inflammatory stimulation may occur because of obesity directly, or in association with infectious processes. Cytokines produced in response to inflammation can further impair insulin sensitivity, increasing the risk of fatty liver.[4]

Infiltration of hepatocytes with fat appears to lead to reduced hepatic function, but there is no clear association between degree of fatty liver and the impairment of specific liver functions. Evidence indicates that gluconeogenic[5] and ureagenic capacities are reduced, although neither of these effects is firmly established. The latter may lead to reduced rates of ammonia detoxification.[6] Amino acid metabolism is also compromised, leading to changes in serum-free amino acid concentrations that, in association with reduced ammonia detoxification, may lead to hepatic encephalopathy.[7] Evidence indicates that fatty liver may lead to reduced immune function, and experts have speculated that clearance of endotoxin from the blood may be impaired because of reduced hepatic blood flow associated with fatty liver. In most cases liver excretory function does not appear to be severely compromised, as evidenced by generally mild increases in serum bilirubin or bile acid concentrations in association with fatty liver.[8]

CLINICAL SIGNS

The clinical signs most consistent with clinical fatty liver disease are depression, extreme anorexia, and ketonuria. The severity of ketonuria may only be moderate. Cows with clinical fatty liver are frequently affected by other common postpartum diseases but do not respond to the usual therapy. These conditions may include retained placenta, metritis, and mastitis. Fatty liver may also be associated with vague central nervous system signs including star-gazing, somnolence, coma, and recumbency. These more severe signs may be evidence of hepatic encephalopathy.[7] Without aggressive treatment, clinical fatty liver frequently progresses to weakness, recumbency, and death. Even if cows survive the initial disease, cows with severe fatty liver are at increased risk of culling. Affected animals are almost always initially obese (body condition score ≥4 on a scale of 1 to 5) at the outset of the dry period. However, weight loss leading to fatty liver is rapid, and at the time of clinical observation and treatment, the cow's body condition may be normal or thin. As clinical fatty liver is frequently a herd-based problem, observation of obese dry cows and thin early-lactation cows is frequently a good clue that there may be some problems with fatty liver in the herd.

In addition to severe clinical fatty liver, subclinical fatty liver in the first 3 to 5 weeks postpartum is a problem in many herds and is associated with economic losses such as delayed postpartum return to estrus and reduced fertility.[9]

Many herd operators can manage even obese cows through the peripartum period reasonably well, until an additional environmental stressor is added. For example, obese cows in a herd may calve and start their lactation in reasonably good health until the weather becomes hot and humid. The addition of heat stress may lead to severe clinical problems with fatty liver and increased rates of concurrent disease and death.

CLINICAL PATHOLOGY

Commonly used tests of hepatic function or integrity are of marginal usefulness in the diagnosis of bovine fatty liver. These include serum activities of hepatic enzymes and serum concentrations of bilirubin and bile acids. The activities of aspartate amino transferase (AST) and ornithine carbamoyl transferase (OCT) are probably the most sensitive predictors of bovine fatty liver,[10] and even in the case of these enzymes the increases in activities are not nearly as marked as in other types of liver disease. Serum AST activity greater than 100 IU/L is consistent with fatty liver, although not specifically diagnostic. It must be considered that serum AST activity is not a specific indicator of fatty liver, and other common conditions such as muscle damage may lead to elevated serum AST activity.

Liver biopsy is currently the most practical means of fatty liver diagnosis. Transthoracic needle biopsies can be taken easily and safely through the tenth intercostal space at the level of the greater trochanter. Biopsy samples so taken should be evaluated quantitatively, either by biochemical or histological means, although biochemical means are most consistent with the most commonly used grading system. Cow-side tests for the estimation of fat concentration in hepatic biopsy samples are available.[11] One drawback in the use of biopsy samples is lack of clear documentation that liver fat is distributed homogeneously. The use of ultrasonography for the diagnosis of bovine fatty liver offers a promising potential for fatty liver diagnosis, but means of estimating fat concentrations from ultrasound images are still under development.[12]

Serum NEFA concentrations are generally elevated in cows with fatty liver, but their measurement is not a specific diagnostic tool in cows with clinical illness because any condition resulting in anorexia can be expected to result in increases in serum NEFA concentrations. Serum NEFA concentrations are best used as a herd screening tool to predict the risk of fatty liver. In cows that develop fatty liver, serum NEFA concentrations are usually elevated several days before calving and spike to high concentrations after calving. Measuring serum NEFA concentrations in groups of cows between 3 weeks prepartum to 3 weeks postpartum is useful in predicting fatty liver risk, and determining the time frame relative to calving at which fatty liver infiltration is beginning. Serum NEFA concentrations greater than 1000 µEq/L in lactating cows and greater than 325 to 400 µEq/L in prepartum cows should be considered evidence of excessive adipose mobilization and fatty liver risk.

Acute phase reactant proteins, particularly haptoglobin, have been used as predictors of fatty liver in cows. The relationship of haptoglobin to fatty liver may result from the association between obesity and chronic inflammation, particularly through the influence of tumor-necrosis factor alpha (TNF-α), the expression of which is elevated in obesity. Increases in TNFa and other cytokines associated with obesity may modulate increased serum concentrations of haptoglobin[4] in cows with fatty liver. Serum haptoglobin concentrations are not specific indicators of fatty liver because they can be affected by any inflammatory process. Their diagnostic use, like that of NEFA, is probably best applied to herd-level assessment of fatty liver risk.

DIAGNOSIS

Clinical ketonuria within 1 week of calving accompanied by depression or other peripartum diseases with death loss, or both, should be considered presumptive evidence of fatty liver. For a definitive diagnosis, analysis of liver tissue for triglyceride or total fat concentration is the most reliable method. A classification of severe fatty liver (>10% triglyceride or > 15% total fat) is necessary to substantiate a diagnosis of the clinical syndrome because subclinical fatty liver, with lesser liver triglyceride or total fat concentrations, is common in cows in early lactation. Moderate fatty liver associated with high production and subsequent poor reproduction may be of importance within a herd, but it should not be viewed as a significant clinical health problem.

Excessive fat mobilization and weight loss is necessary to produce the high serum NEFA concentrations and rapid hepatic triglyceride buildup associated with fatty liver. This usually involves obese cows. However, if weight loss has been rapid, a cow that is no longer obese may be clinically affected with fatty liver. Evidence of obese dry cows and thin early-lactation cows accompanied by high rates of early lactation metabolic disease such as ketosis, retained placenta, and elevated cull rates are strong indications of a herd fatty liver problem. Rate of weight loss is a more important component of the disease syndrome than is weight per se. Liver biopsies or postmortem findings, or both, should be used to verify a presumptive diagnosis. The use of ultrasound measurements of change in subcutaneous fat thickness to assess rates of adipose mobilization is discussed in Chapter 39.

TREATMENT

Treatment of severe cases of fatty liver in cows is often unsuccessful, and the prognosis should be discussed with the owner before initiating treatment. Therapy is focused on reducing further NEFA mobilization and providing a source of glucose and energy until liver function can improve. Treatments discussed in Chapter 36 for ketosis therapy, particularly for peripartum or type II ketosis, are generally the same as those used for fatty liver therapy. Daily administration of 500 mL of a 50% dextrose solution intravenously accompanied by 200 units of long-acting insulin, given once or twice 48 hours apart, can be a practical and effective treatment in mild cases. The inclusion of glucocorticoids such as dexamethasone has been somewhat controversial because of concerns of corticoid-induced increases in lipolysis. Recent evidence indicates that short-term treatment with dexamethasone is not lipolytic in cattle

and probably should be added to the fatty liver treatment regimen.[13] Continuous intravenous infusions of glucose are more effective than bolus injections. Infusion rates of up to 40 g/hr are recommended.[7] The use of orally administered glucogenic agents such as propylene glycol and sodium propionate may be effective and more practical than intravenous glucose therapy, but care should taken not to suppress appetite.

Evidence indicates that oxidative stress and lipoperoxide formation may play a role in the pathogenesis of fatty liver disease, suggesting that antioxidants such as vitamin E and selenium may be useful in therapy.[14]

Promising evidence suggests that administration of glucagon may be effective as fatty liver treatment, but this is still experimental.[12]

Force-feeding the anorexic, depressed cow with clinical fatty liver is an important and useful adjunct treatment. A slurry of a complete feed administered with a large-bore stomach tube has been a useful treatment in extreme cases. Enteral supplements should have high concentrations of rumen available carbohydrates relative to rumen available protein so as not to increase the load of endogenous ammonia. Some clinicians have suggested creating a rumen fistula to permit enteral feeding of cows with fatty liver. All of these treatments are designed to provide energy and glucose to produce an endogenous or exogenous insulin surge and to reduce NEFA mobilization. We have been successful at saving many high-risk cows with these approaches, but many times the productive outcome has been disappointing. Prevention is a much better economic approach.

In herds experiencing a clinical problem with fatty liver, it is important that treatment be initiated early, before hepatic triglyceride accumulation becomes extreme and liver function is irreversibly compromised. Remember that hepatic triglyceride accumulation can occur quickly. In herds with obese dry cows, urine should be monitored for ketone bodies beginning 1 week before calving. If ketonuria occurs, glucose therapy should be initiated. Glucose treatment may be required for 7 to 10 days. Our experience suggests that this aggressive treatment is frequently life-saving, although return to high performance does not often occur. Propylene glycol given orally as a glucose precursor is probably not as effective as parenteral glucose.

PREVENTION

Obesity in dry cows should be avoided. Most obese dry cows do not become obese during the dry period but rather during late lactation. This is particularly true for cows with extended lactation periods such as those in which establishment of pregnancy is delayed. In herds with breeding problems, particular attention needs to be paid to the body condition of late-lactation cows. Dry cows should be fed a diet to maintain weight, not lose weight. A weight-reduction program in late gestation can trigger excessive NEFA mobilization and fatty liver during the dry period.

Herd body condition scoring can be a useful tool to avoid problems with fatty liver. Dry cows and cows 3 to 4 weeks' postpartum can be scored according to body condition. If the difference between condition scores of these two groups is 1 or greater, then excessive fat mobilization is occurring. As discussed in Chapter 39, ultrasound measurement of subcutaneous fat thickness can also be a useful tool with which to monitor rate of adipose mobilization.

Because NEFA mobilization and hepatic triglyceride accumulation are so closely tied to DMI, improving DMI the last 2 to 3 weeks before and the first 2 to 3 weeks after calving should be the top priority. Considerable controversy exists as to what types of diets can best induce maximum DMI. We feel that diets well balanced for fiber and nonfiber carbohydrate and those meeting projected nutrient requirements across the dry period are best suited to maximize feed intake throughout late gestation and early lactation. This strategy usually results in relatively low-energy density diets in the early dry period and a moderate energy density in the last 3 weeks before calving.

Specific feed additives that might be of benefit in prevention of fatty liver include monensin and rumen-protected choline. Monensin increases rumen propionate production relative to acetate and butyrate. Propionate is glucogenic, and monensin feeding generally results in better glucose status and lower serum NEFA and ketone body concentrations when fed to either dry or lactating cows.[15] Previous attempts to use lipotropic agents such as inositol or choline have not proven beneficial in protecting cows from fatty liver. A new rumen-protected form of choline appears to have promise in the management of fatty liver when fed to cows in late gestation and early lactation.[16]

Care to provide the peripartum cow with as stressless an environment as possible is also important. Stress hormones significantly increase NEFA mobilization and have been suggested as a contributing cause in fatty liver. A quiet, clean place for calving is helpful. Providing comfortable, well-designed, well-ventilated stalls is particularly important. Attempts to improve the environment for the cow during the transition period should be helpful in controlling fatty liver.

Fatty liver, both clinical and subclinical, is a disease of excessive NEFA mobilization from adipose tissue. Prevention and treatment efforts must focus on minimizing the adipose mobilization that normally occurs during the periparturient period. The objective is to prevent the downward spiral of declining DMI and increasing NEFA mobilization and hepatic triglyceride accumulation.

References

1. Herdt TH, Wensing T, Haagsman HP et al: Hepatic triacylglycerol synthesis during a period of fatty liver development in sheep, *J Anim Sci* 66:1997-2013, 1988.
2. Gerloff BJ, Herdt TH, Emery RS: Relationship of hepatic lipidosis to health and performance in dairy cattle, *J Am Vet Med Assoc* 188:845-850, 1986.
3. Hayirli A: The role of exogenous insulin in the complex of hepatic lipidosis and ketosis associated with insulin resistance phenomenon in postpartum dairy cattle, *Vet Res Commun* 30:749-774, 2006.
4. Ametaj BN, Bradford BJ, Bobe G et al: Strong relationships between mediators of the acute phase response and fatty liver in dairy cows, *Canad J Anim Sci* 85:165-175, 2005.
5. Murondoti A, Jorritsma R, Beynen AC et al: Activities of the enzymes of hepatic gluconeogenesis in periparturient dairy cows with induced fatty liver, *J Dairy Res* 71:129-134, 2004.
6. Mudron P, Rehage J, Holtershinken M et al: Venous and arterial ammonia in dairy cows with fatty liver and hepatic failure, *Vet Med* 49:187-190, 2004.
7. Rehage J, Starke A, Holtershinken M et al: *Hepatic lipidosis: diagnostic tools and individual and herd risk factors*, Nice, France, 2006, 24th World Buiatrics Congress, pp 69-74.
8. Rehage J, Qualmann K, Meier C et al: Total serum bile acid concentrations in dairy cows with fatty liver and liver failure, *Deutsche Tierarztliche Wochenschrift* 106:26-29, 1999.
9. Jorritsma R, Jorritsma H, Schukken YH et al: Relationships between fatty liver and fertility and some periparturient diseases in commercial Dutch dairy herds, *Theriogenology* 54:1065-1074, 2000.
10. Kalaitzakis E, Roubies N, Panousis N et al: Evaluation of ornithine carbamoyl transferase and other serum and liver-derived analytes in diagnosis of fatty liver and postsurgical outcome of left-displaced abomasum in dairy cows, *J Am Vet Med Assoc* 21:1463-1471, 2006.
11. Herdt TH, Goeders L, Liesman JS et al: Test for estimation of bovine hepatic lipid content, *J Am Vet Med Assoc* 182:953-955, 1983.
12. Bobe G, Young JW, Beitz DC: Invited review: pathology, etiology, prevention, and treatment of fatty liver in dairy cows, *J Dairy Sci* 87:3105-3124, 2007.
13. Jorritsma R, Thanasak J, Houweling M et al: Effects of a single dose of dexamethasone-21-isonicotinate on the metabolism of heifers in early lactation, *Vet Rec* 155:521-523, 2004.
14. Mudron P, Rehage J, Qualmann K et al: A study of lipid peroxidation and vitamin E in dairy cows with hepatic insufficiency, *J Vet Med Series A* 46:219-224, 1999.
15. Petersson-Wolfe CS, Leslie KE, Osborne T et al: Effect of monensin delivery method on dry matter intake, body condition score, and metabolic parameters in transition dairy cows, *J Dairy Sci* 90:1870-1879, 2007.
16. Cooke RF, Rio N-Sd, Caraviello DZ et al: Supplemental choline for prevention and alleviation of fatty liver in dairy cattle, *J Dairy Sci* 90:2413-2418, 2007.

CHAPTER 39

Clinical Use of Ultrasound for Subcutaneous Fat Thickness Measurements in Dairy Cattle

NANDA P. JOSHI and THOMAS H. HERDT

Excessive adipose mass or a high rate of adipose mobilization, or both, have been associated positively with peripartum disease risk in dairy cows. Adipose mass may be estimated by subcutaneous fat thickness. Schröder and Staufenbiel[1] reported the strong relationship between backfat thickness (BFT) and total body fat. High prepartum subcutaneous fat thickness, as estimated by subjective body condition scoring (BCS), has been found to be associated with increased risk of subclinical ketosis,[2] clinical ketosis,[3] and displaced abomasum.[4] Generally, fatter cows are more prone to ketosis and fatty liver. BCS is a subjective estimate of adipose mass. Broring et al.[5] recommended the use of ultrasound measurements of subcutaneous fat in lieu of subjective BCS, especially when comparing cattle across various physiologic states and genotypic body types.

Most evidence suggests that the association between body fat content and disease is related to fat mobilization associated with negative energy balance, rather than the absolute size of the adipose mass. Estimation of fat mobilization by BCS changes may, in the short term, not accurately estimate fat mobilization. Rate of fat mobilization can be accurately estimated by changes in subcutaneous fat thickness in dairy cows using real-time ultrasound. The ultrasound images of subcutaneous fat over the rump are highly repeatable, and the site is easy to access in typical commercial dairy management situations, making the measurements relatively easy to collect and interpret.[6,7] Literature that examines the direct relationship between backfat measurement and disease risk is lacking. One study in Holstein dairy cows demonstrated that larger prepartum BFT (>12 mm) was associated with increased risk of postpartum subclinical ketosis risk.[8]

BACKFAT MEASUREMENT

BCS is a subjective estimate of fat reserve in terms of adipose tissue. It is an evaluation of the appearance of the cow that changes with the changes in energy reserve. In dairy cows, several scoring scales (1-5, 1-8, or 1-10) are being used. However, a BCS scale of 1 to 5 is commonly used in the United States. The correlation between BCS and measured BFT is only moderately strong, ranging from r=0.35 to r=0.86.[9] Moreover, changes of 0.25 BCS units from two consecutive observations could not be

uniformly discerned, even by trained scorers.[1] Therefore there is a need for an objective estimation of adipose mass and mobilization with which to monitor condition and condition changes throughout lactation. Real-time ultrasound measurement of BFT offers this option.

Backfat in the rump or thurl area is measured as the thickness of the layer of subcutaneous fat between the skin and the fascia trunci profunda, located above the gluteus medius muscle. Ultrasound equipment transfers electric pulses into high-frequency sound waves by piezoelectric crystals. The image is generated by the sound waves being reflected from boundaries between adipose, fascia, and muscle. To measure fat thickness at this site, the transducer should be placed vertically to an imaginary line between the pins (tuber ischia) and hooks (tuber coaxe) at the sacral examination site (≈9-11 cm cranial to the pins). The rump region (Fig. 39-1) has the largest amount of subcutaneous adipose tissue of any area along the back of the animal, and the fat thickness there is highly correlated (r=0.90) with body fat content.[1] The site is easy to locate. Domecq and colleagues[9] evaluated the correlation between body fat content in dairy cows and the thickness of adipose tissue at various sites (lumbar, thurl, and tail heads). The highest correlation (r=0.86) was found in the rump or thurl area. To measure subcutaneous fat thickness in this area, the transducer should be held lightly to avoid compression of the fat and orthogonal to the interface of fat and muscle.

Ultrasound images of BFT in a fat cow (Fig. 39-2) and a thin cow (Fig. 39-3) are illustrated. These images were taken using an EasiScan portable ultrasound with a linear transducer with frequency between 5 and 7.5 MHz.

Ultrasound evaluation of backfat is quick, noninvasive, and easy to learn. Numerous portable ultrasound devices are on the market (e.g., SonoSite 180PLUS: *http://www.sonosite.com/home.html*; Tringa linear: *http://www.vetsales.net/*; and Easi-Scan: *http://www.steuartlabs.com/easi_scan.htm*). A linear transducer with a frequency range of 5 to 7.5 MHz is required. To establish good contact with the skin clipping, the use of stand-off pads have been recommended. However, in practice, we do not find these necessary. Vegetable oil works well as a coupling agent to make good contact between the transducer and skin.

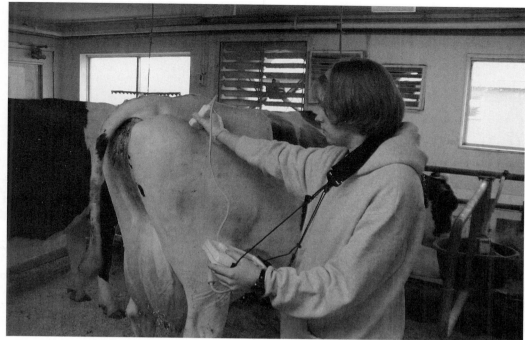

Fig 39-1 Site of backfat measurement.

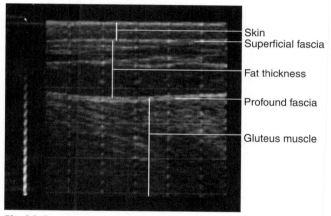

Fig 39-2 Ultrasound image of backfat thickness of a fat cow (18.4 mm).

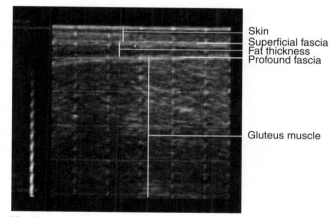

Fig 39-3 Ultrasound image of backfat thickness of a thin cow (4.5 mm).

PORTABLE ULTRASOUND DEVICES

We have used portable ultrasound equipment including the Easi-Scan (Fig. 39-4), Tringa (Fig. 39-5), and SonoSite 180PLUS (Fig. 39-6). These compact units can be easily used in the field. We used transducers with frequencies between 5 and 7.5 MHz. Linear transducers with multifrequency may be used for BFT measurement, as well as for bovine pregnancy determination.

The price of portable ultrasound equipment has reduced considerably since the initial availability of the instruments. Furthermore, many companies sell refurbished portable ultrasound equipment (previously used for human ultrasonography) for veterinary uses. Leasing of ultrasound may be an option for some practitioners.

IMAGE MEASUREMENT AND INTERPRETATIONS

Captured backfat images can be measured for BFT after freezing images using built-in measurement protocols in the instruments. Alternatively, images may be saved in a laptop or desktop PC to be measured using freely available image software like *ImageJ 1.36b (http://rsb.info.nih. gov/ij/)* or *DicomWorks (http://dicom.online.fr/)*. We have found both to be user friendly.

In a large Holstein herd from which we collected backfat data, we found an increased risk of subclinical ketosis (odds ratio: 1.54, $P<0.01$) when BFT was greater than 12 mm. For practical purposes, if the average BFT in a herd is 12 to 14 mm 2 to 3 weeks before calving, cows

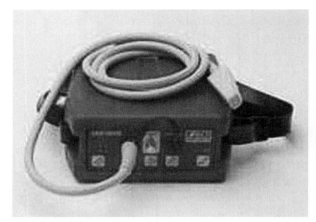

Fig 39-4 Easi-Scan.

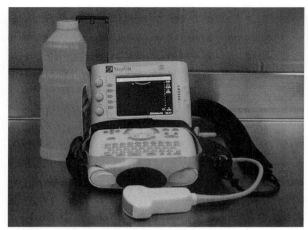

Fig 39-6 SonoSite 180PLUS.

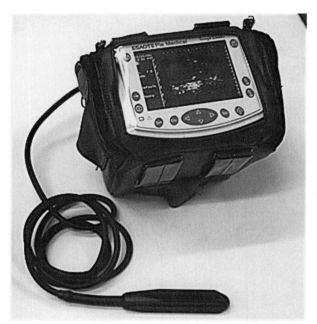

Fig 39-5 Tringa Linear.

should be evaluated for feed intake and diets should be evaluated for energy density.

Schröder and Staufenbiel[10] developed a reference curve for crossbred German Black Pied X Holstein cows using data from 46,000 cows representing 75 farms. It may be used as a reference guide for BFT target until we have a more uniform reference curve for Holstein dairy cows in the United States.

MULTIFUNCTIONAL TRANSDUCERS

The right choice of ultrasound and transducers for veterinary practitioners depends on the type of field practices. Linear, multifrequency transducers (5-7.5 MHz) may work well if backfat and reproductive evaluation are to be

carried out. Effort is under way in the use of ultrasound images for the diagnosis of fatty liver in dairy cows.[11] This potentially could be added benefit for practitioners.

References

1. Schröder UJ, Staufenbiel R: Invited review: methods to determine body fat reserves in the dairy cow with special regard to ultrasonographic measurement of backfat thickness, *J Dairy Sci* 89:1-14, 2006.
2. Duffield T: Subclinical ketosis in lactating dairy cattle, *Vet Clin North Am Food Anim Pract* 16(2):231-253, 2000.
3. Gillund PO, Reksen Y, Grohn T et al: Body condition related to ketosis and reproductive performance in Norwegian dairy cows, *J Dairy Sci* 84:1390-1396, 2001.
4. Cameron RE, Dyke PB, Herdt TH et al: Dry cow diet, management, and energy balance as risk factors for displaced abomasum in high producing dairy herds, *J Dairy Sci* 81:132-139, 1998.
5. Broring NJ, Wilton W, Colucci PE: Body condition score and its relationship to ultrasound backfat measurements in beef cows, *Can J Anim Sci* 83:593-596, 2002.
6. Realini CE, Williams RE, Pringle TD et al: Gluteus medius and rump fat depths as additional live animal ultrasound measurements for predicting retail product and trimable fat in beef carcasses, *J Anim Sci* 79:1378-1385, 2001.
7. Greiner SP, Rouse GH, Wilson DE et al: Prediction of retail product weight and percentage using ultrasound and carcass measurements in beef cattle, *J Anim Sci* 81:1736-1742, 2003.
8. Joshi NP, Herdt THH, Neuder L: *Association of prepartum rump fat thickness and non-esterified fatty acids with subclinical ketosis in Holstein dairy cows,* Proceedings of the 13th International Conference on Production Diseases of Farm Animals, Leipzig, Germany, 2007.
9. Domecq JJ, Skidmore AL, Lloyd JW et al: Validation of body condition scores with ultrasound measurements of subcutaneous fat of dairy cows, *J Dairy Sci* 78:2308-2313, 1995.
10. Schröder UJ, Staufenbiel R: Relationships between backfat thickness, milk yield and fertility traits with resulting standard curves and their application in dairy herd management, *Acta Vet Scand* 44(Suppl 1):P21, 2003.
11. Ametaj BN: A new understanding of the causes of fatty liver in dairy cows, *Adv Dairy Tech* 17:97-112, 2005.

CHAPTER 40

Metabolic Profiling

ROBERT J. VAN SAUN

A "metabolic profile" is defined as a series of specific analytic tests run in combination and used as a herd-based, rather than individual-based, diagnostic aid.[1] Use of a metabolic profile is the result of technologic improvements in analytic instrumentation, which can complete multiple analyses in a short time period. The Compton Metabolic Profile (CMP), first introduced in the early 1970s, has traditionally been used in this approach.[2,3] The original intent of the CMP was to monitor metabolic health of the herd, help diagnose metabolic problems and production diseases, and identify metabolically superior cows. Interpretation issues and a lack of specificity in differentiating normal from problem herds coupled with high inherent costs with little diagnostic returns has limited the application of the CMP test, especially within the United States. Research since the time of CMP development has clarified many metabolic issues of the transition cow and its relationship to periparturient disease.[4-6] In concert with this improved understanding of integrated transition metabolism there has been improvement in technical methods to assess metabolic status. Additionally, the shift to increasing herd size and recognition of significant health, production, and economic consequences of periparturient disease has led to renewed interest in a revised metabolic profile application in monitoring transition cow health and disease risk.[7,8]

INDICATIONS

Blood tests from individual animals are routinely used to diagnose disease problems in dairy cattle. Veterinarians, producers, and nutrition consultants alike seem interested in extracting pertinent information relative to herd nutrition and health status from blood testing. Relationships between nutritional status, metabolic state of the animal, and blood analyte (i.e., collective term for various nutrient and metabolic parameters measured) concentrations have been well documented in experimental research under controlled conditions. Properly applied metabolic profile testing, as defined by appropriate animal selection and sample collection, can potentially provide direct confirmatory evaluation of metabolic health and disease risk or evaluate nutritive status on a herd basis.

Assess nutritional status of feeding group or herd.
Ration evaluation is the cornerstone of herd nutritional assessment, but it can be fraught with uncertainty and difficulty in obtaining a true measure of dry matter or nutrient intake. Metabolic profiling, using specific parameters known to be responsive to dietary intake, can be used to complement dietary evaluation of current feeding program adequacy or a response to a feeding program change.

Identify disease conditions early. Metabolic profiling using defined analytes (β-hydroxybutyrate [BHB], calcium [Ca], magnesium [Mg], rumen pH) can be used to assess prevalence of various subclinical metabolic diseases (ketosis, hypocalcemia, hypomagnesemia, subacute ruminal acidosis [SARA], respectively) in the absence of obvious clinical disease problems.

Identify potential risk for disease problems. Specific blood analytes that are either high or low relative to defined reference or cut point values before calving or immediately postpartum can predict potential for increased risk of experiencing specific or collective periparturient disease events.

Survey for potential causes of disease problems. Broad-based metabolic profiling can be used as a screening tool to direct the focus of a herd investigation. Profile results need to be interpreted relative to diet-specific problems, as well as management and other factors that may secondarily alter animal response to diet.

Recognizing that many factors confound direct interpretation of blood analyte concentrations relative to nutritional status, metabolic profile testing should not be a stand-alone diagnostic test. Metabolic profiles should be part of an integrated complement of diagnostic tools used in evaluating herd nutritional problems.[7,9,10] One should include the following issues in any nutritional diagnostic investigation:

- ***Records analysis.*** Provides historical and current perspectives on the herd relative to animal inventories, clinical disease prevalence, production, milk composition, and dry matter intake.
- ***Animal evaluation.*** Assess general appearance and attitude of the animals, as well as specific indicators (i.e., cud chewing activity, body condition scoring, manure characteristics, and lameness scoring).
- ***Facilities evaluation.*** Assess ventilation adequacy; cow comfort (overcrowding, stall usage); stall design (size and bedding type); feed bunk design (space per animal, surface, width); and water resources (sources, number, availability, and quality).
- ***Feeding management.*** Determine method of feeding (total mixed ration [TMR], conventional feeding, parlor grain); number of feedings and push-ups; timing of feed delivery; and feed availability in bunk over 24 hours. Evaluate feed storage, handling, and preparation procedures.

- *Dietary evaluation.* Evaluate the "four diets" on the farm, namely the formulated diet, mixed and delivered diet, consumed diet, and digested/absorbed diet. Metabolic profiling may be useful in evaluating the latter.

APPLICATION

Although similar samples and analytic methods are used in assessing disease diagnosis or metabolic profiling, the approaches to sample collection and results interpretation are different.[7,11] With disease diagnosis, one selects a small population of representative clinically affected animals for blood analyses. Results are compared with laboratory reference ranges for interpretation. Reference ranges for a given analyte are 95% confidence intervals determined from a population of healthy animals. Disease conditions often induce dramatic changes in analyte variability, much greater than inherent variability because of biologic randomness and other factors.[12,13] Disease diagnosis is based on a recognized pattern to changes in one or more blood analytes. In contrast for metabolic profiling, one collects a greater number of samples from clinically "normal" individuals. A greater number of samples are required to highlight analyte differences caused by the environment, namely nutrition because its contribution to analyte variation is of a smaller magnitude compared with biologic randomness. As a consequence, metabolic profiling should not be a "random" selection process; rather, samples need to be appropriately selected to minimize variation resultant from controllable factors.

Analyte Variation Considerations

Both controllable and uncontrollable factors can introduce variability into blood analyte concentrations and reduce ability to interpret differences relative to nutritional status. Random biologic variation and genetic variation are inherent sources of variation among individual animals and account for the largest source of analyte concentration variability.[12] More controllable, nonnutritional sources of variation are attributed to physiologic state and, more precisely, time relative to calving. Stage of lactation, which reflects level of milk production, also influences analyte variability.[3,14] Many key blood analytes show dynamic changes in concentration, reflective of changing homeorhetic metabolic regulation, around the time of calving and through early lactation until homeostasis can become reequilibrated. This is a critical source of variation but can be managed through appropriate characterization of animal groups to be selected for sampling. Age also influences blood parameters, though the most significant differences seem to be between first pregnancy or lactation and comparative older animals.

Season has been suggested to induce variation in blood analyte concentration.[3,14] However, a more important variation contributor is prandial change throughout a 24-hour period. Blood analyte concentrations significantly altered following feed consumption include nonesterified fatty acids (NEFAs), urea nitrogen (UN), glucose, and BHB. Glucose, BHB, and UN will increase over time, reaching a maximum value between 3 and 5 hours following a primary meal. In contrast, NEFA concentration will decrease following a primary meal. These prandial changes are somewhat tempered over a 24-hour period when a TMR feeding system is used compared with conventional meal feeding programs.[15]

Subclinical disease or any process that activates inflammatory cytokines will initiate a physiologic response that alters a number of blood parameters.[13,16] In this interleukin-1 (IL-1)–mediated response, acute phase proteins (haptoglobin, ceruloplasmin, and others) will be released from the liver while other analyte (albumin, cholesterol, iron, and zinc) concentrations will be reduced independent of nutritive status. With the increased concentration of ceruloplasmin, serum copper concentrations will increase. Cortisol-mediated stress responses can also influence blood analyte concentrations. Animals in negative energy balance will show increased NEFA concentrations when experiencing a stressful event. Similar acute phase protein responses may also be observed in animals exposed to stressful conditions.

Other sources on controllable variation result from sample collection, handling, and analytic methods. Given the effects of time relative to calving and stage of lactation on blood analyte concentrations, any errors in sample labeling in which an inappropriate sample is included within a group will confound interpretation of results. Sample mishandling to the point that hemolysis occurs will alter blood analyte concentrations.[17,18] Specific analytes increase or decrease with hemolysis, though the true effect may be somewhat technique or laboratory dependent.[17,18] Prolonged contact between clot and serum will also induce alterations in blood analyte concentrations, especially glucose (lower). Analytic laboratories can provide detailed information on sample handling artifacts. Analytic techniques can also introduce variation artifacts. Many blood analytes can be determined by more than one method, and results may not be exactly the same. Quality control practices employed by the laboratory can influence consistency in analyte test results. As with forage testing, one should identify a laboratory familiar with metabolic profiling procedures and continue to use the same laboratory for all metabolic profile testing.

Successful outcome to metabolic profile testing can only be realized through strict adherence of practices to reduce these described sources of variation in analyte concentrations to highlight potential nutritional or metabolic differences that might be related to a given herd situation. This is best achieved through careful sample population selection and meticulous sample collection and handling procedures.

Sampling Strategies

For the original CMP test 7 to 10 blood samples were randomly collected from three predefined groups of dairy animals: dry, peak lactation, and midlactation cows.[3] With the random selection process, selected dry cows could have been at any point relative to expected calving. At the time, all dry cows were considered metabolically similar, contrary to current knowledge. Peak and midlactation cows were specifically chosen because they were considered "homeostatically stable" compared with recently fresh cows. However, within the current framework of understanding the relationships between periparturient disease and metabolic status, cows currently experiencing perturbed homeostasis should be selected for analysis. The selected populations of cows preferred for the CMP test may have limited the diagnostic sensitivity of the testing procedure.

Approaches to herd metabolic profiling have evolved since the time of the CMP test, and methods used in sample collection and interpretation will vary by the metabolic profiling procedure used.

Define the Problem to Be Addressed

Metabolic profiling should not be a completely random sample collection process. One should have a plan in mind in approaching a problem. A given herd situation can be assessed by asking a specific question. Are the heifers experiencing subclinical ketosis? Why are mature cows experiencing more retained placenta? Why is the herd experiencing more periparturient disease? One should consider pertinent comparisons of interest relative to the defined problem and identify which cow populations are of concern to be sampled.

Once the herd problem has been defined, a grouping strategy for sample collection can be constructed (Table 40-1). In addressing transition cow problems, blood analyte concentrations from cows just before and immediately following calving are the most diagnostic.[8,12,19] As a result of tremendous individual variation, cows should not be sampled within 3 days before or following calving. Others suggest that samples immediately prepartum and postpartum be avoided, citing large analyte variability, and recommend sampling fresh cows at 25 to 80 days in milk.[9] Although blood analyte concentrations from far-off dry cows (>30 days before calving) are not predictive for postpartum disease risk, results can be used as a reference point for comparison with other groups, or values may be diagnostic within themselves for some disease entity. The group or groups of cows selected for analysis will depend on the problem definition and desired sampling approach.

Cows to be selected within the defined groups for a metabolic profile should be free of obvious clinical disease. By selecting cows defined as "clinically normal," outlier analyte concentrations associated with disease are removed, thus better highlighting potential differences resulting from nutritional or subclinical disease problems. One may elect to sample cows affected with specific diseases for comparison with cows of similar days in milk that are not affected. Differences in blood analyte concentrations between clinically affected and unaffected cows may provide some direction as to underlying problems associated with disease pathogenesis.

Define the Testing Procedure Approach

Metabolic profiling uses the same clinical chemistry tests performed in disease diagnosis. However, testing methods are herd based for metabolic profiling rather than individual based for disease diagnosis. Herd-based testing can be categorized into two approaches: targeted diagnostics and screening tool.

The screening tool approach is consistent with traditional metabolic profiling methods in which multiple analytes are determined within a selected group or groups of cows. Determination of multiple analytes is predicated on the concept that periparturient metabolic disease is a result of the cow's inability to maintain coordinated interrelationships among lipid, glucose, and amino acid metabolism. A screening tool approach to metabolic profiling can be used as a broad-based diagnostic evaluation of herd nutritive status, an assessment of disease risk factors, or an indicator of potential factors responsible for disease conditions. Limitations to the screening tool approach are high testing costs and potential interpretation issues. A pooled-sample process has been advocated to address cost concerns and maintain a wide analyte array in assessing herd nutritional or disease risk status.[11,20-22] Predictive disease risk relationships have been well established with specific analytes, though multiple analyte indices or analyte combinations may provide a better indication of metabolic stability or instability.[23] Unfortunately, few data are available to provide sound reference values for interpretation.

The targeted diagnostic approach uses well-defined diagnostic analytes to determine herd risk for specific "gateway" periparturient diseases. Elevated prepartum

---

Table **40-1**

Suggested Grouping Strategies for Collecting Blood Samples in Completing Metabolic Profile Testing Using Individual or Pooled Samples

Physiologic Groups	Time Relative to Calving	Parity	Disease Status
Far-off dry	>10 days following dry-off and >30 before expected calving	Within any group keep heifers and 2+ lactation animals separate—pool as separate parity groups within physiologic groups	Unknown
Close-up dry	Between 3 and 30 days before calving (7-21 days preferred)		Unknown
Fresh	3-30 days in milk (7-21 days preferred)		Group cows with and without disease within lactational groups—keep days in milk similar within and between groups
Lactation groups	Define as needed based on disease conditions, production level, or other problem		

NEFA concentration and postpartum BHB concentration are recognized risk factors for ketosis and left displaced abomasum.[8,19,24-27] Low blood calcium concentration immediately postcalving is a risk indicator for subclinical hypocalcemia.[8] Blood UN is a potential indicator for assessing herd protein status. In this approach, specific analyte concentration is determined and compared with specific threshold criteria. The percent of individuals above (NEFA and BHB) or below (calcium) is used to interpret herd disease risk. UN values are interpreted as a mean value for the individuals within a defined group. Individual testing, lower testing costs, and ease of interpretation are strengths of this approach. A limitation of this approach is the scope of analytes determined.

Which approach to be used in evaluating a herd will depend on the problem to be addressed, herd size, and cost limitations. Smaller dairy herds (<120 cows) will not have a large enough population of animals to be sampled within defined physiologic groups for the screening tool approach compared with large herds. With limited animal numbers, individual testing and collecting samples over time are possible approaches. Costs are the single most limiting factor to metabolic profiling. Multiple analyte testing services range in cost from $17 to $50 per sample depending on the number of blood analytes measured and laboratory pricing structure. This makes individual testing in multiple groups nearly cost prohibitive, thus the rationale for pooled samples. Using the single analyte approach, the cost may range from $3 to $10 per sample depending on specific analyte of interest and laboratory pricing structure.

Determine Sampling Process and Number
Few would argue the strength of individual analysis in metabolic profile analysis. Indeed, the gold standard for analytic analysis would be to measure a large percent of the population of interest as individuals. Decisions made in grouping and approach strategies will define the suggested number of individuals within a group to be sampled.

Individual sampling. Statistical modeling suggests that at least 8 individuals from a population are representative (mean analysis), though 12 or 13 samples are best for threshold analysis using the targeted diagnostic approach.[3,8,27] Though statistics may show a minimum number of samples needed to represent a population, the best way to truly characterize a population is to obtain more samples. The goal in metabolic profile testing is to appropriately balance quality of information derived from the testing process with analytic costs.

Pooled sampling. In the original protocol for the CMP, mean analyte values within physiologic groupings were used for interpretation. These mean values were arithmetically determined from individual samples. Use of individual sampling resulted in the high associated costs of this procedure. In place of individual analysis, can pooled samples be used to reduce the cost and provide some valid method of herd assessment? In a number of preliminary studies using individual samples, pooled samples from these individuals were found to accurately represent arithmetic means from pool sizes ranging from 5 to 20 animals.[20-22] If sufficient animals are available within a large group, consider taking multiple pooled samples to account for a greater number of animals and provide some degree of variation assessment within the group.

In preparing pooled samples, one must be meticulous in precisely measuring equal amounts of serum from each individual to be included in the pooled sample. Depending on the total number to be included, typically between 100 and 500 μl (0.1-0.5 ml) from each individual are mixed into a new clean test tube (7-10 ml capacity). This process is best completed with use of a micropipette or a 1-ml syringe for precision. Pooled samples should be adequately mixed and then directly submitted to the laboratory or frozen and shipped. Allowing pooled samples to remain at room temperature for a period of time (>1 hour) may result in gel formation that will adversely affect laboratory analysis.

Analyte Selection

Specific analytes determined for any herd metabolic profile are dependent on the metabolic profile sampling strategy described previously. The original CMP test measured 13 different analytes that included packed cell volume, hemoglobin, glucose, blood UN, total protein, albumin, Ca, inorganic phosphorus (P_i), Mg, potassium (K), sodium (Na), copper (Cu), and iron (Fe). The following is a brief overview of possible analytes that could be measured in serum or plasma at most veterinary diagnostic laboratories and their ability to provide either diagnostic or disease risk information.

Energy Balance
Energy balance is by and far one of the most critical nutritional factors affecting animal health, lactation, and reproductive performance. Traditionally, we have monitored changes in energy balance via body weight and condition score changes over time. This procedure may not be a sensitive enough tool when dealing with the transition cow.

NEFAs have become the mainstay in determination of energy balance. Many research studies have shown good correlation between energy balance and serum NEFA concentrations. Concentration of NEFA directly reflects the amount of adipose (fat) tissue breakdown taking place. Excessively high NEFA concentrations because of negative energy balance either prepartum or early postpartum are predictive for increased risk of ketosis, left displaced abomasum, and most other periparturient diseases.[25,28-30]

β-hydroxybutyrate, one of the ketone bodies, is another parameter useful in assessing energy status. However, BHB can come from dietary sources (poorly fermented silage) and not reflect aberrant metabolism. Before calving, BHB concentrations are not predictive for disease risk[31] but may be elevated if the animal is in negative energy balance or consuming ketogenic silage. Following calving, BHB concentrations are diagnostic for disease and predictive for periparturient disease problems.[8,24-27,31-32]

Blood glucose concentration, as an independent test, is not a good indicator of energy status as a result of tight homeostatic control. However, glucose concentrations measured in conjunction with other tests may provide some further insight into underlying mechanisms of disease (type I vs. type II ketosis).

Protein Evaluation

At present there is no single metabolite that can be measured that directly reflects protein status. As a result, multiple parameters are necessary to assess protein status including UN, creatinine, total protein, albumin, and creatine kinase (CK). UN concentrations are influenced by a wide variety of interrelated parameters including dietary protein intake and rumen degradability, dietary amino acid composition, protein intake relative to requirement, liver and kidney function, muscle tissue breakdown and dietary carbohydrate amount, and rumen degradability. Creatinine is used to assess renal function and its impact on UN values. CK is released from muscle when it is injured or catabolized for needed amino acids.

Total protein and albumin reflect availability of amino acids and their concentration decline in the face of protein deficiency. However, this occurs over a period of time. Albumin has a relatively short half-life and can reflect protein deficiency problems over a period of a month or two. Albumin was found to be associated with postpartum disease and can be used to predict disease risk in close-up and fresh periods.[31,32] Other nutrients, namely iron and vitamin A, might also reflect protein status because both require a carrier protein synthesized in the liver. Lower concentrations of either nutrient may be observed when amino acid availability is limited, liver function is compromised, or both.

Liver Function

Liver function can be assessed through a variety of enzymes: gamma-glutamyltransferase (GGT), aspartate aminotransferase (AST), and sorbitol dehydrogenase (SDH) and total bilirubin concentrations in the blood. Unfortunately, an elevation in any of these parameters does not suggest anything more than some insult has occurred to the liver. Muscle catabolism or injury can result in elevated blood AST activities. Bilirubin values are more specific to bile flow problems than overt liver cell damage.

Because these parameters are not specific to liver function, other liver function indices have been advocated. A liver activity index parameter that accounts for changes in albumin, cholesterol, and total bilirubin over the first 28 days following calving has been defined.[23] Although a robust diagnostic tool, it requires multiple samples from the same cow over a period of time. This would preclude its use within a typical metabolic profiling approach.

Calculating the NEFA-to-cholesterol ratio (molar basis) to assess the liver's ability to export incoming NEFA has been advocated.[30] Calculated NEFA-to-cholesterol ratio was predictive for postpartum disease in the close-up dry and fresh cows.[31,32]

Macromineral Evaluation

Macrominerals Ca, P_i, K, Mg, Na, chloride (Cl), and sulfur (S) are of extreme interest as to their status relative to their role in milk fever, alert downer cows, and weak cow syndrome. Unfortunately, most of these minerals are tightly regulated in the body through a variety of homeostatic processes. Blood concentrations of macrominerals are not reflective of dietary status when the homeostatic system is functioning properly.[13] Phosphorus, K, Mg, and S are macrominerals in which blood concentrations are somewhat sensitive to dietary intake.[13] Electrolytes Na, Cl, and K are altered when renal or digestive function is compromised or in extreme dietary deficiency states.

Assessment of Ca concentrations around the time of calving is a useful indicator of how well the Ca regulatory system is working and potential for clinical or subclinical hypocalcemia problems.[8] Despite concerns about homeostatic regulation, prepartum and postpartum concentrations of Ca, Mg, Na, and K were found to be predictive of specific postpartum disease risk.[33-36] Surprisingly, blood P concentrations were not found to be predictive of disease risk, but abnormal values still may provide some diagnostic significance.

Micromineral and Vitamin Evaluation

Assessment of trace mineral and fat-soluble vitamin status is routinely completed using direct blood concentration measurements. Concentrations of Cu, Zn, and Fe are altered by physiologic responses to inflammation,[13] thus confounding their interpretation. Given the additional expense of analyzing for trace elements and vitamins, they are often not included in routine profiling. Associations between trace mineral concentrations and risk of periparturient disease were minimal, though high prepartum iron and low postpartum zinc concentrations tended to be associated with infectious disease problems.[36] Ratios of copper to zinc or iron, potentially reflecting changes indicative of an acute phase inflammatory response, tended to be associated with increased mastitis and metritis risk. In a number of diagnostic situations, analyzing for trace minerals and fat-soluble vitamins has been fruitful in determining potential sources of herd disease problems and should be considered in appropriate situations.

Other Possible Analytes

Research into the role of inflammatory mediators as a contributing factor to periparturient disease pathogenesis has led to interest in measuring markers of an activated inflammatory response as part of metabolic profiling.[16,23] Specific acute phase proteins ceruloplasmin and haptoglobin have been routinely determined by some investigators. Analytic tests for these acute phase proteins are not readily available outside of research laboratories at the current time. Other acute measures of inflammatory mediator activation (i.e., heat shock proteins) and oxidative stress markers may provide further insight but are not currently available for use in metabolic profiling.

Sample Collection, Handling, and Processing Procedures

Blood samples should be taken from either jugular or coccygeal veins with a minimal amount of stress. Lower concentrations of P_i and K have been documented in jugular compared with coccygeal blood samples as a result of salivary gland uptake.[37] Blood samples from the mammary veins are not appropriate given the loss of nutrients into the mammary gland. The following are considerations for sample collection:

Vacuum tubes are color coded for specific diagnostic test procedures based on the specific anticoagulant or additive present in the tube (Table 40-2). Plasma from green-top tubes is generally preferred, but red-top (serum) tubes can be used. It is best to ask the laboratory which sample is preferred.

Meticulous effort should be taken to prevent hemolysis of any sample. All samples should be iced, but not frozen, immediately after collection and kept refrigerated until processed. For serum samples the clot should be removed as quickly as possible (within hours of collection). Although serum separator tubes are convenient, experience suggests that samples are more prone to have some degree of hemolysis and prolonged clot contact.

Recognize that time of sampling relative to feeding and feeding management may also influence metabolite concentrations. If NEFA concentrations are of specific interest, then samples are best collected before the first primary feeding bout. If BHB or UN is of primary interest, then samples are best collected 3 to 5 hours following a primary feeding bout. If both analytes are desired, collect samples when convenient and account for feeding time effects. This is less of a concern in TMR-fed herds. If herds are being repeatedly sampled as a monitoring tool, samples should be taken at approximately the same time of day to minimize diurnal and prandial variation between sampling periods.

All samples should be properly identified with animal and group identification and date of collection. Use herd records to ensure the selected animals fit the defined group parameters, especially relative to parity and days in milk (or time relative to calving). Other pertinent information for interpretation of the metabolic profile includes milk production level, milk composition, pregnancy status, and body condition score. Again, metabolic profiling should only be used as a complement to more traditional diagnostic procedures.

Once the serum or plasma has been harvested from the original sample, it should be frozen and shipped to the laboratory. Alternatively, harvested samples can remain refrigerated and shipped on ice to the laboratory. Most laboratories recommend overnight shipping to minimize any sample deterioration. Contact the laboratory before shipping samples because many laboratories may have specific days of the week that samples can be received for metabolic profiling.

ASSESSMENT AND RESPONSE

Mechanics of metabolic profile testing discussed thus far have focused on obtaining appropriate samples in an effort to control confounding variability to interpretation of test results. The final stage of this process is to integrate test interpretations with other clinical assessments to direct the decision-making process to guide proactive nutritional, management, or environmental change to the current situation. Characterizing interpretation parameters to obtain valid information is the true challenge to metabolic profile testing.

A functional understanding of underlying metabolic and physiologic mechanisms controlling blood metabolite concentrations is necessary to properly interpret metabolic profiles and their application. One must appreciate the fundamental philosophic difference in blood analyte concentration interpretation between disease diagnosis and metabolic profiling paradigms. Disease diagnosis is focused on identifying critical outliers when compared with the population as a whole (i.e., 95% reference range). By definition, individuals sampled for metabolic profiling are expected to be within the 95% reference range for the population because they are "clinically normal." However, "normal" animals can be at risk for experiencing a disease if their metabolic status is trending away from

Table 40-2

Description of Blood Collection Tubes Used for Metabolic Profiles

Stopper Color	Additive	Sample Obtained	Intended Use/Disadvantages
Red	None	Serum	Routine use for all tests; prolonged clot exposure results in errors in glucose, Ca, and phosphorus; hemolysis problems in poorly handled samples
Gray	Na fluoride or K oxalate	Serum	Glycolytic inhibitor for sensitive glucose analysis
Royal blue	Plastic stopper Na heparin	Serum, plasma, or whole blood	Trace mineral analysis, especially Zn
Lavender	EDTA	Whole blood plasma	Routine use for complete blood count/EDTA chelates Ca, Mg, and enzyme activities
Green	Na heparin	Plasma whole blood	Routine analyses for either plasma or whole blood/No effect on metabolites

EDTA, Ethylenediaminetetraacetic acid.

the population central tendency. Blood analyte concentrations measure a continuous spectrum between health and disease and cannot be simply interpreted as "black or white." Metabolic profile criteria are more restrictive than the whole population, and interpretation is based on statistical associations to disease risk. The single most important aspect of metabolic profiling is establishing valid reference values for comparison.[9]

Reference Values

Based on methodology used for the metabolic profiling, reference values can either represent expected values for the equivalent population of healthy animals or specific threshold (cut point) analyte concentrations that have been statistically associated with a specific disease or collective disease risk. Analyte reference values should represent the population mean (or median if not normally distributed) and variation from a defined population of animals clinically evaluated to be free of disease and other health problems and fed an appropriate diet. Reference values for each metabolite need to be refined to minimize inherent variability caused by the effects of age, physiologic state, production level, and other cow-specific factors on analyte concentration and improve sensitivity of analyte to environmental (i.e., nutritional) influences.[31,38] At present, few laboratories have specialized blood analyte reference criteria that are adjusted for age, physiologic state, and time relative to calving effects. Research is currently under way to develop appropriate metabolic profiling reference criteria.

Threshold or cut point criteria are derived from statistical modeling using logistic regression and calculating odds ratios or relative risk. In this process the prevalence of a specific disease (e.g., retained placenta, ketosis, metritis) or any disease event is related to various concentrations of a specific analyte to determine if significant predictive relationships exist. For example, fresh cows with serum BHB concentrations ≥12.5 mg/dl (1200 µmol/L) were eight times more likely to experience a left displaced abomasum.[19] A number of studies have defined disease risk relationships to various blood analyte concentrations.

Expected analyte concentrations for healthy periparturient mature dairy cows are presented in Tables 40-3 and 40-4.[31,38] Standards for defining appropriate reference values for metabolic profiling have been suggested.[38] Greater clinical adoption of metabolic profiling testing is predicated on development of robust reference criteria to improve diagnostic interpretation.

Serum or plasma concentrations of NEFA and BHB have been the most studied in the periparturient dairy cow. Higher NEFA concentrations in either the close-up dry (≥0.4 mEq/L) or fresh (≥0.6 mEq/L) period are associated with increased risk for many periparturient diseases.[8,19,28,29,31] Prepartum BHB concentrations are not predictive of disease, but postpartum concentrations are sensitive indicators of disease risk. Subclinical ketosis diagnosis has been defined by BHB concentrations of 12.5 or 14.5 mg/dl (1200 or 1400 µmol/L).[8,24-27] However, BHB concentrations of 10 mg/dl (0.96 mmol/L) and greater are

Table 40-3

Expected Range (95% Confidence Interval) in Various Blood Analyte Concentrations over the Periparturient Period for Healthy, Mature Dairy Cows

Analyte	Units	Close-up Dry*	Fresh*
Albumin[†]	g/dl	3.3-3.7	3.2-3.6
AST	IU/L	46.5-82.6	61.1-103
BHB[†]	mg/dl	1.25-4.2	1.7-8.9
Cholesterol	mg/dl	65-114	63-253
Glucose	mg/dl	51-74	42-68
NEFA[†]	mEq/L	0.03-0.46	0.01-0.52
Total protein	g/dl	6.9-8.5	7.3-8.9
NEFA-to-cholesterol[†]	Ratio	0.03-0.2	0.03-0.4

Modified from Bertoni G, Calamari L, Trevisi E: New criteria for identifying reference values for specific blood parameters in dairy cows, *La Selezione Vet* Suppl S261-S268, 2000.

*Close-up dry defined as 3-21 days before calving; fresh cows defined as 3-30 days in milk.

[†]Analyte has been shown in one or more studies to be predictive for disease risk.

AST, Aspartate aminotransferase; *BHB,* β-hydroxybutyrate; *NEFA,* nonesterified fatty acid.

Table 40-4

Fresh Cow Mineral Concentrations in Healthy Population and Concentrations That Are of Concern for Potential Disease Risk

Analyte	Adequate Range	Concern Levels
Calcium*	8.7-11 mg/dl (2.17-2.74 mmol/L)	<8 mg/dl (<2 mmol/L)
Phosphorus	4.5-8 mg/dl (1.45-2.58 mmol/L)	<3.5 mg/dl (<1.13 mmol/L)
Magnesium*	2-3.5 mg/dl (0.82-1.43 mmol/L)	<1.5 mg/dl (<0.62 mmol/L)
Sodium*	137-148 mEq/L[†]	<137 mEq/L
Potassium*	3.8-5.2 mEq/L[†]	<3 or >5.5 mEq/L
Copper	0.6-1.5 g/ml (9.4-23.6 mol/L)	<0.45 g/ml (<7.1 mol/L) >4 g/ml (>63 mol/L)
Iron	130-250 g/dl (23.3-44.8 mol/L)	<130 g/dl (<23 mol/L) >1800 g/dl (>322 mol/L)
Zinc	0.8-1.4 g/ml (12.2-21.4 mol/L)	<0.5 g/ml (<7.6 mol/L) >3 g/ml (>45.9 mol/L)
Selenium, serum	70-100 ng/ml (0.89-1.3 mol/L)	<35 ng/ml (<0.44 mol/L) >800 ng/ml (>10.1 mol/L)
Selenium, whole blood	120-250 ng/ml (1.5-3.2 mol/L)	<50 ng/ml (<0.63 mol/L) >1900 ng/ml (>24 mol/L)
Serum vitamin A*	225-500 ng/ml	<150 ng/ml
Serum vitamin E*	3-10 µg/ml	<3 µg/ml
Vitamin E–to-cholesterol ratio[‡]	2.5-6	<1.5

*Analyte has been shown in one or more studies to be predictive for disease risk.

[†]mEq/L=mmol/L.

[‡]Both values in mmol/L, ratio is unitless.

associated with increased risk of a cow experiencing some postpartum disease.[31,32]

Other blood analytes have also been shown to be predictive of disease risk. Albumin concentrations in the close-up (≤3.25 g/dl) and fresh (≤3.4 g/dl) periods have been associated with increased disease risk.[31,32] Low total protein (≤6 g/dl) in fresh cows has also been suggested to indicate disease risk concerns, though hypergammaglobulinemia resulting from inflammatory response can confound total protein interpretations. Calculated NEFA-to-cholesterol ratio was suggested as an index of liver function and indicator of hepatic lipidosis.[30] The ratio is calculated with both measures expressed on a mmol/L basis (mg/dl cholesterol × 0.02586 = mmol/L). Cows with increased NEFA-to-cholesterol ratio in the close-up dry (= 0.2) and fresh (= 0.3) periods were at greater risk for postpartum disease.[32] Other analytes did not show significant disease risk associations, but cows collectively experiencing postpartum disease had lower albumin, UN, glucose, and cholesterol and higher NEFA, BHB, NEFA-to-cholesterol ratio, and AST concentrations compared with healthy cows.[31,32]

Interpretation of Results

As has been emphasized previously, metabolic profile test results must be interpreted in light of animal, dietary, and environmental assessments. This point cannot be over-emphasized because metabolic profile testing results do not always indicate nutrition or diet to be the underlying problem. For example, inadequate dietary energy density is not the only reason for elevated NEFA concentrations. Inadequate dry matter intake as a result of heat stress, overcrowding, poor forage quality, competitive social interactions, inadequate feed availability, or some combination of these could also account for observed negative energy balance. Results of metabolic profiling, depending on the approach chosen, can provide disease diagnosis or insights into how to direct one's diagnostic investigation. The power of metabolic profiling comes from an ability to integrate multiple parameters to determine the scope of metabolic aberrations present. Certain combinations of analyte alterations can provide insight into underlying disease pathogenesis and severity. Optimistically, protocols for disease mitigation and prevention can then be designed appropriately with some increased potential for success.

Individual Samples
Using the *targeted diagnostic* approach, 8 (mean-based analytes) or 12 (threshold-based analytes) individual samples were obtained from a selected group of animals at risk for a disease of interest. Individual analyte results are compared with the reference value, and individual values exceeding (NEFA or BHB) or below (Ca) the defined threshold value are identified as abnormal. Proportion of abnormal results is calculated and compared with defined criteria. Criteria are defined by statistical calculations accounting for desired confidence intervals. The values obtained represent the group sampled and disease prevalence rate (alarm level) that warrants intervention.[8] Clinical decisions require lower confidence intervals, and 70% to 75% is suggested compared with the 95% confidence

interval typically required for research.[8] For a disease with alarm levels of 10% and 25%, abnormal results should exceed 2 of 12 or 4 of 12, respectively.[8] As the proportion of positive abnormal values increases, disease prevalence would be expected to increase. With a positive herd diagnosis, further diagnostics to determine a potential cause can be initiated and disease-specific treatment protocols can be enacted.

Using the *screening tool* approach, a predetermined array of analytes is determined on individual samples collected from a select group or groups of cows. Analyte results from individual cows are compared with reference values for the defined group, and number of abnormal results determined. As the proportion of abnormal values increases, disease risk increases. Response depends on the specific analyte or analytes found to be abnormal. Specific patterns of analyte changes, similar to disease diagnosis, would suggest an associated disease, and defined treatment and prevention protocols can be enacted. If only NEFA concentrations were elevated, then one would be most directed to causes of insufficient energy intake. If, in addition, AST activities were elevated and cholesterol concentrations reduced, then liver dysfunction (fatty infiltration) would be suspected. Reduced UN and albumin concentrations would suggest that protein deficiency were an additional complication in this disease process and might decrease the overall prognosis. Severity of elevation and reduction in concentrations of BHB and glucose, respectively, would provide insight into status of glucose homeostasis and potential for type I or II ketosis being present.

Mean or Pooled Samples
Within the original CMP test, individual analyte values within the three defined groups were averaged and a group mean was compared with herd-based reference values. In comparison with individual samples, mean values lose the measure of individual variability. Mean values need to be compared with appropriate reference values, and these will differ from those used for individual samples. Herd mean reference values should be generated using means of healthy cows within a herd and averaged across herds rather than just an average of all that of individuals.[12] Interpretation of mean values is different from that of individual samples in which you are comparing to the variation of the reference population. Mean values must be compared with variation of the reference population central tendency (median or mean). Criteria for interpreting mean values were not well defined, and this was an interpretation problem with the CMP test. It was recognized that mean values could not span within the 95% confidence range for the reference population. Early adopters of metabolic profiling empirically suggested mean values should range within ±1 or 1.3 standard deviations in the reference population.[2,3,14]

Recent studies further investigated mean sample value interpretation using individual or pooled sampling procedures.[22] Across all analytes measured, mean values of individuals or pooled samples that had less than 10% abnormal values deviated 0.26 standard deviations from the reference population mean (or median). However, the amount of deviation was found to be analyte specific and ranged from 0.11 (glucose) to 0.6 (BHB) standard

Table **40-5**

Proposed Guidelines for Fresh Cow Mean or Pooled Sample Interpretation

Analyte	Units	% ABNORMAL VALUES IN POOL		
		0	20	40
		MEAN ANALYTE VALUE (70% CONFIDENCE INTERVAL)		
Albumin	g/dl	3.85 (3.77-3.92)	3.68 (3.57-3.7)	3.51 (3.38-3.63)
AST	IU/L	93.8 (88.8-98.7)	99.3 (91.8-106.7)	104.7 (94.9-114.6)
BHB	mg/dl	5.21 (4.3-6.2)	9.03 (7.6-10.4)	12.84 (11.0-14.7)
Calcium	mg/dl	9.67 (9.59-9.79)	8.68 (8.37-8.99)	7.68 (7.16-8.2)
Glucose	mg/dl	60.2 (58.6-61.9)	56.9 (54.7-59.1)	53.7 (50.9-56.4)
Magnesium	mg/dl	2.54 (2.49-2.6)	2.33 (2.23-2.42)	2.11 (1.97-2.24)
NEFA	mEq/L	0.299 (.263-.336)	0.454 (.397-.512)	0.609 (.531-.687)
NEFA-to-cholesterol ratio	mmol/L: mmol/L	0.116 (.098-.134)	0.215 (.181-.25)	0.315 (.264-.365)
Urea N	mg/dl	17.83 (16.9-18.8)	15.87 (14.5-17.2)	13.9 (12.2-15.6)

AST, Aspartate aminotransferase; *BHB,* β-hydroxybutyrate; *NEFA,* nonesterified fatty acid.

deviations. A linear association was found between the number of standard deviations that the measured mean or pooled sample moved away from the reference population mean (or median) and percent of abnormal values within the group sample. Using these relationships, analyte concentration guidelines for interpretation of mean or pooled samples can be generated (Table 40-5). At present, interpretation guidelines are available for fresh cow samples. Similar diagnostic interpretations as previously described can be accomplished with the various analytes measured in mean or pooled samples.

If one is using a pooled sample collection process, more than likely samples will be collected from multiple groups of cows (early dry, close-up dry, fresh). Beyond the described analyte concentration evaluation within a cow grouping, comparisons can be made across groups. Patterns in specific blood analyte concentrations across transition cow groups might provide some insightful clues to underlying problems and potential solutions. Measuring analytes across groups might also provide some time dimension as to source and length of a problem. Herds experiencing low protein status in fresh cows typically have low UN and normal albumin concentrations in early dry cows, and these values decline over the close-up dry and fresh periods, indicative of inadequate dietary protein intake.

Another method to diagnostically assess analyte changes over time is to use a variation on statistical process control. Mean group or pooled sample analyte concentrations repeatedly measured over a time frame can be plotted over time. Overall mean and statistical variation within and between time periods can be determined to interpret potential changes in animal performance. Individual test results outside of control limits or three or more consecutive means above or below overall average would indicate significant changes in analyte concentrations. Trends in mean values can then be related back to changes in diet, management, or environment to determine the source of problems or document improvement following changes.

References

1. Ingraham RH, Kappel LC: Metabolic profile testing, *Vet Clin North Am Food Anim Pract* 4:391, 1988.
2. Payne JM, Dew SM, Manston R et al: The use of a metabolic profile test in dairy herds, *Vet Rec* 87:150, 1970.
3. Payne JM, Rowlands GJ, Manston R et al: A statistical appraisal of the results of metabolic profile tests on 75 dairy herds, *Br Vet J* 129:370-381, 1973.
4. Bell AW: Regulation of organic nutrient metabolism during transition from late pregnancy to early lactation, *J Anim Sci* 73:2804-2819, 1995.
5. Grummer RR: Impact of changes in organic nutrient metabolism on feeding the transition dairy cow, *J Anim Sci* 73:2820-2833, 1995.
6. Drackley JK: Biology of dairy cows during the transition period: the final frontier? *J Dairy Sci* 82:2259-2273, 1999.
7. Herdt TH, Dart B, Neuder L: Will large dairy herds lead to the revival of metabolic profile testing? *Proc Am Assoc Bov Pract* 34:27-34, 2001.
8. Oetzel GR: Monitoring and testing dairy herds for metabolic disease, *Vet Clin North Am Food Anim Pract* 20:651-674, 2004.

9. Bertoni G, Trevisi E: *Metabolic profiles in the dairy cows management: a new approach.* Proceedings of the Fifth Congress Internat Soc Anim Clinical Biochem, Sept 2-6, 1992, pp 167-177.

10. Van Saun RJ, Wustenberg M: Metabolic profiling to evaluate nutritional and disease status, *Bov Pract* 31:37-42, 1997.

11. Van Saun RJ: Nutritional profiles: a new approach for dairy herds, *Bov Pract* 31:43-50, 1997.

12. Herdt TH: Variability characteristics and test selection in herd-level nutritional and metabolic profile testing, *Vet Clin North Am Food Anim Pract* 16:387-403, 2000.

13. Herdt TH, Rumbeiha W, Braselton WE: The use of blood analyses to evaluate mineral status in livestock, *Vet Clin North Am Food Anim Pract* 16:423-444, 2000.

14. Rowlands GJ, Little W, Stark AJ et al: The blood composition of cows in commercial dairy herds and its relationships with season and lactation, *Br Vet J* 135:64-74, 1979.

15. Eicher R, Liesgang A, Bouchard E et al: Effect of cow-specific factors and feeding frequency of concentrate on diurnal variations of blood metabolites in dairy cows, *AJVR* 60: 1493-1499, 1999.

16. Bertoni G, Trevisi E, Calamari L et al: The inflammation could have a role in the liver lipidosis occurrence in dairy cows. In Joshi N, Herdt TH, editors: *Production diseases in farm animals: 12th International Conference,* The Netherlands, 2006, Wageningen Academic Publishers.

17. Stokol T, Nydam DV: Effect of hemolysis on nonesterified fatty acid and β-hydroxybutyrate concentrations in bovine blood, *J Vet Diagn Invest* 18:466-469, 2006.

18. Jacobs RM, Lumsden JH, Grift E: Effects of bilirubinemia, hemolysis, and lipemia on clinical chemistry analytes in bovine, canine, equine, and feline sera, *Can Vet J* 33:605-608, 1992.

19. LeBlanc SJ, Leslie KE, Duffield TF: Metabolic predictors of displaced abomasum in dairy cattle, *J Dairy Sci* 88:159-170, 2005.

20. Lehwenich T: *Investigation to the use of metabolic profile test in herd management of dairy cattle,* Berlin University, Germany, 1999 (dissertation).

21. Van Saun RJ: Using a pooled sample technique for herd metabolic profile screening. In Joshi N, Herdt TH, editors: *Production diseases in farm animals: 12th International Conference,* The Netherlands, 2006, Wageningen Academic Publishers, p 47.

22. Van Saun RJ: Use and interpretation of pooled metabolic profiles for evaluating transition cow health status, *Proc Am Assoc Bov Pract* 38:180, 2005.

23. Bertoni G, Trevisi E, Han X et al: The relationship between inflammatory condition and liver activity in the puerperium and their consequences on fertility in dairy cows, *J Anim Sci* 84(suppl 2):84, 2006.

24. Duffield TF: Monitoring strategies for metabolic disease in transition dairy cows. In Proc 23rd World Buiatrics Cong, Quebec, Canada, July 11-16, 2004, pp 34-35.

25. Geishauser T, Leslie K, Duffield T et al: The association between selected metabolite parameters and left abomasal displacement in dairy cows, *J Vet Med* 45:499-511, 1998.

26. Geishauser T, Leslie K, Kelton D et al: Monitoring for subclinical ketosis in dairy herds, *Comp Cont Ed Pract Vet* 23:S65-S70, 2001.

27. LeBlanc SJ: *Monitoring programs for transition dairy cows.* In Proceedings 24th World Buiatrics Congress, October 15-19, Nice, France, pp 460-471, 2006.

28. Cameron REB, Dyk PB, Herdt TH et al: Dry cow diet, management, and energy balance as risk factors for displaced abomasum in high producing dairy herds, *J Dairy Sci* 81:132-139, 1988.

29. Dyk PB, Emery RS, Liesman JL et al: Prepartum nonesterified fatty acids in plasma are higher in cows developing periparturient health problems, *J Dairy Sci* 78(suppl 1):264, 1995 (abstract).

30. Holtenius P, Hjort M: Studies on the pathogenesis of fatty liver in cows, *Bov Pract* 25:91, 1990.

31. Van Saun RJ: *Health status and time relative to calving effects on blood metabolite concentrations.* In Proceedings 23rd World Buiatrics Congress (poster abstracts), Quebec, Canada, July 11-16, 2004, p 87.

32. Van Saun RJ: Metabolic profiling to assess health status of transition dairy cows. In Joshi N, Herdt TH, editors: *Production diseases in farm animals: 12th International Conference,* The Netherlands, 2006, Wageningen Academic Publishers, p 41.

33. Van Saun RJ, Todd A, Varga GA: Serum mineral concentrations and periparturient disease in Holstein dairy cows. In Joshi N, Herdt TH, editors: *Production diseases in farm animals: 12th International Conference,* The Netherlands, 2006, Wageningen Academic Publishers, p 221.

34. Van Saun RJ, Todd A, Varga GA: Serum mineral concentrations and risk of periparturient disease, *Proc Am Assoc Bov Pract* 38:178-179, 2005.

35. Van Saun RJ, Todd A, Varga GA: *Serum mineral concentrations and periparturient health status in Holstein dairy cows.* Proceedings XXIV World Buiatrics Congress, Nice, France, October 15-19, 2006a (abstract #48/OS07-4 [CD-ROM Proceedings]).

36. Van Saun RJ, Todd A, Varga GA: *Serum mineral status and risk of periparturient disease,* Proceedings of the 24th World Buiatrics Congress, Nice, France, October 15-19, 2006b (abstract #49/PS3-016 [CD-ROM Proceedings]).

37. Maas J: Interpreting serum chemistry screens in cattle, *Mod Vet Pract* 64:963-967, 1983.

38. Bertoni G, Calamari L, Trevisi E: New criteria for identifying reference values for specific blood parameters in dairy cows, *La Selezione Vet Suppl* S261-S268, 2000.

SECTION III

Respiratory System

Jeffrey Lakritz **and** *David E. Anderson*

CHAPTER 41

Mannheimia haemolytica– and *Pasteurella multocida*–Induced Bovine Pneumonia

DOUGLAS L. STEP and ANTHONY W. CONFER

In North American cattle, *Mannheimia haemolytica* and *Pasteurella multocida* are primarily associated with severe pneumonia in what is known as the *bovine respiratory disease* (BRD) *complex*. *M. haemolytica* and *P. multocida* are involved in severe fibrinous pleuropneumonia and fibrinopurulent bronchopneumonia in dairy and beef cattle worldwide. Because *M. haemolytica* was formerly named *Pasteurella haemolytica,* bovine respiratory disease associated with these two bacteria have traditionally been called *bovine pneumonic pasteurellosis.* In addition to respiratory disease, these bacteria have sporadically been isolated from bovine diseases such as meningitis, septicemia, localized infections, pericarditis, abortions, and mastitis. *M. haemolytica* and *P. multocida* are ubiquitous in the cattle population as commensals in the nasopharynx. Therefore mechanisms of immunity to them have been difficult to determine, efficacious vaccines have been a challenge to develop, and vaccine efficacy has been difficult to evaluate.

In 1999 *M. haemolytica* became the accepted classification of what was formerly *P. haemolytica* biotype A. The former *P. haemolytica* biotype T (a cause of septicemia in lambs) was reclassified as *Pasteurella trehalosi. M. haemolytica* includes 12 serotypes, 1, 2, 5-9, 10 and 12, 16, and 17. *P. multocida* is classified into 5 serogroups (A, B, D, E, and F) and 16 serotypes (1-16). *M. haemolytica* serotype 1 and *P. multocida* A:3 are the most common serotypes isolated from bovine respiratory disease.[1]

M. haemolytica– and *P. multocida*–induced bovine pneumonia are of substantial economic importance. Severe respiratory disease is the major cause of clinical disease and death loss in stocker and feedlot cattle (shipping fever) and second only to diarrhea as a major disease syndrome in dairy calves. Survey results indicate that more than 80% of cattle deaths in feedlot and stocker operations are caused by shipping fever. In North America alone, bovine respiratory disease results in economic losses to producers estimated at $800 million.

M. haemolytica serotype 1 is the most commonly isolated bacteria in acute fibrinous pleuropneumonia associated with shipping fever (prevalence 65%-75%).[1] *P. multocida* A:3 is the second most common bacteria isolated from acute to subacute fibrinopurulent bronchopneumonia in beef cattle (prevalence 21%-34%)

and the major cause of bronchopneumonia in dairy calves (prevalence >65).[2] The latter condition is part of the enzootic pneumonia complex of dairy calves. In a recent 8-year retrospective study of submissions to the Oklahoma Animal Disease Diagnostic Laboratory, there was a steady decline in the percentage *M. haemolytica* isolates and a proportional increase in the percentage *P. multocida* isolates from beef cattle pneumonia.[1] Therefore *P. multocida* may be emerging as a more important pathogen in shipping fever. In acute pneumonia, *M. haemolytica* or *P. multocida* can be isolated in pure culture; however, as lesions become more chronic with severe necrosis, fibrosis, and abscess formation, multiple bacteria may be isolated, including *M. haemolytica, P. multocida, Arcanobacterium (Actinobacillus) pyogenes, Histophilus (Haemophilus) somni,* or *Mycoplasma bovis.*

The pathogenesis of bacterial pneumonia involves several bacterial-host interactions: nasopharyngeal colonization, inhalation of aerosolized droplets containing bacteria, pulmonary alveolar colonization, host response to colonization, and bacterial evasion of host defenses.[3] Both *M. haemolytica* and *P. multocida* are carried in the nasopharynx and tonsils of cattle in low, often undetectable numbers. In the case of *M. haemolytica,* isolates from the nasal cavity of normal cattle often yield serotypes other than serotype 1, especially serotype 2. Viral infections, commingling of cattle from various sources, inclement weather, overcrowding, poor ventilation, and other causes of stress result in the proliferation of *M. haemolytica* serotype 1 and/or *P. multocida* with subsequent inhalation of bacteria into the lung.

More is known about the host–*M. haemolytica* interactions occurring in the lungs of cattle than the host–*P. multocida* interactions.[4,5] Therefore the following discussion of pathogenesis will concentrate on *M. haemolytica.* Once *M. haemolytica* gain access to the pulmonary alveoli, local host defenses including innate immunity, pulmonary surfactant, alveolar macrophages, the cough reflex, and mucociliary protection must be overcome for pneumonia to result. These local mechanisms, together with cellular and humoral systemic defenses, usually destroy small numbers of bacteria that are inhaled by the uncompromised calf. However, when those responses are insufficient because of stress factors or concurrent infections or overcome by severe bacterial load, several bacterial and host factors (particularly leukocyte products) induce localized tissue damage and incite systemic responses associated with the acute inflammatory process.

Various *M. haemolytica* virulence factors influence the outcome of bacterial-host interactions.[4-6] The bacterium produces a thick polysaccharide capsule that protects the organism from phagocytosis and complement-mediated killing. Endotoxin, which is associated with the outer membrane of *M. haemolytica,* causes alveolar capillary endothelial damage and stimulates cytokine/chemokine production. Endothelial damage results in fluid exudation and neutrophil infiltration into alveoli and activation of the coagulation cascade and stimulation of platelet aggregation resulting in thrombosis. Macrophage activation stimulates the release of pro-inflammatory cytokines such as tumor necrosis factor–α, IL-1β, and IL-8; the latter is a strong neutrophil chemotactant. Leukotoxin (LKT), which is secreted by rapidly growing *M. haemolytica,* causes damage to and activation of neutrophils and macrophages resulting in release of proteolytic enzymes and oxygen radicals with activation of matrix metalloproteases that damage alveoli and inflammatory mediators, which further enhance the inflammatory response in the alveoli. Leukocyte death can occur by causing pore formation and oncotic cell death or by stimulation of death by apoptosis. Endotoxin has also been shown to enhance LKT activity.

In general, clinical signs of shipping fever usually become evident 3 to 10 days after cattle are stressed.[7-9] Occasionally, cattle are found dead with minimal warning signs of disease, but most affected cattle become depressed and are first observed standing alone with their head dropped. Severely affected animals may be found in dorsal recumbency. Respirations are usually shallow, rapid, and accompanied by a slight productive cough, especially when cattle are moved. A mucopurulent nasal discharge may be seen. Most cattle lose their appetite but continue to drink water. Affected cattle are febrile (>104° F [40° C]), and bronchial tones, wheezes, and pleuritic friction sounds may be auscultated. The clinical course usually lasts 2 to 4 days. If treated early, positive clinical responses may be noted within 24 to 36 hours. Treatment failures result in death or chronic pneumonia with continued anorexia, weight loss, and lack of vigor.

The lesion typically observed in shipping fever and attributed to *M. haemolytica* infection is a severe fibrinous pleuropneumonia.[10] Variable amount of fibrin-rich fluid are present in the pleural cavity with abundant fibrin strands adherent to pleural surfaces. The cranioventral lung lobes are dark reddish-black to grayish-brown and firm with marked distention of interlobular septae by gelatinous yellow fluid. On a cut surface, there are sharply demarcated areas of coagulation necrosis within the consolidated parenchyma. Microscopically, alveoli are flooded with fibrin, neutrophils, plump or "streaming" oat-shaped macrophages, animals and necrotic cell debris. Necrotic areas are surrounded by intense inflammatory cell infiltrates, and there are usually numerous bacteria at the margins of the necrotic tissue. Thrombi are frequently found in pulmonary vessels and are thought to account for infarction and subsequent necrosis. Interlobular septae are distended with fibrin-rich edema and neutrophils. Interlobular lymphatics are dilated and often contain fibrin thrombi.

The lesion caused by *P. multocida* in either beef or dairy calves is usually a fibrinopurulent bronchopneumonia that is less fulminating and more chronic than the lesion caused by *M. haemolytica.*[10] The pleural surfaces may have a small to moderate amount of adherent fibrin, which is often concentrated over the cranioventral lung lobes; however, cases are often seen in which pleuritis is absent. The cranioventral lungs are consolidated and dark red to reddish-gray with minimal distention of interlobular septae. On a cut surface, the consolidated areas contain uniformly spaced grayish foci that correspond to bronchioles. Yellow-gray fibrinopurulent exudate can be expressed from bronchioles, and small foci of necrosis or abscesses may be present. Microscopically, lesions center on bronchioles. Bronchiolar epithelial changes vary from necrotic to hyperplastic, and bronchiolar lumens are filled with neutrophils and fibrinonecrotic debris. Alveoli are likewise distended with neutrophils and fibrinonecrotic debris, and these changes are most intense in peribronchiolar alveoli.

TREATMENT

When presented with either an individual animal or group of cattle suffering from BRD, the clinician must be familiar with the treatment goals of the producer. Most producers indicate that reducing or eliminating death loss is their primary goal. Minimizing death loss is an obvious priority; however, although this goal is extremely important, the veterinarian must also focus on the goal of reducing the severity and duration of clinical signs. When clinical signs are decreased, performance reflected in feed intake, feed conversion, gain, and carcass quality improves. Meeting this goal is important from the economic benefit to the producer and also the health and well-being of the cattle.

Producers are interested in reducing the negative economic impact of BRD. Preconditioning programs that stimulate a calf's immune system before exposure to the various respiratory pathogens are a proven method in reducing the incidence of BRD. Even though preconditioning programs benefit the health and performance of cattle, many cattle in the market chain remain unvaccinated to the common respiratory pathogens and are immunologically naive. In the postweaning period, these cattle are at high-risk of developing BRD when commingled and exposed to stressful situations such as shipping. A strategy commonly used to reduce BRD in these high-risk cattle is metaphylaxis, which is the use of antimicrobial drugs for the control of BRD in high-risk cattle. Use of metaphylactic treatments can decrease morbidity and mortality and improve performance in these cattle. Following are guidelines the authors use when determining if prescribing metaphylactic drugs is deemed necessary.

The first criterion involves the producer and individuals caring for the health of the cattle. When personnel are less experienced with early identification of morbid cattle or cannot observe and treat the cattle within a realistic time frame, then metaphylaxis is prescribed and usually has an economic benefit. The time frame guidelines we use are that all cattle requiring an antimicrobial drug be identified and treated by noon or preferably earlier, especially in the hot summer. In the winter the time frame guideline may be extended to 2:00 p.m. This criterion is especially followed for young lightweight cattle weighing less than 400 to 500 lb and is more closely followed in the fall (September through December) than in spring (January through May) cattle because of higher incidence of BRD in the fall. The commonly used commercial products available for metaphylactic use are crystalline ceftiofur free acid (Excede), oxytetracycline 300 mg (Tetradure 300), florfenicol (Nuflor), tilmicosin (Micotil), and tulathromycin (Dra30in). The choice of which drug to choose depends on cost, benefit, quantity of dose administered, season, and the practitioner's experience. To determine the best choice of drugs, a critical evaluation of records is required. Unfortunately, in many operations, sufficient data to evaluate the efficacy of medications are lacking. Communicating with colleagues, university personnel, and critically evaluating refereed scientific literature assists in choosing an appropriate drug.

The cost benefit of the prescribed therapy should thus be remembered when developing a treatment protocol, especially for commercial cattle. In general, in our experience, the broad-spectrum antimicrobials that are currently on the market and used to treat BRD have good clinical efficacy. Any of these can potentially reduce sickness; however, from a production medicine standpoint, one must evaluate the cost benefit of the drugs.

Several FDA-approved drugs are available to treat BRD. Using a drug in an extra-label use to treat BRD must meet the guidelines outlined by the Animal Medicinal Drug Use Clarification Act (AMDUCA). Veterinarians must remember and communicate to their clients that cost is not a valid reason to use an animal drug in an extra-label fashion. The veterinarian that prescribes the extra-label use of a drug is responsible for determining an appropriate withdrawal time.

Evaluation of available scientific literature, findings on postmortem examinations, analysis of records that require animal identification, test results from laboratory submissions, and experience obtained from clinical observations and response to therapy all contribute to prescribing a particular BRD treatment protocol. This section of the chapter discusses the various steps involved in developing a BRD treatment protocol.

Clinical evaluation should involve both subjective and objective components. Early detection and treatment usually results in a more favorable outcome than the approach of "wait and see what the calf looks like in a day or two." Experience is a definite asset for the subjective component of the evaluations. When examining cattle, it is best to observe the cattle from a distance. Because cattle are prey species, they will group together when something is different about their environment or they feel threatened.[11] When an observer enters into close proximity of the cattle environment, whether it is a dry lot pen or a pasture, the animal's flight or fight mechanism is engaged. Frightened cattle may not exhibit any abnormal signs to the observer, or a sick animal may seek a location in the herd so that its weakness is concealed. Cattle exhibiting abnormal signs consistent with BRD may be identified as suspect from a distance. Therefore it is also important to observe cattle before entering and after leaving their usual environment, so that sick animals may feel less threatened and exhibit signs indicative of BRD.

Abnormal clinical signs include depression, abnormal appetite, and altered respirations.[7,8] Lethargy, hanging or droopy head, slow movements, arched back, knuckling at the fetlocks, dragging toes, difficulty rising from a recumbent position, stumbling when moving that is not the result from being bumped by another animal, and paresis are some of the clinical signs evaluated to determine if an animal is depressed. Cattle sometimes just do not appear normal, with no obvious abnormal signs that the evaluator can assign to the individual. These cattle also need further evaluation.

Abnormalities in appetite include anorexia or decreased feed intake, especially if cattle are accustomed to the diet, slow eating if it is considered different from the animal's normal behavior, lack of fill or gaunt, and obvious weight loss. Producers may state that if cattle are still eating, they are not sick and do not need to be further evaluated. This statement is in contrast to our observations in early or mild cases of BRD, whereas cattle still eat early in the disease process. In addition, producers may comment that cattle should be "full" in the left paralumbar fossa within 2 to 4 days following arrival. If the cattle are still gaunt at that time, producers will then treat the cattle for BRD. In our experience, high-risk, exposed, commingled cattle may not "fill in" for 7 days or more; however, they appear clinically normal and perform at the level of their penmates.

Increased respirations and nasal discharge are obvious indications of abnormal respiratory function. However, as most experienced veterinarians and caretakers have observed, these signs alone do not indicate a case of BRD and need for antimicrobial therapy. Increased respirations are a normal response to stress, and thus this sign may be difficult to evaluate for the individual animal in a group or herd situation. Labored breathing, respiratory noise, and extended head and neck combined with other abnormal signs assist the evaluator subjectively to determine that an animal may be suffering from BRD.

For subjective evaluation, one of two scoring systems is generally used. These are as follows: a score of 1 to 4 with 1 = mild, 2 = moderate, 3 = severe, and 4 = moribund or a 1 to 5 scale in which 1 = normal, 2 = mild, 3 = moderate, 4 = severe, and 5 = moribund. In our studies, the simpler scale (1 to 4) works well for us. Subjective scores are combined with an objective evaluation to determine if the animal is to receive an antimicrobial treatment.

For objective evaluation, cattle are restrained and a thorough physical examination is performed. One should attempt to evaluate all body systems as thoroughly as possible including examination for oral erosions, blunted papillae, conjunctivitis, hyphema, and the anatomic location of abnormal lung sounds. A rectal temperature is also helpful. In most field production settings, results of the subjective evaluation plus a rectal temperature exceeding a predetermined value (usually 104° F [40° C]) will result in a diagnosis of BRD and dictate the need for antimicrobial therapy.[12]

Cattle may be suffering from BRD, yet their rectal temperature can be within normal limits or below the predetermined level for treatment. This occurs because the peak febrile response may have been missed or an individual animal may not respond with as elevated a temperature as its cohorts. Therefore the decision to treat is based on a combination of the subjective severity score and the animal's rectal temperature. For example, an animal subjectively scoring a 1 (out of 4) (mild) or 2 (moderate) must have a rectal temperature equal to or greater than 104° F to receive an antimicrobial drug, whereas if the animal's rectal temperature is less than 104° F, it is returned to its pen or to an observation pen for continued evaluation without receiving an antimicrobial treatment. If, however, an animal is subjectively scored a 3 (severe) or 4 (moribund), antimicrobial treatment should be given regardless of rectal temperature.

Antemortem and postmortem tests should be performed to confirm the diagnosis of BRD. Nasal swabs can be submitted for bacterial culture and sensitivity and viral isolation, and transtracheal fluid aspirates and bronchoalveolar lavage samples can be examined cytologically and submitted for culture and sensitivity testing. Endoscopic evaluation, radiographs, and thoracic ultrasound can also be performed antemortem. The results of these diagnostic procedures may support or refute the diagnosis of BRD and potentially yield a more specific morphologic and etiologic diagnosis. Blood submitted for a complete blood cell count with fibrinogen concentrations and haptoglobin analysis can also indicate an active inflammatory process.

Unfortunately for economic reasons, many clients elect not to have a postmortem examination with appropriate diagnostic tests performed. However, many benefits result from conducting postmortem examination and diagnostic procedures. The necropsy can confirm the clinical diagnosis. The severity, extent, and relative duration of the disease can be evaluated. The presence of concomitant diseases such as salmonellosis or bovine viral diarrhea virus infections that may complicate the response of the animal and have herd health implications can be determined. Samples collected at necropsy should be submitted for culture and sensitivity and histopathology. Bacterial culture may yield negative results when collected from animals that were treated previously. Concerns about initial antimicrobial selections and trends in sensitivity patterns can and should be monitored. The results of these tests will also assist the clinician to recommend the most appropriate choice of antimicrobial therapy.

Following these recommendations, the clients can focus on minimizing the negative impact of BRD in production and improving the welfare of the animals. For instance, cattle that die within a few days of arrival and the necropsy findings include multiple thick-walled abscesses and fibrous adhesions indicate that the animal had experienced an episode of BRD before purchase.[8] Obtaining

a health history before purchase would be helpful, and discussing the concerns with the buyer of the cattle may help to reduce these chronic cases. This type of information can also assist the producer to observe newly arrived cattle more closely. If postmortem findings indicate a severe pleuropneumonia and records indicate an acute death without receiving any treatments, criteria for early identification of morbid cattle should be reviewed with the caregivers. If respiratory viral pathogens are identified, the appropriate vaccination protocols and management should be reviewed.

Client communication explaining that laboratory tests are to be used as a guide and are not necessarily the definitive answer is important.[7] In vitro antimicrobial susceptibility results may not reflect the same response in vivo. Antimicrobial testing has practical limitations. For instance, the breakpoints selected for MIC are frequently based on estimates from human isolates and may not be appropriate for bovine pathogens.[13] Although many treatment protocols in the field are based on clinical experience from trial and error, the practitioner should also incorporate data about the drugs including the pharmacokinetics and pharmacodynamics to develop a sound recommendation. A more thorough discussion of applying the pharmacokinetics and pharmacodynamics of medications is presented in the previous edition of the Current Veterinary Therapy. Experience and data may also indicate that a drug with concentrations in lung tissue higher than in plasma or a highly liquid soluble compound may be more beneficial in certain disease situations.

Another valuable resource tool for the clinician to use when developing treatment protocols is the available scientific literature. Clinicians must critically evaluate the study design, type of production system and cattle enrolled in the study, management, product administration, statistical methods used to determine significance, and whether a control group was included in the study. This information will assist the clinician in recommending an appropriate antimicrobial therapy.

Animal identification and accurate records are crucial. Records can consist of simple systems involving paper files such as pocket notebooks to more complex electronic systems with automatic calculations. The information collected is then used to adjust treatment protocols that best meet the needs of the producer and the cattle. Records along with appropriate individual animal identification are necessary to identify animals that may have potential residues as a consequence of administration of an antimicrobial drug. Analysis of the records for case fatality rate, overall mortality, morbidity, relapse rates, response rates, new episodes, days following an event such as days postarrival or weather events including hurricanes or severe winter storms, and treatment costs contribute to a sound scientific evaluation of a treatment protocol.

Another major concern producers and veterinarians have when treating diseased cattle with any antimicrobial agent is resistance of the pathogen to the drug(s).[13,14] Decreased efficacy of the drug can only be truly assessed with a thorough evaluation of records, laboratory results, and an understanding of the pharmacokinetics of the drugs. An abnormal increase in case fatality rates or an increase in retreat rates would dictate an investigation into the cause.[14] Besides a true resistance to the antimicrobial drugs, aspects of the treatment protocol that need to be more thoroughly evaluated include early identification of morbid animals, proper dosing including route of drug administration using an accurate individual weight, and appropriate posttreatment interval.[8,13-15]

The posttreatment interval is the time interval after the drug has been administered until the animal would normally be eligible for evaluation and possible administration of another treatment.[1] Recent evidence and clinical experience have demonstrated that if the interval following drug administration is extended beyond previously accepted time intervals suggested by the manufacturers, fewer animals require a second treatment.[16] The underlying reason for this beneficial response is unclear but may be related to the time required for the animal's immune system to adequately respond and/or the adaptation of an animal to its new environment and reducing stress by not restraining the animal for further evaluation.

Producers frequently want to administer two or more antimicrobial drugs simultaneously, under the premise that if one drug does not kill the bacteria, the other one will. Unfortunately, problems may arise and producers need to be informed of these potential consequences. There could be competition between drugs for binding sites, bacteriostatic drugs may interfere with bactericidal drugs by inhibiting bacterial growth, and injection site blemishes would be increased. Therefore the additional costs would be difficult to justify.[14]

Other frequently asked questions include (1) how many drugs should be used in a treatment protocol? (2) should the same drug be used for the first and second treatment choices or should different classes of drugs be used in a treatment protocol? and (3) which is the best drug to use as the initial treatment? The correct answer to all these questions is that it varies from situation to situation. The veterinarian's experience will influence the answers. With that stated, we provide some guidelines that have worked well for us and others. For the first question, when setting up a treatment protocol, a calf gets three chances to respond to treatment for BRD. If an animal does not respond after three drugs or treatments, then it will be realized (harvested before the desired finish weight) after an appropriate withdrawal period has been followed or euthanized if the clinical condition warrants.

For the second question regarding switching to a different class of drug if an animal needs additional therapy, we have historically rotated classes of antimicrobial drugs between treatments. The rationale is that if the animal did not respond clinically to the first drug, a different drug should be administered for the next treatment, and if the calf failed to respond to the first and second drug, a third was administered. If the calf, however, did not respond to the previous or initial drug, the duration of therapy may not have been long enough for that individual animal. Thus administering the same drug to an animal that did not respond to the first treatment may be appropriate.[7] Controlled studies to support or refute either approach are few. At this point, the veterinarian's clinical experience helps answer whether to rotate classes of drugs or use the same drug two times in a row.

Which is the best drug to use for the initial treatment of cattle with BRD is the most frequently asked question. As mentioned earlier, the broad-spectrum antimicrobials are all clinically performing well in our controlled research studies. Success is reflected by early detection of abnormal signs, most likely as a consequence of BRD and accurate dosing based on body weight using chute scales at the time of treatment.

Determining which drug to choose as the first choice is influenced by the risk category of the cattle and the cost-to-benefit ratio. The treatment protocol for high-risk stressed cattle generally includes a newer generation drug such as ceftiofur, danofloxacin, enrofloxacin, florfenicol, tilmicosin, or tulathromycin. In low-risk cattle, the first choice may be a less expensive broad-spectrum drug such as a long-acting oxytetracycline.

Use of adjunct therapies such as corticosteroids, nonsteroidal antiinflammatory drugs (NSAIDs), or B vitamins along with antimicrobial drugs is widely debated.[8,12,15] The most common medications discussed include dexamethasone, flunixin meglumine or phenylbutazone, and B complex vitamins. Corticosteroids and the NSAIDs decrease inflammation by blocking the enzymes involved in the arachidonic acid cycle and reduce fevers.[15] These medications commonly make the animal feel better, but physiologically this may not be the best choice. Corticosteroids also suppress the immune system. When corticosteroids are used, especially in multiple dosing regimens, the long-term response to antimicrobial therapy is usually less than expected.[12] Additionally, immunosuppression may cause recrudescence of latent bovine herpesvirus 1 infections, which can infect other cattle in a herd or group. NSAIDs do not have the immunosuppressive effects that corticosteroids do, and they do reduce fevers. Early intervention with NSAIDs may be beneficial, but this is not practical in most field situations.[13]

Injectable B vitamins have been administered in conjunction with antimicrobials to stimulate appetite and/or aide the rumen microbes. Scientific controlled research published in refereed literature is scant, if any at all.[7] At present, we do not include any adjunct medications with our choices of antimicrobial drugs for the treatment of BRD.

PREVENTION

The current method of raising, processing, and marketing beef cattle in North America results in severe stress and transmission of numerous respiratory pathogens among cattle. As long as this situation exists, complete prevention of shipping fever is probably not feasible. However, prophylactic treatment and vaccination can reduce morbidity and mortality.

Prophylactic use of antibacterial agents has become increasingly popular and was described earlier. However, the long-term implications of prophylactic use of antibacterial agents have yet to be determined; in particular, the prophylactic use of agents that are frequently used for therapy may promote the establishment of bacterial populations that are resistant to these agents.

Vaccines against *M. haemolytica* and *P. multocida* are available, and there is interest in using them particularly in cow-calf operations.[7,17] Most veterinarians would agree that vaccination of cattle against these bacteria on entry into the feedlot is too late to assist in prevention of shipping fever. Maternal antibodies against these two bacteria are short lived and usually reach undetectable levels by 30 to 90 days of age.[18] Therefore *M. haemolytica* and *P. multocida* vaccines can be given to young calves without fear of interference by maternal antibodies.

When designing a vaccination program for prevention of bovine respiratory disease, four questions should be addressed: (1) Should an *M. haemolytica* or *P. multocida* vaccine be used? (2) What type of *M. haemolytica* or *P. multocida* vaccine should be used? (3) How many doses of *M. haemolytica* or *P. multocida* vaccine should be given? (4) When should a *M. haemolytica* or *P. multocida* vaccine be given?

The specific *P. multocida* immunogens that are important for stimulating immunity in cattle against respiratory disease have not been identified.[17,19,20] Of potential interest as immunogens are purified *P. multocida* capsule, lipopolysaccharide (LPS), outer membrane proteins, and iron-regulated outer membrane proteins. *P. multocida* toxin, which is produced by serotype D *P. multocida*, can stimulate immunity against swine atrophic rhinitis. This toxin, however, is of little importance in preventing bovine pneumonic pasteurellosis because *P. multocida* serogroup D that produces the toxin is rarely isolated from bovine pneumonia. Preliminary experimental evidence favors outer membrane proteins as the major immunogens against *P. multocida*–induced bovine pneumonic pasteurellosis, and experimental vaccination of calves with outer membrane preparations resulted in significant reduction in lesions resulting from *P. multocida* challenge.[21] Two types of *P. multocida* vaccines are currently available for use against pneumonic pasteurellosis: bacterins and a live streptomycin-dependent mutant vaccine. The efficacy of these vaccines has yet to be well documented. However, several studies have documented that production data are better in cattle entering feedlots with anti–*P. multocida* antibodies than in those that had undetectable levels of anti–*P. multocida* antibodies.[22] Therefore vaccination of calves should be considered several weeks before shipment.

The specific *M. haemolytica* immunogens that are important for stimulating immunity in cattle are LKT, surface antigens, and possibly the sialoglycoproteinase that is present in culture supernate.[19,20] Surface antigens could include the capsular polysaccharide, LPS, outer membrane proteins, and iron-regulated outer membrane proteins.[19,20] Experimental data indicate that the most important *M. haemolytica* surface antigens are proteins, and these are most likely outer membrane proteins. Antibodies to capsular polysaccharide and LPS do not appear to play major roles in inducing immunity. Immunity to experimental *M. haemolytica* pneumonia has been induced with *M. haemolytica* vaccines that do not contain LKT; however, to be efficacious, those vaccines require an oil adjuvant.

In the past 15 years, good progress has been made in commercial *M. haemolytica* vaccine technology.[19,23,24] Various formulations of *M. haemolytica* vaccines are currently available including streptomycin-dependent live mutant,

bacterin-toxoids, and culture supernatant vaccines. Efficacy has been demonstrated primarily with experimental challenge methods using direct *M. haemolytica* challenge via intratracheal, intrabronchial, or transthoracic routes or using a combination viral/*M. haemolytica* challenge. Demonstration of efficacy against experimental challenge, however, may not necessarily indicate that the vaccine will be efficacious against natural disease.

In recent years, new approaches are being experimentally tested for improving *M. haemolytica* vaccines. Some of these include vaccines derived from AroA or LKT-mutated *M. haemolytica* or from bacterial ghosts. Use of those mutant vaccine strains of bacteria are in the experimental phases and have not yet been commercialized in North America. In addition, several studies have demonstrated that although vaccination with commercial vaccines can enhance resistance against experimental *M. haemolytica* challenge, addition of one of several *M. haemolytica* recombinant proteins including recombinant LKT, sialoglycoprotease, or outer membrane lipoprotein PlpE can enhance efficacy of the commercial product.[19,23,25-27] At this time, these recombinant proteins are not commercially available in *M. haemolytica* vaccines.

M. haemolytica vaccines should be considered in beef cattle that are to be shipped or to a lesser extent have recently been shipped. Several studies demonstrated an economic advantage to using a *M. haemolytica* vaccine in feedlot or stocker cattle or in cattle that had anti-*M. haemolytica* antibodies at shipment.[28] Even in studies where there was not a clear economic advantage to vaccination, vaccinated cattle usually had reduced morbidity and mortality compared with nonvaccinated cattle.

Determination of which vaccine to use is difficult. In general, traditional *P. multocida*/*M. haemolytica* bacterins that do not contain an LKT toxoid have not been shown to be efficacious. Experimental and field studies with several of the "new-generation" vaccines such as One Shot, Presponse, Pulmoguard, or Once PMH demonstrated efficacy in many of the trials.[24] These vaccines stimulate antibodies to *M. haemolytica* LKT, surface proteins, and in some cases other antigens present in culture supernatants such as sialoglycoprotease. Once PMH contains *P. multocida* and several of the other vaccines can be obtained with *P. multocida* and *H. somni* components. One of these newer vaccines should be considered as part of a bovine respiratory disease prophylaxis program. However, because once PMH is a live bacteria, concurrent use of prophylactic/metaphylactic antibiotics might lower antibody responses to the bacteria.

The use of one dose of *M. haemolytica* vaccine became the industry standard several years ago, when One Shot was introduced. Since then several other vaccines have been introduced or relicensed for use as a single injection. Experimental studies demonstrated that one injection of experimental *M. haemolytica* vaccine stimulated significant protection against challenge, and that protection was no different than that induced by two doses of vaccine administered 1 week apart. The reason that one dose of vaccine stimulates protective immunity, as well as two doses, is that by the time the maternal antibodies decline, most cattle develop *M. haemolytica*– and *P. multocida*–specific antibodies from natural exposure to nasopharyngeal bacteria.[18,20,29] Therefore the first vaccination with a *M. haemolytica* vaccine stimulates an anamnestic response secondary to natural exposure.

Timing of vaccination is a critical issue in management of feedlot and stocker cattle respiratory disease. Evidence indicates that cattle entering a feedlot with preexisting serum antibody titers to *M. haemolytica* have less respiratory disease and fewer deaths than those without serum antibodies. Therefore cattle should be vaccinated against *M. haemolytica* while on the farm of origin, approximately 2 to 3 weeks before shipment. Studies have indicated that one injection of a commercial *M. haemolytica* vaccine stimulates maximum serum antibody titers 2 to 3 weeks after vaccination.[19,30] Those titers, however, rapidly decline to baseline by 6 weeks after vaccination. Vaccination of cattle against *M. haemolytica* and *P. multocida* at the time of shipping or on arrival at the feedlot does not allow enough time for development of immunity, before the period of highest morbidity; however, results in several field trials indicate that this practice may afford some protection against BRD.

References

1. Welsh RD, Dye LB, Payton ME et al: Frequency of isolation and antimicrobial susceptibilities of bacterial pathogens from bovine pneumonia: 1994-2002, *J Vet Diag Invest* 16:426-431, 2004.
2. Aubry P, Warnick LD, Guard CL et al: Health and performance of young dairy calves vaccinated with a modified-live *Mannheimia haemolytica* and *Pasteurella multocida* vaccine, *J Am Vet Med Assoc* 219:1739-1742, 2001.
3. Frank GH, Briggs RE, Loan RW et al: Respiratory tract disease and mucosal colonization by Pasteurella haemolytica in transported cattle, *Am J Vet Res* 57:1317-1320, 1996.
4. Ackermann MR, Brogden KA: Response of the ruminant respiratory tract to *Mannheimia (Pasteurella) haemolytica*, *Microbes Infect* 2:1079-1088, 2000.
5. Czuprynski CJ, Leite F, Sylte M et al: Complexities of the pathogenesis of *Mannheimia haemolytica* and *Haemophilus somnus* infections: challenges and potential opportunities for prevention? *Anim Health Res Rev* 5:277-282, 2004.
6. Jeyaseelan S, Sreevatsan S, Maheswaran SK: Role of *Mannheimia haemolytica* leukotoxin in the pathogenesis of bovine pneumonic pasteurellosis, *Anim Health Res Rev* 3:69-82, 2002.
7. Apley M: Bovine respiratory disease: pathogenesis, clinical signs and treatment in lightweight calves, *Vet Clin North Am Food Anim Pract* 22:399-411, 2006.
8. Hjerpe CA: Clinical management of respiratory disease in feedlot cattle, *Vet Clin North Am Food Anim Pract* 5:119-142, 1983.
9. Jensen R, Pierson RE, Braddy PM et al: Shipping fever pneumonia in yearling feedlot cattle, *J Am Vet Med Assoc* 169:500-506, 1976.
10. Mosier DA: Bacterial pneumonia, *Vet Clin North Am Food Anim Pract* 13:483-493, 1997.
11. Noffsinger T: Lung auscultation and sick calf management, Proc Acad Vet Consult 30XIV:19-34, 2006.
12. Apley M: Ancillary therapy of bovine respiratory disease, *Vet Clin North Am Food Anim Pract* 13:575-592, 1977.
13. Clarke CR, Burrows GE, Ames TR: Therapy of bovine bacterial pneumonia, *Vet Clin North Am Food Anim Pract* 7:669-694, 1991.
14. Apley M: Antimicrobial therapy of bovine respiratory disease, *Vet Clin North Am Food Anim Pract* 13:549-574, 1977.
15. Cusach PMV, McMeniman N, Lean IJ: The medicine and epidemiology of bovine respiratory disease in feedlots, *Aust Vet J* 81:480-487, 2003.
16. Ives S: *Practical application of post-treatment intervals in feedlot, Proc Acad Vet Consult* 30XIV:71-81, 2006.
17. Confer AW, Fulton RW: Evaluation of *Pasteurella* and *Haemophilus* vaccines, *Bov Proceed* 27:136-141, 1995.
18. Prado ME, Confer AW, Prado TM: Maternally- and naturally-acquired antibodies to *Mannheimia haemolytica* and *Pasteurella multocida* in beef calves, *Vet Immunol Immunopathol* 111:301-307, 2006.
19. Confer AW: Immunogens of *Pasteurella*, *Vet Microbiol* 37:353-368, 1993.
20. Shewen PE: Host response to infection with HAP: implications for vaccine development. In Donachie W, Lainson FA, Hodgson JC, editors: Haemophilus, Actinobacillus *and* Pasteurella, London, 1995, Plenum, pp 165-171.
21. Prado ME, Dabo SM, Confer AW: Immunogenicity of iron-regulated outer membrane proteins of *Pasteurella multocida* A:3 in cattle: molecular characterization of the immunodominant heme acquisition system receptor (HasR) protein, *Vet Microbiol* 105:269-280, 2005.
22. Fulton RW, Cook BJ, Step DL et al: Evaluation of health status of calves and the impact on feedlot performance: assessment of a retained ownership program for post weaning calves, *Can J Vet Res* 66:173-180, 2002.
23. Confer AW, Ayalew S, Montelongo M et al: Immunogenicity of *Mannheimia haemolytica* serotype 1 recombinant outer membrane protein PlpE and augmentation of a commercial vaccine, *Vaccine* 21:2821-2829, 2003.
24. Mosier DA, Panciera RJ, Rogers DP et al: Comparison of serologic and protective responses induced by two *Pasteurella* vaccines, *Can J Vet Res* 62:178-182, 1998.
25. Conlon JA, Shewen PE, Lo RY: Efficacy of recombinant leukotoxin in protection against pneumonic challenge with live *Pasteurella haemolytica* A1, *Infect Immun* 59:587-591, 1991.
26. Shewen PE, Lee CW, Perets A et al: Efficacy of recombinant sialoglycoprotease in protection of cattle against pneumonic challenge with *Mannheimia (Pasteurella) haemolytica* A1, *Vaccine* 21:1901-1906, 2003.
27. Confer AW, Ayalew S, Panciera RJ, Montelongo M, Wray JH. Recombinant *Mannheimia haemolytica* serotype 1 outer membrane protein PlpE enhances commercial *M. haemolytica* vaccine-induced resistance against serotype 6 challenge, *Vaccine* 24:2248-2255, 2006.
28. Perino LJ, Hunsaker BD: A review of bovine respiratory disease vaccine field efficacy, *Bov Praction* 31:59-66, 1997.
29. Hodgins DC, Shewen PE: Serologic responses of young colostrum fed dairy calves to antigens of *Pasteurella haemolytica* A1, *Vaccine* 16:2018-2025, 1998.
30. Confer AW, Fulton RW, Clinkenbeard KD et al: Duration of serum antibody responses following vaccination and revaccination of cattle with non-living commercial *Pasteurella haemolytica* vaccines, *Vaccine* 16:1962-1970, 1998.

CHAPTER 42

Viral Diseases of the Bovine Respiratory Tract

ROBERT W. FULTON

Viral infections of the bovine respiratory tract represent significant pathogens. These infections are manifested by various clinical signs and lesions in bovine respiratory disease (BRD) with varying morbidity; mortality; loss of production (treatment costs, reduced weight gain, and carcass value); and lowered economic return to the producer. The principal viruses in BRD have historically and by emphasis on vaccination centered on bovine herpesvirus-1 (also referred to as *infectious bovine rhinotracheitis virus* [IBRV], *parainfluenza-3 virus* (PI-3V), *bovine respiratory syncytial virus* (BRSV), and *bovine viral diarrhea virus* (BVDV).[1-12] Also, bovine adenovirus (BAV) and, more recently, bovine coronaviruses (BCV) have been included.[6,13-15]

Viruses in BRD may cause primary infection with disease, either singly or in combination with other viruses. A significant role for viruses in BRD is their interaction with bacteria and *Mycoplasma* spp. in bacterial pneumonias.[8-12] These severe bacterial pneumonias are caused by *Mannheimia haemolytica, Pasteurella multocida,* and *Histophilus somni. Mycoplasma bovis* represents another agent observed in these severe bacterial pneumonias often initiated by primary viral infections.

Mechanisms by which primary viral infections compromise the host, allowing for severe bacterial pneumonias, are fourfold: (1) upper respiratory tract damage to nasal mucosal epithelial cells and altered mucociliary clearance, as well as bacterial attachment, growth, and colonization; (2) tracheal mucosal epithelial cell damage reducing effectiveness of the mucociliary apparatus, compromising clearance resulting in bacterial attachment, growth, and colonization; (3) innate defenses of the airways and lung are suppressed by viral infections through damage or depletion of macrophages and neutrophils (major phagocytic cells in host defense); and (4) acquired immune system effectors such as the T-cell (cell mediated) and B-cell (humoral) suppression. These immunosuppression effects on the T-cell and B-cell systems are major risk factors caused by selected viruses with BVDV as a prime example.

Bovine respiratory tract infections occur in most types of cattle operations: postweaned beef calves going to stocker operations for forage or to feedlots directly; feeder cattle, often after grazing forage to feedlots; and dairy calves. BRD with infectious etiologies is more often observed in young rather than adult cattle. On occasion, adult cattle with BHV-1 or BRSV disease are reported.

The viruses, except for BHV-1 and BVDV, are primarily surface infections of the epithelial cells throughout the respiratory tract from the nasopharyngeal mucosa to the lungs. BHV-1 and BVDV are often associated with systemic spread of the virus, as manifested by fetal infections in susceptible females. Young calves are especially susceptible to viral infections because their maternally derived immunity from colostrum is reduced with age.[16] Calves held under stressful conditions such as markets, commingling during marketing and shipment, inadequate nutrition, overcrowding, and severe climatic changes are more prone to BRD. Often calves fresh from closed herds of the ranch operation are highly susceptible as they enter the marketing channels and are commingled with other calves, facilitating the spread of the viruses. Viruses are shed primarily in respiratory secretions of the nose, eyes, and sometimes feces. Direct or close contact with animals' infectious secretions are major modes of transmission. The morbidity rate and mortality rate (case fatality) are often low but can be much higher depending on the bacterial agents such as *M. haemolytica, P. multocida, H. somni,* or *Mycoplasma* spp. (*M. bovis*).

The diagnosis of specific etiologic agents requires the use of diagnostic laboratory tests.[7,17] Gross lesions suggest certain etiologies; however, multiple agents may produce similar lesions. In addition, polymicrobial infections may produce the same or similar sets of lesions in affected cattle. Microscopic lesions observed histopathologically sometimes provide strong indications for an agent or perhaps families of viruses. For example, intranuclear inclusions are found in *alphaherpesviruses* such as BHV-1 and intracytoplasmic inclusions are found in paramyxoviruses such as PI-3V. However, absence of these inclusions does not rule out those agents because the inclusions may be minimal in number and tissues submitted may be inappropriate to represent viral tropism.

The clinician should consult with the diagnostic laboratory staff for the tissue submission relative to the clinical syndrome, as well as available tests. It is important that tissue sample collection and shipment be done after discussions with laboratory personnel. Certain tissues and samples require selected conditions such as freezing, fixatives, and collection with anticoagulant for blood cells. Current shipping regulations for formalin must be observed. Adequate identification of samples and submission forms assists diagnostics laboratory personnel by providing recorded history and case records. In cases with potential legal implications, recording animal ID and vaccine serial numbers with expiration dates is useful. Likewise, a precise history of antimicrobial use including dates, dosage used (mg/kg), route of administration, and date/time of last dose should be recorded, especially when culture and antimicrobial susceptibilities are requested. The clinician should also be aware of the appropriate state laboratory, if not the veterinary diagnostic laboratory, providing rabies testing. Ideally and, if feasible, the animal to be examined could be submitted directly to the veterinary diagnostic laboratory. Often collecting samples from multiple animals or submitting multiple animals provides additional information to determine the etiology of involved agents.

VIRUS ISOLATION

Viral isolations in cell cultures are time consuming and often financially expensive to perform. Sample collection and shipment conditions such as freezing are important. Multiple passages (two to three passes) may be required. A limiting factor is the available cell lines in which the viruses are isolated. Some viruses require specific cell lines as evidenced by bovine coronaviruses.[6,15] BRSV isolation by cell culture is difficult, with reduced success associated with freezing and shipment. Ideally the viruses should cause a visible cytopathic effect (CPE) in cell culture somewhat unique for the viral family. Yet common viruses such as most BVDVs (>90%) are noncytopathic (NCP), yielding no visible cytopathologic changes in cell culture. The agent preliminarily identified in cell culture requires confirmation by neutralization with monospecific antiserum/monoclonal antibody or primary binding assays with antiserums/monoclonal antibody such as immunoperoxidase, immunohistochemistry (IHC), enzyme-linked immunosorbent assays (ELISA), fluorescent antibody assays, or immunoelectromicroscopy.

ELECTRON MICROSCOPY

Nasal swabs and fecal samples are often examined by electron microscopy. Viral families may have unique morphologies indicating a viral family. However, confirmatory tests such as immunoelectromicroscopy, as cited earlier, are required to identify the specific agent.

VIRAL ANTIGEN TESTS

Immunofluorescence has been used for several years by the diagnostic laboratory, particularly when monospecific antiserums and proper controls are used. These tests are performed on fresh tissues. More recently the use of immunohistochemistry (IHC) has largely replaced immunofluorescence. The IHC can be performed on fixed formalin tissues. Most diagnostic laboratories have moved to IHC, especially with more available monospecific antiserums or monoclonal antibodies.

In recent years, antigen capture ELISA (ACE) assays have been developed and used both in state/university laboratories and private commercial laboratories. An example is the ACE assay for BVDV using fresh ear notches in PBS for detection of BVDV antigen. The ACE test detects the broad group of BVDV, but confirmation of BVDV types requires neutralization tests or genomic-specific tests such as polymerase chain reaction (PCR).

MOLECULAR DIAGNOSTICS FOR VIRAL GENOMIC MATERIAL

Currently with the known genomic sequences available, the detection of specific viruses can be made by polymerase reaction (PCR) for both RNA and DNA viruses. Initially the reverse transcription-PCR (RT-PCR) was commonly used for BVDV and other RNA viruses. As technology is available to the diagnostic laboratory, procedures such as real-time PCR are now commonplace for viral diagnosis. Viruses difficult to isolate in cell culture such as BRSV are now commonly identified by PCR. Rapid turnaround in hours versus days/weeks in cell culture is an advantage for PCR. The clinician should remain in contact with the diagnostic laboratory on the molecular diagnostic tests available; likewise, the diagnostic laboratory should explore this technology for its service.

SEROLOGIC TESTING

Diagnosis of an active infection with field strains of virus or response to vaccination with killed or modified live virus (MLV) strains can be made by detecting changes in antibody titers in acute to convalescent serum samples. An acute sample should be collected as early as possible in the course of infection/disease, and the convalescent sample 3 to 4 weeks later. It is appropriate to sample multiple animals from the same group, ideally with samples from both apparently healthy and diseased animals. A rise in antibody titer to the specific virus indicates exposure to that agent. A fourfold rise in antibody titer indicates an active infection when the microtiter virus neutralization (VNT) is used. The VNT in cell culture is routinely used for BHV-1, PI-3V, BRSV, and BVDV antibody testing. Recently some laboratories have incorporated ELISA tests for antibodies. The serologic testing for viral infections is both labor and time consuming. Plus time must evolve to get the acute and convalescent samples. Thus serology is retrospective at best and must be well planned to provide useful information. Often both diagnosticians and clinicians are frustrated when only one sample is available for the disease episode.

The prevention and control of viral infections of the respiratory tract focus on biosecurity and vaccination and, where possible, preventing exposure before immunity is established. Few, if any, antivirals are available for treatment of affected animals. When possible, vaccines are used in susceptible calves and selected vaccines are given to cows to boost transfer of immunity to the newborn.

BOVINE HERPESVIRUS-1

Bovine herpesvirus-1 (BHV-1) was first observed in the United States as an acute upper respiratory tract disease in cattle.[18] However, the first description of the disease was from Europe and was a vulvovaginitis in females.[19] Attention is often given to the change in management with large cattle populations in the changing feedlots, along with increased size of dairies resulting in cattle in close proximity, facilitating spread of the virus. Manifestations of the BHV-1 clinical disease include respiratory tract disease, genital tract disease of the superficial surfaces, conjunctivitis, abortion, encephalitis, and generalized disease in the neonate. Researchers readily propagated the virus in cell culture, which led to development of vaccines relatively soon after the disease was characterized in the United States.[20,21] Because of potential losses for BHV-1–induced respiratory disease and abortions, BHV-1 vaccination programs are common in U.S. beef and dairy operations.

Etiology/Epidemiology

BHV-1 is a member of the viral family *herpesviridae,* subfamily *alphaherpesviridae.*[19] Three subtypes exist: BHV-1.1, BHV-1.2a, and BHV-1.2b. The BHV-1.1 are usually associated with respiratory and abortions, and BHV-1.2 is associated with genital tract infections.[19] A third subtype, BHV-1.2b, is not associated with abortion.[19] Experimentally the BHV-1.1 can cause genital infections. Likewise, BHV-1.2a can cause respiratory infections.[19] BHV-1.1, BHV-1.2a, and BHV-1 1.2b share antigenic properties but may be differentiated by restriction enzyme fragment polymorphisms (REFPs). A former term was *BHV-1.3,* which was from encephalitis cases. BHV-1.3 shares antigens with BHV-1.1 and BHV-1.2. Differences in the REFP enzyme profile exist between BHV-1.3 and the other subtypes, so this virus is now referred to as *BHV-5.*

BHV-1 infections are present worldwide in domestic cattle populations, both in beef cattle and dairies.[1] Goats are also susceptible, and other susceptible ruminants include the wild deer family members, water buffalo, and wildebeest. The disease occurs usually after recent additions to a herd, and the virus is transmitted to susceptible cattle.[1] The BHV-1 disease usually occurs after the calves have lost their maternal immunity. The disease is most common in cattle over 6 months of age.[1] The BHV-1 also survives in cattle recovering from primary infections with latency as a hallmark of the BHV-1 ecology.[1,19] The latent virus may be found in trigeminal and sacral ganglia with recrudescence later by stress or administration of corticosteroids.[1,19] After recrudescence/reactivation, the virus may be detected in nasal secretions with potential spread to contacts. Interestingly there may be an effective primary immune response acquired after natural infection or vaccination to control reexcretion (shedding).[19] A secondary immune response boosted by reactivation may also inhibit reexcretion.[19] Animals with high antibody BHV-1 titers (neutralizing) before reactivation did not reexcrete virus after reactivation treatment.[22] Cattle receiving MLV BHV-1 vaccines may also have latent infections with the vaccinal strains.[1,19] The host immunity to BHV-1 has been extensively studied with both T cells (cell-mediated immunity [CMI]) and B cells (humoral/antibodies) important in recovery and prevention on reexposure.[1,19]

Clinical Forms

Respiratory

The respiratory form may range from mild to severe disease. Also, inapparent infections may occur with later potential manifestations as abortions.[1] The respiratory form often occurs after new additions to a herd. The disease can be severe with morbidity up to 100% and a case fatality rate approaching 10%.[1] The disease severity is often due to other infections including *M. haemolytica, P. multocida, H. somni,* and/or *Mycoplasma* spp. The high transmissibility is evident—infectious virus may exceed 10^7 plaque-forming units in the nasal sections at peak shedding.[23] The viral shedding peaks at 3 to 6 days postinfection with clearance by day 12 to 14 after infection.[24] A relatively low dose of 10^3 to 10^4 infectious viral particles may cause infection; thus the virus may spread rapidly among susceptible cattle exposed to the animal shedding virus in close proximity.[25]

Clinical signs include fever, rhinitis, conjunctivitis, inappetence, and labored breathing. In dairy cattle, milk production may drop. Severe hyperemia of the muzzle and external nares may be evident, hence the term "red nose."[1,6,7] Pustules and diphtheritic plaques may be observed in the nasal mucosal of the external nasal passages. The cattle may survive the acute infection and disease, but if the respiratory disease does not resolve in 5 to 10 days, it is likely that secondary invaders may be responsible for severe pneumonia. The resulting death is most likely due to the pneumonia caused by the bacterial invaders. On occasion there can be cases of BHV-1 respiratory disease in feedlot cattle several weeks after the initial processing. Often these cattle had received BHV-1 vaccines at feedlot entry and processing.

The diagnosis of BHV-1 specifically requires laboratory confirmation. The white necrotic plaques observed in the external nares are suggestive of BHV-1. Nasal turbinates and the trachea may have severe inflammation with an adherent necrotic exudate. Primary lung lesions are not a feature normally seen in BHV-1 diseased cattle. The diagnostic testing includes nasal swabs from sick cattle for viral isolation in cell culture. The BHV-1 is one of the most readily/easily isolated viruses in cell culture with distinctive cytopathology. The agent is confirmed by immunofluorescence, neutralization of infectivity, PCR, or ELISA. Lesion material submitted for histopathology, usually from the nasal turbinates and trachea, may have intranuclear inclusions in addition to inflammation and necrosis. The formalin tissues can be examined by IHC to detect the BHV-1 antigen.

Serology is of potential value in surviving cattle with the admonition for both acute and convalescent serums collected 3 to 4 weeks apart to detect rising antibody levels by the VNT.

Conjunctivitis

BHV-1 conjunctivitis can occur as the only organ system involved. Yet it can occur with the respiratory form.[7] The disease is sometimes referred to as "winter pinkeye" because early descriptions were obtained from dairy cattle in the winter months, not normally associated with the time of *Moraxella bovis* induced disease of summer and insect vector involvement. The main signs are conjunctivitis with bilateral hyperemia and discharge. Corneal opacities occur and are in the periphery near the corneal scleral junction.[26] This is in contrast to the central corneal opacities caused by *M. bovis.*[26] The diagnosis can be confirmed by viral isolation in cell culture using swabs from the affected eyes. Although conjunctivitis is the primary clinical sign, abortions can occur 1 or 2 months later.

Abortions

Abortions are relatively common sequelae to inapparent infections, respiratory disease, or the conjunctival form of BHV-1. Although a BHV-1 viremia is not easily detected in circulating leukocyte/monocytes, BHV-1 can infect the fetus in susceptible cows/heifers. The BHV-1 likely does not cause a viremia detected by viral isolation of blood leukocytes, but the virus may be detected by PCR in blood leukocytes.[19] Abortions can occur up to 100 days after initial infection.[1,7] The fetus is susceptible at any gestational age, yet most abortions occur after the fifth month of pregnancy. Abortions are usually observed at 4 to 8 months' gestation.[19] Susceptible females given most parenteral MLV vaccines containing BHV-1 may abort. Clinicians and owners must be aware of label indications because not all MLV BHV-1 vaccines are safe for pregnant female use. Aborted fetuses are usually dead when aborted with blood-tinged pleural and peritoneal fluids. The placental membranes may have to be removed manually. Diagnosis of BHV-1 is difficult in autolyzed fetal material, but when fresh placenta and fetal tissues are available to both histopathology and viral identification, diagnostic attempts can be rewarding. Intranuclear inclusions and focal areas of necrosis in the liver and adrenals are seen in BHV-1 abortions. The virus may be isolated from the placenta, fetal liver, and adrenals. Recently the use of contemporary BHV-1 reagents such as monoclonal antibody and IHC has enhanced BHV-1 abortion diagnosis. Serology using acute serum at time of abortion and a convalescent sample 3 to 4 weeks later in the aborting cow is unrewarding because the initial infection of the dam may have occurred as much as 100 days earlier, and thus she may already have seroconverted. Testing for BHV-1 antibodies in aborted fetuses is not useful because the fetus dies rapidly after infection, precluding immune stimulation with any detectable antibodies.

Genital Tract Infections

The genital tract form occurs in bulls and heifers/cows with the BHV-1.2 subtype.[1] Typically the acute infectious pustular vulvovaginitis (IPV) in the susceptible female occurs within 1 to 3 days of breeding by an infected bull.[1] Vesicles, pustules, ulcers, and plaques are observed on the mucosal surfaces of the vagina and vulva. The animals recover from primary infections in 10 to 14 days. Transient infertility may occur with subsequent bacterial infections causing metritis. The disease in bulls is similar to the female with incubation of 3 days with pustules, vesicles, and plaques on the penile and preputial mucosa (infectious balanoposthitis [IBP]). The virus may be isolated by cell culture using lesion material or swabs of affected lesions. Semen from infected bulls in the artificial insemination industry may contain BHV-1. Thus some AI bull studs may not permit entry of seropositive bulls as a precaution. Clinicians should be aware of such restrictions because BHV-1 vaccinations would likewise induce antibodies to BHV-1, as do natural field BHV-1 strains. Effective control of IPV and IBP because of BHV-1 by use of BHV-1 vaccines is

unclear as to the vaccine efficacy against these genital tract lesions.

Central Nervous System Disease

Both BHV-1.1 and BHV-5 are capable of causing CNS disease, primarily encephalitis.[19,26] A nonsuppurative meningoencephalitis, suggesting viral origin, is observed on histopathologic examination. Clinical signs vary but may include excitement, incoordination, circling, recumbency, coma, and eventually death. Including both BHV-1.1 and BHV-5 in the differential diagnosis with rabies without inclusions is important to distinguish BHV CNS disease from rabies, making viral-specific diagnosis imperative. BHV1.1 or BHV-5 CNS disease is most likely confirmed after rabies diagnosis is negative. Tests such as immunofluorescence or IHC usually do not differentiate BHV-1.1 and BHV-5. Either unique monoclonal antibodies or REPF enzyme differences are required.

Generalized Disease

Typical for *alphaherpesviridae* family members, BHV-1 can also cause generalized disease of neonate calves.[26] Affected calves are either exposed in utero or immediately postpartum. This fatal form is associated with fever, anorexia, respiratory distress, conjunctivitis, and diarrhea. This high-mortality disease is associated with lesions such as necrosis and ulcers of the digestive tract and possible other organs. Microscopic lesions of adrenal necrosis may be evident. It has been suggested that generalized disease among neonate calves may occur simultaneously to the concurrent abortion storms caused by BHV-1.

Prevention and Control

Treatment for any form of primary BHV-1–induced disease is limited by lack of approved antivirals. Use of antimicrobials to minimize bacterial invaders in BHV-1 respiratory diseases is relatively common. Genital tract disease is usually self-limiting, and after recovery, the females return to the breeding program. Affected bulls recovering from IBP are problematic for safe use in the natural breeding herd. The encephalitis and generalized forms are rare in occurrence and are largely dealt with in the differential diagnosis considerations of the respective organ system at necropsy.

Basic control of BHV-1 deals with biosecurity and vaccination. Where possible, cattle with signs of overt BHV-1 should not enter the herd; however, isolation on entry for 30 to 45 days would be compatible with other programs such as Johne's disease or BVDV prevention. Some countries and AI bull studs have moved to monitoring for BHV-1 by serology. Then the seropositive BHV-1 animals may be denied movement into these geographic regions or AI facilities. It is assumed that seropositive status indicates BHV-1 infection such as latency in CNS tissues. Potentially seropositive animals, when stressed or given corticosteroids, may undergo viral recrudescence resulting in viral shedding. However, using serology alone has its drawbacks for detection of potentially infected animals. Many animals have only a low BHV-1 antibody titer or no detectable antibody titer after recovery from field infections or vaccination. Thus relying solely on antibody testing may not be successful to detect latent infections.

In cattle operations and geographic regions (countries) with an already herd level of infection, the approach to controlling the disease is via vaccination.

More than 165 vaccines against BHV-1 are available in the United States for use in cattle.[27] Vaccination protocols for beef and dairy cattle in the United States routinely incorporate use of one or more vaccines against BHV-1. These vaccines are classified into five types: (1) MLV vaccines for parenteral administration (intramuscular and/or subcutaneous); (2) MLV, intranasally administered vaccines; (3) chemically altered, live virus, temperature-sensitive vaccine for parenteral use; (4) inactivated viral vaccines for parenteral use; and (5) a combination of parenteral BHV-1 MLV and inactivated BHV-1 viral vaccine. These vaccines may be single-component (monovalent) vaccines (e.g., BHV-1 alone) or may contain several immunogens including various combinations of BVDV types 1 and 2; PI-3V; BRSV, *Leptospira* spp., *serovars*; *H. somni*; *M. haemolytica*; *P. multocida*; and/or *Campylobacter* spp.

BHV-1 MLV parenteral vaccines induce both B-cell (humoral) and T-cell (cell-mediated) active immune responses after one dose of MLV vaccine.[28] Serum antibodies to BHV-1 along with BHV-1 specific CD4+, CD8+, and γδ T cells were detected after BHV-1 MLV vaccination.[28] Calves born to dams with circulating BHV-1 antibodies may absorb colostrum-derived maternal antibodies to BHV-1 and other viruses.[16] The mean half-life of viral antibodies to BHV-1 in calves receiving maternal immunity was 21.2 days.[16] Potentially, calves receiving passive immunity to BHV-1 may have reduced response to BHV-1.[29] Calves seronegative to BHV-1 were given BHV-1 neutralizing antibody intramuscularly and subsequently given MLV BHV-1 intranasally. The passive BHV-1 immunity via BHV Ig had a reduction on the efficacy of the MLV BHV-1.[29] The passively administered BHV-1 antibodies protected against viral shedding in viral-challenged calves.[29]

The MLV parenteral vaccines were the initially licensed for use in cattle for protection against BHV-1.[30] Vaccines are attenuated by multiple passages in cell culture and/or in heterologous species' cell cultures and often retain their ability to replicate in a susceptible animal, possibly causing a viremia. MLV parenteral vaccines are relatively inexpensive, offer a convenient route of administration, and stimulate a rapid onset of immunity (i.e., within 3 days of administration).[31-33] In general, one dose given to a susceptible animal stimulates protective immunity, which varies in duration depending on the clinical form of the disease challenge. Calves receiving a combination MLV vaccine including BHV-1 were protected for at least 126 days after vaccination as measured by protection against infection.[34] The MLV parenteral vaccines may cross the placenta and infect the fetus, causing abortion.[35] Most MLV BHV-1 parenteral vaccines are not approved for use in pregnant heifers/cows or nursing calves.[27] Recently companies have received label claims for BHV-1 and BVDV MLV vaccine use in pregnant cows providing they vaccinated with that line of vaccines within 12 months and to nursing calves provided their dams were vaccinated within 12 months.[27]

MLV intranasal vaccines generally can be divided into two types, based on the attenuation process: (1) those modified by passage in a cell culture[36,37] and (2) those modified by treatment such that they become "temperature sensitive"[38] (i.e., they do not replicate at internal body temperature). MLV intranasal vaccines stimulate protection in susceptible animals with only one dose, in contrast to the chemically altered MLV parenteral vaccines. The label directions for selected, but not all, MLV intranasal vaccines may indicate that they can be safely used in pregnant cattle.[27] These vaccines induce a rapid onset of protection (within 3 days of administration), possibly through interferon production and release into nasal secretions.[36] One benefit of MLV intranasal vaccines is that they stimulate immunity to mucosal surfaces of the upper respiratory tract, the portal of entry of the virus. Another benefit is their potential to immunize calves that are already seropositive because of maternal (humoral) antibodies passively transferred through the colostrum.[39] Animals vaccinated with the MLV intranasal vaccines may transiently shed virus in the nasal secretions and therefore might infect susceptible contact animals.[40]

The chemically altered BHV-1 vaccine strain for parenteral use was modified by nitrous acid treatment, which caused changes in the viral genome resulting in a strain (temperature sensitive) that is unable to replicate at normal internal body temperature.[41] Presumably, because of the limited viral replication, the vaccine requires two doses to stimulate immunity. Because it is temperature sensitive and should not replicate in the host, the vaccine can be used in pregnant cattle.[27,41,42] In one study heifers received two doses of the vaccine and were challenged with BHV-1 7 months later (at 6 months' gestation). These heifers showed a significant reduction in the number of abortions and stillbirths compared with controls.[42]

Inactivated viral vaccines are prepared by growing virus in cell cultures and then inactivating them with chemicals. An adjuvant is added to the inactivated strain to help stimulate an immune response. Inactivated BHV-1 vaccines require two doses (14-28 days apart) when used for the initial vaccination of susceptible cattle. Historically it has been thought that inactivated vaccines against viruses did not induce as long a duration of immunity as the MLV vaccines, nor did they confer protection against mucosal infections. Controlled studies are required to determine the duration of immunity induced by inactivated BHV-1 vaccines and MLV vaccines, both for respiratory disease and fetal infections. Disadvantages of inactivated vaccines are that the onset of protection may not be as rapid as with MLV parenteral or MLV intranasal vaccines and two doses are required. An advantage of the inactivated vaccines is that they can be used in pregnant cows and nursing calves.

Many vaccines are available for preventing and controlling the different forms of BHV-1 disease, and each vaccine has certain characteristics that should be considered when designing vaccination programs for various types of cattle operations and managements. Each vaccine also has both benefits and limitations. Probably more important is the management of the cattle for which the vaccines are used.

The MLV parenteral vaccines may infect the fetus if pregnant susceptible heifers or cows are vaccinated. Abortions have been reported subsequent to vaccination with MLV parenteral vaccines.[35] The MLV vaccine virus may also result in corpus luteum infection or disease. Experimental studies have indicated a reduced conception rate in susceptible cattle that received an MLV parenteral vaccine 3 to 4 days before or 14 days after breeding.[43,44] Clinical observations indicate that susceptible recipients used in embryo transfer (ET) may have delayed estrous after MLV parenteral (BHV-1 and BVDV) vaccine use and synchronization. It has been reported that pregnant cattle raised in contact with calves recently vaccinated with MLV parenteral vaccines had a greater incidence of BHV-1 abortion than those that did not have contact with vaccinates.[45] Consequently, the labels of MLV parenteral vaccines have usually stated that the vaccine should not be used in calves nursing pregnant cows. Recent studies, however, have shown that calves given an MLV parenteral vaccine did not shed virus in their nasal secretions nor did contact animals become infected with the vaccine virus.[46-48] Multiple companies have received label claims for MLV vaccines containing BHV-1 and BVDV for pregnant cows provided the cows had received the same line of vaccines with the MLV BHV-1 and BVDV within 12 months and/or before breeding. Likewise, these vaccines could be used in nursing calves if cows previously vaccinated with that line of vaccines according to the label. Veterinarians and producers should follow explicitly the label precautions for the respective vaccine. Another concern is that the MLV vaccine virus may recrudesce, with resulting shedding of virus in cattle either stressed or receiving corticosteroids.[49] Realistically, concern about transmission of BHV-1 to animals in contact with those receiving MLV parenteral vaccines would be negligible if the contact animals were properly immunized and immune to BHV-1.

Until the vaccine labels on most MLV parenteral vaccines are changed, MLV intranasal vaccines or the inactivated or chemically altered live virus vaccines are usually recommended for pregnant cattle or those near breeding. The exceptions are the approved vaccines for use in pregnant cattle and nursing calves. Vaccine recommendations should be weighed, with the benefits of vaccination as a guide and especially with the realization that properly vaccinated cattle are better protected when exposed to either field (virulent) or vaccine strains shed by vaccinated animals.

Cattle that are susceptible and likely to be exposed to BHV-1 should receive either an MLV parenteral vaccine or an MLV intranasal vaccine because both types induce immunity within 3 days of the initial dose. Rapid onset of immunity is desirable in such situations as stocker calf and feedlot operations, in which calves are transported long distances to pastures or feedlots, which stresses the animals and makes them more susceptible to infection. Such calves are also exposed to infection with BHV-1 from contact cattle in the markets. The drawback to inactivated vaccines is that two doses are required to obtain good immunity.

Controlled studies on the duration of immunity are limited. A degree of protection against challenge existed at 6 to 9 months after vaccination with an MLV intranasal vaccine or an inactivated vaccine.[50,51] A parenteral MLV BHV-1 MLV vaccine provided protection up to 126 days after vaccination.[34] Challenge studies for licensure are usually performed on calves within days of vaccination, at the time of peak immunity. Also, the challenge may be for only one form of disease, usually the respiratory type. Such challenges may detect only protection against a severe form of the respiratory disease. BHV-1 manifests itself in other forms such as abortions, neonatal disease, genital disease (male and female), and conjunctivitis. Yet little or no data are available about the efficacy of vaccines against these other forms of disease. For example, in one case the genital form of BHV-1 disease (infectious pustular vulvovaginitis) occurred in heifers that had received an MLV parenteral vaccine 5 months earlier.[52] Given the lack of duration of immunity studies for all BHV-1 vaccines individually and the cost of vaccines, breeding animals are usually vaccinated at least annually. In some feedyard situations the animals may be revaccinated during the feeding period. It is industry practice that feedlot cattle receive a monovalent BHV-1 MLV parenteral vaccine at reimplant time at approximately 100 days after arrival. There have been field reports of BHV-1 respiratory disease (IBR) in feedlot cattle after a few months of entry/processing, at which time they received MLV vaccines containing BHV-1.

The possibility exists that maternal BHV-1 antibodies acquired by the calf through ingestion and absorption of colostrum may interfere with vaccination. The level of these serum BHV-1 antibodies in the calf depend on the amount in the colostrum, amount absorbed, and half-life of the particular antibody; for BHV-1, 21.2 days.[16] Some calves receive no BHV-1 antibodies through the colostrum, or they may lose them within 1 month. Some calves, however, may have serum BHV-1 antibodies for up to 6 months after birth.[49]

Vaccination recommendations for neonatal calves include use of multiple doses of an MLV parenteral, an inactivated, or a chemically altered live virus vaccine or administration of an MLV intranasal vaccine. The maternal antibodies may block the parenterally administered MLV or inactivated vaccine. However, the MLV intranasal vaccine may still induce BHV-1 immunity.[39] Calves are often revaccinated at 6 to 8 months of age regardless of their prior vaccination history.

Molecular techniques of biotechnology have been applied to the study of vaccines and the response to vaccination (vaccinology). These advances are especially noted for herpesviruses including BHV-1. In addition to conventional vaccines manufactured via propagation of MLV and inactivated BHV-1 strains, current and future technologies offer opportunities for other vaccines.[53,54] These include subunit vaccines with a portion of the virus, deletion mutants with specific viral genomic fragments deleted, live vectored strains, DNA vaccines using plasmids, and plant-based vaccines. Deletion mutant BHV-1 vaccines as marker vaccines with selected glycoprotein genes deleted along with diagnostic tests for the deleted genes permit identification of vaccinates under control programs.[53] Recently needle-free delivery of vaccines has been developed and implemented.[53] By high-pressure gas delivery, vaccines may penetrate the skin and be administered intradermally, subcutaneously, or intramuscularly.[53] Such delivery is designed to minimize damage resulting from intramuscular injections. Two studies compared needle-free intramuscular injection of multivalent MLV vaccine containing BHV-1 with conventional subcutaneous injection via syringe in dairy calves and feedlot cattle. In both studies antibody titers to BHV-1 were higher at day 21 postvaccination than conventional needle injection.[55,56]

The best possible vaccine provides protective immunity in the host against infection (viral replication) when challenged, protects the animal against all forms of disease including multiple organ and systemic forms, and provides lifelong mucosal and systemic immunity. Ideally the vaccine recommendations would incorporate the results of field trials that are carefully designed to show the efficacy of the vaccine against a pathogen. Unfortunately little information is available, as can be seen by a review of the literature, for evaluating the field efficacy of the respiratory disease vaccines.[57] The summary of results was mixed for BHV-1 vaccines and for other respiratory viral and bacterial vaccines.

Calves may be vaccinated at weaning or 30 days before weaning. Calves vaccinated before 6 months of age should be revaccinated because the earlier vaccination may have been blocked by maternal antibodies. The MLV parenteral and intranasal vaccines require only one dose in susceptible calves, whereas the chemically altered live virus or inactivated vaccines require two doses. Although the labels for most MLV parenteral vaccines state that the vaccine should not be used if the calf is nursing a pregnant cow, the likelihood of infection of the pregnant cow may be minimal, especially if she is already immune. Yet as described earlier, MLV parenteral vaccines are available for use in pregnant cows and nursing calves.

Yearling heifers (12-14 months of age) should be vaccinated at least 1 month before breeding. Any of the vaccines may be used, but if two doses are required, the second dose should be given at least 1 month before breeding.

Pregnant cows may be vaccinated with a vaccine that has a label description permitting such use; these include MLV intranasal vaccines, chemically altered live virus vaccines, inactivated vaccines, and approved MLV parenteral vaccines. Generally one dose is used, primarily because of management considerations. Administering booster doses of the BHV-1 vaccines may have two conflicting outcomes as a result of booster dose stimulation of an increase in colostral BHV-1 antibodies, which are transferred to the newborn calf in the colostrum; consequently, (1) it may be beneficial to the calf to have increased BHV-1 serum antibodies for protection against BHV-1 disease, or (2) the calf may have longer duration of BHV-1 antibodies, which may block BHV-1 immunization. No multiyear-duration-of-immunity studies in vaccinated cattle challenged with virulent BHV-1 have been published. Because of the relatively low cost of BHV-1 vaccines and the need to vaccinate against other pathogens, many breeding cows are given BHV-1 vaccine annually.

Cattle to be shipped to forage pasture after weaning (wheat pasture or native grass) or to feedyards should be vaccinated 2 to 3 weeks before shipment. However, management practices and marketing may only permit vaccination at the initial collection point, market site, or stocker/feedlot delivery. All the major types of BHV-1 vaccines may be used, but those that require only one dose have two advantages: rapid onset of immunity and less handling required (one dose vs. two).

Cattle presented for purchase immediately before shipment, with no known vaccination history, pose a challenge. Presumably healthy cattle may be candidates for the one-dose MLV parenteral or MLV intranasal vaccines because these calves may benefit from rapid immunity. Cattle already infected with BHV-1 may not be protected by vaccination.

Cattle entering the feedyard usually receive either the MLV parenteral or MLV intranasal vaccine, particularly for the rapid onset of immunity. Cattle in the feedlot are routinely revaccinated later during the feeding period (at reimplant time) to ensure protection against possible BHV-1 disease occurring several weeks late in the feeding period.

Veterinarians should consult the breeding bull center for vaccination requirements of bulls, especially relating to export shipment and collection for artificial insemination (AI). Potentially the MLV BHV-1 vaccines including intranasal vaccines could induce latent infections and also stimulate antibody production.[58] Surveillance for BHV-1 includes serotesting, and potentially antibody-positive bulls could be disqualified for AI purposes.

BOVINE RESPIRATORY SYNCYTIAL VIRUS

Bovine respiratory syncytial virus (BRSV) is one of several viruses causing respiratory tract infection and disease in cattle. The BRSV infections range from inapparent and mild to severe respiratory tract disease.[2] The BRSV can be a single etiologic agent; participate with other viruses; and/or damage the respiratory tract disease, allowing secondary invaders entry and environment for more severe BRD with pneumonia. BRSV appears limited to the respiratory tract with no effects on reproduction and/or fetal disease.

Etiology/Epidemiology

The BRSV is a member of the genus *Pneumovirus* of the family Paramyxoviridae.[2] The virus replicates in cell culture, permitting cell culture propagation for serology, viral isolation, and vaccine production. Because this is an enveloped virus, it is susceptible to the environment and disinfectants. Sheep and goats are susceptible to BRSV but are not likely important as a reservoir for exposing cattle. An RSV for goats exists. Although there are possible antigenic differences among BRSV strains, they are believed to have one major antigenic type. Cattle are the reservoirs of infection serving as the source of exposure to susceptible cattle.[2,7] Numerous serosurveys indicate that BRSV antibody-positive cattle had not received BRSV vaccinations. In general the disease occurs in the younger cattle, 3- to 12-month-old calves. Aged/adult cattle with BRSV disease, either in feedlots or dairy cows, have been reported.[2,7] Spread of the virus is via infected respiratory tract secretions, and the virus can move quite rapidly in a susceptible population.

Clinical Disease

Infections with BRSV may be inapparent, cause primary respiratory tract disease, or cause damage to the respiratory tract with bacteria such as *M. haemolytica, P. multocida, H. somni,* and *Mycoplasma* spp.[2,7,8,12,59] Often in epizootics of BRD there will be seroconversions in both healthy and diseased cattle with no difference in seroconversion rates of both groups.[8,12,59] The BRSV infects epithelial cells from the nasal mucosa to the bronchi including the type II pneumocytes and alveolar macrophages.[2] Loss of cilia and necrosis of bronchial and bronchiolar epithelial cells occurs with BRSV infection. Similar to human RSV in infants, a hypersensitivity causing bovine respiratory disease has been suggested. Because of widespread use of killed and MLV vaccines, this hypothesis for severe disease was advanced. However, despite numerous experiments, this has not been conclusively determined to be a hypersensitivity affecting the bovine respiratory tract that results in clinical disease in cattle.

The clinical signs are limited to those of respiratory disease with fever, coughing, nasal discharge, and ocular discharges.[2,7] Severely affected cattle may have severe respiratory distress. Mouth breathing along with subcutaneous emphysema is observed on occasion. In some instances BRSV disease has been observed in late feeding periods in the feedlots. Attempts were made to implicate BRSV as a severe respiratory disease problem occurring late in the feedlot, atypical interstitial pneumonia (AIP). So far a clear connection of BRSV and AIP has not been established. Necropsy lesions in affected BRSV cases reveal a diffuse interstitial pneumonia with subpleural and interstitial edema.[2,7] Pulmonary emphysema may be present as well. Microscopic lesions may reveal multinucleated (syncytia) in the bronchiolar epithelium and lung parenchyma. Intracytoplasmic inclusions may also be present.[2,7] Often the bacterial secondary invaders may cause severe pathology resulting in bronchopneumonia or fibrinous pneumonia.

Diagnosis

The lesions, although suggestive of those caused by *paramyxovirus* family viruses, are not by themselves diagnostic for BRSV. The virus must be identified by viral isolation in cell culture from nasal swabs or lesion materials. However, the virus is quite labile and rarely isolated in cell culture. PCR tests in infected nasal swabs can detect BRSV.[60] However, better reagents assist use of immunofluorescence in tissues. More recently, IHC testing of lung tissues has increased the diagnostic capability for BRSV. Some laboratories have used human RSV ELISA kits to detect BRSV antigens. Serology using acute and convalescent serums may detect active infections as supported by a fourfold rise in titers in neutralization tests. Clinicians submitting samples to diagnostic laboratories should inquire beforehand about samples to be collected and shipping conditions.

Prevention and Control

Antibiotics to lessen effects of bacterial infections, and sometimes antihistamines, have been used for treatment.

The prevention of BRSV relies heavily on use of MLV and killed BRSV vaccines, and there are numerous vaccines in the United States, usually in combination with BHV-1, PI-3V, BVDV, and bacterial immunogens.[27] These multicomponent vaccines with BHV-1, PI-3V, BVDV, and BRSV are standard for vaccination programs in both beef and dairy operations. These BRSV vaccines are parenterally administered vaccines. No licensed intranasal BRSV vaccines are available in the United States. Most initial vaccine regimens use two doses, 1 to 4 weeks apart. Annual revaccinations are included in both beef and dairy operations. BRSV protection for both beef stocker operations and feedlot entry by routine vaccination is standard industry practice.

BOVINE PARAINFLUENZA-3 VIRUS

Bovine parainfluenza-3 virus (PI3V) is a relatively common infection in domestic cattle.[4,6,7] Similar to BRSV, BVDV, and other viruses, the PI-3 infections are both inapparent and sometimes associated with clinical signs and mortality with respiratory tract disease. The PI-3V should be considered both as a primary invader, but likely more importantly as a virus capable of compromising the bovine respiratory tract for secondary invaders. The PI-3V is limited to the respiratory tract causing no other diseases for the digestive tract, CNS, or fetal infections. The PI-3 virus immunogen is included in almost all killed and MLV bovine vaccines.

Etiology/Epidemiology

PI-3V is a member of the *Paramyxovirus* genus of the viral family Paramyxoviridae.[4,7] This RNA virus also contains an envelope and is thus susceptible to the environment and disinfectants. Cattle are the major host, although sheep, goats, and wild ruminants are susceptible.[4,6] This virus followed BHV-1 in its initial isolation in cell culture and characterization from cattle with BRD. This *paramyxovirus* is readily propagated in cell cultures with cytopathology, and it also causes hemagglutination with RBC. Virus neutralization tests and hemagglutination inhibition tests are used for serology.

Clinical Disease

The PI-3V is limited to respiratory tract infections with epithelial cells from the trachea bronchi and alveoli affected.[4,6,7] The ciliated epithelial cells are necrosed with resulting altered mucociliary clearance. Clinical signs include fever, coughing, nasal and ocular discharges, and altered lung sounds suggesting pneumonia. An incubation of between 24 and 36 hours with a subsequent fever with the previously mentioned clinical signs in a primary PI-3V infection with the calf usually recovering is the norm. However, as with other bovine viruses altering the respiratory tract, secondary invaders complicate the disease with often severe bacterial pneumonia. Interestingly, it is not unusual for healthy calves to seroconvert without BRD signs after arrival in facilities directly from the ranch. PI-3V infections often occur in both healthy and diseased cattle (unvaccinated) commingled for

30 to 35 days after sale barn acquisition and entering the feedlot.[8,9,12]

Diagnosis

Lesions in primary PI-3V respiratory disease are minimal with mild pneumonic lesions, interstitial pneumonia, and intracytoplasmic inclusion in various regions of the nasal mucosa to developing syncytia in the lung.[4,6,7]

The virus may be isolated in cell cultures from nasal swabs and lung tissues at necropsy. Immunofluorescence and IHC are also available to detect the viral antigen in affected tissues. VNT tests and hemagglutination inhibition antibody tests are available to detect rising antibody levels in acute and convalescent serums.

Prevention and Control

Prevention involves both killed and MLV vaccines using parenteral administered vaccines.[27] A limited number of MLV vaccines are given intranasally.[27] Experts have mixed attitudes about the pathogenic potential of PI-3V, with some referring to PI-3V as limited to inapparent infections or minimal signs or lesions. Yet PI-3V has been isolated from sick cattle and severe pneumonias at necropsy, albeit with secondary bacteria. The PI-3V vaccine immunogens were readily incorporated into the BHV-1 vaccines and subsequently with BVDV in the 1960s and remain there today along with BRSV. No adverse effects of PI-3 immunogens are apparent, and some proponents feel that the PI-3V vaccines may be beneficial.

BOVINE ADENOVIRUSES

Bovine adenoviral infections are likely evident in cattle populations worldwide.[13] Bovine adenoviruses (BAVs) have been found in both the respiratory and/or digestive tract in either inapparently infected or diseased cattle.

Etiology/Epidemiology

BAVs are members of DNA viral family Adenoviridae.[13] Ten recognized serotypes of bovine adenoviruses are available.[61] These are divided into two genera, *Mastadenovirus* and *Atadenovirus*. *Mastadenovirus* genus contains BAV1, 2, 3, 9, and 10 serotypes and *Atadenovirus* 4, 5, 6, 7, and 8 serotypes. These serotypes are based on viral neutralization tests. The Adenoviridae family is well known for infections in affected organs with intranuclear inclusion bodies. Based on serosurveys for viral antibodies, the BAV are quite common in cattle. As with BRSV and PI-3V, it is not unusual for calves held after shipment and commingled to seroconvert with no apparent disease and BAVs may be found in cattle with other viruses such as BVDV.[14]

Clinical Infections

Experts believe that with BAVs causing respiratory and digestive tract infections, respiratory secretions and feces could have infectious virus for transmission.[1] BAVs have been found in inapparently infected healthy calves, as well

as in selected cattle with respiratory disease or digestive tract disease.[13] Reports on field studies trying to establish disease potential for BAV are mixed. Experimental studies with BAV challenges have resulted in no lesions or limited respiratory or digestive tract disease lesions.[13]

Diagnosis

The diagnostic laboratory may find an occasional cell culture isolate with viral cytopathology in affected cells with both samples from healthy or diseased animals at necropsy, or possibly from nasal swabs or fecal samples. The lack of envelope on the agent showing resistance to ether or chloroform as lipid solvents points to adenoviruses, which lack an envelope. Sometimes antisera to BAV are available to confirm the virus, or electron microscopy may detect morphology of adenoviruses.

Prevention and Control

No licensed or marketed BAV vaccines are available in North America, nor does there appear to be justification to develop the BAV vaccines.

BOVINE CORONAVIRUS

Bovine coronaviruses (BCVs) were initially associated with neonatal calf diarrhea.[15] Then BCVs were identified with "winter dysentery" in adult dairy cattle.[7,15] Later BCVs were detected in respiratory secretions of infected calves with subsequent isolation from cattle with BRD signs. This isolation of BCVs from calves with "shipping fever" pneumonias led to the assumption that BCVs were a major etiology for BRD. In some studies other agents such as BRSV, BVDV, and PI-3V along with bacteria were also found in these severely ill cattle. No doubt BCVs are found in conjunction with other respiratory tract infections, yet their sole or primary BRD role has not been clearly established. Including BCV along with other bovine respiratory tract viruses contributing to BRD is best. Clearly, experimental reproduction of detectable and severe respiratory tract disease such as pneumonia would better make the case for BCV as a significant primary pathogen in respiratory tract disease in cattle.

Etiology/Epidemiology

BCVs are RNA viruses of the viral family Coronaviridae.[6,15] They are enveloped viruses, thus sensitive to disinfectants and the environment. It is not unexpected that cattle would have a coronavirus with tropism for the respiratory tract. Coronaviruses infect the respiratory tract of other species including humans, pigs, turkeys, and chickens. BCV infections in cattle are worldwide. Initially implicated in neonatal calf diarrhea, BCVs were also reported with etiology in "winter dysentery" of adult cattle. Subsequently BCVs have been isolated from the nasal samples of cattle undergoing respiratory tract disease.[62-66] Thus this virus has a purported role in both respiratory tract disease and enteric diseases. Only one serotype is recognized, but likely there is some antigenic variability.[15] The dilemma for working with BCV experimentally and diagnostic laboratories attempting to isolate the virus is that BCV replicates poorly or is quite difficult to isolate in standard cell cultures. A specialized cell line, a human rectal adenocarcinoma line, is permissive for BCV and has been used for virus isolation from feces and nasal swabs by selected laboratories.

The BCV is considered relatively common in enteric infections in both beef and dairy operations. The virus has been isolated from cells with disease including calf pneumonias, as well as beef cattle entering feedlots in various U.S. regions. The BCV was isolated from both healthy and sick cattle in these BRD episodes. And BCV was detected by seroconversions during the first month in feedlots in transported cattle.

Clinical Disease

The association of BCV with BRD has been primarily by the isolation of virus from nasal swabs of cattle with BRD signs and seroconversions to BCV. The virus has been found in healthy calves as well. Likewise, antibody testing has detected seroconversions in cattle in BRD cases. The clinical signs in the BRD cases are not unlike other BRD cases with viral etiologies present such as BVDV; PI-3V; BRSV; and other viruses with fever, nasal and ocular discharges, anorexia, and coughing. Typically these BCV isolations and seroconversions occur soon after arrival to the feedlot. As expected there is often involvement of secondary bacteria such as *M. haemolytica* and/or *P. multocida.*

Attempts have been made to demonstrate the pathogenicity of BCV for the bovine respiratory tract. After experimental challenge in young calves, the virus could be found in feces of diarrheic calves and nasal swabs for up to 5 days.[15] Respiratory disease signs occurred in only a few calves. Lesions of emphysema and interstitial pneumonia were evident in only a few calves.[67,68] For other studies, there are mixed reports of BCV detected in lung tissues of cattle with BRD, one report with no BCV detection in lungs of cattle with BRD,[6] and another detecting BCV antigen by immunofluorescence in respiratory tissues.[69]

Diagnosis

The virus can be isolated in cell culture provided that a unique cell culture is available to the diagnostic laboratory, the human rectal adenocarcinoma line (HRT-18).[15] The nasal swabs collected appear to be the choice of collections from live cattle for testing. An antigen capture ELISA originally used for detecting BCV antigen in fecal samples is also used by some diagnostic laboratories for BCV detection in respiratory disease samples. Also, BCV immunofluorescence is available to detect BCV antigen. Selected diagnostic laboratories and research units have used PCR to detect BCV in diagnostic samples. Use of electron microscopy could detect BCV in respiratory samples similar to the use of EM for fecal samples. Selected research laboratories have used ELISA tests for BCV antibodies, and in some selected studies they found seroconversions when paired samples were available. Clinicians should consult with their respective diagnostic laboratory for their testing for BCV.

Prevention and Control

Although there are licensed BCV vaccines for enteric disease protection, there are no licensed BCV vaccines in the United States to control respiratory tract disease in cattle. Treatment focuses on the use of antimicrobials to control the bacterial secondary infections. As in prevention of the neonatal enteric disease, it is assumed that adequate colostrum is available to provide protection in the young calf.

BOVINE VIRAL DIARRHEA VIRUS

Bovine viral diarrhea viruses (BVDVs) are a diverse group of viruses that cause infections in domestic ruminants worldwide. The virus is responsible for considerable economic losses from morbidity, mortality, loss of production (milk), reproduction losses, reduced feedlot performance, cost of treatments and prophylaxis, and cost of control measures. The infections range from inapparent to severe, with pathology involving single or multiple organ systems.

Two major aspects of BVDVs have brought the group of BVDVs to the forefront: (1) the presence of persistently infected (PI) cattle as the reservoir of infection; and (2) availability of tests such as the immunohistochemistry (IHC) and antigen capture ELISA (ACE) to detect PI cattle. These diagnostic tests permit more effective and timely identification and removal of PI cattle, minimizing virus exposure in susceptible cattle.

BVDVs often interact with other infectious agents contributing to substantial respiratory and digestive tract diseases. Together with fetal infections, these manifestations of disease have focused continual scrutiny for BVDVs in several forms.

Numerous detailed reviews/books of BVDV are available with considerable detailed information on BVDV. These references should benefit all clinicians, diagnosticians, researchers, and producers interested in BVDV.[3,70-73] For extensive and specific citations and references to the BVDV following coverage, readers should consult these extensive reviews/books.[3,70-73]

Etiology/Epidemiology

BVDVs are members of the Flaviviridae family, *Pestivirus* genus along with classical swine fever/hog cholera virus and border disease virus of sheep.[74-76] The BVDV is a single-stranded RNA of 12.5-kb length, translated into a polyprotein.[74-76] The protein is cleaved into individual proteins by cellular and viral proteases.

The four viral structural proteins are the capsid protein (C) and three glycoproteins of the envelope (Erns [ribonuclease], E1, and E2) at the 5' region of the viral genome (Fig. 42-1). These three glycoproteins (GP) are involved with the induction of neutralizing antibodies. The E2 (GP53) glycoprotein is considered the principal epitope for viral neutralizing antibodies. The nonstructural proteins (NS) are toward the 3' region of genome. The biotypes of BVDV are based on presence or absence of cytopathology in cell cultures, cytopathic (CP) or noncytopathic (NCP).[3,70-73] The NCP strains encode for an

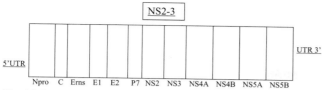

Fig 42-1 Bovine viral diarrhea virus genome and proteins encoded.

intact NS2-3 protein; however, the CP strains have the NS2-3 cleaved into separate NS2 and NS3 proteins. This is a molecular event separating the CP and NCP biotypes. Although not part of the assembled virion, the individual NS proteins may have functions including protease and polymerase activity. Genomic variabilities encode for these proteins, and there is diversity noted by monoclonal binding studies.[77]

The BVDVs are a diverse group, both by antigenic and genomic properties.[78-84]

Until recently in the United States, BVDVs were divided into two major genotypes, BVDV1 and BVDV2. In the United States there are three major subtypes: BVDV1a, 1b, and 2a. One isolate of BVDV2b in the United States has been reported from a feedlot case of fatal pneumonia.[11] Reports indicate that there are 11 subgenotypes of BVDV1.[85] The phylogenetic analysis of BVDV can be performed by analyzing genomic sequences of five different regions: 5'-UTR, Npro, E2, NS3, and NS5B-3'UTR.[86] Based on homology using a 5'-UTR region, there was 67.1% homology between BVDV1 (including BVDV1a and BVDV1b) and BVDV2a strains.[81] And there was 85.3% homology between BVDV1a and BVDV1b strains.[81]

BVDVs cause important and commonplace infections in domestic cattle worldwide.[3] In addition, other susceptible domestic species include sheep (also susceptible to the related border disease virus), goats, pigs, and a wide range of wild ruminants, as well as camelidae and cervidae species.[3] The most important reservoirs of the virus are the PI cattle. PI cattle are the result of susceptible pregnant cattle becoming infected between 42 and 125 days of gestation.[87] The infected fetuses are carried to term, born infected and immunotolerant to the BVDV strain causing the infection. The calves are lifelong shedders of the virus in all body excretions/secretions including feces. Animals with acute, transient infections shed virus at far smaller amounts and for a shorter time than PI cattle.[3]

The distribution of the BVDV subtypes in the United States has been reported in two groups of livestock: BVDV isolates from cases submitted to diagnostic laboratories and from PI cattle in various management schemes. The prevalence of BVDV biotypes and subtypes was determined in BVDV-positive samples from diagnostic laboratory accessions.[88] The results were 89.3% NCP strains, 8.4% CP strains, and 2.3% in which both CP and NCP were isolated. The distribution of the BVDV subtypes was 45.8% BVDV1b, 28.2% BVDV1a, and 26% BVDV2a. In a survey of Northwestern U.S. diagnostic laboratory accessions, there were 18.5% BVDV1a, 40.7% BVDV1b, and 40.7% BVDV2.[89] A survey of BVDV-positive samples from bulk milk and infected cattle indicated 49.1% BVDV1b, 11.3% BVDV1a, and 39.3% BVDV2a. [90] Thus it appears

that in the United States, BVDV1b is the predominant subtype in diagnostic laboratory cases.

The prevalence of PI cattle in the United States was reported in two surveys.[91-93] In a multistate study of 18,931 cattle, there was a PI positive rate of 0.17%.[91] Studies of prevalence of PI cattle entering feedlots indicated 0.3% and 0.4% BVDV PI.[92,93] The PI strains from a feedlot study indicated that BVDV1b was the predominant subtype; BVDV1b, 77.9%; BVDV1a, 11.6%; and BVDV2a, 10.5%.[93]

Transmission of BVDV is by direct or close contact with infected cattle (horizontal transmission).[3] Direct contact with infectious secretions or aerosols from PI cattle are the most likely sources of infection. In PI animals, BVDV is present in the serous secretory and ductular epithelium from the nasal mucosa to the lung, along with infected respiratory tract leukocytes.[94] The potential for iatrogenic mechanical transmission via infected veterinary instruments and rectal palpation was also suggested as a possible role for biting insects.[3] In reality, the large amount of virus continually shed by PI cattle is considered the most important source of BVDV.[3,93,95]

The BVDV may also be transmitted via infected semen or embryo transfer.[3] An important reason for monitoring the safety and purity of MLV bovine vaccines is that NCP strains, accidentally introduced into vaccines, have induced BVDV disease in susceptible vaccinates. The movement of BVDV in viremic heifers/cows to the developing fetus/oocyte or to the uterus can result in disruption of the fertilized oocyte's implantations in addition to causing developmental defects or PI individuals.

Clinical Manifestations

BVDV infections occur in cattle in various forms. Creating unique disease categories is therefore nearly impossible. The BVDV can cause single organ infections, involve several systems, and/or work in concert with numerous other infectious agents to cause disease. The BVDV has tropism for many organs including respiratory, digestive, lymphoid, reproductive tract, and fetus. Therefore it is overly simplistic to classify infections into specific diseases for BVDV, except for mucosal disease (MD) and PI calves resulting from fetal infections.

The role of BVDV in either synergistic or mixed infections is most likely due to its well-known immunosuppression. In the review by Potgeiter,[3] there are numerous references to the effects on the lymphoid organs and reduction in B cells, T cells, and neutrophils. Likewise, there may be a decline in T-helper and T-cytotoxic lymphocytes. In addition to immunosuppression in the bovine acquired immune system (humoral and cell mediated), the innate immune system of the bovine respiratory tract can be impaired by BVDV.[96]

Acute Transient Infections

As with many viruses, BVDV infections in the postnatal susceptible calf are most often inapparent. Numerous serologic surveys indicate the presence of antibody-positive cattle in the unvaccinated population. The young calf is usually the target of the BVDV after the loss of maternal antibodies. The mean half-life of passively acquired antibodies for BVDV is approximately 23 days.[16] The actual age the calf becomes susceptible to infection is thus dependent on the amount of BVDV antibodies absorbed from the colostrum and dose of virus.

Respiratory Disease

BVDV may cause primary respiratory infection.[97-99] Bovine viral diarrhea viruses may also occur in conjunction with other agents such as BHV-1, PI-3V, BRSV, bovine coronavirus, bovine adenoviruses, *M. P. multocida, H. somni,* and *Mycoplasma* spp.[8,9,11,99-103] BVDV infections can occur as inapparent infections in healthy cattle, as well as cause disease during episodes of respiratory tract disease.[9,12,104] The role of PI calves in respiratory disease, particularly in feedlots, is illustrated by the study with PI calves and their effect on calves in adjacent pens. The risk of treatment was placed at 43% due to exposure to a PI calf, and 15.9% of initial cases of respiratory disease were attributed to PI calves.[92] BVDV can be transmitted quite easily following exposure to a PI calf with 70% to 100% of susceptible, nonvaccinated cattle becoming infected with BVDV under feedlot conditions.[12,104] Also, the beneficial effects of BVDV immune cattle were shown where cattle with higher BVDV circulating antibody levels had lower respiratory disease morbidity rates, lower treatment costs, and lower treatment rates.[105]

Recently attention has been focused on the interaction of *M. bovis* and BVDV in Canadian feedlots including animals with joint disease.[102,103] Samples of lung and joint tissues from feedlot animals that failed to respond to antibiotic therapy were tested by IHC for several antigens including BVDV, *M. bovis, H. somni,* and *M. haemolytica. M. bovis* was found in 80% of the cases including 45% of the joints and 71% of the lungs. Infection with BVDV was found in more than 40% of the cases. *M. bovis* and BVDV were the most common pathogens persisting in the tissues of animals failing to respond to therapy.

Digestive Tract Infections

The digestive tract disease associated with BVDV may occur in almost any age group from neonate to adult. As described earlier, the postnatal calf after decay of colostral immunity appears most susceptible. The acute form is manifested by fever, anorexia, and depression along with ulcers/erosions in oral mucosa and tongue and, possibly, diarrhea.[3,70] Mixed infections with other enteric agents such as *E. coli, Salmonella* spp., Johne's disease, rotavirus, coronavirus, and cryptosporidia may exist. Lesions may be noted throughout the digestive tract but are not disseminated in all regions of the digestive tract in every case. Ulcers and erosions in the digestive tract occur frequently with the acute forms. Because of the affinity of BVDV for lymphoid tissues, Peyer's patches in the intestine are often involved.

The acute digestive tract diseases are most likely caused by the NCP strains of BVDV with exposure to the virus occurring in the postnatal animal. This is in contrast with MD discussed later.

Thrombocytopenia/Hemorrhagic Form

Another acute form of BVDV is the hemorrhagic syndrome.[106] This form is characterized by thrombocytopenia, bloody diarrhea, hemorrhages on visible mucosa surfaces, bleeding from injection sites, and death.[3,106,107] The NCP strains are the biotype involved. The mechanism of thrombocytopenia and bleeding is not clear. The hemorrhagic form is usually fatal and occurs in both calves and adults. Hemorrhagic syndrome is not believed to be a manifestation of persistent infection with BVDV.

Mucosal Disease

MD was thought by several investigators to be the "classical" form of BVDV with low morbidity and high mortality. MD is the result of a PI calf (by definition infected with NCP strain) developing disease (MD) after infection with a CP strain (closely related to the NCP strain). Infection with a CP strain may occur via exposure to CP strains circulating in cattle, but it most likely occurs when the NCP PI strain mutates to form the related CP strain.[70] The disease is characterized by severe digestive tract disease with ulcers and erosions throughout the tract, skin lesions, and hoof lesions (interdigital). The disease is uniformly fatal. Concern was that MLV BVDV vaccination may have contributed to MD. However, with such a low PI rate (<1% of cattle entering the feedlot) and almost all cattle at the feedlot receiving the MLV BVDV vaccines, there is an extremely low incidence of MD to support that connection to BVDV vaccine. Also, one study demonstrated that vaccination of PI calves with different MLV vaccines did not induce MD.[108]

Reproductive Tract Infections/Fetal Infections

The outcome of infection in the susceptible heifer/cow depends on the stage of the pregnancy. An excellent review of BVDV reproductive consequences gives numerous references to field studies, diagnostic laboratory reports, and experimental studies.[72,109]

Exposure to BVDV in the susceptible female shortly before breeding or early in gestation does have negative effects on conception and/or implantation of the fertilized ovum.[109] The mechanisms for the decreased conception rates are not clearly understood, but they may depend on the time of infection with respect to reproductive stage.[109] The ovary may become infected with BVDV, as has been noted in heifers receiving CP MLV vaccine, acutely infected cattle, or PI cattle.[110-112]

BVDV abortions may also result after infection during the embryonic stage of 45 to 175 days.[109] Other outcomes of fetal infections may occur during this interval, and abortions can occur after this as well. Both NCP and CP strains have been isolated from aborted fetuses.[109] Label indications for several current NCP and CP MLV BVDV vaccines in the United States indicate these products may not be safe in pregnant cows/heifers.[27] With a limited number of exceptions such as females being vaccinated before breeding and/or within the past 12 months, there are a few MLV vaccines approved for use in pregnant cattle.[27] Clinicians and cattle producers should follow the label indications explicitly for each MLV vaccine.

Fetal infections—persistently infected calves. Fetuses infected by an NCP BVDV between days 42 and 125 may survive and be carried to term, be born alive, and survive as a lifetime shedder of virus.[71,87] Not all fetuses exposed in this time frame will result in persistent infection; some may be aborted or develop congenital defect(s).[109] The CP strains cannot cause PI infections. The PI calf is the most important cattle reservoir of virus, shedding virus in all secretions/excretions. PI calves are immunotolerant to the infecting NCP strain and may respond by developing antibodies to heterologous BVDV strains including MLV vaccine strains.[108] However, infection of a PI calf with a closely related CP strain of virus could lead to MD and the eventual death of the calf.

Congenital effects. The fetus exposed between days 100 and 150 of gestation may develop congenital defects.[109] The defect depends on organ development when infected. A wide variety of defects may occur, with cerebellar hypoplasia in newborn calves the most documented or observed.[109] The affected calves usually die soon after birth or are euthanized. Diagnosis requires examination for gross and microscopic lesions. Other defects may include microencephaly, hydrocephalus, hydranencephaly, porencephaly, hypomyelination, cataracts, microphthalmia, retinal degeneration, optic neuritis, thymic hypoplasia, hypotrichosis, deranged osteogenesis, brachygnathism, and growth retardations.[109] Cerebellar hypoplasia calves have difficulty becoming ambulatory and may be ataxic with other neurologic signs, often resulting in death or euthanasia.[109] Clinicians should be aware of potential congenital defects because a variety of sequelae may occur if BVDV circulates among pregnant females. Not all pregnant females will be in the same gestational stage and, therefore, may not result in a specific outcome.

Late gestation infections. Fetal infections in late gestation may occur after organogenesis is complete and after development of the immune system (last trimester). These infections in the last trimester result in calves born with BVDV antibodies in the precolostral serum and without detectable virus as the fetal immune system clears the virus.[109] The term "congenitally infected" (CI) has been used for these virus-negative, BVDV-seropositive calves (at birth), and they appear to be at greater risk for severe illness than calves born antibody negative.[113] The extent/prevalence of these CI calves remains to be determined in cattle operations. Some years ago, the use of MLV BVDV vaccines in the last trimester (off label) was advocated by some to boost colostral antibodies in the dam. However, reports indicate negative effects of vaccine virus infecting the fetus when the dam was vaccinated with MLV BVDV in the last trimester.

Infections of the Bull

Semen of bulls, either from acutely or PI infected, may contain BVDV.[114-120] Bulls with BVDV in semen may sire calves, but their breeding efficiency may be reduced.[114,118] These bulls and their semen could infect susceptible females.[118,120]

Recently in the United States, BVDV was detected in testicular tissues by PCR up to 7 months after the seronegative bulls were infected with NCP BVDV.[121] The bulls recovered from the acute infection and subsequently became seropositive. Persistent testicular infection will have to be studied further to determine its role in transmitting BVDV to susceptible females. More recently, susceptible postpubertal bulls given an NCP MLV vaccine had prolonged testicular infection after recovery from the acute vaccinal infection.[122] The clinical implication of persisting vaccine virus (NCP) in the testes and its role in fertility remains to be determined. A commercial CP MLV BVDV vaccine protected bulls against the persistent testicular infection when exposed to an NCP BVDV strain.[123]

Diagnosis of BVDV Infection

The definitive diagnosis of BVDV in disease requires extensive use of specific laboratory tests. Although necropsy and histopathology may give strong indications of BVDV, other agents (predominantly viruses) such as foot-and-mouth disease virus, Rinderpest, and MCF may have features similar to BVDV. With keen awareness of exotic diseases, practitioners must consider these diseases along with BVDV as part of foreign animal disease surveillance in the United States. Bovine viral diarrhea virus infections may occur together with other bacterial agents with the pathologic changes often more representative of those other agents.

Lesions caused by BVDV may be present in some, but not necessarily all, affected organ systems.[3,70-73] Animals with digestive tract disease may have ulcers and erosions involving the oral mucosa, tongue, esophagus, rumen, omasum, abomasum, and the small and large intestines. Peyer's patches may be necrotic and hemorrhagic. Skin lesions may be seen in some MD cases with patchy hyperkeratosis around the neck, shoulder, and perineal regions.[70] Erosive lesions in the perineal area, prepuce, interdigital space, and coronary band may be evident in MD cases. Fetal lesions in abortions are difficult to detect because the fetus is often autolytic. Congenital defects are detected by characteristic gross and microscopic lesions.

Virus Isolation

Even with many available molecular diagnostic tests, virus isolation remains a standard laboratory technique. The challenge for viral isolation is to provide definitive answers in a timely manner. Often multiple passages in cell cultures are required. Thus an interval of 2 to 3 weeks may pass before the results are known from the viral isolation attempts. Acutely infected animals are best detected when peripheral leukocytes are collected in blood tubes with anticoagulant. The serums from acutely infected animals had virus in only 38.1% of cattle with virus in the blood leukocytes.[12] Thus the PBL/buffy coat is the preferred blood sample for diagnosis of acute infections using viral isolation. Nasal swabs from cattle with BVDV respiratory disease are often used for submission to the diagnostic laboratory to identify BVDV as an etiologic agent in BRD. In addition to BVDV, other viral agents could be isolated as well from the nasal swabs. Selected organ tissues collected at necropsy can be used as inoculum for viral isolation. Most BVDV are NCP: thus agent identification in positive cell culture cases is confirmed for BVDV antigen by fluorescent antibody tests, ELISA, or immunoperoxidase staining. Neutralization tests with monospecific BVDV antisera or monoclonal antibody are sometimes used. Likewise, CP agents are confirmed by these same tests.

Antigen Detection

Until recently immunofluorescent antibody was used to detect BVDV antigen, especially in necropsy tissues and infected cell cultures. The use of immunofluorescence and other antigen detection systems have been greatly enhanced by monoclonal antibodies. This holds true for various ELISA tests and IHC. Modifications of ELISA tests can confirm BVDV in cell cultures.

An antigen capture ELISA (ACE) test for BVDV has recently been developed and is being used worldwide. Originally designed to detect BVDV antigen in serum from PI calves, it is now used to detect BVDV antigen in the fluid from fresh ear notch samples collected in PBS.

The IHC test is also used for PI diagnosis but additionally can be used to detect BVDV antigen in formalin fixed tissues. The IHC test is widely used to diagnose acute BVD in postnatal cattle and fetal infections in addition to PI animal identification.

Polymerase Chain Reaction

Both reverse transcriptase polymerase chain reaction (RT-PCR) and real-time PCR are available in most diagnostic laboratories for detecting BVDV genomic material.[72] These tests are both sensitive and specific for BVDV. By definition, these PCR tests detect by amplification specific regions of the viral genome of BVDV. The PCR tests are completed in hours compared with several days for viral isolation. The PCR tests are used for bulk milk testing; nasal swab tests; and, most recently, for detecting BVDV in fluid from ear notches of PI calves collected in PBS.

Serology-Antibody Tests

The use of serology for BVDV antibodies is usually performed as a virus neutralization test (VNT) in cell culture. An active immune response to a virus, either as exposure to the agent or by vaccination, is quantitated by a rise in antibody levels. In the VNT a rise of fourfold or greater is an indication of infection. This measurement of the active infection requires an acute and convalescent set of samples 3 to 4 weeks apart. The acute sample should be collected as soon as possible in the disease. Most U.S. diagnostic laboratories use both BVDV1a and BVDV2a viral strains in their VNT. A growing number of laboratories include VNT testing for BVDV1b antibodies because it is the predominant BVDV subtype in several regions.

The use of serology is not helpful when only one sample is available in the postnatal animal. Likewise, paired sera from aborting cows are not rewarding because the infection may have occurred several weeks or months prior. Thus the so-called acute sample in abortion cases would likely already contain high antibody levels, which would not increase in the convalescent sample. When selecting animals to test in a disease outbreak, it is suggested that multiple animals be tested including both healthy and diseased animals.

In fetal infections the collection of a single serum sample may have diagnostic value. If a calf's precolostral serum is positive for antibodies to an infectious agent, it is presumed those antibodies were the result of an active infection by the fetus. Likewise, if fetal fluids are collected from an aborted bovine fetus and are positive for antibodies for the agent, it is considered that the fetus was infected with that agent. These assumptions are based on the understanding that the transfer of maternal antibodies in cattle is via colostrum and not transplacental during pregnancy.

The PI calf will be seronegative to the infecting BVD virus during its gestational life, but it could respond with an active immune response to a heterologous BVDV such as a natural field strain or vaccine.[108] Use of serology cannot be used as the sole criteria for PI status.

Attempts have been made to equate high antibody levels with natural infections as compared with antibody levels induced by vaccination. Experiences of our laboratory have indicated that the two types of exposure (vaccination versus natural infection) cannot be differentiated by antibody levels.[12,104]

Diagnosis of the PI Animal

Control programs for BVDV center on the identification and removal of the major source/reservoir of the virus, the PI animal. Numerous tests for BVD infectious virus and antigen are available. The applications for BVDV testing were summarized in a recent review article.[124] When attempts were made to diagnose PI calves several years ago, the virus isolation test was used with two samples collected 4 weeks apart. The criteria for PI status were that both samples had to be positive for infectious virus. Calves that were only virus positive in the first sample were considered acutely infected.

The presence of BVDV antigen detected by IHC in the epidermis of skin samples such as ear notches has been used as criteria for PI status.[125] These samples were from those submitted for IHC in formalin fixed tissues. Selected diagnostic laboratories may request a second sample for IHC after the first positive IHC test. However, in at least three studies one positive IHC from fixed notches was suitable criteria for PI status.[92,93,126] This approach was confirmed when acutely infected animals were tested by the IHC and found to be IHC negative.[104]

The use of the ACE test detecting BVDV antigen in the fluids of the fresh notches is available now in state diagnostic and commercial laboratories. Recently, a variety of tests were evaluated in PI cattle entering a feedlot.[93] Positive ACE samples were detected in PI calves when compared with concurrent samples for IHC.[93] A limited number of low ACE positives (<5%) were IHC negative. Such low ACE positives should be retested. The ACE test for BVDV was negative in fresh notches in all acutely infected animals.[104] Thus a negative ACE test is expected for acutely infected cattle. In another study of five diagnostic methods for BVDV, only PI calves were positive in skin samples by IHC and ACE test.[127]

In some studies pooling of samples and screening either by ACE in fresh notches or RT-PCR will detect a positive in a pool of several samples.[128-130] The positive pool members were then tested individually by the ACE test to identify the individual positive animals.[129,130] The number of individual samples present in the pooled samples with positive PCR assay results ranged from 50 to 100.[130] Screening cattle using pooled samples is an attempt to reduce the cost of testing. The sensitivity of the ACE test using pooled saline from two notches was less than 100%.[128] Increasing the pool size for the ACE test will decrease the sensitivity.[128] Likewise, another study reported that pooling with 10 samples, 1 positive and 9 negative (1:10), could result in failure to detect 10% of the PI samples and pooling of 100 samples could result in 50% failure to detect a positive.[131]

Veterinarians electing to test for PI cattle should consult their diagnostic laboratory for the tests being offered. Most state diagnostic laboratories offer both the IHC and ACE on notches. Most laboratories adhere strictly to the U.S. Department of Agriculture (USDA)–approved protocol of one animal, one test for the ACE test. A limited number of state diagnostic laboratories and commercial laboratories offer pooled ear notch testing using PCR.

Prevention and Control

The principles for controlling BVDV are similar to those for other diseases such as BHV-1 and Johne's disease. No antiviral treatments are used for BVDV for PI or acutely infected cattle. This section centers on biosecurity and appropriate use of vaccines.

Biosecurity

The introduction of BVDV into a susceptible herd is often by addition of infected cattle. The principal source of virus is a PI animal. Thus a PI animal such as a bull, cow/heifer, or stocker animal could be the source of infection entering a susceptible operation. Direct fence line contact with PI animals has been reported. PI cattle in a feedlot can affect cattle in adjacent pens.[92] In addition to an untested PI animal entering the herd, a heifer/cow could be BVDV test negative yet acutely infected, resulting in a PI calf. Importantly, all new cattle entering the herd must be tested negative (by IHC or ACE) for BVDV and, if female, remain isolated until they calve, with the calves then tested for BVDV.

If a PI animal is found, it should be isolated from other animals, particularly on breeding farms. The disposition of a PI animal includes euthanasia or feeding until market weight for processing. PI cattle cannot enter the marketing system as unidentified. In selected operations, PI cattle could be fed to market weight. However, although some reach adult age, most die of natural disease by 6 months to a year.

More than 140 vaccines against BVDV are available in the United States for use in cattle.[27] These vaccines are MLV and killed, often in combination with BHV-1, PI-3V, BRSV, *M. haemolytica*, *P. multocida*, *H. somni*, *Leptospira serovars*, and *Campylobacter* spp. Vaccine programs for beef and dairy cattle in the United States routinely incorporate use of one or more doses against BVDV. These licensed vaccines are classified as modified live virus (MLV) for parenteral administration (intramuscular and/or subcutaneous [IM or SC] and inactivated (killed [KV] for parenteral use. The parenteral routes include both IM and SQ; however, several vaccines are approved/recommended for SQ to reduce tissue damage, as stressed in beef quality assurance programs. No USDA-licensed intranasal BVD vaccines are available in the United States. Worldwide there have been attempts to use other technologies for BVD vaccine including viral subunit, DNA vaccines,

and, more recently, an equine herpesvirus vector expressing BVDV structural proteins.[132,133]

Cattle respond to the MLV and KV by development of a humoral (B-cell) response with neutralizing antibodies.[12,80,104,134] Passively acquired antibodies from BVDV antibody-positive dams have been shown to provide protection.[135,136] Also, calves fed colostrums from vaccinated dams were protected against BVDV disease.[137] In addition, high maternal antibody concentrations blocked a protective response to MLV BVDV1a vaccine.[138] Vaccination with MLV BVDV vaccine will also induce activated T-cell subsets after vaccination.[139] Cattle can also have an activated T-cell system in situations where the calves have maternal antibodies to BVDV.[140] The total protection against BVDV is not likely limited to either T-cell or B-cell function. One must consider, however, the potential for maternal antibodies to inhibit the active immune response following vaccination. With the half-life of approximately 23 days, the date the calf responds to vaccination will depend on the quality and quantity of antibodies absorbed. One study indicated some calves could retain colostral antibodies up to 299 days based on half-life calculations,[16] whereas other calves maintained antibody levels for a much shorter time (mean of 192 days).

The requirements for U.S. vaccines are set forth in the Code of Federal Regulations (CFR) 113.311 "Live virus vaccines" and 113.215 "Killed virus vaccines." Initially, viral vaccines were evaluated by acute challenge with virulent virus 2 to 4 weeks after vaccination. In recent years there have been additions to the regulations relating to efficacy studies and label claims concerning BVDV vaccines for protecting the fetus. The current USDA APHIS CVB regulations for the BVDV reproductive efficacy and label claims are noted at that website.

The BVDV strains in the MLV and KV are predominantly the CP BVDV1a and BVDV2a strains (Tables 42-1 and 42-2). A limited number of vaccines have NCP strains. Both MLV and KV vaccines induce antibodies to a wide range of BVDV strains including the three predominant subtypes in the United States: BVDV1a, 1b, and 2a.[80,141]

For many years the BVDV vaccines contained only BVDV1a strains. A severe acute disease outbreak of BVDV in North America caused by BVDV2a focused attention on another BVDV subtype.[142] The outbreaks occurred in herds with partial or incomplete BVDV vaccinations. BVDV type 2 disease was identified in beef herds receiving BVDV1 vaccines.[143] Attention was given to whether the BVDV1a vaccines induced protection against BVDV2a. Studies showed protection in cattle receiving BVDV1 vaccine and challenged with BVDV.[137,144,145] Yet there was a drive by some companies to add the BVDV2 strains to their vaccines and receive USDA approval. Today, almost all marketed MLV and KV vaccines in the United States have BVDV1a and BVDV2a strains (see Tables 42-1 and 42-2).

Considerable emphasis has been placed on preventing fetal BVD infections, especially PI calves. Vaccination with the BVDV1a MLV vaccine induced protection, preventing calves from becoming PI when an NCP BVDV1a strain was given to the pregnant vaccinates and nonvaccinates.[146] Eighty-three percent (83.3%) of the calves carried to term were protected from challenge with BVDV1a.

Table 42-1

MLV Vaccines with BVDV Strain and Genotype/Biotype

MLV	Company	Strain	Genotype/Biotype
Express 5	Boehringer Ingleheim Vetmedica	Singer 296	1a CP 2a CP
Pyramid 5 Pyramid 10	Fort Dodge	Singer 5912	1a CP 2a CP
Pyramid 4	Fort Dodge	Singer	1a CP
BoviShield 4	Pfizer	NADL	1a CP
BoviShield Gold 5	Pfizer	NADL 53637	1a CP 2a CP
BoviShield Gold FP5			
Titanium 5	AgriLabs	C24V 296	1a CP 2a CP
Vista 5	Intervet	Singer 125A	1a CP 2a CP
Reliant Plus	Merial	NADL	1a CP
Arsenal 4.1	Novartis	GL760	1a NCP
Jencine 4	Schering Plough	WRL	1 NCP

BVDV, Bovine viral diarrhea virus; MLV, modified live virus.

Table 42-2

Killed Vaccines with BVDV Strain and Genotype/Biotype

Killed	Company	Strain	Genotype/Biotype
Elite 4	Boehringer Ingleheim Vetmedica	Singer	1aCP
MasterGuard 5	AgriLabs	C24V 125C	1aCP 2aCP
Triangle 4+II BVD	Fort Dodge	Singer 5912	1aCP 2aCP
CattleMaster Gold	Pfizer	5960 53637	1aCP 2aCP
CattleMaster 4	Pfizer	5960 6309	1aCP 1 NCP
ViraShield 6	Novartis	K22 GL 760 TN 131	1aCP 1a NCP 2 NCP
Respishield	Merial	Singer	1aCP

BVDV, Bovine viral diarrhea virus.

When that protocol was used with the same BVDV1a MLV vaccine and vaccinates/nonvaccinates challenged with BVDV2, there was 57.9% protection against BVDV2 causing PI fetuses.[147] The addition of an MLV BVDV2a component to the BVDV1a MLV vaccine in the previously mentioned studies protected all vaccinated heifers' (challenged with BVDV type 2a during pregnancy) calves against PI, while the BVDV1 vaccinates' calves became PI in 6/18 and 7/19 from heifers receiving one or two doses of the vaccine.[148] Another MLV BVDV vaccine containing types 1 and 2 protected gestating fetuses against both type 1 infection (100%) and type 2 (95%).[149] An NCP BVDV MLV type 1 MLV vaccine protected heifers and their fetuses against both BVDV1 and BVDV2 challenge.[150] A duration of immunity study using MLV vaccine in heifers demonstrated protection 370 days after vaccination, and all fetuses/calves were negative for BVDV.[151]

Most susceptible heifers/cows are exposed to BVDV via direct or close contact with PI cattle. In three studies, one in the United Kingdom[152] and two in the United States, PI calves were used to challenge vaccinates and controls with fetal protection as the goal.[153,154] In the United Kingdom, PI cattle with BVDV1a were used to measure the efficacy of KV vaccine.[152] In that study vaccinated and control heifers were exposed to PI heifers with BVDV1a.[152] Vaccination with the KV BVDV vaccine containing BVDV1a provided protection against the PI heifer challenge.[152] In another study in the United States, MLV vaccine with BVDV types 1 and 2 protected pregnant heifers and their fetuses at 149 to 217 days' gestation against exposure to calves PI with a BVDV 2a virus.[153] A KV BVDV vaccine containing BVDV1a and BVDV2a protected fetuses (but not 100% of fetuses) against infection after exposure to PI calves.[154]

The risk of cattle shedding MLV BVDV vaccine virus and infecting contacts appears minimal. A transient viremia may occur in susceptible cattle for a few days after vaccination with MLV BVDV vaccines.[48,155] No shedding in the nasal secretions of the vaccinates has been noted,[48] nor was there infection of susceptible calves housed with vaccinates.[155]

Vaccination programs for cattle depend on the livestock management systems for the beef and dairy operations. One set regimen is unlikely because management will vary.

Breeding Herds for Beef and Dairy

Annual vaccination of the adult breeding herds for BVDV is recommended as part of a herd health vaccine program. BHV-1 and BVDV vaccines are often given to adult breeding beef herds at pregnancy check. This is a management decision, not related to the pathogenesis of BVDV or BHV-1. Vaccinations at pregnancy check for BHV-1 and BVDV have little or no benefit for the fetus, and in some cases, if the dam is susceptible, the fetus may become infected. Ideally vaccination should occur before breeding to maximize protection against fetal infection. USDA-licensed vaccines, both MLV and killed, are used before breeding.[27] For the MLV, it is generally recommended that the vaccines be given 30 to 60 days before breeding or exposure to bulls in natural breeding operations. Certain MLV virus vaccines can be used safely in pregnant cows and are labeled as such.[27] Generally, these vaccines require vaccination prebreeding and/or within a time frame such as the preceding 12 months. Caution must be given to each vaccine label's inserts for those requirements. The same requirements apply to the vaccination of nursing calves. Some MLV vaccines are approved for nursing calves, but label restrictions should be followed, especially as they relate to the vaccination status of the dam.

Calf Vaccinations in Beef Breeding Operations

Generally, it is recommended that calves receive two doses of BVDV vaccines. These are usually done as part of a preconditioning program for beef calves entering stocker and/or feedlot operations. Two doses are given in that maternal antibodies may persist blocking the first dose[16] or, in some cases, a seronegative calf will not respond to vaccination and does respond after a second dose.[155] The initial dose could be given before weaning such as at branding. Other cattle operations may wait until weaning for the first dose and give the second dose 3 to 4 weeks later. Industry practices in beef are moving toward MLV vaccines, although some veterinarians and producers elect to use KV vaccines. One approach is to use KV for the first dose followed by MLV.[156]

Stocker Operations and Feedlots

Cattle for stocker operations are traditionally vaccinated with MLV vaccines containing BVDV, BHV-1, PI-3V, BRSV, and bacterial immunogens. Some cattle operations and veterinarians will elect-to use KV vaccine in selected highly stressed calves. Likewise, at commercial feedlots, the MLV vaccines are standard vaccination protocol. Most feedlots may use only one dose of the MLV BVDV and other viral components, given at entry, but many will give an MLV BHV-1 at reimplanting.

Calf Raising Units

Heifer raising units and veal operations use both modified live and killed vaccines.

Summary

Bovine virus diarrhea viruses (BVDV) are a group of viruses causing both primary disease and/or acting in concert with numerous other agents to produce disease. The PI animal is the central figure as the principal reservoir exposing susceptible cattle. BVDV disease and its impact on cattle are evident in many management situations, from breeding herd to the stocker and feedlot operations. The emphasis should be to recognize that the BVDV PI begins with infection in the breeding herd. Controlling BVDV fetal infections will reduce and, ideally, eliminate the PI animal. The detection and removal of the PI animal is the goal of BVDV control along with biosecurity and effective vaccination. With the diagnostic tests available to detect PI cattle, BVDV impact on cattle production can be greatly diminished with the removal of these individuals.

References

1. Babiuk LA, van Drunen Littel-van den Hurk S, Tikoo SK: Infectious bovine rhinotracheitis/infectious pustular vulvovaginitis and infectious pustular balanoposthitis. In Coetzer JAW, Tustin RC, editors: *Infectious diseases of livestock*, ed 2, Oxford, England, 2004, Oxford University Press, pp 875-886.
2. Van Vuuren M: Bovine respiratory syncytial virus infection. In Coetzer JAW, Tustin RC, editors: *Infectious diseases of livestock*, ed 2, Oxford, England, 2004, Oxford University Press, pp 677-680.
3. Potgeiter LND: Bovine viral diarrhea and mucosal disease. In Coetzer JAW, Tustin RC, editors: *Infectious diseases of livestock*, ed 2, Oxford, England, 2004, Oxford University Press, pp 946-969.
4. Van Vuuren M: Parainfluenza type 3 infection. In Coetzer JAW, Tustin RC, editors: *Infectious diseases of livestock*, ed 2, Oxford, England, 2004, Oxford University Press, pp 673-676.
5. Campbell JR: Effect of bovine viral diarrhea virus in the feedlot, *Vet Clin North Am Food Anim Pract* 20:39-50, 2004.
6. Kapil S, Basaraba RJ: Infectious bovine rhinotracheitis, parainfluenza-3, and respiratory coronavirus, *Vet Clin North Am Food Anim Pract* 13:455-469, 1997.
7. Ames TR, Baker JC, Wikse SE: Lower respiratory tract diseases. In Smith BP, editor: *Large animal internal medicine*, ed 3, St Louis, 2002, Mosby, pp 556-562.
8. Fulton RW, Purdy CW, Confer AW et al: Bovine viral diarrhea infections in feeder calves with respiratory disease: interactions with *Pasteurella* spp., parainfluenza-3 virus and bovine respiratory syncytial virus, *Can J Vet Res* 64:151-159, 2000.
9. Fulton RW, Ridpath JF, Saliki JT et al: Bovine viral diarrhea virus (BVDV)1b: predominant subtype in calves with respiratory disease, *Can J Vet Res* 66:181-190, 2002.
10. Step DL, Confer AW, Kirkpatrick JG et al: Respiratory tract infections in dairy calves from birth to breeding age: detection by laboratory isolations and seroconversions, *Bov Pract* 39:44-53, 2005.
11. Fulton RW: *Respiratory disease in cattle: isolation of infectious agents and lesions in fatal feedlot cases and diversity of bovine viral diarrhea viruses in cattle: impact on diagnosis and vaccination,* Academy of Veterinary Consultants Meeting, Denver, 2003.
12. Fulton RW, Briggs RE, Ridpath JF et al: Transmission of bovine viral diarrhea virus 1b to susceptible and vaccinated calves by exposure to persistently infected calves, *Can J Vet Res* 69:161-169, 2005.
13. Thomson GR: Adenovirus infections. In Coetzer JAW, Tustin RC, editors: *Infectious diseases of livestock*, Oxford, England, 2004, Oxford University Press, ed 2, pp 819-821.
14. Fent GM, Fulton RW, Saliki JT et al: Bovine adenovirus-7 infections in postweaning calves, *Am J Vet Res* 63:976-978, 2002.
15. Saif LJ: Bovine coronavirus infection. In Coetzer JAW, Justin RC, editors: *Infectious diseases of livestock*, ed 2, 2004, pp 795-802.
16. Fulton RW, Briggs RE, Payton ME et al: Maternally derived humoral immunity to bovine viral diarrhea virus (BVDV)1a, BVDV1b, BVDV2, bovine herpesvirus-1, parainfluenza-3 virus, bovine respiratory syncytial virus, *Mannheimia haemolytica* and *Pasteurella multocida* in beef calves, antibody decline by half-life studies and effect on response to vaccination, *Vaccine* 22:644-650, 2004.
17. Goyal SM: Diagnosis. In Goyal SM, Ridpath JF, editors: *Bovine viral diarrhea virus, diagnosis, management, and control,* Boston, 2005, Blackwell Publishing, pp 197-208.
18. Schroeder RJ, Moys MD: An acute respiratory infection of dairy cattle, *J Am Vet Assoc* 125:471-472, 1954.
19. Muylkens B, Thiry J, Kirten P et al: Bovine herpesvirus 1 infection and infectious bovine rhinotracheitis, *Vet Res* 38:181-209, 2007.
20. Madin SH, York CJ, McKercher DG: Isolation of the IBR virus, *Science* 124:721-722, 1956.
21. Schwartz AJF, York CJ, Zirbel LW et al: Modification of infectious bovine rhinotracheitis (IBR) virus in tissue culture and development of a vaccine, *Proc Soc Experimental Biol* 96:453-458, 1957.
22. Bosch JC, DeJong MCM, Franken P et al: An inactivated gE-negative marker vaccine and an experimental gD-subunit vaccine reduce the incidence of bovine herpesvirus 1 infections in the field, *Vaccine* 16:265-271, 1998.

23. Babiuk LA, L'Itaben J, van Drunen Little-van den Hurk S et al: Protection of cattle from bovine herpesvirus type 1 (BHV-1) infection by immunization with individual viral glycoproteins, *Virology* 159:57-66, 1987.

24. Lupton HW, Reed DE: Clearance and shedding of infectious bovine rhinotracheitis virus from nasal mucosa of immune and non-immune calves, *Am J Vet Res* 124:721-722, 1980.

25. Schroyer EL, Easterday BC: Studies on the pathogenesis of infectious bovine rhinotracheitis following aerosol exposure, *Cornell Vet* 58:442-461, 1968.

26. Osorio FA: Infectious bovine rhinotracheitis and other clinical syndromes caused by bovine herpesvirus types 1 and 5. In Howard JL, Smith RA, editors: *Current veterinary therapy: food animal practice*, ed 4, St Louis, 1999, Saunders, pp 283-286.

27. *Compendium of veterinary products*, ed 9, Port Huron, Mich, 2006, North American Compendiums, pp 302–310.

28. Endsley JJ, Quade MJ, Terharr B et al: BHV-1 specific CD4+, CD8+, and γδ T cells in calves vaccinated with one dose of a modified live BHV-1 vaccine, *Viral Immunol* 15:385-393, 2002.

29. Patel JR, Shilletto RW: Modification of active immunization with live bovine herpesvirus 1 vaccine by passive viral antibody, *Vaccine* 23:4023-4028, 2005.

30. Kendrick JW, York CJ, McKercher DG: A controlled field trial of a vaccine for infectious bovine rhinotracheitis, *Proc US Livestock Sanitary Assoc* 60:155-158, 1956.

31. Bordt DE, Thomas PC, Marshall RF: Early protection against infectious bovine rhinotracheitis with intramuscularly administered vaccine, *Proc 79th Ann Mtg U S Anim Health Assoc* 79:50-60, 1975.

32. Sutton ML: Rapid onset of immunity in cattle after intramuscular injection of a modified live virus IBR vaccine, *Vet Med/SAC* 75:1447-1456, 1980.

33. Fairbanks K, Campbell J, Chase CL: Rapid onset of protection against infectious bovine rhinotracheitis with a modified live virus multivalent vaccine, *Vet Ther* 5:17-25, 2004.

34. Ellis J, Waldner C, Rhodes C et al: Longevity of protective immunity to experimental bovine herpesvirus-1 infection following inoculation with a combination modified-live virus vaccine in beef calves, *J Am Vet Med Assoc* 227:123-128, 2005.

35. Kennedy PC, Richards WPC: The pathology of abortion caused by the virus of infectious bovine rhinotracheitis, *Pathol Vet* 1:7-17, 1964.

36. Todd JD, Volenec FM, Paton IM: Interferon in nasal secretions and sera of calve after intranasal administration of a virulent infectious bovine rhinotracheitis virus: association of interferon in nasal secretions with early resistance to challenge with virulent virus, *Infect Immun* 5:699-706, 1972.

37. Todd JD, Volenec FM, Paton IM: Intranasal vaccination against infectious bovine rhinotracheitis studies on early onset of protection and use of the vaccine in pregnant cows, *J Am Vet Med Assoc* 159:1370-1374, 1971.

38. Kucera CJ, White RG, Beckenhauer WH: Evaluation of the safety and efficacy of an intranasal vaccine containing a temperature-sensitive strain of infectious bovine rhinotracheitis virus, *Am J Vet Res* 39:607-610, 1978.

39. Todd JD: Intranasal vaccination of cattle against IBR and PI-3: field and laboratory observations in dairy, beef, and neonatal populations, *Dev Biol Stand* 33:391-395, 1976.

40. Baker JC, Rust SR, Walker RD: Transmission of a vaccinal strain of infectious bovine rhinotracheitis virus from intranasally vaccinated steers commingled with nonvaccinated steers, *Am J Vet Res* 50:814-816, 1989.

41. Talens LT, Beckenhauer WH, Thurber ET et al: Efficacy of viral components of a nonabortagenic combination vaccine for prevention of respiratory and reproductive system diseases in cattle, *J Am Vet Med Assoc* 194:1273-1280, 1989.

42. Cravens RL, Ellsworth MA, Sorensen CD et al: Efficacy of a temperature-sensitive, modified live bovine herpesvirus type 1 vaccine against abortion and stillbirth in pregnant heifers, *J Am Vet Med Assoc* 208:2031-2034, 1996.

43. Chiang BC, Smith PC, Nusbaum KE, Stringfellow DA: The effect of infectious bovine rhinotracheitis vaccine on reproductive efficiency in cattle vaccinated during estrus, *Theriogenology* 33:1113-1120, 1990.

44. Miller JM, Van Der Maaten MJ, Whetstone CA: Infertility in heifers inoculated with modified live infectious bovine rhinotracheitis on postbreeding day 14, *Am J Vet Res* 50:551-554, 1989.

45. Kelling CL, Schipper IA, Strum GE et al: Infectious bovine rhinotracheitis (IBR) abortion: observations on incidence in vaccinated and nonvaccinated and exposed cattle, *Cornell Vet* 63:383-389, 1973.

46. Gatewood DM, Sprino PJ, Ohnesorge WC et al: *Evaluation of IBR vaccine virus shedding after parenteral administration to suckling calves*. Proceedings of the Twenty-Ninth Annual Convention of the American Association of Bovine Practitioners, 1996, p 178.

47. Roth JA, Vaughn MB: Evaluation of viral shedding and immune response following vaccination with a modified live BHV-1 vaccine, *Bov Pract* 32:1-4, 1998.

48. Kleiboecker SB, Sang-Myeong L, Jones CA et al: Evaluation of shedding of bovine herpesvirus 1, bovine viral diarrhea virus 1, and bovine viral diarrhea virus 2 after vaccination of calves with a multivalent modified live virus vaccine, *J Am Vet Med Assoc* 222:1399-1403, 2003.

49. Kahrs RF: Infectious bovine rhinotracheitis, In *Viral diseases of cattle*, Ames, Iowa, 1981, Iowa State University Press.

50. Savan M, Angulo AB, Derbyshire JB: Interferon, antibody responses, and protection induced by an intranasal infectious bovine rhinotracheitis vaccine, *Can Vet J* 20:207-210, 1979.

51. Sibbel RL, Bass EP, Thomas PC: How long will a killed IBR vaccine protect against challenge? *Vet Med* 83:90-92, 1988.

52. Trueblood MS, Swift BL, McHolland-Raymond LE: An outbreak of infectious pustular vulvovaginitis, *Vet Med/SAC* 72:1622-1624, 1977.

53. van Drunen Little-van den Hurk S: Rationale and perspectives on the success of vaccination against bovine herpesvirus-1, *Vet Microbiol* 113:275-282, 2006.

54. Henderson LM: Overview of marker vaccine and differential diagnostic test technology, *Biologicals* 33:203-209, 2005.

55. Hollis LC, Smith JF, Johnson BJ et al: A comparison of serological responses when modified live infectious bovine rhinotracheitis virus vaccine, *Mannheimia haemolytica* bacterin-toxoid and *Leptospira pomona* bacterin are administered with needle-free versus conventional needle-based injection in yearling feedlot steers, *Bov Pract* 39:106-109, 2005.

56. Hollis LC, Smith JF, Johnson BJ et al: A comparison of serological responses when modified live infectious bovine rhinotracheitis virus vaccine, *Mannheimia haemolytica* bacterin-toxoid and *Leptospira pomona* bacterin are administered with needle-free versus conventional needle-based injection in Holstein dairy calves, *Bov Pract* 39:110-114, 2005.

57. Perino LJ, Hunsaker BD: A review of bovine respiratory disease vaccine field efficacy, *Bov Pract* 31:59-66, 1997.

58. Jones C, Newby TJ, Holt T et al: Analysis of latency in cattle after inoculation with a temperature sensitive mutant of bovine herpesvirus 1 (RLB106), *Vaccine* 18:3185-3195.

59. Fulton RW, Briggs RE, Ridpath JF et al: Bovine viral diarrhea virus (BVDV)1b: predominant subtype in calves with respiratory disease, *Can J Vet Res* 66:181-190, 2002.

60. West K, Bogdan J, Hamel A et al: A comparison of diagnostic methods for the detection of bovine respiratory syncytial virus in experimental clinical specimens, *Can J Vet Res* 62:245-250, 1998.

61. Horner GW, Hunter R, Bartha A et al: A new subgroup 2 bovine adenovirus proposed as the prototype strain 10, *Archiv Virol* 109:121-124, 1989.

62. Storz J, Stine L, Liem A et al: Coronavirus isolation from nasal swab samples in cattle with signs of respiratory tract disease after shipping, *J Am Vet Med Assoc* 208:1452-1455, 1996.

63. Storz J, Purdy CW, Lin X et al: Isolation of respiratory bovine respiratory coronavirus, other cytocidal viruses, and *Pasteurella* spp. from cattle involved in two natural outbreaks of shipping fever, *J Am Vet Med Assoc* 216:1659-1604, 2000.

64. Storz J, Lin XQ, Purdy CW et al: Coronavirus and *Pasteurella* infections in bovine shipping fever pneumonia and Evans criteria for causation, *J Clin Microbiol* 38:3291-3298, 2000.

65. Thomas CJ, Hoet AE, Sreevatsan S et al: Transmission of bovine coronavirus and serologic responses in feedlot calves under field conditions, *Am J Vet Res* 67:1412-1420, 2006.

66. Hasoksuz M, Hoet AE, Loerch SC et al: Detection of respiratory and enteric shedding of bovine coronaviruses in cattle in an Ohio feedlot, *J Vet Diagn Invest* 14:308-313, 2002.

67. Kapil S, Pomeroy KA, Goyal SM et al: Experimental infection with a virulent pneumoenteric isolate of bovine coronavirus, *J Vet Diagn Invest* 3:88-89, 1991.

68. Saif LJ, Redman DH, Theil KW: Experimental coronavirus infections in calves: viral replication in respiratory and intestinal tracts, *Am J Vet Res* 47:1426-1432, 1986.

69. Reynolds DJ, Debney TG, Hall GA et al: Studies on the relationship between coronaviruses from the intestinal and respiratory tracts of calves, *Arch Virol* 85:71-83, 1985.

70. Grooms D, Baker JC, Ames TR: Diseases caused by bovine diarrhea virus. In Smith BP, editor: *Large animal internal medicine*, ed 3, St Louis, 2002, Mosby, pp 707-714.

71. Baker JC: The clinical manifestations of bovine viral diarrhea infection, *Vet Clin North Am Food Anim Pract* 11:425-445, 1995.

72. Brock KV: Bovine viral diarrhea virus: persistence is the key, *Vet Clin North Am Food Anim Pract* 20:1-180, 2004.

73. Goyal SM, Ridpath JF: *Bovine viral diarrhea virus, diagnosis, management, and control*, Boston, 2005, Blackwell Publishing, pp 1-243.

74. Collett MS, Anderson DK, Retzel E: Comparisons of the pestivirus bovine viral diarrhea virus with members of the, *Flaviviridae*, *J Gen Virol* 69:2637-2643, 1988a.

75. Collett MS, Larson R, Belzer SK et al: Proteins encoded by bovine viral diarrhea virus: the genomic organization of a pestivirus, *Virology* 165:200-208, 1988b.

76. Collett MS, Wiskerchen M, Weiniak E et al: Bovine viral diarrhea virus genomic organization, *Arch Virol* 3:19-27, 1991.

77. Corapi W, Donis RO, Dubovi EJ: Characterization of a panel of monoclonal antibodies and their use in the study of the antigenic diversity of bovine viral diarrhea virus, *Am J Vet Res* 51:1388-1394, 1990.

78. Pellerin CJ, van den Hurk J, Lecomte J et al: Identification of a new group of bovine viral diarrhea virus strains associated with severe outbreaks and high mortalities, *Virology* 203:260-268, 1994.

79. Ridpath JF, Bolin SR, Dubovi EJ: Segregation of bovine viral diarrhea virus into genotypes, *Virology* 205:66-74, 1994.

80. Fulton RW, Saliki JT, Burge LJ et al: Neutralizing antibodies to type 1 and 2 bovine viral diarrhea viruses: detection by inhibition of viral cytopathology and infectivity by immunoperoxidase assay, *Clin Diagn Lab Immunol* 4:380-383, 1997.

81. Fulton RW, Ridpath JF, Confer AW et al: Bovine viral diarrhea antigenic diversity: impact on disease and vaccination programmes, *Biologicals* 31:89-95, 2003.

82. Ridpath JF, Bolin SR: Differentiation of types 1a, 1b, and 2 bovine viral diarrhea virus (BVDV) by PCR, *Mol Cell Probes* 12:101-106, 1998.

83. Ridpath JF, Neill JD, Frey M: Phylogenetic, antigenic and clinical characterization of type 2 BVDV from North America, *Vet Microbiol* 77:145-155, 2000.

84. Flores EF, Ridpath JF, Weiblen R et al: Phylogenetic analysis of Brazilian bovine viral diarrhea virus type 2 (BVDV-2) isolates: evidence for a subgenotype within BVDV-2, *Virus Res* 87:51-60, 2002.

85. Vilcek S, Durkovic B, Kolesarova M et al: Genetic diversity of BVDV: consequences for classification and molecular epidemiology, *Prev Vet Med* 72:31-35, 2005.

86. Nagai M, Hayashi M, Sugita S et al: Phylogenetic analysis of bovine viral diarrhea viruses using five different regions, *Virus Res* 99:103-113, 2004.

87. McClurkin AW, Littledike ET, Cutlip RC et al: Production of cattle immunotolerant to bovine viral diarrhea virus, *Can J Comp Med* 48:156-161, 1984.

88. Fulton RW, Ridpath JF, Ore S et al: Bovine viral diarrhoea virus (BVDV) subgenotype in diagnostic laboratory accessions: distribution of BVDV1a, 1b, and 2a subgenotypes, *Vet Microbiol* 111:35-40, 2005.

89. Evermann JF, Ridpath JF: Clinical and epidemiologic observations of bovine viral diarrhea virus in the northwestern United States, *Vet Microbiol* 89:129-139, 2002.

90. Tajima M, Dubovi EJ: Genetic and clinical analyses of bovine viral diarrhea virus isolates from dairy operations in the United States of America, *J Vet Diagn Invest* 17:10-15, 2005.

91. Wittum TE, Grotelueschen DM, Brock KV et al: Persistent bovine viral diarrhoea virus infection in US beef herds, *Prev Vet Med* 49:83-94, 2001.

92. Loneragan GH, Thomson DU, Montgomery DL et al: Prevalence, outcome, and health consequences associated with bovine viral diarrhea virus in feedlot cattle, *J Am Vet Med Assoc* 226:595-601, 2005.

93. Fulton RW, Hessman B, Johnson BJ et al: Evaluation of diagnostic tests used for detection of bovine viral diarrhea virus and prevalence of BVDV subtypes 1a, 1b, and 2a, in persistently infected cattle entering a feedlot, *J Am Vet Med Assoc* 228:578-584, 2006.

94. Confer AW, Fulton RW, Step DL et al: Viral antigen distribution in the respiratory tract of cattle persistently infected with bovine viral diarrhea virus subtype 2a, *Vet Pathol* 42:192-199, 2005.

95. Brock KV, Redman DR, Vickers ML et al: Quantitation of bovine viral diarrhea virus in embryo transfer flush fluids collected from a persistently infected heifer, *J Vet Diagn Invest* 3:99-100, 1991.

96. Al-Haddawi M, Mitchell GB, Clark ME et al: Impairment of innate immune responses of airway epithelium by infection with bovine viral diarrhea virus, *Vet Immunol Immunopathol* 116:153-162, 2007.

97. Potgieter LND, McCracken MD, Hopkins FM et al: Comparison of the pneumo-pathogenicity of two strains of bovine viral diarrhea virus, *Am J Vet Res* 46:151-153, 1985.

98. Potgieter LND, McCracken MD, Hopkins FM et al: Effect of bovine viral diarrhea virus infection on the distribution of infectious bovine rhinotracheitis virus in calves, *Am J Vet Res* 45:687-690, 1984.

99. Potgieter LN, McCracken MD, Hopkins FM et al: Experimental production of respiratory tract disease with bovine viral diarrhea virus, *Am J Vet Res* 45:1582-5, 1984.

100. Brodersen BW, Kelling CL: Alteration of leukocyte populations in calves concurrently infected with bovine respiratory syncytial virus and bovine viral diarrhea virus, *Viral Immunol* 12:323-334, 1999.

101. Brodersen BW, Kelling CL: Effect of concurrent experimentally induced bovine respiratory syncytial virus and bovine viral diarrhea virus infection on respiratory tract and enteric disease in calves, *Am J Vet Res* 59:1423-1430, 1998.

102. Haines DM, Martin KM, Clark EG et al: The immunohistochemical detection of *Mycoplasma bovis* and bovine viral diarrhea virus in tissues of feedlot cattle with chronic unresponsive disease and/or arthritis, *Can Vet J* 41:857-860, 2001.

103. Haines DM, Moline KM, Sargent RA et al: Immunohistochemical study of *Hemophilus somnus, Mycoplasma bovis, Mannheimia haemolytica,* and bovine viral diarrhea virus in death losses due to myocarditis, *Can Vet J* 45:231-234, 2004.

104. Fulton RW, Johnson BJ, Briggs RE et al: Challenge with bovine viral diarrhea virus by exposure to persistently infected calves: protection by vaccination and negative results of antigen testing in acutely infected calves, *Can J Vet Res* 70: 121-127, 2006.

105. Fulton RW, Cook BJ, Step DL et al: Evaluation of health status of calves and the impact on feedlot performance: assessment of a retained ownership program for postweaning calves, *Can J Vet Res* 66:173-180, 2002.

106. Corapi WV, Elliot RD, French TW et al: Thrombocytopenia and hemorrhages in viral calves infected with bovine viral diarrhea virus, *J Am Vet Med Assoc* 196:590-596, 1990.

107. Corapi WV, French TW, Dubovi EJ: Severe thrombocytopenia in young calves experimentally infected with noncytopathic bovine viral diarrhea virus, *J Virol* 63:3934-3943, 1989.

108. Fulton RW, Step DL, Ridpath JF et al: Response of calves persistently infected with noncytopathic bovine viral diarrhea virus (BVDV) subtype 1b after vaccination with heterologous BVDV strains in modified live viral vaccines and *Mannheimia haemolytica* bacterin-toxoid, *Vaccine* 21: 2980-2985, 2003.

109. Grooms DL: Reproductive consequences of infection with bovine viral diarrhea virus, *Vet Clin North Am Food Anim Pract* 20:5-19, 2004.

110. Grooms DL, Brock KV, Ward LA: Detection of cytopathic bovine viral diarrhea virus in the ovaries of cattle following immunization with a modified live bovine viral diarrhea vaccine, *J Vet Diagn Invest* 10:130-134, 1998.

111. Grooms DL, Ward LA, Brock KV: Morphologic changes and immunohistochemical detection of viral antigen in ovaries from cattle persistently infected with bovine viral diarrhea virus, *Am J Vet Res* 57:830-833, 1996.

112. Grooms DL, Brock KV, Ward LA: Detection of bovine viral diarrhea virus in the ovaries of cattle acutely infected with bovine viral diarrhea virus, *J Vet Diagn Invest* 10:125-129, 1998.

113. Munoz-Fanzi CA, Hietala SK, Thurmond MC et al: Quantification, risk factors, and health impact of natural congenital infection with bovine viral diarrhea virus in dairy calves, *Am J Vet Res* 64:358-365, 2003.

114. Kirkland PD, Macintosh SG, Moyle A: The outcome of widespread use of semen from a bull persistently infected with pestivirus, *Vet Record* 135:527-529, 1994.

115. Paton DJ, Goodey R, Brockman S et al: Evaluation of the quality and virological status of semen from bulls acutely infected with BVDV, *Vet Rec* 124:63-64, 1989.

116. Kirkland PD, Richards SG, Rothwell JT et al: Replication of bovine viral diarrhea virus in the bovine reproductive tract and excretion of virus in semen during acute and chronic infections, *Vet Rec* 128:587-90, 1991.

117. Kommisrud E, Vatn T, Lange-Ree JR et al: Bovine virus diarrhea virus in semen from acutely infected bulls, *Acta Vet Scand* 37:41-47, 1996.

118. Paton DJ, Brockman S, Wood L: Insemination of susceptible and preimmunized cattle with bovine viral diarrhea virus infected semen, *Br Vet J* 146:171-174, 1990.

119. McClurkin AW, Coria MF, Cutlip RC: Reproductive performance of apparently healthy cattle persistently infected with bovine viral diarrhea virus, *J Am Vet Med Assoc* 174:1116-1119, 1979.

120. Wentink GH, Remmen JL, van Exsel AC: Pregnancy rate of heifers bred by an immunotolerant bull persistently infected with bovine viral diarrhea virus, *Vet Q* 11:171-174, 1989.

121. Givens MD, Heath AM, Brock KV et al: Detection of bovine viral diarrhea virus in semen obtained after inoculation of seronegative postpubertal bulls, *Am J Vet Res* 64:428-434, 2003.

123. Givens MD, Riddell KP, Walz PH et al: Noncytopathic bovine viral diarrhea virus can persist in testicular tissue infection after vaccination of peri-pubertal bulls but prevents subsequent infection, *Vaccine* 25:867-876, 2007.

123. Givens MD, Riddell KP, Zhang X et al: Use of a modified live vaccine to prevent persistent testicular infection with bovine viral diarrhea virus, *Vet Ther* 7:305-318, 2006.

124. Larson RL, Brodersen RW, Grotelueschen DM et al: Considerations for bovine viral diarrhea (BVDV) testing, *Bov Pract* 39:96-100, 2005.

125. Njaa BL, Clark EG, Janzen E et al: Diagnosis of persistent viral diarrhea virus infection by immunohistochemical staining of formalin-fixed skin biopsy specimens, *J Vet Diagn Invest* 12:393-399, 2000.

126. Larson RL, Miller RB, Kleiboeker SB et al: Economic costs associated with two testing strategies for screening feeder calves for persistent infection with bovine viral diarrhea virus, *J Am Vet Med Assoc* 226:249-254, 2005.

127. Hilbe M, Stalder H, Peterhans E et al: Comparison of five diagnostic methods for detecting bovine viral diarrhea virus infections in calves, *J Vet Diagn Invest* 19:28-34, 2007.

128. Cleveland SM, Salman MD, Van Campen H: Assessment of a bovine viral diarrhea virus antigen capture ELISA and microtiter virus isolation ELISA using pooled ear notch and serum samples, *J Vet Diagn Invest* 18:395-398, 2006.

129. Kennedy JA, Mortimer RG, Powers B: Reverse transcription-polymerase chain reaction on pooled samples to detect bovine viral diarrhea virus by using fresh ear-notch sample supernatants, *J Vet Diagn Invest* 18:89-93, 2006.

130. Kennedy JA: Diagnostic efficacy of a reverse transcriptase-polymerase chain reaction assay to screen cattle for persistent bovine viral diarrhea virus infection, *J Am Vet Med Assoc* 229:1472-1474.

131. Ridpath JF, Hessman BE, Neill JD et al: Parameters of ear notch samples for BVDV testing: stability, size requirements, and viral load, *Proc Am Assoc Bov Pract* 39:269-270, 2006.

132. Fulton RW: Vaccines. In Goyal SM, Ridpath JF, editors: *Bovine viral diarrhea virus, diagnosis, management and control,* Boston, Blackwell Publishing, 2005, pp 209-222.

133. Rosas CT, Konig P, Beer M et al: Evaluation of the vaccine potential of an equine herpesvirus type I vector expressing bovine viral diarrhea virus structural proteins, *J Gen Virol* 88:748-757, 2007.

134. Fulton RW, Confer AW, Burge LJ et al: Antibody responses by cattle after vaccination with commercial viral vaccines

containing bovine herpesvirus-1, bovine viral diarrhea virus, parainfluenza-3 virus and bovine respiratory syncytial virus immunogens and subsequent revaccination at day 140, *Vaccine* 13:725-733, 1995.

135. Howard CJ, Clarke MC, Brownlie J: Protection against respiratory infection with bovine virus diarrhea virus by passively acquired antibody, *Vet Microbiol* 19:195-203, 1989.

136. Bolin SR, Ridpath JR: Assessment of protection from systemic infection or disease afforded by low to intermediate titers of passively acquired neutralizing antibody against bovine viral diarrhea virus in calves, *Am J Vet Res* 56:755-759, 1995.

137. Cortese VS, West KH, Hassand LE et al: Clinical and immunological responses of vaccinated and unvaccinated calves to infection with a virulent type II isolate of bovine viral diarrhea virus, *J Am Vet Med Assoc* 213:1312-1319, 1998.

138. Ellis J, West K, Cortese V et al: Effect of maternal antibodies on induction and persistence of vaccine-induced immune responses against bovine viral diarrhea virus type II in young calves, *Am J Vet Res* 219:351-356, 2001.

139. Endsley JJ, Quade MJ, Terhaar B et al: Bovine viral diarrhea virus type 1- and type 2-specific bovine T lymphocyte subset responses following modified-live virus vaccination, *Vet Ther* 3:364-372, 2002.

140. Endlsey JJ, Ridpath JF, Neill JD et al: Induction of T lymphocytes specific for bovine viral diarrhea virus in calves with maternal antibody, *Viral Immunol* 17:13-23, 2004.

141. Fulton RW, Burge LJ: Bovine viral diarrhea virus type 1 and 2 antibody response in calves receiving modified live virus or inactivated vaccines, *Vaccine* 19:264-274, 2000.

142. Carman S, vanDreumel T, Ridpath J et al: Severe acute bovine viral diarrhea in Ontario, *J Vet Diagn Invest* 10:27-35, 1998.

143. Van Campen H, Vorpahl P, Huzurbazar S et al: A case report: evidence for type 2 bovine viral diarrhea virus (BVDV) associated disease in beef herds vaccinated with modified live type 1 BVDV vaccine, *J Vet Diagn Invest* 12:263-265, 2000.

144. Dean HJ, Leyh R: Cross-protective efficacy of a bovine viral diarrhea virus (BVDV) type 2 challenge, *Vaccine* 17:1117-1124, 1999.

145. Fairbanks K, Schnackel J, Chase CL: Evaluation of a modified live virus type 1a bovine viral diarrhea virus vaccine (Singer strain) against a type 2 (Strain 890) challenge, *Vet Ther* 4:24-34, 2003.

146. Cortese VS, Grooms DK, Ellis J et al: Protection of pregnant cattle and their fetuses against infection with bovine viral diarrhea virus type 1 by use of a modified live virus vaccine, *Am J Vet Res* 59:1409-1413, 1998.

147. Brock KV, Cortese VS: Experimental fetal challenge using type II bovine viral diarrhea virus in cattle vaccinated with modified live virus vaccine, *Vet Ther* 2:354-360, 2001.

148. Ficken MD, Ellsworth MA, Tucker CM et al: Effects of modified live bovine viral diarrhea virus vaccines containing either type 1 or type 1 and 2 BVDV on heifers and their offspring after challenge with noncytopathic type 2 BVDV during gestation, *J Am Vet Med Assoc* 228:1559-1564, 2006.

149. Fairbanks KK, Rinehart CL, Ohnesorge WC et al: Evaluation of fetal protection against experimental infection with type 1 and type 2 bovine viral diarrhea virus after vaccination of the dam with a bivalent modified-live virus vaccine, *J Am Vet Med Assoc* 225:1898-1904, 2004.

150. Brock KV, McCarty K, Chase CCL, Harland R: Protection against fetal infection with either bovine viral diarrhea virus type 1 or type 2 using a noncytopathic type 1 modified live vaccine, *Vet Ther* 7:29-34, 2006.

151. Ficken MD, Ellsworth MA, Tucker CM: Evaluation of the efficacy of a modified live combination vaccine against bovine viral diarrhea virus types 1 and 2 challenge exposures in a one year duration of immunity fetal protection study, *Vet Ther* 7:283-294, 2006.

152. Patel JR, Shilleto DW, Williams J, Alexander DCS: Prevention of transplacental infection of bovine fetus by bovine viral diarrhea virus, *Arch Virol* 147:2453-2463, 2002.

153. Ellsworth MA, Fairbanks KK, Behan S et al: Fetal protection following exposure to calves persistently infected with bovine viral diarrhea virus type 2 sixteen months after primary vaccination of the dams, *Vet Ther* 7:295-306, 2006.

154. Grooms DL, Bolin SR, Coe PH et al: Fetal protection against continuous exposure to bovine viral diarrhea virus following administration of a vaccine containing an inactivated BVDV fraction, *Proc Am Assoc Bov Pract* 39:266, 2006.

155. Fulton RW, Saliki JT, Burge LJ et al: Humoral immune response and assessment of vaccine virus shedding in calves receiving modified live virus vaccines containing bovine herpesvirus-1 and bovine viral diarrhea virus 1a, *J Vet Med B*, 50:31-37, 2003.

156. Grooms DL, Coe P: Neutralizing antibody responses in preconditioned calves following vaccination for respiratory viruses, *Vet Ther* 2:119-128, 2002.

CHAPTER 43

Mycoplasmas in Bovine Respiratory Disease

RICARDO F. ROSENBUSCH

The role of mycoplasmas in bovine respiratory disease has been the subject of controversy. Because nine pathogenic species of mycoplasmas have been reported to be recovered from pneumonic infections,[1] discrimination between these species is of importance. For North America, two species have been reported as common and significant agents to consider. In young dairy calves, pneumonia is often seen shortly after grouping dairy calves that have been raised individually in hutches. *Mycoplasma dispar* is a prevalent agent implicated in these infections, often with limited mortality.[2] Nevertheless, it should be noted that this mycoplasma can occasionally produce lobar bronchopneumonia with severe peribronchial cuffing, primarily in highly stressed young calves.[3]

In contrast, *Mycoplasma bovis* is not as ubiquitous but is often involved in more severe presentations. Introductions of this mycoplasma into stocker or feedlot operations occur through apparently normal cattle,[4,5] and it spreads rapidly among commingled cattle.[6,7] Although cattle are the primary hosts affected, there have been reports of American bison and white-tailed deer infected with *M. bovis* and presenting classical disease symptoms and lesions at necropsy.[8] A characteristic presentation with *M. bovis* is that referred to as "pneumonia-arthritis syndrome"[1] and involves calves presenting with upper respiratory signs at 2 to 4 weeks after arrival, often refractory to antimicrobial therapy. Some or most of the affected calves may also present polyarthritis and tenosynovitis involving large joints such as shoulder, elbow, carpal, hip, stifle, and hock. Lesions at necropsy include a suppurative bronchopneumonia, edematous pulmonary septa, and pleuritis. The appearance of multiple small round coagulative necrosis lesions disseminated throughout the lung is also often reported.[9,10] Affected joints may be swollen, and abundant yellow-tinted clear to turbid synovial fluid can be obtained from them. Joint capsules will be thickened. Tendon sheaths and joint capsules may present small coagulative necrosis lesions similar to those seen in lung.[4] Histologically, the coagulative necrosis lesions present as a purulent center arising from an affected bronchiole, surrounded by a histiocytic and mononuclear infiltrate layer with minimal encapsulation. The lesions are characteristic of *M. bovis* and distinct from those produced by other bacterial agents involved in bovine respiratory disease.[11] Variation in pathogenicity among strains of *M. bovis* is significant, and the strain-specific attributes of *M. bovis* to destroy tracheal epithelium, disseminate systemically, or cause coagulative necrosis can be demonstrated on experimental inoculation of cattle.[12] A wide variation in *M. bovis* strain pathogenicity is also suspected in field outbreaks, although correlations between field virulence and strain pathogenicity phenotype have not been done.[9,10] Even though there is systemic dissemination, localizations are primarily in joints and lung, targeting the vascular linings of these sites.[1] Localizations in various viscera, skin, or brain have been reported either in very young calves or mature cattle sporadically.[13,14] In addition to localized lesions, *M. bovis* infections can lead to rapid loss of body condition. This is assumed to be caused by the high levels of tumor necrosis factor alpha released from lung macrophages when exposed to chronic infection with the mycoplasma.[15] Cachexia is a common terminal syndrome in calves with severe *M. bovis* lung burden.[16]

Morbidity and mortality in pneumonia-arthritis syndrome can reach 80% and 10% of those affected, respectively.[5] No wide-scale studies on overall incidence of this syndrome are available, although there is evidence that the condition is becoming more prevalent and more severe.[17] In a Kansas survey, producers responded that clinical signs of antibiotic-resistant respiratory disease occurred in 34% of the lots of stocker calves they processed, with one out of five of these affected lots presenting calves with classical pneumonia-arthritis syndrome.[18] Retrospective data from cases submitted to diagnostic laboratories have been used to estimate incidence. Of 99 cases of pneumonia submitted, 16 were found to yield *M. bovis,* and in 6 of these, *M. bovis* was the only pathogen.[12] In contrast, 59 of 64 cases of feedlot respiratory disease in Saskatchewan province involved *M. bovis* as noted by immunohistochemistry.[19] Most of the *M. bovis* positive lungs were also found to be positive for bovine viral diarrhea virus (BVDV) antigen, suggesting synergy between these two agents. This tight association of BVDV and *M. bovis* infection was not observed in more recent studies.[17] Other studies reported that a high proportion of cases submitted for diagnosis yielded *Mycoplasma* spp. from lungs.[20] Seroconversions to *M. dispar* and *M. bovis* after arrival at feedlots provided evidence that these mycoplasma species spread among the commingled calves.[21] Similar to other bacterial pathogens involved in bovine respiratory disease, *M. bovis* can act as a primary agent in highly stressed calves, although most commonly it plays a secondary agent role in multiagent infections.[1,17]

Immune responses to infection vary among the respiratory mycoplasmas of cattle. Maternal immunity protects calves from mucosal colonization with *M. dispar* for a few weeks after birth, whereas no such protection is seen in calves against *M. bovis*. Protection against *M. dispar* is mediated by antibodies to a conserved capsular polysaccharide of this mycoplasma.[22] In contrast, immune responses against *M. bovis* confront a rapidly changing surface expression of *M. bovis* variable surface proteins.[23] Response to lower respiratory tract infection with *M. bovis* also results in a Th-2 biased immune response.[24] Vaccination with bacterins, on the other hand, results in a high interferon gamma and Th-1 biased immune response with enhanced lung damage.[25] This supports observations on vaccine-enhanced disease when mammary gland protection against *M. bovis* is attempted.[26] Federally licensed *M. bovis* bacterins are available in the United States for use in calves before commingling, and field assessment of their effectiveness awaits peer-reviewed reports. Experimental vaccines have been shown to elicit protection against challenge as measured by decreased lung lesions and decreased lung *M. bovis* burden.[27]

Control approaches to mycoplasmal infections have been controversial. Mycoplasmal mastitis is not treated, and segregation and culling are the main methods of control.[28] In contrast, treatment is often attempted in calves affected with pneumonia-arthritis syndrome, even though this is unrewarding in advanced cases.[1] Treatment regimens should ideally focus on antimicrobial agents active against *M. bovis*[29] and provide coverage over 7 to 14 days.[30] Positive treatment responses can be obtained using antimicrobial agents known to lack in vitro effectiveness against *M. bovis* strains used in experimental infections.[31] At this time it is unknown if this is because of poor correlation of in vitro data with in vivo activity for specific drugs or if therapeutic suppression of other important respiratory pathogens results in reduced pathogenic impact by *M. bovis*.

Given the multifactorial nature of bovine respiratory disease, diagnosis of *M. bovis* pneumonia requires laboratory detection and speciation of the mycoplasma. Immunohistochemistry of lung sections is a method of choice because it only gives a positive lung signal in the presence of large concentrations of antigen, and the characteristic coagulative necrosis lesions can also be evaluated.[32] Detection of the mycoplasma in joint fluid is also of value. Highly sensitive detection methods such as culture and PCR should be used with caution because a low-level presence of *M. bovis* in respiratory tract sites may not be significant.[6] The application of quantitative PCR techniques to detect high lung burden of the mycoplasma could provide the needed specificity to diagnose involvement of *M. bovis* in calf pneumonia.[33]

References

1. Step DL, Kirkpatrick JG: Mycoplasma infection in cattle. I. Pneumonia—arthritis syndrome, *Bov Pract* 35:149, 2001.
2. Virtala AK, Mechor GD, Grohn YT et al: Epidemiologic and pathologic characteristics of respiratory tract disease in dairy heifers during the first three months of life, *J Am Vet Med Assoc* 208:2035, 1996.
3. Tinant MK, Bergeland ME, Knudtson WR: Calf pneumonia associated with *Mycoplasma dispar* infection, *J Am Vet Med Assoc* 175:812, 1979.
4. Adegboye DS, Halbur PG, Nutsch RG et al: *Mycoplasma bovis*-associated pneumonia and arthritis in cattle complicated with pyogranulomatous tenosynovitis, *J Am Vet Med Assoc* 209:647, 1996.
5. Rosenbusch RF: *Cow-calf sessions—bovine mycoplasmosis*. In Proceedings of the 34th Annual Conference of the American Association of Bovine Practitioners, 2001, p 49.
6. Allen JW, Viel L, Bateman KG et al: Changes in the bacterial flora of the upper and lower respiratory tracts and bronchoalveolar lavage differential cell counts in feedlot calves treated for respiratory disease, *Can J Vet Res* 56:177, 1992.
7. Rosenbusch RF: *Transmission of Mycoplasma bovis and the syndromes that result in beef and dairy cattle*. In Proceedings of the 38th Annual Conference of the American Association of Bovine Practitioners, 2005, p 1.
8. Dyer NW, Krogh DF, Schaan LP: Pulmonary mycoplasmosis in farmed white-tailed deer (*Odocoileus virginianus*), *J Wildlife Dis* 40:366, 2004.
9. Adegboye DS, Rasberry U, Halbur PG et al: Monoclonal antibody-based immunohistochemical technique for the detection of *Mycoplasma bovis* in formalin-fixed paraffin-embedded calf lung tissues, *J Vet Diagn Invest* 7:261, 1995a.
10. Khodakaram-Tafti A, Lopez A: Immunohistopathological findings in the lungs of calves naturally infected with *Mycoplasma bovis*, *J Vet Med Sci* 51:10, 2004.
11. Gagea MI, Bateman KG, van Dreumel T et al: Diseases and pathogens associated with mortality in Ontario beef feedlots, *J Vet Diagn Invest* 18:18, 2006a.
12. Rosenbusch RF: Should *Mycoplasma bovis* be a concern in feedlots? *Proc Acad Vet Consult* 28:20, 2000.
13. Maeda T, Shibahara T, Kimura K et al: *Mycoplasma bovis*-associated suppurative otitis media and pneumonia in bull calves, *J Comp Pathol* 129:100, 2003.
14. Ayling R, Nicholas R, Hogg R et al: *Mycoplasma bovis* isolated from brain tissue of calves, *Vet Rec* 156:391, 2005.
15. Jungi TW, Krampe M, Sileghem M et al: Differential and strain-specific triggering of bovine alveolar macrophage effector functions by mycoplasmas, *Microb Pathogenesis* 21:487, 1996.
16. Rosenbusch R: *What we know about mastitis and systemic disease*. Proceedings of the Minnesota Dairy Health Conference, 2003, p 8.
17. Gagea MI, Bateman KG, Shanahan RA et al: Naturally occurring *Mycoplasma bovis*-associated pneumonia and polyarthritis in feedlot beef calves, *J Vet Diagn Invest* 18:29, 2006.
18. Spire M, Sargent J, Blasi D et al: Kansas survey on *Mycoplasma* in stockers, *Bov Vet* May-June:12, 2002.
19. Shahriar FM, Clark EG, Janzen E et al: Coinfection with bovine viral diarrhea virus and *Mycoplasma bovis* in feedlot cattle with chronic pneumonia, *Can Vet J* 43:863, 2002.
20. Welsh RD: Bacterial and *Mycoplasma* species isolated from pneumonic bovine lungs, *Agri Pract* 14:12, 1993.
21. Rosendal S, Martin SW: The association between serological evidence of mycoplasma infection and respiratory disease in feedlot calves, *Can J Vet Res* 50:179, 1986.
22. Bansal PL, Adegboye DS, Rosenbusch RF: Immune responses to the capsular polysaccharide of *Mycoplasma dispar* in calves and mice, *Comp Immunol Microbiol Infect Dis* 18:259, 1995.
23. Lysnyansky I, Sachse K, Rosenbusch R et al: The vsp Locus of *Mycoplasma bovis*: gene organization and structural features, *J Bacteriol* 181:5734, 1999.
24. Vanden Bush TJ, Rosenbusch RF: Characterization of the immune response to *Mycoplasma bovis* lung infection, *Vet Immunol Immunopathol* 94:23, 2003.
25. Ball HJ, Bryson D, Finlay D et al: Investigation into the host immune response in the vaccine primed experimental Mycoplasma bovis calf pneumonia model. In *Mycoplasmas of ruminants: pathogenicity, diagnostics, epidemiology and molecular genetics*, vol. 5, Brussels, 2001, European Commission, pp 158-161.

26. Boothby JT, Shore CE, Jasper DE et al: Immune responses to *Mycoplasma bovis* vaccination and experimental infection in the bovine mammary gland, *Can J Vet Res* 52:355, 1988.

27. Nicholas RAJ, Ayling RD, Stipkovits LP: An experimental vaccine for calf pneumonia caused by *Mycoplasma bovis*: clinical, cultural, serological and pathological findings, *Vaccine* 20:3569, 2002.

28. Judge L: Mycoplasma mastitis: an emerging disease in Michigan dairy cattle. Michigan State University Veterinary Extension Articles and bulletins: dairy, *Mich Dairy Rev* 2:4, 1997.

29. Rosenbusch RF, Kinyon JM, Apley M et al: In-vitro antimicrobial inhibition profiles of Mycoplasma bovis isolates recovered from various regions of the United States from 2002 to 2003, *J Vet Diagn Invest* 17:436, 2005.

30. Skogerboe TL, Rooney KA, Nutsch RG et al: Comparative efficacy of tulathromycin versus florfenicol and tilmicosin against undifferentiated bovine respiratory disease in feedlot cattle, *Vet Ther* 6:180, 2005.

31. Godinho KS, Rae A, Windsor GD et al: Efficacy of tulathromycin in the treatment of bovine respiratory disease associated with induced *Mycoplasma bovis* infections in young dairy calves, *Vet Ther* 6:96, 2005.

32. Adegboye DS, Halbur PG, Cavanaugh DL et al: Immunohistochemical and pathological study of Mycoplasma bovis-associated lung abscesses in calves, *J Vet Diagn Invest* 7:333, 1995b.

33. Cai HY, Bell-Rogers P, Parker L et al: Development of a real-time PCR for detection of Mycoplasma bovis in bovine milk and lung samples, *J Vet Diagn Invest* 17:537, 2005.

CHAPTER **44**

Ovine and Caprine Respiratory Disease: Infectious Agents, Management Factors, and Preventive Strategies

SHERRILL FLEMING

In 2004 respiratory diseases in lambs and breeding sheep were the third highest category of identified death losses, behind lambing losses and digestive disorders.[1] These death losses represented 0.36% of the national sheep inventory ($\approx$53,000 sheep deaths). Pneumonia losses in lambs were highest in the central United States. Despite documented losses, the 1996 Sheep Health and Productivity Needs Assessment survey did not identify respiratory disease as a high or moderate concern of producers.[2]

A variety of infectious agents, alone or in combination, have been identified from cases of sheep respiratory disease (Table 44-1) and goat respiratory disease (Table 44-2).[3-5] Many of these agents can be isolated from the nasal passages, pharynx, and tonsillar areas of normal, adult sheep. Individually, these agents cause mild respiratory disease when inoculated into susceptible animals. More severe respiratory disease occurs when a combination of agents are sequentially introduced to naive animals.[6]

Parainfluenza type 3, adenoviruses, and respiratory syncytial virus are frequently isolated from sheep and goats.[7-16] However, the inoculation of these viruses into susceptible animals usually results in mild catarrhal inflammation of the upper respiratory tract or subclinical respiratory disease.[6] Seroconversion occurs in most animals, and antibodies in the general population are widespread. Although more commonly associated with abortion and balanoposthitis, caprine herpes virus has been isolated from cases of conjunctivitis and respiratory disease.[13,14] Ovine herpes virus classically is known to cause malignant catarrhal fever in other ruminants. Studies on the disease transmission demonstrate that the virus is shed in the respiratory and nasal secretions and is associated with mild respiratory disease.[15] Introducing *Mannheimia haemolytica* several days after any respiratory viral exposure results in more severe clinical disease and possible mortality.[6,11,12] *M. haemolytica* is often the bacteria isolated from "quick" pneumonia, which causes sudden death with few premonitory signs in neonatal lambs. *Mycoplasma* spp. are reported from

Table **44-1**

Summary of Infectious Causes of Sheep Respiratory Diseases by Clinical Signs

Coughing	Serous Nasal Discharge	Mucopurulent Nasal Discharge
Mannheimia haemolytica*	Mannheimia haemolytica*	Mannheimia haemolytica*
Pasteurella spp.*	Pasteurella spp.*	Pasteurella spp.*
Lungworm infection/verminous pneumonia	Lungworm infection/verminous pneumonia	Lungworm infection/verminous pneumonia
Mycoplasma ovipneumoniae*	Mycoplasma ovipneumoniae spp.*	Mycoplasma ovipneumoniae spp.*
Mycoplasma arginini*	Mycoplasma arginini*	Mycoplasma arginini*
Ovine progressive pneumonia	Ovine progressive pneumonia	Ovine progressive pneumonia
Ovine adenovirus*	Ovine adenovirus*	—
Ovine herpes virus	Ovine herpes virus	—
Reovirus type 3	Reovirus type 3	—
Chlamydia spp.	Chlamydia spp.	—
Pulmonary adenomatosis, jaagsiekte	Pulmonary adenomatosis, jaagsiekte	Pulmonary adenomatosis, jaagsiekte
—	Oestrus ovis, nose bots*	Oestrus ovis, nose bots*
—	Early bacterial pneumonia*	Chronic bacterial pneumonia*
—	Bluetongue	Bluetongue
—	Border disease, hairy shaker disease	—
—	—	Postviral bacterial infection of respiratory tract*
—	—	Abscesses/caseous lymphadenitis*
—	—	Ovine nasal granuloma

*Common.

Table **44-2**

Summary of Infectious Causes of Goat Respiratory Diseases by Clinical Signs

Coughing	Serous Nasal Discharge	Mucopurulent Nasal Discharge
Mannheimia haemolytica*	Mannheimia haemolytica*	Mannheimia haemolytica*
Pasteurella spp.*	Pasteurella spp.*	Pasteurella spp.*
Lungworm infection/verminous pneumonia	Lungworm infection/verminous pneumonia	Lungworm infection/verminous pneumonia
Mycoplasma ovipneumoniae*	Mycoplasma ovipneumoniae spp.*	Mycoplasma ovipneumoniae spp.*
Mycoplasma arginini*	Mycoplasma arginini*	Mycoplasma arginini*
Mycoplasma mycoides ssp. mycoides	Mycoplasma mycoides ssp. mycoides	Mycoplasma mycoides ssp. mycoides
Caprine arthritis and encephalitis virus	Caprine arthritis and encephalitis virus	Caprine arthritis and encephalitis virus
Respiratory syncytial virus	Respiratory syncytial virus	—
Caprine herpesvirus	Caprine herpesvirus	Caprine herpesvirus
Chlamydia spp.	Chlamydia spp.	—
Pulmonary adenomatosis, jaagsiekte	Pulmonary adenomatosis, jaagsiekte	Pulmonary adenomatosis, jaagsiekte
—	Oestrus ovis, nose bots*	Oestrus ovis, nose bots*
—	Early bacterial pneumonia*	Chronic bacterial pneumonia*
—	—	Postviral bacterial infection of respiratory tract*
Abscesses/caseous lymphadenitis*	—	Abscesses/caseous lymphadenitis*

*Common.

respiratory outbreaks and chronic pneumonia problems, particularly in areas that confine sheep and goats during winter months.[17-23] M. ovipneumoniae and M. arginini have been reported from chronic respiratory disease in lambs and goats in North America.[20-22] Catastrophic outbreaks of Mycoplasma mycoides sspp. mycoides have been reported in goats associated with mastitis, arthritis, pneumonia, pleuritis, and abortion.[19] Recently M. mycoides ssp. capri was isolated from an outbreak of high mortality respiratory disease in goats in Mexico that resembles contagious caprine pleuropneumonia (M. capricolum ssp. capripneumoniae).[23]

Retroviral infections are slow viral diseases that can involve the respiratory tract and are of major importance to the economics of sheep and goat production.[24] Ovine progressive pneumonia (OPP) and caprine arthritis and encephalitis (CAE) viruses affect sheep and goat, respectively. These diseases limit the productive life of sheep and goats, as well as decrease the milk production and weaning weights of offspring.[25] The presence of retroviral infection predisposes to chronic bacterial pneumonia.[26] Producers that attempt to control these diseases have significant investment in testing and culling of infected animals.

Caseous lymphadenitis caused by *Corynebacterium pseudotuberculosis* is another chronic infection that may involve the respiratory tract with abscess formation in the lungs and/or mediastinal or retropharyngeal lymph nodes. This disease is a major concern of producers, particularly meat goat producers. High rates of condemnation and carcass trimming are caused by the presence of abscesses in internal organs and peripheral lymph nodes. The respiratory tract is an important reservoir for spreading the bacteria to other animals. Abscessation of lungs affects individual production.[27] Both chronic retroviral pneumonia and caseous lymphadenitis represent a drain on the individual animal's resources, which makes them more susceptible to other respiratory diseases.

RISK FACTORS

Stress, heat, overcrowding, exposure to inclement weather, poor ventilation, handling, and transportation predispose small ruminants to respiratory disease.[6] Outbreaks of respiratory disease are multifactorial processes that are affected by the interplay of individual animals, the entire flock, infectious agents, and environmental conditions. The immunity of the individual to infectious agents is determined by previous exposure/passive immunity, nutritional status, vitamin/mineral deficiencies, environmental stressors, level of exposure, and possibly genetic factors. Younger animals are at higher risk because they are initially dependent on colostral immunity and have had limited opportunities to develop immunity. Young animals are also limited in their resources to withstand extremes in environmental conditions.

A wide range of environmental conditions across the United States result in major regional differences in farm management. In the northeast, sheep are in smaller flocks, with more confinement and more dependence on stored feeds. Confinement during cold weather may result in decreased ventilation and increased humidity and ammonia levels, thus predisposing animals to respiratory disease. The Southeast is greatly dependent on grazing and provides minimal housing. Flock size is small, and gastrointestinal parasitism is a major problem. Hot, humid conditions are experienced during the summer, which results in animals crowding into shaded areas.[28] Mountainous areas have large flocks that must be grazed in extensive pastures high on the mountains during the summer and moved to more sheltered areas during the winter. Housing is virtually nonexistent for these large flocks. However, inclement weather can result in severe stress in lambs and adults. Lamb feedlots are located in the Western United States and often have dry and dusty environments. Grain supplements in all types of production tend to contain cracked or ground grain, which can be dusty unless pelletized or added to dried molasses.

Times of particular stress for sheep and goats are at lambing/kidding; weaning; processing (e.g., castration, shearing); prolonged transportation or moving between ranges; overcrowding; and extremely hot, cold, wet, or humid weather. Provision of shade and fans during hot and humid weather, windbreaks, or open-sided sheds during cold weather can help decrease the adverse effects of the weather. Adequate ventilation and protection from drafts during winter housing are crucial. Limiting the time that groups are held in overcrowded conditions is accomplished by planning in advance. Attention to proper nutrition and consideration of prophylactic antibiotic treatment (chlortetracycline in feed) will help to minimize the incidence of respiratory disease under adverse conditions.

DIAGNOSIS OF RESPIRATORY DISEASE

Physical examination of affected animals should include observation of the attitude and appetite. Depression, listlessness, separation from the flock and decreased to absent appetite are common presentations. The rectal temperature (normal 101.5° F-103.5° F) and respiratory rate are usually elevated. Elevated respiratory rates in sheep and goats can also be caused by handling and high environmental temperature. Auscultation of the lung fields demonstrates an increase in breath sounds, and if secondary bacterial infections are present, squeaks and wheezes may be audible in the peripheral lung fields. Radiographs of the thorax may be helpful in assessing the degree of consolidation present and the prognosis. Radiographs can also be diagnostic of abscesses in the lungs. Transtracheal washes for viral/bacterial isolation and cytology may be attempted if the animal is not dyspneic and overly stressed. In the event of a flock outbreak of disease, one or two representative cases should be selected for euthanasia and necropsy. Collection of a serum sample from affected animals on the initial presentation for follow-up serology is a wise precaution. Producers should be encouraged to submit any animals that die, as promptly as possible, for necropsy examinations.

TREATMENT

Viral diseases alone do not usually require treatment other than nursing care (provision of shade, shelter, fresh water, and palatable feed within easy reach). Few antimicrobials are labeled for use in small ruminants, and veterinarians must rely on extralabel use. Antibiotic susceptibility patterns in small ruminant bacterial isolates tend to be relatively sensitive to most antibiotics.[29-31] Prophylactic antibiotics are often administered during viral outbreaks in an attempt to prevent secondary bacterial infections.[29] A variety of antibiotics are routinely used including procaine penicillin G, amoxicillin, ampicillin, oxytetracycline, ceftiofur, tylosin, erythromycin, flufenicol, and tilmicosin (sheep only).[30,31] Tilmicosin should *not* be used in goats because a high percentage of goats may have an adverse reaction that results in acute death. Oxytetracycline, tylosin, and flufenicol are often chosen because of their efficacy against chlamydial and mycoplasmal agents. Care must be taken to recommend appropriate withdrawal periods for slaughter in small ruminants that are treated with extralabel antibiotics. Supportive therapy includes the use of nonsteroidal antiinflammatory drugs. Flunixin meglumine and ketoprofen in the acute stages can be useful in combating the toxic effects of bacterial pneumonia and making animals more comfortable. Monitoring of temperature, pulse, respiration, appetite, and attitude during therapy is important. Treatment with antibiotics should continue for at least 48 hours after the animal returns to normal.

MANAGEMENT OF RESPIRATORY DISEASE

During an acute outbreak within a flock or group of small ruminants, isolation of affected individuals should be attempted. Rectal temperatures in contact sheep or goats can be used to identify those animals that are in the early stages of infection, depending on the facilities of the producer and the numbers of animals involved. In flocks that have tendencies for annual respiratory outbreaks, inclusion of chlortetracycline in the feed before problem time periods has been successful in reducing morbidity and mortality in many herds. The immediate postweaning period appears to be a high-risk period for respiratory problems in sheep.

Producers reporting repeated bouts of respiratory disease are anxious to attempt vaccination programs. Currently there are no licensed vaccines to address commonly encountered pathogens in ovine or caprine respiratory disease.[32] The use of modified live intranasal parainfluenza type 3 vaccines, which also include infectious bovine rhinotracheitis (IBR) virus, have been popular among producers.[33] Cattle *Pasteurella* vaccines have been used in sheep, but cross protection against the serotypes found in small ruminant disease are unlikely. Other than anecdotal testimonials, there is little documentation that these products are effective in reducing morbidity and mortality from respiratory disease. The ability to produce ovine adenoviral vaccines is available but has not been attempted by vaccine companies because of limited markets.[34] Several commercial vaccines for caseous lymphadenitis have been produced.[35,36] Currently, Colorado Serum Company markets a vaccine for use in sheep that is reasonably effective. Adverse reactions in goats that have received this vaccine have been reported.[37] Several commercial companies offer production of autogenous vaccines from individual farm isolates of *Corynebacterium pseudotuberculosis*.

Biosecurity is an area that is not well understood or practiced by many producers. Buyer beware is commonly encountered when purchases of breeding animals are made. Producers should be aware of diseases that can be introduced into their flocks by purchased additions. Testing programs for CAE and OPP are relatively common so that seronegative sheep and goats can be purchased.[24] The synergistic hemolysis-inhibition (SHI) serology test for caseous lymphadenitis is available and makes recommendations on whether individuals have active abscesses or residual titers.[38,39] Others report difficulty in interpreting tests depending on the vaccination status.[40,41] A receiving protocol should be instituted on farms for any new arrivals and for reintroducing individuals that have participated in shows. These protocols should include an isolation area that has no contact with sheep and/or goats on the farm. After 30 days on the farm with no observed disease, several sentinel sheep or goats from the farm may be introduced to the purchased group. If no illnesses are noted in either group after 2 weeks, the flock additions may be commingled with the main flock. Receiving protocols can include control programs for Johne's disease, anthelmintic resistant nematodes, soremouth (also known as orf), and foot rot, as well as reduce upper respiratory disease when introducing new animals to a farm.

References

1. *Sheep and lamb nonpredator death loss in the United States, 2004* USDA:APHIS:VS,CEAH, National Animal Health Monitoring System, Fort Collins, Colo, #N445.0906, 2005.
2. *1996 Sheep Health and Productivity Needs Assessment, Centers for Epidemiology and Animal Health, USDA:APHIS:VS,* Attention NAHMS, Fort Collins, Colo, 80521, 1996.
3. Wilson WD, Lofstedt J: Alterations in respiratory function. In Smith BP, editor: *Large animal internal medicine*, ed 3, St Louis, 2002, Mosby, pp 46-69.
4. Smith MC, Sherman DM: Respiratory system. In Smith MC, Sherman DM: *Goat medicine*, Philadelphia, 1994, Lea & Febiger, pp 247–274.
5. Belknap EM: Diseases of the respiratory system. In Pugh DG, editor: *Sheep and goat medicine*, Philadelphia, 2002, Saunders, pp 107-128.
6. Brogden KA, Lehmkuhl HD, Cutlip RC: *Pasteurella haemolytica* complicated respiratory infections in sheep and goats, *Vet Res* 29:233-254, 1998.
7. Lamontagne L, Descoteaux JP, Roy R: Epizootiological survey of parainfluenza-3, reovirus-3, respiratory syncytial and infectious bovine rhinotracheitis viral antibodies in sheep and goat flocks in Quebec, *Can J Comp Med* 49: 424, 1985.
8. Lemkuhl HD, Cutlip RC, Brogden KA: Seroepidemiologic survey for adenovirus infection in lambs, *Am J Vet Res* 54: 1277, 1993.
9. Pommer J, Schamber G: Isolation of adenovirus from lambs with upper respiratory syndrome, *J Vet Diagn Invest* 3:204, 1991.
10. Whetstone CA, Evermann JF: Characterization of bovine herpesviruses isolated from six sheep and four goats by restriction endonuclease analysis and radioimmunoprecipitation, *Am J Vet Res* 49:781, 1988.
11. Trigo FJ, Breeze RG, Liggitt HD et al: Interaction of bovine respiratory syncytial virus and Pasteurella haemolytica in the ovine lung, *Am J Vet Res* 45:1671, 1984.
12. Davies DH, Long DL, McCarthy AR et al: The effect of parainfluenza virus type 3 on the phagocytic cell response of the ovine lung to *Pasteurella haemolytica*, *Vet Microbiol* 11: 125, 1985.
13. Buddle BM, Pfeffer A, Cole DJW et al: A caprine pneumonia outbreak associated with caprine herpesvirus and *Pasteurella haemolytica* respiratory infection, *N Z Vet J* 38:28-31, 1990.
14. Tempesta M, Pratelli A, Corrente M et al: A preliminary study on the pathogenicity of a strain of caprine herpesvirus-1, *Comp Immuno Microbiol Inf Dis* 22:137-143, 1998.
15. Li H, Taus NS, Lewis GS et al: Shedding of ovine herpesvirus 2 in sheep nasal secretions: the predominant mode for transmission, *J Clin Microbiol* 42:5558-5564, 2004.
16. Tempesta M, Greco G, Camero M et al: Virological and histological findings in goats infected by caprine herpesvirus 1, *New Microbiol* 25:281-284, 2002.
17. Brogden KA, Rose D, Cutlip RC et al: Isolation and identification of mycoplasmas from the nasal cavity of sheep, *Am J Vet Res* 49:1669, 1988.
18. Brandão E: Isolation and identification of Mycoplasma mycoides subspecies mycoides SC strains in sheep and goats, *Vet Rec* 136:98, 1995.

19. DaMassa AJ, Brooks DL, Holmberg CA et al: Caprine mycoplasmosis: an outbreak of mastitis and arthritis requiring the destruction of 700 goats, *Vet Rec* 120:409, 1987.

20. Niang M, Rosenbusch RF, Lopez-Virella J et al: Differential serologic response to *Mycoplasma ovipneumoniae* and *Mycoplasma arginini* in lambs affected with chronic respiratory disease, *J Vet Diagn Invest* 11:34-40, 1999.

21. Goltz JP, Rosendal S, McCraw BM et al: Experimental studies on the pathogenicity of *Mycoplasm ovipneumoniae* and *Mycoplasma arginini* for the respiratory tract of goats, *Can J Vet Res* 50:59-67, 1986.

22. Niang M, Rosenbusch RF, Andrews JJ et al: Occurrence of autoantibodies to cilia in lambs with a "coughing syndrome," *Vet Immunol Immunopath* 64:191-205, 1998.

23. Hernandez L, Lopez J, St-Jacques M et al: *Mycoplasma mycoides* subsp. capri associated with goat respiratory disease and high flock mortality, *Can Vet J* 47:366-369, 2006.

24. Madewell BR, Gill DB, Evermann JF: Seroprevalence of ovine progressive pneumonia virus and other selected pathogens in California cull sheep, *Prev Vet Med* 10:31, 1990.

25. Pekelder JJ, Veenink GJ, Akkermans JPWM et al: Ovine lentivirus induced indurative lymphocytic mastitis and its effect on the growth of lambs, *Vet Rec* 134:348, 1994.

26. Myer MS, Huchzermeyer HFAK, York DF et al: The possible involvement of immunosuppression caused by a lentivirus in the aetiology of jaagsiekte and pasteurellosis in sheep, *Onderstepoort J Vet Res* 55:127, 1988.

27. Paton MW, Rose IR, Hart RA et al: New infection with *Corynebacterium pseudotuberculosis* reduces wool production, *Aust Vet J* 71:47, 1994.

28. Gomez da Silva R, LaScala N, Filho AE et al: Respiratory heat loss in the sheep: a comprehensive model, *Int J Biometeorol* 46:136-140, 2002.

29. Appleyard WT, Gilmour NJL: Use of long-acting oxytetracycline against pasteurellosis in lambs, *Vet Rec* 126:231, 1990.

30. Diker KS, Akan M, Haziroglu: Antimicrobial susceptibility of *Pasteurella haemolytica* and *Pasteurella multocida* isolated from pneumonic ovine lungs, *Vet Rec* 134:597, 1994.

31. Berge AC, Sischo WM, Craigmill AL: Antimicrobial susceptibility patterns of respiratory tract pathogens from sheep and goats, *JAVMA* 229:1279-1281, 2006.

32. Council Report: Vaccination guidelines for small ruminants (sheep, goats, llamas, domestic deer, and wapiti), *J Am Vet Med Assoc* 205:1539, 1994.

33. Salsbury DL: Assessing the effectiveness of bovine respiratory vaccines for treating sheep with rhinitis, *Vet Med* 79:1520, 1984.

34. Lehmkuhl HD: Personal communication, 1996.

35. Eggleton DG, Middleton HD, Doidge CV et al: Immunization against ovine caseous lymphadenitis: comparison of *Corynebacterium pseudotuberculosis* vaccines with and without bacterial cells, *Aust Vet J* 68:317, 1991.

36. Menzies PI, Muckle CA, Brogden KA et al: A field trial to evaluate a whole cell vaccine for the prevention of caseous lymphadenitis in sheep and goat flocks, *Can J Vet Res* 55:362, 1991.

37. Bretzlaff KN: Personal communication, 1996.

38. Glenn JS: *Caseous lymphadenitis in goats with supplemental notes about sheep* (website) *http://cahfs.ucdavis.edu/disease_pdfs/caseous_lymphadenitis.pdf*. Accessed November 14, 2007.

39. Brown CC, Olander HJ, Alves SF: Synergistic hemolysis-inhibition titers associated with caseous lymphadenitis in a slaughterhouse survey of goats and sheep in northeastern Brazil, *Can J Vet Res* 51:46-49, 1987.

40. ter Laak EA, Bosch J, Bijl GC et al: Double-antibody sandwich enzyme-linked immunosorbent assay and immunoblot analysis used for control of caseous lymphadenitis in goats and sheep, *Am J Vet Res* 53:1125, 1992.

41. Menzies PI, Muckle CA, Hwang YT et al: Evaluation of an enzyme-linked immunosorbent assay using an *Escherichia coli* recombinant phospholipase D antigen for the diagnosis of *Corynebacterium pseudotuberculosis* infection, *Small Rum Res* 13:193, 1994.

CHAPTER 45

Disorders of the Upper Respiratory Tract in Food Animals

JEFFREY LAKRITZ, D. MICHAEL RINGS, and BRUCE L. HULL

Upper airway disorders are relatively uncommon in livestock, but several disorders occur frequently enough to warrant discussion. These disorders often require immediate attention because of life-threatening dyspnea. In addition, early recognition and appropriate treatment of upper airway problems provides greater likelihood of recovery, reduction of chronic scarring, and permanent dysfunction.

Historical information such as recent dehorning or weaning, as well as vaccinations status, may provide differentials helpful in narrowing the potential causes of dysfunction. In calves, historical information regarding dystocia delivery and early neonatal problems may also shed light onto upper airway disorders.

EXAMINATION OF UPPER AIRWAY

Initial examination of the upper airway patient includes observation of the animal at a distance, followed by careful auscultation and percussion of the respiratory system (including the chest, head, and neck). After thorough evaluation of the thorax, abnormal lung sounds should be compared with sounds (if any) ausculted at the level of the larynx.

Evaluation of the cardiovascular system and body temperature is also warranted to further characterize these respiratory disorders. Elevated heart rate with fever in an animal with marked inspiratory dyspnea is compatible with toxemia associated with some bacterial infections of the upper airway, head, and neck. Further, in hot climates, the respiratory system is critical to regulation of body temperature, especially in young animals.

Examination of the animal should begin by observing the animal's demeanor and attitude, as well as the respiratory rate and character. Increased work of breathing, coughing, open mouth, and the presence of noises on inspiration or expiration are all suggestive of upper airway dysfunction (such as obstruction); however, chest disease may often be involved. A honking cough in an animal displaying marked inspiratory dyspnea may also support upper airway dysfunction with reduced pharyngeal clearance of saliva and debris. Modification of the respiratory cycle to rapid, shallow breathing is sometimes observed in both pulmonary and extra-thoracic respiratory diseases.

Evaluation of the symmetry of airflow from each nostril, as well as odor from the nares or mouth, should provide information as to the location of airflow obstruction (cranial to nasal septum—unilateral; caudal to nasal septum—bilateral reduction in airflow) and whether or not necrosis of nasal or nasopharyngeal/laryngeal tissues (putrid odor) has occurred. Evaluation of the nasal mucosa at the nares is also indicated to determine whether ulcerations or erosions are noted. Ulcerations or erosions of the oral and ocular mucosae may also be assessed at this point. The presence of exudates and debris on the nares may indicate malaise and reduced cleaning by the animal's tongue. Further, dryness, chapping, and cracking of the nares may be indicative of toxemia with fever. Unilateral nasal discharge may indicate a problem rostral to the pharynx, whereas bilateral nasal discharge usually indicates lung inflammation; however, it may also indicate bilateral nasal or sinus problems.

Palpation of the trachea, larynx, and submandibular lymphoid tissue should provide information relative to airway inflammation and irritation, as well as response to the inflammation (lymphadenopathy). Animals with respiratory disease often display easily elicited coughing and pain and are generally reluctant when the head and neck are examined. This reluctance may result in fatality to the animal and potential injury to the examiner. Often two halters (on either side of the head) tied so that the head is immobilized provides efficient evaluation. Abnormalities of the larynx and throat latch can be appreciated visually and palpably if enlargement, swelling, heat, or pain are present. Evaluation of the trachea may also be performed to determine the presence of inflammation or injury of the extra-thoracic trachea or stenosis. Evaluation of submandibular lymphoid tissue is important to evaluate the severity of inflammation and for potential abscesses in this region.

Endoscopic and radiographic evaluation of the upper respiratory system, although less practical in the field, may provide much-needed information regarding the nature and severity of the problem(s) in the upper respiratory tract. Endoscopy is helpful in diseases of the nasal cavity and pharynx/larynx to observe both the anatomy and function/dysfunction of the airway. Importantly, structures rostral to the caudal aspect of the nasal septum are bilateral and passage of the endoscope up both nostrils is useful to evaluate symmetry or lack thereof. Furthermore, abnormalities of the larynx can be directly visualized including lack of mobility of the arytenoids and the presence of asymmetry or mass lesions.

Radiographic evaluation of the skull is complicated by the complexity of the bony structures in the nasal cavity and sinuses. The tremendous overlap of paired structures such as the mandibular rami, dental arcades, makes a minimum of four views necessary to highlight one side of the skull in comparison with the opposite side. In most instances several additional views may be required to help differentiate laterality, extent of lesion, and precise location. Various obliquities and rostral-to-caudal views of the poll may be helpful in evaluation of sinuses. The utility of bony structures encompassing air-filled cavities improves radiographic evaluation of these structures. The advent of digital radiography using portable radiographic equipment may make these evaluations more practical than in the past; however, cost remains prohibitive for most farm animals.

Ultrasound evaluation of the respiratory system is inherently limited by the amount of air present in these tissues. However, ultrasound evaluation of the pharynx and larynx provide valuable information regarding the location and extent of abscesses in relation to vital structures of this area. Careful study of the ventral larynx, dorsal pharynx may provide much-needed information on masses including abscesses, enlarged lymph nodes, and other abnormalities.

NASAL PASSAGES

Evaluation of the nasal planum, facial, and periorbital bones for function, symmetry, swelling, or deformation will provide external clues to problems in this anatomic location. Obvious discharges from the head (such as after dehorning) with or without facial deformation should provide clues as to the cause of depression, change in behavior, unilateral nasal discharge, or reduced productivity (Fig. 45-1). Animals with sinusitis may squint their eyes, hold their heads in unusual positions, press their heads against immovable objects, and be reluctant when the examiner approaches their heads.

The nasal cavity and sinuses may be easily evaluated by percussion of the sinuses. In a quiet environment, digital percussion over the nasal cavity and frontal/maxillary sinuses should be performed by repeatedly tapping first on one side of the face and then the other to compare the resonance of these areas. Because they are normally filled with air, percussion of these areas should have a markedly dull sound compared with nasal cavities with large space-occupying masses or sinuses full of purulent exudate. Normal sinuses sound hollow, whereas sinuses containing exudate or tissue have a remarkably dull resonance to them.

Endoscopic and radiographic imaging of the nasal passages is often rewarding in livestock in cases where treatment options are required. Although it is not possible to pass an endoscope into the sinus from the nares in livestock, one may observe changes in the architecture and/or discharges emanating from the naso-maxillary openings, suggesting sinusitis is involved. Furthermore,

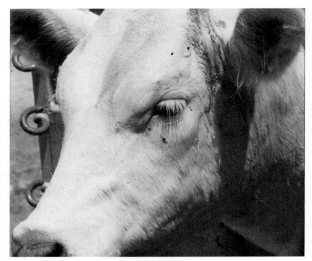

Fig 45-1   Sinusitis in a beef cow. Chronic unilateral drainage from the poll after dehorning.

rigid or flexible endoscopes may be helpful after surgical drainage of a sinus has been performed to determine the nature of residual exudates and/or presence of foreign bodies (bone sequestra, desiccated exudates).

NASAL OBSTRUCTION

Nasal obstruction in cattle may occur in association with foreign bodies, trauma, neoplasia, and various inflammatory disorders. Nasal granulomas caused by a variety of fungal agents are reported, but they are not common.[1-6] Clinical signs include unilateral or bilateral reduction of airflow, upper airway stridor, nasal discharge, objectionable odor, epistaxis, and facial deformation.[7]

Nasal masses are often unnoticed until associated with behavioral changes, dyspnea, discharge, or facial deformation. The discharge may be opaque without odor, malodorous, or with facial deformation. Nasal masses in ruminants often cause variable respiratory dysfunction (reduced airflow) and may present as unilateral airflow deficit and respiratory stridor or demonstrate severe dyspnea with open mouth breathing caused by bilateral obstruction.

For masses present in the pharynx caudal to the nasal septum, reduced airflow should be appreciated from both nostrils. For masses localized rostral to the pharynx, airflow is generally reduced on the side of the lesion assuming that enlargement of the mass has not compromised airflow to the opposite nasal passage.

Diagnostic evaluation should include radiographic and endoscopic evaluation before attempting to remove these surgically. Transendoscopically guided nasal biopsy in conjunction with sodium iodide therapy or surgical removal of these masses via a variety of approaches (laser, trephine, nasal flap) and provision of a patent airway have been recommended.[7] Alternatively, after confirmation of etiology either through demonstration of fungal elements or eosinophilia in cytologic or biopsy preparations, intravenous sodium iodide (70 mg/kg IV every 10-14 days) may be helpful in early cases.[8] Nasal obstruction associated

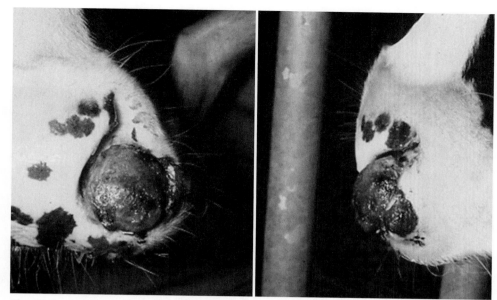

Fig 45-2   Atypical actinobacillosis in a Holstein cow. Granulomatous mass protruding from the left nares in a cow with nasal obstruction, stridor, discharge, and odor.

with *Actinobacillosis* and *Nocardiosis* have also been associated with obstructive nasal lesions[4-6,9] (Fig. 45-2). The severity of dysfunction caused by nasal obstruction in ruminants often depends on location of the mass and chronicity of the lesion. Bilateral airflow reduction is generally associated with more severe lesions or lesions involving the caudal nasal and pharyngeal regions.

Nasal tumors are rare in cattle; however, squamous cell carcinoma, liposarcoma, chondrosarcoma, lymphosarcoma, and osteomas have all been reported in cattle[10-14] (Fig. 45-3).

Nasal obstruction in sheep can occur with nasal bot *(Oestrus ovis)* infestation and a variety of tumors. The most frequently observed nasal tumor of sheep and goats clinically is the enzootic nasal adenocarcinoma.[15-17]

This tumor is associated with the presence of an endogenous beta retrovirus and is most common in younger sheep. These masses form in the ethmoidal region of the nasal turbinates and are cystic, nodular masses (Fig. 45-4). Clinical signs include nasal discharge, inspiratory dyspnea, open mouth breathing, decreased airflow, and head shaking or sneezing.

PARANASAL SINUSES

Sinusitis is most common in cattle and less common in sheep and goats. Sinusitis is commonly observed after dehorning or trauma to the skull or horn and less commonly occurs in animals postviral infection (see Fig. 45-1). Sinusitis also most commonly occurs in the frontal sinus, with the maxillary sinus (tooth root abscesses, fractures) being next most common (Fig. 45-5). Sinusitis may also occur after facial trauma, neoplasia and nasal bot infestation in sheep.

Sinusitis may occur immediately after or months after dehorning.[14] Sinusitis often involves trauma or contamination during the surgical procedure or postdehorning fly

strike or hemorrhage. In some cases the wound produced during dehorning has not yet healed or has broken open, resulting in the presence of purulent exudates draining from the wound. In the case of chronic sinusitis, facial deformation may occur because of long-standing accumulation of exudates within the sinus (Fig. 45-6).

Typical clinical signs in cases of sinusitis may include normal to elevated body temperature, discharge from a wound, unilateral or bilateral nasal discharge, reduced productivity associated with reduced appetite, depression, and increased apprehension when the animal's head is examined. Animals may lower their heads, press heads against immovable objects, and extend their heads and necks, suggesting skull discomfort.

Management of sinusitis relies on establishing open drainage and lavage of the sinus to remove exudate. Antimicrobial therapy in conjunction with antiinflammatory drugs are of use to reduce the discomfort and inflammation to improve the animal's appetite. However, drainage and lavage is most critical to resolution and prevention of further disfigurement or more severe consequences (Fig. 45-7). Drainage of the frontal and maxillary sinuses has been described elsewhere; however, several key features are worth mentioning.[7,18] First, normal bone in the skull is difficult to trephine, whereas bone overlying an infected sinus is relatively soft and easy to cut into with standard instruments. Small holes, as drilled with a 14-gauge needle, are useful to obtain diagnostic specimens. However, because of the nature of the exudates, larger-diameter (trephine) holes are necessary to drain the sinus and promote healing. Recurrent sinusitis after adequate drainage and lavage should indicate the need for radiographic evaluation. Inspissated exudates or sequestered bone may both result in recurrence of sinusitis. Radiographic evaluation of the sinuses should also be performed after drainage and lavage of the affected sinus in cases where resolution of the problem is not observed (see Fig. 45-7).

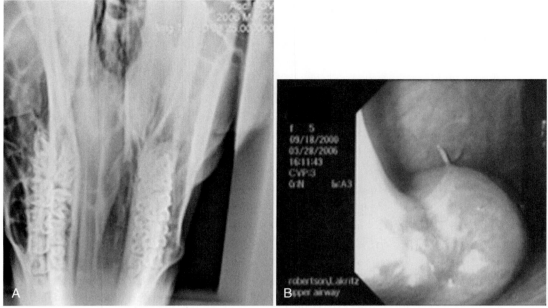

Fig 45-3   Nasal obstruction caused by lymphosarcoma in an adult Brown Swiss cow. Nasal lymphoma in a 6-year-old Brown Swiss cow presented for upper airway stridor, open mouth breathing, and odor. On placement of a tracheotomy tube, the cow's demeanor and respiratory effort improved dramatically. After removal of the mass via nasal flap and partial nasal septum removal, the cow was able to breath without the help of a tracheotomy tube. Unfortunately, the cow died 4 months later because of a gastrointestinal disturbance later diagnosed as abomasal lymphoma. **A,** Dorso-ventral radiograph of the nasal passages of the cow. The nasal septum deviates laterally on the left side near the caudal aspect of the septum. **B,** Endoscopic appearance of the nasal septum from the left nostril demonstrating a mass protruding into the nasal cavity, partially obstructing the flow of air.

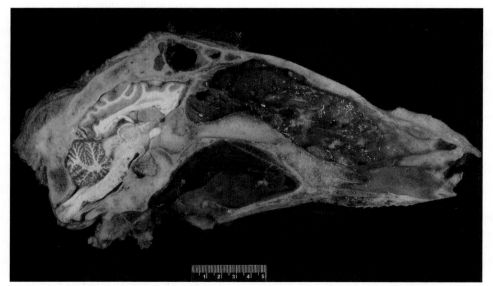

Fig 45-4   Sagittal section of the skull of a ram presenting for dyspnea, upper airway obstruction, nasal discharge, and chronic weight loss. The nasal passages and pharynx are nearly completely obstructed by an edematous, cystic, and nodular mass.

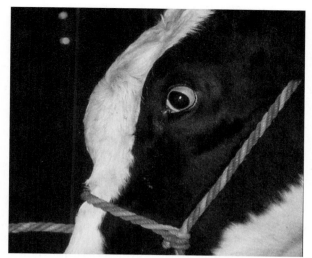

Fig 45-5 Frontal sinusitis in a Holstein heifer. Note the marked distortion of the face of this animal.

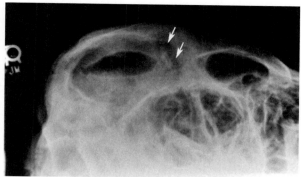

Fig 45-7 Rostral to caudal radiographic view of the frontal sinus of the yearling Guernsey heifer shown in Figure 45-6. This radiographic view is produced by placement of the cassette caudal to the poll to demonstrate the caudal portions of the frontal sinuses. Note the significant deformation of the skull, amount of exudate and granulation tissue present within the left sinus, and sequestered bone near the midline in the sinus cavity (arrows). After removing the bone fragment and débriding the granulation tissue present within the sinus and repeated lavage, the sinusitis was resolved.

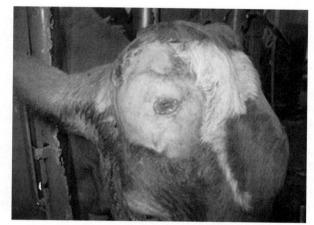

Fig 45-6 Standing photograph of yearling Guernsey heifer with frontal deformation caused by fluid-filled sinus several months postdehorning. The dehorning site never completely healed over and periodically produced exudate. At the time of initial evaluation, this animal was reluctant to have the skull examined and demonstrated marked unilateral dullness on percussion and deformation of the right side of the skull. This photograph was made several days after a cornual opening was débrided and a ventral trephine hole was produced to facilitate drainage. The heifer continued to drain material from the sinus despite daily saline lavage.

PHARYNX

Pharyngeal/retropharyngeal abscessation occurs most commonly through inappropriate use of oral dosing equipment, stomach tubes, or potentially coarse feedstuffs. Indiscriminant consumption of foreign bodies in cattle leading to pharyngeal infections is infrequently observed. Coarse feeds or foreign body punctures may damage the pharyngeal mucosa, allowing deep inoculation of infectious material in the peripharyngeal tissues and resulting in abscessation. Pharyngeal abscesses usually reduce airflow bilaterally from the nares. The bacteria most frequently involved include *Archanobacter pyogenes* and anaerobic bacteria. In sheep and goats, retropharyngeal abscessation is associated with oral trauma and may result from *Corynebacterium pseudotuberculosis* infection of the submandibular or retropharyngeal lymph nodes, leading to airway compromise.

History and clinical signs often include prior oral medications or magnets, hasty use of stomach tubes, poor quality forage, and forage containing foreign bodies (such as wire). Clinical signs include pharyngeal swelling, head and neck extension, excessive salivation, increased water consumption, and decreased feed consumption. The respiratory signs may include dyspnea on inspiration and may be severe. Animals with pharyngeal puncture often have extremely malodorous breath. Palpation of the dorsal pharyngeal and laryngeal areas may elicit severe pain, and the animal may attempt to escape vigorously.

Diagnostics should include complete oral examination and careful external palpation. If the pharyngeal mass is obstructing the flow of air significantly, one may consider placement of a tracheotomy tube before performing further diagnostics. Endoscopic, ultrasonographic, and radiographic imaging are extremely helpful in these cases (Figs. 45-8 to 45-10).

Treatment may include intraoral lancing and drainage of abscesses and local wound care or a lateral or ventral cervical approach to these abscesses. Animals that cannot swallow feed may benefit from placement of a rumen fistula to provide feed and water in conjunction with surgical drainage. Antimicrobial drugs should include penicillin G (20,000-40,000 IU/kg IM once daily) or tetracyclines (6.6 mg/kg IV twice daily or 11 mg/kg IV once daily).

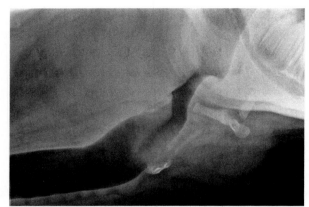

Fig 45-8   Retropharyngeal abscessation in a yearling heifer with unknown etiology. Notice the reduction in the size of the laryngeal opening and the enlargement of the submandibular lymph nodes bilaterally. Surgical drainage of the abscess was effected by placement of a 6-inch spinal needle into the abscess and blunt dissection down into the abscess cavity to facilitate drainage. A second opening was made ventrally to allow placement of a Penrose drain to ensure resolution. Daily lavage and removal of debris resulted in complete recovery and return to normal airway function.

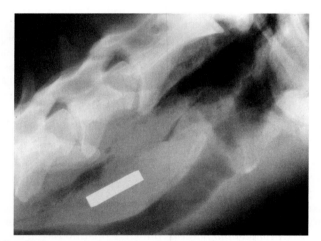

Fig 45-9   Standing lateral radiograph of a heifer with dorsal pharyngeal soft tissue gas accumulation and swelling associated with inappropriate administration of a magnet. The magnet punctured the dorsal pharyngeal wall, inducing cellulitis and abscessation.

Antimicrobial treatment for approximately 5 days is generally sufficient for responsive cases. Flunixin meglumine (0.5-1.1 mg/kg IV once to twice daily) may help improve the animals' comfort enough to resume feed consumption. A cheaper alternative to flunixin meglumine is aspirin (100 mg/kg orally twice daily), although bolusing aspirin to animals with pharyngeal trauma is not recommended. In granulomatous infections, the use of sodium iodide at 70 mg/kg IV once weekly may help to reduce the duration of dysfunction.

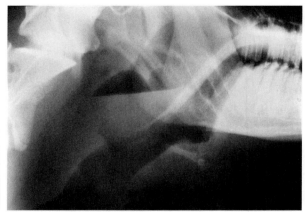

Fig 45-10   Standing lateral radiographic appearance of a cow with dorsal retropharyngeal abscessation demonstrating gas accumulation with a fluid line. The animal presented with her head and neck extended.

LARYNX

Laryngeal dysfunction most commonly occurs secondary to chondritis of the laryngeal cartilages with or without pharyngeal involvement. Necrosis of the laryngeal cartilages with abscessation most commonly occurs after a viral infection or injury to the laryngeal or perilaryngeal mucosa with subsequent infection associated with anaerobic bacteria. One reference suggested that anaerobic bacterial invasion occurs most commonly secondary to gram-negative, nonenteric, bacterial perilaryngeal vasculitis associated with *Histophilus somnus*.[19] In most cases in our practice, treatment has been attempted for 1 to 3 weeks or more without success. Most cases are in respiratory distress when examined, with loud, harsh respiratory sounds emanating from the upper airway. Recently weaned calves may develop dysfunction of the pharynx and larynx because of persistent vocalization. Older calves and cattle are more reluctant when the head and neck are manipulated or examined than younger suckling calves. Rapid and efficient management of these cases is prudent.

Some have moderate swelling of the pharyngeal area observed on the ventral aspect of the throat-latch area. Calves with necrotic laryngitis are most often febrile with rectal temperatures exceeding 104° F to 106° F (40°-41.1° C), display head and neck extension with open mouth breathing, and are generally mildly to moderately dehydrated. Some animals have extremely malodorous breath associated with pyogenic bacterial abscessation of the laryngeal cartilages.

Auscultation of the thorax reveals loud, harsh inspiratory sounds that, when the larynx and proximal trachea are ausculted, reveal the location of the sounds as the upper airway. When these cases are further evaluated by tracheotomy, the immediate response to provision of a patent airway of suitable diameter is generally diagnostic. In the absence of response, our experience suggests that tracheal stenosis/collapse or unresponsive bronchopneumonia causes the clinical signs.

Endoscopic examination of the upper airway is recommended in cases where additional handling is thought to

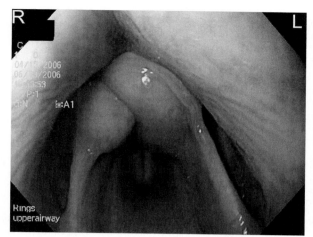

Fig 45-11 Endoscopic appearance of the larynx in a 4-month-old Holstein heifer demonstrating swelling and edema of the arytenoids, marked increase in the size of the left arytenoid, and inability to abduct the arytenoids bilaterally. Notice the vocal folds are closely apposed. In video examination they did not move during inspiration.

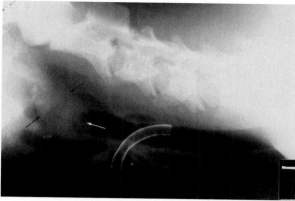

Fig 45-12 Lateral radiograph of a 6-month-old Holstein heifer with upper airway obstruction. After placement of a temporary tracheotomy tube, marked improvement in ventilation was evident. Note the large, soft tissue mass obscuring the larynx (arrows). Resected mass from larynx of calf via laryngotomy approach was malignant lymphoma.

produce minimal additional distress to the animal (Fig. 45-11). However, initial tracheotomy with placement of a temporary tracheotomy tube is usually preferred, before further examination.

After proper placement of a temporary tracheotomy tube, the respiratory effort generally decreases dramatically. Auscultation of the thorax will confirm the reduced effort and referred sounds, although a fair number of calves will have aspiration pneumonia before initial examination. In addition to endoscopic examination, radiographic evaluation of the severity of aspiration pneumonia and a single standing lateral radiograph of the larynx and pharyngeal region should be sufficient to determine the extent of laryngeal narrowing, perilaryngeal/pharyngeal compression, or other lesions. In our opinion, after careful thoracic examination, loud upper airway sounds are suggestive of proximal airway stenosis and placement of a tracheotomy tube is both diagnostic and therapeutic. Assumptions such as aspiration pneumonia are valid in many cases, but the antimicrobial agent and ancillary therapy should cover the infectious processes present: namely, anaerobic bacterial laryngitis with chronic aspiration pneumonia.

Other proximal airway lesions may be observed from time to time. Subepiglottic cysts or abscesses and laryngeal neoplasia have been reported (Fig. 45-12).[20,21] In one case examined, radiographic evaluation revealed a large subepiglottic mass extending rostrally and dorsally, obscuring the view of the laryngeal opening (Fig. 45-13). Ultrasound imaging revealed a mass with mixed echogenicity surrounded by a dense capsule suggestive of an abscess. Aspiration of the mass revealed purulent exudate, which resolved once surgical drainage was established (Fig. 45-14). Culture of abscess material revealed growth of large numbers of *Mycoplasma bovis*.

Early treatment of these cases involves steroidal or nonsteroidal antiinflammatory drugs, in addition to broad-spectrum antimicrobial therapy. In our experience, procaine penicillin G (22,000-44,000 U/kg, IM or SQ) twice daily in conjunction with 0.25 to 0.5 mg/kg dexamethasone (IV, IM) once to twice daily reduces swelling, allowing more effective treatment of the bacterial infections. If laryngeal abscessation is suspected, drainage of the abscess is usually required for more rapid recovery and return of function. In more chronic cases, laryngotracheotomy or permanent tracheostomy is the preferred means of providing a patent airway. Some authors have demonstrated suitable clinical response with relatively long-term use of lincomycin (3-8 mg/kg IV/IM; q 24 hr) for intervals of up to 3 weeks; however, this drug is not approved for use in cattle in North America.

Careful management of the tracheotomy tube is required to prevent asphyxiation. First, the tube should be cuffless or not inflated in case of accumulation of hemorrhage or exudates over the end of the tracheotomy tube (see Fig. 45-13). In animals in which the cuff is inflated, obstruction of the tube with debris will result in asphyxiation. Second, the tube should be removed and cleaned twice daily. Some temporary tracheotomy tubes are made with indwelling inserts, allowing removal of the inner tube for cleaning and replacement. The tracheotomy tube is generally secured to the neck with umbilical tape, roll gauze, or twine to prevent expulsion of the tube during coughing frequently observed in these animals.

TRACHEAL STENOSIS IN CALVES

Tracheal stenosis is uncommon in calves. When observed, it is frequently associated with fractured ribs that occurred during delivery of the calf. The rib fractures develop a bony callous that enlarge, deform, and eventually compress the intrathoracic trachea (Fig. 45-15). Vigorous extraction of the calf (generally posterior presentation, dorso-sacral position) during dystocia results in significant compression of its thorax because of the impact of

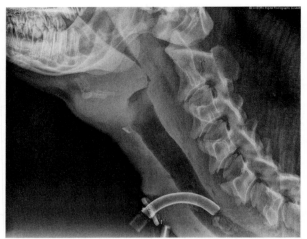

Fig 45-13 Lateral radiograph of a 2-month-old Holstein heifer with upper airway obstruction. Placement of a temporary tracheotomy tube resulted in immediate clinical improvement. Note that a large, soft tissue density below the epiglottis retroflexes the epiglottis caudally and over the laryngeal opening. Note also the presence of exudates near the distal opening of the tracheotomy tube within the trachea.

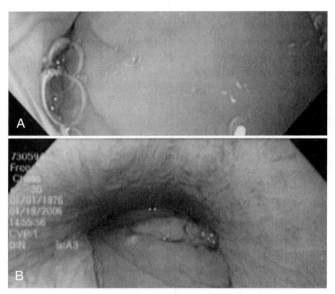

Fig 45-14 Endoscopic appearance of the larynx of the calf shown in Figure 45-13. **A,** The mass protrudes upward to the dorsal pharyngeal wall and completely obscures the laryngeal opening. **B,** Two days post-drainage of the subepiglottic mass, the soft palate and tip of the epiglottis are visible. The mass lesion had not completely resolved at this time.

the calf sternum on the floor of the dams pelvis. This may result in fractures of the cranial-most ribs, which form a callous during healing. Historical information such as dystocia with or without fetal extraction involving the rear limbs first is generally helpful information. Animals

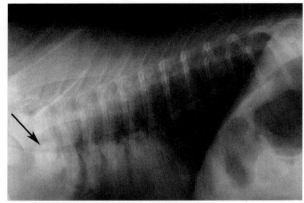

Fig 45-15 Radiographic appearance of 3-week-old Limousin calf with chronic rib fractures demonstrating marked bony proliferation and tracheal narrowing *(arrow)*.

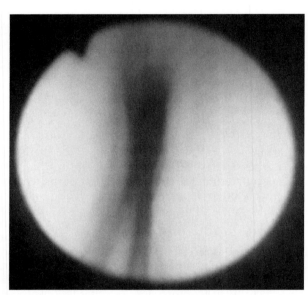

Fig 45-16 Endoscopic appearance of trachea of calf with tracheal stenosis. Marked reduction of the diameter of the trachea is evident.

with rib fractures are often not exceptionally vigorous immediately after birth, and this information may also help to confirm the diagnosis. Palpation of the thorax for deformation of the thoracic cage, irregularities in the contour of external surface, and endoscopic documentation of tracheal narrowing are helpful in the diagnosis of tracheal stenosis (Fig. 45-16).

TRACHEAL COLLAPSE IN SHEEP/GOATS

Tracheal collapse is sometimes observed in goats and sheep. Most cases are associated with dysplasia and may be the result of maternal consumption of toxic plants during gestation. Administration of *Veratrum californicum* by gavage to ewes at gestational days 31 to 33 of pregnancy is associated with tracheal stenosis in their lambs.[22,23]

References

1. Conti DI, Vargas R, Apolo A et al: Mycotic bovine nasal granuloma, *Rev Inst Med Trop Sao Paulo* 45:163-166, 2003.
2. De Bosschere H, Audenaerde P, Ducatelle R: Seasonal variation in the morphology of a bovine nasal granuloma, *Vet Rec* 146:322-323, 2000.
3. Penrith ML, Van der Lugt JJ, Henton MM et al: A review of mycotic nasal granuloma in cattle, with a report on three cases, *J S Afr Vet Assoc* 65:179-183, 1994.
4. Rebhun WC, King JM, Hillman RB: Atypical actinobacillosis granulomas in cattle, *Cornell Vet* 78:125-130, 1988.
5. Shibahara T, Mitarai Y, Ishikawa Y et al: Bovine nasal eosinophilic, granuloma with blood eosinophilia caused by *Nocardia* species, *Aust Vet J* 79:363-365, 2001.
6. Takahashi K, Toda N, Kakiichi N et al: Nasal nocardiosis in a calf, *J Vet Med Sci* 61:421-423, 1999.
7. Gaughan EM, Provo-Klimek J, Ducharme NG: *Farm animal surgery*, St Louis, 2004, Saunders, pp 141-159.
8. Baker JC, Smith JA: *Large animal internal medicine*, St Louis, 2002, Mosby, pp 541-550.
9. Anderson KL, Fairley RA, Duncan D: Suspected actinobacillosis manifested by facial enlargement in a heifer, *J Am Vet Med Assoc* 197:1359-1360, 1990.
10. Beytut E, Kilic E, Ozturk S et al: Nasal chondrosarcoma in a Simmental cow, *Can Vet J* 47:349-351, 2006.
11. Pycock JF, Pead MJ, Longstaffe JA: Squamous cell carcinoma in the nasal cavity of a cow, *Vet Rec* 114:542-543, 1984.
12. Rumbaugh GE, Pool RR, Wheat JD: Atypical osteoma of the nasal passage and paranasal sinus in a bull, *Cornell Vet* 68:544-554, 1978.
13. Shive H, Mohammed F, Osterstock J et al: Liposarcoma in the nasal cavity of a cow, *Vet Pathol* 43:793-797, 2006.
14. Ward JL, Rebhun WC: Chronic frontal sinusitis in dairy cattle: 12 cases (1978-1989), *J Am Vet Med Assoc* 201:326-328, 1992.
15. DeMartini JC, Carlson JO, Leroux C et al: Endogenous retroviruses related to jaagsiekte sheep retrovirus, *Curr Top Microbiol Immunol* 275:117-137, 2003.
16. DeMartini JC, York DF: Retrovirus-associated neoplasms of the respiratory system of sheep and goats. Ovine pulmonary carcinoma and enzootic nasal tumor, *Vet Clin North Am Food Anim Pract* 13:55-70, 1997.
17. Sharp JM, DeMartini JC: Natural history of JSRV in sheep, *Curr Top Microbiol Immunol* 275:55-79, 2003.
18. Honnas CM, Pascoe JR, East NE: *Large animal internal medicine*, St Louis, 2002, Mosby, pp 543-545.
19. Baker JC, Smith JA: Diseases of the pharynx, larynx and trachea. In Smith BP, editor: *Textbook of large animal internal medicine*, St Louis, 2002, Mosby, pp 545-550.
20. Mattoon JS, Andrews D, Jones SL et al: Subepiglottic cyst causing upper airway obstruction in a neonatal calf, *J Am Vet Med Assoc* 199:747-749, 1991.
21. Willoughby RA: Case report. Laryngeal obstruction due to lymphosarcoma, *Can Vet J* 8:291-293, 1967.
22. Keeler RF, Binns W: Teratogenic compounds of Veratrum californicum (Durand). II. Production of ovine fetal cyclopia by fractions and alkaloid preparations, *Can J Biochem* 44:829-838, 1966.
23. Keeler RF, Young S, Smart R: Congenital tracheal stenosis in lambs induced by maternal ingestion of *Veratrum californicum*, *Teratology* 31:83-88, 1985.

CHAPTER 46

Surgery of the Larynx and Trachea

DAVID E. ANDERSON

ARYTENOID CHONDRITIS AND LARYNGEAL GRANULOMA

Arytenoid chondritis is rarely diagnosed, but it is not uncommonly seen in cattle affected with necrotic laryngitis. Arytenoid swelling may cause inspiratory dyspnea and respiratory noise ("honker" calves). The narrowed glottis causes increased airway turbulence that may cause the arytenoid swelling to persist. Medical treatment (antibiotics and antiinflammatory drugs) is usually curative. Administration of steroids is indicated when acute swelling with severe dyspnea is found. I have performed temporary tracheostomy in calves when chronic arytenoid swelling caused sufficient inspiratory dyspnea to limit activity and feed intake. Partial or subtotal arytenoidectomy via a laryngotomy is only indicated when necrosis of the arytenoid cartilage is found. Scar tissue formation causing reduced glottic diameter ("webbing") may require ventral laryngotomy and surgical reduction of the scar tissue.[1] Excessive scar tissue is usually formed on the vocal cords (vocal process of the arytenoid cartilage); excessive granulation is usually formed on the medial aspect of the arytenoid cartilages. For débridement of the larynx and removal of necrotic cartilage, a ventral midline incision centered over the larynx is made; the sternohyoideus muscles are separated; and the thyroid cartilage, cricothyroid ligament, cricoid cartilage, and first two tracheal rings are incised.[2] Volkmann retractors are helpful to expose the larynx. Necrotic tissues are débrided and excised. The laryngotomy may be closed primarily, partially closed with implantation of a Penrose drain, or left open for second intention healing. A tracheostomy may be required for intubation of the trachea when general anesthesia is used, and the tracheostomy should be maintained after surgery until laryngeal swelling has diminished sufficiently for adequate breathing.

Laryngeal granuloma may be formed as a result of trauma to the arytenoid cartilage or vocal cords (rough feeds, balling gun, orogastric tube), infection (necrotic laryngitis), infectious bovine rhinotracheitis, laryngeal ulcers, and foreign bodies.[3] Differential diagnoses should include laryngeal abscess, hematoma, neoplasia, and papilloma. When inspiratory dyspnea is present, surgical removal of the granulation tissue is indicated. This may be performed transorally using a wire loop, transendoscopically with cautery or laser, or via a ventral laryngotomy. Endoscopy-guided transoral removal of an extensive laryngeal granuloma was curative in a 5-year-old Hereford bull.[3] A temporary tracheostomy tube was used, and aspiration of small quantities of food into the trachea was observed as a short-term complication.

SURGICAL APPROACH TO LARYNX AND PHARYNX

Surgery of the larynx and pharynx may be performed transnasally using a flexible endoscope, transorally using a mouth speculum, or via ventral midline pharyngotomy or laryngotomy. Transnasal endoscopy is limited to surgery amenable to transendoscopic instruments (biopsy, wire loops, electrocautery, laser). Therefore manipulation and dissection are minimal. Transoral surgery has limited access to the pharynx and larynx because the mouth can only be opened approximately 30 degrees. Usually surgery is limited to the use of a single hand. Ventral midline pharyngotomy or laryngotomy is the approach of choice when transnasal and transoral approaches are not adequate. Ventral laryngotomy can be performed with the animal standing in a restraint chute. Sedation and use of halters or a nose lead may be required. Tissues are locally anesthetized with 2% lidocaine HCl immediately before surgery. When extensive débridement is anticipated, I prefer to perform laryngotomy with the animal under general anesthesia.

It is recommended that all feed and water be withheld from mature cattle for 24 and 12 hours before surgery, respectively, to minimize the risks of regurgitation during surgery. An 8-cm incision is made along the ventral midline, centered over the thyroid cartilage. The thyroid cartilage of cattle does not have a large V-shaped indentation on its ventral aspect, as is found in horses. Therefore incision through the thyrocricoid ligament provides inadequate exposure to the larynx. Division of the ventral midline of the thyroid, cricoid, and cranial tracheal cartilages may be necessary to achieve adequate exposure.[1,2] Alternatively, the incision may be centered rostral to the thyroid cartilage and a pharyngotomy performed. This involves deeper tissue dissection but provides exposure to the pharynx without incising the laryngeal cartilages.

TRACHEOSTOMY

Tracheostomy may be performed on an emergency or an elective basis. Tracheostomy is required in cattle to bypass a life-threatening obstruction of the upper respiratory tract or prophylactically for extensive upper respiratory tract surgeries in which postoperative swelling could be severe or in which tamponade of the nasal passages is required to control hemorrhage. Some examples are necrotic laryngitis, actinobacillosis, neoplasm of the pharyngeal or nasal region, cystic nasal conchae, foreign bodies in the upper respiratory tract, and laryngeal spasm.[4] Tracheostomy is usually performed with the animal in a standing position. Using a halter and a nose lead is recommended. Both the lead rope and nose lead should be attached to the overhead frame of the head gate or chute. This will extend the head dorsally and renders the cervical areas available for surgery. Bow knots should be used in case quick release is necessary.

Sedation should be administered only if absolutely necessary because sedation can produce more upper airway collapse. The surgical site is approximately at the junction of the middle and rostral third of the neck.[5] Ideally, if time allows, the operative site is clipped and the incision site is shaved and aseptically prepared. Local anesthesia is achieved by infiltrating the proposed incision area with 15 ml of 2% lidocaine HCl. With the head extended upward so that the skin over the trachea is taut, the trachea is stabilized with the thumb and index finger of one hand. An 8-cm incision is made on the ventral midline and is extended through the cutaneous coli muscle and the septum of the paired sternothyroideus and sternohyoideus muscles. The trachea is gently freed by blunt dissection from the surrounding fascia, and with a scalpel a stab incision is made horizontally in the annular ligament between two tracheal rings. Scissors can be used to enlarge the opening, but the incision of the annular ligament should not extend more than half the circumference of the trachea. A tracheostomy tube can then be inserted. Another method is to remove an elliptical piece of cartilage from each of the two adjacent rings. The tracheal rings should not be severed completely to avoid tracheal collapse.

The tracheostomy tube is anchored in position. The tracheostomy tube should be changed and cleaned once or twice daily, depending on the amount of accumulated secretions. The tube is removed permanently when the upper airway is patent. The tracheostomy site usually heals uneventfully by secondary intention healing. Complications of tracheostomy are cellulitis, subcutaneous abscess, subcutaneous emphysema, and tracheal stenosis. Tracheal stenosis often depends on the length of time the tracheostomy tube was left in place or if tracheal cartilage were incised or damaged by tubes. A permanent tracheostomy may be indicated for certain conditions like severe necrotic laryngitis. To create a permanent tracheostomy, portions of three or four tracheal rings are removed and the mucosa of the trachea is apposed to the skin.[6] Some of the complications with this technique are closure of the tracheal stoma, tracheal collapse, and chronic obstructive pulmonary disease.

References

1. Fischer W: Experiences with surgical treatment of the larynx in cattle with special consideration of calves, *Dtsch Tierarztl Wschr* 82:137-146, 1975.
2. Gamboa Je, Angel KL, Shoemaker RS et al: Laryngeal granuloma in a bull, *J Am Vet Med Assoc* 201:460-462, 1992.
3. Kersjes AW, Nemeth F, Rutgers LJE: The neck: larynx and trachea. In Kersjes AW, Nemeth F, Rutgers LJE, editors: *Atlas of large animal surgery*, Utrecht, The Netherlands, 1985, Wetenschappelijke uitgeverij Bunge, p 23.
4. Lekeux P, Art T: Functional changes induced by necrotic laryngitis in double muscled calves, *Vet Rec* 121:353, 1987.
5. Krypan MK: Tracheostomy in the horse: a photo essay, *Mod Vet Pract* 65:9-12, 1984.
6. Shappel KK, Stick JA, Derksen FJ et al: Permanent tracheostomy in Equidae: 47 cases (1981-1986), *J Am Vet Med Assoc* 192:939-942, 1988.

CHAPTER 47

Thoracic Surgery in Cattle

DAVID E. ANDERSON

PULMONARY ABSCESS

Lung abscesses are usually caused by chronic pneumonia or septicemia, or they are secondary to trauma or parasite infestation. Often, these abscesses are multiple and spread throughout the lung parenchyma. Therefore surgical treatment is not practical; however, lung abscess secondary to foreign body penetration of the lung (including traumatic reticulopleuritis/pneumonitis) may be amenable to surgery. Surgical treatment of pulmonary abscesses may include partial lung lobectomy or marsupialization of a large abscess. A large abscess within the right caudal lung lobe of a 2-year-old Simmental heifer was marsupialized to the thoracic wall. The abscess was caused by a wire penetrating through the reticulum and into the caudal aspect of the lung. The abscess was identified using ultrasonography and evaluated by thoroscopy. Six centimeters of the overlying seventh rib were resected, and the capsule of the abscess marsupialized to the thoracic wall and skin. These abscesses may contain *Arcanobacter pyogenes*, *Fusobacterium necrophorum*, *Clostridium* spp., and mixed populations of gram-positive and gram-negative bacteria.

LUNG BIOPSY

Percutaneous lung biopsy has been used in some species to obtain specimens for cytology, histopathology, bacterial and fungal culture, or for virus isolation. In my experience, this technique has limited usefulness compared with transtracheal wash or bronchoalveolar lavage. Pulmonary disease must be regionally diffuse to ensure that a diagnostic specimen is obtained. Also, lung biopsy has the risk of inducing tension pneumothorax or hemothorax. Lung biopsy can be done through the fifth, sixth, seventh, or eighth intercostal space at a point approximately 10 to 15 cm dorsal to the costochondral junction. I recommend ultrasound guidance or thoroscopy to increase the chances of obtaining a diagnostic specimen. Once the site has been selected, the hair is clipped, the skin aseptically prepared, and local anesthesia induced with 2% lidocaine HCl. Care should be taken not to lacerate the lung with the tip of the needle in case of sudden movement by the animal. Cattle should be observed for respiratory distress (pneumothorax, hemothorax) for 6 to 12 hours after biopsy.

SURGICAL APPROACH TO LUNG AND MEDIASTINUM

Surgery of the lung or mediastinal structures is rarely indicated in cattle. Lung abscesses or congenital anomalies in calves may be removed by lung lobectomy. Collapsing trachea in calves, tracheal foreign body, or intrathoracic esophageal obstruction may require surgical approach to the mediastinum. The cranial rib cage of cattle has limited compliance; therefore exposure to the cranioventral thorax requires rib resection. Fifth or sixth rib resection and thoracotomy are described under surgery of the thorax.

Exposure of the cranial portion of the thoracic trachea is done by resection of the first two ribs from a caudal cervical approach. This procedure is described under surgery of the trachea. Exposure to the caudal lung lobes and mediastinum is done by making a 15-cm vertical incision into the pleural space through the seventh, eighth, or ninth intercostal space. The incision is begun approximately 10 cm dorsal to the costochondral junction and extended dorsally. The caudal lung lobes are immediately accessible. The mediastinum is approached by cranial displacement of the lungs and careful dissection. Histologic diagnosis of esophageal adenocarcinoma was made from the surgical biopsies and confirmed after necropsy. Disruption of the vagus and phrenic nerves, the caudal vena cava, descending aorta, or esophagus is undesirable. Positive-pressure ventilation is required when performing thoracotomy with the animal in lateral recumbency. Rib resection can be performed in standing cattle and cattle restrained on an inclined table without mechanical ventilation because of the intact mediastinum; however, I recommend that immediate access to tracheal intubation and ventilation be available before standing thoracotomy is attempted. The intercostal muscles and pleura are closed together with absorbable suture material (No. 1 polydioxanone or polymerized caprolactam) and subcutaneous tissues, and skin closure is routine.

THORACIC WOUNDS, RIB FRACTURE

Thoracic wounds causing compromise of the thoracic cavity are infrequently found in cattle. Puncture wounds, such as from homed cattle, gunshot, fence posts, or other foreign bodies can cause tension pneumothorax and pyothorax. Tension pneumothorax is created when a wound in the thoracic wall or lung allows movement of air into the pleural space but does not allow exiting of the air. Thus intrathoracic pressure increases cause collapse of the lung and diminished movement of the diaphragm and thoracic wall. Tension pneumothorax is immediately life threatening. Placement of a chest tube or suction tube into the affected side of the thorax is followed by immediate improvement in respiratory effort. Open thoracic wounds (allowing two-way movement of air) are usually not immediately life threatening because of the complete mediastinum of cattle. Cattle can adequately oxygenate their blood with one healthy lung; however, productivity is markedly compromised. Open wounds may be treated by surgical closure (which may require use of a myocutaneous flap) and reestablishment of normal thoracic pressure by use of a suction tube or one-way valve (Heimlich) attached to a chest tube.

Rib fracture occurs most commonly in calves born with dystocia. Excessive traction during manual extraction of the calf can cause fracture of ribs 1, 2, 3, 4, or 5, or any combination of these. Multiple rib fractures may cause a flail chest breathing pattern. The rib cage caudal to rib 5 is more compliant, and trauma is less likely to cause fracture during dystocia. Trailer accidents may result in rib fracture, but fracture in the appendicular skeleton is more common. Although calves usually do well in the immediate postparturient period after rib fracture, these calves

may succumb to pneumonia or septicemia or develop progressive tracheal collapse.

PLEURITIS AND PERICARDITIS

In cattle, pericarditis is most commonly caused by penetrating foreign bodies originating in the reticulum. Pleuritis may be caused by pneumonia, pulmonary abscess, extension of a liver abscess through the diaphragm, and penetrating reticular foreign bodies.[1,2] Nonseptic pleural effusion is most commonly caused by heart failure or thoracic neoplasia. Septic pericarditis has a poor to grave prognosis for life, and septic pleuritis has a guarded to poor prognosis for life. In one retrospective study, cattle with pericarditis ($n = 7$) or unilateral pleuritis ($n = 7$) had thoracotomy performed.[1] Of seven cattle with pericarditis, one survived to discharge from the hospital. Of seven cattle with unilateral pleuritis, five survived to discharge from the hospital. One year after discharge, five cows were productive and one had been culled because of infertility. Although death after foreign body penetration of the pericardium is usually caused by progressive fibrosing constrictive pericarditis and epicarditis, cardiac tamponade from perforation of the coronary artery also has been found.[3] Prognosis may be better for cattle in good body condition, with relatively normal appetite, ability to ambulate, and age younger than 5 years.[4]

DIAPHRAGMATIC HERNIA

Diaphragmatic hernias are infrequently diagnosed in cattle. The most common clinical signs are recurrent rumen tympany (bloat), abdominal pain, diarrhea, dyspnea, anorexia, and weight loss.[5-8] Diaphragmatic defects have been diagnosed in young calves and adults.[8] Although traumatic reticuloperitonitis and congenital defects are thought to be the most common causes of diaphragmatic hernia in cattle, trauma (in calves from dystocia and in bulls from bull fights) and increased preparturient and parturient abdominal pressure should be considered.[9-12] The severity of clinical signs is related to the severity of visceral displacement into the thorax. Surgical correction has been described in cattle. A 10 cm × 8 cm defect in a 5-month-old heifer was closed using a nylon mesh implant via a right paramedian incision.[8] A 12-cm defect in an 18-month-old heifer was repaired via seventh rib resection and thoracotomy.[5] After closure of the diaphragmatic defect, pneumothorax was resolved by suctioning the remaining air from the thorax.

THORACOCENTESIS

I prefer to perform pleurocentesis with ultrasound guidance. This minimizes the risk for accidental puncture of the lung, heart, and major vessels and maximizes the opportunity to obtain a diagnostic sample. Most commonly, pleurocentesis is performed through the fifth or sixth intercostal space at or immediately dorsal to the costochondral junction (level of the point of the elbow). A large chest trocar (20-36 Fr) can be used when evacuation of large volumes of fluid is anticipated. These trocars also are useful when maintenance of an indwelling drain is desired. I have used a 28-Fr chest trocar for catheterization of the pericardial sac for treatment of septic pericarditis. The trocar is placed with ultrasonography guidance and secured to the skin using a "Chinese finger trap" suture. Daily lavage of the pleural cavity or pericardial sac with isotonic saline (with or without antibiotics) is performed through the trocar. This procedure may be a safer alternative to fifth rib resection and pericardial sac marsupialization.

THOROSCOPY

Thoroscopy is infrequently performed in cattle; however, the complete separation of the thorax by the mediastinum allows examination with creation of hemopneumothorax. Examination of the thorax and collection of diagnostic specimens (fine-needle aspirates, biopsy) is performed, and the carbon dioxide gas removed by suction. Thoroscopy has been done for evaluation of pulmonary abscesses and pleuritis in an adult cow. Widespread use of this technology is limited because specialized equipment is required and treatment of specific lesions is rare.

SURGICAL APPROACH TO THORAX

Surgery of the thorax of cattle is most commonly done for treatment of traumatic reticulopericarditis or reticulopleuritis[3,4]; however, thoracotomy has been reported for attempted treatment of stenosis of the pulmonary artery in a 10-month-old Holstein heifer.[13] Thoracotomy also has been used for treatment of pyothorax.[1] The surgical approach of choice is partial resection of the fifth or sixth rib to create a window into the cranioventral thorax. This surgery may be performed standing with local anesthesia, restrained on an inclined table with local anesthesia, or with the cow under general anesthesia. I prefer to perform this surgery with the animal on an inclined table. Reticulopericarditis causes a progressive restrictive pericarditis resulting in limited ventricular filling and reduced cardiac output. Therefore the cardiovascular side effects of general anesthesia may result in death. In one report of cattle having thoracotomy, fewer cattle on which surgery was performed under general anesthesia (one of five cattle survived; three deaths were attributed to anesthetic complications) survived the procedure compared with cattle having surgery performed on an inclined table (nine of nine cattle survived).[1] The animal is placed on its right side on a tilt table at no more than a 45-degree angle.[14]

Alternatively, a right thoracotomy may be performed.[1] The left (or right) front limb is pulled forward as far as possible, and the fifth rib resected. An area extending from the sternum to the middle region of the thorax is clipped and prepared for aseptic surgery. The fifth or sixth rib is identified by counting forward from the last rib, and 2% lidocaine infused in a line block along the rib. Additional lidocaine is infused into the cranial and caudal intercostal spaces proximal and distal to the proposed surgery site. A linear incision is made along the fifth rib extending from the costochondral junction (at the level of the elbow) dorsally for approximately 15 cm. The lateral periosteum of the rib is incised, and the periosteum elevated for the circumference of the rib. Obstetrical wire is passed around the rib at the proximal and distal aspects of the incision. This portion of the rib is transected and removed. Next, the medial periosteum and parietal pleura are incised to expose the cranioventral thorax. Often with pericarditis the pericardium is adhered to the pleura. If the pericardium is not adhered to the pleura, the pericardial sac should be isolated from the pleural cavity before being opened. One author recommends decompression of the pericardial sac before pericardiotomy to avoid sudden decompression of the pericardium and cardiac arrest.[4] The pericardial sac is entered and drained. If the wire or foreign body can be found, it is removed. Often the foreign body has returned to the reticulum after penetrating the thorax. In my experience, laparotomy and rumenotomy cause excessive stress on affected cattle and may contribute to the demise of the animal. I prefer to place a magnet into the reticulum until the survival of the patient has been determined. Alternatively, an instrument for removal of metallic foreign bodies has been developed and is useful for removal of those foreign bodies that can be attracted to a magnet.[15] The pericardium is marsupialized to the thoracic wall and skin using interrupted sutures (e.g., No. 3 Braunamid, No. 2 PDS), and the pericardial sac is lavaged with isotonic saline. Belt loop sutures are placed in the skin along the cranial and caudal margins of the incision, a stent bandage is placed over the wound, and umbilical tape is threaded through the belt loop sutures in a boot lace pattern to secure the bandage in place. Daily wound care involves lavage of the pericardial sac until the wound is closed. Alternatively, the pericardium and pleura may be closed in one layer and then the intercostal muscles and skin closed individually. An indwelling drain may be placed into the pericardial sac before closure.

A similar approach is made for septic pleuritis or pulmonary abscess without entry into the pericardial sac, but the sixth or seventh rib is resected. After débridement and thorough lavage of the hemithorax has been performed, a drainage tube may be placed into the hemithorax through an adjacent stab incision and the thoracotomy wound closed primarily. The pleura, periosteum, and intercostal muscles are closed in one layer (interrupted or continuous pattern, No. 1 PDS), the muscles overlying the thoracic wall (latissimus dorsi, serratus ventralis thoracis, superficial pectoral, external abdominal oblique) are closed in one layer (interrupted or continuous pattern, No. 1 PDS), and the skin is closed routinely. The air remaining in the thorax is removed via the drainage tube, and a Heimlich valve is placed on the open end of the tube. Use of a Heimlich valve (one-way valve) allows continued drainage without compromise of thoracic pressure. A convenient way to construct a one-way valve is to attach a 15-cm, 1.25-cm diameter Penrose drain onto the end of the chest tube. When the inner surface of the drain is wet, the sides of the Penrose drain will collapse and provide a sufficient seal for the tube.

References

1. Ducharme NG, Fubini SL, Renhun We et al: Thoracotomy in adult dairy cattle: 14 cases (1979-1991), *J Am Vet Med Assoc* 200: 86, 1992.
2. McLennan MW, McGowan MR: Pyothorax in a Friesian bull, *Aust Vet J* 72:115-116, 1995.
3. Awadhiya RP, Kolte GN, Vegad JL: Cardiac tamponade: a fatal complication of traumatic reticulitis in cattle, *Vet Rec* 95:260-262, 1974.
4. Noordsy JL: Pericardiotomy: surgically correcting traumatic pericarditis in cattle. In Noordsy JL, editor: *Food animal surgery*, Lenexa, Kansas, 1989, Veterinary Medicine Publishing Co, p 77.
5. DeMoor A, Verschooten F, Desmet P: Thoracic repair of a diaphragmatic hernia in a heifer, *Vet Rec* 85:87, 1969.
6. Done SH, Drew RA: Aperture in the diaphragm with protrusion of abnormal liver tissue: a report of three cases in the ox, *Br Vet J* 128:553, 1972.
7. Hesselink JW: Rupture in the diaphragm of a cow, *Tijdschr Diergeneeskd* 114:1109, 1989.
8. Troutt HF, Fessler JF, Page EH et al: Diaphragmatic defects in cattle, *J Am Vet Med Assoc* 151:1421, 1967.
9. Deore PA, Jahagirdar SS: Incidence of diaphragmatic hernia in cattle and buffaloes: case record of 16 cases, *Indian Vet J* 48:1172-1176, 1971.
10. Dhablania De, Tyagia RPS, Nigam JM: A study on diaphragmatic hernia in bovines, *Indian Vet J* 48:91-98, 1971.
11. Homey FD, Cote J: Congenital diaphragmatic hernia in a calf, *Can Vet J* 2:422-424, 1961.
12. Hutchins DR, Blood DC, Hyne R: Residual defects in stomach motility after traumatic reticuloperitonitis of cattle: pyloric obstruction, diaphragmatic hernia, and indigestion due to reticular adhesions, *Aust Vet J* 33:77-82, 1957.
13. Shiroya K, Saitoh Y, Muto M, et al: Crossed fat embolism in a cow with tetralogy of Fallot, *J Vet Med Sci* 56:969-971, 1994.
14. Rings DM: Surgical treatment of pleuritis and pericarditis, *Vet Clin North Am Food Anim Pract* 11:177, 1995.
15. Hekmati P, Bakshodeh GA, Poulsen JSD: Traumatic reticulitis, the Comet naso reticular instrument for withdrawal of foreign bodies from the reticulum of cattle, *Nord Vet Med* 37:338-348, 1985.

SECTION IV

Cardiovascular Diseases

Kathryn M. Meurs

CHAPTER 48

Examination of the Bovine Patient with Heart Disease

KATHRYN M. MEURS

Cardiovascular disease is uncommon in the bovine patient and, when diagnosed, is most commonly a form of acquired heart disease as opposed to congenital heart disease. The most commonly diagnosed acquired cardiac diseases include traumatic reticulopericarditis, bacterial endocarditis, and occasionally myocardial diseases (e.g., lymphosarcoma, myocarditis, cardiomyopathy).

Many of the clinical signs in cattle with cardiac disease are fairly nonspecific and can include lethargy, weight loss, anorexia, ascites, and diarrhea. However, the majority of cattle with heart disease have at least one of the following symptoms: a cardiac murmur, peripheral subcutaneous edema of the mandible, brisket or ventral abdomen, milk vein distension, jugular venous distention or abnormal jugular pulsations, muffled heart sounds, or a cardiac arrhythmia.

PHYSICAL EXAMINATION

Examination of the patient may give additional information on the origin or extent of cardiac disease. A hunched appearance and abducted elbows can be suggestive of the pain associated with traumatic reticulopericarditis. Intermandibular and brisket edema can be suggestive of right heart failure.

The jugular veins should be evaluated for distension and/or abnormal pulsation by palpating and briefly holding off and releasing. A normal jugular vein should be easily compressible, fill rapidly when held off, and empty rapidly. In the standing cow with head parallel to the ground, pulsations should not be observed beyond one third of the way up the jugular furrow. A distended jugular vein or the observation of abnormal pulses can be highly suggestive of elevated right ventricular filling pressures that could be observed with pericardial effusion and traumatic reticulopericarditis, obstruction to normal cardiac flow from a cardiac mass, tricuspid insufficiency associated with endocarditis, an arrhythmia, or right heart failure.

Auscultation

Adult resting cattle should have a regular sinus rhythm with a heart rate between 48 and 84 beats per minute (bpm). Increased heart rates can be associated with physiologic responses to fever, stress, and excitement among other things, but highly elevated rates (>120 bpm) are highly suggestive of heart failure.

Heart murmurs are never a normal auscultatory finding, although they can be physiologic (functional). When trying to determine the etiology of the murmur it is extremely helpful to describe the location, timing, and intensity of the murmur. Physiologic murmurs such as those observed with anemia (PCV < 20%), fever, and excitement in cattle are generally located at the left base of the heart in the aortic valve area (left fourth intercostal space), systolic, and quite soft (1-2 on a 1-6 grading scheme). Murmurs associated with cardiac disease are often, but not always, louder (>2/6), and the localization can help one to generate a differential list. For example, a systolic murmur over the tricuspid valve area (right third intercostal space) in an adult may be associated with bacterial endocarditis and in a calf may be associated with a ventricular septal defect. A murmur over the mitral valve (left fifth intercostal space) would be more frequently observed with cardiomyopathy or myocarditis. Murmurs over the pulmonic valve (left third intercostal space) are uncommon.

Muffled heart sounds may be associated with either pericardial or pleural effusion. However, obesity and thoracic masses (neoplasia, abscess) can also result in muffled heart sounds.

A pericardial friction rub can sometimes be ausculted in cases with traumatic reticulopericarditis. Friction rubs are higher-pitched sounds that can vary in sound from beat to beat.

ELECTROCARDIOGRAM

As stated earlier, the normal rhythm in adult cattle is a regular (sinus) rhythm. If cardiac auscultation identifies an arrhythmia, an electrocardiogram may be necessary to verify the type of arrhythmia. Because the conduction system of the ventricle in ruminants is more diffuse than that of small animals, observation of the normal ventricular conduction is optimized when a base apex electrocardiogram is performed. A base apex is performed by placing the LA electrode at the left apex of the heart (left axillary area, behind the point of the elbow) and the RA lead in the right jugular furrow (midcervical level). A chest lead can be attached on the right side as a ground lead. However, it is often possible to get a reasonable QRS complex for evaluation of cardiac rhythms by placing the leads on the limbs with LA at the left elbow, RA at the right elbow, and LL at the left hock with a ground lead on the right leg.

ECHOCARDIOGRAPHY

Cardiac ultrasonography, echocardiography, allows the clinician an opportunity to visualize the cardiac valves, myocardium, pericardium, and myocardial function. The most common indications for echocardiography include the evaluation of the valves or myocardium to determine the etiology of a murmur, to evaluate the pericardium in suspect reticulopericarditis cases, and to evaluate for cardiac disease if jugular venous distention or a tachyarrhythmia has been identified.

However, echocardiography can be challenging in adult cattle because of the large size of the animal and the narrow intercostal spaces, which prevent easy ultrasound probe manipulation. A reasonable amount of strength and patience are necessary on the part of the echocardiographer to push the echo probe up under the elbow (scapulohumeral joint) and angle it back to image the heart. Additionally, many ultrasound machines have a depth limitation of 25 centimeters. This may make it difficult to visualize all of the cardiac structures from one side in a large animal. Sometimes the depth limitation may be compensated for by imaging from both sides of the chest. With persistence, in the majority of adult cattle the atria, ventricles, and heart valves can be imaged with a 3.5 MHz or lower probe if approached between the fourth and fifth intercostal spaces of both the left and right sides.

Recommended Readings

Braun U, Schweizer T, Pusterla N: Echocardiography of the normal bovine heart: technique and ultrasonographic appearance, *Vet Record* 148:47, 2001.

Callan RJ, McGuirck SM, Step DL: Assessment of the cardiovascular and lymphatic systems, *Vet Clin North Am Food Anim Pract* 8:257, 1992.

McGuirck SM: Treatment of cardiovascular disease in cattle, *Vet Clin North Am Food Anim Pract* 7:729, 1991.

CHAPTER **49**

Congenital Heart Disease in Cattle

KATHRYN M. MEURS

Congenital heart diseases are relatively uncommon in cattle compared with acquired heart disease. The ventricular septal defect is the most commonly reported congenital heart defect; however, atrial septal defects and complex defects such as a double outlet right ventricle and transposition of the great vessels have been reported.

Indications of a congenital heart defect in a calf may include vague clinical signs such as poor growth, exercise intolerance, failure to nurse, or dyspnea. Physical examination may demonstrate tachypnea; tachycardia; and in the majority of cases, a heart murmur. Some calves have a soft (usually<3 on a 1-6 grading scale) physiologic heart murmur at the left base of the heart (aortic valve area [fourth intercostal space]). Murmurs at locations other than the left base, or at the left base but louder, should be more thoroughly evaluated if possible with echocardiography.

Dyspnea, peripheral edema, distended jugular veins, cyanosis, and arrhythmias suggest the development of heart failure or the presence of a complex cardiac defect with right to left shunting and are indications for echocardiography or discussion with the owners of a likely poor prognosis.

VENTRICULAR SEPTAL DEFECT

The ventricular septal defect (VSD) is the most common congenital heart defect in cattle. A hereditary transmission is suspected in Herefords, Limousines, and possibly Jerseys. Additionally, Holsteins and Aryshires were reported to be overrepresented in one study of 25 calves with VSDs, which could suggest a heritable trait in these breeds but could also just be an indication of the regional prevalence of these breeds.

Calves with a VSD frequently present for respiratory signs (dyspnea, tachypnea) but may be asymptomatic. In some cases, vague clinical signs including anorexia and poor growth may be observed.

Physical examination findings may include tachycardia and/or tachypnea. A heart murmur is typically present over the right apical area (approximately the right fifth intercostal space). The location of the murmur on the right side of the chest is inconsistent with a physiologic murmur and should suggest that cardiac disease is present.

Radiographs may help verify pulmonary edema and heart failure and, in some cases, cardiac enlargement. Echocardiography should be used to verify the presence of the VSD, determine the size of the defect, and evaluate for other congenital heart defects.

If echocardiography is available to evaluate the size of the defect, the information may be used to develop a prognosis for the owners. Some animals with small defects can have loud murmurs but remain asymptomatic for years. On the other hand, some calves with large VSDs may progress into heart failure fairly rapidly. In most cases, VSDs shunt blood from the left ventricle to the right ventricle. In a left-to-right shunting VSD, most of the shunted blood is directed from the left ventricle into the right ventricle and the pulmonary artery. This results in a volume overload to the left side and left heart failure (tachypnea, pulmonary edema). Some animals with VSDs do not develop signs of heart failure but are small and may have difficulties becoming pregnant.

Recommended Readings

Buczunski S, Fecteau G, DiFruscia R: Ventricular septal defects in cattle: a retrospective study of 25 cases, *Can Vet J* 47:246, 2006.

Michaelsson M, Ho SY: *Congenital heart malformations in mammals,* London, 2000, Imperial College Press.

CHAPTER 50

Acquired Heart Diseases in Cattle

KATHRYN M. MEURS

The most commonly acquired heart diseases in cattle include bacterial endocarditis, traumatic reticulopericarditis, arrhythmias, and, in some cases, myocardial disease (lymphosarcoma, cardiomyopathy, myocarditis).

BACTERIAL ENDOCARDITIS

Bacterial endocarditis is the most common form of valvular disease in cattle. The tricuspid valve is most frequently affected, although infection of the mitral, aortic, and pulmonic valves is also reported. The most common etiologic agents include *Streptococcus* organisms, *Corynebacterium pyogenes, Escherichia coli, Staphylococcus aureus, Pseudomonas* organisms, *Klebsiella pneumonia,* and *Proteus mirabilis.*

The history and clinical signs associated with endocarditis can be quite vague and include weight loss, decreased milk production, recurring fever, anorexia, lameness, weight loss, and inappetence. Some animals have a past history of pneumonia or traumatic reticulopericarditis.

Physical examination findings most often include a heart murmur, but sinus tachycardia and other tachyarrhythmias are frequently observed. In one report the most consistent findings were tachycardia (80% of cases), weight loss, lameness (50% of cases), heart murmur, and fever. Signs of congestive heart failure including peripheral edema and distended jugular veins and/or mammary veins were observed in about one third of the cases. Although a heart murmur is not always heard, it is in many of the cases. Because cattle rarely, if ever, suffer from degenerative valve disease, a murmur over the tricuspid valve area (right apex, fifth intercostal space) in an adult cow is highly suggestive of endocarditis. In some cases, a heart murmur may not be ausculted due to the environment in which the auscultation is performed, the large size of the animal, or the animal's discomfort and dyspnea and restlessness, all of which can make an accurate auscultation difficult. Thus the absence of a murmur should not rule out a diagnosis of endocarditis.

Laboratory findings can support a diagnosis of bacterial endocarditis and may include a normocytic, normochromic anemia, a neutrophilic leukocytosis, and hyperfibrinogenemia.

An electrocardiogram may demonstrate a normal rhythm or sinus tachycardia, but other tachyarrhythmias including atrial or ventricular premature complexes (described more thoroughly below) or atrial fibrillation may be observed.

Echocardiography, if available, can be used to confirm the irregular, thickened, and hyperechoic appearance of one, or sometimes more, of the heart valves, typically the tricuspid valve.

If a diagnosis of bacterial endocarditis is suspected based on history; physical examination; and, if possible, echocardiographic findings, a blood culture should be performed to try to determine the causative bacteria. Confirming the type of bacteria by blood culture is ideal but practically difficult. In many cases, blood cultures do not result in growth of any bacteria or the only growth is from bacteria thought to be contaminants from the skin. However, the benefits achieved by being able to select antibiotic therapy based on the type of bacteria infecting the valve are great enough that blood cultures are still highly recommended. Current recommendations include pulling three 10-mL samples of blood over a 3- to 6-hour period and placing them into both aerobic and anaerobic growth bottles. Ideally blood cultures are obtained before any antibiotics are given. The best evidence that one has successfully grown the bacteria of interest is the growth of the same bacteria in at least two of the three samples.

Bacterial endocarditis is rarely, if ever, a curable disease. The bacteria create permanent damage to the valve and often become walled off from antibiotic penetration by layers of fibrin and platelets. Affected animals generally progress into congestive heart failure because of the damage to the heart valve or develop more systemic signs (dyspnea, lameness, fever) from continual showering of bacterial thrombi from the valve to the lungs or the rest of the body. At the time of diagnosis, decisions about treatment will need to be based on the value of the animal and possible benefits of palliative therapy to provide increased comfort and survival for a limited period of time. Antibiotics and heart failure medications, if necessary, may provide some improvement for a period of time. If a decision to treat is made, initial selection of antibiotics should be based on the list of common bacteria known to be associated with bacterial endocarditis. If blood cultures are successful at isolating a likely bacterial agent, the antibiotic can be changed when the culture and sensitivity results are available. Antibiotics should be given for at least 4 to 6 weeks.

MYOCARDIAL DISEASE

Two forms of myocardial disease are seen in cattle: dilated cardiomyopathy and myocarditis. The clinical signs associated with myocardial disease can include nonspecific findings such as lethargy, decreased milk production, and tachycardia. A heart murmur, arrhythmia, and jugular venous dissention may also be observed. Occasional ventricular premature complexes may be observed on an electrocardiogram. The best test for confirming myocardial disease is an echocardiogram. Echocardiography should demonstrate dilation of the left and/or right ventricle, atrial dilation, and myocardial dysfunction (decreased fractional shortening percentage).

Dilated cardiomyopathy is a primary myocardial disease characterized by ventricular dilation and myocardial systolic dysfunction that may result in congestive heart failure and sudden death. It is thought to be familial disease in Canadian Holsteins, among others. It is commonly a familial disease in human beings and dogs, so a familial etiology should strongly be considered even if not yet proven in a specific breed. Although the pattern of inheritance is not known, an eradication strategy that culled carrier sires was successful in reduction of the disease prevalence in Canadian Holsteins in Switzerland.

Digoxin may be used as a positive inotrope to treat cattle with decreased myocardial systolic function. However, digoxin is really quite a weak inotrope and is unlikely to make a significant difference in the outcome of the case, although some improvement in clinical status may be observed. Digitalis is destroyed by the ruminal contents in cattle and can cause muscle necrosis if given intramuscularly, so it should be given intravenously. Given intravenously, it has a half-life of about 7.8 hours in adult cattle, so it should be given frequently or continuously.

Digoxin has tremendous patient-to-patient variability. Ideally serum levels should be monitored. The therapeutic serum level for cattle is not known, but based on the suggested serum level in other species, a level of 0.5 to 1.25 ng/ml could be used. Digoxin toxicities are well reported, particularly if loading doses are used including depression, anorexia, diarrhea, and arrhythmias. Avoiding use of a loading dose and monitoring the serum level should help reduce the risk of toxicity. If signs of toxicity develop, the drug should be discontinued.

Myocarditis is an inflammatory myocardial disease that can be caused by bacterial, viral, and protozoal agents. Sudden cardiac death in feedlot cattle has been associated with myocarditis defined by focal myocardial infarcts, necrosis, and fibrosis. In one report, *Haemophilus somnus* antigen was demonstrated within the areas of necrosis in the heart tissue of most affected calves.

Adult bovine lymphosarcoma can also involve the myocardium, and the clinical signs will depend on the location of the mass. Typically the mass starts in the right atrium and can infiltrate additional areas of the myocardium, resulting in the development of congestive heart failure and/or arrhythmias including ventricular premature complexes. Echocardiography can be used to identify the mass and rule out other causes of heart failure and arrhythmia, but it cannot confirm the diagnosis of lymphosarcoma.

TRAUMATIC RETICULOPERICARDITIS

The most common form of pericardial disease in cattle is traumatic reticulopericarditis. Traumatic reticulopericarditis is the result of a sharp foreign object penetrating the reticulum, diaphragm, and pericardium, inducing a bacterial infection into the pericardial sac.

Typical clinical signs are lethargy, loss of appetite, decreased milk production, and reluctance to move. A mild fever may be observed. The effect of the constriction of the pericardium and pericardial fluid on right ventricular filling pressure generally results in jugular venous distention or abnormal pulsation. Muffled heart sounds are typically observed. Friction rubs, a transient, higher-pitched sound, may be ausculted, especially in the early stages of the disease. Some cattle will be quite painful and may stand with a hunched appearance and abducted elbows.

The best diagnostic test for reticulopericarditis is an echocardiogram that demonstrates fluid within the pericardial sac and, possibly, visualization of the foreign object. Radiographs may also demonstrate the object within the pericardial sac. A tentative diagnosis can be made based on history, physical examination findings, and pericardiocentesis with culture and sensitivity of the septic pericardial fluid, although it would be ideal to see the fluid by echocardiography before pericardiocentesis.

The pericardium can be tapped by clipping and prepping the fifth intercostal space on the left side about 2.5 to 10 cm above the olecranon. A local anesthetic such as lidocaine can be used to block an approximately 1 cm area, and a small cut is made into skin to make it easier to advance the needle into the chest. A 14- to 16-gauge over the needle catheter with a length of at least 15 cm is slowly advanced into the pericardium. Once a fluid flash is evident in the hub of the catheter, the catheter is advanced and the needle withdrawn. The fluid should be submitted for both anaerobic and aerobic cultures and drained as completely as possible. In many cases of pericarditis, the patient may have pleural, as well as pericardial, fluid. In these cases the flash of fluid in the catheter may be pleural fluid, and the catheter may not yet have penetrated the pericardium. One should actually feel the needle push up against the distended pericardium and may need to give a sharp push to penetrate the inflamed pericardial sac. Once the pericardium is penetrated and fluid removed, the heart rate should begin to fall and the patient should begin to appear more comfortable. If palliative, short-term treatment may be achieved by pericardiocentesis and lavage. Pericardiotomy may also be considered. A combination of antibiotics that provide gram-negative and gram-positive, as well as anaerobic and aerobic, coverage should be selected, ideally based on culture and sensitivity of the pericardial fluid. A combination of amoxicillin or ampicillin with an aminoglycoside may be considered while waiting for the culture results.

The prognosis for traumatic reticulopericarditis is guarded to poor, although the prognosis may be slightly better for patients diagnosed in the early stages of the disease. Cases that are diagnosed early in the stage of the disease may respond, at least for a short time, to pericardiocentesis, prolonged antibiotic therapy, and removal of the foreign object. Chronic disease often results in fibrosis and constriction of the diseased pericardium onto the myocardium and permanent impairment of the ability of the right ventricle to fill normally. Therefore the best treatment is prevention, through decreased exposure to metal objects and a magnet.

TREATMENT OF CONGESTIVE HEART FAILURE

In the majority of cases of congestive heart failure in cattle the primary disease (endocarditis, myocarditis, traumatic reticulopericarditis) is not curable. Therefore treatment of heart failure is performed to achieve short-term goals for survival (e.g., to get an animal to parturition). Animals in heart failure should be removed from stressful situations if possible and should either be on sodium-restricted diets or have the sodium in their diet monitored. Diuretics can be given for reduction of fluid retention and edema. Diuretics potentiate the loss of sodium, chloride, and potassium and can result in acid/base imbalances, so these values should be monitored. This is especially important if the patient is also on cardiac drugs like quinidine and digitalis because electrolyte and acid/base imbalances can increase the toxicity of these drugs. The most commonly used diuretic is furosemide, 500 mg q12-24h or 2 to 4 mg/kg q12-24h intravenously.

ARRHYTHMIAS IN CATTLE

The presence of an arrhythmia in cattle is most often associated with systemic, often gastrointestinal, disease rather than primary cardiac disease. Therefore, if an arrhythmia is present, evaluation of the whole animal is warranted, as opposed to immediate focus on the cardiovascular system.

Bradyarrhythmias

Sinus bradycardia and sinus arrhythmia are most often associated with decreased feed intake in cattle, generally after 12 to 48 hours. These sinus rhythms are characterized by a slow heart rate with a normal appearance to both the P wave and the QRS. A sinus bradycardia, defined by a slow, regular heart rate may be associated with anorexia and high vagal tone. Sinus arrhythmias should be regularly irregular in rhythm with pauses that correlate with the phase of respiration. Both of these rhythms should resolve with a return to normal dietary habits.

Tachyarrhythmias

Atrial fibrillation is characterized by a rapid, irregularly irregular rhythm. P waves are not present, and irregularly spaced fibrillation waves, "f" waves, may be present (Fig 50-1). Atrial fibrillation is typically associated with acid/base and electrolyte imbalance and gastrointestinal disease.

Atrial premature beats are complexes that come closer to the previous QRS than expected and are thus premature. Atrial premature complexes have a normal QRS shape. The P wave should have a slightly different shape in comparison with the normal complexes, although this can be subtle (Fig 50-2). Both atrial premature complexes (APC) and atrial fibrillation are most often associated with metabolic imbalances and gastrointestinal diseases.

Ventricular premature beats are characterized by complexes that are premature but have an abnormal QRS shape, indicating that their origin is from the ventricle. Ventricular premature complexes are more suggestive of true cardiac disease.

Because the most common arrhythmias in cattle are associated with systemic issues that will resolve once those issues are addressed, treatment of arrhythmias is generally not performed unless serious hemodynamic alterations are present. If the heart rate with the arrhythmia is in the normal range, immediate therapy is not necessary.

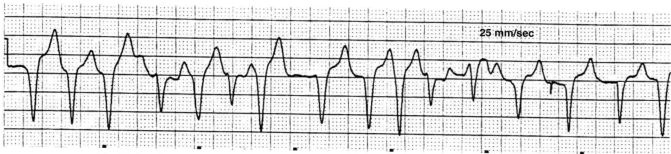

Fig 50-1   Electrocardiogram of a cow in atrial fibrillation. Heart rate is 140 beats per minute and the rhythm is irregularly irregular. P waves are not seen.

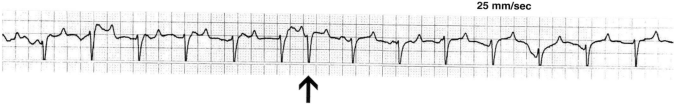

Fig 50-2   Electrocardiogram of a cow with sinus tachycardia and an atrial premature beat *(arrow)*. Heart rate is 100 beats per minute. Note the normal shape of the QRS with this premature beat.

Quinidine is the drug of choice for supraventricular tachyarrhythmias including sustained atrial fibrillation if the heart rate is fast enough to have a hemodynamic consequence or does not improve with treatment of the systemic issues. Additionally, it can be used for ventricular tachyarrhythmias. Because of bioavailability issues, quinidine should be given intravenously. However, it is not without side effects (diarrhea, disorganized ruminal activity, sinus tachycardia). Additional signs of toxicity include supraventricular and ventricular tachycardia and prolongation of the QRS complex (>50% of complex width at the start of therapy). Signs of toxicity can be reduced with a decreased rate of infusion or if discontinued.

Recommended Readings

Callan RJ, McGuirk SM, Step RL: Assessment of the cardiovascular and lymphatic system, *Vet Clin North Am Food Anim Pract* 8:257, 1992.

Haines DM, Moline KM, Sargent RA et al: Immunohistochemical study of *Hemophilus somnus, Mycoplasma bovis, Mannheimia hemolytica* and bovine viral diarrhea virus in death losses due to myocarditis in feedlot cattle, *Can Vet J* 45:231, 2004.

Leifsson PS, Agerholm JS: Familial occurrence of bovine dilated cardiomyopathy in Denmark, *J Vet Med* 51:332, 2004.

McGuirk SM: Treatment of cardiovascular disease in cattle, *Vet Clin North Am Food Anim Pract* 7:729, 1991.

Roussel AJ, Kasari TR: Bacterial endocarditis in large animals. Part II. Incidence, causes, clinical signs and pathologic findings, *Compend Cont Ed Pract Vet* 11:769, 1989.

SECTION V

Musculoskeletal System Medicine

André Desrochers

CHAPTER 51

Noninfectious Disorders of the Foot

SAREL R. VAN AMSTEL

LAMINITIS (PODODERMATITIS ASEPTICA DIFFUSA) (CORIITIS; CLAW HORN DISRUPTION)

Laminitis in the cow involves all parts of the dermis, not only the sensitive laminae but other components of the suspensory system for the third phalanx found in cattle. Thus the term *pododermatitis aseptica diffusa* is more appropriate.

Suspensory System of Third Phalanx (P_3)

The sensitive laminae (laminar corium) in the cow are not as extensive as in the horse and only provide support for the front half to two thirds of the third phalanx. For this reason cattle have an alternate support structure for the back part of the third phalanx. This support is provided by connective tissue attachments between the bone and the inside of the wall, as well as the digital cushion, which provides additional support and consists of loose connective tissue and varying amounts of adipose tissue. The digital cushions are arranged in a series of three parallel cylinders and extend from the skin/horn junction at the heel toward the tip of the third phalanx. The amount of fat (and thus cushioning capacity) increases with age and is believed to have significant implications for animals relative to the development of sole lesions (e.g., sole ulcers following disruption of the suspensory and support system of the third phalanx as a consequence of laminitis).

Forms and Presentation

Subclinical laminitis is the most important claw condition of dairy cattle. Other stages of the condition include acute, subacute, and chronic forms. In the acute and subacute form there is no time lapse between the inciting cause and the development of clinical signs, which are associated with pain caused by vascular and inflammatory changes within the claw. The acute form occurs sporadically, with the incidence highest for first lactation animals within 60 to 90 days of lactation. Animals with acute laminitis are reluctant to walk; have an arched back when standing (Fig 51-1) or walking; spend most of their time lying down; and, depending on the predisposing cause, may show signs of systemic disease. The coronary band may be red, tender, swollen, and warm to the touch with a palpable

digital pulse. At this stage the claw horn shows little visible change.

With subclinical laminitis there is a definite time lapse of several weeks before clinical signs may be seen. Such signs relate to claw horn disruption resulting from impaired keratogenesis. Sole horn hemorrhages and yellow discoloration of sole horn and white line are the most common findings (Fig 51-2). Other claw lesions such as sole ulcers, white line separation, and heel erosion are also common.

Repeated episodes of acute or subacute or subclinical laminitis will result in the chronic form characterized by claw horn deformities, which include widened and flattened claws with horizontal grooves (hardship grooves) (Fig 51-3) that may form fissures and progress to a full-thickness break in the wall (thimble). The dorsal wall may deviate and become concave (buckled claw), and the toe often has an axial deviation. The heels are often shallow. The sole horn is soft and may be powdery in parts. Typically the white line is widened and often has a yellow discoloration. Recurring heel and sole ulcers and white line defects are common. Animals with chronic laminitis are usually not lame unless the hooves are overgrown, which may cause discomfort when walking, or the claws have lesions involving the corium.

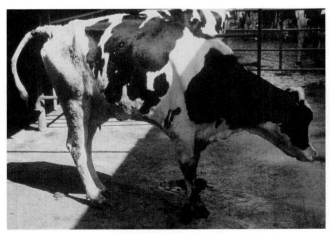

Fig 51-1 Acute laminitis. (Courtesy Dr. Jan Shearer, University of Florida, Gainesville, Fla.)

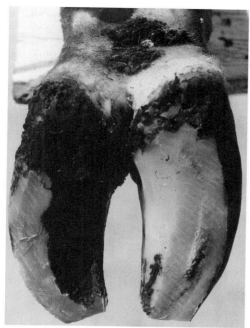

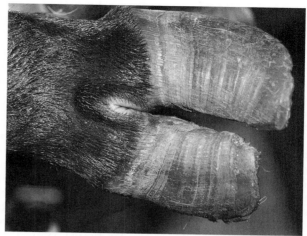

Fig 51-3 Hardship grooves denoting repeated interruption of horn growth. (Courtesy Greg Hirshoren, College of Veterinary Medicine, University of Tennessee.)

Fig 51-2 Subclinical laminitis. Note hemorrhage and yellow discoloration of sole horn and white line. Separation of the abaxial white line exists.

Predisposing Causes

Endotoxin released from gram-negative organisms associated with coliform mastitis or rumen acidosis is implicated in several biochemical pathways leading to vascular and tissue changes within the claw.

Rations high in carbohydrate may lead to acute/subacute rumen acidosis with accumulation of lactic acid. The acidic environment in the rumen causes bacteriolysis of gram-negative organisms with release of endotoxin. Both endotoxin and lactic acid have been shown experimentally to cause vascular and inflammatory changes in the claw. Barley is rapidly fermented, resulting in increased volatile fatty acid concentration in the rumen including lactic acid and histamine as one of the breakdown products. Rations containing 18% digestible protein levels and lush growing rye grass pasture with high protein and energy have been implicated as a trigger for laminitis. However, the mechanism by which protein initiates laminitis is not clear. The quantity and quality of the roughage is a major factor in rumination and saliva production, which is the major source of buffers to keep rumen pH within acceptable limits. At least one third of the total dry matter intake (DMI) should consist of roughage of adequate quality and particle length (≥2.5 cm).

In areas with high environmental temperatures and humidity, dairy cattle may develop heat stress, which can cause respiratory alkalosis because of increases in respiratory rate in an effort to control body temperature. A compensatory mechanism is increasing urinary bicarbonate excretion. In addition, animals with heat stress commonly exhibit open-mouth breathing, resulting in loss of saliva with further bicarbonate losses, which leads to inadequate buffering of rumen contents. Animals with heat stress also tend to select more energy-dense feeds rather than roughage with rumen acidosis as a consequence.

Inadequate cow comfort is an important factor, which may predispose to laminitis. This includes sudden introduction to concrete flooring, poorly designed free stalls and lack of bedding, poor stockmanship, and commingling of different age groups, all of which affect standing or lying time and cow behavior. Adequate sole thickness is necessary to protect the underlying corium. In situations in which sole horn wear exceeds growth, such as with abrasive walking surfaces and overtrimming, overly thin soles may be a consequence and mechanically induced laminitis may result. Overtrimming should be avoided by applying proper trimming techniques.

Both a familial and genetic predisposition to laminitis has been reported. An inherited tendency toward laminitis has been demonstrated in Jerseys. Claw and body conformation characteristics are heritable, and this may be the reason for the observed difference in susceptibility to laminitis between breeds of cattle.

Normal biomechanics lead to overgrowth of outer claw of the hind leg, which results in increasing the total weight-bearing and concussive forces within the foot. This can lead to mechanical injury and inflammatory changes within the solar corium, particularly in the axial heel/sole or heel areas.

Pathogenesis

Both inflammatory and noninflammatory events play a role in the pathogenesis of laminitis.

Noninflammatory Pathway

Hormonal and biochemical changes around calving such as the production of matrix metalloproteases of noninflammatory origin and the effect of the hormone relaxin on collagen fiber attachments can both lead to instability or breakdown of connective tissue in the suspensory apparatus of the claw, resulting in sinking of the third phalanx (particularly its caudal aspect) with disruption of horn production in the basal layer of the epidermis through direct trauma.

Other hormonal and biochemical changes such as low insulin levels and insulin resistance and inhibition of epidermal growth factor can result in defective keratogenesis with further disruption of epidermal growth.

Inflammatory Pathway

Triggering factors such as endotoxin, hormones (epinephrine and norepinephrine), and inflammatory mediators such as prostanoids (prostaglandins and thromboxanes TXA_2) can cause vasoconstriction of the main arterial supply to the claw, thus diverting blood away from the ventral parts of the wall, as well as the sole. This is complicated by the fact that there are fewer primary arterial branches and inter-arterial connections in the ventral wall and sole. In addition, recent work has found an increase in capillary pressure and postcapillary resistance, which will assist transvascular fluid movement and an increase in tissue pressure with digital venous constriction, possibly the initiating step. The reduced arterial blood flow may be further compromised by thrombosis associated with endotoxin-induced disseminated intravascular coagulation (DIC), developing arteriosclerosis and an increase in the number of direct arteriovenous anastomoses (AVAs), which further divert blood away from the corium and basal layers of the epidermis. Arteriosclerosis and AVAs are prominent features in subacute and chronic cases.

The resulting changes in blood flow including congestion, edema, and thrombosis will result in tissue hypoxia of the corium, connective tissue attachments between the third phalanx and the claw wall, the dermal epidermal interface, and basal layers of the epidermis, which will result in failure of the suspensory system of the third phalanx and epidermal proliferation and differentiation. These pathologic changes are further enhanced by the formation of matrix metalloproteinases associated with inflammation.

Pathologic Lesions

In acute/subacute laminitis, microscopic changes in the corium include hyperemia, congestion, edema, cellular infiltration, and hemorrhage. Cellular infiltrate consisted mainly of macrophages and neutrophils. The number of side and secondary papillae (vascular pegs) are increased and show a more irregular and convoluted capillary network. Degenerative changes are present in the epidermis, particularly in areas adjacent to vessels occluded with thrombosis.

In chronic laminitis, arteriosclerosis, as well as sclerosis in small arterioles, is a common finding. Arteriosclerosis is more pronounced at ulcer sites as compared with other parts of the sole. There is a marked increase in arteriovenous shunts with neocapillary formation (regarded as newly induced arteriovenous shunts) in all areas of the corium. Hyperkeratosis and parakeratosis are present in epidermal lamellae. The number of tubules can be significantly reduced in animals with laminitis, resulting in poor horn quality.

Macroscopic pathologic changes include downward rotation of tip of the third phalanx in some cases. In cases of sole ulcers the flexor tuberosity of the claw is displaced downward and the palmar dermis and subcutis thinner as compared with normal controls. The digital cushions contained less fat and had been replaced by collagenous connective tissue, resulting in less shock absorbency and further damage to the sole microstructures.

Treatment

Treatment of laminitis is based on identification and management of the risk factors.

The use of pain medication and coldwater hydrotherapy may be considered in the treatment of acute laminitis. Pain relief could be provided in the form of systemic or oral analgesics such as opioids and antiinflammatory drugs. Aspirin (15-100 mg/kg bid) is commonly used, but its efficacy is questionable. Morphine could be used in selected cases at 0.25 to 0.5 mg/kg intramuscularly (IM) every 4 to 6 hours or butorphanol at 0.05 to 0.01 mg/kg IM. The analgesic effects of these drugs may be enhanced with the combined use of nonsteroidal antiinflammatory drugs such as flunixin at 1.1 mg/kg.

In cases of chronic laminitis with claw horn deformities, an upward deviation of the dorsal wall is usually present (Fig 51-4). The abaxial wall is usually deviated (flared) to the outside, and the abaxial white line becomes widened because of poor-quality horn being produced. Corrective trimming consists of reducing the toe to the required length (7.5 cm or 3 inches), after which the dorsal walls of both claws are straightened. In normal claws the abaxial wall is normally not trimmed because the wall constitutes an important part of the normal weight-bearing surface. However, in the case of laminitic claws, an attempt should be made to trim the claw back to what its normal conformation should be, which may require removing some of the deviated abaxial wall (Fig 51-5).

Laminitis is commonly associated with sole ulcers and white line disease. The treatment for these entities is discussed in the appropriate sections.

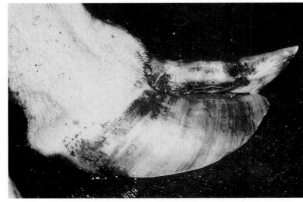

Fig 51-4 Chronic laminitis showing upward deviation of the dorsal wall of the claw.

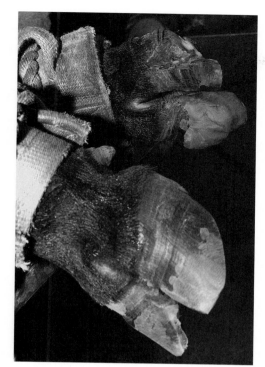

Fig 51-5 Corrective trimming of chronic laminitis involves straightening the dorsal wall and removing some of the deviated (flared) abaxial wall. (Courtesy Greg Hirshoren, College of Veterinary Medicine, University of Tennessee.)

It has been reported that supplemental dietary biotin and trace minerals may have a beneficial effect on claw health in intensively managed primiparous dairy cows.

SOLE HEMORRHAGES

Background

The solar corium consists of a rich vascular network, which terminates in dermal papillae or vascular pegs. A vascular peg consists of a main arteriole, which connects directly to a venule at the tip. Between the arteriole and venule is an extensive capillary network. The epidermal layer overlying the vascular pegs produces horn cells in the form of tubules (tubular horn). Cells within the tubules are arranged in a steep spiral around the center axis. Approximately 20/mm^2 tubules are in the sole. Intertubular horn is produced between the papillae and interconnects the tubular horn. Intertubular horn consists of sheets of elongated polygonal cells arranged parallel with the bearing surface.

Pathogenesis

Vascular changes associated with laminitis such as increases in capillary pressure and permeability caused by inflammatory mediators can lead to various degrees of hemorrhage, the extent of which depends on the severity of the primary insult. Blood seeps into the horn tubules and intertubular horn and appears on the surface of the

sole after a time lapse, the length of which depends on the severity of the hemorrhage and the rate of wear of the solar horn. Because blood seems to penetrate tubular horn at a more rapid rate, sole hemorrhage may have a paintbrush appearance.

In more severe cases ecchymotic or splash hemorrhages may occur on the sole surface. Severe hemorrhage of the solar corium may result in a temporary cessation of horn production. Cells in the basal layer of the epidermis undergo degeneration and slough, which, together with blood cells, fill the space created by the temporary interruption in horn formation. Once normal horn formation is resumed, the claw develops a false sole. Repeat damage to the solar corium may result in the presence of multiple false soles.

Incidence and Presentation

The incidence can be high. One study reported an incidence of 94% in primiparous and 66% in multiparous cows. Hemorrhages may be present in heifers for up to 4 months before calving. Factors that may play a role include rapid weight gain, commingling with older and dominant cows, and housing on concrete in a zero-grazing cubicle system. In another study the prevalence of sole hemorrhages was found to be 37.9% when the hind feet of 1141 female dairy calves between 2.5 and 12 months of age were examined. Hemorrhage scores were found to be higher in cows on a high-concentrate diet and kept on concrete in a cubicle system. Hemorrhage scores were found to be higher in cows on a high-concentrate diet and kept on concrete in a cubicle system.

Sole hemorrhages occur most commonly in association with subclinical laminitis and usually becomes visible 2 to 4 months after calving. Hemorrhages that occur after calving in first lactation cows tend to disappear later in the lactation, whereas in some multiparous cows such hemorrhages may remain throughout the lactation, indicating permanent damage to the corium.

Hemorrhages may occur randomly on the sole surface, often in association with hemorrhages involving the white line, or occur in specific locations. One of the common locations is generally referred to as hemorrhage in the "typical place." Hemorrhage in this location is often a sign of a developing sole ulcer (also known as *Rusterholtz ulcer*) and occurs most commonly on the outer claw of the hind leg (Fig 51-6). Other specific locations include hemorrhage at the apex of the toe, usually in association with rotation of the third phalanx. Hemorrhage at the heel-sole junction may be associated with sinking of the flexor tuberosity (area of insertion of the deep flexor tendon) of the third phalanx or with thin soles due to contusion of the solar corium and may precede a heel ulcer. In cows with overly thin soles, hemorrhage along the sole junction with the abaxial white line is quite common due to extreme wear of the sole in that area (Fig 51-7).

Treatment

Nutritional, management, and housing factors that predispose to sole hemorrhages should be identify and corrected when possible. In individual cases in which sole hemorrhages are associated with lameness, corrective

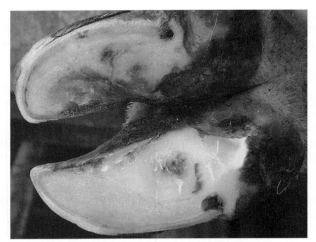

Fig 51-6 Hemorrhage in the "typical place" indicative of a developing sole ulcer, Rusterholtz ulcer.

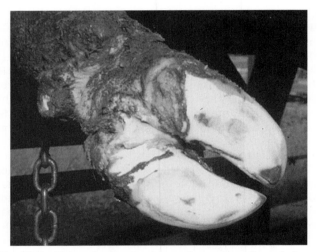

Fig 51-7 Thin sole showing hemorrhage along the sole junction with the abaxial white line in the outer claw of the hind leg.

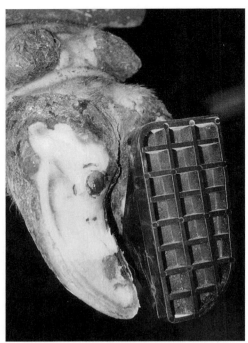

Fig 51-8 Sole ulcer with full-thickness horn defect and protruding sole corium.

Depending on the degree of damage to the sole corium, the hemorrhage may grow out without a defect in horn development and growth. Sole hemorrhage associated with pain is a sign of a developing ulcer in the preclinical stage. Such lesions often progress to a full-thickness horn defect (Fig 51-8). The surface of the sole horn around the ulcer appears damaged and is often loose and underrun. Protrusion of the solar corium becomes evident once the loose horn has been pared away. In early cases the exposed corium shows little damage but becomes traumatized by the horn edges of the defect and the walking surface, resulting in the formation of granulation tissue.

Clinical Presentation

Animals with preclinical or fully developed sole ulcers may show different degrees of lameness and may have an obvious cow-hocked stance in an effort to place more weight on the inner claws. Sole ulcers can become infected and involve the deeper structures of the heel or toe. In the case of typical sole and heel ulcers, infection may progress to involve the distal interphalangeal joint. In the case of toe ulcers the apex of the third phalanx may become infected, resulting in a septic osteitis and pathologic fracture. Animals with such complicated lesions are severely lame, reluctant to move, lie down most of the time, and show severe weight loss.

In complicated cases of typical sole or heel ulcers there is usually unilateral swelling of the affected digit, particularly in the area of the heel, and the swelling may extend along the coronary band. The toe of the affected claw may become overextended due to avulsion of the deep flexor tendon at its insertion. The presence of concurrent tenosynovitis is indicated by a fluctuant swelling proximal

trimming and relief of weight bearing should be carried out. More specific information regarding treatment is provided in the relevant sections on sole ulcers, white line disease, and thin soles.

ULCERATION OF THE SOLE
(pododermatitis circumscripta, sole ulcer/Rusterholtz ulcer, heel ulcer, toe ulcer/toe abscess)

An ulcer is defined as a full-thickness break in the epidermis. In the sole there are three types of sole ulcers commonly recognized including typical sole ulcer or "Rusterholtz ulcer," which occur at the axial heel-sole junction; toe ulcer near the apex of the toe; and heel ulcer, which is centrally located on the heel. Typical sole and heel ulcers occur more commonly on the outer claw of the rear leg, whereas toe ulcers occur commonly on front feet. Sole hemorrhage is the early clinical sign of sole ulcer but only becomes visible several weeks after the initial injury.

and plantar to the metatarsophalangeal joint. A draining tract extending from the ulcer site into the heel and/or another tract from the skin of the dorsal coronary band to the distal interphalangeal joint may also be present in chronic cases and indicates involvement of the joint.

In cases of toe ulcer with complications there is usually no swelling of the digit, although some bulging of the sole is sometimes present due to the formation of a subsolar abscess. The horn lesion may be small and only present as a small black defect in the sole or white line at the apex of the toe. Hoof tester applied to this area provokes a pain response. Any animal showing severe lameness and a heel-first foot placement should be suspected of having a toe ulcer.

Treatment

One of the most important treatment considerations is to relieve all weight bearing from the affected claw by application of a claw block. This provides both pain relief and aids healing. To achieve this, the sound claw should be pared flat to provide a stable weight-bearing surface for application of the claw block. The block should be placed back far enough to provide proper heel support (Fig 51-9). Blocks that have been applied incorrectly or left on longer than 5 to 6 weeks can cause damage to the sound claw because of mechanical pressure or overstretching of the flexor tendons. Horn covering and surrounding the ulcer is often loose and necrotic and can trap dirt. The loose horn should be pared in the form of a gradual slope around the ulcer until only a thin layer of normal horn surrounds the exposed corium. This prevents further entrapment and damage to exposed corium by the horn edges. Avoid creating deep holes around the ulcer because this predisposes to manure becoming trapped and retard healing. Protruding corium showing exuberant granulation tissue should be surgically removed to the level of the surrounded pared horn. Application of antibiotic dressings such as oxytetracycline may be necessary if the exposed corium has become complicated with papillomatous digital dermatitis. Application of protective bandages is not necessary and does not improve the rate of healing of sole ulcers unless used for hemostasis or application of specific treatment.

In cases of a developing ulcer characterized by hemorrhage and pain as indicated by means of pressure with either a hoof tester or the handle of a hoof knife, lowering the affected heel transfers sufficient weight to the healthy claw to assist in healing.

Complicated and infected sole ulcers may require invasive surgical intervention and other treatments including intravenous regional antibiotic therapy.

Prevention

Overgrowth of the outer claw of the hind leg occurs commonly and is associated with the normal biomechanics of weight bearing. This asymmetry between the two claws of the hind leg is progressive, leading to excessive weight bearing and concussion of the sole corium, which in turn predisposes to sole ulcer formation. Reestablishing balance in heel height between the two claws of the hind

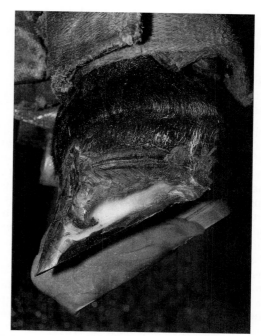

Fig 51-9 Correct block placement showing good heel support. (Courtesy Greg Hirshoren, College of Veterinary Medicine, University of Tennessee.)

leg is an important step during routine claw trimming to minimize the effects of weight bearing in the development of typical sole and heel ulcers.

Vascular and inflammatory changes associated with laminitis play an important role in weakening or breakdown of the support system of the third phalanx within the claw, resulting in the sinking or rotation of the bone with damage to the sole corium. Hormonal or biochemical changes associated with calving have similar effects. The etiology of laminitis is primarily nutritionally based, and factors leading to subacute rumen acidosis should be identified and properly managed.

Supplementation with trace minerals, particularly zinc, copper, and manganese, as well as biotin, may be beneficial in the control and prevention of sole ulcers by improving horn quality.

DOUBLE SOLE

Double sole results from interrupted sole horn formation following laminitis-induced vascular and inflammatory changes with congestion, edema, and extravasation of fluid and hemorrhage of the solar corium. Once healing of the solar corium has occurred, horn production is restored with formation of a space filled with blood and cellular debris between the old and new sole, thus creating a double sole. Repeated insults may result in a number of double soles within the same claw. The size of the double sole depends on the severity and size of the affected area of the solar corium. Double sole is usually not associated with lameness and may be found as an incidental finding during routine claw trimming. The treatment consists of paring away the overlying double sole. The exposed new sole may be hard and inflexible on finger pressure, thus ready for normal weight bearing. Elevation of the unaffected claw is usually only necessary where there are other lesions of the corium present such as a sole ulcer.

SOLE ABSCESS (pododermatitis septica and pododermatitis septica [traumatica], subsolar abscess)

Subsolar abscess is not a primary condition but usually occurs as a complication or manifestation of another lesion, most frequently white line disease, but it can also follow toe or sole ulcers and foreign body penetration. The sole becomes separated from the underlying solar corium and the space filled with pus. The abscess may be formed from the outside, in which case it will be septic, or from the inside with laminitis when the laminar corium becomes separated from the wall, forming a sterile abscess.

The approach to the treatment of subsolar abscess depends on the inciting cause (refer to later section on white line disease and earlier section on sole/toe ulcers) but should include removal of all the loose sole horn until the point of reattachment between the solar horn and the corium is reached. A thin layer of new horn may already be present, in which case careful manipulation of the hoof knife is necessary to avoid injury to the newly formed horn. In some animals the whole inner surface of the sole may be underrun, and rupture of the abscess at the horn skin junction at the back of the heel may have occurred. In other cases a sinus tract may be present on the abaxial wall (see later section on white line disease). Removal of weight bearing of the affected claw is necessary. A protective bandage is usually not required and no antibiotic treatment should be necessary except where severe damage to the corium is present. Necrosis of the corium may extend to the ventral surface of the distal phalanx resulting in sequestrum formation, which should be surgically removed. Because of damage to the corium, healing takes place with formation of very soft dyskeratotic horn or scar tissue. Non-healing or a persistent draining tract in the granulation bed on the solar surface is an indication of possible septic osteitis, septic bursitis and pathological fracture of the third phalanx.

WHITE LINE DISEASES (white line disease/ separation, white line abscess, white line fissure, white line hemorrhage, white line lesions)

Eighty percent of the white line consists of laminar horn produced by the epidermis overlying the laminar corium (sensitive laminae). The white line consists of three zones, of which the outer and middle zones are uniform and contain no tubules while the most inner part of the white line (adjacent to the sole) consists of large, loosely arranged tubules. This soft, flexible, heterogeneous structure of the white line makes it more susceptible to mechanical shearing, the corrosive effects of manure and slurry, and penetration by bacteria and foreign bodies such as coarse dirt and gravel. Laminar horn cells thus have a high turnover rate, placing relative immature cells on the outside in contact with the walking surface. The integrity of the

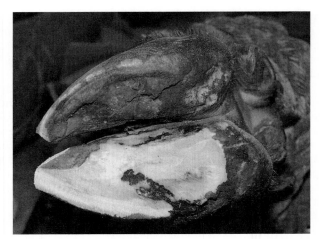

Fig 51-10   White line separation with impacted dirt. (Courtesy Greg Hirshoren, College of Veterinary Medicine, University of Tennessee.)

white line is particularly challenged at the heel wall junction of the outer claw of the hind leg because most of the weight-bearing force is concentrated in this area during the heel strike phase of the stride. The outer claw of the hind leg, particularly at the heel, becomes progressively overgrown, which exacerbates the problem. Small cracks running obliquely across the abaxial white line near the heel wall junction are often seen in early cases. Further separation allows dirt to become impacted within the separated portion of the white line (Fig 51-10). Infection may follow, and once the separation between sole and wall has progressed to the level of the solar corium, subsolar abscess formation is a common consequence. The separation may also progress farther dorsally between the wall and the laminar and coronary corium, forming a wall abscess (white line abscess) that ruptures and forms a sinus tract at the skin horn junction. Sinus tracts associated with white line disease are most commonly located on the coronary band at the junction between the abaxial wall and heel or further forward at the curve of the abaxial wall (Fig 51-11). In some cases the infection may penetrate into the heel, affecting deeper structures, which may include the deep flexor tendon, flexor tendon sheath, distal sesamoid bursa, distal sesamoid bone, and distal interphalangeal joint.

Animals suffering white line disease may in some cases be severely lame but without visible lesions in all areas of the white line. The outer claw is usually overgrown, particularly at the heel. The animal may show a pain response to pressure with a hoof tester in the area of the white line at the heel wall junction. Trimming of the abaxial wall at an angle to expose the white line at the heel wall junction may show a yellowish discoloration of the laminar horn. Further trimming of the laminar horn often opens a white line abscess. Such a lesion may follow alterations in the microcirculation, which could be mechanical due to overgrowth or metabolic (laminitis) in origin. This results in hemorrhage often visible within the white line, sloughing of necrotic epidermal cells, and interruption in laminar horn production with formation of a sterile abscess.

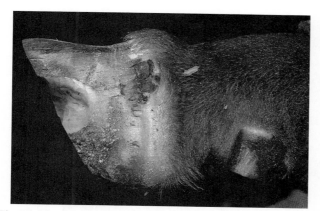

Fig 51-11 White line separation with tract opening at the coronary band. (Courtesy Greg Hirshoren, College of Veterinary Medicine, University of Tennessee.)

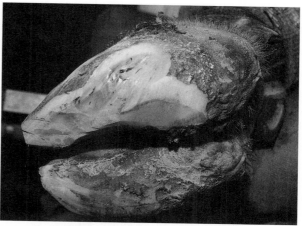

Fig 51-12 Corrective trimming of white line separation should involve full exposure of the undermined wall and sole horn. (Courtesy Greg Hirshoren, College of Veterinary Medicine, University of Tennessee.)

Treatment for white line disease includes sloping the wall at a 45-degree angle over the area of the white line separation, the full extent of which should be exposed and can involve a large part of the sole, as well as the abaxial wall (Fig 51-12). With small lesions lowering of the heel may provide enough relief from weight bearing on the affected claw. However, in more severe cases application of a claw block to the healthy claw is necessary. Swelling above the coronet or at the heel may indicate that the infection had penetrated the deeper structures such as the flexor tendons, flexor tendon sheath, navicular bursa and navicular bone, and retro-articular space. Infection may also enter the distal interphalangeal joint and is usually associated with severe lameness. Such cases require invasive surgical intervention, which may include aggressive débridement of the affected area, resection of the necrotic portion of the flexor tendon, and flushing of the tendon sheath followed by the insertion of a drain in some cases. Surgical ankylosis of the distal interphalangeal joint may be necessary if the joint is involved in the septic process. Regional limb perfusion with antibiotics such as ceftiofur (1 g) or ampicillin (1 g) or sodium benzyl penicillin (10 million units) may be beneficial in combination with antiinflammatory (flunixin 1.1 mg/kg bid) and analgesic drugs (morphine 0.5 mg/kg IM every 6-8 hours).

VERTICAL WALL FISSURE (fissura ungulae longitudinalis) (crack, sand cracks, quarter cracks)

Sand cracks are more common in beef cattle compared with dairy cattle, in which the incidence is low. An incidence of 28% to 59% has been reported in problematic beef herds. In Western Canada the incidence of sand cracks in beef cattle averages 37.2%.

Classification of vertical wall cracks by type include the following:

- Type 1. Associated with coronary band. Usually not recognized.
- Type 2. Extend from the coronary band to halfway down the dorsal wall. Can be associated with horizontal wall crack.
- Type 3. Involve the entire length of the dorsal wall.
- Type 4. Extend from the middle of the dorsal wall to the level of the sole. Could represent a wall crack that is healing and growing out or may have originated from the level of the bearing surface.
- Type 5. Confined to the middle of the dorsal wall.

Vertical cracks can occur in two anatomic locations, the most common being the dorsal wall of the front outer claw. Less commonly a vertical wall crack develops at the junction of the abaxial and axial walls.

Sand cracks relate to factors influencing fracture toughness (horn quality) of the claw wall. Microscopic cracks (fractures), which initiate the problem, develop adjacent to horn tubules. Progression of the crack is slowed or arrested by the intertubular horn, which diverts the direction of the crack away from the tubules. The extent of the crack may be confined to the perioplic horn and coronary band or extend all the way to the bearing surface and depends on the predisposing cause, which may include diet, trace minerals and vitamins, and moisture content of the horn. Lush grass high in soluble sugars can cause laminitis (grass founder) and has been associated with development of vertical wall cracks resulting from the production of inferior-quality horn. Dry and desiccated horn is more predisposed to development of vertical wall cracks because of the loss of normal moisture-dependent flexibility. Deficiency of biotin; sulfur containing amino acids, calcium, and phosphorus; and trace minerals including zinc, copper, and manganese necessary for normal keratinization of horn cells or excessive selenium may contribute to the development of sand cracks. Sulfate, iron, and nitrates in water sources such as well water may bind zinc and copper, making them less available. The incidence is also reported to be higher in heavy animals. Animals with vertical wall cracks often show other changes in claw conformation and structure indicative of subclinical laminitis including concave dorsal wall, soft powdery sole horn, widening of the white line, and horizontal grooves (hardship grooves).

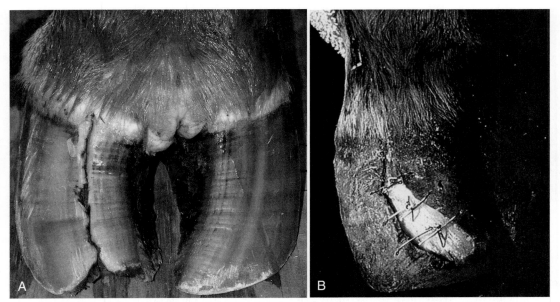

Fig 51-13 **A,** Type 3 vertical wall crack. **B,** Wire support of vertical wall crack as part of the corrective trimming procedure. (**A,** Courtesy Dr. Jan Shearer, University of Florida, Gainesville.)

No treatment is necessary if the animal is not showing any signs of lameness, but natural resolution is rare. Larger cracks may have ragged and thickened edges because of excess horn growth. Dirt may become trapped in the fissure. Any removal of underrun horn in the wall should be done with care to avoid cutting into the corium, and it should be pared in a V shape along its entire length to stop further entrapment of dirt. Wire support across the vertical wall crack to provide additional support has been used (Fig 51-13, *A* and *B*). The use of acrylics for support of a wide crack is questionable because it may trap dirt and bacteria, which may exacerbate the problem, particularly if the depth of the crack is close to or has reached the corium. The heat generated by the methyl methacrylate may also damage the corium. Fissures that do not extend through the full thickness of the wall usually do not result in lameness. However, once the fissure extends to the depth of the corium, lameness will result. Lameness can be severe, and trauma to the corium can have serious consequences including necrosis of the dorsal aspect of the corium extending to the third phalanx, resulting in a septic osteitis and pathologic fracture. Or the corium may proliferate with the formation of abundant granulation tissue growing over the horn edges, particularly if the coronary corium is involved. Histopathologically the protruding corium consists of typical granulation tissue. In such cases surgical excision of the granulation tissue, as well as thinning of the horn around the lesion, is important in combination with freezing the area with a cryoprobe and application of topical agents, which may inhibit the formation of granulation tissue such as a steroid. A mixture of oxytetracycline powder and dexamethasone appears to be helpful in suppressing formation of granulation tissue. Large lesions with abundant granulation tissue have a poor prognosis and tend to recur even after several treatments. Claw amputation may be the only option in nonresponsive cases.

HORIZONTAL WALL GROOVES (fissura ungulae transversalis) (hardship grooves, fissures, thimble)

Horizontal wall grooves (hardship grooves) result from interruption of horn growth of the basal layer of the epidermis overlying the coronary corium, which provides vascular and nutritional support to the horn of the wall. Full-thickness defects in horn growth are referred to as *fissures*, which may fracture or partially break away from the claw, resulting in a "thimble" (Fig 51-14). Fissures may extend to the corium, resulting in lameness. Horizontal grooves or fissures are commonly associated with disease-related "stresses" such as metritis or coliform mastitis or laminitis, all of which may be associated with either fever and/or endotoxemia.

Horizontal wall fissures, even thimbles not involving the sensitive laminae, can be left untreated and will eventually grow out. Those that do reach the corium and cause lameness need to be treated by removing all the loose and underrun horn. Care must be taken not to cause trauma to the underlying corium. A foot block to the healthy claw should be applied in such cases.

CORKSCREW CLAW

Corkscrew claw is observed most commonly in the lateral claws of the hind leg in cattle older than 3.5 years of age. It is reported to be heritable, although other factors such as claw disease, inappropriate claw care nutrition, and

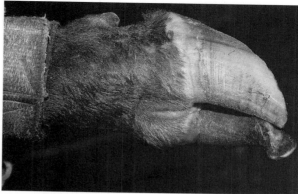

Fig 51-15   Corkscrew claw. Note the rotation of the toe with displacement of the sole, white line, and axial wall. (Courtesy Greg Hirshoren, College of Veterinary Medicine, University of Tennessee.)

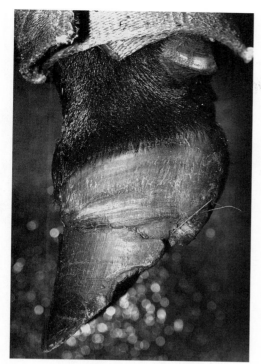

Fig 51-14   Full-thickness horizontal wall crack (thimble). (Courtesy Greg Hirshoren, College of Veterinary Medicine, University of Tennessee.)

management may play a role. It is more likely to be heritable if claw changes occur at a young age, whereas other factors are more likely to play a role in older animals.

A misalignment of the second and third phalanges within the digit occurs, and the third phalanx may have an abnormal structure including being narrower and having an abaxial to axial curve. This may lead to inappropriate weight bearing within the claw with excessive weight distribution at the abaxial sole and white line junction, resulting in white line lesions. Such lesions, which start from inside the claw, may become exposed during trimming. Overgrowth of the corkscrew claw, which in some cases may be pronounced, is another predisposing factor for development of claw horn lesions. Growth rates of the mid and caudal walls may be faster with corkscrew claw as compared with normal claws and may predispose to lameness because of increased weight bearing. Lesions within the horn capsule associated with overgrowth include hemorrhage of the sole and white line, sole ulcers, and white line separation, particularly at the heel wall sole junction.

Corkscrew claw is characterized by the following abnormalities in claw conformation and growth:

- The mid and caudal abaxial walls curve ventrally and often become part of the bearing surface of the claw.
- Axial displacement of the sole and axial white line and rotation of the toe result in loss of its weight-bearing function (Fig 51-15). The sole and white line at the toe may be perpendicular to the weight-bearing surface. In addition, the axial wall becomes displaced and a fold may develop in the axial wall.

- The corkscrew claw becomes overgrown compared with the normal claw, particularly at the heel and axial heel sole junction. In some instances the claw opposite to the corkscrew claw may become virtually non–weight bearing and appears to undergo disuse atrophy. In such instances the opposite claw appears smaller, the sole is sunken with a marked slope toward the interdigital space, and the abaxial wall shows little or no sign of wear.

Correction of the height difference (imbalance) between the two claws is one of the primary concerns during the corrective trimming procedure, the approach for which is the following:

- The toe length of the claw opposite the corkscrew claw is reduced to 3 inches (7.5 cm) in length for Holstein dairy cattle. In beef cattle the overgrown wall at the toe is removed by using the white line as a guide. No further trimming of this claw should be done at this point.
- Next, the toe length of the corkscrew claw is reduced to the same length as that of the already trimmed opposite claw.
- To align the dorsal wall of the screw claw with that of the opposite claw, the upward deviation and rotation of the dorsal wall is removed (straightened) with the use of an angle grinder (Fig 51-16). Use finger pressure during this procedure to assess thickness of the wall because overthinning of the dorsal wall with hemorrhage may result. However, this usually does not result in any complications provided it is limited to a small confined area.
- Balance the bearing surface including the heel of the corkscrew claw with that of the opposite claw. The wall is often hard, and an angle grinder or nippers can facilitate this procedure.
- Slope the sole of the corkscrew claw at the interdigital space and simultaneously remove the fold in the axial wall. The trimmed corkscrew claw often has a small, narrow weight-bearing surface.

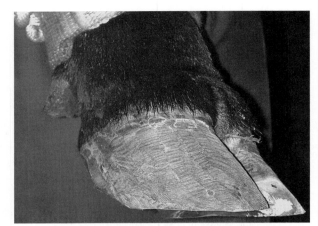

Fig 51-16 Corrective trimming of corkscrew claw involves straightening the dorsal wall. Note small area of hemorrhage along the displaced sole/white line border, which occurred during the trimming procedure and is of no consequence.

- If enough sole horn thickness remains on the corkscrew claw, both claws can be further trimmed to increase the stability of the weight-bearing surfaces.
- Specific corrective trimming procedures including the application of a claw block to the healthy claw to relieve weight bearing may be required if other claw horn lesions such as sole ulcers and white line disease are present.
- Corkscrew claw should preferably be trimmed at 3 to 4 month intervals.

Claw Horn Changes Resembling Corkscrew Claw

Claw Rotation of the Inner Claw of the Rear Leg in Heifers

Abaxial to axial deviation of the abaxial wall and rotation of the toe of the rear leg's inner claw similar to that seen with screw claw has been observed in heifers in Europe, where prevalence rates of up to 50% have been reported. The inner claw is usually longer than the outer claw. Trimming consists of correcting the abnormal length and creating a stable weight-bearing surface for the affected claw.

Claw Rotation of the Inner Claw of the Front Legs in Cows (acquired corkscrew claw)

A common condition seen in dairy cows kept in partial and total confinement housing is axial rotation of the toe of the inner claw of the front leg. The abaxial wall has an abaxial to axial curve and is somewhat overgrown. The sole is sloped toward the interdigital space (Fig 51-17). Corrective trimming is done by removing the axial curve at the toe without penetrating the axial white line and creating a stable weight-bearing surface for the inner claw by balancing it with that of the outer claw.

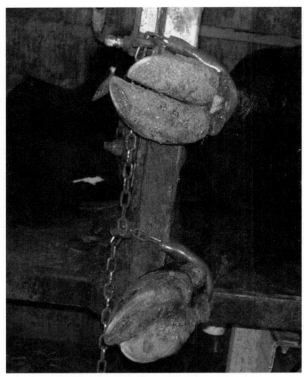

Fig 51-17 Acquired screw claw. (Courtesy Dr. Jan Shearer, University of Florida, Gainesville.)

THIN SOLES IN CATTLE

Thin soles are an important cause of lameness in large dairies and result from an increase in sole horn wear, the causes of which are multifactorial: moisture content of sole horn, long distances cows have to walk on concrete to be milked, sharp turns and sloped walkways, aggregates in new concrete, subacute laminitis that reduces horn quality, forcing cows to move at a faster pace on hard walking surfaces, poor cow comfort caused by overcrowding, poor stall design, insufficient bedding, and heat stress, all of which increase the time cows remain standing; commingling of different age groups; and overtrimming.

Clinical Signs

The outer claw of the hind leg is most commonly affected, although in severe cases the claws of all four feet may be affected, with the back feet usually affected to a greater degree than those of the front. The soles are usually flat and flexible on finger pressure, and the heels are shallow and soft. Separation between the sole and abaxial white line and sole hemorrhage and extreme thinning of the sole occur at the heel sole junction. More severe complications include exposure of the corium between the sole and abaxial white line. This may be further complicated by penetration of dirt and bacteria into the corium and apex of the third phalanx, resulting in osteitis and pathologic fracture of the third phalanx and formation of a subsolar abscess. Heel and sole ulcers are also common. One study found 30% of rear feet in cows with thin soles had pathologic claw horn lesions including sole/white line separation (72%) and sole ulcers (28%). Of the affected claws, 13% had more than one lesion. Seventy percent of claw lesions occurred in the lateral claw of the hind leg.

Treatment and Control

The mechanical abrasiveness of new concrete can be reduced by using a wood-float finish in combination with grooving. Grooves should be 12 mm wide and 10 mm deep and placed 5 to 7.5 cm apart and be placed in the same direction as that in which the manure scraper travels. This provides good traction and a stable weight-bearing surface. Sharp edges and protruding aggregate can be removed by dragging a heavy concrete block or steel scraper along the floor. The use of conveyor belting in feed alleys and walkways appears to be helpful in limiting mechanical abrasion of solar horn.

Once a thin-soled problem has developed, care should be taken in removing additional solar horn during maintenance trimming procedures. Cows with thin flexible soles should preferably be taken off concrete and kept in a dirt lot close to the milking parlor. If sole horn thickness of the inner hind claw allows, a claw block can be applied to elevate the affected outer claw.

Recommended Readings

Acuna R, Scarci R: *Toe ulcer: the most important disease in first-calving Holstein cows under grazing conditions.* Proceedings of the 12th International Symposium on Lameness in Ruminants, Orlando, Fla, 2002, pp 276-279.

Belknap EB, Cochran A, Schwartzkopf E et al: *Digital expression of isoforms of cyclooxygenase in a model of bovine laminitis.* Proceedings of the 36th Annual Convention of the American Association of Bovine Practitioners, 2003, p 191.

Bergsten C, Frank B: Sole hemorrhages in tied primiparous cows as an indicator of periparturient laminitis: effects of diet, flooring and season, *Acta Vet Scand* 37:383, 1996.

Bergsten C, Herlin AH: Sole hemorrhages and heel horn erosion in dairy cows: the influence of housing system on their prevalence and severity, *Acta Vet Scand* 37:395, 1996.

Blowey RW, Watson CL, Green LE et al: *The incidence of heel ulcers in a study of lameness in five UK dairy herds.* Proceedings of the 11th International Symposium on Disorders of the Ruminant Digit and 3rd International Conference on Bovine Lameness, Parma, Italy, 2000, pp 163-164.

Budras KD, Mülling C, Horowitz A: The rate of keratinization of the wall segment of the cattle hoof and its relationship to width and structure of the zona alba (WL) with respect to claw disease, *Am J Vet Res* 57:444, 1996.

Christmann U, Belknap EB, Lin HC et al: *Evaluation of hemodynamics in the normal and laminitic bovine digit.* Proceedings of the 12th International Symposium on Lameness in Ruminants, Orlando, Fla, 2002, pp 165-166.

Eggers T, Mülling C, Lischer CH et al: *Morphological aspects on wound healing of Rusterholtz ulcer in the bovine hoof.* Proceedings of the 11th International Symposium on Disorders of the Ruminant Digit and 3rd International Conference on Bovine Lameness, Parma, Italy, 2000, pp 203-205.

Enevoldsen C, Gröhn YT, Thysen I: Sole ulcers in dairy cattle: associations with season, cow characteristics, disease, and production, *J Dairy Sci* 74:1284, 1991.

Frankena K, van Keulen KAS, Noordhuizen JP et al: A cross-sectional study into prevalence and risk indicators of digital hemorrhages in female dairy calves, *Prevent Vet Med* 14:1, 1992.

Hendry KA, Knight CH, Galbraith H et al: *Basement membrane role in keratinization of healthy and diseased hooves.* Proceedings of the 11th International Symposium on Disorders of the Ruminant Digit and 3rd International Conference on Bovine Lameness, Parma, Italy, 2000, pp 128-129.

Hendry KA, MacCullum AJ, Knight CH, Wilde CJ: Effect of endocrine and paracrine factors on protein synthesis and cell proliferation in bovine hoof tissue culture, *J Dairy Res* 66:23, 1999.

Hendry KA, MacCullum AJ, Knight CH, Wilde CJ: Laminitis in the diary cow: a cell biological approach, *J Dairy Res* 66:213, 1999.

Hirschberg RM, Mülling C: *Preferential pathways and haemodynamic bottlenecks in the vascular system of the healthy and diseased bovine claw.* Proceedings of the 12th International Symposium on Lameness in Ruminants, Orlando, Florida, 2002, pp 223-226.

Hirschberg RM, Plendl J: *Pododermal angiogenesis—new aspects of development and function of the bovine claw.* Proceedings of the 11th International Symposium on Disorders of the Ruminant Digit and 3rd International Conference on Bovine Lameness, Parma, Italy, 2000, pp 67-69.

Hoblet KH, Weiss W: Metabolic hoof horn disease. Claw horn disruption, *Vet Clin North Am Food Anim Pract* 17:111, 2001.

Knott L, Webster AJ, Tarlton JF: *Biochemical and biophysical changes to connective tissues of the bovine hoof around parturition.* Proceedings of the 11th International Symposium on Disorders of the Ruminant Digit and 3rd International Conference on Bovine Lameness, Parma, Italy, 2000, pp 88-89.

Lischer ChJ, Koller U, Geyer H et al: Effect of therapeutic dietary biotin on the healing of uncomplicated sole ulcers in dairy cattle: a double blinded controlled study, *Vet J* 163:51, 2002.

Lischer CJ, Ossent P: *Pathogenesis of sole lesions attributed to laminitis in cattle.* Proceedings of the 12th International Symposium on Lameness in Ruminants, Orlando, Florida, 2002, pp 83-89.

Midla LT, Hoblet KH, Weiss WP et al: Supplemental dietary biotin for prevention of lesions associated with aseptic subclinical laminitis (pododermatitis aseptica diffusa) in primiparous cows, *Am J Vet Res* 59:733, 1998.

Mülling C, Lischer CJ: *New aspects on etiology and pathogenesis of laminitis in cattle.* Proc Internatl Buiatrics Conference, Hanover, Germany, 2002, pp 236-247.

Mülling C: *Theories on the pathogenesis of white line disease—an anatomical perspective.* 2002 Proceedings of the 12th International Symposium on Lameness in Ruminants, Orlando, Fla, pp 90-98.

Ossent P, Lischer CJ: Bovine laminitis: the lesions and their pathogenesis, *Practitioner* 20:415, 1998.

Russell AM, Rowlands GJ, Shaw SR, Weaver AD: Survey of lameness in British dairy cattle, *Vet Rec* 111:155, 1982.

Sangues Gonzalez A: *The biomechanics of weight bearing and its significance with lameness.* Proceedings of the 12th International Symposium on Lameness in Ruminants, Orlando, Fla, 2002, pp 117-121.

Shearer JK, van Amstel SR: Functional and corrective claw trimming, *Vet Clin North Am Food Anim Pract* 17:53, 2001.

Tarlton JF, Webster AJF: *A biochemical and biomechanical basis for the pathogenesis of claw horn lesions.* Proceedings of the 12th International Symposium on Lameness in Ruminants, Orlando, Fla, 2002, pp 395-398.

Tarlton JF, Webster AJF: *A biochemical basis for the pathogenesis of claw horn lesions.* Proceedings of the 12th International Symposium on Lameness in Ruminants, 2002, pp 395-398.

Toussaint Raven E: Structure and functions (Chapter 1) and trimming (Chapter 3). In Toussaint Raven E, editor: *Cattle foot care and claw trimming,* Ipswich, UK, 1989, Farming Press, pp 24-26 and 75-94.

van Amstel SR, Shearer JK: Abnormalities of hoof growth and development, *Vet Clin North Am Food Anim Pract* 17:73, 2001.

van Amstel SR, Shearer JK, Palin FL: Moisture content, thickness and lesions of sole horn associated with thin soles in dairy cattle, *J Dairy Sci* 87:757, 2004.

Vermunt JJ: *Risk factors of laminitis—an overview.* 11th International Symposium on Disorders of the Ruminant Digit and 3rd International Conference on Bovine Lameness, Parma, Italy, 2000, pp 34-42.

Vermunt JJ, Greenough PR: Lesions associated with subclinical laminitis of the claws of dairy cows in two management systems, *Br Vet J* 151:391, 1995.

Vermunt JJ, Greenough PR: Predisposing factors of laminitis in cattle, *Br Vet J* 150:151, 1994.

CHAPTER **52**

Infectious Disorders of the Foot Skin

JAN K. SHEARER

INTERDIGITAL DERMATITIS (stinky foot, stable foot rot)

Interdigital dermatitis has been a source of controversy among researchers. Based on clinical and histopathologic findings, it shares a number of similarities with digital dermatitis (e.g., superficial dermatitis, heel horn erosion, presence of bacterial spirochetes). This has caused some researchers to question whether these disorders are in fact one and the same. Although this issue remains unresolved, for the purposes of this discussion, interdigital and digital dermatitis are described as distinct and separate diseases.

Interdigital dermatitis tends to be a mild inflammatory condition of the interdigital skin, most commonly observed in confinement-housed cattle where feet are continuously exposed to manure slurry and moisture. Lesions have a characteristic foul odor, which accounts for the term "stinky foot" in reference to this disease. Although painful to the touch, lesions rarely seem to cause lameness. Chronic inflammation of the interdigital skin is one of the hallmarks of this disease. Therefore it is believed to be a predisposing cause of interdigital hyperplasia or corns. Interdigital dermatitis is also associated with heel horn erosion because the infection often extends to the heel, where organisms, equipped with keratinolytic enzymes, erode the relatively softer horn of the heel bulb (Fig 52-1). Initially, erosion of the heel horn appears as a diffuse pitting on the axial surface of the heel. Over time, erosion progresses to a more severe stage, resulting in multiple fissures and undermining of heel horn (Fig 52-2).

Although heel erosion does not appear to be a direct cause of lameness, it may be important as an indirect cause of lameness due to sole and heel ulcers because of its effects on weight bearing and claw horn overgrowth in affected digits. The erosive loss of heel horn leads to an abnormal displacement of weight within the digit that is countered by an acceleration of sole horn growth anterior to the eroded horn of the heel. These effects are usually greatest on the lateral claw as a consequence of weight-bearing dynamics that generally result in greater weight bearing on the lateral claw of the rear foot. Balance between the weight-bearing surfaces of each digit is severely disrupted by accelerated overgrowth of the lateral claw and the formation of a wedge of abnormal horn that develops in the axial region of the heel-sole junction. The combination of these horn growth abnormalities leads to contusion of the corium and eventually the development of a sole or heel ulcer.

Early reports suggest *Dichelobacter nodosus* as the primary causative agent of interdigital dermatitis and heel horn erosion. Current thought is that, in addition to *D. nodosus*, bacterial spirochetes belonging to the genus *Treponema* sp. may be involved as well. *Fusobacterium necrophorum* is also frequently observed in the lesions of interdigital dermatitis, where it is believed to be responsible for necrosis of the interdigital skin lesions.

In individual animals with severe lesions of interdigital dermatitis that may be causing lameness, topical antibiotic preparations under a loose wrap are generally recommended. Herd-level control is best accomplished with a footbath containing either a 3% to 5% concentration of

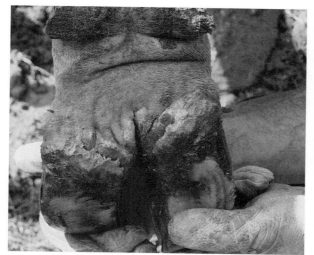

Fig 52-1 Interdigital dermatitis with a mild form of heel erosion.

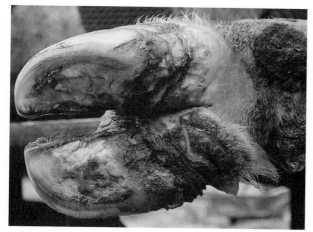

Fig 52-2 Heel horn erosion (fissure-type) secondary to digital and interdigital dermatitis. Note undermining of the heel horn on the claw with the digital dermatitis lesion.

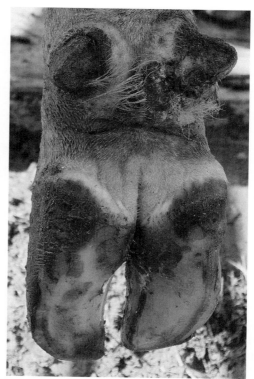

Fig 52-3 An ulcerative lesion of digital dermatitis adjacent to the dew claws.

formalin or 5% to 10% copper sulfate. Depending on prevalence and other considerations, herds may be required to operate their footbaths three to five times per week for optimal control. In individual animals where heel erosion has led to the formation of rough, irregular horn on the bulbar surfaces, careful paring of horn ridges to provide a smooth surface is advised. This may be followed by the topical application of an astringent or antibacterial spray, which will provide additional protection to the newly exposed horn.

DIGITAL DERMATITIS (Mortellaro's disease, papillomatous digital dermatitis, hairy heel warts, footwarts)

"Mortellaro's disease," better known as *digital dermatitis,* was first reported by Italian researchers Cheli and Mortellaro in 1974. One anecdotal report and at least one scientific report of the occurrence of papillomatous digital

lesions in dairy cows and beef bulls suggest that digital dermatitis (DD) was also present during the same period in the United States. Since these early reports, the disease has been recognized throughout much of the developed world.

Clinical Signs

The lesions of DD typically occur on the skin of the plantar aspect of the rear foot adjacent to the interdigital cleft, or at the skin-horn junction of the heel bulbs. On occasion lesions may be found adjacent to the dew claws or bordering the dorsal interdigital cleft (particularly on front feet) (Figs 52-3 and 52-4). Most lesions are circular or oval with clearly demarcated borders. Hypertrophied hairs surround the lesion borders and should be distinguished from epithelial filiform papillae, which often extend from the surface of chronic lesions. Chronic lesions without filiform papillae are generally thickened and have a granular surface. Histologically, lesions demonstrate a range of ulcerative and proliferative changes including ulceration of the dermal papillae, epidermal hyperplasia with parakeratosis and hyperkeratosis, and inflammation along with the presence of numerous spirochetes invading the stratum spinosum.

Even a mild disturbance of the inflamed tissue tends to result in extreme discomfort and mild to moderate bleeding. Therefore, cows will alter their posture and/or gait to avoid direct contact between lesions and the floor or other objects. These pain avoidance adaptations also lead to abnormal wear of the weight-bearing surface of affected

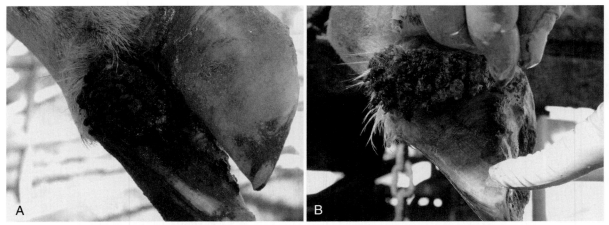

Fig 52-4 **A,** Large chronic lesion of digital dermatitis with filiform papillae protruding from the dorsal interdigital cleft. **B,** Spreading the digits apart reveals the extent of the lesion in the interdigital space.

claws. Lesions associated with the plantar interdigital cleft usually cause the cow to shift weight bearing toward the toe. This results in increased wear at the toe, decreased wear in the heel, and an overall reduction in the weight-bearing surface of the affected claw. When lesions occur on the dorsal aspect of the foot, cows respond by altering posture and weight bearing, resulting in overgrowth at the toe and greater wear in the heel. These alterations in shape of the claw generally require correction at the time of trimming.

Etiology

Stained sections from infected tissues typically yield large numbers of bacterial spirochetes. This has led researchers to conclude that these organisms are likely involved in the pathogenesis of this disease either as primary causative agents or secondary invaders. One report of a study involving experimentally induced infection, followed by sequential tissue sampling in calves, suggested that spirochetes were likely the first organisms to invade and colonize the epidermal and dermal tissues. Spirochetes most commonly observed are from the genus *Treponema* and apparently similar to those associated with periodontal disease in humans.

Epidemiology

The prevalence of DD in herds is variable and usually underestimated by herd owners. Rates of 20% to more than 50% have been reported. Despite the severe pain that animals seem to experience when lesions are disturbed, lameness associated with this disease is inconsistent and often lower than might be expected. It appears that pain resulting in lameness is often due to an extension of the lesion to the horny structures of the claw.

The housing, environment, and management conditions most consistently identified as predisposing causes of DD include large herd size, wet and muddy corrals, and the purchase of replacement animals. Other risk factors cited in a national U.S. study were use of a footbath, housing

on grooved concrete, use of a trimmer who trimmed feet at other farms, and failure to clean and sanitize equipment between uses on cows. Although the latter study suggested important epidemiologic relationships, it did not distinguish between cause and effect. In other words, considering the relationship of footbaths and DD as cited in this study, analysis of the data did not establish that DD was caused by footbaths or that herds with DD were more likely to use footbaths. One would have concluded, however, that housing and environmental hygiene are important factors in control of this disease. Furthermore, based on these studies, the importance of hygiene could be extended to those who provide foot care services (veterinarians and/or trimmers) on dairy farms. Knives and nippers may be cleaned and disinfected initially with a brush and antibacterial dish detergent. These items are inexpensive and readily available and may be useful for other procedures such as a pre-scrub for initial cleaning to remove organic material from surgical sites and for general cleaning of other items such as boots. This permits the judicious use of more expensive and, in some cases, more corrosive types of disinfectants for those applications where they may be specifically required.

The highest incidence of DD is often observed in early lactation. In most cases this is due to extremely high rates of DD in prefresh, home-grown or off-site, custom-raised heifers. Herds that purchase replacements usually do not request DD-free animals, nor do they normally inspect purchased animals for the presence of DD lesions before introducing them into their herds. Researchers have suggested that one of the potential causes of a higher incidence of DD in the early postpartum period may be due to periparturient immune suppression. However, another reason for a higher incidence of DD in prefresh heifers may be because these animals are not usually accessible by the normal modes of control used in lactating cows (i.e., footbaths).

Possible reservoirs and mode of transmission of DD are largely unknown but assumed to be clinically and subclinically infected cows and fomites. For example, the heel bulbs adjacent to the plantar interdigital cleft are closely apposed, creating a "pocket" that serves as an ideal microenvironment for the harboring of bacteria (presumably spirochetes) that are presumed to be the cause of this disease. Despite the application of control measures, this area is difficult if not impossible to disinfect and thus likely serves as a reservoir of infection. Precise mechanisms of fomite involvement through contamination of the animal's environment are poorly understood but presumed to be a part of the disease reservoir and mode of transmission.

Attempts to reproduce the disease under controlled conditions have proved difficult, but it has been accomplished in calves. Experimental transmission was achieved by the placement of scrapings from DD lesions under a wrap designed to create an oxygen-depleted and moist microenvironment in the intended anatomic site. Typical lesions were observed after a period of several weeks.

Effects of Digital Dermatitis on Performance

Few studies have attempted to assess the effects of DD on performance. A U.S. study found that cows affected with DD produced less milk (153.3 kg) than healthy cows, although the difference was not significant. Another earlier study conducted on a 600-cow dairy in Mexico had similar results. Cows affected with DD produced 121.6 kg less milk than their unaffected herd mates. But, as in the previous study this difference was not significant. Significant effects on reproductive performance occurred, however. For cows affected with DD, the calving-to-conception interval was increased from 93 to 113 days. Average days open were increased by approximately 14 days as compared with noninfected herd mates.

Treatment and Control of Digital Dermatitis

Numerous studies have demonstrated a response to antibiotic treatment applied topically as a spray or under a loose bandage. Residue violations are always a concern with antibiotic treatment; however, this does not appear to be a significant problem with topical treatment. Several nonantibiotic preparations have been evaluated as well. In general, nonantibiotic preparations have shown reduced efficacy with one exception—Victory (Westfalia-Surge, Inc.), a triplex formulation containing soluble copper, a peroxide compound, and a cationic agent. Studies of parenteral therapy for DD have shown mixed results. The literature offers no reports on the effectiveness of oral antibiotic therapy in feed or water.

The use of a walk-through footbath has been a popular approach to treatment of DD. However, there is little information in the scientific literature to support its efficacy. Products suggested for use usually include $CuSO_4$, $ZnSO_4$, formalin, and various antibiotics. Arkins reported on two controlled field studies using 5% formalin. Both studies demonstrated improvements in claw health from reduced incidence of interdigital lesions and severity of heel horn erosion. Disadvantages to the use of footbaths include human health concerns from exposure to formalin, environmental and claw health concerns from the use of $CuSO_4$ and $ZnSO_4$, and potential antimicrobial resistance from the use or overuse of antibiotics. Regardless of the method

chosen for treatment of DD, recurrence rates are high, requiring some form of continued treatment for optimal control.

Compounds or products used in footbaths should make good biologic sense with regard to the condition being treated or prevented. Furthermore, benefits must be weighed against risks to animal and human health, environmental contamination, and potential for antimicrobial resistance.

The following compounds are commonly used in footbaths*:

Copper Sulfate
5%—requires 8 lb copper sulfate in 20 gallons of water
10%—requires 16 lb copper sulfate in 20 gallons of water
Formalin
5%—requires 1 gallon of 36% formaldehyde in 19 gallons of water
Zinc Sulfate
10%—requires 16 lb of agricultural grade zinc sulfate monohydrate (36%) in 20 gallons of water

Many other commercial footbath products are on the market. Few have research data verifying efficacy. Other options include the soluble powder formulations of tetracycline or oxytetracycline and lincomycin or the combination product lincomycin-spectinomycin at concentrations ranging between 0.1 and 1 g/L. Although these formulations are normally used for oral medication purposes, because of their reduced cost relative to injectable forms, they are often used in extra-label fashion for footbath applications.

Proper formulation of footbath solutions is important. The excessive use of footbath compounds is needlessly expensive and in some cases may even cause harm. On the other hand, footbath solutions that are too dilute are likely to be ineffective. Therefore one of the first steps in footbath management is to determine the footbath's capacity or volume so that compounds intended for use may be accurately diluted. Most footbaths are rectangular, thus permitting calculation of the volume by application of the following simple formula:

$$\text{Length (feet)} \times \text{width (feet)} \times \text{depth (feet)} \times 7.46$$
$$= \text{volume in gallons}$$

So, to calculate the number of gallons of water in a footbath 6 foot long by 3 foot wide and 6 inches deep, one would multiply:

$$6 \text{ ft} \times 3 \text{ ft} \times .5 \text{ ft} \text{ (½ foot deep)} \times 7.46 = 67 \text{ gallons}$$

Because there are 3.8 L in 1 gallon, all one needs to do to determine the total number of liters in the previous example is simply multiply the total number of gallons (67 gallons) by 3.8.

$$67 \text{ gallons} \times 3.8 \text{ (liters in 1 gallon)} = 255 \text{ L}$$

The use of these simple calculations for volume of a footbath and conversion to metric terms in combination with the suggested use rates or concentrations helps to avoid potential damage to cows and the environment.

One challenge in using footbaths for treatment of infectious foot skin disorders is that although only 10% of cows in a herd may be affected, all cows must traverse the bath in order to expose those affected with disinfectant solutions. Contamination and neutralization of footbath solutions becomes a significant complication in the achievement of therapeutic benefit for the smaller number of animals affected. Better results may be achieved by finding ways to limit footbath access to only those cows affected. Because this may not be practical under some conditions, another option for the treatment of small numbers of animals might be use of a stand-in footbath. As the name implies, a stand-in footbath is used to provide prolonged exposure to footbath solutions. These may be designed to accommodate multiple animals or as simple as a 5-gallon bucket. If formalin is used, the bath should be in an outdoor location or where there is adequate ventilation to avoid irritation to the eyes and mucus membranes from fumes.

In recent years alternatives to walk-through footbaths have been marketed. These include footbath mats and foot foams. Footbath mats are made of an absorbable compressible material enclosed in a porous shell or cover. These are usually positioned in parlor exit lanes. As cows exit the parlor and place their feet on the mat, footbath solutions are expressed from the mat and bathe the feet. The cover prevents direct contamination of the mat and foot bath solutions, thereby, in theory, reducing the neutralization rate of footbath solutions. Foot foams, on the other hand, are often applied at the entrance to milking parlors. As cows enter the holding area, they walk through the foam, which adheres to their feet, providing exposure to the disinfectant properties of the foam during the premilking, milking, and immediate postmilking period. One of the potential advantages of this system is prolonged exposure of feet to disinfectant solutions. Despite claims of efficacy by persons who market these devices, data from well-controlled studies are lacking.

Vaccination for Control of Digital Dermatitis

Because of high recurrence rates and the inability to conveniently treat high-risk groups of animals (such as growing heifers), an effective vaccine for control of DD is highly desirable. Results from early studies of a *Treponema* bacterin for control of DD in cattle concluded that immunization could reduce clinical disease. In contrast, German researchers found no benefit from a vaccine containing herd-specific pathogens including *Treponema* sp. Similar results were observed in a recent U.S. field trial that found no therapeutic or prophylactic benefit from vaccination with a *Treponema* bacterin. At the present time, there are no vaccines commercially available for control of digital dermatitis.

INTERDIGITAL PHLEGMON (foot rot, interdigital necrobacillosis, interdigital pododermatitis, acute foot rot, and foul in the foot)

Interdigital phlegmon is occasionally confused with interdigital dermatitis because both conditions are associated with lesions of the interdigital skin. However, interdigital phlegmon is an infection of the interdigital skin that extends into the deeper underlying soft tissues of the foot. The disease is characterized by swelling of the foot, severe lameness, and in most cases a necrotic lesion of the interdigital skin. Although occurrence is generally sporadic, epidemics are known to occur in confinement-housed cattle. Secondary complications associated with foot rot include infectious arthritis of the distal interphalangeal joint, necrotic tendinitis, navicular bursitis, and abscessation of the retro-articular space.

Etiology

Although evidence is inconclusive, most believe that the disease occurs subsequent to injury or abrasion of the interdigital skin. Lesions of the interdigital skin are secondarily infected by two gram-negative anaerobic bacteria, *Fusobacterium necrophorum* ssp. *necrophorum* and *Porphyromonas levii*. Both organisms are considered to be normal flora of the bovine gastrointestinal tract and are readily isolated from the rumen and, to a lesser extent, feces of cattle. Experimental inoculation of *F. necrophorum* alone into the skin of cattle is reportedly sufficient to create the typical lesion of foot rot. Other workers suggest that consistent experimental reproduction of the disease requires both *F. necrophorum* and *P. levii*.

Clinical Signs and Diagnosis

Foot rot is characterized by swelling of the foot, the presence of a necrotic lesion in the interdigital skin, and severe lameness. The highest incidence occurs in rear feet, and normally only one foot is affected. Inflammation of the foot is generally symmetrical and frequently extends to the region of the fetlock. Swelling of the foot is usually sufficient to result in separation of the digits. Body temperature is normally elevated (39°-40° C) with feed intake, and performance significantly reduced. Closer inspection of the foot and interdigital skin usually reveals a swollen necrotic lesion of the skin that may extend the length of the interdigital cleft. This necrotic lesion yields exudates with a characteristic foul odor that is one of the diagnostic features of this disease. On occasion, particularly early in the course of the disease, cases are encountered where there is no interdigital lesion. *Blind foot rot* or *blind foul* are terms used to describe this condition.

Lameness varies from moderate to severe depending on the involvement of deeper structures within the foot. One of the more common secondary complications is extension of the infection into the distal interphalangeal joint. This is accompanied by extreme lameness, a preference for lying down, and rapid weight loss. On occasion, the infection may extend into the distal sesamoid bursa, flexor tendon sheath, ligaments, and retro-articular space. Extension of the infection into these deeper tissues lessens the likelihood of a successful medical treatment, and surgical correction should be considered.

Treatment

The administration of parenteral antibiotics early in the course of the disease is necessary for optimal results from therapy. In fact, antibiotic selection is probably less important than treatment duration and time to initiation of therapy. Sulfadimethoxine given by intravenous injection at the rate of 55 mg/kg is effective. Also, procaine penicillin G (22,000 IU/kg body weight) and oxytetracycline (10 mg/kg) by either an intramuscular or subcutaneous route (according to label instructions) are frequently recommended. Ceftiofur at the rate of 1 to 2 mg/kg of body weight at 24-hour intervals for 3 consecutive days offers effective therapy without the threat of antibiotic residue when used according to label directions. A few newer, long-acting products are not only effective but also offer the convenience of single-dose treatment. Noticeable improvement (i.e., reduced swelling and improved gait) should be observed within 3 to 5 days of the onset of treatment.

Local treatment of the lesion should include cleaning and careful débridement of necrotic tissue in the interdigital skin. Because this can be a painful procedure, xylazine or preferably intravenous regional anesthesia is recommended. Once the lesion has been cleaned and all necrotic tissue removed, it may be treated with a topical antimicrobial ointment and secured with a bandage, if desired. Bandages should be applied carefully (not too tight) so that they do not cause additional damage to the interdigital skin as a result of the migration or contraction of bandage material into the interdigital space. When a bandage is used, it should be removed in approximately 3 days or sooner if necessary. When at all possible, affected animals should be housed in a clean and dry area where they can be monitored during the recovery period for signs of improvement or deterioration that may indicate a need for reexamination.

Control

The use of walk-through footbaths are generally recommended for control of foot rot during outbreaks. Footbaths containing 3% to 5% formalin, 5% to 10% copper sulfate, or 10% zinc sulfate are often recommended. In addition, it is advised that cow lanes, walkways, floors, and/or lots be inspected for items that could cause interdigital skin injuries. Areas where mud and standing water accumulate should be fenced off or drained so that debris which may cause interdigital lesions can be found and removed. Some experts recommend isolating or moving infected animals to separate lots or areas to avoid further contamination of the environment of unaffected cows. This may or may not be a practical control measure for most operations because space is often limited.

The efficacy of vaccines for foot rot has not been conclusively established from well-controlled trials and therefore cannot be recommended for control and prevention at this time.

SUPER FOOT ROT

Super foot rot is, as the name implies, a much more severe form of interdigital phlegmon. It is observed most commonly in dairy cattle and characterized by a peracute onset, rapid progression of clinical signs (i.e., severe interdigital lesion and swelling), and a poor response to therapy. Secondary complications associated with

treatment failure include deep digital sepsis often involving the distal interphalangeal joint and retroarticular space and, in the worst-case scenario, death. Successful therapy and control requires heightened surveillance and aggressive treatment at the earliest stages possible in order to affect a desirable outcome from treatment. Organisms involved in this form of foot rot may be more resistant to commonly used antibiotics. Therefore it may be necessary to consider extra-label treatment options.

MUD FEVER

Mud fever is a generalized dermatitis of the lower leg that is often associated with cold, wet, and muddy conditions. Occurrence is sporadic and seems to be associated with the accumulation of muddy debris on the skin of the lower leg. Rear legs seem to be affected more so than front legs. In some cases the dermatitis may extend as high as the hock joint. There is usually significant hair loss, and the skin appears reddened and thickened in response to inflammation. Although mud fever does not cause lameness, it does cause significant skin irritation. The precise cause or etiologic agent is unknown, but *Dermatophilus* sp. may be involved. Teat dip solutions containing emollients as a topical spray are recommended for treatment.

Recommended Readings

Allenstein LC: Wart-like foot lesions caused lameness, *Hoard's Dairyman* 137:696-697, 1992.

Argaez-Rodriguez FJ, Hird FJ, Hernandez de Anda J et al: Papillomatous digital dermatitis on a commercial dairy farm in Mexicali, Mexico: incidence and effect on reproduction and milk production, *Prev Vet Med* 32:275-286, 1997.

Arkins S, Hannan J, Sherington J: Effects of formalin footbathing on foot disease and claw quality in dairy cows, *Vet Rec* 118:580-583, 1986.

Bargai U: Excessive dietary protein as the cause of herd outbreaks of "Mortellaro's disease," *Proc Int Symp Dis Ruminant Digit* 8:183, 1994.

Basset HF, Monaghan ML, Lenham P: Bovine digital dermatitis, *Vet Rec* 126:164-165, 1990.

Berg JN, Franklin CL: *Interdigital phlegmon a.k.a. interdigital necrobacillosis a.k.a. acute foot rot of cattle: considerations in etiology, diagnosis and treatment.* Proceedings of the 11th International Symposium on Disorders of the Ruminant Digit & International Conference on Bovine Lameness, Parma, Italy, 2000, pp 27-30.

Berg JN, Loan RW: Fusobacterium necrophorum and *Bacteroides melaninogenicus* as etiologic agents of foot rot in cattle, *Am J Vet Res* 36:1115-1122, 1975.

Berry SL, Ertze RA, Read DH: *Field evaluation of prophylactic and therapeutic effects of a vaccine against (papillomatous) digital dermatitis of dairy cattle in two California dairies.* Proceedings of the 13th International Symposium on Ruminant Lameness, 2004.

Berry SL, Graham TW, Mongini A: The efficacy of *Serpens* spp. bacterin combined with topical administration of lincomycin hydrochloride for treatment of papillomatous digital dermatitis (footwarts) in cows on a dairy in California, *Bov Pract* 33:6-11, 1999.

Berry SL, Maas J: *Clinical treatment of papillomatous digital dermatitis (footwarts) on dairy cattle.* Proceedings of the Hoof Health Conference, Batavia, NY, 1997.

Berry SL, Maas J, Reed BA, et al: The efficacy of five topical spray treatments for control of papillomatous digital dermatitis in dairy herds, *Proc Am Assoc Bov Pract* 29:188, 1996a (abstract).

Berry SL, Read DH, Walker RL: Recurrence of papillomatous digital dermatitis (foot-warts) in dairy cows after treatment with lincomycin HCI or oxytetracycline HCI, *J Dairy Sci* 82:34, 1999b (abstract).

Berry SL, Read DH, Walker RL: *Topical treatment with oxytetracycline or lincomycin HCl for papillomatous digital dermatitis: gross and histological evaluation.* Proceedings of the 10th International Symposium on Lameness in Ruminants, Lucerne, Switzerland, 1998, pp 291-292.

Blowey RW: *Cattle lameness and hoofcare,* Ipswich Ip1,4LG, United Kingdom, 1993, Farming Press.

Blowey RW: Control of digital dermatitis, *Vet Rec* 146:295, 2000.

Blowey RW: *Interdigital causes of lameness.* Proceedings of the 8th International Symposium on Disorders of Ruminant Lameness & International Conference on Bovine Lameness, Banff, Canada, 1994, pp 142-154.

Blowey RW, Done SH, Cooley W: Observations on the pathogenesis of digital dermatitis in cattle, *Vet Rec* 135:115-117, 1994.

Blowey RW, Sharp MW: Digital dermatitis in dairy cattle, *Vet Rec* 122:505-508, 1988.

Blowey RW, Sharp MW, Done SH: Digital dermatitis, *Vet Rec* 131:39, 1992.

Blowey RW, Weaver AD: *Cattle lameness and hoofcare, an illustrated guide,* Ipswich, United Kingdom, 1998, Farming Press, pp 54-55.

Borgmann IE, Bailey J, Clark EG: Spirochete-associated bovine digital dermatitis, *Can Vet J* 37:35-37, 1996.

Britt JS, Carson MC, von Bredow JD et al: Antibiotic residues in milk samples obtained from cows after treatment for papillomatous digital dermatitis, *J Am Vet Med Assoc* 215:833-836, 1999.

Britt JS, Gaska J, Garrett EF et al: Comparison of topical application of three products for treatment of papillomatous digital dermatitis in dairy cattle, *J Am Vet Med Assoc* 209:1134-1136, 1996.

Britt JS, McClure J: Field trials with antibiotic and nonantibiotic treatments for papillomatous digital dermatitis, *Bov Pract* 32:25-28, 1998.

Brizzi A: Bovine digital dermatitis, *Bov Pract* 27:33-37, 1993.

Cheli R, Mortellaro C: *La dermatite digitale del bovino.* Proceedings of the VIII International Meeting on Diseases of Cattle, Milan, Italy, 1974, pp 208-213.

Choi BK, Nattermann H, Grund S et al: Spirochetes from digital dermatitis lesions in cattle are closely related to treponemes associated with human periodontitis, *Int J Sys Bacteriol* 47:175-181, 1997.

Clark BL, Stewart DJ, Emery DL: The role of *Fusobacterium necrophorum* and *Bacteroides melanogenicus* in the etiology of interdigital necrobacillosis in cattle, *Aus Vet J* 62:47-49, 1985.

Collighan RJ, Woodward MJ: *Spirochaetes* and other bacterial species associated with bovine digital dermatitis, *FEMS Microbiol Lett* 156:37-41, 1997.

Cruz C, Driemeier D, Cerva C et al: Bovine digital dermatitis in southern Brazil, *Vet Rec* 148:576-577, 2001.

David GP: Severe foul-in-the-foot in dairy cattle, *Vet Rec* 132:567-568, 1993.

Demirkan I, Carter SD, Hart A, et al: Isolation and cultivation of a *Spirochaete* from bovine digital dermatitis, Vet Rec 145:497-498, 1999a.

Demirkan I, Carter SD, Murray RD, et al: The frequent detection of a treponeme in bovine digital dermatitis by immunocytochemistry and polymerase chain reaction, *Vet Microbiol* 60:285-292, 1998.

Demirkan I, Murray RD, Carter SD: Skin diseases of the bovine digit associated with lameness, *Vet Bull* 70:149-171, 2000.

Demirkan I, Walker RL, Murray RD et al: Serological evidence of spirochaetal infections associated with digital dermatitis in dairy cattle, *Vet J* 157:69-77, 1999b.

Doherty ML, Bassett HF, Markey B et al: Severe foot lameness in cattle associated with invasive spirochetes, *Irish Vet J* 51:195-198, 1998.

Döpfer D, Koopmans A, Meijer FA et al: Histological and bacteriological evaluation of digital dermatitis in cattle, with special reference to *Spirochaetes* and *Campylobacter faecalis, Vet Rec* 140:620-623, 1997.

Edwards AM, Dymock D, Jenkinson HF: From tooth to hoof: treponemes in tissue-destructive diseases, *J Appl Microbiol* 94:767-780, 2003a.

Edwards AM, Dymock D, Woodward MJ et al: Genetic relatedness and phenotypic characteristics of *Treponema* associated with human periodontal tissues and ruminant foot disease, *Microbiology* 149:1083-1093, 2003b.

Esslemont RJ, Peeler EJ: The scope for raising margins in dairy herds by improving fertility and health, *Br Vet J* 149:537-547, 1993.

Gourreau JM, Scott DW, Rousseau JF: La dermatite digitee des bovins, *Le Point Vet* 24:49-57, 1992.

Gradle CD, Felling J, Dee AO: *Treatment of digital dermatitis lesions in dairy cows with a novel nonantibiotic formulation in a foot bath.* Proceedings of the 12th International Symposium on Lameness in Ruminants, Orlando, Fla, 2002, pp 363-365.

Graham PD: *A survey of digital dermatitis treatment regimens used by veterinarians in England and Wales.* Proceedings of the 8th International Symposium Disorders Ruminant Lameness & International Conference on Bovine Lameness, Banff, Canada, 1994, pp 205-206.

Greenough PR: *Lameness in cattle,* ed 3, Philadelphia, 1997, Saunders.

Guard C: Recognizing and managing infectious causes of lameness in cattle, *Proc Am Assoc Bov Pract* 27:80-82, 1995.

Guterbock W, Borelli C: Footwart treatment trial report, *West Dairyman* 76:17, 1995.

Hartog BJ, Tap SHM, Pouw HJ et al: Systemic bioavailability of erythromycin in cattle when applied by footbath, *Vet Rec* 148:782-783, 2001.

Hernandez J, Shearer JK, Elliott JB: Comparison of topical application of oxytetracycline and four nonantibiotic solutions for treatment of papillomatous digital dermatitis in dairy cows, *J Am Vet Med Assoc* 214:688-690, 1999.

Hernandez J, Shearer JK: Therapeutic trial of oxytetracycline in dairy cows with papillomatous digital dermatitis lesions on the interdigital cleft, heels, or dewclaw, *J Am Vet Med Assoc* 216:1288-1290, 2000.

Hernandez J, Shearer JK, Webb DW: Effect of lameness on milk yield in dairy cows, *J Am Vet Med Assoc* 220:640-644, 2002.

Hultgren J, Bergsten C: Effects of a rubber-slatted flooring system on cleanliness and foot health in tied dairy cows, *Prev Vet Med* 52:75-89, 2001.

Keil DJ, Liem A, Stine DL: *Serological and clinical response of cattle to farm-specific digital dermatitis bacterins.* Proceedings of the 12th International Symposium on Lameness in Ruminants, Orlando, Fla, 2002, p 385.

Kempson SA, Langridge A, Jones JA: *Slurry, formalin, and copper sulphate: the effect on the claw horn.* Proceedings of the 10th International Symposium on Lameness in Ruminants, Lucerne, Switzerland, 1998, pp 216-217.

Kimura Y, Masahiro T, Matsumoto N et al: Verrucose dermatitis and digital papillomatosis in dairy cows, *J Vet Med Jpn* 46:899-906, 1993.

Laven RA: Control of digital dermatitis in cattle, *In Pract* 23:336-341, 2001.

Laven RA: The environment and digital dermatitis, *In Pract* 7:349-356, 1999.

Laven RA, Hunt H: Comparison of valnemulin and lincomycin in the treatment of digital dermatitis by individually applied topical spray, *Vet Rec* 149:302-303, 2001.

Laven RA, Hunt H: Evaluation of copper sulphate, formalin and peracetic acid in footbaths for the treatment of digital dermatitis in cattle, *Vet Rec* 151:144-146, 2002.

Laven RA, Proven MJ: Use of an antibiotic footbath in the treatment of bovine digital dermatitis, *Vet Rec* 147:503-506, 2000.

Lindley WH: Malignant verrucae of bulls, *Vet Med Agric Pract* 69:1547-1550, 1974.

Manske T, Hultgren J, Bergsten C: The effect of claw trimming on the hoof health of Swedish dairy cattle, *Prev Vet Med* 54: 113-129, 2002b.

Manske T, Hultgren J, Bergsten C: Prevalence and interrelationships of hoof lesions and lameness in Swedish dairy cows, *Prev Vet Med* 54:247-263, 2002a.

Manske T, Hultgren J, Bergsten C: Topical treatment of digital dermatitis associated with severe heel-horn erosion in a Swedish dairy herd, *Prev Vet Med* 53:215-231, 2002c.

Moeller MR, Waters WR, Goff JP et al: Papillomatous digital dermatitis (PDD): Immune responses of Iowa dairy cattle with PDD to California-isolated PDD spirochetes, *Proc 80th Conf Res Workers Anim Dis* 80:5P, 1999 (abstract).

Moore DA, Berry SL, Truscott ML: Efficacy of a nonantimicrobial cream administered topically for treatment of digital dermatitis in dairy cattle, *J Am Vet Med Assoc* 219:1435-1438, 2001.

Mortellaro CM: *Digital dermatitis*. Proceedings of the 8th International Symposium on Disorders of Ruminant Lameness & International Conference on Bovine Lameness, Banff, Canada, 1994, pp 137-141.

Moter A, Leist G, Rudolph R et al: Fluorescence in situ hybridization shows spatial distribution of as yet uncultured treponemes in biopsies from digital dermatitis lesions, *Microbiology* 144:2459-2467, 1998.

Murray RD, Downham DY, Demirkan I et al: Some relationships between spirochaete infections and digital dermatitis in four UK dairy herds, *Res Vet Sci* 73:223-230, 2002.

Nowrouzian I: Risk factors in the development of digital dermatitis in dairies in Tehran, Iran, *Proc Int Symp Dis Ruminant Digit* 8:155, 1994.

Oliver KH: *The efficacy of a vaccine developed for papillomatous digital dermatitis (footwarts) in dairy cattle*, MS Animal Science California Polytechnic University, Pomona, 1999.

Radostitts OM: *Veterinary medicine*, ed 8, London, United Kingdom, 1994, Baillere Tendall.

Read DH: *Pathogenesis of experimental papillomatous digital dermatitis (PDD) in cattle: bacterial morphotypes associated with early lesion development*. Proc Seventy-Eighth Conf Res Workers Anim Dis, Chicago, No. 32, 1997 (abstract).

Read DH, Berry SL, Hird DW et al: *Papillomatous digital dermatitis (footwarts) of cattle: research review and update*. Proceedings of the 1999 Hoof Health Conference, Modesto, Calif, 1999, pp 45-46.

Read DH, Walker RL, Castro AE et al: An invasive spirochete associated with interdigital papillomatosis of dairy cattle, *Vet Rec* 130:59-60, 1992.

Read DH, Walker RL: *Comparison of papillomatous digital dermatitis and digital dermatitis of cattle by histopathology and immunohistochemistry*. Proceedings of the 10th International Symposium on Lameness in Ruminants, Lucerne, Switzerland, 1998a, pp 268-269.

Read DH, Walker RL: Experimental transmission of papillomatous digital dermatitis (footwarts) in cattle, *Vet Pathol* 33:607, 1996 (abstract).

Read DH, Walker RL, Hird DW et al: *Footwarts of cattle—papillomatous digital dermatitis*, UC Davis, Calif Vet Diag Lab (pamphlet), 1995a.

Read DH, Walker RL: *Papillomatous digital dermatitis and associated lesions of dairy cattle in California: pathologic findings*. Proceedings of the 8th International Symposium on Disorders of Ruminant Lameness & International Conference on Bovine Lameness, Banff, Canada, 1994a, pp 156-158.

Read DH, Walker RL: *Papillomatous digital dermatitis of dairy cattle in California: clinical characteristics*. Proceedings of the 8th

International Symposium on Disorders of Ruminant Lameness & International Conference on Bovine Lameness, Banff, Canada, 1:59-163, 1994b.

Read DH, Walker RL: Papillomatous digital dermatitis (footwarts) in California dairy cattle: clinical and gross pathologic findings, *J Vet Diagn Invest* 10:67-76, 1998b.

Read DH, Walker RL: *Research update: etiology of papillomatous digital dermatitis (footwarts) in dairy cattle*, Wild West Veterinary Conference Veterinary Syllabus, Reno, Nev, 1997, pp 105-109.

Read DH, Walker RL, Van Ranst M et al: *Studies on the etiology of papillomatous digital dermatitis (footwarts) of dairy cattle*. Proceedings of the 38th Annual Meeting of the American Association of Veterinary Laboratory Diagnostics, Sparks, Nev, 68, 1995b (abstract).

Rebhun WC, Payne RM, King JM et al: Interdigital papillomatosis in dairy cattle, *J Am Vet Med Assoc* 137:437-440, 1980.

Reed B, Berry SL, Maas JP et al: Comparison of five topical spray treatments for control of digital dermatitis in dairy herds, *J Dairy Sci* 79:189, 1996.

Rodriguez-Lainz A, Hird DW, Carpenter TE et al: Case-control study of papillomatous digital dermatitis in Southern California dairy farms, *Prev Vet Med* 28:117-131, 1996a.

Rodriguez-Lainz A, Hird DW, Walker RL, et al: Papillomatous digital dermatitis in 458 dairies, *J Am Vet Med Assoc* 209:1464-1467, 1996b.

Rodriguez-Lainz A, Melendez-Retamal P, Hird DW et al: Papillomatous digital dermatitis in Chilean dairies and evaluation of a screening method, *Prev Vet Med* 37:197-207, 1998.

Rodriguez-Lainz A, Melendez-Retamal P, Hird DW et al: Farm- and host-level risk factors for papillomatous digital dermatitis in Chilean dairy cattle, *Prev Vet Med* 42:87-97, 1999.

Scavia G, Sironi G, Mortellaro CM et al: *Digital dermatitis: further contribution on clinical and pathological aspects in some herds in northern Italy*. Proceedings of the 8th International Conference on Bovine Lameness, Banff, Canada, 1994, pp 174-176.

Schrank K, Choi BK, Grund S et al: "*Treponema brennaborense*" sp. nov., a novel spirochete isolated from a dairy cow suffering from digital dermatitis, *Int J Sys Bacteriol* 49:43-50, 1998.

Schütz W, Metzner M, Pijl R et al: *Evaluation of the efficacy of herd-specific vaccines for the control of digital dermatitis (DD) in dairy cows*. Proceedings of the 11th International Symposium on Disorders of the Ruminant Digit & 3rd International Conference on Bovine Lameness, Parma, Italy, 2000, pp 183-185.

Seymour J, Durkin J, Bathina H et al: *Footbathing in the management of digital dermatitis*. Proceedings of the 12th International Symposium on Lameness in Ruminants, Orlando, Fla, 374-376, 2002.

Seymour J, Durkin J, Bathina H et al: Footbathing in the management of papillomatous digital dermatitis, *Proc Am Assoc Bov Pract* 34:200, 2001.

Shearer JK, Elliott JB: Papillomatous digital dermatitis: treatment and control strategies—part I, *Compend Cont Educ Pract Vet* 20:S158-S173, 1998.

Shearer JK, Elliott JB: *Preliminary results from a spray application of oxytetracycline to treat control, and prevent digital dermatitis in dairy herds*. Proceedings of the 8th International Symposium on Disorders of Ruminant Lameness & International Conference on Bovine Lameness, Banff, Canada, 1994, p 182.

Shearer JK, Hernandez J: Efficacy of two modified nonantibiotic formulations (Victory) for treatment of papillomatous digital dermatitis in dairy cows, *J Dairy Sci* 83:741-745, 2000.

Shearer JK, Hernandez J, Elliott JB: Papillomatous digital dermatitis: treatment and control strategies—part II, *Compend Cont Educ Pract Vet* 20:S213-S223, 1998.

Somers JGC, Frankena JK, Noordhuizen-Stassen EN et al: Prevalence of claw disorders in Dutch dairy cows exposed to several floor systems, *J Dairy Sci* 86:2082-2093, 2003.

Thomas ED: Foot bath solutions may cause crop problems, *Hoard's Dairyman* 458-459, 2001.

Toussaint Raven E: Cattle footcare and claw trimming, Ipswich, United Kingdom, 1989, Farming Press.

Trott DJ, Moeller MR, Zuerner RL et al: Characterization of *Treponema phagedenis*-like spirochetes isolated from papillomatous digital dermatitis lesions in dairy cattle, *J Clin Microbiol* 41:2522-2529, 2003.

van Amstel SR, Bemis D: *Aspects of the microbiology of interdigital dermatitis in dairy cows*. 10th International Symposium on Lameness in Ruminants, Lucerne, Switzerland, 1998, pp 274-275.

van Amstel SR, van Vuuren S, Tutt CL: Digital dermatitis: report of an outbreak, *J S Afr Vet Assoc* 66:177-181, 1995.

Vokey FJ, Guard CL, Erb HN et al: Effects of alley and stall surfaces on indices of claw and leg health in dairy cattle housed in a free-stall barn, *J Dairy Sci* 84:2686-2699, 2001.

Walker RL, Berry SL, Rodriguez-Lainz A et al: *Prospective study on foot conformation characteristics predisposing to the development of papillomatous digital dermatitis*. Proceedings of the 12th International Symposium on Lameness in Ruminants, Orlando, Fla, 2002, p 370.

Walker RL, Read DH, Hird DW et al: *Vaccine against papillomatous digital dermatitis (PDD)*. The Regents of the University of California. 08/943,571[6,287,575 B1], 1-42. 2001. Oakland, Calif, q.v. patent. 10-3-1997. Patent.

Walker RL, Read DH, Loretz KJ et al: Humoral response of dairy-cattle to spirochetes isolated from papillomatous digital dermatitis lesions, *Am J Vet Res* 58:744-748, 1997.

Walker RL, Read DH, Loretz KJ et al: *Spirochetes associated with papillomatous digital dermatitis and interdigital dermatitis in dairy cattle*. Proceedings of the 37th Annual Meeting of the American Association of Veterinary Laboratory Diagnostics, Grand Rapids, Mich, 1994.

Walker RL, Read DH, Loretz KJ et al: Spirochetes isolated from dairy cattle with papillomatous digital dermatitis and interdigital dermatitis, *Vet Microbiol* 47:343-355, 1995.

Walker RL, Read DH, Sawyer SJ et al: Phylogenetic analysis of spirochetes isolated from papillomatous digital dermatitis lesions in cattle, *Proc Ann Mtg Conf Res Workers Anim Dis* 79:17, 1998 (abstract).

Wells SJ, Garber LP, Wagner BA et al: *Papillomatous digital dermatitis on U.S. dairy operations (footwarts)*, National Animal Health Monitoring System (NAHMS), 1-28, 1997.

Wells SJ, Garber LP, Wagner BA: Papillomatous digital dermatitis and associated risk factors in US dairy herds, *Prev Vet Med* 38:11-24, 1999.

Zemljic B: *Current investigations into the cause of dermatitis digitalis in cattle*. Proceedings of the 8th International Symposium on Disorders of Ruminant Lameness & International Conference on Bovine Lameness, Banff, Canada, 1994, pp 164-167.

Zemljic B: *Pathophysiological features and possible infective reasons for papillomatous digital dermatitis on dairy farms in Slovenia*. Proceedings of the 11th International Symposium on Disorders of the Ruminant Digit & 3rd International Conference on Bovine Lameness, Parma, Italy, 2000, pp 186-189.

CHAPTER 53

Surgery of the Bovine Digit

KARL NUSS

SURGICAL MANAGEMENT OF DEEP INFECTION OF THE CLAW

Lameness has an immense impact on the welfare, production performance, and fertility of dairy cows.[1,2] Severe lameness caused by digital disease results in the most significant losses. The prevalence of lameness ranges from 20% to 30% in one lactation period but can exceed 70% in some dairy operations.[3,4] Diseases of the foot account for 80% to 90% of all cases of lameness in cattle. Deep infections develop when the barriers provided by the corium and subcutis are compromised, and tendons, synovial structures, or bones become involved. These so-called complicated claw diseases can result from several different claw conditions such as sole ulcers, white line diseases,

and toe infections. Complicated claw diseases constitute an estimated 0.5% to 2% of all claw diseases, but in referral centers they may comprise 3% to 10% of cases. Clinical signs include severe lameness, swelling of the coronet, and a fistulous tract. The diagnosis is based on clinical signs but can be characterized further by nerve blocks, synoviocentesis, and medical imaging techniques such as radiography or ultrasonography. These ancillary tests aid in the selection of the best surgical approach. For surgery, intravenous regional anesthesia of the affected limb distal to a tourniquet or a palmar/plantar and dorsal digital nerve block in the proximal metacarpus/metatarsus is carried out. Treatment options for deep infections include digital salvage techniques (resections) and removal of the affected digit (amputation).

Digital Salvage Techniques

Resection of the Insertion of the Deep Digital Flexor Tendon, Removal of the Distal Sesamoid Bone, and Resection of the Distal Interphalangeal Joint

Infection in the retro-articular area, which in many cases originates from a sole ulcer or white line disease, can be approached from the heel and pastern region.[5-7] The surgery is performed under sedation and intravenous regional anesthesia. Cattle are restrained in a trimming chute or in lateral recumbency. After anesthesia, the sole and bulb horn is pared away until it can be indented easily and incision with a scalpel is possible. The distal limb is prepared aseptically. The procedure starts with a vertical incision extending from the dewclaw to the area in the posterior part of the sole where ulcers typically occur. The incision is extended around the sole or wall lesion, and the fistulous tract is located and removed. Then a self-retaining retractor is inserted in the vertical incision, and the tendon sheath is opened along the length of the incision (Fig 53-1) with a sterile scalpel. This allows aseptic removal of the distal part of the deep digital flexor tendon and, at the same time, minimizes the risk of ascending infection. Subsequent removal of the infected insertion of the deep digital flexor tendon, the infected podotrochlear bursa, and the osteolytic distal sesamoid bone can be carried out with a good view of the surgical field. Alternative approaches via an incision restricted to the sole and not extending proximally to the bulb,[8] or via a horizontal incision in the bulb area,[9] have the disadvantage of poorer visibility of the surgical field and therefore can make resection more difficult. These latter approaches also involve a greater risk of unintentional contamination of more proximal tissues such as the digital flexor tendon sheath.

The distal sesamoid bone is usually removed with a scalpel and a sharp periosteal elevator, but it can also be split into two parts with a chisel or pared out with a rongeur. If the synovia of the distal interphalangeal joint shows signs of infection or the joint cartilage is damaged, resection of the pedal joint is carried out. First, the tuberculum flexorum is curetted thoroughly or, preferably, removed with a drill to eliminate the site of the bone infection and to ensure good ventral drainage of the wound. Thereafter, a channel of approximately 1.5 cm is drilled through the distal interphalangeal joint, exiting at the dorsal wall of the claw, to remove infected cartilage and ensure bony fusion of the pedal joint. Thorough rinsing during drilling is necessary to prevent thermal damage to the bones. If the origin of infection is located in the interdigital space, the same plantar approach can be used, but the port of entry of the infection in the interdigital space is also drilled out (Fig 53-2). The wound is not sutured but packed with dilute iodine-soaked gauze and bandaged. Topical antibiotics or local intravenous antibiotics may be used alternatively. A wooden block is glued to the sole of the contralateral claw, and the toe of the operated claw is fixed to the toe of the other claw with a steel wire, a metal clip, or a similar device.

The surgical technique described earlier can also be used to preserve the claw after an open fracture of the distal phalanx, which is usually characterized by an axial

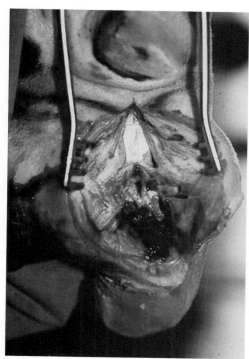

Fig 53-1 Longitudinal approach to the deep digital flexor tendon, sesamoid bone, and distal interphalangeal joint from the palmar/plantar pastern area. An elliptical incision is made around the ulcer to excise it, and the tendon sheath is incised with a sterile scalpel. Retractors allow good visualization of the deep digital flexor tendon and its infected insertion site on the tuberculum flexorum of the pedal bone.

fragment and joint communication (Fig 53-3). In such cases the smaller axial fragment is extracted, and the joint surfaces of the middle phalanx and the remaining distal phalanx are removed with a drill.[10]

The bandage is changed regularly after surgery. On day 3, the foot is prepared aseptically and the gauze is removed and not replaced. Flushing off the area is not necessary and may even interfere with wound healing and granulation. The bandage is changed every 3 to 5 days. Weight bearing improves 10 to 12 days after joint resection, and 2 to 3 weeks later, patients are sound at a walk provided there are no complications. Complications involve persistence of infection after incomplete removal of infected tissue or bone necrosis caused by drilling. By 8 to 10 weeks postoperatively, the wound is covered with new horn and the block is removed from the contralateral claw. Based on radiographic follow-up studies, complete bony fusion of the joint occurs by 7 to 12 months.[11] The procedure is ideal for young valuable animals but can also be used successfully in heavier and older cows and breeding bulls.[12,13] Ankylosis of the joint after drilling provides better long-term stabilization than removal of the sesamoid bone without drilling. Based on the findings of various studies, it appears that joint resection produces better long-term results than amputation. Cows remained in the herd for an average of 18 to 22 months after joint resection[11,14] and on average 15 to 17 months after

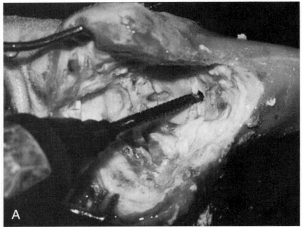

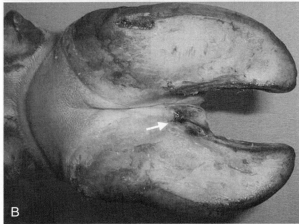

Fig 53-2 **A** and **B,** Plantar approach for drilling of the distal interphalangeal joint. The deep digital flexor tendon and sesamoid bone have been removed, and the drill is directed toward the distal interphalangeal joint. When the port of entry of infection is in the interdigital cleft (*arrow*) or in another location, the direction of drilling is adjusted accordingly.

amputation.[15] However, other studies showed no difference in the long-term outcome of the two procedures and cows remained in the herd for an average of 20 months postoperatively after digit amputation.[16]

A number of alternative techniques for digital salvage are available. When the infection does not originate from a sole ulcer, one can use a dorsal or abaxial approach for curettage or drilling of the joint.[17] However, compared with the previously described procedure, visualization of the site of infection is not as good and resection is usually less complete when a dorsal or abaxial approach is used. Postoperative treatment is labor intensive, prolonged, and costly and includes installation of drains and lavage. Residual lameness may be apparent for up to 4 months after surgery. Abaxial fenestration is another method in which excision of the claw wall provides a good view of the abaxial side of the joint.[18] Disadvantages include lack of postoperative drainage and risk of damage to the distal sesamoid bone. If the osteolytic area is small, it can be curetted and packed with cancellous bone to promote healing.[19]

Resection of the Apex of the Distal Phalanx

Damage to the tip of the claw is most commonly caused by overtrimming or excessive wear on abrasive surfaces. Occasionally, it is caused by an injury to the claw with an open fracture of the tip of the pedal bone or it can be a sequel of diffuse aseptic pododermatitis (laminitis). Infection can spread rapidly into the distal phalanx because there is no subcutis at the tip of the pedal bone to protect the cancellous bone surface.[20-22] Early treatment is critical, especially when more than one claw is affected, to prevent the animal from becoming recumbent because of pedal osteitis. For resection of an infected pedal bone tip, the phalanx is accessed from the apex of the sole. Osteolytic bone is then drilled away, parallel to the dorsal wall of the claw, until only healthy bone is visible (Fig 53-4). Flushing with sterile Ringer's solution helps remove debris and prevent thermal bone damage. Alternatively, the tip of the distal phalanx can be removed with a wire saw or nippers. After application of topical antibiotics and bandaging, a wooden block is applied to the sole of the contralateral claw. During the postsurgical period, bandage changes are necessary every 3 to 5 days. By 8 weeks the defect is usually covered with newly formed horn.[21]

If more than the distal third of the pedal bone is affected, it is likely that the marrow cavity of the pedal bone is involved and that the entire bone will become infected; in these cases, digit amputation should be considered. In addition, amputation should be considered after the removal of more than one third of the pedal bone because the claw horn tends to grow in a corkscrew fashion and lameness is a possible sequel.[21] The long-term outcome for resection of the tip of the pedal bone is good if only one claw is affected. Often, several claws are affected and when treatment is not instituted within the first few hours of trauma, the animal becomes recumbent because of the pain resulting from pedal osteitis, which makes therapy difficult.

Resection of the Superficial and Deep Digital Flexor Tendons within the Common Digital Sheath

The digital flexor tendon sheath may require treatment if ascending infection from a sole ulcer or puncture wound occurs.[23] Although needle lavage of the infected sheath is an option, it is only successful early in the course of the disease. Tenosynoviotomy with placement of an indwelling multifenestrated silicone rubber drain has been used successfully for the repeated lavage of the flexor tendon sheaths.[24,25] However, in more advanced cases the pouches of the tendon sheath may harbor pockets of fibrin and purulent debris. Therefore removal of debris by opening the tendon sheath is indicated.[26] In cattle with purulent tenosynovitis, there may be tendon abscesses, which can be removed only by resection of both flexor tendons.[27] For this operation the skin of the affected digit is incised in a vertical direction starting 5 cm proximal to the dewclaw.[28] The incision axially curves closely around the dewclaw to prevent damaging blood vessels and nerves. Distal to the dewclaw the incision extends into the coronet of the affected digit. After careful preparation of the subcutis, the dewclaw is reflected abaxially to allow a straight incision of the underlying fascia, annular ligament, and tendon sheath (Fig 53-5). The tendons

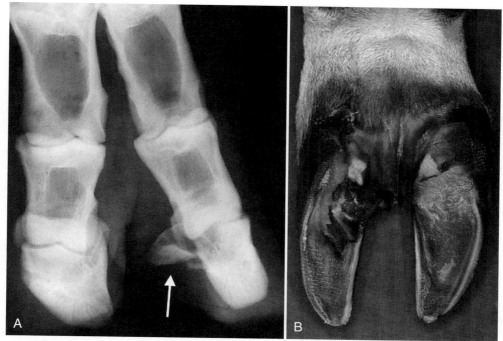

Fig 53-3   **A,** Plantarodorsal radiograph of the digit of the left hind limb in a young heifer showing a fracture of the pedal bone of the lateral claw after injury on a slatted floor. Mild abaxial dislocation of the lateral claw occurs. An axial fragment *(arrow),* which is attached to the second phalanx by the collateral ligament, is seen in the interdigital cleft. **B,** Left hind digit of a calf 5 weeks after open fracture of the pedal bone of the lateral claw and resection of the distal interphalangeal joint. Wound in granulation.

are subsequently removed along with the entire length of the sheath, and care is taken not to incise the sheath of the contralateral tendons. The incision can be left open to heal by second intention or partially sutured to prevent formation of proud flesh. In both instances a bandage is applied to the operated digit, and a block is glued to the sole of the contralateral claw. As with resection of the insertion site of the deep digital flexor tendon and the distal interphalangeal joint, the tip of the operated claw is fixed to the tip of the contralateral claw to prevent overextension.

With concurrent infection of the fetlock joint, the plantar pouch of the fetlock joint can be accessed via an incision, 3 cm long and 0.5 cm wide, between the two branches of the suspensory ligament (Fig 53-6). This allows easy access to the plantar joint pouch, removal of fibrin clots, and effective joint lavage.[29]

Resection of the Proximal Interphalangeal Joint and the Fetlock Joint

Infection of the proximal interphalangeal joint may result from an injury and primary infection or from cellulitis or hematogenous spread. If the primary cause is interdigital cellulitis, other synovial structures such as extensor/flexor tendon sheaths may be affected and treatment may not be indicated. The affected joint is drilled out via a dorsal approach or a dorsal approach combined with a second approach from the axial side. Reports about the success rate and prognosis are sparse.[13]

Postoperative treatment is similar to that for resection of the distal interphalangeal joint. If resection is not economically feasible or not possible for medical reasons, digit amputation is the only viable alternative.[25,30]

In acute cases, septic arthritis of the fetlock joint can be treated with joint lavage. Because the lateral and medial pouches communicate,[31] the joint can be successfully lavaged from the dorsomedial to the dorsolateral pouch.[32] When fibrin is seen on ultrasonograms, arthrotomy and lavage are indicated. Longitudinal incisions into the dorsal and plantar pouches (Fig 53-7) allow access to the joint cavity and removal of fibrin. Resection of the fetlock joint and arthrodesis are indicated if there are radiographic changes in the subchondral bone as a result of infectious arthritis. Because the lateral and medial compartments of the fetlock joint communicate, it can be assumed that both are infected. However, a fibrin clot can partially occlude the communication site and one compartment may be less severely affected. The joint is opened dorsally by making a semicircular incision at the level of the articular surface of the proximal phalanx. The incision is extended to the collateral ligaments, and separate incisions are made into the palmar/plantar pouches (see Fig 53-7). In advanced cases the collateral ligaments are transected to gain complete access to the palmar/plantar joint cavities and the proximal sesamoid bones (Fig 53-8). The joint is maximally flexed, and all of the articular cartilage and infected subchondral bone are removed.[33,34] The skin is closed, and a full limb cast or a transfixation pin cast is applied.

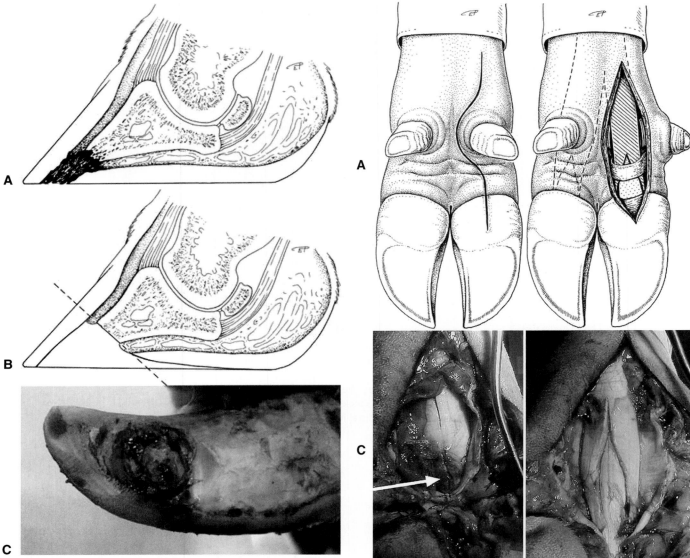

Fig 53-4 **A** and **B,** Schematic representation of infection and resection of the tip of P3. Resection of the infected P3 can be achieved with a wire saw or a drill. A milling drill is used to remove thin layers of bone until healthy, well-perfused **(C)** bone with a normal white color is seen. (From Fiedler A, Maierl J, Nuss K: *Erkrankungen der klauen und zehen des rindes,* Stuttgart, 2004, Schattauer [jeweilige Seitenzahl], with permission.)

Fig 53-5   Incision of the common tendon sheath. The skin incision curves axially to, and closely around, the dewclaws **(A)** to avoid damaging the nerves and blood vessels. After careful dissection, the dewclaw is reflected abaxially to allow a straight incision of the tendon sheath **(B).** Tendovaginotomy to repair an injury to the superficial and deep digital flexor tendons after a puncture with a pitchfork *(arrow).* The tendon sheath has been opened, and the puncture wound in the superficial digital flexor tendon is visible **(C).** The damaged sections of the tendons have been removed. The photo was taken before final wound lavage. (Schematic from Fiedler A, Maierl J, Nuss K: *Erkrankungen der klauen und zehen des rindes,* Stuttgart, 2004, Schattauer [jeweilige Seitenzahl] with permission.)

Resection of Infected Epiphyseal Plates of the Phalanges or the Metacarpal/Metatarsal Bones

In fattening bulls, but also in heifers, the epiphyseal plates of the metacarpus/metatarsus and, rarely, those of the phalanges may become infected hematogenously.[35,36] Medical treatment consists of parenteral antibiotics and NSAIDs. A tourniquet is applied to the affected limb, and antibiotics such as cephalosporins or penicillin are administered intravenously. A bandage or splint is then applied to the leg. If medical treatment fails, surgical excision involving curettage of the affected parts of the physis can be attempted. Half-limb casts are indicated to stabilize the physis. In advanced cases it may be necessary to drill out the entire epiphyseal growth plate.[37] After radical surgery, a transfixation pin cast must be applied for limb stabilization (see Fig 53-8, *B* and *C*).

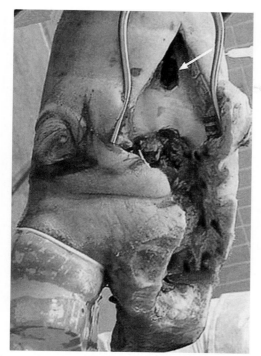

Fig 53-6 Plantar approach to the infected fetlock joint with concurrent infection of the common digital flexor tendon sheath. Both flexor tendons have been removed. An incision *(arrow)* has been made in the medial branch of the suspensory ligament to remove fibrin from the fetlock joint in a plantar direction. Healing was complete in this case. (Courtesy Johann Kofler, University of Vienna, Austria.)

Digital Fractures and Luxations

Fracture of the pedal bone is the most common digital fracture in cattle,[38] occurring preferably at the medial claws of a front limb in pasture animals. Pedal fractures may be open (see Fig 53-3) or closed. Fractured lateral claws of cattle housed on slatted floors are more susceptible to be opened. Closed fractures are best treated with a wooden block glued to the contralateral claw for 8 to 10 weeks. This is usually sufficient for clinical healing, whereas radiographic resolution of the fracture takes 6 to 8 months (Fig 53-9). Open fractures of the pedal bone can be treated conservatively in rare instances but often require pedal joint resection or amputation of the digit because of treatment delay. Fractures of the first and the second phalanx are rare. In cattle they are usually treated conservatively. A wooden block is glued to the contralateral claw and/or a half limb cast is applied to the foot for 6 weeks. During this time the patient must be carefully monitored for cast sores and overloading of the healthy claw. In rare cases fractures of the first phalanx are amenable to repair by internal fixation.

Subluxation and luxation of the digits, especially of the first phalanx, have been reduced successfully, and torn collateral ligaments replaced with a synthetic prosthesis.[39] With extensive soft tissue trauma in a valuable animal, resection of the fetlock joint and application of a transfixation pin cast is an option (see Fig 53-8). A cast is required for several weeks after surgery.

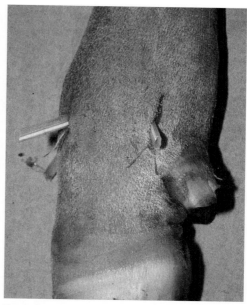

Fig 53-7 Arthrotomy of the fetlock joint via dorsal and lateral longitudinal incisions. The joint has been opened at four locations, which allows the complete removal of fibrin. Drains were inserted into this joint, and the foot was immobilized with a splint.

Amputation Techniques

Digit Amputation

Lameness usually resolves more quickly after amputation than after resection techniques. Digit amputation is the treatment of choice when infection does not permit salvage of the claw or in animals destined for slaughter. Many techniques of amputation have been described in the literature.[30] The advantage of digit amputation is that all infected tissue is removed completely. Recovery after surgery is usually rapid, and pain and lameness subside within a week.[40] For amputation of a digit, "high" amputation at the level of the proximal interphalangeal joint is the most common technique. With high amputation, complete removal of infected tissue can be achieved in most cases, even when the second phalanx or second interphalangeal joint and the first phalanx are affected. In addition, resolution of pain appears to be more rapid compared with low amputation because the wound is located further from the ground, which also helps prevent ascending infection. On the other hand, low amputation may provide some more lateral stability to the digits provided the distal interdigital or cruciate ligament can be preserved. In a study comparing high and low amputation,[41] the former technique was found to be superior. A commonly used high amputation technique involves the creation of a lateral and a medial skin flap by incising the dorsal and palmar/plantar skin from the coronet to the level of the dewclaws.[42] The lateral flap is lifted, and the digital structures are exposed. The distal part of the proximal phalanx is then transected with wire or an amputation saw (Fig 53-10). The distal part of the first phalanx, the second phalanx, and the claw are then removed by careful preparation. By doing this,

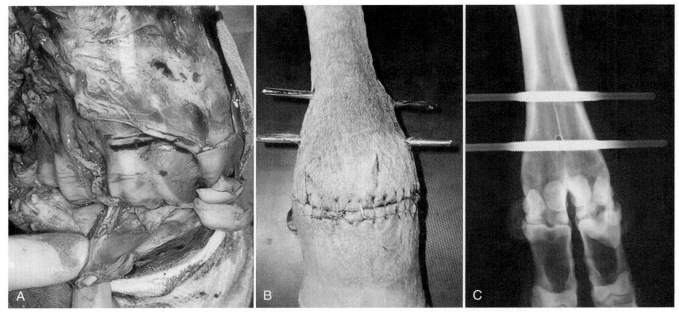

Fig 53-8   **A,** Resection of the fetlock joint in a calf. Semicircular incision and separation of the extensor tendons, nerves, blood vessels, and collateral ligaments to allow complete exposure of the fetlock joint. **B,** Walking cast for immobilization of the fetlock joint after resection of the articular surface and infected bone in a 6-year-old Holstein cow; the picture was taken when the cast was changed 12 days postoperatively. **C,** Dorsoplantar radiograph of this foot. (*A,* Courtesy Ann Martens, University of Ghent, Belgium.)

infected parts of the digit and flexor and extensor tendons are removed. Major vessels are ligated. If no abscess is present in the coronary area and no contamination has occurred during surgery, the wound can be closed with single interrupted sutures to achieve first intention healing. Otherwise, the wound is only partially sutured and the remaining cavity packed with gauze. Regular bandage changes are necessary until granulation tissue covers the wound and reepithelialization has occurred, which usually takes 4 to 6 weeks.[43]

Alternatively, an amputation can be carried out at the level of the proximal interphalangeal joint. The second phalanx is then removed with a strong double-edged knife via a distal approach,[40] after removing the claw with a wire saw at the level of the coronary band. Alternatively, the middle phalanx can be drilled out entirely with a large drill bit via a distal approach.[6] Another method is amputation at the level of the proximal interphalangeal joint by making a circular skin incision 2 cm proximal to the coronet and transecting the tendons and ligaments, which conveniently requires only a few instruments.[25] Exarticulation is followed by removal of the articular cartilage of the distal end of the proximal phalanx. Another practical method of amputation involves introducing a wire saw in the interdigital space and obliquely removing the digit in the area of the distal interphalangeal joint and part of the proximal phalanx. With this technique, complete removal of the second phalanx must be ensured.

The level of aftercare depends on the technique used but may also be dictated by financial restraints.

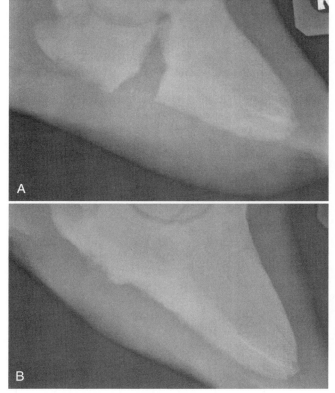

Fig 53-9   Closed fracture of P3 **(A)** of the medial claw of the right front limb in a 5-year-old Simmental cow. Complete bony healing 6 months after the fracture **(B).**

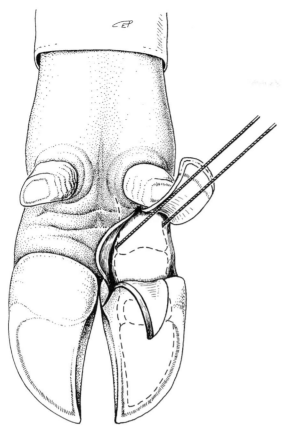

Fig 53-10   Amputation of the claw at the level of the first phalanx. The skin is incised at the dorsal and palmar/plantar aspects to create two flaps. After transection of P1 in an oblique plane, the skin is partially or completely closed. (Schematic from Fiedler A, Maierl J, Nuss K: *Erkrankungen der klauen und zehen des rindes,* Stuttgart, 2004, Schattauer [jeweilige Seitenzahl] with permission.)

Surgery of Interdigital Hyperplasia

Interdigital hyperplasia occurs in the median of the interdigital space and probably has a hereditary component. It can also result from chronic trauma to the interdigital space, for instance with slippery floors or inadequate claw trimming. In the hind limbs, corns are often more closely associated with the lateral claw, which suggests overloading of that claw and concussion of the soft tissue of the axial wall as possible causes.[44] Smaller lesions usually do not cause lameness. Interdigital fibromas that are large and infected or necrotic should be removed surgically. Local interdigital anesthesia at the level of the diaphysis of the first phalanx is achieved by injecting 20 ml of lidocaine, and the claws are spread apart by an assistant. All infected and undermined tissue is removed using a scalpel or, if available, a thermocautery sling, which helps control hemorrhage (Fig 53-11). When the infection has spread distally along the axial walls of the claws, the loose and undermined horn must be removed. The collateral and interdigital ligaments, as well as the capsule of the distal interphalangeal joint, should be spared. Abscesses

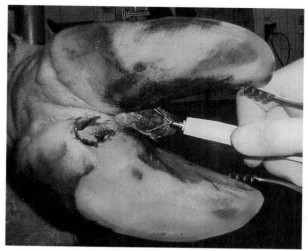

Fig 53-11   Removal of an interdigital fibroma using a thermocautery sling.

in the interdigital area should be drained. Systemic antibiotics and pain medication are often necessary. Confining the patient to a clean pen and bandaging for the first 10 to 12 days after surgery help improve the outcome. If applied properly, the bandage prevents the claws from spreading. Alternatively, the toes can be held together with wire. The prognosis is usually good. For healing of a surgically treated hyperplasia and prevention of reoccurrence, functional claw trimming that keeps the heels as high as possible and the sole surface perpendicular to the limb axis is essential.

References

1. Sogstad AM, Osteras O, Fjeldaas T: Bovine claw and limb disorders related to reproductive performance and production diseases, *J Dairy Sci* 89:2519-2528, 2006.
2. Whay HR, Waterman AE, Webster AJ: Associations between locomotion, claw lesions and nociceptive threshold in dairy heifers during the peri-partum period, *Vet J* 154:155-161, 1997.
3. Cook NB, Bennett TB, Nordlund KV: Effect of free stall surface on daily activity patterns in dairy cows with relevance to lameness prevalence, *J Dairy Sci* 87:2912-2922, 2004.
4. Smits M, Frankena K, Metz J et al: Prevalence of digital disorders in zero-grazing cows, *Livestock Prod Sci* 32:231-244, 1992.
5. Assmus G: Erfahrungen mit der resektion des klauensesambeines beim rind, *Nordisk Veterinaermedicin* 16:326-334, 1964.
6. Clemente CH: [Surgery on the hoof in cattle], *Tieraerztliche Praxis* 7:153-206, 1979.
7. Kostlin RG, Nuss K: [Treatment of purulent hoof joint inflammation in cattle by joint resection—results], *Tierarztl Prax* 16:123-131, 1988.
8. Kersjes AW, Németh F, Rutgers L et al: *A colour atlas of large animal surgery,* St Louis, 1985, Mosby, pp 96-97.
9. Greenough PR, Ferguson JG: Alternatives to amputation, *Vet Clin North Am Food Anim Pract* 1:195-203, 1985.
10. Köstlin R, Petzoldt F: [Pedal bone fractures in cattle], *Tierärztl Umsch* 40:864-874, 1985.

11. Nuss K, Weaver MP: Resection of the distal interphalangeal joint in cattle: an alternative to amputation, *Vet Rec* 128:540-543, 1991.

12. Bicalho R, Cheong S, Warnick L et al: The effect of digit amputation or arthrodesis surgery on culling and milk production in Holstein dairy cows, *J Dairy Sci* 89:2596-2602, 2006.

13. Kofler J, Feist M, Starke A et al: Digital amputation and resection of the distal interphalangeal joint in heavy breeding bulls—outcome and long-term follow-up, *Slov J Vet Res* 43:210-213, 2006.

14. Grisiger M, Martig J: [Follow-up studies of resections of claws in cattle], *Dtsch Tierärztl Wochenschr* 103:454-457, 1996.

15. Ziffer A: Untersuchungen über verbleib und milchleistung von rindern nach klauenamputation. Inaugural-dissertation. Hannover, 1980, Tierärztliche Hochschule.

16. Pejsa TG, St Jean G, Hoffsis GF et al: Digit amputation in cattle: 85 cases (1971-1990), *J Am Vet Med Assoc* 202:981-984, 1993.

17. Desrochers A, St-Jean G, Anderson DE: Use of facilitated ankylosis in the treatment of septic arthritis of the distal interphalangeal joint in cattle: 12 cases (1987-1992), *J Am Vet Med Assoc* 206:1923-1927, 1995.

18. Zulauf M, Jordan P, Steiner A: Fenestration of the abaxial hoof wall and implantation of gentamicin-impregnated collagen sponges for the treatment of septic arthritis of the distal interphalangeal joint in cattle, *Vet Rec* 149:516-518, 2001.

19. Kasari TR, Taylor TS, Baird AN et al: Use of autogenous cancellous bone graft for treatment of osteolytic defects in the phalanges of three cattle, *J Am Vet Med Assoc* 201:1053-1057, 1992.

20. Kofler J: *Clinical study on toe abscess and necrosis of the apex of the distal phalanx in cattle*. In 9th International Symposium on Disorders of the Ruminant Digit, Mizpeh Rachel, Jerusalem, p 22, 1996a.

21. Nuss K, Kostlin RG, Bohmer H et al: [The significance of ungulocoriitis septica (traumatica) at the toe of the bovine claw], *Tierarztl Prax* 18:567-575, 1990.

22. Taylor J: The applied anatomy of the bovine foot, *Vet Rec* 72:1212-1215, 1960.

23. Kofler J: [New possibilities for the diagnosis of septic tenosynovitis of the digital flexor tendon sheath in cattle using sonography—therapy and long-term results], *Dtsch Tierärztl Wochenschr* 101:215-222, 1994.

24. Anderson DE, Allen D, St-Jean G et al: Use of a multifenestrated indwelling lavage system for treatment of septic digital tenosynovitis in cattle, *Aust Vet J* 75:796-799, 1997.

25. Desrochers A, Anderson DE, St-Jean G: Surgical treatment of lameness, *Vet Clin North Am Food Anim Pract* 17:143-158, vii, 2001.

26. Kofler J: Ultrasonographic imaging of pathology of the digital flexor tendon sheath in cattle, *Vet Rec* 139:36-41, 1996b.

27. Nuss K, Hanichen T: [Fibrino-purulent flexor tendon tendinitis in infected tendovaginitis of the digital flexor tendon sheath in cattle], *Tierarztl Prax* 23:565-569, 1995.

28. Illing K: Ein beitrag zur operativen behandlung der tendovaginitis purulenta der gemeinschaftlichen sehnenscheide der oberflächlichen und tiefen beugesehne des rindes, *Mh Vet Med* 19:932-935, 1964.

29. Kofler J, Martinek B: New surgical approach to the plantar fetlock joint through the digital flexor tendon sheath wall and suspensory ligament apparatus in cases of concurrent septic synovitis in two cattle, *Vet J* 169:370-375, 2005.

30. Desrochers A, St-Jean G: Surgical management of digit disorders in cattle, *Vet Clin North Am Food Anim Pract* 12:277-298, 1996.

31. Desrochers A, St-Jean G, Cash WC et al: Characterization of anatomic communications of the fetlock in cattle, using intra-articular latex injection and positive-contrast arthrography, *Am J Vet Res* 58:710-712, 1997.

32. Nuss K, Hecht S, Maierl J et al: Zur punktion der gliedmabengelenke beim rind. Teil I: schultergliedmabe, *Tierärztliche Praxis (G)* 30:226-232, 2002.

33. Van Huffel X: Surgical treatment of joint and tendon disease in calves and cattle, *Cattle Pract* 4:187-192, 1996.

34. Verschooten F, De Moor A, Steenhaut M et al: Surgical and conservative treatment of infectious arthritis in cattle, *J Am Vet Med Assoc* 165:271-275, 1974.

35. Barneveld A: Cancellous bone grafting in the treatment of bovine septic physitis, *Vet Quart* 16:104-107, 1994.

36. Firth E, Kersjes A, Dik K, et al: Haematogenous osteomyelitis in cattle. *Vet Rec* 120:148-152, 1987.

37. De Kesel A, Verschooten F, De Moor A et al: Bacterial osteitis-osteomyelitis of the growth plates in cattle, *Vlaams Diergeneeskd Tijdschr* 51:397-422, 1982.

38. Numans S, Wintzer HJ: Gedeckte klauenbeinfrakturen während des weidegangs beim rind, *Dtsch Tierärztl Wschr* 65:201, 1958.

39. Rothlisberger J, Schawalder P, Kircher P et al: Collateral ligament prosthesis for the repair of subluxation of the metatarsophalangeal joint in a Jersey cow, *Vet Rec* 146:640-643, 2000.

40. Starke A, Heppelmann M, Kehler W et al: *Septic arthritis of the distal interphalangeal joint in HF cows: controlled clinical study comparing the efficacy of digital amputation and resection of the coffin joint*. 13th International Symposium and 5th Conference on Lameness in Ruminants, Maribor, Slovenija, 2004, pp 124-125.

41. Osman MA: A study of some sequelae of amputation of the digit using three operative techniques, *Vet Rec* 87:610-615, 1970.

42. Pfeiffer W, Williams W: A course in surgical operations for veterinary students and practitioners, Ballière, London, 1900.

43. Funk KA: [Late results after toe and claw amputation in cattle], *Berl Munch Tierarztl Wochenschr* 90:152-156, 1977.

44. Nuss K, Steiner A: Spezielle diagnostik und therapie. In Fiedler A, Maierl J, Nuss K, editors: *Erkrankungen der klauen und zehen des rindes*, Schattauer, Stuttgart, 2004, pp 77-125.

CHAPTER 54

Small Ruminant Infectious Disease of the Foot

PASCAL DUBREUIL

FOOTROT

Footrot, an infectious disease caused by the bacterium *Dichelobacter nodosus,* is the leading cause of lameness in sheep around the world. The goat is the only species other than sheep in which footrot has long been recognized as a serious clinical problem. Studies to define the etiology and pathogenesis of this disease have been mainly limited to sheep, but the same strains of *D. nodosus* can affect both species. However, footrot in goats is less severe than in sheep. *D. nodosus* is the essential causative agent. The disease is characterized by a mixed bacterial infection that creates an anaerobic environment allowing multiplications of the agent. Protease production results in the separation of the horn of the hoof from the underlying soft tissue. Virulent, intermediate, and benign footrot are the recognized forms and are associated with the nature of the isolate. Sheep susceptibility associated with the major histocompatibility complex has been reported.

Etiology and Pathogenesis

Footrot is caused by the association of *D. nodosus* and *Fusobacterium necrophorum.* Both bacteria are gram-negative rods. *D. nodosus* isolates can show a marked variation in inherent virulence, which appears to be related to the nature of the fimbriae (pili) and proteases produced by the bacteria. *D. nodosus* cannot survive longer than a few days outside the feet of the small ruminants, and the strains causing virulent footrot do not readily establish persistent subclinical infections. Inversely, strains that cause mild and benign footrot may persist for prolonged periods in the stratum corneum without detectable lesions.

Environmental conditions such as wet weather, lush pastures, and a moderate climate (>10° C) can favor transmission of the causative agents. Usually summer and fall seasons are at higher risk. However, transmission can occur at any time on warm and moist bedding.

Environmental and host factors are closely related to the development of the disease. The attachment of *D. nodosus* to the interdigital skin is predisposed by the pili of the bacteria and also by prolonged exposure to wet conditions. Environmental bacteria such as *F. necrophorum* establish first the ovine interdigital dermatitis, which is by itself a relatively mild condition, providing the necessary conditions to *D. nodosus* colonization. *F. necrophorum* and *D. nodosus* are essential for the invasion of the epidermal matrix of the hoof and neither bacteria alone

can cause footrot lesions. In fact, following the colonization of the *stratum corneum* by *F. necrophorum,* *D. nodosus* can infect the tissue, allowing *F. necrophorum* to deeply penetrate and destroy the epidermal tissue. The hoof separation is secondary to the protease production by *D. nodosus.* Hoof separation is first seen at the axial aspect of the heel and then spreads laterally and cranially to the abaxial wall and the toe of the hoof.

Transmission of the disease is caused by contaminated soil. The infection may persist in a proportion of the flock in cool and moist conditions where persistent lesions are clinically detectable as pockets of infected tissue in sole defects or as interdigital skin abrasion and inflammation. Usually this benign form has no negative impact on body condition. Dry and cool climates reduce the prevalence of new cases.

Morbidity can approach 100% in virulent cases. Lameness associated with extensive necrosis underrunning the hoof leads to emaciation as the animal reduces its displacement while grazing. The animal may remain in sternal recumbency and may develop sternal skin ulceration and necrosis. In extreme cases, mortality results from emaciation and secondary systemic infection.

Diagnosis

Clinical signs, high morbidity, and examination of the hoof with characteristic lesions of footrot are usually sufficient to establish the diagnosis. However, culture of the causative bacteria, Gram stain of exudates (gram-negative, barbell-shaped bacteria), and serologic classification by agglutination tests following culture or by evaluation of the proteolytic activity of the isolate may help to confirm the diagnosis or the virulence of the agent.

Treatment

Therapeutic approach depends on the severity of the clinical signs.

Benign Footrot

A foot bath (without trimming) containing 10% to 15% zinc sulfate is preferred to copper sulfate (5%) or formalin (3%) because it is less hazardous than Cu SO$_4$, causes less discomfort than formalin, and does not stain the wool. The addition of lauryl sulfate enhances the penetration of Zn SO$_4$. Ideally the procedure should be a prolonged soaking time (0.5-1 hour), and then the animals should be kept in a dry place for a few hours before being moved to a separate pasture that has been free of sheep for 7 to 10 days. This procedure should be repeated every 7 to 10 days until conditions improve or signs of lameness abate.

Virulent Footrot

Cases with separation of either soft or hard horn should receive topical and parenteral treatments.

The mainstay of therapy is proper hoof trimming. Trimming all overlying necrotic tissue is laborious and painful for the animal. However, a good trimming followed by topical treatment with tetracycline, Cu SO$_4$, Zn SO$_4$, or formalin may cure the animals. Foot baths as previously described may be performed following an appropriate paring. However, different authors report that paring will not improve the success rate of a foot bath when lesions are not advanced.

Parenteral treatment using procaine penicillin G (20,000-30,000 IU/kg IM, bid for 3 days), long-acting oxytetracycline (20 mg/kg IM, SC every 72 hours), erythromycin (3-5 mg/kg IM, bid for 3 days), lincomycin, spectinomycin, and florfenicol (20 mg/kg IM, every 48 hours) have been reported to be successful, especially in dry weather conditions. These treatments are not approved in all countries.

Both topical and parenteral treatments when properly applied will cure 90% to 95% of the animals within 3 to 4 weeks. The remaining affected animals should be eliminated.

Prevention

Eradication of virulent footrot is difficult but possible, especially in wet areas because *D. nodosus* does not persist in the environment. Treating affected animals, culling of chronic or recurrent cases, isolation of newly affected animals, and stopping foot baths should be performed during an eradication program of virulent footrot. Eradication of benign footrot in commercial flocks does not necessarily warrant the expense involved.

Vaccination with multivalent bacterin vaccines can prevent transmission and accelerate healing. Two doses of the vaccine 4 to 6 weeks apart are recommended as a first vaccination because it is reported that the duration of the immunity lasts 4 to 12 weeks. Only one booster shot is necessary thereafter annually. For this reason, animals should be vaccinated before the risky period of the year. If the transmission period is long, a single dose of vaccine may be required. Severe local reactions to the vaccines have been reported.

OVINE INTERDIGITAL DERMATITIS

This condition is of minor clinical importance and is associated with *F. necrophorum*. This condition occurs in sheep chronically exposed to wet conditions. The interdigital skin may become eroded and may even ulcerate. This condition is the first step toward footrot, but in the absence of *D. nodosus*, only a mild and transient lameness may be observed and does not warrant treatment.

CONTAGIOUS OVINE DIGITAL DERMATITIS

Cases of unusually severe footrot may have been misdiagnosed in this situation. Spirochetes similar to those found in the bovine digital dermatitis of cattle have been isolated. Molecular information suggests that these spirochetes belong to the genus *Treponema*. Initial lesions are observed at the coronet, followed by extensive underrunning of the horn with possible loss of the hoof. The interdigital lesion of footrot is usually absent. Further research on the etiology is necessary to confirm the exact causative agent, as well as the relationship of this disease to the bacteria *D. nodosus*. Topical, parenteral, or foot bath therapy with tetracycline may be used to control the infection.

Recommended Readings

Abbott KA, Lewis CJ: Current approaches to the management of ovine footrot, *Vet J* 169:28, 2005.

Casey RH, Martin PA: Effect of foot paring of sheep affected with footrot in response to zinc sulfate/sodium lauryl sulphate foot, bathing treatment, *Aust Vet J* 65:258, 1988.

Colligan RJ, Naylor RD, Martin PK et al: A spirochete isolated from a case of severe virulent ovine foot disease is closely related to a treponeme isolated from human periodontitis and bovine digital dermatitis, *Vet Microbiol* 74:249, 2000.

Escayg AP, Hickfoid JG, Bullock DW: Association between alleles of the ovine major histocompatibility complex and resistance to footrot, *Res Vet Sci* 63:283, 1997.

Ghimire SC, Egerton JR, Dhungyel OP: Transmission of virulent footrot between sheep and goats, *Aust Vet J* 77:450, 1999.

Lewis C: Update on footrot in sheep, *State Vet J* 8:4, 1998.

Moore LJ, Woodward MJ, Grogono-Thomas R: The occurrence of treponemes in contagious ovine digital dermatitis and the characterisation of associated *Dichelobacter nodosus*, *Vet Microbiol* 111:199, 2005.

Reed GA, Alley DV: Efficacy of a novel copper-based foot bath preparation for the treatment of ovine footrot during the spread period, *Aust Vet J* 74:375, 1996.

CHAPTER 55

Fracture Management in Cattle

ADRIAN STEINER and DAVID E. ANDERSON

GENERAL CONSIDERATIONS

Fractures are common in food animals. They involve most frequently the long bones; occasionally the ribs, mandible, and pelvis; and rarely the scapulae and vertebrae. Long bone fractures occur mainly in young stock and often as a consequence of forced extraction during dystocia. Fractures of metacarpus III/IV (MC) and metatarsus III/IV (MT) comprise about 50% of all long bone fractures. Less frequently occur fractures of the tibia (12%); radius/ulna (7%); femur, humerus, and pelvis (<5% each); and P1 and P2 (<1%).[1] Food animals are considered to be excellent patients for fracture treatment because they spend a majority of time lying down, have a tremendous osteogenic potential, are more resistant to limb breakdown and laminitis than horses, and usually do not resist having appliances on their limbs. The decision to treat a fracture in a food animal is made by considering the cost and success rate of the treatment, the perceived or potential economic or genetic value of the animal, and the location and type of fracture.

EMERGENCY AND FIRST AID TREATMENT

Before the decision for treatment, a thorough physical examination must be conducted on all animals suspected of having a fracture. First, the patient must be made safe from continued trauma. If the animal is recumbent, it should be allowed to remain recumbent until the physical examination and fracture assessment have been conducted. Assessment of hydration and cardiopulmonary and shock status is of utmost importance. Adequate passive antibody transfer to newborn calves is critical to preoperative preparation and success of the procedure. If colostrum ingestion is unknown, serum immunoglobulin or total protein should be determined. Calves that are hydrated and have a serum protein of less than 5 g/dl should be considered to have poor colostral antibody transfer and receive a plasma transfusion before attempting repair. Assessment of skin integrity at the fracture site is of crucial importance. Open fractures generally do have a markedly less favorable prognosis than closed fractures. Open fractures should be treated immediately with local wound débridement, irrigation, antimicrobial dressing, and administration of broad-spectrum antimicrobials given systemically or preferably by retrograde intravenous route after temporary administration of a tourniquet.

Temporary stabilization of limb fractures may be performed before moving the animal or attempting to get the animal to stand. As a general rule, fractures below the level of the midradius or midtibia may be temporarily stabilized with splints or casts. Field stabilization of fractures proximal to this level should not be attempted. These efforts often result in the creation of a "fulcrum effect" at the fracture site and also in increased soft tissue trauma, damage to neurovascular structures, or compounding of the fracture. Cattle with these fractures should be carefully loaded into the trailer and allowed time to lie down before beginning transport. Because these animals usually do not try to get up once they are down, sedation is not indicated. External coaptation for temporary stabilization of the fracture may be done by using two splints or a cast. Two boards, placed 90 degrees to each other (e.g., caudal and lateral aspect of the limb), or one piece of a large polyvinyl chloride (PVC) pipe cut in half, create a stable external coaptation. A padded bandage is placed on the limb, the splints positioned, and elastic tape applied firmly. All external coaptation devices should incorporate and immobilize the carpus/tarsus and extend to the ground (below the sole). For injuries proximal to the carpus or hock and distal to the midradius or midtibia, the lateral splint should extend to the level of the proximal scapula or pelvis, respectively (Fig. 55-1).

PRINCIPLES AND TECHNIQUES OF FRACTURE MANAGEMENT

Good radiographs, taken in two planes, are an indispensable prerequisite for adequate fracture evaluation. Configuration and location of the fracture, the presence of soft tissue and neurovascular trauma, closed or open fracture environment, behavioral nature of the animal, and experience of the veterinarian are important factors in considering what type of treatment is chosen.[2] Fractures of the axial skeleton are often treated by stall rest alone because external or internal fixation is neither required nor feasible. For fractures involving the appendicular skeleton, the following questions must be answered: Is treatment required? Is the fracture open? If yes, for how long? Can the fracture be acceptably reduced closed or is internal reduction required? Can the fracture be adequately immobilized using external coaptation alone, or is use of internal fixation required or advantageous? What is the cost-benefit analysis?

Walking Block for Bovine Digit

Cattle have two weight-bearing digits for each limb and therefore may stand on one digit during convalescence of the paired digit (e.g., phalangeal fracture). A wooden,

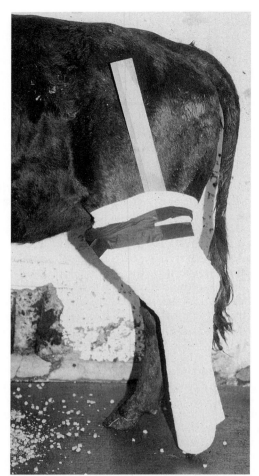

Fig 55-1 External coaptation for temporary fixation of a tibia fracture. The lateral splint extends to the level of the pelvis.

rubber, or plastic block (2-2.5 cm in height and formed to the size and shape of the healthy claw) can be applied to the sole of the healthy digit. The animal is confined to a stall or small pen for 6 to 10 weeks while fracture healing proceeds and the block is removed. Blocks that break away before expected healing time has passed have to be replaced.

Casting

Half-limb casts can be used for immobilization of phalangeal and distal physeal fractures of MC and MT. The cast is placed from a point immediately distal to the carpus or hock extending to the ground and encasing the foot. The interdigital space, coronary band, dewclaws, and top of the cast are slightly padded, but only stockinette or foam padding (3M Custom Support Form, 3M Animal Care Products) is placed on the remainder of the limb. Thick padding placed along the limb will quickly become compressed, leaving room for the limb to move within the cast and displacement of the fracture to occur. Full-limb casts are placed similarly to half-limb casts, but the prominences of the accessory carpal bone, styloid process of the ulna, calcaneus, and medial and lateral malleolus of the tibia must be padded.

Placement of the cast is facilitated by use of rope restraint and deep sedation or general anesthesia as needed. An assistant should help to maintain alignment of the limb during application, being sure to check the position of the limb in the cranial to caudal and lateral to medial planes. Tension on the limb during casting may be obtained by placing wires through holes drilled in the hoof through the abaxial wall close to the heel and tightening them. The hoof should be positioned in a normal to slightly flexed position. Fiberglass casting tape should be used, but the thickness of the cast is usually based on clinical judgment; casts six to eight layers thick may be used for calves less than 150 kg body weight, but adult cattle may require 12 to 16 layers' thickness. Each layer should be applied quickly to avoid any lamination of the casting material. Generally, casts used on the hind limbs must be thicker because of stress concentration by the angulation of the hock. Because fiberglass is weak in compression, a thin cast will break at the dorsal aspect of the hock. Incorporation of metal rods within the cast (two rods placed 90 degrees to each other) may be necessary in extremely large patients. The bottom of the cast is protected with PMMA to avoid excessive wearing. Scheduled cast changes at 3-week intervals may be required for rapidly growing calves or for calves that become lame during convalescence. In adult cattle the cast is changed once during the healing period. Physeal fractures are usually healed within 3 to 4 weeks, but nonphyseal fractures often require 4 to 6 weeks to reach clinical union (defined as sufficient bridging callus to allow weight bearing without additional support to the limb) in calves. Fractures in adult cattle often heal within 8 to 10 weeks but may require 12 to 16 weeks for clinical union to occur. Radiographic union of the fracture (defined as bone union with resolution of the fracture line) is not seen for weeks to months after clinical union has been reached.

Transfixation Pinning and Casting and External Skeleton Fixation

Transfixation pinning and casting may be applied either as a "hanging-limb pin-cast" or as an external skeletal fixator[2] (Fig. 55-2). Hanging-limb pin-cast refers to placement of transfixing, or transcortical, pins through the bone proximal to the injury, followed by application of a full-limb cast (i.e., walking cast).[3] The body weight is transferred to the cast by the pins and transmitted through the cast to the ground. Therefore the distal limb "hangs" inside the walking cast. Pin-casts may be used for external skeletal fixation (ESF) by placing transfixation pins proximal and distal to the injury. The advantages of using pin-casts for ESF compared with walking casts are that the fracture is more stable, the fracture fragments are unable to move within the pin-cast after the swelling within the limb resolves, and the pin-cast may not need to span adjacent joints (in cattle weighing <300 kg). Pin selection is based on the body weight of the animal, size of the bone involved, and configuration of the fracture. The diameter of the pin should not exceed 20% to 30% of the diameter of the bone.

Defects larger than 30% of the diameter of the bone cause marked loss of the bone's resistance to torsion

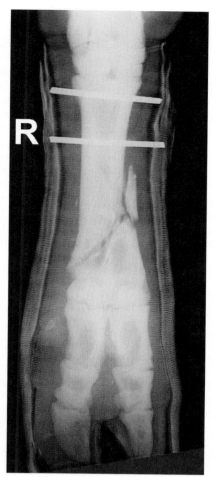

Fig 55-2 Hanging-limb, pin-cast fixation of a metatarsal fracture in a 600-kg cow.

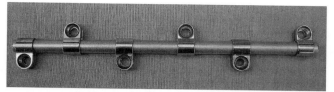

Fig 55-3 Clamp rod internal fixator with six standard clamps.

in the limb becomes concentrated at the defect in the cast. Preferably, metal or acrylic sidebars should be used. These sidebars must be made large enough to sustain the weight of the patient.

Internal Fixation (plate, Clamp Rod Internal Fixator, intramedullary interlocking nail)

Internal fixation may be the treatment of choice for certain fractures in cattle of high perceived economic value. Dynamic compression plates or the newly developed Clamp Rod Internal Fixator (CRIF) may be used for treatment of simple or wedge fractures that tend to override[4] (Fig. 55-3). Early mobilization of the active and passive parts of the musculoskeletal apparatus and optimal anatomic alignment of the fragments with minimal callus formation are the main advantages of these internal fixation techniques. Techniques for application of bone plates in cattle are similar to those for horses. Recently developed implants such as intramedullary interlocking nails (IINs) and the CRIF may prove to be useful for management of fractures with historically poor success with bone plating (e.g., humerus and femur fracture).

Closed versus Open Fractures

Overall, closed fractures without damage to the blood supply to the limb have a good to excellent prognosis for healing in cattle. The prognosis is less good for older cattle, cattle of high body weight, and fractures of the proximal long bones. Open long-bone fractures generally have a guarded to poor prognosis for healing in cattle. The success rate depends on the severity of soft tissue damage, the bone affected, the age of the patient, the duration and degree of contamination of the wound, and the economic limitations placed on fracture management. Prolonged antibiotic therapy is indicated, and open wound management is preferable to enclosing the wound within a cast.

TREATMENT AND PROGNOSIS OF SPECIFIC FRACTURES

Mandible

Mandibular fractures occur during dystocia or direct trauma. Repair of mandible fractures is indicated if the patient has difficulty eating. Fractures of the mandibular symphysis occur frequently in skeletally immature cattle and are best treated with orthopedic wires placed around the incisors. In calves with fractures occurring in the rostral half of the body of the mandible, intramedullary

loading. In general, ³⁄₃₂- to ⅛-inch (2.4-3.2 mm) pins are used in calves weighing less than 100 kg, ⅛- to ³⁄₁₆-inch (3.2-4.8 mm) pins are used in cattle weighing 100 to 300 kg, ³⁄₁₆- to ¼-inch (4.8-6.4 mm) pins are used in cattle weighing 300 to 600 kg, and ¼-inch (6.4 mm) pins are used in cattle weighing more than 600 kg. Pins should not be placed parallel to each other. The distance between pins should be such that they are separated by a minimum of four times the diameter of the pin. These measures will minimize the risk of the concentration of mechanical forces between the two pins ("stress riser effect"). Before pin insertion, a hole should be predrilled through the bone to accommodate the pin. This hole should not be smaller than 0.5 mm less than the diameter of the pin (e.g., 2.7-mm hole for a 3.2-mm pin). Veterinary orthopedic pins are not designed to be drilled while being inserted. Therefore significant thermal and mechanical injury occurs in the bone during insertion. Predrilling using an orthopedic drill bit limits this injury.

For management of open fractures, daily access to the wound is desired. This may be accomplished by leaving a hole in the cast ("window cast") at the site of the injury, but this often gives unsatisfactory access to the wound and is uncomfortable to the patient because the swelling pins placed from the rostral to the caudal aspect of the body of the mandible may provide adequate stabilization. Fractures occurring rostral to the ramus of the mandible may be treated by application of an external skeletal fixator anchored to the bone with either pins or clamps.[5,6] Bone plates may be used for fixation of closed fractures of the mandibular body and represent the option of choice for fractures occurring in the ramus of the mandible. The presence of an open wound does not significantly worsen the prognosis of mandibular fractures if bone plating is avoided.

Vertebrae

Vertebral fractures happen during handling for vaccination, when mounting for breeding, or when excessive traction occurs during dystocia. Vertebral fractures causing paralysis of the limbs have a grave prognosis, and euthanasia is indicated. Minimally displaced fractures associated with minor neurologic deficits may be treated by stall confinement. However, progressive neurologic deficits may be seen weeks to months after the injury because of compression of the spinal cord by fibroplasias or callus. Treatment of fracture of the sacrum or caudal vertebrae may be done for cosmetic purposes. Application of a four- or five-hole bone plate or a pinless external fixator allows restoration of normal anatomy. These injuries are often associated with tail paralysis, and the prognosis for return to normal function is guarded.

Pelvis

Fractures involving the acetabulum, wing of the ilium, or sacroiliac junction are the most common pelvic fractures in cattle. These injuries occur because of falls during mounting or on slippery flooring. Fractures involving the acetabulum carry a poor prognosis because of osteoarthrosis formation. Fractures of the wing of the ilium respond well to stall confinement but may become open, with bone projecting through the skin. Infection rapidly becomes established, and bone sequestration occurs. Surgical removal of the detached fragment and the spiky projecting aspects of the wing of the ilium is indicated when sepsis or debilitating lameness is present. Fractures of sacroiliac junction may respond favorably to strict stall confinement, but prognosis for return to normal productive use is usually poor.

Rib

Rib fractures usually occur during manual extraction for dystocia but may be caused by rough handling in restraint chutes. Treatment of rib fractures is not indicated unless flail chest is present or lung injury is imminent. Owners should be warned that fracture of the first three ribs, as sometimes encountered in calves, may cause progressive tracheal collapse weeks to months after injury. Tracheal collapse is caused by compression of the trachea by the forming callus or by the fibrous tissue response to the injury. When this occurs, rib resection or slaughter/euthanasia is indicated.

Humerus

Nonarticular, minimally displaced fractures of the humerus are best treated by stall confinement and carry a guarded to good prognosis for return to normal productive use. Open reduction and internal fixation of the humerus with an IIN or through a cranial approach[7] with bone plates or application of a CRIF is indicated in moderately to severely displaced fractures. In fractures older than 24 hours, anatomic reduction of the fragments may be difficult because of increasing muscular contraction. Care has to be taken not to cause permanent radial nerve injury during internal fixation. The fixation with an IIN may allow rigid fixation with minimal risk of radial nerve injury. The prognosis after successful internal fixation of closed fractures is guarded to favorable, for articular fractures; however, the prognosis for return to productive life is poor.

Radius and Ulna

Closed fractures of the distal physis of the radius may be treated by a full-limb cast and have a good prognosis for success. Fractures of the midradius and ulna require transfixation pinning and casting or internal fixation with bone plates or the CRIF. Implants for internal fixation are applied at the cranial and/or craniolateral aspects of the radius. The ulna is anatomically reduced, but fixation is not required in combined fractures. After successful internal fixation of closed fractures, the prognosis for healing is good.

Femur

Femoral fractures most often occur in calves during forced extraction for dystocia but occasionally are found in adult cattle after falling during mounting or on slippery flooring. Femoral fractures in mature cattle have a grave prognosis because of high body weight and an inability to reduce the fracture. Capital physeal fractures (fracture through the physis of the head of the femur) in mature cattle may be successfully repaired using cross-pins or cannulated screws.[8,9] Selected minimally displaced femoral fractures may respond to stall rest for 8 to 10 weeks. These cattle may require assistance in standing during the first 2 to 4 weeks after the injury. Simple oblique or spiral fractures may be treated successfully with a CRIF in animals up to 300 kg (Fig. 55-4). In calves, stack pinning of the femur has a good prognosis for success.[10] Open reduction of the fracture is performed, and two to five intramedullary pins are placed into the femur. If large cortical defects are present, then an external skeletal fixator may be applied in addition to the intramedullary pins. These fractures are usually healed by 6 weeks after surgery.

Tibia

Although fractures of the tibia have been seen as a result of forced extraction during dystocia, tibia fractures are usually caused by direct trauma. Fracture of the distal physis of the tibia may be treated with a full-limb cast, but these fractures are uncommon. Fractures of the middle portion

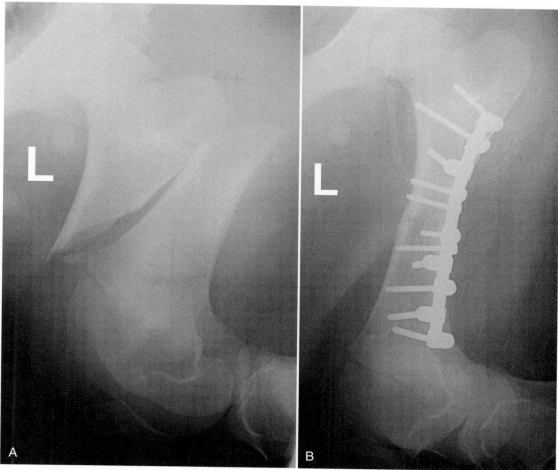

Fig 55-4   Simple spiral fracture of the femur of a 140-kg heifer before (**A**) and after (**B**) open reduction and internal fixation with a clamp rod internal fixator.

of the tibia are treated similarly to fractures of the radius and have a similar prognosis and encounter similar complications.

Metacarpus and Metatarsus III/IV

Fractures involving the MC or MT are the most common fractures to occur in food animals.[11,12] Closed fractures of the distal physis (Salter-Harris types I and II) of the MC or MT may be treated using a half-limb cast (Fig. 55-5). Physeal fractures involving the joint (Salter-Harris types III and IV), although rare, require optimal reduction of the joint surface and internal fixation with screws applied in lag fashion. If the fracture configuration is such that overriding of the fragments or collapse of the fracture is unlikely to occur after closed reduction, closed fractures of the middle or proximal portions of the MC or MT may be treated with a full-limb cast. To avoid fracture collapse and sepsis after secondary perforation of the skin

within the cast, application of a walking cast is indicated in compound diaphyseal fractures. Internal fixation with bone plates may be used for repair of simple or wedge diaphyseal fractures to achieve an optimal cosmetic result. Alternatively, minimal internal fixation of the fragments may be reinforced by application of a full-limb cast to achieve a similar result. Because the CRIF implants are voluminous and the amount of soft tissues present between skin and MC/MT is low, the CRIF is rarely used for fixation of fractures distal to the carpus and tarsus. In valuable cattle and young calves, treatment of open fractures of MC or MT may be aimed at using an external skeletal fixator and daily wound care until healed. Bone sequestra are often present in open fractures, and healing may not occur until these have been removed. If prolonged sepsis has been present, cancellous bone grafts may facilitate bone union. The optimal sites for harvesting cancellous bone grafts are the wing of the ilium and the proximal tibia.

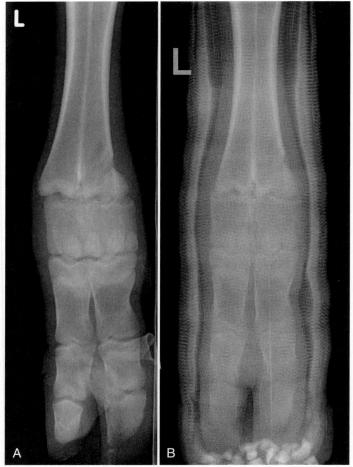

Fig 55-5 Salter-Harris type II fracture of a 5-week-old calf before **(A)** and after **(B)** closed reduction and external fixation with a half-limb cast.

References

1. Ferguson JG: Management and repair of bovine fractures, *Compend Contin Educ Pract Vet* 4:S128, 1982.
2. Anderson DE, St-Jean G: External skeletal fixation in ruminants, *Vet Clin North Am Food Anim Pract* 12:117, 1996.
3. Németh F, Back W: The use of the walking cast to repair fractures in horses and ponies, *Eq Vet J* 23:32, 1991.
4. Gamper S, Steiner A, Nuss K et al: Clinical evaluation of the CRIF 4.5/5.5 system for long-bone fracture repair in cattle, *Vet Surg* 35:361, 2006.
5. Lischer CJ, Fluri E, Kaser-Hotz B et al: Pinless external fixation of mandible fractures in cattle, *Vet Surg* 26:14, 1997.
6. Reif U, Lischer CJ, Steiner A et al: Long-term results of bovine mandibular fractures involving the molar teeth, *Vet Surg* 29:335, 2000.
7. Rakestraw PC, Nixon AJ, Kaderly RE et al: Cranial approach to the humerus for repair of fractures in horses and cattle, *Vet Surg* 20:1, 1991.
8. Wilson DG, Crawford WH, Stone WC et al: Fixation of femoral capital physeal fractures with 7.0 mm cannulated screws in 5 bulls, *Vet Surg* 20:240, 1991.
9. Hull BL, Koenig GJ, Monke DR: Treatment of slipped capital femoral epiphysis in cattle. 11 cases (1974-1988), *J Am Vet Med Assoc* 197:1509, 1990.
10. St-Jean G, DeBowes RM, Hull BL et al: Intramedullary pinning of femoral diaphyseal fractures in neonatal calves: 12 cases (1980-1990), *J Am Vet Med Assoc* 200:1372, 1992.
11. Steiner A, Iselin U, Auer JA et al: Physeal fractures of the metacarpus and metatarsus in cattle, *Vet Comp Orthop Traumatol* 6:131, 1993.
12. Steiner A, Iselin U, Auer JA et al: Shaft fractures of the metacarpus and metatarsus in cattle, *Vet Comp Orthop Traumatol* 6:138, 1993.

CHAPTER 56

Septic Arthritis in Cattle

DAVID FRANCOZ

Joint diseases are reported to be the second most important cause of lameness in cattle.[1] Among them, septic arthritis is by far the most frequent. In Sweden the incidence rate of arthritis was reported to be 0.002 cases per calf-months at risk.[2]

ETIOLOGY

In adult animals, direct inoculation of a microorganism into the joint (primary septic arthritis) and extension from periarticular infection (secondary septic arthritis) are at the origin of septic arthritis. In such cases, only one joint is generally involved and joints particularly susceptible to traumatic injury (fetlock, carpus, and tarsus) are most frequently affected. In young animals, most cases of septic arthritis are due to blood dissemination of bacteria from a primary site of infection (tertiary septic arthritis). Primary foci of infection include umbilical structures, lungs, and digestive tract. One or multiple joints could be involved, and high motion joints (stifle, carpus, and tarsus) are most frequently affected.

Numerous microorganisms have been implicated in septic arthritis, but in ruminants, bacteria are essentially at the origin of the infection. *Arcanobacterium pyogenes* is the most frequent bacteria isolated in cattle and represents approximately 40% of positive culture. *Streptococci, Staphylococci,* and Enterobacteriaceae can also be isolated. Anaerobic bacteria are important bacteria to consider. Because their culture requires specific media, they are frequently underestimated.[3] Recently, mycoplasma has been emerging as an important cause of septic arthritis in calves.[4] Mycoplasma septic arthritis should be suspected, particularly in animals with a history of pneumonia or otitis media. Mycoplasma culture also requires specific media and is probably underestimated.

An acute inflammatory response occurs after bacterial contamination of the joint. This reaction initiates a rapid influx of inflammatory cells, mostly neutrophils, as well as activation of synoviocytes and chondrocytes, release of many inflammatory mediators, and finally decreased proteoglycan synthesis. This cascade of events ultimately leads to a reduction in joint lubrication and an increase in cartilage destruction, thus contributing to the process of joint disease. Chronic septic arthritis may develop and may be attributed to persistent bacterial infection, presence of bacterial wall materials, or an immune-mediated process.

CLINICAL SIGNS AND DIAGNOSIS

Diagnosis of septic arthritis is based on the clinical signs, medical imaging examination, bacterial culture, and cytologic analysis of synovial fluid. Prompt diagnosis of septic arthritis is important because delay in the initiation of treatment worsen the prognosis.

Clinical signs of septic arthritis include acute non–weight-bearing lameness, joint swelling, and pain and heat on palpation and manipulation of the joint. The animal may be febrile and anorexic. Complete physical examination is essential to find the origin of the infection: wounds in adult animals and umbilical structure infection, pneumonia, or diarrhea in young animals.

Cytologic synovial fluid examination is a useful ancillary test for the diagnosis of joint diseases and the differentiation among them. In septic arthritis the synovial fluid appears macroscopically cloudy and without viscosity. Cytologic analysis revealed elevated total protein and total nucleated cell count, predominantly neutrophils. Free or phagocyted bacteria may be seen. Cutoff points for the differentiation between inflammatory and infectious joint diseases in cattle are reported to be more than 25,000 total nucleated cells/µl, more than 20,000 neutrophils/µl, more than 80% of neutrophils, and total protein concentration more than 45 g/L.[5]

Positive bacterial culture confirms the diagnosis of joint infection and provides information for the antimicrobial treatment. Unfortunately, bacterial culture is only positive in 60% of cases.[3] Negative culture results can be explained by chronic infection and isolation of bacteria in synovial membrane villosity or prior treatment with antibiotics or absence of specific culture request (anaerobic and mycoplasma culture). The use of blood culture bottle (associated or not with villosity biopsy or fibrin culture) could increase the rate of positive culture. Blood culture bottles enhance bacterial culture using a rich medium, additives to eliminate endogenous and exogenous antimicrobial factors, and a large inoculum to ensure against a low microbial density. They allow culture of anaerobic bacteria. However, most blood culture bottles inhibit mycoplasma growth. In cases for which mycoplasma is suspected, a synovial sample in a sterile tube must be submitted for specific mycoplasma culture.

Radiographic examination may help to rule out fracture and osteomyelitis from the differential diagnosis. It can also provide useful information about joint damage associated with infection and help determine the prognosis. Most osseous lesions associated with joint infection (subchondral bone lysis, osteomyelitis, osteosclerosis, periosteitis) cannot be radiographically visible before 1 to 2 weeks after the beginning of the diseases.

Ultrasonography can be useful for the diagnosis of septic arthritis by evaluation of the joint distension; the character of the joint liquid (presence or absence of fluid, presence or absence of floating debris); and the appearance of cartilage. But most of all, ultrasonography provides important information on the integrity of periarticular tissue (particularly ligaments) that can be affected primarily or secondarily to the joint infection.[6] It also helps to choose the appropriate treatment. If fibrin is observed in the joint, arthrotomy should be favored instead of through-and-through lavage with a needle.

TREATMENT

Treatment of septic arthritis in cattle consists of eliminating the causative agents; controlling the inflammatory process; and removing deleterious enzymes and their cellular sources, which can damage the cartilage.

Early institution of treatment, less than 48 hours after the beginning of the disease, is necessary to prevent development of irreversible lesions. Consequently, antibiotic treatment must be initiated before the knowledge of bacterial culture and sensibility results. In adult animals an antimicrobial drug effective against *Arcanobacterium pyogenes* (e.g., one in the β–lactam family) should be used first. In young animals an antimicrobial drug effective against gram-positive and gram-negative bacteria, as well as mycoplasma, should be favored. However, knowing the primary course of the hematogenous spread could help to determine which antimicrobial drugs should be used in first intention. The antimicrobial treatment regimen should then be based on bacterial culture and sensitivity results when available. Intravenous administration of antibiotic is favored for the first days of treatment. Intravenous regional injection under tourniquet can be used to increase local concentration of the antimicrobial drugs and decrease costs of treatment (Fig. 56-1). However, little data on its efficacy are available.[7] The usefulness of intra-articular administration of antibiotic remains uncertain. Some antibiotics (tetracycline) are reported to induce synovitis and must not be used for intra-articular administration.[8] The successful use of intra-articular implants (polymethylmethacrylate [PMMA] or collagen sponges) impregnated with antimicrobial drugs has been reported.[9,10] Duration of antibiotic treatment in cattle remains empirical. It should be at least 15 days. However, duration of clinical signs before the institution of an adequate treatment, bacteria involved in the diseases, and response to treatment should be taken in consideration when deciding the treatment duration.[11]

Joint lavage and drainage are important steps in the treatment of septic arthritis in order to remove the potential deleterious enzymes and their cellular sources (Fig. 56-2). Different methods could be used for joint lavage: tidal irrigation, through-and-through lavage, arthroscopy and lavage, and arthrotomy. Joint lavage is repeated every 24 or 48 hours until improvement of cytologic modification. Knowledge of joint communications and boundaries is essential before flushing complex joints.[12]

Through-and-through lavage is the technique of choice in first intention. The procedure can be performed while the animal is standing or recumbent. The animal is sedated, and regional or intraarticular anesthesia is performed if possible. After preparation of the joint for aseptic surgery, two or three 14- to 18-gauge hypodermic needles are inserted into the joint. One or two liters of a balanced polyionic solution (Ringer's solution, lactated Ringer's solution, or 0.9% NaCl solution) are then infused under pressure. Needles are frequently closed to allow joint distension and disruption of adherence and fibrin. The addition of antibiotics or iodine in the irrigation solution has no clear advantages.

Joint lavage associated with arthroscopy provides diagnostic information, visualization of joint damage, possibility of joint débridement, and lavage with a large amount of fluid. However, this procedure is more expensive and requires specific materials, specialized surgical training, and general anesthesia. Epidural anesthesia may

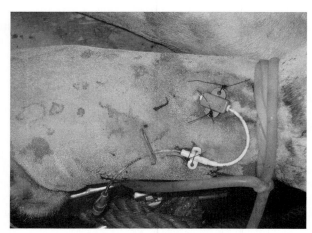

Fig 56-1 An 18-gauge polyurethane catheter was inserted intravenously at the lateral and distal aspect of the metatarsus to treat a chronic septic arthritis of the metatarsophalangeal joint.

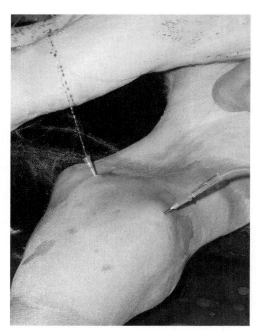

Fig 56-2 A through-and-through lavage is performed on a tarsus with 16-gauge needles.

be used on young animals when hind limbs are treated by arthroscopy and even through-and-through lavage. For the front limbs, a brachial plexus block can be attempted but it is more difficult to achieve successfully.

Arthrotomy should be considered if a large amount of fibrin was observed at ultrasound or the hypodermic needles are obstructed constantly by it while performing a lavage. Joint lavage and débridement, as well as removal of necrotic tissue, fibrin clots, necrotic bone, and/or affected cartilage can be performed. The arthrotomy sites are the same as the arthrocentesis sites. Arthrotomy incisions are left open and allowed to drain but covered with a protective bandage.

Arthrodesis may be a solution of treatment in chronic or severely affected joint. Arthrodesis of articulations of the distal limbs can be performed with minimal consequences for the animal locomotion and has a good prognosis. Arthrodesis of carpus and tarsus can be successful, but the impact on the animal living conditions should be considered and discussed thoroughly with the owner before attempting the procedure.

The role of nonsteroidal antiinflammatory drugs must not be underestimated in the treatment of septic arthritis. Their analgesic effect renders the animal more comfortable, and it will therefore stand up more frequently and return to normal function more rapidly. Their antiinflammatory effects contribute to fight against the inflammatory process associated with joint infection. This inflammatory process seems to persist days to weeks after the elimination of bacteria from the joint,[11] meaning that it can be potentially and solely responsible for the clinical signs.

Joint movements are an important part in the cure of septic arthritis. Small movements are necessary for cartilage nutrition and removal of waste products. Large movements can increase cartilage damage because of inadequate lubrication of septic joints. Absence of movement can lead to reduction in the range of motion of the affected joint. Consequently, movements of the animal must be encouraged but restrained (e.g., rest in a small stall) and the articulation must not be immobilized in order to allow the small movements necessary for the joint cure.

PROGNOSIS

The main factors affecting the prognosis include duration of clinical signs before institution of treatment (see comments earlier), joints involved, number of joints involved, and the etiologic agent. Because treatment alternatives are both more numerous and easier to perform on distal joints than on proximal joints, prognosis is better for distal joints. Involvement of more than one joint implicates the presence of factors allowing important blood dissemination of the pathogen (e.g., immunodepression, virulence of the pathogen) and affecting the efficacy of treatment. Moreover, adequate treatment is more difficult and more expensive to institute when all joints are involved. In cases of mycoplasma septic arthritis, prognosis is always guarded. In such cases, response to treatment cannot be predicted and relapses can be observed.

References

1. Russel AM, Rowlands GJ, Shaw SR et al: Survey of lameness in British dairy cattle, *Vet Rec* 111:155, 1982.
2. Svensson C, Lundborg K, Emanuelson U et al: Morbidity in Swedish dairy calves from birth to 90 days of age and individual calf-level risk factors for infectious diseases, *Prev Vet Med* 58:179, 2003.
3. Francoz D, Desrochers A, Fecteau G, et al: *A retrospective study of joint bacterial culture in 172 cases of septic arthritis in cattle.* Proceedings of the 20th Annual ACVIM Forum 774, Dallas, 2002 (abstract).
4. Gagea MI, Bateman KG, Shanahan RA et al: Naturally occurring *Mycoplasma bovis*–associated pneumonia and polyarthritis in feedlot beef calves, *J Vet Diagn Invest* 18:29, 2006.
5. Rhode C, Anderson DE, Desrochers A et al: Synovial fluid analysis in cattle: a review of 130 cases, *Vet Surg* 29:341, 2000.
6. Kofler J: Arthrosonography—the use of diagnostic ultrasound in septic and traumatic arthritis in cattle: a retrospective study of 25 patients, *Br Vet J* 152:683, 1996.
7. Fajt VR, Apley MD: Antimicrobial issues in bovine lameness, *Vet Clin North Am Food Anim Pract* 17:159, 2001.
8. Trent AM, Plumb D: Treatment of infectious arthritis and osteomyelitis, *Vet Clin North Am Food Anim Pract* 7:747, 1991.
9. Butson RJ, Schramme MC, Garlick MH et al: Treatment of intrasynovial infection with gentamicin-impregnated polymethylmethacrylate beads, *Vet Rec* 138:460, 1996.
10. Hirsbrunner G, Steiner A: Treatment of infectious arthritis of the radiocarpal joint of cattle with gentamicin-impregnated collagen sponges, *Vet Rec* 142:399, 1998.
11. Francoz D, Desrochers A, Fecteau G et al: Synovial fluid changes in induced infectious arthritis in calves, *J Vet Intern Med* 19:336, 2005.
12. Anderson DE, Desrochers A: Musculoskeletal examination in cattle. In Fubini SL, Ducharme NG, editors: *Farm animal surgery,* St Louis, 2004, Elsevier.

CHAPTER 57

Osteochondrosis in Cattle

PIERRE-YVES MULON

Osteochondrosis is a skeletal disorder of growing animals that takes place in the physis or in the articular-epiphyseal cartilage complex. Osteochondrosis is a miscellaneous cause of lameness described in cattle compared with its incidence in other species (horses, pigs, and dogs).

PATHOGENESIS

Osteochondritis is a focal disturbance of the endochondral ossification, for which the exact underlying disease mechanisms remain unknown. The course of the disease is separated into different phases. Chondrocytes into the hypertrophic zone failed to pursue differentiation and mineralization of the extracellular matrix, inducing a failure in neoangiogenesis and subsequent new bone formation. The consequence is an abnormal thickening of the cartilage known as cartilage retention. Failure of invasion by sinusoidal loops into the calcifying zone combined with the increased cartilage thickness that reduces diffusion of nutrients from the synovial fluid can lead to cartilage degeneration and necrosis. Evolution of the lesion is highly dependent on the type of forces applied to the dysplastic cartilage area. Fissures or fractures of the cartilage occur in areas subjected to shear forces. Those fractures and focal cartilage weakness can evolve to a complete separation of the cartilage from the underlying subchondral bone to form a typical osteochondritis dissecans (OCD) lesion. Osteochondral fragments are formed when cartilage flaps separate entirely. In contrast, high compressive loading on dysplastic cartilage areas create cartilage infolding and resorption evolving to a subchondral bone cyst (SBC).

Predisposing factors are not well established. High-energy and protein diets have been investigated and suspected as a cause of osteochondrosis. Animals on high-intensity diets were more affected, and the lesions more severe. Low concentration of calcium was also suspected. Other nutrients like phosphorus and vitamins A and D may play a role in osteochondrosis as well. Inheritance has been suspected in grazing beef cattle when affected animals, the males, shared a common ancestral sire. Hard flooring was shown to exacerbate metaphyseal osteochondrosis lesions in calves.

CLINICAL SIGNS AND DIAGNOSIS

Onset of the lameness is gradual, and early stages can be missed, especially in large herds. Affected animals become stiffer and more reluctant to walk. Body condition is unchanged at the beginning of the disease but can deteriorate if not addressed. However, some animals do present osteochondrosis lesions at the postmortem examination without any history of lameness. Affected animals are young, with an average age ranging from 10 to 24 months.

Joint distention is variable. Lesions are bilateral in the majority of cases, although there are no obvious clinical signs (Fig. 57-1). Synovial fluid analysis is characterized by an elevated nucleated cell count, predominantly macrophages and lymphocytes and mild elevation of the proteins, which is compatible with degenerative joint diseases.

In cattle, joints commonly affected are the stifle (Fig. 57-2) and the tarsus. But osteochondrosis lesions have been diagnosed in the carpus, shoulder, and distal interphalangeal joint. In a study in which 28,235 atlanto-occipital joints were examined, 3.8% had lesions compatible with osteochondrosis. In the same study 8.5% of the 106 lame cattle had lesions of osteochondrosis, mostly in the stifle. Final diagnosis is often based on radiographic findings. Osteochondrosis dissecans, bone cysts, and physitis can be observed. In one study 79% of the lesions were considered osteochondritis dissecans,

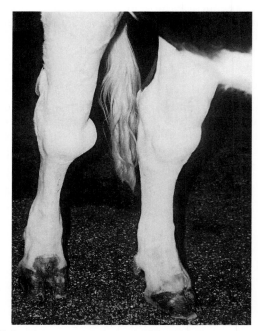

Fig 57-1 This young Holstein bull has bilateral tarsus distention because of osteochondrosis.

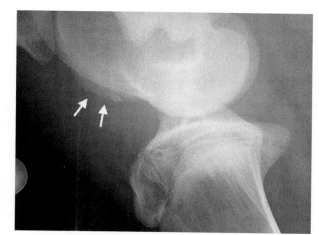

Fig 57-2 Lateromedial radiographic viewing of a stifle. Flattening of the lateral trochlear ridge of the femur *(arrows)* occurs.

and 21% of the lesions were subchondral bone cysts. Bilateral lesions of the same joint were present in 88% of the animals. Preferential sites on the stifle are the trochlear ridges of the distal femur (OCD), lateral femoral condyle (OCD), and the tibial plateau (SBC). Preferential sites in the tibiotarsal joint are the distal intermediate ridge of the tibia and the lateral and medial trochlear ridges of the talus (OCD). Both tibial malleoli are less common sites of osteochondrosis. The atlanto-occipital joint has a lesion on the occipital condyles. Those lesions were diagnosed postmortem without premortem clinical signs. The distal physis of long bones may also show signs of osteochondrosis.

TREATMENT

Analysis of feed intake and mineral supplementation should be verified when outbreaks of lameness occur in young cattle receiving a fattening ration. On an individual standpoint, animals can be treated conservatively or surgically.

Conservative treatment consists of stall rest for 1 to 3 months, and flooring should be soft to avoid cartilage while standing. Nonsteroidal antiinflammatory drugs can be administered to control the pain and decrease the swelling. In one study conservative treatment was associated with a poor prognosis. If the animal is of some value, surgical treatment should be performed rapidly before the osteoarthritis process starts. Arthroscopy is the treatment of choice for osteochondrosis lesions. Thorough evaluation of the joint and débridement of affected cartilage can be performed to promote joint surface healing with a new formation of fibrocartilage.

Surgical approaches are the same as described in horses. However, some anatomic particularities should be considered before doing arthroscopy in cattle. Skin and synovial membrane is thicker in cattle compared with horses. It may impair the arthroscope's motion amplitude into the joint. Skin incision should be slightly larger to allow free movement. Postoperatively affected animals are stall rested for 4 to 6 weeks. Nonsteroidal antiinflammatory drugs can be administered as needed. In one study, surgery was associated with a better prognosis than conservative treatment. Five of six animals treated surgically were functional in the herd compared with only 3 out of 16 treated conservatively.

Recommended Readings

Baxter GM, Hay WP, Selcer BA: Osteochondrosis dissecans of the medial trochlear ridge of the talus of a calf, *J Am Vet Med Assoc* 198:669, 1991.

Gaughan EM: Arthroscopy in food animal practice, *Vet Clin North Am Food Anim Pract* 12:233, 1996.

Hill BD, Sutton RH, Thompson H: Investigation of osteochondrosis in grazing beef cattle, *Aust Vet J* 76:171, 1998.

Jensen R, Park RD, Lauerman LH et al: Osteochondrosis in feedlot cattle, *Vet Pathol* 18:529, 1981.

Reiland S, Strömberg B, Olsson SE et al: Osteochondrosis in growing bulls: pathology, frequency and severity on different feeding, *Acta Radiologica* 358:179 (suppl), 1978.

Scott PR, Rhind S, Brownstein D: Severe osteochondrosis in two 10-month-old beef calves, *Vet Rec* 147:608, 2000.

Trostle SS, Nicoll RG, Forrest LJ et al: Clinical and radiographic findings, treatment, and outcome in cattle with osteochondrosis: 29 cases (1986-1996), *J Am Vet Med Assoc* 211:1566, 1997.

Tryon KA, Farrow CS: Osteochondrosis in cattle, *Vet Clin North Am Food Anim Pract* 15:265, 1999.

White SL, Rowland GN, Whitlock RH: Radiographic, macroscopic, and microscopic changes in growth plates of calves raised on hard flooring, *Am J Vet Res* 45:633, 1984.

CHAPTER 58

Ligament Injuries of the Stifle

ANDRÉ DESROCHERS

The most common pathologies associated with the stifle are septic arthritis, osteochondrosis, and ligament injuries. The common ligament injuries are cranial cruciate ligament rupture, lateral patellar luxation, meniscal tears, and upward fixation of the patella.

ANATOMY OF THE STIFLE

The stifle is composed of the lateral femorotibial (LFT), medial femorotibial (MFT), and femoropatellar (FP) joints. The joint capsule is attached about 1 cm proximally to the articular surface of the femoral condyles and distally to the articular margin of the tibia. The synovial membrane and the cruciate ligaments between the femoral condyles separate the joint into lateral and medial synovial sacs. The LFT joint extends distad by a projection of its synovial sac in the extensor sulcus of the tibia around the tendinous portion of the long digital extensor and peroneus tertius muscles. The FP joint is composed of the patella, which glides proximally and distally within the intertrochlear groove at the craniodistal aspect of the femur. Its synovial sac is large and extends proximad under the quadriceps muscles. The distal portion is in contact with the femorotibial joints. The medial femorotibial and the FP joint always communicate. Fifty-seven percent of the lateral femorotibial joint communicates with the other joints.

CLINICAL PRESENTATION AND DIAGNOSIS

The degree of lameness is variable depending on the condition and duration of the disease. Septic arthritis causes a non–weight-bearing lameness. This is more frequent in young animals and often secondary to a systemic infectious disease. Gait and posture of animals affected with noninfectious stifle conditions may be highly suggestive of a specific condition. Palpation of the stifle should be performed with the animal standing and in motion. Collateral ligaments and patella and joint spaces should be clearly identified and evaluated. Specific manipulation of the affected leg like adduction or abduction may help to diagnose meniscal injuries.

Complementary tests are essential to make a precise diagnosis. Radiographs, ultrasound, and arthrocentesis are frequently used. Radiographic views of the stifle are sometimes difficult to achieve, especially on adult animals because of the difficulty in inserting the cassette medially and the need for a powerful x-ray machine. Ultrasonography is helpful to evaluate the echogenicity of the synovial fluid and, more specifically, the presence of fibrin. Experienced ultrasonographers can evaluate articular cartilage, collateral ligament tears, and meniscus injury.

CRANIAL CRUCIATE LIGAMENT RUPTURE

Cranial cruciate ligament (CCL) rupture can be caused by an acute trauma like hyperextension or progressive tears secondary to degenerative joint disease (DJD). Reportedly, the cranial cruciate ligament is more likely to rupture acutely in dairy cattle, whereas DJD causes chronic fraying of the ligament with complete rupture in beef cattle.

Cranial cruciate ligament (CCL) rupture can be difficult to diagnose. The animal stands and bears weight on its toe with the stifle rotated outward and the hock inward. While walking or standing on the affected leg, crepitus or a popping sound can be heard or felt with hands on the upper leg from the stifle to the hip. Typically, the stifle is swollen and painful to palpation. A "drawer" test can be performed with the animal standing. This is easier to perform when weight is being borne on the injured limb. The examiner should stand immediately behind the affected leg and place both hands on the tibial crest by encircling the limb. Next, the examiner's knee is placed on the back of the calcaneus. A drawer test is positive if displacement or a crepitation can be felt after firm caudal traction on the tibial crest followed by a sudden release. The anatomy and function of the rear limb of cattle is such that the tibia is already displaced cranial to the femur when the CCL is ruptured. Thus movement of the tibia caudal is a sign of "positive drawer."

Radiographic images are important to confirm the diagnosis and evaluate the presence of DJD or other radiographic lesions. Radiographs should be taken with the animal standing in full weight bearing. Radiographic diagnosis of CCL rupture is based on the abnormal cranial positioning of the tibia whereabouts the intercondylar eminences of the tibia are seated cranially to the femoral condyles (Fig. 58-1). Bone fragments, soft tissue mineralization, and osteophytes can also be observed depending on the severity, chronicity, and other ligament injuries. Severe DJD is associated with a poor prognosis, so culling the animal should be considered. Meniscal injury can be associated or not to cranial cruciate ligament injuries.

Treatment options are based on the weight of the animal, radiographic findings, and value of the animal. Conservative treatment consisting of stall rest has never been associated with a good prognosis, especially on heavy animals. Therefore surgical treatment is recommended if the owner wants a productive animal for a longer period.

Different surgeries are described to correct CCL rupture. All surgeries must be performed under general anesthesia. Whichever technique is used, the heavier the animal, the

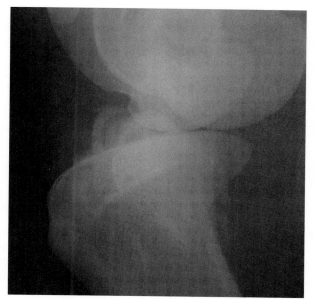

Fig 58-1 Radiographic image of the stifle, lateral view, of an adult Holstein cow. The intercondylar eminences of the tibia are seated cranially to the femoral condyles. Small bone fragments are present on the intercondylar eminences. These lesions are compatible with a rupture of the cranial cruciate ligament.

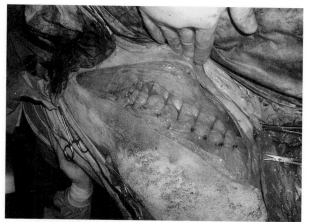

Fig 58-2 Intraoperative view of an imbrication of the joint capsule on a cow with a cranial cruciate ligament rupture.

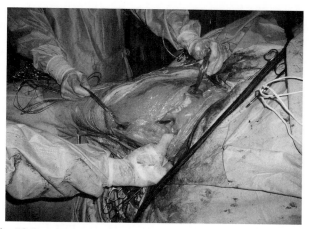

Fig 58-3 Intraoperative view of a replacement of a ruptured cranial cruciate ligament with a prosthesis made of nylon fishing line.

poorer the prognosis. On animals weighing less than 500 kg, an imbrication of the joint capsule and deep fascia has been successfully used. The imbrication is achieved with two rows of Lembert suture with nonabsorbable large-diameter suture material on the lateral and medial sides of the patella (Fig. 58-2). The overall rate of improvement after the surgery was 52%. In this study, when cattle with preoperative DJD were eliminated, the rate increased to 70.5%.

Intraarticular replacement of the cranial cruciate ligament is currently the technique of choice, especially on valuable and heavy animals. Different techniques have been described in the literature. Crawford described the use of an autogenous fascial graft from the gluteobiceps tendon. The success rate was reportedly 43% in bulls and 88% in cows. Hamilton described a different technique in which different suture materials, skin, and fascia were used to replace the CCL by tunneling them through the femur and tibia (Fig. 58-3).

Postoperatively, it is imperative that the animal should have stall rest for 6 to 8 weeks.

Supporting the leg with a splint or a Robert-Jones does not improve the prognosis. Complete failure of the implant, septic arthritis, surgical wound dehiscence, and DJD are the most common complication following this surgery. Radial paralysis has been reported on heavy animals secondary to prolonged lateral recumbency under general anesthesia.

MENISCAL INJURIES

Menisci are commonly involved simultaneously to other ligament injuries of the stifle in all species. In cattle, literature is sparse regarding the frequency of menisci lesions and cruciate or collateral ligament injuries. These injuries are most likely underestimated because they are clinically difficult to diagnose. Young or older animals can be affected. In a study reporting cattle with meniscal injuries without cruciate ligament rupture, 76% were younger than 2 years old. Lameness is variable from stiff gate to weight bearing on the toe with the leg slightly abducted. At palpation the joint is swollen. The medial collateral ligament is frequently simultaneously involved. A stretched or ruptured collateral ligament will increase the joint space at palpation, whereas a varus/valgus stress test is applied to the stifle. The medial meniscus is attached to the synovial membrane and the medial collateral ligament. Its detachment will allow axial movement while the distal limb is abducted or will protrude between the joint space when a varus stress test is applied. The same manipulations can be performed on the lateral collateral ligament, but the lateral meniscus is difficult to palpate because of the muscles covering it. Ultrasound examination may be used effectively to evaluate the menisci and the collateral ligaments damages (Fig. 58-4). However, radiographic examinations have been inconclusive to evaluate meniscal injuries.

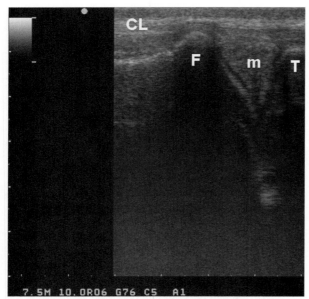

Fig 58-4 Ultrasound image of a normal medial meniscus on an adult Holstein cow. A 10-mHz ultrasound linear probe was used to obtain this image. *CL,* Collateral ligament; *F,* femur; *T,* tibia; *m,* medial meniscus.

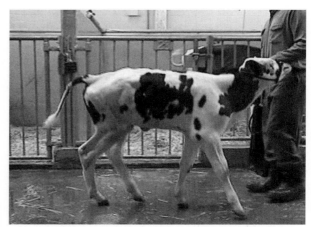

Fig 58-5 One-month-old Holstein heifer with right femoral nerve paralysis. The gait is typical of this condition, with the stifle overly flexed because of the quadriceps weakness.

If the cranial cruciate ligament is ruptured at the same time, appropriate joint stabilization of the stifle should be performed. Meniscopexy has been described to reattach the medial meniscus to its collateral ligament in animals without cruciate ligament injuries. Seventy-four percent of the animals that underwent a meniscopexy were slightly lame or sound postoperatively compared with 9% without surgery.

UPWARD FIXATION OF THE PATELLA

This is characterized by an intermittent or permanent medial and dorsal dislocation of the patella. Affected animals have a locked, hyperextended hind limb and drag it while walking. Affected animals are between 2 and 6 years of age and mostly female around parturition. Other risk factors include poor body score, rest after strenuous exercise (ox), dry season in Brazil, and type of pasture. According to some authors, Brahman-type breeds have an increased risk of upward fixation of the patella. The condition can be bilateral (27%-45%). The treatment is surgical and consists of a medial patellar ligament desmotomy standing or on lateral recumbency. Some authors combine a tenotomy of the vastus medialis muscle at its insertion on the patella. Improvement of the condition is immediate after the surgery. The success rate is reported to be 89% to 99.7%. Some cattle treated unilaterally have developed upward fixation of the patella in the untreated leg a few months after surgery.

FEMORAL NERVE PARALYSIS AND LATERAL PATELLAR LUXATION IN CALVES

Femoral nerve paralysis and lateral patellar luxation are closely related in young calves following dystocia or assisted calving. In both conditions the quadriceps muscle is ineffectual biomechanically with the incapacity to extend the stifle. Therefore the clinical signs are similar, and it is somehow difficult to differentiate each other. The femoral nerve gets damaged by being overstretched, while the extended hind limbs are engaged in the pelvic canal over the cranial border of the pelvic rim. The nerve is damaged at its entry in the quadriceps muscle. Experimental femoral nerve sections reproduced the clinical conditions.

Patellar luxation is lateral in calves. Its origin is still unclear. Femoral nerve paralysis, trauma, or congenital weakness of surrounding patellar ligaments have all been evocated as a cause of luxation. Laxity of the patella is found on calves with femoral paralysis. However, spontaneous luxation in calves with femoral nerve paralysis rarely appears.

The gait of affected animals is typical. The stifle flexes and collapses rapidly when the animal attempts to bear weight on it because of the quadriceps femoris muscle weakness (Fig. 58-5). At the same time, the hock flexes as well with the leg positioned slightly backward. Hypometria is also observed. While standing, the hip of the affected limb is lower and the lower joints flexed. No knuckling of the fetlock occurs. Muscle atrophy appears faster, and it is more severe on calves with femoral nerve paralysis. Research has shown experimentally and in clinical cases that atrophy may appear as early as 2 days after the nerve was injured and significant atrophy after 6 days. Lack of skin sensitivity may be present at the medial aspect of the tibia if the saphenous nerve has been involved in the trauma. In one study on 30 calves suffering from femoral nerve trauma, 57% had lack of skin sensitivity. The right leg is more commonly affected than the left for unknown reasons. Chronically affected animals have a prominent femur because of the atrophy (Fig. 58-6). After a while, the neurogenic atrophy may lead to patellar luxation. A complete physical examination must be performed to identify other traumatic injuries related to the dystocia (e.g., long bone fractures). Calves with bilateral femoral paralysis carry a poor prognosis.

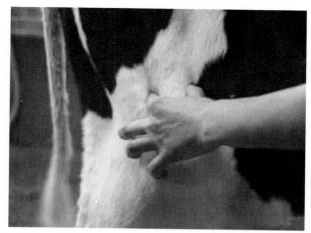

Fig 58-6   Calf with a right femoral nerve paralysis. The femur is prominent because of severe muscle atrophy.

Calves with unilateral femoral nerve paralysis need assistance to stand and nurse. After a few days they will adapt their stance. It is not possible to predict the final outcome based on the clinical signs. Depending on the severity of nerve damage, clinical signs may improve in 2 weeks to 6 months. Muscle atrophy will improve with time but rarely returns to normal.

Luxation of the patella is treated surgically under epidural or general anesthesia. If femoral nerve paralysis is the primary cause, surgery can be performed as well. It will improve the biomechanics of the stifle and recovery speed while the nerve heals and muscles strengthen. Different surgical stabilization techniques for lateral patellar luxation have been described. Medial patellar ligament prosthesis combined with a joint capsule imbrication can be performed easily without invading the stifle and without specialized orthopedic equipment. Another technique consists of shortening of the intermediate patellar ligament and the use of prosthesis between the patella and the tibial crest to keep it aligned in the trochlear ridge. Sulcoplasty is a technique of choice in other species and can also be used in calves. However, special orthopedic knowledge and equipment are necessary to accomplish this technique. Finally, in some rare cases the lateral connective tissues must be released to allow reduction of the lateral patellar luxation. If the femoral nerve is normal, clinical improvement postoperatively is rapid.

Recommended Readings

Baird AN, Angel KL, Moll HD et al: Upward fixation of the patella in cattle: 38 cases (1984-1990), *J Am Vet Med Assoc* 202:434, 1993.

Bartels JE: Femoro-tibial osteoarthrosis in the bull: I. Clinical survey and radiologic interpretation, *J Am Vet Radiol Soc* 16:151, 1975.

Crawford WH: Intra-articular replacement of bovine cranial cruciate ligaments with an autogenous fascial graft, *Vet Surg* 19:380, 1990.

Decante F: Traitement chirurgical de la laxité patellaire traumatique du veau, *GTV* March:47, 1998.

Desrochers A, St-Jean G, Cash WC et al: Characterization of anatomic communications between the femoropatellar joint and lateral and medial femorotibial joints in cattle, using intra-articular latex, positive contrast arthrography, and fluoroscopy, *Am J Vet Res* 57:798, 1996.

Ducharme NG: Stifle injuries in cattle, *Vet Clin North Am Food Anim Pract* 12:59, 1996.

Hamilton GF, Adams OR: Anterior cruciate ligament repair in cattle, *J Am Vet Med Assoc* 158:178, 1971.

Healy A: Dystocia and femoral nerve paralysis in calves, *Compend Contin Educ* 19:1299, 1997.

Hofmeyr CF: Reconstruction of the ruptured anterior cruciate ligament in the stifle of a bull, *Veterinarian* 5:89, 1968.

Huhn JC, Kneller SK, Nelson DR: Radiographic assessment of cranial cruciate ligament rupture in the dairy cow: a retrospective study, *Vet Radiol* 27:184, 1986.

Kim NS, Alam R, Lee JI et al: Trochleoplasty in lateral patellar luxation in two calves, *J Vet Med Sci* 67:723, 2005.

Kofler J: Ultrasonographic examination of the stifle region in cattle: normal appearance, *Vet J* 158:21, 1999.

Nelson DR, Huhn JC, Kneller SK: Peripheral detachment of the medial meniscus with injury to the medial collateral ligament in 50 cattle, *Vet Rec* 127:59, 1990.

Nelson DR, Koch DB: Surgical stabilisation of the stifle in cranial cruciate ligament injury in cattle, *Vet Rec* 111:259, 1982.

Silva da LAF, Fioravanti MCS, Eurides D et al: Dorsal patellar fixation in cattle: desmotomy on lateral recumbency, *Israel J Vet Med* 59:43, 2004.

Silva da OC, Silva da LAF, Fioravanti MCS et al: Occurrence and epidemiological aspects of dorsal patellar fixation in cattle, *Ciencia Animal Brasileira* 5:149, 2004.

CHAPTER 59

Coxofemoral Luxation

ANDRÉ DESROCHERS

Any condition affecting the coxofemoral joint in cattle is always serious. Although well protected by a large muscular mass, trauma can still happen. The bovine coxofemoral joint is shallow compared with other species, but there is a larger marginal cartilage of the acetabulum to compensate. Conditions affecting the hip in cattle are luxation of the coxofemoral joint, fracture of the femoral head, septic arthritis, and dysplasia. Among those, luxation of the coxofemoral joint is the most commonly diagnosed. Hip dysplasia has been reported in Charolais, Hereford, Jersey, Angus, and other breeds.

Lameness originating from the hip is difficult to diagnose because the joint cannot be seen or palpated directly. Anamnesis, stance, examination, and manipulation of the rear limb are essential to confirm or rule out a coxofemoral problem. Luxation of the coxofemoral joint occurs mainly when an animal splays on a slippery floor; when it is weak around parturition because of metabolic, neurogenic, or muscular problems; and when it is mounted while in heat. In calves, luxation occurs during a difficult calving. The luxations are mostly craniodorsal (48%-73%) or caudoventral (23%-53%). When luxated in the caudoventral position, the femoral head will be located in the obturator foramen, damaging muscles and nerves of this area and aggravating the prognosis.

PHYSICAL EXAMINATION

Complete examination of the limb from the digit to the hip helps eliminate any obvious cause of lameness. An animal with a hip problem can be standing with moderate lameness or incapable of raising or standing. If the joint is septic, the lameness is severe, or the gait quite stiff, the greater trochanter and limb are normally positioned and manipulations of the limb provoke pain. An animal affected with a dorsal luxation has a shorter-looking leg, a stifle rotated outward and looking larger, and the hock rotated inward. Although specific manipulation of the limb to diagnose luxation can be performed standing, a better examination is achieved with the animal on lateral recumbency with the affected limb uppermost. The relative position of the greater trochanter to that of the tuber coxae and the tuber ischii should be determined before the animal is laid down. The normal position of the greater trochanter is ventral to both of these bony prominences, and imaginary lines drawn between them create a "triangle." Positioning of the greater trochanter in line with the tuber coxae and tuber ischii suggests dorsal luxation of the coxofemoral joint (Fig. 59-1). Differentiating a dorsal luxation from a femoral head fracture with only the physical examination is difficult.

Radiographic imaging is necessary to confirm the diagnosis. If a ventral luxation is present, the greater trochanter cannot be seen or palpated as usual because of its abnormal medial positioning. The limb will be abducted, and most likely the animal will be down (Figs. 59-2 and 59-3). After the animal is laid down with the affected leg uppermost, the foot or the metatarsus III/IV is grasped and the entire limb rotated while performing repeated abduction and adduction motions. Fracture of the physis of the head of the femur (capital physeal fracture) should elicit crepitation of the hip that can be felt and occasionally heard. Coxofemoral joint luxation should elicit more crepitation, excessive movement of the greater trochanter, and ease of abduction if the luxation is cranioventral. Palpation and location of the femoral head per rectum can also be performed if limb manipulation is inconclusive. As reported in the literature, most cows affected with ventral luxation are presented down (68%-83%) compared with dorsal luxation (6%-43%).

MEDICAL IMAGING

Radiographic examination of the hips, when available, helps to confirm the diagnosis or identify other lesions. A powerful radiographic unit is essential to achieve readable diagnostic images. The animal has to be on dorsal

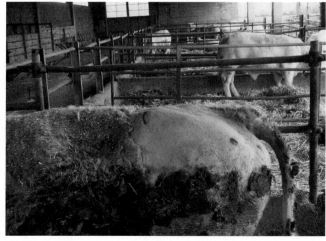

Fig 59-1 Cross-bred bull with a left coxofemoral luxation. Prominent bony surfaces of the hip are marked. The greater tubercle of the femur is aligned with the tuber coxae and the ischium, which is compatible with a dorsal luxation of the coxofemoral joint. (Courtesy Dr. Michele Ballotin, Miega, Italy.)

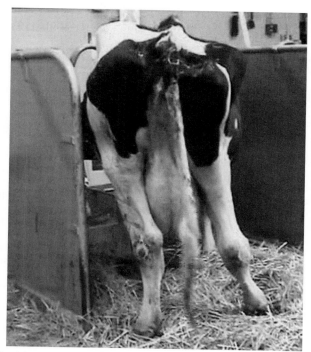

Fig 59-2   Right ventral coxofemoral luxation on a Holstein cow. The leg is abducted, and the greater trochanter cannot be seen.

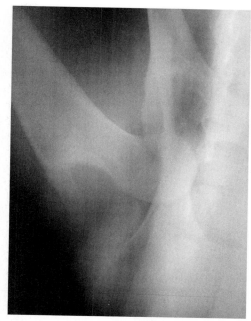

Fig 59-4   Radiographic imaging, ventro-dorsal view, of a luxated coxofemoral joint on a Holstein cow. The femoral head is caudal to the acetabulum. With this view, we cannot tell if the luxation is dorsal or ventral.

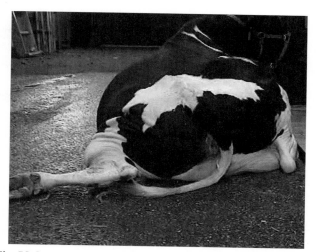

Fig 59-3   Left ventral coxofemoral luxation on a Holstein cow. She was unable to stand. The left hind limb is severely abducted with an abnormal angle.

recumbency with the hind limbs extended caudally. The examination is performed under sedation with xylazine (0.05-0.1 mg/kg IV), depending on the behavior and general status of the animal (Fig. 59-4). Recently, ultrasound examination of the normal coxofemoral joint has been described and potentially could be used to evaluate joint congruency. Arthrocentesis of the coxofemoral joint is difficult but possible. A good knowledge of the anatomy and a long needle (10-15 cm) are necessary to realize it. Arthrocentesis is more indicated if a septic process is suspected. The synovial fluid will spill out the torn joint capsule caused by luxation, rendering aspiration of fluid difficult.

TREATMENT OPTIONS

Coxofemoral luxation can be reduced by a closed or open approach, depending on the position of the femoral head and duration of clinical signs. Closed reduction is favored if the luxation occurred less than 24 hours and the luxation is dorsal. The reduction is performed with the animal on lateral recumbency under deep sedation with the affected limb uppermost, well tied to allow traction on the affected limb. Closed reduction was reported to be successful in 43% to 75% of cases. If the duration is reported to be more than 24 hours, open reduction under general anesthesia should be considered. Ventral luxation always carries a poor prognosis, whichever technique is used for reduction. Recovering animals should be kept in a small stall with deep bedding on a nonslippery floor for 2 months. Hobbles are used to prevent excessive abduction and recurrence of the luxation after reduction. In calves a modified Ehmer sling has been applied for 2 to 4 weeks, providing joint stability and allowing healing of the joint capsule (Fig. 59-5). According to one study, the prognosis factors for successful outcome were (1) standing at admission, (2) being younger than 3 years old, (3) having body weight less than 400 kg, and (4) enduring luxation less than 12 hours.

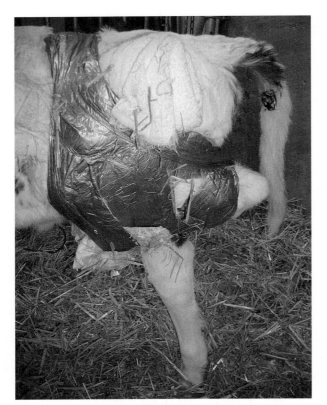

Fig 59-5   Ayrshire heifer with an Ehmer sling to prevent recurrence of a reduced dorsal coxofemoral luxation.

Recommended Readings

Agerholm JS, Basse A: Hip dysplasia in a nine-month-old male Jersey calf, *Vet Rec* 133:273, 1993.

Grubelnik M, Kofler J, Martinek B et al: [Ultrasonographic examination of the hip joint region and bony pelvis in cattle], *Berl Munch Tierarztl Wochenschr* 115:209, 2002.

Hull BL: Fractures and luxations of the pelvis and proximal femur, *Vet Clin North Am Food Anim Pract* 12:47, 1996.

Jubb TF, Malmo J, Brightling P et al: Prognostic factors for recovery from coxo-femoral dislocation in cattle, *Aust Vet J* 66:354, 1989.

Keller AM, Nuss KM, Schmid T et al: [Surgical treatment of coxofemoral luxation in two cattle], *Schweiz Arch Tierheilkd* 148:657, 2006.

Larcombe MT, Malmo J: Dislocation of the coxo-femoral joint in dairy cows, *Aust Vet J* 66:351, 1989.

Squire KR, Fessler JF, Toombs JP et al: Femoral head ostectomy in horses and cattle, *Vet Surg* 20:453, 1991.

Tulleners EP, Nunamaker DM, Richardson DW: Coxofemoral luxations in cattle: 22 cases (1980-1985), *J Am Vet Med Assoc* 191:569, 1987.

CHAPTER 60

Hygroma of the Carpus and Tarsus

PIERRE-YVES MULON

Carpal and tarsal hygromas are defined as fluid accumulation in a circumscribed cavity in the subcutaneous tissue.

ETIOLOGY

The origin of the lesion is most likely caused by repeated trauma resulting from inadequate housing conditions like sparse bedding and poorly designed cubicles. Repeated trauma over a bony surface poorly covered by soft tissue traumatizes underlying structures, resulting in a true or acquired bursitis. Olecranon, calcaneum, carpus, sternum, and tarsus are commonly affected. A true bursitis is the inflammation of an anatomic or congenital bursa. Acquired or false bursitis is formed by accumulation of fluid in subcutaneous tissue. The cavity of the acquired bursitis is lined with a synovial-like membrane without basal lamina covered by a thick connective tissue capsule. Serous fluid, blood, fibrin, and pus can be found in the cavity. *Brucella abortus* has been isolated in bursitis, but direct implication of the bacteria has never been well established.

CLINICAL SIGNS AND DIAGNOSIS

Carpal and tarsal hygromas are the most frequently diagnosed in cattle (Figs. 60-1 and 60-2). Their dimensions vary from 5 to 25 cm in diameter. Before the fluids accumulate, there is hair loss at the trauma site and skin thickening with subsequent inflammation and swelling of adjacent soft tissue. Skin can become ulcerated, predisposing the animal to infection. Lameness is rarely observed except in large hygromas because of reduced range of joint motion or if an adjacent joint gets infected. Therefore assessment of the joint is important before starting a treatment and giving an accurate prognosis.

Joint distention is rarely observed unless it is infected. Diagnosis is mostly based on physical examination. If the animal is severely lame, radiographic images of the affected area should be performed to evaluate bone and joint infection. Otherwise, ultrasonography of the mass and puncture are usually used. Puncture could be used if a septic process is suspected; otherwise, it should be avoided or performed aseptically to avoid any contamination. Ultrasound images vary depending on the cavity content. Generally the content is hypoechoic, with floating fibrin filaments associated or not with spongelike appearance areas. Fluid appears more hyperechoic in case of infection or blood. Ultrasound findings may help to decide the treatment approach.

Before establishing a treatment approach, joint cavities, tendons, tendon sheath, and natural bursa should be evaluated carefully.

TREATMENT

The cause of trauma should be identified and corrected before treating the animal. Treatment is considered if the animal is lame, the hygroma is infected, or it is for cosmetic reasons. Otherwise, the animal can live with it and be productive. Drainage and injection of the cavity with prednisolone or iodine have been used successfully in small, noninfected hygroma. If the hygroma is infected, surgical drainage, lavage with or without drains, and compressive bandages are favored instead. The same treatment can be applied on large, noninfected hygromas if en-bloc surgical resection is not possible. However, recurrences and complications are frequent. Systemic antibiotics are administered for a few days, if the capsule is surgically drained.

En-bloc resection is the treatment of choice for valuable animals and is highly successful, with a low recurrence

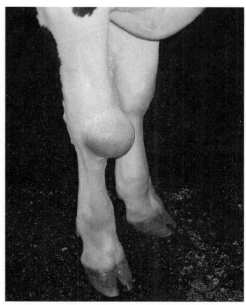

Fig 60-1 Holstein heifer with a right carpal hygroma.

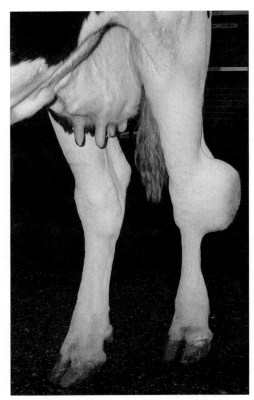

Fig 60-2   Holstein cow with a left tarsal hygroma.

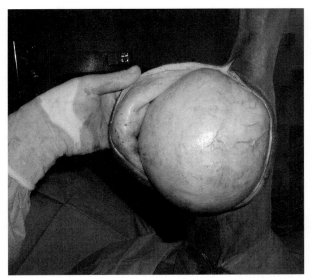

Fig 60-3   Intraoperative view of en-bloc resection of a carpal hygroma. Subcutaneous dissection is completed.

rate. Tarsal hygroma en-bloc resection is more challenging compared with carpal hygroma. The cow is positioned in dorsal or lateral recumbency with the affected limb uppermost under general anesthesia. An Esmark bandage associated with a pneumatic tourniquet can be used to reduce bleeding during the procedure. The mass is incised with a curvilinear or S-shaped incision starting 3 cm proximally and ending 3 cm distally. Curved Metzenbaum or Mayo scissors are used to bluntly dissect subcutaneous tissue surrounding the mass (Fig. 60-3). Sharp dissection between the mass and the cranial side of the carpus or the lateral side of the tarsus should be done carefully because of the presence of tendon sheets and joint capsule. After removal of the hygroma, the tourniquet is gradually loosened and hemostasis performed with USP 2-0 absorbable suture material and electrosurgery. Redundant skin is excised until skin edges can be sutured. Positive suction drain or Penrose drain can be placed if dead space could not be prevented by suturing the defect. Subcutaneous dead space is reduced by using multiple rows of sutures between skin and the underlying tissue with USP 2-0 absorbable suture material. Simple or cruciate interrupted suture pattern is used for skin closure. To decrease the chance of surgical wound dehiscence, the limb is immobilized in a compressive bandage with a polyvinyl chloride splint or a full limb cast for 15 days to limit the joint motion.

Prognosis associated with the surgical en-bloc resection of hygroma is excellent.

Complications associated with the surgical procedure are perforation of the hygroma during the dissection and subcutaneous hematoma during the postoperative period. Perforation of the mass should be considered as a major contamination of the surgical site. Dissection of the rest of the hygroma is therefore more difficult.

Recommended Readings

Anderson DE, Desrochers A, St-Jean G et al: Use of hock bandages for prevention of tarsal cellulitis (tarsal bursitis) in dairy cattle housed in a tie-stall barn, *Agri-Practice* 17(7):23-28, 1996.

Fathy A, Radad K: Surgical treatment and histopathology of different forms of olecranon and presternal bursitis in cattle and buffalo, *J Vet Sci* 7:287, 2006.

Greenough PR, Weaver DA: *Lameness in cattle*, ed 3, Philadelphia, 1997, WB Saunders.

Jann H, Slusher SU, Courtney Q: Treatment of acquired bursitis (hygroma) by en-bloc resection, *Equine Pract* 12:8, 1990.

Lemay A, Couture Y, Babkine M: Traitement chirurgical des hygromas du carpe et du tarse chez la vache laitière: 11 cas (1992-1998), *Médecin vétérinaire du Québec* 30:173, 2000.

Piguet M, Steiner A, Eicher R et al: Traitement chirurgical de l'hygroma du carpe chez les bovins: 17 cas (1990-1994), *Schweiz Arch Tierheilkd* 139:210, 1997.

Saikia B, Sarma KK: Therapeutic efficacy of prednisolone with and without ampicillin in acute carpal hygroma of bovine, *Indian Vet J* 78:635, 2001.

Seyrek-Intas D, Celimli N, Gorgul O et al: Comparison of clinical, ultrasonographic, and postoperative macroscopic findings in cows with bursitis, *Vet Radiol Ultrasound* 46:143, 2005.

SECTION VI

Neurologic Diseases of Cattle, Sheep, and Goats

Gilles Fecteau and Lisle W. George

CHAPTER 61

Clinical Examination

JOANE PARENT

NEUROLOGIC EXAMINATION OF THE RUMINANT

A neurologic examination should be performed whenever the history, complaint, or physical finding suggests involvement of the nervous system. The objective of the neurologic examination is to localize the area of the nervous system that is affected. Too often, and especially in neurology, clinicians try to fit a clinical sign to a specific disease overlooking significant abnormalities. A neurologic examination form should be used to ensure that all nerves and reflexes are evaluated, record the findings, and more adequately monitor the animal's improvement or deterioration. The list of possible causes is established based on the patients' signalment and history. Unfortunately, as is often the case in food animals, a thorough history is often unavailable. One cannot overemphasize the power of observation in food animal neurology.

The neurologic examination has six parts:

1. Mental status
2. Cranial nerves
3. Gait and posture
4. Postural reactions
5. Spinal reflexes
6. Response to pain

Of these, (1) the mental status and (2) gait and posture evaluation are the most important in terms of lesion localization.

Mental Status

The mental status evaluation offers the most important clue in differentiating intracranial from extracranial disease. Abnormalities of the mental status relate to the brainstem, or to the thalamocortex.

Brainstem: Arousal

The bulk of the brainstem parenchyma is made of the reticular formation or the so-called Ascending Reticular Activating System (ARAS). This formation is responsible for the state of arousal of the animal. When affected, the animal becomes somnolent. As the disease progresses, there is stupor, then coma. Somnolence is what is most often present at the time of examination in animals with brainstem involvement. This is characterized by an animal that is quieter but aware of its surroundings, responding adequately to stimuli in the environment. Critically assessing the behavior of the animal is of utmost importance; this is done first when the patient is nonstimulated, then when it is approached. *If a cranial nerve deficit is associated with a diminution of the state of arousal, the disease is localized to the brainstem.*

Thalamocortex: Behavior

The thalamocortex involves cognitive function. It is the center for goal-directed behavior. Abnormalities may be obvious such as in patients circling compulsively or head pressing. However, in most cases, these signs are not present. The animal is subdued, reacting poorly if at all to its environment. It may stay away from the herd. Disinterest in and disconnection from the surroundings may be evident. The animal may bump into things. In cortical disease the blindness is centrally mediated. The pupillary reflexes are normal in the light of bilateral absence of menace responses. From the veterinarian's point of view, it is frequently difficult to separate mental status abnormalities related to the cerebrum from those related to the brainstem. The information gathered during history taking and observation of the animal during examination must be critically appraised, keeping in mind the function of each of these two major parts of the brain.

The four tests of the neurologic examination that evaluate the thalamocortex include the evaluation of the mental status, menace responses, responses to nasal septum stimulation, and proprioceptive positioning. The results may be altered in the fearful animal, but the abnormalities should then be bilateral and symmetric.

Cranial Nerves

Twelve pairs of cranial nerves (CNs) exist, numbered I to XII, from the most rostral to the most caudal. Cranial nerves I (olfactory) and II (optic) are associated with the thalamocortex and are located rostrally at the base of the thalamocortex (cranial fossa). The nuclei of nerves III (oculomotor) to XII (hypoglossal) are located in the brainstem. Remembering the location of the nucleus of each of the cranial nerves greatly helps lesion localization in the presence of a centrally mediated cranial nerve deficit.

The cranial nerves are described as follows:

THALAMOCORTEX:
    I—OLFACTORY N.
    II—OPTIC N.
MIDBRAIN:
    III—OCULOMOTOR N.
    IV—TROCHLEAR N.

PONS:
   V—TRIGEMINAL MOTOR N.
ROSTRAL MEDULLA:
   V—TRIGEMINAL SENSORY N.
   VI—ABDUCENT N.
   VII—FACIAL N.
   VIII—VESTIBULOCOCHLEAR N.
CAUDAL MEDULLA:
   IX—GLOSSOPHARYNGEAL N.
   X—VAGAL N.
   XI—ACCESSORY N.
   XII—HYPOGLOSSAL N.

No reliable clinical test to evaluate nerve I (olfactory) is available. Nerve XI (accessory) has axonal inputs from the first three cervical spinal nerves, and its deficit is masked if the other nerves are intact. As a consequence, nerves I and XI are not examined.

Cranial Nerve II: Optic Nerve and Visual Pathways (Menace Response)

The role of the optic nerve is to carry the image from the retina to the visual cortex. The menace responses evaluate not only the optic nerves but also the visual pathways in their entirety (retinas, optic nerves, optic chiasm, optic tracts, optic radiations, occipital cortices). The optic nerve also requires intact facial nerves and cerebellum. All these structures must be intact to obtain a response. The visual pathways include two parts: an extra-parenchymal part in the retinas, optic nerves, and optic chiasm; and an intra-parenchymal part made of the optic tracts, optic radiations, and occipital cortices. The menace gesture must be performed adequately to obtain a reliable response. This is not a reflex because it involves the cerebrum. The presence of the menace response parallels the maturity of the cerebellum. It should be present by the end of the first week of life in food animals.

How to perform the test. The "menacing" gesture must be done at least one and a half feet from the animal's head. Avoid fanning the animal. In this instance, it is the sensory part of the trigeminal nerve that is stimulated. The hand that does not menace holds the opposite side of the animal's head while covering the eye that is not examined. The responses from each side are compared. In the cow, there is no need to obstruct the eye that is not examined because the eyeballs are positioned laterally.

Cranial Nerve III: Oculomotor Nerve: Pupillary Light Reflexes

The retinas, optic nerves, and optic chiasm represent the afferent pathways of the pupillary light reflexes, whereas the oculomotor nerves (III) are the efferent pathways. The menace gesture, when present, assuming that facial nerve and cerebellum are intact, indicates integrity of the visual pathways. If the pupil is dilated and nonresponsive to light, then this indicates dysfunction of or damage to ipsilateral CN III (oculomotor). If the menace gesture is absent, assuming the animal can blink and there are no cerebellar signs, a dysfunction along the visual pathways has occurred. If the pupillary light reflexes are present, the blindness is centrally mediated, above the optic chiasm, at the level of the thalamocortex.

How to perform the test. The pupils are observed for (1) size at rest, (2) symmetry, and (3) pupillary light reflexes.

Size at rest. The normal animal has larger than normal pupils on examination due to the fear created by the examination or hospital environment. In progressive cerebral disease, the pupils may be smaller than normal. This finding should not be overlooked because it may be an indication of increased intracranial pressure.

Symmetry. The pupils are evaluated for symmetry before stimulation with a light source. The evaluation for symmetry is best done with the animal in a relatively dark environment using a direct ophthalmoscope. The examiner holds the animal's head at arm's reach with one hand, directing the light source equally toward the animal's eyes with the other. This allows equal stimulation of each pupil simultaneously. The pupil size is examined through the ophthalmoscope. The impression is as "a deer in the headlight."

Pupillary light reflexes. A strong light source must be used to overcome the stress response of the pupils. The use of a transilluminator is strongly recommended. The light beam is directed in a naso-temporal direction toward the temporal region of the retina, where the concentration of rods and cones is at its highest. In the normal animal the pupils should constrict down to 3 to 5 mm.

CN III: Oculomotor; CN IV: Trochlear; CN VI: Abducent

These three nerves are examined as a functional unit. They are responsible for conjugate eye movements. Look first for presence of strabismus (permanent abnormal position of the eyeball). The oculomotor nerve is the major nerve controlling eye movements. In my experience, the "down-and-out" strabismus associated with CN III paralysis is an uncommon occurrence. Instead, the eyeball on the affected side appears immobile in the orbit when the physiological nystagmus is induced. In CN IV deficit, the medial aspect of the pupil deviates dorsally causing a dorsomedial strabismus. The CN VI is responsible for the retraction of the globe and its deficit causes the eyeball to be more forward. Deficits of CN VI are easily missed.

How to perform the test. Nerves III, IV, and VI are evaluated as a functional unit by observing for presence of a strabismus and indirectly by inducing the physiological nystagmus. In the ruminants, it is best to look at the eye position with the head in a normal position. The best is to not touch the head while the observation is done. Elevating the head often causes aberrant eyeball positions; commonly, there is a ventral and dorsomedial strabismus.

Physiologic nystagmus. The test is performed with the examiner facing the animal and moving the animal's head horizontally from side to side, observing for coordinated conjugate eye movements. The nystagmus should be brisk. The physiologic nystagmus involves the eye muscles; cranial nerves III, IV, and VI; the medial longitudinal fasciculus (MLF); and cranial nerves VIII. It is by the MLF that the information travels from the vestibular apparatus (proprioception for the head) to cranial nerves III, IV, and VI. All these structures must be intact for coordinated conjugate eye movements to occur.

CN V: Trigeminal Nerve; Ophthalmic, Maxillary, and Mandibular Branches

The trigeminal nerve has two functions: (1) innervation of the masticatory muscles (mandibular nerve) and (2) sensation for most of the head.

How to perform the test. The masticatory muscles are palpated for symmetry and atrophy. A unilateral involvement is represented by unilateral atrophy, whereas bilateral involvement leads to a dropped jaw. The sensory part of the nerve is assessed through the palpebral reflexes. In these reflexes the trigeminal nerve is the afferent limb (sensory), while the facial nerve is the efferent limb (motor). The ophthalmic branch is assessed by touching the medial canthus and observing for a blink reflex. The maxillary branch is assessed by touching the lateral canthus and observing for a blink reflex. The mandibular branch is assessed by touching the base of the ear and observing for a blink reflex. The indicated areas to touch are the only ones that consistently give a blink reflex in the normal animal. The canthus is the region where the lid margins meet.

Touching the canthi and the ear assesses all three parts of the reflex but **does not** assess if the information reaches the cerebral cortex. This is evaluated by stimulating the nasal septum. The animal may or may not blink, but the head is pulled away as a pain response. This test should be done gently using cotton swabs or the small finger so as to reveal subtle differences between sides. Start with a gentle stimulus and gradually increase the strength of the stimulus going from side to side, until a consistent response (normal or not) is obtained. The nasal septum is the only area that consistently elicits a cortical response in the domestic species. For this test, it is best not to restrain the animal's head.

Cranial Nerve VII: Facial Nerve

At this stage of the examination, the examiner has some knowledge of the function of the facial nerves because the nerves were involved in the menace responses and the palpebral reflexes.

How the test is performed. The ears, eyelids, lip commissures, and nostrils are observed for symmetry and function. To evaluate the symmetry of the lip commissures, it is helpful to lift the animal's head with a finger on the mandibular symphysis. Then the strength of the palpebral closures is evaluated. The normal animal closes his eyelids completely on the first gentle stroke of a finger on the upper and lower lids at once.

Cranial Nerve VIII: Vestibulo-Cochlear Nerve

The **cochlear** part of the nerve can be objectively assessed only with the use of electrodiagnostic testing (brain auditory evoked responses).

The **vestibular** part is evaluated by observing for the presence of a head tilt (salient feature of vestibular dysfunction) and abnormal nystagmus. The presence of a head tilt is best assessed when the animal's head is facing the examiner, by pulling an imaginary line through both eyes. The line should be horizontal. If a pathologic nystagmus is observed with the head at rest (resting), its direction should be noted. The fast phase of the nystagmus is usually directed away from the side of the lesion.

The head should then be elevated, and the eyes observed for induction of a nystagmus (positional) or a change in the direction of the nystagmus. Vertical nystagmus and a nystagmus that changes in direction indicate brainstem disease at the level of the eighth cranial nerve nucleus.

CN IX: Glosso-Pharyngeal and CN X: Vagal Nerves

These nerves are evaluated together as a functional unit. Their abnormalities are disclosed on observation alone. Airway compromise (larynx) leads to difficulty breathing, dyspnea (noisy respirations), snoring, and voice change. Pharyngeal problems lead to dysphagia clinically characterized by choking, gagging, drooling from an inability to swallow saliva, and food coming out of the nostrils.

Cranial Nerve XII: Hypoglossal Nerve

At this stage an experienced examiner has already observed the animal licking its lips during the examination. If not, pull the tongue out of the mouth and observe the tongue. Look for deviation and atrophy. Tongue tone may appear decreased in the sick animal from the overall ill-being state of the animal. Motor neuron disease may be associated with difficulty in food prehension, tongue atrophy ± deviation, and fasciculations of the tongue.

Gait and Posture

The cow is allowed to walk freely in an enclosed area, or in the goat, sheep, and calf, it is relatively easy to make them walk with a lead using a food item or milk bottle. The owner should walk the animal at slow pace, back and forth, in the direction of the examiner. The clinician should observe the front limb gait as the animal approaches, and the hind limb gait should be evaluated as the animal walks away. Particular attention is given to the foot placement as the animal turns or changes direction and speed. A series of questions are then answered.

1. Is the animal able to walk?
2. Is the gait normal?
3. Which limb(s) is/are affected? One limb, both hind limbs, the hind and front limbs, or the ipsilateral limbs?
4. Is there presence of ataxia?
5. If there is ataxia, of which type? Vestibular, cerebellar, or proprioceptive?
6. Is there postural abnormality? Hunching of the back, low head carriage, or opisthotonus?

These questions should not be left unanswered. The evaluation of the gait is extremely important in lesion localization. If unsure, the gait should be examined for a longer period.

There are three types of ataxia: vestibular, cerebellar, and proprioceptive.

Vestibular Ataxia

The vestibular ataxia is *always* associated with a head tilt. The animal leans, falls or turns on itself toward the side the head is tilted. Be aware of the animal that circles without a head tilt. In most cases where circling is observed, it is associated with thalamocortical lesion and does not have a vestibular in origin. With bilateral vestibular dysfunction, the head tilt is often subtle on the side that is more affected but there is a characteristic striking head carriage. The head moves with wide excursions.

Cerebellar Ataxia

Strength is preserved, and there are no proprioceptive deficits. The ascending proprioceptive pathways from the limbs to the cerebrum and the descending motor pathways (upper motor neurons [UMNs]) from the cerebrum to the limbs are intact. Consequently with cerebellar ataxia, there are no proprioceptive deficits (no knuckling) or weakness. All four limbs are affected if the lesion is bilateral, or the ipsilateral front and rear limbs if the disease is unilateral. Clinically, diffuse involvement of the cerebellum is more frequent than unilateral involvement.

Proprioceptive Ataxia

This ataxia is also called *spinal ataxia* because it is usually observed with spinal cord disease. Although proprioceptive pathways are part of the brainstem and thalamocortex, it is unusual to have proprioceptive ataxia with head disease even though proprioceptive positioning test is delayed to absent unilaterally in these patients. Proprioceptive ataxia is secondary to damage of the ascending proprioceptive pathways. A concomitant weakness always occurs because of the simultaneous involvement of the descending motor pathways (UMNs). It is the concomitant presence of weakness that helps in differentiating this ataxia from the cerebellar ataxia. Proprioceptive ataxia is the most difficult of the three types of ataxia to recognize, especially in its early stage. Ruling out the two others is often easier.

How the test is done. The evaluation of the gait is by far the best proprioceptive test. Observing the cerebrospinal axis in relation to the foot placement while the animal walks freely, putting its head down to sniff and elevating the head to look around while walking, and changing direction, are all great ways to evaluate proprioception. The animal can be made to circle or be pulled by the tail while the examiner observes the foot placement. Moreover, lower motor neuron (LMN) deficits are present in the gait. In the cow the gait evaluation is all that is possible to assess if there are proprioceptive deficits or LMN disease. One cannot overemphasize the keen observation necessary during evaluation of the gait.

Postural Reactions

The postural reactions complement the evaluation of the gait. By themselves, they are of little localizing value. Their usefulness is best in identifying asymmetry between sides and front and hind limbs. Proprioceptive positioning (knuckling) and hopping are the only two postural reactions that I perform. Proprioceptive positioning, if done appropriately, evaluates proprioception. Hopping as done in canine neurologic examination is not usually performed because of the size of the large animal patient.

How to perform the tests. Postural reaction testing can be performed in the goat, sheep, and calf as it is done in large dogs. To evaluate proprioceptive positioning of the hind limbs, the clinician is positioned behind the animal. The animal's weight must be supported with the forearm and hand placed between and behind the hind limbs. For the evaluation of the front limbs, the examiner is positioned on the side of the animal, down on one knee while the other is bent under the animal thorax. With the back of his or her forearm and hand on his or her knee, the animal's chest is supported while the hoof is slowly knuckled. This test cannot be performed appropriately in wild or aggressive animals. The examiner looks for asymmetry between sides or between front and hind limbs.

Hopping is evaluated with each limb and can only be performed on smaller-sized animals. The animal is kept on the same plane. With the examiner positioned on the left side of the animal, the animal's right front limb is hopped laterally, while the examiner holds the left front limb off the ground and pushes the animal gently toward the right side. The left limb is held off the ground with the animal's shoulder joint. Avoid performing the test folding the limb over because most animals resent it. The left front limb is evaluated in a reverse manner. For the hind limbs, the front end of the animal acts naturally as a pivot. The examiner is positioned behind the patient. The right hind limb is hopped *laterally*, pushing the animal sideways with its left hind limb. This left limb is held off the ground by the tibia while the examiner pushes the animal toward the right side. The left hind limb is evaluated in a reverse manner.

Spinal Reflexes

Flexor and extensor reflexes are evaluated for the front and the hind limbs. In the sheep, goat and calf, the spinal reflexes are examined with the animal in lateral recumbency, the side being evaluated in the upper position.

Extensor Reflex of Front Limb

The extensor reflexes of the front limb assess the radial nerves and are evaluated by observing if the animal can bear weight on either of the front limbs. The radial nerve is responsible for weight bearing in the front limb. If the animal is down and too heavy to be made to stand, the extensor reflex is evaluated by observing if extensor tone can be raised in the limb. This is done putting a hand under the foot of the animal and pushing the limb gently toward the animal until extensor tone appears.

Patellar Reflex

The patellar reflex evaluates the motor and sensory components of the femoral nerve. The femoral nerve is responsible for hip flexion and stifle extension. It is the nerve responsible for weight bearing in the hind limb. The patellar reflex is a tendinous reflex. The reflex is elicited by tapping the patellar tendon and observing an extension of the stifle. The limb should be in a relaxed flexion. The flexion should be just enough so that the tendon is tight. The tendon is first palpated. Then while keeping the fingers on the tendon, the limb is flexed until the tendon feels tight. It helps raise tension in the tendon by putting a hand under the foot while extending the digits. The tapping on the tendon is done with a pendulum motion. If the limb is tense, the reflex will not be elicited. By tapping the tendon rhythmically, the animal relaxes with time. The strength of the reflex is proportional to the force applied to the tendon. The plexor used in large dogs is adequate in the goat, sheep, and smaller calf, but larger instruments must be used in heavier animals.

In LMN disease affecting the femoral nerve, the animal walks dragging the affected limb behind and is unable to bear weight on the limb and with the foot knuckled over.

Withdrawal (Flexor) Reflexes
In the front limbs the flexor reflex evaluates the axillary, median, and ulnar nerves. In the hind limb the reflex evaluates the motor part of the sciatic nerve. However, the sensory function of the lateral part of the limb is provided by the sciatic nerve and the medial part by the femoral nerve. Consequently, for the flexor reflex to occur, the sensory part of both nerves, femoral and sciatic, must be intact. The flexor reflex is examined by pinching (a hemostat is often necessary to elicit a reliable reflex response) the lateral digit while observing a flexion of the limb. Then the medial digit is pinched, and the examiner observes again for a flexion of the limb. Because of secondary myopathy from prolonged recumbency, flexor reflexes may be difficult to interpret. With loss of the LMN to the limb, there is weak or absence of flexion of one or more joints. In UMN disease, the joints flex, but the overall strength with which this is done may be decreased.

Animals that have lesions in the distal sciatic nerve walk with a plantigrade (or palmigrade in the front limb) stance in the limb affected. If the lesion involves the proximal part of the sciatic nerve, the affected limb has an exaggerated hip flexion accompanied by a nonflexion of the hock.

Perineal Reflex
The perineal region is delineated by a change in the growth of the hair surrounding the anus. This reflex is assessed by gently touching with a finger or a cotton swab the perineal region of the animal under its tail. Avoid manipulating the tail because this causes a contraction of the anus, preventing the examiner from assessing the sensory part of the reflex because the anus is already contracted.

The reflex is evaluated on each side, separately. The expected response is a downward contraction of the tail and an accompanying anal sphincter contraction. Performed in this manner, the afferent limb of the tail movement reflex is the sensory part of the pudendal nerve while the efferent limb consists of the caudal nerves. To evaluate the motor part of the pudendal nerve, a rectal examination observing the anal sphincter strength is preferable.

Cutaneous Trunci Reflex
Applying stimulation multiple times is sometimes necessary to elicit this reflex. The afferent limb of this reflex is made of the regional spinal nerves, which carry the impulse to the eighth cervical and first thoracic spinal segments by way of the spinal cord white matter. The

impulses created by pinching the skin on one side ascend the spinal cord bilaterally. The efferent limb is the lateral thoracic nerve, which causes the skin to flinch. The reflex is elicited by pinching the skin with a hemostat, from the level of the wing of the ilium to T2, approximately 1 inch on either side of the dorsal processes. The reflex is evaluated on both sides. If the reflex is present at the level of the wing of the ilium, there is no need to assess its presence any farther along the animal's back because the afferent limb must be intact all the way to allow the contraction of the cutaneous trunci muscles by the lateral thoracic nerve (which originates from the C8 and T1 spinal segments but mainly from C8).

Pain Perception

Response to pain is evaluated at the end of the examination so as to keep the patient's cooperation. With experience, one realizes that it does not always need to be examined because many clues are gleaned during the examination to inform the clinician about the presence of pain perception. Because of the nature of our patients, the expressions "deep" and "superficial" pain should probably not be used in veterinary medicine. Decreased, increased, or absence of pain perception occurs.

Neck/Back Pain
The animal posture is observed during the gait evaluation. Animals with neck pain move as a block, avoiding turning their head/neck as they change direction. They look up with their eyes only, avoiding lifting their head. Animals with back pain have a hunched back. The back is palpated for presence of back pain. The palpation is performed from the upper thoracic to the lumbosacral region.

CONCLUSION

The neurologic examination of the ruminant is an exercise in observation. Even if the animal cannot be approached, the behavior, gait, posture, and most cranial nerves can be evaluated at a distance. A neurologic form should always be completed. Although the examination when performed on a regular basis becomes routine, the form is a legal document and serves as a checkpoint ensuring that all tests have been done. More importantly, it is an invaluable document in the follow-up and monitoring of the neurologic patient.

Recommended Readings
DeLahunta A: *Veterinary neuroanatomy and clinical neurology,* ed 2, Philadelphia, 1983, Saunders, pp 389-406.
Mayhew IG: *Large animal neurology: a handbook for veterinary clinicians,* Philadelphia, 1989, Lea & Febiger, pp 15-47.
Parent J: *The canine and feline neurological examination CD ROM* (website): www.neuroexamination.com. Accessed December 5, 2007.

CHAPTER 62

Ancillary Tests

DAVID FRANCOZ

Neurologic examination may lead to the localization of the lesion and establishment of a differential diagnostic list. Based on the results, different diagnostic tests may be performed to determine a precise diagnosis. Because of cost and availability and the requirements for general anesthesia, electrophysiologic diagnostic tests that are available in neurologic investigation of small animals are not performed routinely in ruminant medicine. However, the veterinary practitioner should be aware of the diagnostic tests that are useful in the diagnosis of neurologic diseases. Indeed, this will allow an adequate decision based on the cost-benefit ratio of these tests in order to provide the best service to their clients. The following tests are recommended for evaluation of neurologic patients.

COMPLETE BLOOD COUNT AND SERUM BIOCHEMISTRY PROFILE

A baseline workup should include a complete blood count (CBC) and serum biochemistry profile (SBP), the general health status of the animal, and the integrity of particular body systems. This information is useful for diagnostic purposes and for the establishment of a therapeutic plan including supportive treatments. The anomalies observed may be primary or secondary to the neurologic disorder. Hematologic findings range from normal to those consistent with an inflammatory process, lymphocytosis, platelet disorders, and coagulopathy. The SBP provides information on the integrity of the musculoskeletal, hepatic, and renal systems and may also reveal electrolyte imbalances.

In most situations results are not specific, but they can strengthen the suspicion of a precise diagnosis. For example, hepatic encephalopathy is strongly suspected when hepatic failure is documented in association with clinical signs of central nervous system (CNS) disorders. Salt toxicity may be confirmed by the finding of hypernatremia (>160 mEq/L).[1] Hypomagnesemia is diagnosed when serum concentration of magnesium is less than or equal to 1.2 mg/dl.[2]

CEREBROSPINAL FLUID ANALYSIS

Analysis of cerebrospinal fluid (CSF) is easily performed and is relatively inexpensive. The test provides useful information about the type of neurologic lesion that is present. The CSF is located within the subarachnoidal space, where it surrounds the central nervous system. Consequently, diseases involving the brain or spinal cord may lead to modifications of the CSF. However, CSF analysis may remain normal even in the case of advanced and severe CNS lesions. The CSF may be evaluated for gross physical appearance, total nucleated cells count and differential, red blood cell count, total protein concentration and fractioning, and biochemical composition (electrolytes, enzymes).

Collection of Cerebrospinal Fluid

CSF can be collected at either the atlanto-occipital or lumbosacral space. In ruminants the CSF can be easily and safely collected at the lumbosacral space.[3-5] However, one should also be concerned about the risk of tentorial herniation when performing CSF tap on an animal with suspected highly increased intracranial pressure, as in cases of salt poisoning or polioencephalomalacia. In such cases the animal should be stabilized first. Lumbosacral CSF tap requires minimal immobilization and, in rare cases, sedation. It can be performed on a standing or recumbent animal. The procedure and necessary materials are described in Figs. 62-1 and 62-2. Collection of CSF from the atlanto-occipital is more hazardous. This procedure must be performed on animals under general anesthesia or at least heavily sedated.[6] Theoretically, CSF should be collected as near as possible to the suspected lesion. However, in ruminants, apart from some rare cases of focal spinal compression, it seems that there are no substantial differences between the composition of CSF collected from the atlanto-occipital and the lumbosacral spaces.[7]

Examination of Cerebrospinal Fluid

Gross Physical Appearance

Normal CSF is clear, colorless, and does not clot. Inflammatory CSF is cloudy and clots after collection. A red-colored CSF is a consequence of blood contamination, which can result from the collection procedure or from a preexisting hemorrhage. The two conditions can be differentiated by noting the timing of the hemorrhage appearance during sample collection.[8-10] In the case of a preexisting hemorrhage, the CSF is uniformly red and does not clot. In the case of blood contamination, the CSF is heterogeneous, with redness often decreasing in intensity as further CSF is withdrawn, and may clot. After centrifugation of the CSF, the supernatant of samples with blood contamination appears clear and colorless. If previous hemorrhage is present, the sample remains red or xanthochromic. Finally, in cases of previous hemorrhage, erythrophagy (presence of phagocyted red blood cells in macrophages)[9] is usually seen.

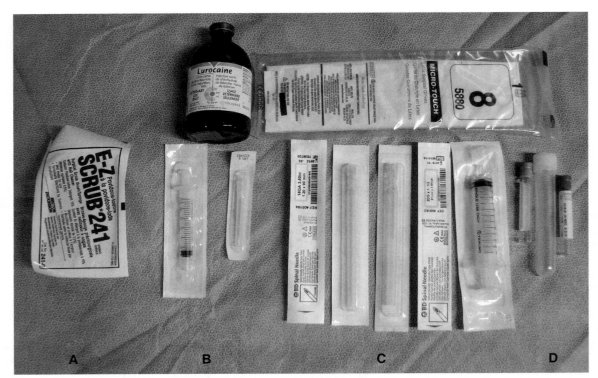

Fig 62-1   Necessary materials for collection of cerebrospinal fluid (CSF) in cattle. The site for aspiration is first clipped and surgically prepared **(A)**. The skin is anesthetized with 2% lidocaine **(B)**. Spinal needles that are 18 gauge and 3.5 to 8 inches and 20 gauge and 1.5 to 3.5 inches are used in adult and young animals, respectively **(C)**. Sterile gloves must be used **(C)**. The CSF collected is transferred into an EDTA tube for cytology, dry tube for biochemistry analysis, and/or sterile tube for culture **(D)**.

Xanthochromia is a slight orange to yellow coloration of the CSF. Xanthochromia may be due to the presence of pigment secondary to red blood cell lysis, increased content of protein, or bilirubin.[6,8,9]

Cytologic Examination

Because cells in the CSF degenerate rapidly, cytologic examination should be performed rapidly after collection, ideally within 30 minutes, but within 2 hours is considered acceptable.[5,8] This is an important limitation to the realization of cytologic analysis of CSF under field conditions. However, cells may be preserved by mixing the CSF samples with an equal volume of 40% to 50% ethanol.[8,11] A sedimentation chamber can also be used for the preparation of slides that can be stained and analyzed at the clinic or sent to a diagnostic laboratory for analysis.[5,12] A total nucleated cell count is first performed using a hemacytometer. Morphologic cell evaluations and differential counts are then determined on cytocentrifuged or decanted samples stained with a Romanovsky-type (e.g., Wright-Giemsa) stain. In normal CSF, only mononuclear cells are present and neutrophils are detected in small numbers. Normal values have been reported in ruminants.[1,3] The normal CSF is also free of red blood cells. Minor blood contamination should be expected when lumbosacral taps are performed. Depending on the amount, the contamination may influence the total nucleated cell and differential[3] counts. An accepted formula that allows accurate correction of the total nucleated cells for the amount of blood contamination does not exist.[3,13] However, studies have demonstrated that minimal blood contamination does not interfere with adequate interpretation of the CSF analysis.[3,13]

Total nucleated cells count and differential. An increase in the number of nucleated cells indicates inflammation. Which cellular population predominates may help in determining the cause. Viral diseases are usually characterized by a lymphocytic pleocytosis, whereas bacterial diseases are manifested by a neutrophilic pleocytosis.[6,14] One exception is *Listeria monocytogenes* infection, which is associated with increased numbers of mononuclear cells.[15,16] Duration of the disease and treatments may alter the result. In cases of bacterial meningitis, neutrophils predominate in the acute phase, whereas chronic or treated cases are reflected by a predominance of macrophages and mononuclear cells.[17,18] Mild mononuclear pleocytosis can also be associated with degenerative diseases, hemorrhagic processes, neoplasia, idiopathic myelopathy, and polioencephalomalacia.[6,14,19]

Cellular morphologic changes can also provide useful information. Degenerative changes of neutrophils or neutrophils phagocyting bacteria may be observed in cases of bacterial infection.[12,18] Atypical and large lymphocytes may be present in the CSF of cows suffering from lymphosarcomas. These tumors are extradural. However, CSF analysis may provide the final diagnosis secondary to

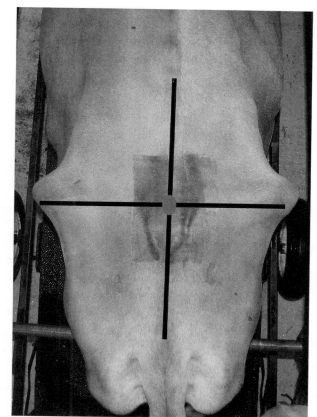

Fig 62-2 Anatomic site for collection of cerebrospinal fluid (CSF) at the lumbosacral space. The spinal needle is slowly inserted perpendicularly to the point where a line drawn between the caudal aspects of the two tuber coxae intersects the midline (between the L6 vertebra and S1 vertebra). The animal may react (twitching) when the spinal needle passes through the interacuate ligament and penetrates the extradural space. At this time a loss of resistance is felt. The needle is further inserted to reach the subarachnoid space. A gentle negative pressure can be applied to withdraw the CSF into a syringe.

exfoliation of tumoral cells within the CSF, concurrent involvement of the spinal cord,[19] or needle aspiration through a tumor located in the lumbosacral area.[20]

Red blood cells and pathologic hemorrhage. Pathologic hemorrhage, characterized by the presence of red blood cells, erythrophagocytosis and xanthochromia, occurs after CNS trauma, inflammation, degenerative diseases, and neoplasia.[6,9]

Protein Concentrations and Fractioning

The normal concentrations of protein in the CSF are low. Increased CSF protein concentrations are associated with intradural inflammation or hemorrhage. Protein fractioning or determination of the presence of specific proteins does not appear to provide useful information in ruminants, whereas it may provide useful information in other species.[7]

Biochemical Assays

Cerebrospinal fluid glucose, electrolyte, and enzyme (CK and LDH) concentrations are not routinely evaluated in ruminant medicine. Reported normal concentrations of glucose in the CSF are approximately 80% of the contemporary blood glucose concentrations. Decreases in CSF glucose concentrations have been associated with bacterial infections.[12,21] Increased CK and LDH CSF concentrations have been associated with neurologic diseases.[21,22] However, they provide little additional information in the establishment of a precise diagnosis.

In some cases of salt poisoning (hypernatremia) and hypomagnesemia, animals may present neurologic signs despite normal serum electrolyte values.[1,2] In such cases, determination of Na and Mg CSF concentrations may help. Sodium CSF concentrations above 160 mEq/L or a CSF/serum-sodium ratio greater than 1 is diagnostic for salt poisoning.[1] Likewise, a magnesium CSF concentration below 1.45 mg/dl is sufficient for diagnosis of hypomagnesemia.[2] However, CSF is difficult to obtain on animals with clinical signs of hypomagnesemia.

Bacteriologic Examination

Bacteriologic culture of CSF can be performed. In cases of meningitis in calves, success rates of culture have been reported to be 50% to 60%.[18,19,23] Centrifugation of the CSF sample before culture may increase bacterial culture rate.[12] Although bacteriologic culture of CSF provides little additional diagnostic information,[9,19] the results may influence the antibiotic treatment. Because these procedures require time, empirical antibiotic treatment may be instituted first based on Gram stain coloration of the CSF or likelihood of a disease.

In some cases of bacterial infection of the CNS, bacterial culture may be disappointing. For example, culture of *Histophilus somni* requires special media. *Listeria monocytogenes* is rarely cultured from the CSF, even if special culture techniques are used.

MEDICAL IMAGING

Radiography and Myelography

Radiology is indicated for the diagnosis of skull trauma, spinal cord trauma (vertebral fracture), vertebral malformation or vertebral osteomyelitis. Rigorous clinical examination must be performed first to localize the affected region of the CNS.

Myelography can provide useful information for compressive lesions of the spinal cord. However, this is rarely used in farm animals. The technique is limited to referral centers, is expensive, and requires general anesthesia. Furthermore, results of myelography rarely affect the treatment options and prognosis.

Computed Tomography and Magnetic Resonance Imaging

In small animals, computed tomography (CT) and magnetic resonance imaging (MRI) are the most useful ancillary tests for the diagnosis of CNS disorders. Unfortunately, they are rarely used in farm animal medicine.

These tests are expensive, must be performed under general anesthesia, and are limited to calves and small ruminants in referral centers. As examples, CT has been used for the diagnosis and the management of otitis media in calves and a heifer[24,25] and discospondylitis,[26] a cerebral abscess,[27] and a glioma[28] in goats. Case reports of MRI diagnosis of brainstem abscess and hydrocephalus,[29] cerebellar hypoplasia,[30] or spinal cord compression by a mass[31] have been described.

Ultrasonography

Because of the bone structures that surround the CNS, ultrasonography is of limited value for the diagnosis of CNS diseases. However, transorbital echoencephalography has been reported for the diagnosis of hydranencephaly.[32]

ELECTROPHYSIOLOGY— ELECTRODIAGNOSTIC

Tests that evaluate the abnormal changes in cellular electrical activity include electromyography, electroencephalography, electroretinography, brainstem auditory evoked potentials, and somatosensory evoked potentials.[33-40] However, the necessity for highly specialized equipment limits their use to referral and research centers.

Electromyography is used for the detection of lower motor neuron or motor unit disorders (myopathies, peripheral nerves disorders). Electroencephalography is useful for the diagnosis of diffuse or local intracranial diseases (polioencephalomalacia, hydrocephaly, transmissible spongiform encephalopathy, epilepsy). Brainstem auditory evoked potentials are useful for the evaluation of the cranial nerve VIII and the auditory pathway along the brainstem (otitis media, listeriosis). Electroretinography and visual evoked response are used for the differentiation between retinal and central blindness, as well as the evaluation of the central visual pathway (polioencephalomalacia, listeriosis). Somatosensory-evoked potentials evaluate the functional capacity of the sensory pathway.[41]

PERIPHERAL NERVE AND MUSCULAR BIOPSIES

Peripheral nerve and muscular biopsies can be performed when a neuropathy is suspected and differentiation from a myopathy is required. It must be noted, however, that diagnostic accuracy is increased when the tissues are examined by a neuropathologic specialist.[41]

OTHER SPECIFIC DIAGNOSTIC TESTS

Specialized tests that may be indicated for the diagnosis of specific diseases include erythrocyte transketolase activity for the diagnosis of polioencephalomalia,[42] fecal examination for the presence of coccidia, and toxicologic sampling.

In cases of suspected congenital defects of the CNS (hydranencephaly or cerebellum hypoplasia) in calves secondary to fetal infection by bovine virus diarrhea virus, precolostral antibody titers and viral detection may be performed.[1]

References

1. Smith MO: Diseases of the nervous system. In Smith BP, editor: *Large animal internal medicine*, St Louis, 2002, Mosby, pp 873-1017.
2. Blackwelder JT, Hunt E: Disorders of magnesium metabolism. In Smith BP, editor: *Large animal internal medicine*, St Louis, 2002, Mosby, pp 1256-1261.
3. Welles EG, Tyler JW, Sorjonen DC, Whatley EM: Composition and analysis of cerebrospinal fluid in clinically normal adult cattle, *Am J Vet Res* 53:2050-2057, 1992.
4. Scott PR: Collection and interpretation of cerebrospinal fluid in ruminants, *Practitioner* 15:298-300, 1993.
5. Ferrouillet C, Fecteau G, Lanevschi A: Prélèvement et analyse du liquide céphalo-rachidien chez les bovins, *Point Vet* 29:15-20, 1998.
6. DeLahunta A: Cerebrospinal fluid and hydrocephalus. In DeLahunta A, editor: *Veterinary neuroanatomy and clinical neurology*, Philadelphia, 1983, Saunders, pp 30-52.
7. Scott PR: The collection and analysis of cerebrospinal fluid as an aid to diagnosis in ruminant neurological disease, *Br Vet J* 151:603-614, 1995.
8. Hayes TE: Examination of cerebrospinal fluid in the horse, *Vet Clin North Am Equine Pract* 3:283-291, 1987.
9. Tvedten HW: Clinical pathology of bovine neurologic disease, *Vet Clin North Am Food Anim Pract* 3:25-44, 1987.
10. Scott PR: Diagnostic techniques and clinicopathologic findings in ruminant neurologic disease, *Vet Clin North Am Food Anim Pract* 20:215-230, 2004.
11. Holbrook TC, White SL: Ancillary tests for assessment of the nervous system, *Vet Clin North Am Food Anim Pract* 8:305-316, 1992.
12. Jamison JM, Prescott JF: Bacterial meningitis in large animals, *Comp Contin Educ Pract Vet* 9:F399-F406, 1987.
13. Wilson JW, Stevens JB: Effects of blood contamination on cerebrospinal fluid analysis, *J Am Vet Med Assoc* 171:256-258, 1977.
14. Howard RJ: Neurologic disease differentiation, *J Am Vet Med Assoc* 154:1174-1175, 1969.
15. Braun U, Stehle C, Ehrensperger F: Clinical findings and treatment of listeriosis in 67 sheep and goats, *Vet Rec* 150:38-42, 2002.
16. Schweizer G, Ehrensperger F, Torgerson PR, Braun U: Clinical findings and treatment of 94 cattle presumptively diagnosed with listeriosis, *Vet Rec* 158:588-592, 2006.
17. Nye FJ: Partial treatment and partial diagnosis in pyogenic meningitis, *J Antimicrob Chemother* 12:300-301, 1983.
18. Green SL, Smith LL: Meningitis in neonatal calves: 32 cases (1983-1990), *J Am Vet Med Assoc* 201:125-128, 1992.
19. Ferrouillet C, Fecteau G, Higgins R, Lanevschi A: Analyse du liquide céphalorachidien pour le diagnostic des atteintes du système nerveux des bovins, *Point Vet* 29:783-788, 1998.
20. Divers TJ: Acquired spinal cord and peripheral nerve disease, *Vet Clin North Am Food Anim Pract* 20:231-242, 2004.
21. Nazifi S, Rezakhani A, Badran M et al: Evaluation of hematological, serum biochemical and cerebrospinal fluid parameters in experimental bacterial meningitis in the calf, *Zentralbl Veterinarmed A* 44:55-63, 1997.
22. Wilson JW: Clinical application of cerebrospinal fluid creatine phosphokinase determination, *J Am Vet Med Assoc* 171:200-202, 1977.
23. Scott PR, Penny CD: A field study of meningoencephalitis in calves with particular reference to analysis of cerebrospinal fluid, *Vet Rec* 133:119-121, 1993.
24. Braun U, Scharf G, Blessing S, Kaser-Hotz B: Clinical and computed tomographic findings in a heifer with vestibular syndrome caused by bullous empyema, *Vet Rec* 155:272-273, 2004.

25. Van Biervliet J, Perkins GA, Woodie B et al: Clinical signs, computed tomographic imaging, and management of chronic otitis media/interna in dairy calves, *J Vet Intern Med* 18:907-910, 2004.
26. Levine GJ, Bissett WT, Cole RC et al: Imaging diagnosis: bacterial diskospondylitis in a goat, *Vet Radiol Ultrasound* 47:585-588, 2006.
27. Gerros TC, Mattoon JS, Snyder SP: Use of computed tomography in the diagnosis of a cerebral abscess in a goat, *Vet Radiol Ultrasound* 39:322-324, 1998.
28. Marshall CL, Weinstock D, Kramer RW, Bagley RS: Glioma in a goat, *J Am Vet Med Assoc* 206:1572-1574, 1995.
29. Tsuka T, Taura Y: Abscess of bovine brain stem diagnosed by contrast MRI examinations, *J Vet Med Sci* 61:425-427, 1999.
30. Gordon PJ, Dennis R: Magnetic resonance imaging for the ante mortem diagnosis of cerebellar hypoplasia in a Holstein calf, *Vet Rec* 137:671-672, 1995.
31. Gygi M, Kathmann I, Konar M: [Paraparesis in a dwarf goat: clarification by means of magnetic resonance imaging], *Schweiz Arch Tierheilkd* 146:523-528, 2004.
32. Tsuka T, Okamura S, Nakaichi M et al: Transorbital echo-encephalography in cattle, *Vet Radiol Ultrasound* 43:55-61, 2002.
33. Strain GM, Olcott BM, Hokett LD: Electroretinogram and visual-evoked potential measurements in Holstein cows, *Am J Vet Res* 47:1079-1081, 1986.
34. Strain GM, Claxton MS, Turnquist SE, Kreeger JM: Evoked potential and electroencephalographic assessment of central blindness due to brain abscesses in a steer, *Cornell Vet* 77:374-382, 1987.
35. Strain GM, Olcott BM, Turk MA: Diagnosis of primary generalized epilepsy in a cow, *J Am Vet Med Assoc* 191:833-836, 1987.
36. Strain GM, Graham MC, Claxton MS, Olcott BM: Postnatal development of brainstem auditory-evoked potentials, electroretinograms, and visual-evoked potentials in the calf, *J Vet Intern Med* 3:231-237, 1989.
37. Strain GM, Olcott BM, Thompson DR, Graham MC: Brainstem auditory-evoked potentials in Holstein cows, *J Vet Intern Med* 3:144-148, 1989.
38. Strain GM, Claxton MS, Olcott BM, Turnquist SE: Visual-evoked potentials and electroretinograms in ruminants with thiamine-responsive polioencephalomalacia or suspected listeriosis, *Am J Vet Res* 51:1513-1517, 1990.
39. Strain GM: Antemortem diagnosis of scrapie and bovine spongiform encephalopathy, *J Am Vet Med Assoc* 198:360, 1991.
40. Strain GM, Kraus-Hansen AE, Tedford BL, Claxton-Gill MS: Cortical somatosensory evoked potentials in cows, *Am J Vet Res* 53:1627-1630, 1992.
41. Lorenz MD, Kornegay JN: Confirming a diagnosis. In Lorenz MD, Kornegay JN, editors: *Handbook of veterinary neurology*, St Louis, 2004, Saunders, pp 91-109.
42. Edwin EE, Markson LM, Shreeve J et al: Diagnostic aspects of cerebrocortical necrosis, *Vet Rec* 104:4-8, 1979.

CHAPTER 63

Muscular Tone and Gait Abnormalities

MARIE-EVE FECTEAU and RAYMOND W. SWEENEY

INCREASED MUSCULAR TONE

TETANUS

Definition/Etiology

Clostridium tetani is a gram-positive, anaerobic, spore-forming rod. Tetanus results when *C. tetani* organisms proliferate in an anaerobic site within the animal and elaborate toxins, which have their effects in the spinal cord. Although wound infection (surgical or traumatic) occurs, tetanus can also occur because of proliferation of organisms in the uterus (in association with postpartum metritis),[1] the intestinal tract, or through lesions induced by elastrator bands. Cattle are more resistant to the toxin produced by *C. tetani* than horses, but tetanus prophylaxis is less commonly used in cattle than in horses.[2] Cases are usually sporadic, although outbreaks are occasionally observed in young ruminants following castration, shearing, docking, vaccinations, or injections of pharmaceuticals.

Pathogenesis

Following inoculation and proliferation under anaerobic conditions, *C. tetani* organisms elaborate at least two toxins. Tetanolysin causes local tissue necrosis that may serve to decrease tissue oxygenation and facilitate proliferation of the bacteria.[3] Tetanospasmin (TeNT) is responsible for the clinical signs.[4] The toxin is transported centripetally (via axons of motor neurons) from the site of introduction to the spinal cord. TeNT then inhibits the function of Renshaw cells (inhibitory neurons), resulting in uninhibited contraction of motor neurons and spasmodic tetany. The binding of TeNT to the nerve tissue is considered irreversible, with recovery occurring only with the growth of new nerve terminals.

Clinical Signs

Wounds do not need to be obviously contaminated for tetanus to develop, and the source of infection may not be apparent. The first clinical signs reported are often related to a change in gait with the animal appearing stiff at the walk. Other common clinical signs in cattle include bloat because of failure of eructation, rigid extension of the limbs, raised tail head, and tetany of facial muscles resulting in trismus, dysphagia, and retraction of the lips and ears.[5] Inability to open the mouth ("locked jaw") may develop due to masseter muscle spasms. Prolapse of the third eyelid occurs because of spasm of the retractor oculi muscle, which pulls the globe into the orbit and allows passive prolapse of the nictitating membrane. Signs are exacerbated when the animal is startled or excited. As the disease progresses, muscular tetany increases and the animal may become recumbent. Affected animals then lie on their side and adopt the characteristic appearance of tetanus with the head and legs in full extension accompanied by increased tonic muscular activity, which results in hyperthermia. Aspiration pneumonia may develop secondary to impaired swallowing function. Death is usually caused by respiratory paralysis. The mortality rate from tetanus is high in young ruminants, but the recovery rate is significantly better in adult cattle.[2] This could perhaps be explained by a shorter incubation period and duration of disease in young ruminants. Similarly, the duration of fatal illness in cattle is usually 5 to 10 days, but sheep usually die on about the third or fourth day.[2]

Diagnosis

The presence of typical clinical signs of muscular spasm, erect head posture, trismus, flashing third eyelid, along with a wound or history of recent surgical intervention or calving, are often sufficient to make a diagnosis of tetanus. Isolation of *C. tetani* is not usually attempted, and there are no specific abnormalities in blood or cerebrospinal fluid analysis. There are no gross or histologic findings by which a diagnosis can be confirmed, although direct smears prepared from the wound site or spleen may reveal the presence of large gram-positive rods with terminal spores ("tennis-racket morphology") and help confirm the diagnosis.[2] Differential diagnoses for muscular spasms may include hypomagnesemia, hypocalcemia, meningitis, rabies, nervous coccidiosis, enterotoxemia, toxins (e.g., strychnine), and congenital abnormalities/inherited abnormalities.

Treatment

The principles of treatment of tetanus are (1) elimination of the causative bacteria, (2) neutralization of the residual toxins, (3) relief of muscle spasms, (4) provision of good nursing care, and (5) establishment of active antitoxic immunity. Elimination of the organism involves parenteral administration of penicillin in large doses and aggressive cleaning and surgical débridement of the wound. Wounds may also be irrigated with hydrogen peroxide or injected with penicillin. Administration of tetanus antitoxin (100 IU/kg), subcutaneously, may neutralize unbound toxin and halt progression of the disease. Administration of tetanus antitoxin may be repeated daily for 3 to 5 days.[4] Intrathecal administration of equine-origin antitoxin should not be performed in cattle because severe anaphylactic reactions can occur.[5] Providing an environment with minimal stimulation is important. Sedation may be required to prevent muscle spasms and hyperesthesia associated with excitement. Acepromazine (0.5 mg/kg IM or IV q4-6h) is especially useful for this purpose.[4-5] In addition to providing sedation, acepromazine may also activate some descending inhibitory tracts that are resistant to tetanus toxins.[4] Diazepam (0.01-0.4 mg/kg IV q4-6h) may also provide sedation and muscle relaxation, but its use may be precluded by cost.[5] Other drugs that have been used to provide muscular relaxation include guaifenesin and mephenesin given to effect as a 5% solution.[4] These drugs interfere with the nerve transmission at the level of the interneurons of the spinal cord. Magnesium sulfate has recently been used for sedative and muscle relaxant in human tetanus patients.[6] Nursing care consists of maintaining hydration and nutritional status, as well as managing the recumbent patient. Water and alfalfa gruel can be force-fed by repeated ororuminal intubation. Alternatively, a temporary rumenostomy can be performed, alleviating bloat and providing access for direct intraruminal feeding. Feeding through a rumenostomy is preferred over force-feeding because repeated ororuminal intubation may carry an increased risk of aspiration pneumonia. Because recovery from clinical tetanus is not associated with active immunity, affected animals should be immunized with tetanus toxoids at the time of treatment and a booster should be administered 4 to 6 weeks later.

Prevention

Tetanus prophylaxis is not usually prescribed in cattle because of the low incidence of the disease. However, inoculation with tetanus toxoid may be recommended if individual farms have had multiple cases. In small ruminants, tetanus is a disease of importance and vaccination should be recommended. Because lambs and kids are likely to be exposed early in life through docking and castration, protection is important. The annual vaccination of ewes and does late in gestation should provide enough colostral antibodies to protect the lambs and kids until the age of 6 weeks when a two-dose course of toxoid should be administered, followed by annual vaccination. If the vaccination status of the dam is unknown or inadequate, administration of tetanus antitoxin (200 IU/ lamb or kid) at the time of docking or castration is recommended.

SPASTIC PARESIS (ELSO HEEL)

Definition/Etiology

Spastic paresis is a progressive condition that is characterized by intermittently increased extensor tonus in one or both pelvic limbs of young animals. The etiology and pathogenesis are unknown. Elso Heel affects the Holstein, Angus, Hereford, Charolais, and other breeds of cattle,[5] and has been reported in pygmy goats.[7] Experts disagree about the heritability of this condition.[8-10]

Clinical Signs

Spastic paresis is characterized by periodic spastic contraction of the gastrocnemius and superficial digital extensor muscles in cattle younger than 1 year of age.[5,11-13] Unilateral or bilateral involvement may exist. The extensor tone is typically normal when the animal is recumbent, but clinical signs are typically exhibited when the animal stands. The hock is extended in an uncontrolled fashion, and the affected limb is extended caudally, which gives the impression the leg is too short. The limb is held straight, and thus the calf has difficulty advancing the limb when walking. Manipulation of the limb is not resented, and both the hock and stifle are flexed. The spinal reflexes are intact, with possible increased patellar reflex. Chronic hyperextension from Elso Heel also results in remodeling of the affected tibiotarsal joint. The proximal portion of the tail is often held in an elevated position. If left untreated, calves with Elso Heel will usually fail to grow and will become recumbent.

Treatment

Medical treatment with lithium gluconate (40 mg/kg) administered orally or intramuscularly daily for 10 to 30 days has been recommended early in the course of disease.[5,13] Surgical interruption of the tibial nerve fibers supplying the gastrocnemius muscle (partial tibial neurectomy) or tenotomy/tenectomy of the two insertions of the gastrocnemius muscle on the calcaneus is often successful.[14,15] The advisability of introducing these animals to the breeding herd has been questioned in light of the possible heritability of this condition. Treatment should only been considered to allow the animal to grow normally for slaughter purposes.

INHERITED PERIODIC SPASTICITY

Definition/Etiology

Spastic syndrome, or periodic spasticity ("barn cramps"), is similar to spastic paresis except that it occurs in animals older than 3 years of age and is more episodic.[5-12] Although the onset of the disease is later in life, the condition is thought to be inherited as an autosomal recessive trait.[16] The condition has been reported in many dairy breeds including Holstein, Ayrshire, Jersey, Brown Swiss, and Guernsey.[17] It is a particular problem in mature bulls maintained in artificial insemination centers.[5]

Clinical Signs

This progressive syndrome is characterized by episodic muscle spasms of one or both hind limbs. The spasticity is worse when the animal arises. The affected leg is lifted and held in flexion, accompanied by muscle tremors and kyphosis. Episodes usually last for a few seconds up to 1 minute but may eventually last for up to 30 minutes as the disease progresses. Initially the episodes are mild and do not interfere with production, but they may progress over 2 to 3 years to become a debilitating condition.

Treatment

No specific treatment for periodic spasticity is available, and the condition is progressive. It has been suggested that mephenesin (30-40 mg/kg) administered orally once per day for 3 days could reduce the severity of clinical signs, but treatment efficacy has not been established.[18] Genetic screening, especially of bulls used for artificial insemination, is recommended.[8]

DECREASED MUSCULAR TONE

Marie-Eve Fecteau, Raymond W. Sweeney, and Simon F. Peek

DISEASES OF THE PERIPHERAL NERVOUS SYSTEM

Simon F. Peek

Peripheral nerve disorders of ruminants are predominantly caused by trauma, but inflammatory and neoplastic conditions also occur.[19,20] Peripheral nerve dysfunction in cattle may also accompany myopathy secondary to recumbency because of metabolic disease or poor footing.[19,21] A myriad of potential traumatic causes exist, but some of the more common ones are dystocia associated with parturition,[22] mechanical damage during handling, and improper injection techniques.[19] Educating lay personnel with respect to correct injection technique and the risks associated with the overzealous use of force during dystocia is important if peripheral nerve injuries are to be avoided. Farmers and lay personnel should also be informed of the risks of ill-fitting devices for head restraint, prolonged recumbency on poorly padded tilt tables or concrete flooring, and the overaggressive use of hydraulic chutes in an effort to minimize traumatic injuries causing peripheral nerve damage.[23] The increase in the construction and use of free stall housing for dairy cattle in the United States has brought with it an obligation to ensure that stall design and facility engineering are conducted so as to minimize the chances for injury to cattle. Stall dimensions need to vary between breeds and ages of animal, and a thorough understanding of the mechanics of how cows lie down and rise is important in the installation of partitions at the side and front of cattle in free stall barns. Too frequently traumatic injuries to the back and limbs of cattle become the consequence of ignorance and/or a "one-size-fits-all" approach to stall construction. Spinal cord, distal limb, and peripheral nerve injuries are all potential consequences.

The peripheral nerves of the thoracic and pelvic limbs are individually discussed here alongside a detailed explanation of the specific signs associated with the dysfunction of each nerve.

Suprascapular Nerve Injury

The suprascapular nerve provides motor innervation to the supraspinatus and infraspinatus muscles. The nerve winds distally around the head of the scapula and is most susceptible to trauma at this site. Damage to the suprascapular nerve can occasionally be seen following blunt injury to this region in cattle chutes or following the subcutaneous injection of irritating compounds in the caudal cervical region.

Suprascapular nerve paralysis causes loss of motor innervation to the scapular musculature and leads to limb abduction at rest and circumduction of the affected limb during protraction. Affected cattle have a shortened stride and an abnormal posture, as well as an outward bow in the scapulo-humeral joint during weight bearing. Atrophy of the infraspinatus and supraspinatus muscles occurs if the denervation is permanent. The condition is known as "sweeney."

Radial Nerve Injury

The radial nerve provides motor innervation to the extensor muscles of the forelimb and is particularly susceptible to injury as it courses close to the skin surface over the lateral aspect of the elbow joint. Damage to this nerve is most commonly seen following prolonged lateral recumbency from anesthesia or on tilt tables for foot trimming. Direct trauma to the nerve or damage associated with humeral fractures is also possible.

Radial nerve injury and associated loss of forelimb extensor function typically lead to the animal's being unable to bear weight on the affected limb and the toe being dragged. The toe is knuckled over at rest, and the limb cannot be protracted properly. The elbow may be carried lower than in the opposite limb. On the rare occasions when the nerve is damaged distal to the elbow joint, the elbow may not be significantly "dropped" and partial weight bearing may be possible if the distal limb is extended. In chronic cases extensor muscle atrophy and significant soft tissue abrasions on the dorsum of the pastern and fetlock are potential complications.

Brachial Plexus Injury

Brachial plexus injuries are most commonly encountered following excessive traction on the forelimbs of a neonate during parturition. Severe soft tissue shoulder injuries or deep soft tissue lacerations of the axilla may also cause brachial plexus injury in animals of any age.

The clinical signs of brachial plexus injury reflect a complete inability to support weight on the affected limb. The elbow is dropped to an even lower position than that typically seen with radial nerve paralysis, and the animal is completely unable to protract the affected limb. Affected animals may attempt to compensate for the lack of support in the forequarters by standing with the hind limbs in a more cranial position.

Femoral Nerve Injury

The femoral nerve innervates the iliopsoas and quadriceps muscles and is sensory to the medial part of the thigh. The nerve is most commonly injured following overextension of the coxofemoral or stifle joints. Excessive traction on a posteriorly presented fetus with the stifles in a locked position is probably the most common cause of traumatic femoral nerve injury.[24] The nerve is rarely injured by external blows to the limb, but femoral nerve paralysis can occasionally be seen in down cows that have repeatedly struggled to rise on slippery surfaces. Direct injury to the femoral nerve may occur when one or both hind limbs are retracted caudally, and there is subsequent tearing of the iliopsoas and quadriceps femoris muscles through which the femoral nerve passes distal to the hip.[23,24] Involvement of these muscles in compartment syndrome and ischemic myopathy in down cows provides another opportunity for femoral nerve paresis.

Femoral nerve paralysis is associated with an inability to support weight on the affected limb. In cases of unilateral nerve injury the stifle of the affected limb is flexed, as are all distal limb joints, because of a loss of normal stay apparatus function. However, femoral nerve injury does not cause the toe to knuckle over onto the dorsum of the digit, as would be seen with peroneal nerve paralysis. The affected limb is unable to bear weight and cannot be advanced normally. Complete bilateral femoral nerve paralysis results in recumbency and accordingly carries a poor prognosis in both adult cattle and newborn calves. Occasionally, partial bilateral femoral nerve paralysis is seen in down cows. The affected animal struggles to rise with all the hind limb joints in a continuously flexed position, creating a creeping posture. Femoral nerve paralysis of greater than 2 weeks' duration is accompanied by significant quadriceps femoris muscle atrophy.

When examining a calf with absent patellar reflexes, clinicians must differentiate between femoral nerve paralysis and thrombosis of the aorta or iliac arteries. Calves with bilateral thromboses have cold extremities that lack sensation over the dorsal and lateral aspects of the limb.

Sciatic Nerve Injury

The sciatic nerve and its terminal branches, the tibial and peroneal nerves, are the most commonly injured peripheral nerves of the hind limb. Proximal sciatic nerve damage can occasionally result from pelvic and femoral injuries but is more commonly seen following iatrogenic injury due to poor injection technique or the intramuscular administration of irritating compounds in the gluteal region of calves and small ruminants. Iatrogenic sciatic nerve damage can also result from injections that are directed too laterally into the biceps femoris muscle. Excessive traction of an oversized or malpresented fetus can result in intrapelvic damage to the sciatic nerve and is a significant cause of calving paralysis in postparturient cattle.

The sciatic nerve innervates the extensors of the hip and flexor muscles of the stifle, as well as all the distal limb musculature. Sciatic nerve paralysis is therefore associated with a dropped hip, stifle, and hock. The stifle is extended, and the fetlock knuckles over dorsally, but the limb is usually able to bear partial weight because of the reciprocal apparatus. Complete sciatic nerve paralysis causes constant knuckling onto the dorsum of the digit, but this may not be seen with partial paralysis. Chronic sciatic nerve paralysis is associated with neurogenic atrophy of the caudal thigh and all muscles distal to the stifle.

Tibial Nerve Injury

The sciatic nerve branches into the tibial and peroneal nerves at the level of the distal third of the femur. Injury to the tibial nerve is rarer than injury to the peroneal nerve but may follow the injection of irritant compounds into the caudal thigh close to the stifle joint. Occasionally, tibial nerve deficits are observed in recumbent or downer cattle. Traumatic tibial nerve injury has also been reported in small ruminants following dog attacks.

The tibial nerve supplies motor innervation to the flexors of the digit and extensors of the hock, and paralysis is associated with overflexion of the hock, knuckling of the fetlock, and an asymmetric appearance to the pelvis with the affected side held lower than normal. The limb can usually bear weight, and the toe is not knuckled as with peroneal and complete sciatic nerve paralysis. Neurogenic atrophy of the gastrocnemius muscle is a feature of chronic tibial nerve damage. Complete or partial rupture of the gastrocnemius muscle or tendon can produce clinical signs similar to those seen with tibial nerve paralysis. Recumbent cattle that make repeated efforts to stand on slippery surfaces are also at risk of traumatic gastrocnemius muscle injury. Gastrocnemius rupture also produces an overflexed hock and may be associated with extreme difficulty in rising, particularly if the condition is bilateral. The two conditions can be easily differentiated by palpation of the gastrocnemius muscle and tendon proximal to the point of the hock.

Although it is strictly speaking a progressive muscular disorder, spastic paresis is a condition that can be alleviated in some cases by tibial neurectomy. Spastic paresis (also known as *Elso heel* in Holstein calves) is covered in greater detail elsewhere in this book.

Peroneal Nerve Injury

The peroneal nerve is most susceptible to traumatic injury as it courses superficially over the lateral aspect of the proximal fibula. Peroneal nerve deficits are an unfortunate but common sequela to recumbency in down cattle.[25]

The peroneal nerve innervates the flexors of the hock and extensors of the digit such that damage to this nerve results in hyperextension of the hock and flexion of the fetlock and pastern. The straightened hock makes the limb appear stiff during protraction. Typically the limb is knuckled over onto the dorsum, even at rest. Incomplete paralysis may allow the animal to stand with the foot positioned normally at rest, but the fetlock should characteristically knuckle when the limb is advanced.

Obturator Nerve Injury

Historically, obturator nerve injury has been incriminated as the major cause of unilateral or bilateral adductor dysfunction in the postparturient cow. However, calving paralysis is more likely to result in combined obturator and intrapelvic sciatic nerve injury, particularly when the loss of adductor function is accompanied by knuckling of the distal hind limb joints.[26] Anatomic differences in the relative size of the pelvic bones between species make obturator nerve injury rare except in cattle. The obturator nerve is susceptible to damage as it courses along the medial aspect of the ilium, and paralysis is a potential complication of dystocia, especially in first-calf heifers. The sixth lumbar spinal nerve, which contributes to the sciatic nerve, is also susceptible to injury as it runs ventral to the prominent sacral ridge. Injudicious use of force to deliver an oversized or malpresented fetus is an unfortunate but rather common cause of obturator and intrapelvic sciatic nerve injury in cattle.[27]

Cattle retain their ability to stand and walk after bilateral sectioning of obturator nerves are severed.[26] The gait is only mildly affected following bilateral injury of the nerve. Denervated animals develop a hopping gait. Adductor function is maintained provided the animal is not placed on a slippery surface. However, combined obturator and sciatic nerves damage results in more severe clinical signs. Cattle with bilateral sciatic nerve injuries are unable to rise and sit in a froglike position with the hind limbs simultaneously flexed and abducted. Unilateral damage to these nerves results in impaired limb adduction and knuckling of the distal limb joints as described for proximal sciatic nerve paralysis. Cattle may still be able to rise following unilateral injury if good footing and assistance are provided. Unfortunately, cattle with obturator and/or sciatic nerve damage are at greater risk of life-threatening musculoskeletal injuries such as femoral neck or shaft fractures, coxofemoral luxations, and severe hind limb myopathy should they repeatedly struggle to rise on slippery surfaces. Therapeutic or even prophylactic use of cloth, canvas, or leather hobbles can be useful in preventing initial or worsening traumatic upper limb and pelvic injuries in cattle with mild deficits. Heifers and adult cows can ambulate and rise without difficulty when such devices are applied appropriately, and the restraints can be helpful in preventing sudden, potentially disastrous limb abduction in high-risk cattle. The potential for secondary compartment syndrome will also increase with the duration of recumbency and the weight of the affected animal.

Other Peripheral Nerve Injuries

Although traumatic forelimb or hind limb peripheral nerve injury is the most common form of peripheral neuropathy encountered in ruminants, veterinarians may occasionally observe neurologic deficits associated with injury to other peripheral nerves. In small ruminants the nasal philtrum is deviated away from the affected side. Peripheral facial nerve injury is occasionally encountered in cattle and small ruminants. Iatrogenic damage from poorly fitted halters, particularly those with metal rings that apply pressure to the facial nerve branches on the caudodorsal aspect of the mandibular ramus, can result in facial nerve paresis. Goats that are dragged by the neck chain may develop facial nerve paralysis. The neurologic disease can occur as a cluster epidemic if the goats are handled poorly as a group.

For prevention of facial paralysis, appropriate padding and loosely fitting halters should be used when animals are restrained on tilt tables or in lateral recumbency for any significant period of time, to prevent facial nerve injury on the down side. The clinical signs of facial nerve paresis include ptosis, lack of menace response on the affected side, ear droop, and an ipsilateral loss of lip tone.

Facial nerve deficits can also be seen as a complication of otitis media or interna in calves and small ruminants. This particular syndrome is covered elsewhere in the text.

Specific bilateral auriculopalpebral nerve dysfunction has also occasionally been observed in dairy cattle that are restrained in stanchions. If an animal is startled and makes a sudden movement backward, the head can become lodged within the device just caudal to the orbit, thereby applying severe pressure to the auriculo-palpebral nerve in the region of the zygomatic arch. The clinical signs of auriculopalpebral nerve injury reflect a loss of motor function to the frontalis and the levator and depressor auriculi muscles. The palpebral response is absent, the ears are drooped, and the animal may be observed to tear excessively. Although it is unlikely that sufficient force will be generated to cause an orbital or zygomatic fracture, cattle may be transiently anorectic as a result of generalized pain in the area of the temporo-mandibular joint. Discomfort during palpation and soft tissue swelling in the affected area often assist in making the diagnosis.

On rare occasions, Horner's syndrome may be observed in cattle subsequent to perivascular leakage of irritating solutions intended for jugular administration.[23] Solutions such as 50% dextrose, as well as some commonly used pharmacologics or merely the act of venipuncture itself, can injure and/or irritate the ocular sympathetic pathways in the cervical region, resulting in ipsilateral ptosis and a dry muzzle on the affected side. Enophthalmos often results in mild third eyelid prolapse on the affected side, and cutaneous hyperthermia may be appreciated on that side also. Most cases resolve in the immediate days following the inciting event, but persistent signs beyond this time period carry an unfavorable prognosis for return to function. The low frequency of Horner's syndrome in cattle despite the large number of perivascular injections that occur because of inadequate restraint and technical expertise suggest that this it is a much harder condition to induce than in horses.

Peripheral Nerve Injury and the Downer Cow

It is of particular importance to consider peripheral nerve injuries as a complication of prolonged recumbency in the downer cow syndrome.[21,28] Large animal practitioners are only too aware of the frustrations and economic losses that can accompany recumbency of even relatively short duration in adult cattle, and although the continued inability of a downer cow to rise may be due to a number of causes, peripheral nerve dysfunction can undoubtedly contribute to the problem. Recumbency of even a few hours' duration can be associated with significant myopathy in cattle.[29] Reported values for overall survival rates for downer cows vary widely among authors, but there is a consensus that survival rates decrease in animals with prolonged recumbency.[30] Although antecedent peripheral nerve damage, particularly following dystocia, may occasionally be directly responsible for a cow being unable to rise, most peripheral nerve deficits in downer cows develop secondary to pressure necrosis. Metabolic, endotoxic, and musculoskeletal conditions can result in recumbency and significant secondary muscle and nerve damage. Sciatic and peroneal nerve deficits are particularly common in recumbent cattle, in part because of their anatomic location. Ischemic damage to the caudal and lateral thigh musculature in downer cows can implicate sciatic and peroneal nerve branches and add varying degrees of hind limb paresis to an already challenging clinical picture. A number of devices are available to assist downer cows to stand, but

hoisting adult cattle is physically and technically challenging and a time-consuming task. Hip slings, hip clamps, inflatable bags, and mobile flotation tanks are all available, but no single technique is without its drawbacks. Personal preference and the availability of help and required equipment will dictate which approach is chosen because there is no categorical research to validate any one technique over another. The value of immersion hydrotherapy for the treatment of severe musculoskeletal and neurologic conditions in other species would intuitively lead one to believe that flotation, if available, would be an excellent choice,[31] and indeed, flotation tanks represent the best and safest option for recumbent cattle. Whatever technique is chosen, there is little doubt that early and aggressive assistance in standing and good-quality nursing care are important if therapy is to stand a reasonable chance of success.

Although botulism is, strictly speaking, a neuromuscular disorder, it is worth considering in the differential diagnosis of weakness and recumbency in adult cattle. In recent years the incidence of *Clostridium botulinum* type B toxicosis has increased in association with the feeding of contaminated silage to cattle in the northeastern United States. The clinical signs, diagnosis, and treatment of botulism are covered in another section.

Peripheral Nerve Neoplasia

Clinically relevant peripheral nerve neoplasms are rarely encountered in ruminant practice. It is more common to see peripheral nerve deficits as a complication of other primary or metastatic neoplasms that impinge on peripheral nerve branches. Although more common in a spinal location, lymphosarcoma can occasionally be associated with peripheral nerve deficits that will vary according to the nerve or nerves involved.[32]

The most common primary neoplasm of nervous tissue origin in cattle is the schwannoma, and it is usually seen in cattle older than 5 years of age.[32] This neoplasm can arise in both peripheral and spinal locations. Abattoir surveys have reported on schwannomas involving the brachial plexus, cardiac nerves, intercostal nerves, cervical spinal nerve rootlets, visceral nerves to the abdomen and thorax, as well as the peripheral nerves to skeletal muscles. However, most accounts of clinically relevant schwannomas in older cattle relate to animals with caudal spinal cord involvement and resultant paraparesis. Current management practices make it unlikely that many beef or dairy animals will live long enough to develop these tumors. A putative hereditary neoplastic disorder involving cells of Schwannian descent has also been reported in adult Holstein cattle.[33] Affected cattle had multiple cutaneous nodules involving the skin of the head, neck, brisket, and thorax but were otherwise clinically normal. The condition resembles cutaneous neurofibromatosis type 1 of human beings. The condition is in an autosomal dominant disorder.

Familial Peripheral Neuropathy of Gelbvieh Calves

Recently, a familial peripheral neuropathy and glomerulopathy has been described in the Gelbvieh breed.[34] Clinically affected calves usually manifest in the first year of life (reported cases have been between 5 weeks and 13 months of age) with rear limb ataxia that progresses to generalized paresis and recumbency over just a few days to several weeks. Diminished hind limb reflexes, hypotonia, muscle atrophy, and loss of anal tone have also been reported. Both sexes can be affected, but calves typically remain bright, alert, and appetent even when recumbent. Proteinuria and histologic evidence of glomerular disease are also prominent features. Affected individuals should be humanely euthanized. Prominent histologic features of the nervous system include degenerative lesions in both the spinal cord and peripheral nerves. Pedigree analysis has indicated a probable hereditary basis to the condition.

Miscellaneous

The involvement of the peripheral nervous system in several other important diseases of cattle is worth mentioning. Although the predominant clinical features of several diseases such as bovine spongiform encephalopathy (BSE); bovine herpes encephalitis; and the storage diseases such as the mannosidoses (alpha and beta), gangliosidosis, and glycogenosis involve the central nervous system (CNS), histologic abnormalities can be seen within the peripheral nervous system. Distribution of the protease-resistant prion protein of BSE has been detected in low amounts in peripheral nerves and myenteric plexi,[35] and latency-associated transcripts of BHV1[36] and BHV5[37] have been documented in trigeminal ganglia and trigeminal nerves. The clinically relevant neurologic signs associated with each of these diseases, however, reflect the overwhelming CNS disease in each case.

BOTULISM

Marie-Eve Fecteau and Raymond W. Sweeney
Etiology/Pathogenesis

Botulism is caused by the consumption of the toxin produced by *Clostridium botulinum*, which prevents release of acetylcholine from the presynaptic membrane of the neuromuscular junction. Loss of neuromuscular junctional function results in flaccid paralysis. Botulism in cattle usually occurs as a herd outbreak, often following feeding of silage (e.g., ryelage) stored in plastic bags. Improper or incomplete fermentation may lead to conditions that favor sporulation of *C. botulinum* and production of toxin. Other sources of toxin include other spoiled forages, consumption of carrion particularly in animals with pica, carcass contamination of feeds, and poultry litter.

Clinical Signs

Botulism in cattle should be considered in cases of generalized motor weakness and recumbency. In dairy cattle the index case is often mistaken as hypocalcemic paresis, with inadequate and temporary response to calcium treatment.

Hypokalemic myopathy may also resemble botulism because cows may be recumbent and show severe muscular weakness. Careful examination of other cattle in the herd will often reveal early clinical signs of botulism. Typical clinical signs of botulism include weak tongue tone

progressing to pharyngeal paralysis with dysphagia and drooling; generalized muscle weakness; tremors, progressing to recumbency; and dilated pupils or poor pupillary light response.

Diagnosis

No practical laboratory diagnostic test is available for botulism. The diagnosis is established based on clinical signs and exclusion of other differentials. A postfacto diagnosis can be established by identification of toxin or botulinum spores in feedstuffs, feces, or gastrointestinal contents. Mouse bioassay techniques may help identify the presence of *C. botulinum* toxins from serum and tissues of clinical animals.[38,39] Animals that die of botulism do not have detectable pathologic lesions.

Treatment

A bovine origin antitoxin is available by special arrangement on a limited basis (RH Whitlock, U of PA). Toxin administration does not reverse clinical signs but may halt progression of the disease and allow recovery, which often requires 1 to 2 weeks. Supportive treatments include nutritional support for dysphagic animals, consisting of intraruminal feeding (via orogastric tube or rumenotomy) of a feed gruel such as alfalfa meal in water, and nursing care to prevent complications from recumbency. Orogastric tubes must be passed carefully to prevent aspiration pneumonia in the dysphagic patient. The prognosis for animals with gradual onset of signs (several days) and that can remain standing is good. Rapid progression to recumbency in less than 24 hours suggests consumption of a large quantity of toxin and a poor prognosis. Death occurs secondary to respiratory paralysis.

Prevention

A toxoid is commercially available. Although most herds are not normally vaccinated, three doses of toxoid 2 to 4 weeks apart should provide protection for 1 year.

TRIARYL PHOSPHATE ESTER POISONING

Marie-Eve Fecteau and Raymond W. Sweeney
Etiology/Pathogenesis

Triaryl phosphate ester poisoning (chronic organophosphate poisoning, dying back axonopathy, organophosphate-induced delayed polyneuropathy [OPIDP]) is caused by accidental ingestion of chemicals containing triaryl phosphates.[5] Common chemicals include industrial solvents, automotive brake fluid and other lubricating oils, certain herbicides and insecticides, and plasticizers. Chronic organophosphate poisoning also occurs idiosyncratically in some families of sheep after treatment with organophosphorus anthelmintics.[40] Oral ingestion is most common, but dermal exposures have also been reported.[41] OPIDP is characterized by distal degeneration of axons of both the peripheral and CNS, occurring 2 to 25 days after single or short-term exposure.[42] Neurotoxicity is profound for the longest axons as the fibers degenerate first at the distal, nonterminal areas. The degenerative lesions then spread proximally from the terminal nerve rootlets into the spinal cord until the cell body dies (dying back axonopathy). Calves are less susceptible to OPIDP than cows.[41] A single dose of 500 mg of triaryl phosphate/kg body weight will produce complete paralysis in a mature cow in 26 days.[41]

Clinical Signs

The clinical signs of chronic organophosphate toxicity usually have slow and progressive onset. Muscular weakness and incoordination of the hind limbs may progress to recumbency. Muscular tone and flexor reflexes may range from normal to flaccid paralysis. The tail, bladder, and rectum are often paralyzed, and affected animals show signs of incontinence such as urine dribbling and perineal staining. Affected animals may have laryngeal paralysis and display the attendant signs of dyspnea, bloat, or aphonia. Most animals remain bright and alert and are appetent. Clinical signs of cholinesterase inhibition (hypersalivation, lacrimation, diarrhea, bradycardia, and pupillary constriction) observed with acute toxicity to organophosphates and carbamates are usually not seen with chronic organophosphate poisoning.

Diagnosis

Presumptive diagnosis of triaryl phosphate ester toxicosis is based on the clinical signs and history of exposure. The levels of cholinesterase are low or undetectable at the time of clinical onset but may return to normal concentrations by the time the animals display advanced clinical signs. Confirmation of the condition is usually based on histopathologic detection of a dying back axonopathy in the peripheral nervous tissues. Nerve biopsies performed in human cases have shown axonal degeneration with secondary demyelination.[42]

Treatment

Delayed organophosphate toxicity is not treatable and is irreversible.

OTHER CONDITIONS CAUSING DECREASED MUSCULAR TONE

Marie-Eve Fecteau and Raymond W. Sweeney

Enzootic ataxia of lambs and kids (swayback) is caused by copper deficiency during the prenatal/neonatal period.[43] This condition is caused by bilateral, symmetric loss of myelin in the dorsolateral spinal cord tracts and the cerebral white matter.[44] The pathogenesis of the disease is thought to be related to abnormal mitochondrial function in the CNS, leading to oxidative degeneration with secondary Wallerian degeneration.[45] Clinical signs may vary from tetraparesis at birth to hind limb ataxia at 2 to 4 months of age. Diagnosis is based on clinical signs, histologic findings on the nervous tissue, and low liver copper concentrations. Treatment with copper is usually unsuccessful in restoring neurologic function. Copper, molybdenum, sulfur, and iron concentrations in the diet should be determined to prevent other cases.

Cauda-equina neuritis associated with tail docking can be observed in cattle and sheep secondary to severe infection of the surgical site following a tail amputation. In addition to the obvious signs of infection of the surgical site and the signs of generalized sepsis, animals may present with loss of tail tone, swelling of the tail-head area, hind limb weakness, and recumbency.[44] Prognosis is guarded, but treatment should include surgical drainage of the infected area, high doses of penicillin, and supportive treatments for septic shock. Tail docking should not be performed in adult cattle. Tetanus antitoxin should also be administered to lambs, as well as tetanus toxoids depending on the age of the lamb at the time of surgery.

Fibrocartilaginous embolization has been described in mixed-breed lambs.[46] The emboli are believed to originate from the nucleus pulposus of the intervertebral disks. The pathogenesis of the syndrome is unknown. Affected animals present with acute to peracute onset of asymmetric myelopathy. Paresis to paralysis of the limbs caudal to the lesion occurs, and lambs may develop diffuse tremors that resemble truncal ataxia of cerebellar disease. No treatment is available for the condition.

ATAXIA AND GAIT ANOMALIES

Marie-Eve Fecteau and Raymond W. Sweeney

SPINAL FRACTURES, LUXATIONS, AND SPINAL CORD TRAUMA

Etiology/Pathogenesis

Spinal cord injuries may occur following handling of the animals in a chute or in heifers that have been mounted by other cattle while in estrus. Thoracolumbar fractures may occur in calves during forced extraction, and luxation of the sacroiliac joint in the dam may occur with the use of excessive force during extraction of a calf.[47,48] In small ruminants, trauma to the spinal cord can result from injuries caused by other animals (e.g., predators, other goats or sheep, horses); cars; and hunting accidents. Traumatic luxations or fractures of the atlanto-occipital and atlanto-axial joints may occur in goats when the horns are held during restraint.[5] Spinal cord compression may result from pressure applied by hemorrhage within the spinal canal or by direct compression from vertebral fracture fragments.[44] Pathologic vertebral fractures, secondary to nutritional osteopenia, should be suspected in young animals presented with an acute onset of paralysis. Typically, this occurs in weaned calves, kids, or lambs younger than 1 year of age when their diets are inadequate in calcium, vitamin D, or copper.[5] Multiple animals are often affected. Compression fractures of the thoracic or lumbar vertebrae result in paraplegia. Many animals may also have pathologic fractures of long bones or ribs. Bulls with spondylosis deformans may spontaneously fracture a lumbar vertebrae during breeding. Cows with cystic ovaries and resultant nymphomania may fracture the sacral and coccygeal vertebrae from being mounted excessively by the herdmates.

Clinical Signs

The clinical signs of spinal cord trauma vary depending on the neuroanatomic site of the lesion and severity of the spinal cord compression. Typically, there is an acute onset of signs with variable rates for progression after 24 hours. Neurologic signs include paraparesis, paraplegia, tetraparesis, tetraplegia, sensory deficits, conscious proprioceptive deficits, and changes in spinal reflexes. In addition to the neurologic examination, palpation of the vertebrae (externally and per rectum) or overlying soft tissue may reveal evidence of trauma that includes swelling, asymmetry, or pain elicited on palpation.

Diagnosis

Diagnosis of spinal cord injury caused by vertebral fracture or luxation is based on history, clinical signs, and radiographic confirmation of the fracture or luxation. Myelography, MRI, or CT may be necessary to confirm a diagnosis of spinal cord injury resulting from internal concussion or soft tissue compression. Nuclear scintigraphy may be useful for the detection of spondylitis in bulls that are not destined for the food chain.[49]

In young stock, radiographs of the spine may be diagnostic, but in adult cattle, often only the cervical vertebrae may be imaged well. In cases of pathologic fractures, radiographs may reveal generalized reduced mineralization of bone and thin cortices of the long bone diaphysis. CSF analysis may reveal a higher than normal red blood cell count, depending on the location of the lesion and the site from which the CSF is collected. The CSF may have a xanthochromic discoloration beginning approximately 24 hours after the injury. In cases of potential pathologic fracture, ration analysis should be performed to determine dietary intake of essential minerals (especially calcium and phosphorus), trace minerals (copper and molybdenum), and vitamin D.

Treatment

Treatment of spinal cord edema and hemorrhage caused by contusion injury should focus on reducing edema in the spinal canal. Although commonly employed, corticosteroids such as dexamethasone or methylprednisolone have not been shown to improve outcome.[50] Nevertheless, dexamethasone (0.2 mg/kg, IV or IM q12-24h) and other steroids are occasionally used by some clinicians. Mannitol, hypertonic saline, and dimethyl sulfoxide (DMSO) (1 mg/kg diluted in 5% dextrose or 0.9% saline to a 30% DMSO solution) have also been used for their osmotic potential.[5] Guidelines for extra-label use of these compounds should be followed. Nonsteroidal antiinflammatory agents may be administered if analgesia is required. Appropriate nursing care for recumbent animals is necessary to prevent secondary problems such as decubitus and muscle ischemic damage.

Prognosis

The prognosis for cattle with spinal cord trauma is guarded. Animals that have contusions of the spinal cord without vertebral fractures may recover if they can stand. However, animals that are unable to stand or those that have spinal cord compression associated with a vertebral fracture have a poor prognosis. Calves with pathologic vertebral fractures secondary to nutritional osteopenia have a poor prognosis.

ANKYLOSING SPONDYLITIS OF HOLSTEIN BULLS

Ankylosing spondylitis is a degenerative intervertebral arthritis of Holstein bulls. Bridging ossification of the ventral ligaments of the thoracolumbar vertebrae may result in a stiff or stilted gait, reluctance to move, and dragging of the toes of the hind limbs. Spinal cord compression does not occur in all cases, but if it occurs will result in progressive hind limb ataxia and paresis. The ankylosed area of the spine may fracture, leading to acute recumbency. In bulls, diagnosis is based on signalment, clinical signs, and radiographic findings. Nonsteroidal antiinflammatory drugs may alleviate the early clinical signs associated with lumbar pain, but there is no successful treatment. The condition appears to be hereditary because bulls with the condition possess the class I MHC-BoLA A8 phenotype.[51]

SPINAL ABSCESSES AND VERTEBRAL OSTEOMYELITIS

Etiology/Pathogenesis

Vertebral body osteomyelitis or spinal cord abscesses usually occur by spread of bacteria to vertebrae hematogenously. Embolization of septic thrombi into the metaphyseal vessels is thought to be related to the bilateral and sluggish blood flow in these torturous vessels.[52] Affected animals are usually younger than 3 years old.[52,53] Chronic infections such as pneumonia in other sites of the body may serve as the source of bacteria, but occasionally infected foci cannot be found in cattle presented with this lesion. Neonates may develop vertebral abscesses secondary to septicemia or omphalitis. In lambs, infection at the tail docking site may predispose to vertebral body infection. Some of the agents that are commonly isolated from these lesions include *Arcanobacterium pyogenes* or *Fusobacterium necrophorum* in cattle and *Corynebacterium pseudotuberculosis* (the agent of caseous lymphadenitis) in small ruminants.[52,54] If the infectious agent remains localized in the vertebral body, the patient usually shows spinal neurologic signs.[5] Extension of the infection into the spinal canal may result in secondary problems that include meningitis, spinal cord compression, or pathologic fracture of the infected vertebra.

Clinical Signs

Clinical signs are compatible with a focal spinal cord lesion, with the specific deficits depending on the location of the lesion. In the author's opinion, thoracolumbar lesions are most common, resulting in paraplegia. Additionally, animals with vertebral osteomyelitis often exhibit marked stiffness or reluctance to flex the spine, walk, or lower the head to graze.[5] Patients with cervical abscesses may exhibit a stiff neck and resist passive flexion. These animals often eat by kneeling and lapping the food with their tongues.

Diagnosis

In many cases, radiographs of the spine will exhibit findings characteristic of osteomyelitis such as osteolysis, osteoproliferation, and pathologic fracture. Lesions of the lumbar vertebrae in larger cattle may not be apparent. Myelography, CT, or scintigraphy can be used to detect the specific site of spinal cord compression or confirm the diagnosis. Although nuclear scintigraphy has the potential to be a useful diagnostic aid for this condition, use of radionuclides in cattle may obviate their future use as food-producing animals. Clinical laboratory findings may indicate the presence of a chronic active inflammation with elevations of the plasma fibrinogen and globulin concentration, as well as a chronic anemia.[5] If infection has extended into the subarachnoid space, results of CSF analysis may show evidence of inflammation such as neutrophilic pleocytosis and high protein concentration. The CSF is normal because the meninges are not involved.[44]

Treatment

If spinal abscessation is recognized early, treatment may be attempted with prolonged antimicrobial therapy (at least 4 weeks). Selection of the appropriate antimicrobial agents may be based on the results of cultures from the patient's CSF or from blood culture results. When bacteriologic cultures are inconclusive, penicillin (22,000 IU/kg IM BID), or florfenicol (20 mg/kg IM q48h) should be administered. Nonsteroidal antiinflammatory drugs such as flunixin meglumine may be administered for pain relief. Surgical drainage of the abscess and curettage of the necrotic bone may be attempted but are difficult because of the size of the epaxial musculature and the inaccessibility of the spine in large animals.[5] Treatment is often unsuccessful once neurologic signs are manifested.

SPINAL TUMORS

Etiology/Pathogenesis

Spinal lymphosarcoma is less common in small ruminants than in cattle.[32] Spinal lymphosarcoma of cattle is caused by the bovine leukosis virus (BLV). Tumors are usually extradural within the spinal canal and are most frequently located in the lumbar or sacral area, resulting in hind limb paresis.[44] As with other forms of lymphosarcoma, cattle older than 4 years of age are more commonly affected. Sporadic lymphosarcoma of small ruminants is not considered to be virally induced. Neurofibromas occur rarely in cattle and sheep but may be clinically indistinguishable from lymphosarcoma.[55] Both neurofibroma and lymphosarcoma can compress the spinal cord or the peripheral nerve roots.

Clinical Signs

The onset of neurologic signs is usually gradual over a 1- to 2-week period but occasionally may be acute. Affected cattle show clinical signs of a focal spinal cord lesion. These signs include knuckling of the fetlocks, hypermetria, paraparesis, paraplegia, tetraparesis, tetraplegia, proprioceptive deficits, and hyporeflexia or hyperreflexia. Generally the neurologic signs are indistinguishable from those caused by trauma or vertebral osteomyelitis. However, neurologic signs are usually not progressive in cases of trauma, whereas lymphosarcoma usually results in continued progression of signs after initial detection. Careful physical examination may reveal additional evidence of enzootic lymphosarcoma such as lymphadenopathy or involvement of other sites (heart, abomasum, and uterus).

Diagnosis

Laboratory confirmation of the diagnosis is often not straightforward. Because lymphosarcoma tumor masses are often extradural, finding neoplastic lymphocytes on cytologic evaluation of CSF may not be possible in all cases. Neoplastic cells may be found if the tumor is exfoliated in the cerebrospinal fluid or if the spinal needle passes directly through the tumor mass when lumbosacral puncture is performed. A positive agar gel immunodiffusion (AGID) test result for antibodies to BLV provides evidence that the cow is infected with the BLV and could have lymphosarcoma, but it does not confirm the diagnosis because most infected cows never develop lymphosarcoma. Similarly, finding persistent lymphocytosis only provides evidence that the cow is infected with BLV, not that lymphosarcoma is present. Finding other clinical signs compatible with lymphosarcoma such as lymphadenopathy, pyloric obstruction, abomasal ulceration, or heart failure would strengthen the diagnosis. If peripheral lymph nodes are involved, cytologic evaluation of a needle aspirate or histopathologic examination of a biopsy specimen may confirm the diagnosis. However, even when other supporting evidence is lacking, posterior paralysis in an adult cow older than 4 years of age with no history of trauma is highly suggestive of lymphosarcoma.

Prognosis

Long-term success following treatment of bovine spinal lymphosarcoma has not been reported. Temporary palliation of signs can be achieved in some cases by administration of dexamethasone or L-asparaginase.[44,56] This may permit recovery of genetic potential through superovulation and embryo transfer or recovery of ova for in vitro fertilization.

CEREBROSPINAL NEMATODIASIS IN RUMINANTS

Cattle

Etiology/Pathogenesis

Spinal cord disease associated with parasite migration in cattle is primarily caused by larvae of *Hypoderma bovis* (warble flies). *H. bovis* has a worldwide distribution, although many European countries have eradicated the fly through treatment programs.[57] Larvae burrow through the skin, migrate to the spinal canal, and lie dormant in the epidural fat for several months. Under normal circumstances, this does not result in neurologic disease. However, if the larvae are killed by systemic administration of an organophosphate or an avermectin dewormer, the dying larvae release proteins that cause edema and inflammation of the spinal cord.[58,59] In North America the disease is usually seen between July and October, when *H. bovis* typically inhabits the epidural space.

Clinical Signs

The onset of neurologic signs first occurs 24 to 72 hours after administration of an anthelmintic. Although all four limbs may be affected, more commonly just the hind limbs are affected because of a predilection of the larvae for the lumbosacral region. Clinical signs include ataxia, weakness, conscious proprioceptive deficits, and altered reflexes in affected limbs. Clinical signs must be distinguished from those of organophosphate toxicosis. For example, pour-on chlorpyrifos treatment of bulls has resulted, 2 to 7 days after treatment, in signs of depression, weakness, and muscle fasciculations, which could be mistaken for cerebrospinal nematodiasis.[60]

Diagnosis

Presumptive diagnosis can be made based on the presence of characteristic clinical signs in an animal that was recently treated outside the recommended season for grubs. Because of the epidural location of the grub, most affected animals have normal CSF values. Definitive diagnosis can be made only by demonstrating larvae and characteristic lesions at necropsy.

Treatment

Treatment is symptomatic. Steroids (dexamethasone 0.1 to 0.2 mg/kg IV, q12-24h) and nonsteroidal antiinflammatory agents may ameliorate the inflammatory response to dying grub larvae. In most cases the neurologic signs will resolve, but some animals with severe damage to the spinal cord may remain recumbent, necessitating euthanasia.

Prevention

The disease may be prevented by appropriate timing of systemic anthelmintic grub treatments to precede the migration of the larvae into the epidural space (i.e., July in North America) or after they leave the spinal canal.[61] There have been concerns with the use of organophosphate compounds because of their small margin of safety.[61] Avermectin has been shown to be extremely efficacious against hypoderma larvae.[62,63]

Small Ruminants

Etiology/Pathogenesis

Spinal cord disease caused by migrating larvae in small ruminants and camelids is primarily caused by *Parelaphostrongylus tenuis*. The disease is endemic in the Northeastern United States and Canada, where white-tailed deer are common. It is possible to see clinical disease in susceptible species outside this area if they are housed with or have access to translocated white-tailed deer. Although migration of the parasite in the CNS of deer is usually innocuous, aberrant migration of the larvae in small ruminants results in severe signs of spinal cord and brainstem disease. The life cycle of the worm encompasses the white-tailed deer as primary host and a snail or slug as intermediate host. The adult parasite resides in the subarachnoid space of the deer, and eggs are removed from the CNS through venous sinuses, where they embryonate into first-stage larvae. First-stage larvae then enter the pulmonary parenchyma, undergo tracheal migration, and are coughed up, swallowed, and passed in the feces of the deer. The larvae then burrow into a slug or snail and develop for some time (3-4 weeks) into infectious third-stage larvae. When an infected snail or slug is ingested during grazing, the larvae are released in the abomasum of the goat or sheep and begin to migrate to the subarachnoid space through the dorsal nerve roots. In aberrant hosts the migrating larvae and the resulting inflammatory response damage the spinal cord or brainstem and induce disease.

Clinical Signs

Because of the complex life cycle of the parasite, the disease occurs most commonly during the late autumn and winter in most climates. Clinical signs typically develop 4 to 8 weeks postinfection. Asymmetric signs of spinal cord or brainstem disease usually present acutely. The initial clinical signs observed in affected small ruminants often include paraplegia, paraparesis, tetraplegia, tetraparesis, recumbency, alteration of spinal reflexes, and one or more cranial nerve signs. Posterior ataxia that progresses to recumbency often follows if left untreated. Affected animals are typically alert and responsive and continue to eat and drink normally unless the brainstem is affected. Animals with brainstem disease develop clinical signs of depressed sensorium, conscious proprioceptive deficits, and one or more asymmetrical cranial nerve deficits.

Diagnosis

Presumptive diagnosis of CNS parelaphostrongylosis is made based on clinical signs and the result of CSF evaluation. The CSF of animals with *P. tenuis* infection contains increased concentration of protein, red blood cells, and white blood cells. The differential cell counts contain a large number of eosinophils (7%-97%). Definitive diagnosis can only be made at necropsy by demonstrating the parasites in the spinal cord.

Treatment

Prognosis for complete recovery varies greatly among cases, but early diagnosis and institution of treatment greatly affects the prognosis. Even if given early and at an appropriate dose, a lack of efficacy of an appropriate anthelmintic may be observed because of the impermeability of the blood-brain barrier to most anthelmintics.[63] Treatment protocols, usually consisting of multiple high doses of anthelmintics (ivermectin, fenbendazole, or moxidectin) alone or in various combinations have been described.[64-67] For example, a treatment protocol could consist of oral fenbendazole (10-50 mg/kg) given on days 2 to 7 and subcutaneous ivermectin (200-400 µg/kg) as a single injection on days 1, 3, and 7.[67] Diethylcarbamazine (50 mg/kg PO SID for 7 days) has also been used successfully in combination with fenbendazole (50 mg/kg PO SID for 5 days).[67] Nonsteroidal antiinflammatory agents and dexamethasone have been used as adjunctive therapy because of the concerns that the inflammatory response to the parasite may account for most of the clinical signs. Finally, supportive care including providing nutritional support and appropriate nursing care of a recumbent patient are essential. Recovery depends on the site of the lesion(s), the onset of treatment with respect to the occurrence of clinical signs, and the diligence of nursing care.

Prevention

Minimizing contact with white-tailed deer, as well as removing animals from low-lying or moist pastures, is most important for preventing cases of parelaphostrongylosis but is difficult to accomplish. Therefore most recommended prevention protocols involve frequent deworming during periods of gastropod activity to kill migrating larvae before they reach the CNS. Monthly administration of an avermectin dewormer during the months of late fall to winter is recommended.

NEOSPOROSIS

Etiology/Pathogenesis
Neospora caninum can cause clinical neurologic disease and abortions in ruminants.[61] The definitive host of *N. caninum* is currently believed to be the dog.[68-70] Dogs pass unsporulated, noninfectious oocysts in the feces. The oocysts then sporulate and become infectious within 3 days. The intermediate host (e.g., cattle) ingests oocysts by way of contaminated food and water, and after ingestion tissue cysts form. Infected cattle remain infected for life. Tachyzoites can be passed through the placenta and infect the fetus.[61] The stage of gestation in which a fetus is exposed to the parasite determines the outcome for that fetus. The time of fetal infection to produce congenital neurologic disease is unknown.[61] The most common repercussions of fetal infection are mid- to late-term abortion and in utero vertical transmission.[5]

Clinical Signs
Neurologic signs associated with *N. caninum* in ruminants are confined to congenitally infected neonates. The clinical signs may include recumbency, lethargy, difficulty rising, ataxia, opisthotonus, and seizures. Strabismus, cranial nerve deficits, abnormal reflexes, flaccid paralysis of the pelvic limbs, and spastic paresis of the pelvic limbs have also been reported. Other congenital defects such as flexural contractions of the forelimbs, scoliosis, domed skull, and exophthalmos may be observed. Affected calves are also usually smaller than expected. Calves are usually born with the clinical signs but may initially be mild and progress after birth.

Diagnosis
Little information on antemortem diagnostics in calves with neurologic lesions is available. Serologic testing of calves before ingestion of colostrum may help determine their serologic status. Final diagnosis is usually made at necropsy. Protozoa can be seen in microscopic sections of the stained CNS tissues. Serologic titers for *N. caninum* can be determined on the dams to know their infection status.

Treatment
No treatment is available for CNS neosporosis, and animals are usually euthanized for humane reasons.

Prevention
Canid exposure to placentas and aborted fetuses should be avoided, and access of canids to the livestock feed should be restricted. Definitive prevention protocols for neosporosis have not been identified, but this is an active area of research. Additional areas of research include vaccination and ionophores efficacy.[71-74] In addition, assuming the efficiency of vertical transmission of *N. caninum* from cow to calf, culling of seropositive cows will decrease the incidence of *Neospora* within the herd. Embryo transfer into seronegative recipients is an effective way to prevent vertical transmission of *N. caninum*.[75]

PROGRESSIVE ATAXIA OF CHAROLAIS CALVES

Progressive ataxia is a syndrome of pure and mixed breed Charolais calves between 6 and 36 months of age.[76] The disease is thought to be caused by a recessive genetic defect of both males and females. Progressive ataxia of Charolais calves is characterized by posterior paresis followed by recumbency when the animal reaches 2 years of age. Additional clinical signs include stiffness of the neck, aggressiveness, dragging of the rear toes, stumbling, and loss of conscious proprioception. The gait deficits typically worsen with exercise. Affected animals may have muscular tremors of the limbs and tail when attempting to rise and may show difficulty in assuming and maintaining urination posture. Some animals nod their heads from side to side when excited. Presumptive diagnosis is made based on signalment and clinical signs. The major histopathologic lesion is the formation of eosinophilic plaques in the cerebrocortical white matter. No cure for this disease exists, so affected animals should be humanely destroyed.

WEAVER SYNDROME

Weaver syndrome (bovine progressive degenerative myeloencephalopathy) is a hereditary progressive neurodegenerative disease of Brown Swiss cattle. Males are more commonly affected than females.[77] An association between Weaver syndrome and high milk production is apparent, which may have favored retention of carrier animals within a herd.[78] Neurologic signs usually develop by 6 months of age, consisting of ataxia, proprioceptive deficits, muscle tremors, and eventually recumbency. Some animals may show hypermetria in the limbs, and infertility of both males and females has been reported. The disease may be diagnosed based on signalment and clinical signs. CSF of affected animals may show increased concentration of protein and creatinine phosphokinase.[79] Histopathologic findings include, but are not restricted to, axonal degeneration, vacuolation of the white matter, spheroids, phagocytosis of myelin debris, and gliosis of the thoracic spinal cord. The responsible gene has been mapped, which may offer the possibility for genetic screening to eliminate the disease.[80] Carrier bulls identified by the American Brown Swiss registry are designated by the suffix "W."[5] No effective treatment is available for this hereditary condition.

OTHER HEREDITARY CONDITIONS CAUSING ATAXIA AND GAIT ANOMALIES

Bovine spinal muscular atrophy (SMA) is a heritable disorder of Brown Swiss cattle that is characterized by motor neuron degeneration of the ventral horn cells of the spinal cord.[5] This syndrome clinically resembles Weaver syndrome except that the age of onset is different, with SMA first seen at a much younger age (2-5 weeks of age), and the degree of muscular atrophy is much greater with this syndrome than with Weaver syndrome. Progressive spinal myelinopathy of beef cattle is a progressive disorder of possible genetic origin reported in Murray Grey calves.[81] Affected animals develop ataxia of the hind limbs, swaying of the hindquarters, and collapse of one hind leg when falling to one side. Spinal dysmyelination of Braunvieh-Brown Swiss calves is a congenital spinal condition characterized by dysmyelination of the dorsal tracts of the spinal cord.[82] Calves are recumbent from birth; have coarse tremor of the head, neck, and body; and generalized muscle atrophy. Doddler syndrome is a congenital defect of Jersey cattle that is thought to be inherited as an autosomal recessive trait.[83] Calves are recumbent from birth but appear bright and alert. They can stand with assistance and show severe head tremor when forced to stand.

OTHER CONGENITAL CONDITIONS CAUSING ATAXIA AND GAIT ANOMALIES

Congenital spinal cord diseases are rare in cattle. Occipitoatlantoaxial malformation is a congenital deformation of the cranial cervical spinal column, resulting in progressive tetraplegia in newborn calves, lambs, and kids.[84-86] Spina bifida (failure of closure of a vertebral neural arch) and hemivertebrae (unilaterally incomplete vertebral segment) are vertebral malformations that are usually apparent at birth.[5] Although affected animals may be asymptomatic, often paraplegia or tetraplegia develops. These conditions can be easily diagnosed by examination of plain radiographs.

TREMORS

David Francoz

CEREBELLAR DISEASES

Cerebellar diseases are most commonly diagnosed in young animals. Clinical signs are characterized by hypermetria (excessive movement of the limb during the protraction phase), base-wide stance, truncal ataxia (poorly controlled swaying of the body), and intention tremor (tremor that is more pronounced when a movement is initiated). Intention tremor is usually more pronounced in the head and most obvious when the animal intends voluntary movements such as eating or drinking. In severe cases the animal may fall and be unable to stand or walk. Despite normal vision and facial nerve function, the menace response may be impaired in animals with extensive cerebellar disease. Head tilt may be present if the vestibular components of the cerebellum are affected. Abnormal nystagmus may also be present. The animal is usually alert, responsive, and has normal proprioceptive positioning.[87] In acute, severe, and diffuse cerebellar lesion, the animal may have a decerebellate posture characterized by opisthotonos and rigid extension of the limbs.

According to DeLahunta,[87] cerebellar diseases may be classified into three categories: (1) in utero or neonatal viral infection; (2) malformations of genetic or unknown cause; and (3) degenerative diseases referred to as *abiotrophies*. The first two categories occur in the neonatal period. Clinical signs are present at birth or by the time they become ambulatory. In the opposite, animals with cerebellar abiotrophy develop clinical signs after a variable period of normal neurologic function.

In Utero Viral Infection

Different viruses have been implicated naturally or experimentally with in utero infection and development of cerebellar hypoplasia.

Bovine Viral Diarrhea Virus

Cerebellar hypoplasia has been associated with bovine virus diarrhea virus (BVDV) in utero infection in calves, lambs, and kids. In calves the exposure may occur from 90 to 170 days of gestation.[88,89] The viral infection and inflammatory response lead to massive destruction of Purkinje cells in the granular layer and secondary development arrest.[88,90] Other congenital defects may be observed including hydranencephaly, as well as musculoskeletal and ocular malformations. Diagnosis is based on viral isolation or viral antigen detection from blood samples or fetal tissues and/or detection of antibodies in precolostral blood samples.

Border Disease Virus

Midgestation infection has been reported to induce CNS malformation such as cerebellar hypoplasia in lambs and kids.[91] Description of border disease neurologic signs and diagnosis is performed elsewhere.

Bluetongue Virus

After fetal exposure in cattle and sheep, the mainly reported CNS congenital defect is hydranencephaly. However, in severely affected animals, cerebellar lesions may develop.[87]

Aino Virus

Cases of arthrogryposis, hydranencephaly, and cerebellar hypoplasia have been reported in calves in Japan and Australia.[92,93] The lesions were reproduced experimentally by inoculation of the virus to pregnant cows between 122 and 162 days of gestation.[94]

Kasba (Formerly Chuzan) Virus

A syndrome characterized by hydranencephaly and cerebellar hypoplasia has been associated with Kasba virus infection in Japan.[95,96]

Wesselsbron Disease Virus

The Wesselsbron disease is an acute arthrop-borne infection of sheep, goats, and cattle mainly reported in South Africa. Congenital malformations of the CNS and arthrogryposis have been described in calves and lambs. Porencephaly and cerebellar hypoplasia has been observed following experimental inoculation of cows at 115 days in gestation with the wild Wesselsbron disease virus.[97]

Cache Valley Virus

A report of an outbreak of congenital malformations due to in utero infection with the Cache Valley virus was described in Texas. Malformations included arthrogryposis, hydranencephaly, hydrocephalus, micrencephaly, porencephaly, micromelia, and cerebellar hypoplasia.[98]

Cerebellar Hypoplasia of Genetic or Unknown Causes

Hereditary encephalopathy including cerebellar hypoplasia caused by an autosomal recessive trait has been reported in Hereford,[99] Shorthorn,[100] and Aberdeen Angus.[101] A similar phenomenon was suspected in Ayrshire[102] and Jersey calves,[103] but the possible role of BVDV infection was not thoroughly investigated.

Cerebellar Abiotrophy

Cerebellar abiotrophy is defined as the premature death of cerebellar tissues.[87] In cattle, clinical signs usually appear at 3 to 9 months of age. When the degeneration occurs rapidly, onset of clinical signs is acute. They remain constant or slowly progressing. On the opposite, destruction of cerebellar tissues may be progressive. In such cases, clinical signs develop as the destruction advances.[87] In cattle, it has been reported in Holstein, Charolais, Limousine, and Angus breeds. A recessive mode of inheritance has been implicated in Holstein and strongly suspected in other species. Cerebellar abiotrophy has also been described in Merino, Corriedale, Welsh, Border Leicester, and Charolais lambs. It is suspected to be hereditary.

BORDER DISEASE

Border disease (BD) is a worldwide viral infection that affects mainly sheep. The disease was first reported in 1959[104] as an endemic condition of sheep in the border counties of England and Wales, which leads to its name. The condition is also known as hairy shaker disease or fuzzy-lamb syndrome according to the typical clinical signs observed in lambs. The disease has also been reported in goats. Clinical signs associated with BD virus infection have not been reported in cattle under natural conditions.

The border disease virus belongs to the pestivirus, family Flaviridae. The BD virus is closely related to BVDV and more distantly related to the swine fever virus. The virus is transmitted by oronasal or transplacental routes.[91,105,106] Similarly to what is described with the BVDV infection in cattle, animals may be persistently infected (PI) and continuously spread the virus in their nasal secretion and saliva. PI animals constitute the main reservoir of infection and play an important role in the persistence and transmission of the infection within a herd.[91,105,106]

Clinical signs associated with BD virus depend on the age of the infected animals. Infection of adult sheep, as well as newborn lambs, is usually asymptomatic.[91] A mild fever may develop in some animals. Clinical signs are observed on newborn lambs that were affected in utero between 16 and 80 days of gestation.[105,106] Central nervous system and dermatologic disorders are the predominant clinical signs of BD virus. Lambs are born with a subtle head tremor with only fine trembling of the head, tail, and ears to violent tonic clonic contractions. The severity of the clinical signs decreases progressively during the first weeks of life, and in some cases they disappear.[91,106] However, fine trembling may reoccur with stressful conditions.[91] Affected lambs have fleece anomalies that consist of hairy fleeces (mainly observed in smooth-coated breed) and abnormal pigmentation (observed in pigmented breeds). These anomalies also progressively return to normal. Midgestational (54-71 days) infections of fetuses may result in CNS malformations that include cerebellar hypoplasia, hydranencephaly, and porencephaly. At birth, these infected lambs show severe nervous disorders. Skeleton malformations are also a common feature.

Confirmation of clinical diagnosis is based on viral detection to identify the persistent infection. Virus isolation, viral antigen detection by ELISA, and nucleic acid detection by polymerase chain reaction are possible tests to confirm the diagnosis. High plasma levels of colostral antibodies can mask the detection of persistent viremia or lead to false-negative results in neonates.[91] To exclude the possibility of a transient viremia associated with an acute infection, persistent infection should be confirmed by a convalescent sample from the animal 3 weeks later.[91] Postmortem diagnosis is mainly performed by antigen detection in the tissues. PI animals are usually born without antibody titer against BD virus. However, they can become positive secondary to ingestion of colostral antibodies (for 2-3 months) or develop an immune response to a virus strain different from the strain that infected them in utero.[91,107]

No treatment is available. The control of border disease is based on the identification and elimination of PI animals and prevention of introduction of a new carrier in the flock.[91]

MAPLE SYRUP URINE DISEASE (BRANCHED CHAIN KETOACID DECARBOXYLASE DEFICIENCY)

Calves affected by branched chain ketoacid decarboxylase deficiency (BCKAD) may be born dead or develop clinical signs shortly after birth (1-3 days). It is an inherited autosomal recessive fatal disorder principally affecting Poll Hereford and Poll Shorthorn cattle. The absence of branched chain ketoacid decarboxylase caused an accumulation of branched chain amino acids (valine, leucine, and isoleucine). The clinical signs include dullness, tremors, recumbency and opisthotonos, blindness, and severe hyperthermia. The urine has a particular burnt sugar smell. A severe spongiform encephalopathy is present postmortem.

References

1. Bretzlaff KN, Whitmore HL, Spahr SL et al: Incidence and treatments of postpartum reproductive problems in a dairy herd, *Theriogenology* 17:527-535, 1982.
2. Radostits OM, Gay CC, Blood DC et al: Diseases caused by *Clostridium spp*. In *Veterinary medicine: a textbook of the diseases of cattle, sheep, pigs, goats, and horses*, ed 9, Philadelphia, 2000, Saunders, pp 753-777.
3. Pinder M: Controversies in the management of severe tetanus, *Intensive Care Med* 14:129-143, 1997.
4. Rings DM: Clostridial disease associated with neurologic signs: tetanus, botulism, and enterotoxemia. In Constable PD, editor: *Vet Clin North Am Food Anim Pract: Ruminant neurologic diseases*, 20:379-391, 2004.

5. Smith MO: Diseases of the nervous system. In Smith BP, editor: *Large animal internal medicine*, ed 3, St Louis, 2002, Mosby, pp 873-1018.

6. James MF, Manson ED: The use of magnesium sulphate infusions in the management of very severe tetanus, *Intensive Care Med* 11:5-12, 1985.

7. Baker J, Ciszewski D, Lowrie C et al: Spastic paresis in pygmy goats, *J Vet Intern Med* 3:113, 1989.

8. Sponenberg DP, Van Vleek LD, McEntree K: The generics of the spastic syndrome in dairy bulls, *Vet Med* 80:92-94, 1985.

9. Leipold HW, Huston K, Guffy MM et al: Spastic paresis in beef shorthorn cattle, *J Am Vet Med Assoc* 151:598-601, 1967.

10. Wijeratne WVS: Heritability of spastic paresis, *Vet Rec* 98:139-140, 1976.

11. Radostits OM, Gay CC, Blood DC, Hinchcliff KW: Inherited defects of the nervous system. In *Veterinary medicine: a textbook of the diseases of cattle, sheep, pigs, goats, and horses*, ed 9, Philadelphia, 2000, Saunders, pp 1733-1742.

12. Scarratt WK: Cerebellar disease and disease characterized by dysmetria or tremors. In Constable PD, editor: *Vet Clin North Am Food Anim Pract: Ruminant neurologic diseases*, 20:275-286, 2004.

13. Mayhew IG: Opisthotonus, tetanus, myoclonus, tetany, tremor and other localized muscle spasms and movement disorders. In *Large animal neurology: a handbook for veterinary clinicians*, Philadelphia, 1989, Lea & Febiger, pp 243-333.

14. Ducharme NG: Spastic paresis (Elso Heel). In Fubini SL, Ducharme NG, editors: *Farm animal surgery*, St Louis, 2004, Saunders, pp 349-350.

15. Weaver AD: Spastic paresis (Elso heel). In Greenough PR, editor: *Lameness in cattle*, ed 3, Philadelphia, 1997, Saunders, pp 213-215.

16. Becker RB, Wilcox CJ, Pritchard WR: Crampy or progressive posterior paralysis in mature cattle, *J Dairy Sci* 54:542-547, 1964.

17. Furie WS: Inherent nervous system disorders of cattle. III. Disorders lacking light microscopic lesions, *Agric Pract* 4:25-28, 1983.

18. Roberts SJ: Hereditary spastic diseases affecting cattle in New York State, *Cornell Vet* 55:637-644, 1965.

19. Ciszewski DK, Ames NK: Diseases of the peripheral nerves, *Vet Clin North Am Food Anim Pract* 3:193-312, 1987.

20. George LW: Peripheral nerve disorders. In Smith BP, editor: *Large animal internal medicine*, ed 2, St Louis, 1995, Mosby.

21. Cox VS: Understanding the downer cow syndrome, *Compend Contin Educ Pract Vet* 3:5472-5478, 1981.

22. Cox VS, Breazile JE, Hoover TR: Surgical and anatomic study of calving paralysis, *Am J Vet Res* 36:427-430, 1975.

23. Rebhun WC: *Diseases of dairy cattle*, Philadelphia, 1995, Lea & Febiger.

24. Tryphonas L, Hamilton GF, Rhodes CS: Perinatal femoral nerve degeneration and neurogenic atrophy of quadriceps femoris muscle in calves, *J Am Vet Med Assoc* 164:801-807, 1974.

25. Cox VS: Peroneal nerve paralysis in a heifer, *J Am Vet Med Assoc* 167:142-143, 1975.

26. Cox VS, Breazile JE: Experimental bovine obturator paralysis, *Vet Rec* 93:109-110, 1973.

27. Hallgren W: Studies of parturient paresis in dairy cows, *Nord Vet Med* 7:433, 1955.

28. Cox VS, McGrath CJ, Jorgensen SE: The role of pressure damage in pathogenesis of the downer cow syndrome, *Am J Vet Res* 43:26-31, 1982.

29. Vaughan LS: Peripheral nerve injuries: an experimental study in cattle, *Vet Rec* 76:1293-1301, 1964.

30. Cox VS, Marsh WE, Sterernagel GR et al: Downer cow occurrence in Minnesota dairy herds, *Prev Vet Med* 4:249, 1982.

31. Smith BP, Angelos J, George LW et al: *Down cows and hot tubs*. Proceedings of the 12th ACVIM Forum, American College of Veterinary Internal Medicine, San Francisco, 1994, pp 652-655.

32. Rebhun WC, deLahunta A, Baum KH et al: Compressive neoplasms affecting the bovine spinal cord, *Compend Contin Educ Pract Vet* 6:S396-400, 1984.

33. Sartin EA, Doran SE, Gatz Riddell M et al: Characterization of naturally occurring cutaneous neurofibromatosis in Holstein cattle, *Am J Pathol* 145:1168-1174, 1994.

34. Panciera RJ, Washburn KE, Streeter RN et al: A familial peripheral neuropathy and glomerulopathy in Gelbvieh calves, *Vet Pathol* 40:63-70, 2003.

35. Iwata N, Sato Y, Higuchi Y et al: Distribution of PrP(Sc) in cattle with bovine spongiform encephalopathy slaughtered at abattoirs in Japan, *Jpn J Infect Dis* 59:100-107, 2006.

36. Perez SE, Lovato L, Zhou J et al: Comparison of inflammatory infiltrates in trigeminal ganglia of cattle infected with wild-type Bovine herpesvirus 1 versus a virus strain containing a mutation in the LR (latency-related) gene, *J Neurovirol* 12:392-397, 2006.

37. Perez SE, Bretschneider G, Leunda MR et al: Primary infection, latency, and reactivation of bovine herpesvirus type 5 in the bovine nervous system, *Vet Pathol* 39:437-444, 2002.

38. Jean D, Fecteau G, Scott D et al: *Clostridium botulinum* type C intoxication in feedlot steers being fed ensiled poultry litter, *Can Vet J* 36:626-628, 1995.

39. Galey FD, Terra R, Walker R et al: Type C botulism in dairy cattle from feed contaminated with a dead cat, *J Vet Diagn Invest* 12:204-209, 2000.

40. Williams JF, Dade AW: Posterior paralysis associated with anthelmintic treatment of sheep, *J Am Vet Med Assoc* 169:1307-1309, 1976.

41. Coppock RW, Mostrom MS, Khan AA et al: A review of non-pesticide phosphate ester-induced neurotoxicity in cattle, *Vet Hum Toxicol* 37:576-579, 1995.

42. Lotti M, Moretto A: Organophosphate-induced delayed polyneuropathy, *Toxicol Rev* 24:37-49, 2005.

43. Suttle E, Field A, Barlow R: Experimental copper deficiency in sheep, *J Com Pathol* 80:151-162, 1970.

44. Divers TJ: Acquired spinal cord and peripheral nerve disease. In Constable PD, editor: *Vet Clin North Am Food Anim Pract: Ruminant neurologic diseases*, 20:231-242, 2004.

45. Alleyne T, Adogwa A, Lalla A et al: Novel mitochondrial proteins and decreased intrinsic activity of cytochrome-c oxydase. Characteristic of swayback in sheep, *Mol Chem Neuropathol* 28:285-293, 1996.

46. Jeffrey M, Wells GAH: Multifocal ischaemic encephalomyelopathy associated with fibrocartillaginous emboli in the lamb, *Neuropathol Exp Neurobiol* 12:415-424, 1986.

47. Schuijt G: Iatrogenic fractures of ribs and vertebrae during delivery in perinatally dying calves: 235 cases (1978-1988), *J Am Vet Med Assoc* 197:1196-1202, 1990.

48. Edwards JF, Wiske SE, Loy JK et al: Vertebral fracture associated with trauma during movement and restrain of cattle, *J Am Vet Med Assoc* 207:934-935, 1995.

49. Laflin SL, Steyn PF, VanMetre DC et al: Evaluation and treatment of decreased libido associated with painful lumbar lesions in two bulls, *J Am Vet Med Assoc* 224:533, 565-570, 2004.

50. Olby N: Current concepts in the management of acute spinal cord injury, *J Vet Intern Med* 13:399-407, 1999.

51. Park CA et al: Association between the bovine major histocompatibility complex and chronic posterior spinal paresis: a form of ankylosing spondylitis in Holstein bulls, *Anim Genet* 24:53-58, 1993.

52. Finley GG: A survey of vertebral abscesses in domestic animals in Ontario, *Can Vet J* 16:114-117, 1975.

53. Sherman DM, Ames TR: Vertebral body abscesses in cattle: a review of five cases, *J Am Vet Med Assoc* 188:608-611, 1986.

54. Radostits OM, Gay CC, Blood DC et al: Diseases of the spinal cord. In *Veterinary medicine: a textbook of the diseases of cattle, sheep, pigs, goats, and horses*, ed 9, Philadelphia, 2000, Saunders, pp 542-547.

55. Helfer DH, Stevens DR: Spinal neurofibroma in a sheep, *Vet Pathol* 15:784-786, 1978.

56. Masterson MA, Hull BL, Vollmer LA: Treatment of bovine lymphosarcoma with L-asparaginase, *J Am Vet Med Assoc* 192:1301-1302, 1988.

57. Boulard C: Durably controlling bovine hypodermosis, *Vet Res* 33:455-464, 2002.

58. Keck G, Combier L, Boulard C et al: Adverse effects in cattle treated against *Hypoderma, Point Veterinaire* 23:927-931, 1992.

59. Boulard C, Argente G, Hillion E: Undesirable effects of antiparasitic agents (hypersensitivity), *Recueil de Medecine Veterinaire* 167:1127-1132, 1991.

60. Rich GB: Post-treatment reactions in cattle during extensive field tests of systemic organophosphate insecticides, *Can J Comp Med Vet Sci* 29:30-37, 1965.

61. Nagy DW: *Parelaphostrongylus tenuis* and other parasitic diseases of the ruminant nervous system. In Constable PD, editor: *Vet Clin North Am Food Anim Pract: Ruminant neurologic diseases*, 20:231-242, 2004.

62. Lonneux JF, Losson BJ: The efficacy of mocidectin 0.5% pour-on against *Hypoderma bovis* in naturally infested cattle: parasitological and serological data, *Vet Parasitol* 52:313-320, 1994.

63. Alva-Valdes R, Wallace DH, Holste JE et al: Efficacy of ivermectin in a topical formulation against gastrointestinal and pulmonary nematode infections and naturally acquired grubs and lice, *Am J Vet Res* 47:2389-2392, 1996.

64. Kopcha M, Marteniuk JV, Sills R et al: Cerebrospinal nematodiasis in a goat herd, *J Am Vet Med Assoc* 194:1439-1442, 1989.

65. Brown TT, Jordan HE, Demorest CN: Cerebrospinal parelaphostrongylosis in llamas, *J Wildl Dis* 14:441-444, 1978.

66. Nagy DW, Lakritz J, Tyler JW et al: The treatment of suspected cerebrospinal nematodiasis with moxidectin in 3 llamas, *(llama glama), J Camel Pract Res* 9:145-149, 2002.

67. Lunn DP, Hinchcliff KW: Cerebrospinal fluid eosinophilia and ataxia in five llamas, *Vet Rec* 124:302-305, 1989.

68. Lindsay DS, Dubey JP, Duncan RB: Confirmation that the dog is the definitive host for *Neospora caninum, Vet Parasitol* 82:327-333, 1999.

69. McAllister MM, Dubey JP, Lindsay DS et al: Dogs are definitive hosts of *Neospora caninum, Int J Parasitol* 28:1473-1478, 1998.

70. Dijkstra T, Barkema HW, Hesselink JW et al: Point source exposure of cattle to *Neospora caninum* consistent with periods of common housing and feeding and related to the introduction of a dog, *Vet Parasitol* 105:89-98, 2002.

71. O'Handley RM, Morgan SA, Parker C et al: Vaccination of ewes for prevention of vertical transmission of *Neospora caninum, Am J Vet Res* 64:449-452, 2003.

72. Barling KS, Lunt DK, Graham SL et al: Evaluation of an inactivated *Neospora caninium* vaccine in beef feedlot steers, *J Am Vet Med Assoc* 222:624-627, 2003.

73. Lindsay DS, Rippey NS, Cole RA et al: Examination of the activities of 43 chemotherapeutic agents against *Neospora caninum* tachyzoites in cultured cells, *Am J Vet Res* 55:976-981, 1994.

74. Lindsay DS, Dubey JP: Evaluation of anti-coccidial drugs' inhibition of *Neospora caninum* development in cell cultures, *J Parasitol* 75:990-992, 1989.

75. Baillargeon P, Fecteau G, Paré J et al: Evaluation of the embryo transfer procedure proposed by the International Embryo Transfer Society as a method of controlling vertical transmission of Neospora caninum in cattle, *J Am Vet Med Assoc* 218:1803-1806, 2001.

76. Palmer AC, Blakemore WF, Barlow RM et al: Progressive ataxia of Charolais cattle associated with a myelin disorder, *Vet Rec* 91:592-593, 1972.

77. Stuart LD, Leipold HW: Lesions in bovine progressive degenerative myeloencephalopathy "weaver" of Brown Swiss cattle, *Vet Pathol* 22:13-23, 1985.

78. Hoeshechele I, Meinert TR: Association of genetic defects with yield and type traits: the weaver locus effect upon yield, *J Dairy Sci* 73:2503-2515, 1990.

79. Oyster R, Leipold HW, Trove D et al: Laboratory studies in bovine progressive degenerative myeloencephalopathy in Brown Swiss cattle, *Bov Pract* 26:77-83, 1991.

80. Georges M, Dietz AB, Mishra A et al: Microsatellite mapping of the gene causing weaver disease in cattle will allow the study of and associated quantitative trait locus, *Proc Natl Acad Sci U S A* 90:1058-1062, 1993.

81. Edwards JR, Richards RB, Carrick MJ: Inherited progressive spinal myelinopathy in Murray Grey cattle, *Aust Vet J* 65:108-109, 1988.

82. Hafner A, Dahme E, Obermaier G et al: Spinal dysmyelination in newborn Brown Swiss-Braunvieh calves, *J Vet Med* 40:413-422, 1993.

83. Gregory PW, Mead SW, Regan WM: Hereditary congenital lethal spasms in Jersey cattle, *J Hered* 35:195-200, 1944.

84. Watson AG, Wilson JH, Cooley AJ et al: Occipitoatlantoaxial malformation with atlantoaxial subluxation in an ataxic calf, *J Am Vet Med Assoc* 187:740-742, 1985.

85. Schmidt SP, Forsythe WB, Cowgill HM et al: A case of congenital occipitoatlantoaxial malformation (OAAM) in a lamb, *J Vet Diagn Invest* 5:458-462, 1993.

86. Robinson WF, Chapman HM, Grandage J et al: Atlantoaxial malarticulation in Angora goats, *Aust Vet J* 58:105-107, 1982.

87. DeLahunta A: Comparative cerebellar disease in domestic animals, *Comp Contin Educ Pract Vet* 2:8-19, 1980.

88. Brown TT, DeLahunta A, Bistner SI et al: Pathogenetic studies of infection of the bovine fetus with bovine viral diarrhea virus. I. Cerebellar atrophy, *Vet Pathol* 11:486-505, 1974.

89. Done JT, Terlecki S, Richardson C et al: Bovine virus diarrhoea-mucosal disease virus: pathogenicity for the fetal calf following maternal infection, *Vet Rec* 106:473-479, 1980.

90. Straver PJ, Journee DL, Binkhorst GJ et al: Neurological disorders, virus persistence and hypomyelination in calves due to intra-uterine infections with bovine virus diarrhoea virus. II. Virology and epizootiology, *Vet Q* 5:156-164, 1983.

91. Nettleton PF, Gilray JA, Russo P, Dlissi E: Border disease of sheep and goats, *Vet Res* 29:327-340, 1998.

92. Coverdale OR, Cybinski DG, St George TD et al: Congenital abnormalities in calves associated with Akabane virus and Aino virus, *Aust Vet J* 54:151-152, 1978.

93. Kitano Y, Yamashita S, Makinoda K et al: Congenital abnormalities in calves suggesting Aino virus infection in Kagoshima Prefecture, *J Japan Vet Med Assoc* 46:469-471, 1993.

94. Tsuda T, Yoshida K, Ohashi S et al: Arthrogryposis, hydranencephaly and cerebellar hypoplasia syndrome in neonatal calves resulting from intrauterine infection with Aino virus, *Vet Res* 35:531-538, 2004.

95. Goto Y, Miura Y, Kono Y: Serologic evidence for the etiologic role of Chuzan virus in an epizootic of congenital abnormalities with hydranencephaly-cerebellar hypoplasia syndrome of calves in Japan, *Am J Vet Res* 49:2026-2029, 1988.

96. Miura Y, Kubo M, Goto Y, Kono Y: Hydranencephaly-cerebellar hypoplasia in a newborn calf after infection of its dam with Chuzan virus, *Nippon Juigaku Zasshi* 52:689-694, 1990.

97. Coetzer JA, Theodoridis A, Herr S, Kritzinger L: Wesselsbron disease: a cause of congenital porencephaly and cerebellar hypoplasia in calves, *Onderstepoort J Vet Res* 46:165-169, 1979.

98. Edwards JF, Livingston CW Jr, Chung SI, Collisson EC: Ovine arthrogryposis and central nervous system malformations associated with in utero Cache Valley virus infection: spontaneous disease, *Vet Pathol* 26:33-39, 1989.

99. Innes JR, Russel DS, Wilsdon AJ et al: Familial cerebellar hypoplasia and degeneration in Hereford calves, *J Pathol Bacteriol* 50:455-461, 1940.

100. O'Sullivan BM, McPhee CP: Cerebellar hypoplasia of genetic origin in calves, *Aust Vet J* 51:469-471, 1975.

101. Edmonds L, Crenshaw D, Selby LA: Micrognathia and cerebellar hypoplasia in an Aberdeen Angus herd, *J Hered* 64:62-64, 1973.

102. Howell JM, Ritchie HE: Cerebellar malformations in two Ayrshire calves, *Pathol Vet* 3:159-168, 1966.

103. Allen JG: Congenital cerebellar hypoplasia in Jersey calves, *Aust Vet J* 53:173-175, 1977.

104. Hughes LE, Kershaw GF, Shaw IG: "B" or border disease. An undescribed disease of sheep, *Vet Rec* 71:313-316, 1959.

105. Sawyer MM: Border disease of sheep: the disease in the newborn, adolescent and adult, *Comp Immunol Microbiol Infect Dis* 15:171-177, 1992.

106. Loken T: Border disease in sheep, *Vet Clin North Am Food Anim Pract* 11:579-595, 1995.

107. Cebra C, Cebra M: Diseases of the hematologic, immunologic, and lymphatic systems (multisystem diseases). In Pugh DG, editor: *Sheep and goat medicine*, Philadelphia, 2002, Saunders, pp 359-391.

CHAPTER 64

Cranial Nerve Abnormalities

DAVID FRANCOZ

LISTERIOSIS

Listeriosis is the designated term for infections associated with *Listeria monocytogenes*. In ruminants, *L. monocytogenes* causes neurologic disorders (encephalitic listeriosis), keratoconjunctivitis (silage eye), septicemia, mastitis, and abortion.[1] Encephalitic listeriosis and silage eye are the most common forms of listeriosis. One study in dairy cattle reported that silage eye accounted for 79.7% of cases of listeriosis; encephalitic listeriosis for 9%; a combination of silage eye and encephalitic listeriosis for 5.4%; and abortion, mastitis, sudden death, and diarrhea for the rest of the clinical presentation.[2] Even though all ruminants can be affected, encephalitic listeriosis is more frequently reported in cattle and sheep than in goats.[3] The clinical cases of listeriosis are characterized by unilateral clinical signs of cranial nerve and brainstem lesions. *L. monocytogenes* is considered a major food-borne pathogen in human beings.

Etiologic Agent

L. monocytogenes is a nonsporulating, facultative, anaerobic gram-positive rod. This worldwide pathogen is dispersed in soil; silage; water; and the digestive tract of mammals, birds, and fish.[1] *L. monocytogenes* is resistant to adverse environmental conditions and may persist for months to years in soil and contaminated food. *L. monocytogenes* can grow at low temperatures (4°-6° C), but the optimal growth temperature is 30° to 37° C. *L. monocytogenes* can multiply within a wide range of pH (5.6-9.6) but is inhibited by a pH less than 5.6.[1] *L. monocytogenes* is sensitive to common disinfectants.[4]

L. monocytogenes is a facultative intracellular pathogen that is capable of multiplying in macrophages and monocytes. Bacterial virulence factors that are produced by *L. monocytogenes* include hemolysin, listeriolysin O, phospholipases, the protein ActA, and internalins.[5]

Incidence and Prevalence

One study reported that the incidence of clinically apparent listeriosis in cows and heifers was 11 and 67 per 1000 cows per year, respectively, in affected herds and was 0.25 and 0.31 per 1000 cows per year, respectively, in all herds.[2]

Within a herd, the encephalitic form of listeriosis is typically sporadic, with a morbidity rate less than 5%.[6,7] Outbreaks of encephalitic listeriosis are usually observed in sheep, in which the clinical attack rates may range between 12% and 17%.[8,9]

Risk Factors

Animals of all ages and breeds may develop encephalitic listeriosis. Older animals are more frequently affected than the younger animals. Clinical cases of encephalitic listeriosis are more frequent during winter.[2,10] Moreover, in cattle, goat, and sheep, prevalence of *L. monocytogenes* in fecal samples peaks during winter.[3,10] Reasons to explain this seasonal variation include increased animal density; immune suppression associated with adverse weather conditions; and poor quality of stored feed.

Development of encephalitic listeriosis in ruminants may be influenced by stress and immune system deficiencies.[11,12] However, this remains controversial.[1]

Consumption of malfermented and bacteriologically contaminated silage is an accepted risk factor for the development of encephalitic listeriosis. All forage types of silage are equally prone to *Listeria* contamination. The quality of the silage is also important. Even if *L. monocytogenes* can be isolated from high-quality silage (pH 4-4.5), the culture rate is much higher in inadequately preserved silage that has a pH greater than 5.[13-15] Indeed, the bacteria can proliferate in silage with a pH greater than 5 and/or when anaerobic conditions are not achieved.[14] Silages with poor nutritional value have also been associated with the development of clinical listeriosis.[3] Even though improperly preserved silage usually looks grossly abnormal, it is difficult to identify the contaminated source. In some instance, only part of the silage may be contaminated. Moreover, the delay between contamination and development of clinical signs is usually long (2-6 weeks),[1] so all the contaminated silage may have been consumed when clinical signs develop. Clinical listeriosis may occur with all types of silage storage, but baylage and bunkers have been reported to be particularly at risk.[10] Encephalitic listeriosis has also been reported with a wide variety of feed (pasture, hay, soybean products, and grains).[16-18]

Pathogenesis

The primary source of *L. monocytogenes* infection is the ingestion of contaminated feed or materials. The pathogenesis of encephalitic listeriosis in ruminants is not completely elucidated. According to the most widely accepted theory, *L. monocytogenes* enters the terminal roots of the trigeminal nerve through small wounds in the oropharyngeal cavity and then migrates intra-axonally to the trigeminal nucleus in the pons of the brainstem.[19,20] Involvement of adjacent cranial nerve nuclei results from local spread of *L. monocytogenes*. Ipsilateral nuclei are infected first, but contralateral nuclei may also be infected with time as demonstrated by bilateral clinical lesions and signs in advanced cases.[21,22] Such phenomena may occur with other nerve rootlets.[21]

One particularity of *L. monocytogenes* is that it may survive phagocytosis and spread from cell to cell without any contact within the extracellular environment.[5]

Clinical Signs

Experimental models suggest that clinical signs of encephalitic listeriosis develop 3 to 6 weeks after bacterial inoculation into the oral cavity.[20,23] Typically, unilateral deficits of the cranial nerves V (trigeminal), VII (facial), VIII (vestibulocochlear), and/or IX (glossopharyngeal) are observed. However, other cranial nerves may be affected and deficits may be bilateral in advanced cases.[22,24]

Animals are usually anorectic and depressed. Heart and respiratory rates may be normal, decreased, or increased. Fever is usually present for the first few days but may be normal once clinical signs are well established.[22,24] Animals may be dehydrated secondary to their inability to swallow. They become unable to drink, and the salivary loss exacerbates the degree of dehydration. Rumen motility and filling are usually decreased.[22,24]

Deficits of the trigeminal nerve are characterized by the loss of superficial sensitivity of the face, poor jaw tone, and inability to eat. These deficits are ipsilateral to the lesion. Lesions of the facial nerve result in ipsilateral ptosis, ear and lip drop, and drooling from the affected side of the mouth. Deviation of the nasal philtrum to the normal side may be observed. Decreased palpebral reflex, menace response, and exposure keratitis occur secondary to decreased motor function of the facial nerve. Head tilt, pathologic nystagmus (mainly horizontal nystagmus with the slow phase toward to the side of the lesion), turning in circles, falling or drifting toward the side of the lesions, and vestibular ataxia reflect vestibulocochlear nerve lesions. The major clinical sign of lesions involving the glossopharyngeal and vagus nerves is dysphagia. Dysphagia is principally manifested by salivary loss, retention of food or rumination bolus in the mouth, and reflux of feed into the nostrils. Involvement of the other cranial nerves may be manifested by decreased tongue tone (hypoglossal nerve) and strabismus (oculomotor, trochlear, or abducens nerves).

In advanced cases the animals become recumbent and unable to rise. Opisthotonos and convulsions may be observed. In such cases, prognosis is fatal and animals die despite intensive treatments.[22,24]

A central nervous system form of the disease (listerial myelitis) has been described in sheep and cattle. The pathologic lesions and clinical signs are restricted to the spinal cord. Animals affected by listerial myelitis have normal mental status and cranial nerve function but demonstrate paresis or paralysis of one or several limbs.[25,26]

Diagnosis

History (consumption of silage) and classical clinical signs (unilateral deficits of several cranial nerves) are usually sufficient for a presumptive diagnosis of encephalitic listeriosis and initiation of treatment.

Complete blood count and serum biochemistry profile are of little diagnostic value. CBC only reflects a stress response and an inflammatory condition. Dehydration and prerenal azotemia may be evaluated by measurement of the hematocrit, serum creatinine, and blood urea nitrogen values. Electrolyte and venous blood gas analysis helps to quantify the severity of the imbalance associated with anorexia and the salivary loss.

Cytologic analysis of the CSF is the most useful diagnostic test to support a presumptive diagnosis of encephalitic listeriosis. Cytologic modifications observed are an increase in total protein concentration and nucleated cells, predominantly mononuclear.[22,24,27,28] Because *L. monocytogenes* rarely reaches the meningoventricular system, detection of the bacteria by culture or PCR in the CSF is frequently negative.[29] Cytologic modifications of the CSF observed in cases of listeriosis may be observed in other neurologic disorders. Consequently, CSF analysis supports the presumptive diagnosis but does not provide a definitive diagnosis. Analysis of CSF does not seem to provide information on the outcome of the disease.[27] Some animals with encephalitic listeriosis shed the bacteria in the feces. *Listeria* genomes may be detected in feces by PCR.

Definitive diagnosis can only be made postmortem. Macroscopically, no lesions are observed except a mild to moderate meningitis. However, histologic lesions are typical. They are principally located in the pons and the medulla oblongata and consist of focal meningitis, disseminated microabscesses, gliosis, malacia, and perivascular infiltration of lymphocytes and monocytes.[24] Gram-positive rods may or may not be seen in stained sections of the brainstem, and culture results of the tissues are inconsistent. Listeria-specific immunochemical testing of brainstem tissues is reported to be a much more efficient and rapid tool for confirmation of the histologic diagnosis of encephalitic listeriosis than Gram stain or culture.[30]

Treatment

Specific treatment of listeriosis is based on antimicrobial therapy. *L. monocytogenes* has been demonstrated to be sensitive in vitro to a wide range of antibiotics including penicillin, ampicillin, amoxicillin, aminoglycosides, macrolides (erythromycin), and chloramphenicol (florfenicol).[31] Cephalosporins are considered ineffective.[31] Sporadic antimicrobial resistance of clinical isolates to erythromycin, chloramphenicol, tetracycline, and streptomycin has been described.[1] Recently, an increase in antimicrobial-resistant strains of *L. monocytogenes* isolated from different sources has been reported.[32] The proportion of isolates from a dairy environment that were resistant to penicillin, ampicillin, tetracycline, or florfenicol were 40%, 92%, 45%, and 66%, respectively.[32] Theoretically, effective antibiotics used for the treatment of listeriosis should penetrate the intracellular space, cross the blood-brain barrier, and be bactericidal. In human medicine the recommended treatment for listeriosis is a combination of amoxicillin (or ampicillin) and an aminoglycoside (gentamicin).[33] In ruminants, little data are available to determine the best antimicrobial treatment. Retrospective studies of clinical cases of encephalitic listeriosis showed no significant differences in the survival rates of cattle treated with different antibiotic treatments.[22,24] Antibiotics that have been most frequently used for the treatment of encephalitic listeriosis include penicillin and tetracycline. One of the suggested penicillin treatments is 40,000 to 80,000 IU/kg, IV, four times daily for 3 to 5 days and then 20,000 IU/kg, IM, twice daily for another 14 to 21 days. However, administration of penicillin at 40,000 IU/kg, twice daily IM may be sufficient when administered early in the course of the disease.[34] Recommended dosages for tetracycline are 20 mg/kg IV, once daily or 10 mg/kg, IV twice daily. Because of the extra-label use of the antibiotics (no antibiotics are approved for the treatment of encephalitic listeriosis in North America), the high dosage used, and the long duration of treatment, prolonged antibiotic withdrawal times must be applied.

The survival rates reported in small ruminants and cattle are 26% and 70%, respectively.[22,24] The major explanation for the low success rate is that *L. monocytogenes* is inaccessible to antibiotics because it is an intracellular pathogen. Additionally, infection is localized to a site (brainstem) where antibiotics diffuse with difficulty. To be effective, antimicrobial treatment must also be instituted early in the disease. Prognosis is guarded for advanced cases despite institution of adequate treatment. An antibiotic treatment of long duration (2-4 weeks) is recommended to ensure a complete cure and prevent relapse.[12]

Administration of nonsteroidal antiinflammatory drugs (NSAIDs) is recommended to relieve the pain caused by the leptomeningitis.[35] However, their adverse effects (renal insufficiency and gastrointestinal ulceration) are exacerbated in dehydrated and anorexic animals. Corticosteroids should not be administered to patients with listeric encephalitis because one experimental study demonstrated an increase of the shedding of *L. monocytogenes* in milk of dexamethasone-treated, intramammarily infected cows.[36]

Supportive therapy for patients with encephalitic listeriosis should also include fluid, to restore hydration and correct electrolyte and acid-base disturbances. Adequate treatment of exposure keratitis and nursing care to prevent secondary musculoskeletal injury are also important. Transfaunation and administration of feed orally (alfalfa meal via a stomach tube) or using a rumenostomy may contribute to maintain nutritional support during recovery.[37]

Prevention

Because *L. monocytogenes* is widely distributed in the environment, prevention of listeriosis is based on reducing the exposure to *L. monocytogenes*. Although it is impossible to prepare silage without *Listeria*, adequate silage preparation is nonetheless essential in maintaining the level of silage contamination as low as possible. Adequate animal hygiene and access to pasture are reported to be preventive measures against listeriosis.[10]

OTITIS MEDIA AND INTERNA

Otitis (inflammation of the ear) is classified according to the affected part of the ear: otitis externa, otitis media, and otitis interna for the external ear, middle ear, and inner ear, respectively. Otitis media and interna are associated with clinical signs of cranial nerves VII (facial) and VIII (vestibulocochlear) deficit. Otitis media have been reported in multiple domestic ruminant species: cattle,[38] llamas,[39,40] sheep,[41,42] and goats.[43] In humans, acute otitis media is the most common childhood bacterial infection and the most common reason for antibiotic prescription in children.[44] In calves, otitis media is relatively common, but it is believed to remain subclinical in several cases.

Etiology

Numerous pathogens have been isolated from cases of otitis media and interna. They include *Haemophilus somnus*,[45,46] *Pasteurella multocida*,[47,48] *Mannheimia haemolytica*,[49] *Streptococcus* spp.,[50] *Arcanobacterium pyogenes*,[49,50]

Mycoplasma bovis,[38] *Listeria monocytogenes*,[39] as well as the ear mites *Raillietia auris*,[51] *Psoroptes cuniculi*,[43,52] and the nematode *Rhabditis bovis*.[53]

The relative importance of these pathogens in the etiology of otitis media/interna in cattle is difficult to evaluate. However, recent reports in dairy calves in North America[38,54,55] demonstrated an increasing number of *M. bovis*–associated otitis media. Because *Mycoplasma* sp. are difficult to culture, they may have been overlooked in the past or their relative prevalence has truly increased recently.

Pathogenesis

Otitis media may result from the extension of an otitis externa infection, colonization of the middle ear from the auditory tube (Eustachian tube), or hematogenous spreading.

Several risk factors associated with otitis media indicate that the main route of infection may be the colonization of the middle ear from the auditory tube, which links the nasopharynx to the middle ear (Fig. 64-1).[56] In humans, viral infection of the nasopharynx and subsequent functional disruption of the eustachian tubes is believed to be part of the pathophysiology of otitis media.[57] Subsequently, bacteria from the nasopharynx may colonize the middle ear and proliferate.[57] The role of viral infection in otitis media/interna is not known.

Pharyngeal inflammation and colonization of the nasopharynx by a pathogenic bacteria with extension into the middle ear have been implicated in numerous studies.[54,58] Bottle feeding[41] and feeding of contaminated milk or colostrum[50,54] have been associated with the development of otitis media. A direct relationship between the occurrence of otitis media and the presence of concurrent respiratory infections exists.[38,41,47,55]

Extension of external otitis infection is probably the main route of infection in cases of otitis media associated with ear mites. *R. auris* and *P. cuniculi* may be found in healthy and sick cattle and goats, respectively.[43,51,59] Parasitic infection may lead to inflammation of the external acoustic meatus and damage or rupture of the tympanic membrane.[43] Secondary bacterial infection of the middle ear may then occur.[43] The importance of hematogenous spreading in the development of otitis media is probably minimal. However, otitis media have been reported in animals with an intact tympanic membrane and no respiratory diseases.[38]

Some cases of otitis media/interna develop osteomyelitis, which extends into the calvarium. Invasion of the infection through the dura mater leads to brain abscessation or to disseminated meningitis.

Epidemiology

Otitis media/interna occurs in all domestic ruminant species throughout the world. Sporadic cases, as well as outbreaks, have been described.[46,49,60,61] All ages and sexes may be affected, but young animals appear to be particularly susceptible.

The incidence of otitis media/interna in ruminants is not known. Herd morbidity estimates in dairy cattle range from 1% to as high as 80% in individually housed calves.[48,62] In feedlots, morbidity estimates range from 1% to 20%.[45,47] Otitis media has been predominantly identified in beef cattle, but the frequency of the condition in dairy cattle appears to be increasing. This increase in dairy production animals is thought to be due to a rising rate of *M. bovis* infections.[38,54,55]

Otitis media/interna occurs more frequently during the autumn and winter.[47] Feeding contaminated colostrum or milk have been identified as risk factors for the development of otitis media.[41,54] However, the main risk factor associated with the development of otitis media is the presence of a coincidental respiratory infection. Most studies on otitis media in calves demonstrated that pneumonia is the most frequent concurrent disease observed in affected animals.[38,47,48,55]

Clinical Signs

The clinical signs of otitis media/interna are attributable to dysfunction of cranial nerves VII and VIII. Because of the anatomic location of these nerves, lesions of the facial

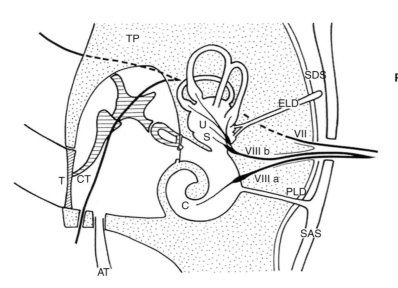

Fig 64-1 Middle and inner ear in ruminants. *T,* Tympanic membrane; *CT,* tympanic cord; *AT,* auditory tube; *TB,* temporal bone; *C,* cochlea; *U,* utricle; *S,* saccule; *ELD,* endolymphatic duct; *PLD,* perilymphatic duct; *SDS,* subdural space; *SAS,* subarachnoidal space; *VII,* facial nerve; *VIIIa,* cochlear portion of the vestibulocochlear nerve; *VIIIb,* vestibular portion of the vestibulocochlear nerve. (From Wilkie HC: The auditory organ of the ox, *Proc Zool Soc* 106:985-1009, 1936.)

nerve develop with infection of the middle ear, whereas lesions of the vestibulocochlear nerve appear with extension of the infection into the inner ear (see Fig. 64-1).

Lesions of the facial nerve produce ptosis and ear drop. Epiphora and exposure keratitis may develop secondarily to the paresis of the eyelid. Lip drop may also be observed. Head tilt is the most common clinical sign associated with lesions of the vestibulocochlear nerve. Nystagmus, circling, falling, or drifting toward the side of the lesions and vestibular ataxia may also reflect vestibulocholear nerve involvement in some cases. In most cases, clinical signs are unilateral. Affected animals have extensor hypertonia and hyperreflexia on the limbs on the ipsilateral side of the lesion and extensor hypotonia and hyporeflexia on the contralateral limbs.

In early disease and cases of uncomplicated otitis media, the animals remain alert with a good appetite. However, they become febrile and lose their appetite as the disease progresses.[12,61] Purulent aural discharge may be present if the tympanic membrane is ruptured. It is reported to develop 2 to 3 days after appearance of clinical signs.[49,63] Clinical signs of pneumonia are frequently observed in calves with otitis media. In advanced cases of otitis interna, clinical signs of meningitis (depression, convulsion) may develop.

Diagnosis

Diagnosis of otitis media/interna is based on clinical signs of vestibulocochlear disease and history. The main differential diagnosis is encephalitic listeriosis, which is characterized by unilateral involvement of multiple cranial nerves and attacks adult ruminants that are eating silage. The CSF analysis is abnormal in encephalitic listeriosis.

Complete blood count and serum biochemistry profile are of little diagnostic value. Radiographic images of the tympanic bulla of calves have been reported to be useful for the diagnosis of otitis media/interna[64] (Fig. 64-2). Evaluation of the tympanic bulla is best achieved with a lateral oblique view. Calves' mouth opening does not allow open-mouth projections to compare the two tympanic bullae. Increased opacity or thickening of the osseous bulla is suggestive of otitis media. However, radiographs of the tympanic bulla should be considered as a specific but not sensitive diagnostic tool. In small animals, computed tomographic and magnetic resonance imaging are reported to be superior to conventional radiographs for the diagnosis of middle and inner ear diseases.[65] Computed tomographic imaging has been reported for the diagnosis of otitis media/interna in calves.[66] However, such procedures are restricted to referral centers and valuable animals.

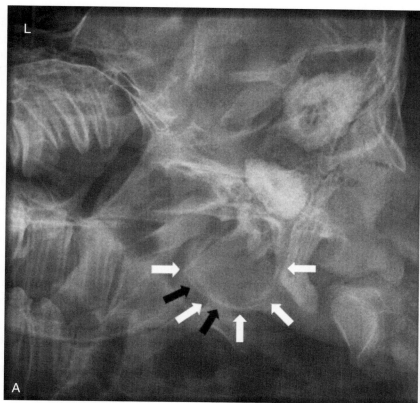
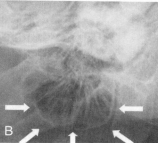

Fig 64-2   Lateral oblique projection of the left tympanic bulla of a calf with left otitis media/interna. **A,** Opacification of the normal air-filled bullae and lysis of the trabeculae of the tympanic bullae. *Black arrows,* thickening of the osseous bulla; *white arrows,* increased size of the tympanic bullae. **B,** Lateral oblique projection of a normal tympanic bulla of a calf. (From Francoz D, Fecteau G, Desrochers A, Fortin M: *Can Vet J* 45:661-666, 2004.)

Unless complicated by meningitis, cytologic CSF analysis is normal in cases of otitis media/interna. In one retrospective study[38] the results from the CSF analysis were compatible with an inflammation of the CNS in two out of five calves. These two cases presented clinical signs of CNS disease.

In animals affected with otitis media/interna, it can be difficult to identify the etiologic agent. Because the tympanic membrane is not ruptured in all cases, purulent secretion may or may not always be sampled in the external auditory canal. Also, because of the length and tautness of the bovine canal, samples may be easily contaminated by external ear bacterial flora. Some pathogens reported to induce otitis media such as parasites or *Mycoplasma* sp. may be isolated from the external ear of normal ruminants.[67] When pneumonia is associated with otitis media/interna, the same etiologic agent may be responsible for both diseases.[38] Consequently, culture of a transtracheal lavage may be useful to identify the pathogens and recommend adequate antimicrobial treatment.

Treatment

Treatment of otitis media/interna is based on the institution of antimicrobial therapy. Antimicrobial drugs used for the treatment of otitis media/interna must be effective against the most frequently isolated pathogens (i.e., *Mycoplasma* sp.) and diffuse into the middle and the inner ear. Antimicrobial drugs that could be used to treat mycoplasma infections in cattle are tetracycline, spectinomycin, tylosin, tilmicosin, florfenicol, and fluoroquinolones. Resistance to several of these drugs has been reported with *M. bovis*.[68-70] Successful treatment of otitis media/interna has been reported with enrofloxacin,[38,49] but that drug is only approved by the U.S. Food and Drug Administration for the treatment of respiratory disease in beef cattle. Optimal therapy of otitis media in cattle remains to be determined. Proposed duration of treatment ranges from 5 days to several weeks.[38,49,63] The duration of the treatment is influenced by the chronicity of the disease, as well as the implicated pathogens.

Nonsteroidal antiinflammatory drugs can be administered to increase the animal's comfort. Although local treatment does not appear necessary, local irrigation of the middle ear may be performed when the tympanic membrane is ruptured.[12]

Surgical treatment of chronic cases has been reported to be successful in calves[60,66] and goats.[43] On the other hand, surgical approach was unsuccessful in a llama.[40]

Prognosis

The prognosis appears to depend on the chronicity of the disease and the etiologic agent involved. Prognosis was reported to be poor in yearlings (12-13 months of age) and good in calves (5-7 months of age).[47] Full clinical recovery was observed in 60% to 100% of cases in cattle, even if some recurrences were reported.[38,45,64] However, according to others, antimicrobial therapy is commonly unsuccessful and the prognosis should be considered as guarded.[71] Our clinical impression is that the prognosis is good even in chronic cases with long-term antimicrobial therapy.[38]

VITAMIN A DEFICIENCY

In ruminants, vitamin A mainly originates from the conversion of green plants' carotenoid pigments (β-carotene) in the liver or the intestinal epithelium. Concentration of carotenoid in feed decreases with the duration of storage. Vitamin A is necessary for night vision, normal bone and epithelial tissue growth, normal reproductive functions, and embryonic development. Because vitamin A is stored in the liver, deficiency can be tolerated for 12 to 24 days.[72]

Vitamin A deficiency may be primary or, rarely, secondary. Primary deficiency results from inadequate feed intake. It principally affects cattle that graze on dry pastures for a long period of time or in cattle housed inside and fed improperly stored feed that has inadequate vitamin supplementation.[72,73] Secondary deficiency occurs consequently to inadequate intestinal absorption or inhibition of intestinal or liver conversion.[72,73]

Neurologic signs of vitamin A deficiency result from poliomalacia caused by increased intracranial pressure (ICP). They include blindness, convulsions, and depression.[72,74,75] The increased ICP develops secondary to thickening of the dura mater and impairment of CSF absorption.[75] In calves, alteration of the skull growth and narrowing of the bony foramina has also been implicated in the development of increased ICP. Blindness is bilateral and results from decreased regeneration of rhodopsin, a pigment that is necessary for night vision, degenerative changes in the outer retinal layers, and optic nerve compression secondary to narrowing of the optic foramen[72] in combination with the hydrocephalus-related pressure changes. The first two causes occur early in the disease and are reversible, whereas the compression occurs late and appears to be irreversible. Pupillary light reflex and response menace are absent, which can help to differentiate vitamin A deficiency from polioencephalomalacia.[75] Ophthalmoscopic examination reveals bilateral papilledema with bilateral dilated and unresponsive pupils in most affected cases.[75] Papilledema is a consistent and early clinical finding that results from chronic increased ICP in adults and optic nerve compression in the stenotic optic canal.[75] Retinal changes may also be seen in advanced cases.[75] Usually, there is no other ocular anomaly. Pneumonia, diarrhea, skin and reproductive disorders, as well as reduced growth rate may be associated clinical signs.[72]

Confirmation of vitamin deficiency A may be performed by concomitant measurement of vitamin A and/or β-carotene concentration in the feed, plasma, or liver. Deficient animals usually have vitamin A and β-carotene plasma concentrations that are less than 10 and 70 mg/dl, respectively,[73,76] and hepatic concentrations of vitamin A and β-carotene that are less than 14 and 32 mg/dl, respectively.[76]

Treatment consists of parenteral administration of aqueous vitamin A (440 UI/kg).[73] If the treatment is instituted early in the disease, the prognosis may be good. However, the treatment is ineffective in advanced cases.

References

1. Low JC, Donachie W: A review of *Listeria monocytogenes* and listeriosis, *Vet J* 153:9-29, 1997.
2. Erdogan HM, Cetinkaya B, Green LE et al: Prevalence, incidence, signs and treatment of clinical listeriosis in dairy cattle in England, *Vet Rec* 149:289-293, 2001.
3. Wilesmith JW, Gitter M: Epidemiology of ovine listeriosis in Great Britain, *Vet Rec* 119:467-470, 1986.
4. Euzéby JP: Listeria. *Abrégé de Bactériologie Générale et Médicale*, from http://www.bacteriologie.net/. Accessed December 16, 2007.
5. Kathariou S: Listeria monocytogenes virulence and pathogenicity, a food safety perspective, *J Food Prot* 65(11):1811-1829, 2002.
6. Green LE, Morgan KL: Descriptive epidemiology of listerial meningoencephalitis in housed lambs, *Prev Vet Med* 18:79-87, 1994.
7. Molsan PG, Andrews GA, DeBey BM et al: Listeriosis associated with silage feeding in six Midwest cattle herds, *Large Anim Pract* 19:40-46, 1999.
8. Blenden DC, Kampelmacher EH, Torres-Anjel MJ et al: Listeriosis, *J Am Vet Med Assoc* 191:1546-1551, 1987.
9. Vazquez-Boland JA, Dominguez L, Blanco M et al: Epidemiologic investigation of a silage-associated epizootic of ovine listeric encephalitis, using a new *Listeria*-selective enumeration medium and phage typing, *Am J Vet Res* 53:368-371, 1992.
10. Nightingale KK, Fortes ED, Ho AJ et al: Evaluation of farm management practices as risk factors for clinical listeriosis and fecal shedding of Listeria monocytogenes in ruminants, *J Am Vet Med Assoc* 227:1808-1814, 2005.
11. Cooper J, Walker RDL: Listeriosis, *Vet Clin North Am Food Anim Pract* 14:113-125, 1998.
12. Morin DE: Brainstem and cranial nerve abnormalities: listeriosis, otitis media/interna, and pituitary abscess syndrome, *Vet Clin North Am Food Anim Pract* 20:243-273, vi, 2004.
13. Irvin AD: The effect of pH on the multiplication of Listeria monocytogenes in grass silage media, *Vet Rec* 82:115-116, 1968.
14. Gronstol H: Listeriosis in sheep. Isolation of *Listeria* monocytogenes from grass silage, *Acta Vet Scand* 20:492-497, 1979.
15. Sargisson N: Health hazards associated with the feeding of big bale silage, *In Pract* 15:291-297, 1993.
16. Smith HC, Sundquist E: Listeriosis in a herd of cattle, *Vet Med* 55:70-73, 1960.
17. Wood JS: Encephalitic listeriosis in a herd of goats, *Can Vet J* 13:80-82, 1972.
18. Wesley IV, Larson DJ, Harmon KM et al: A case report of sporadic ovine listerial meningoencephalitis in Iowa with an overview of livestock and human cases, *J Vet Diagn Invest* 14:314-321, 2002.
19. Asahi O, Akiyama Y, Hosoda T et al: Studies on the mechanism of infection of the brain with *Listeria* monocytogenes, *Am J Vet Res* 18:147-157, 1957.
20. Asahi O: *Pathogenesis of encephalitic listeriosis: invasion of nerve fibers by* Listeria monocytogenes. Proceedings of the 2nd Symposium on Listeric Infection, Bozeman (MT), Aircraft Printers, 1963.
21. Antal EA, Loberg EM, Bracht P et al: Evidence for intraaxonal spread of *Listeria monocytogenes* from the periphery to the central nervous system, *Brain Pathol* 11:432-438, 2001.
22. Schweizer G, Ehrensperger F, Torgerson PR et al: Clinical findings and treatment of 94 cattle presumptively diagnosed with listeriosis, *Vet Rec* 158:588-592, 2006.
23. Barlow RM, McGorum B: Ovine listerial encephalitis: analysis, hypothesis and synthesis, *Vet Rec* 116:233-236, 1985.
24. Braun U, Stehle C, Ehrensperger F et al: Clinical findings and treatment of listeriosis in 67 sheep and goats, *Vet Rec* 150:38-42, 2002.
25. Seaman JT, Carter GI, Carrigan MJ et al: An outbreak of listerial myelitis in sheep, *Aust Vet J* 67:142-143, 1990.
26. Schweizer G, Fuhrer B, Braun U et al: Signs of spinal cord disease in two heifers caused by *Listeria monocytogenes*, *Vet Rec* 154:54-55, 2004.
27. Scott PR: A field study of ovine listerial meningo-encephalitis with particular reference to cerebrospinal fluid analysis as an aid to diagnosis and prognosis, *Br Vet J* 149:165-170, 1993.
28. Ferrouillet C, Fecteau G, Higgins R, Lanevschi A: Analyse du liquide céphalorachidien pour le diagnostic des atteintes du système nerveux des bovins, *Point Veterinaire* 29:783-788, 1998.
29. Peters M, Pohlenz J, Jaton K et al: Studies of the detection of *Listeria monocytogenes* by culture and PCR in cerebrospinal fluid samples from ruminants with listeric encephalitis, *Zentralbl Veterinarmed B* 42:84-88, 1995.
30. Loeb E: Encephalitic listeriosis in ruminants: immunohistochemistry as a diagnostic tool, *J Vet Med A Physiol Pathol Clin Med* 51:453-455, 2004.
31. Hof H: Therapeutic activities of antibiotics in listeriosis, *Infection* 19(Suppl 4):S229-S233, 1991.
32. Srinivasan V, Nam HM, Nguyen LT et al: Prevalence of antimicrobial resistance genes in *Listeria monocytogenes* isolated from dairy farms, *Foodborne Pathog Dis* 2:201-211, 2005.
33. Hof H: An update on the medical management of listeriosis, *Expert Opin Pharmacother* 5:1727-1735, 2004.
34. Divers TJ: Infectious causes of meningitis and encephalitis in cattle. In Howard JL: *Current veterinary therapy: food animal practice*, vol 2, Philadelphia, 1986, Saunders, pp 852-855.
35. Lorenz MD, Kornegay JN: Pain. In Lorenz MD, Kornegay JN: *Handbook of veterinary neurology*, St Louis, 2004, Saunders, pp 345-353.
36. Wesley IV, Bryner JH, Van der Maaten MJ et al: Effects of dexamethasone on shedding of *Listeria monocytogenes* in dairy cattle, *Am J Vet Res* 50:2009-2013, 1989.
37. Chigerwe M, Tyler JW, Dawes ME et al: Enteral feeding of 3 mature cows by rumenostomy, *J Vet Intern Med* 19:779-781, 2005.
38. Francoz D, Fecteau G, Desrochers A et al: Otitis media in dairy calves: a retrospective study of 15 cases (1987 to 2002), *Can Vet J* 45:661-666, 2004.
39. Van Metre DC, Barrington GM, Parish SM et al: Otitis media/interna and suppurative meningoencephalomyelitis associated with *Listeria monocytogenes* infection in a llama, *J Am Vet Med Assoc* 199:236-240, 1991.
40. Koenig JB, Watrous BJ, Kaneps AJ et al: Otitis media in a llama, *J Am Vet Med Assoc* 218:1582, 1619-1623, 2001.
41. Macleod NS, Wiener G, Barlow RM et al: Factors involved in middle ear infection (otitis media) in lambs, *Vet Rec* 91:360-361, 1972.
42. Jensen R, Pierson RE, Weibel JL et al: Middle ear infection in feedlot lambs, *J Am Vet Med Assoc* 181:805-807, 1982.
43. Wilson J, Brewer B: Vestibular disease in a goat, *Comp Contin Educ Pract Vet* 6:S179-S182, 1984.
44. Rovers MM, Glasziou P, Apelman CL et al: Antibiotics for acute otitis media: a meta-analysis with individual patient data, *Lancet* 368:1429-1435, 2006.
45. Nation P, Frelier P, Gifford GA et al: Otitis in feedlot cattle, *Can Vet J* 24:238, 1983.
46. McEwen SA, Hulland TJ: Haemophilus somnus-induced otitis and meningitis in a heifer, *Can Vet J* 26:7-8, 1985.
47. Jensen R, Maki LR, Lauerman LH et al: Cause and pathogenesis of middle ear infection in young feedlot cattle, *J Am Vet Med Assoc* 182:967-972, 1983.

48. Rademacher G, Schels H, Dirksen G: [Enzootic otitis in a herd of calves], *Tierarztl Prax* 19:253-257, 1991.

49. Yeruham I, Elad D, Liberboim M et al: Clinical and microbiological study of an otitis media outbreak in calves in a dairy herd, *Zentralbl Veterinarmed B* 46:145-150, 1999.

50. Baba AI, Rotaru O, Raputean G: Middle ear infection in suckling and weaned calves, *Morphol Embryol (Bucur)* 34:271-275, 1988.

51. Ladds PW, Copeman DB, Daniels P et al: Raillietia auris and otitis media in cattle in Northern Queensland, *Aust Vet J* 48:532-533, 1972.

52. Rollor EA III, Nettles VF, Davidson WR, Gerrish RR: Otitis media caused by *Psoroptes cuniculi* in white-tailed deer, *J Am Vet Med Assoc* 173:1242-1243, 1978.

53. Msolla P, Semuguruka WD, Kasuku AA et al: Clinical observations on bovine parasitic otitis in Tanzania, *Trop Anim Health Prod* 25:15-18, 1993.

54. Walz PH, Mullaney TP, Render JA et al: Otitis media in preweaned Holstein dairy calves in Michigan due to *Mycoplasma bovis*, *J Vet Diagn Invest* 9:250-254, 1997.

55. Lamm CG, Munson L, Thurmond MC et al: Mycoplasma otitis in California calves, *J Vet Diagn Invest* 16:397-402, 2004.

56. Wilkie HC: The auditory organ of the ox, *Proc Zool Soc* 106:985-1009, 1936.

57. Hendley JO: Clinical practice. Otitis media, *N Engl J Med* 347:1169-1174, 2002.

58. Duarte ER, Hamdan JS: Otitis in cattle, an aetiological review, *J Vet Med B Infect Dis Vet Public Health* 51:1-7, 2004.

59. Heffner RS, Heffner HE: Occurrence of the cattle ear mite (*Raillietia auris*) in southeastern Kansas, *Cornel Vet* 73:193-199, 1983.

60. Mahin L: Symptoms and treatment of unilateral labyrinthitis in a calf, *Vet Rec* 107:448, 1980.

61. Gawthrop JC: *Practitioners experience with* Mycoplasma bovis *outbreaks—dairy calves*. The 38th Annual Convention Proceedings of the American Association of Bovine Practitioners, Salt Lake City, Utah, American Association of Bovine Practitioners, 2005.

62. De Chant G, Donovan GL: *Otitis media in dairy calves: a preliminary case report*. The 28th Annual Convention Proceedings of the American Association of Bovine Practitioners, 1996.

63. Henderson JP, McCullough WP: Otitis media in suckler calves, *Vet Rec* 132:24, 1993.

64. Vestweber JG: Otitis media/interna in cattle, *Comp Contin Educ Pract Vet* 21:S34-S38, 1999.

65. Garosi LS, Dennis R, Schwarz T et al: Review of diagnostic imaging of ear diseases in the dog and cat, *Vet Radiol Ultrasound* 44:137-146, 2003.

66. Van Biervliet J, Perkins GA, Woodie B et al: Clinical signs, computed tomographic imaging, and management of chronic otitis media/interna in dairy calves, *J Vet Intern Med* 18:907-910, 2004.

67. Hazell SL, Greenwood PE, Adams BS et al: Isolation of mycoplasmas from the external ear canal of a cow, *Aust Vet J* 63:129-130, 1986.

68. Nicholas RA, Ayling RD: *Mycoplasma bovis:* disease, diagnosis, and control, *Res Vet Sci* 74:105-112, 2003.

69. Francoz D, Fortin M, Fecteau G, Messier S: Determination of *Mycoplasma bovis* susceptibilities against six antimicrobial agents using the E test method. *Vet Microbiol* 105(1):57-64, 2005.

70. Rosenbusch RF, Kinyon JM, Aply M et al: In vitro antimicrobial inhibition profiles of *Mycoplasma bovis* isolates recovered from various regions of the United States from 2002 to 2003, *J Vet Diagn Invest* 17:436-441, 2005.

71. Radostits OM, Gay CC, Blood DC et al: Otitis media. In Radostits OM, Gay CC, Blood DC et al: *Veterinary medicine: a textbook of the diseases of cattle, sheep, pigs, goats and horses*, London, UK, 2000, Saunders, pp 535-536.

72. Nielsen SW, Mills JH, Woelfel CJ et al: The pathology of marginal vitamin A deficiency in calves, *Res Vet Sci* 7:143-150, 1966.

73. Kopcha M: Nutritional and metabolic diseases involving the nervous system, *Vet Clin North Am Food Anim Pract* 3:119-135, 1987.

74. Van der Lugt JJ, Prozesky L: The pathology of blindness in newborn calves caused by hypovitaminosis A, *Onderstpoort J Vet Re* 56:99-109, 1989.

75. Anderson WI, Rebhun WC, DeLahunta A et al: The ophthalmic and neuro-ophthalmic effects of a vitamin A deficiency in young steers, *Vet Med* 86:1143-1148, 1991.

76. Smith MO: Diseases of the nervous system. In Smith BP (editor): *Large animal internal medicine*, St Louis, 2002, Mosby, pp 873-1017.

CHAPTER 65

Mentation Abnormality, Depression, and Cortical Blindness

GILLES FECTEAU and LISLE W. GEORGE

POLIOENCEPHALOMALACIA

Etiology

Polioencephalomalacia (PEM), or cerebrocortical necrosis, is a disease of ruminants responsive to thiamine therapy. However, the precise cause of PEM remains uncertain. Because feeding antimetabolites of thiamine reproduces the disease, it is generally accepted that thiamine deficiency plays an important role in the pathophysiology of the disease.

Epidemiology

PEM occurs sporadically or may affect several animals in the same group. Calves are considered at greater risk, particularly during the 2 to 12 months of age window. Some risk factors are associated with feeding practice: low amount of dietary roughage, high-sulfate ration,[1] molasses-urea diet, and cobalt-deficient diet.[2,3] Feeding cattle with a high level of amprolium may cause a similar clinical entity. Uses of acepromazine sedation, as well as deworming with levamisole or thiabendazole, are recognized risk factors associated with PEM.

Pathophysiology

Normal rumen microbial activity allows an adequate level of thiamine to be produce. Thiamine is necessary in the synthesis of red blood cell transketolase, the rate-limiting enzyme in the pentose phosphate pathway. Glucose metabolism of the brain depends largely on the pentose pathway. Altered glucose metabolism in the brain leads to cerebral edema and necrosis. Different clinical situations (exposure to risk factors) may lead to either a reduction in thiamine production or an increase in thiamine destruction.

Clinical Signs

Affected animals are depressed and anorexic. Rapidly, neurologic signs appear with possibly cortical blindness being the first to be recognized (no menace response despite intact pupillary light reflex). Neurologic signs, most often symmetrical, reflect cerebrocortical involvement (edema, elevated intracranial pressure, and necrosis).

Ataxia and proprioceptive deficits are present if the animal is capable of walking. Head-pressing and episode of excitement may arise. Cranial nerve evaluation remains normal except for a dorso-medial strabismus associated with the "stretching" of cranial nerve V. As the disease progresses, recumbency, opisthotonus, extensor rigidity, abnormal nystagmus, and convulsions occur. The disease is most often fatal in a few days.

Clinical Pathology and Diagnosis

Clinical signs and in some situations the response to treatment are often the basis to establish a presumptive diagnosis. The CSF analysis from acute cases is usually considered normal except for a slight elevated protein concentration. As the cortical necrosis progresses, protein concentration and the nucleated cells number become elevated. Nevertheless, CSF analysis helps to rule out diseases with marked changes (listeriosis and meningitis).

Postmortem examination, especially histopathology allows the definitive diagnosis to be made. Macroscopic examination reveals edema and yellow discoloration of the cerebral gyri, and, when exposed to an ultraviolet light, the cerebral cortex shows some fluorescence.[4] In severe cases the cerebellum may be pushed caudally into the foramen magnum, and/or tentorial herniation may be present. Histopathology of the cerebral cortex reveals the most prominent lesions. Edema (cellular and extracellular), necrosis of the gray matter, and gliosis are the most frequently observed.

Specific tests exist and include the following: erythrocyte transketolase activity,[5] blood thiamine levels,[6] tissue thiamine levels,[7] thiamine pyrophosphate,[5] erythrocyte concentration of thiamine,[6] and rumen or fecal thiaminase activity.[4,7] All of these tests may not be offered by all laboratories.

Treatment

As usual, early treatment is more rewarding and in most situations effective. A response to treatment is usually observed within hours (2-12 hours). As the severity of the case increases, the time to response increases, as well as the risk of permanent sequela. Specific therapy requires thiamine hydrochloride (10 mg/kg IV, SC, or IM) given 2 to 4 times a day until response to treatment and evidence of adequate rumen function (rumination). One should pay attention not to follow the recommended dosage from the bottle because it is often labeled for preventive purposes.

Supportive care is indicated and includes maintaining the animal in a safe, calm, and comfortable stall. Cerebral edema may have to be specifically treated. Corticosteroids and mannitol can be used. If convulsions are present, diazepam (Valium) should be given. When the animal improves and can swallow and stand on its own, rumen transfaunation may help restore the normal rumen flora, especially in cases where diet changes seem to be involved in the apparition of the disease.

Improvement is in some cases spectacular. I personally recommend administering thiamin to all patients with clinical signs of cerebral edema before completing a thorough neurologic examination. In many cases, by the time the examination is finished, the patient has already shown signs of improvement. Blindness may persist a few days after the animal has recovered.

Prevention

Reducing the exposure to the risk factors contributes to prevention and is especially important when multiple cases within a group are diagnosed. The caretaker can maintain a healthy rumen flora and activity in the animal by ensuring that its diet contains enough fiber.

When an animal from a group has been diagnosed, it may be suitable to preventively treat with thiamine injection the other animals from the same group until the risk factor is identified and the appropriate changes made. Addition of thiamine into the ration has been recommended as well.

SALT POISONING/WATER DEPRIVATION

Definition and Etiology

Water deprivation is almost a necessary condition for salt poisoning to occur. The common presentation relates to several days of excessive intake of dietary salts while water intake is restricted, followed by free access to water, but various circumstances may lead to salt poisoning in cattle. The precise toxic dose associated with salt poisoning depends on the availability of free water. As an example, ingestion of water with salt concentrations greater than 1% results in clinical signs if no access to free water was provided.[8,9]

Epidemiology

Risk factors associated with salt poisoning often relate to management errors: cows given access to a pasture without any source of water, cattle fed a protein supplement with an excessive amount of salt, cattle offered access to salty water as an only source of drinking water, and calves given improperly formulated milk replacers or oral electrolyte replacements.

Pathophysiology

The pathogenesis of salt poisoning involves the accumulation of sodium ions in the central nervous system (CNS) (tissue and CSF). The resulting changes in osmolarity disturb the normal energy-dependant sodium ion transport mechanisms, as well as the anaerobic glycolytic pathways. Lack of efficiency of these mechanisms prevents sodium ions from being removed from the neural cell. Because the thirst receptors are triggered by the increased osmolality, if the animal gains access to free water, the fluid absorbed from the gastrointestinal tract creates some expansion of the extracellular fluid. Water then diffuses from the blood into the relatively hyperosmolar CNS, resulting in edema, increased intracranial pressure, and its consequences.

Clinical Signs

Clinical signs are associated with digestive and CNS involvement. Depression, weakness, and ataxia are observed in most cases. Facial muscle fasciculation has been observed by some authors.[10] Excessive thirst and diarrhea may be seen in some cases. Eventually, the neurologic signs evolve toward recumbency, opisthotonus, convulsions, and death.

Diagnosis

The clinical diagnosis of salt poisoning is based on the exposure to the recognized risk factors (feeding high salt concentrations and/or water deprivation), and the serum or cerebrospinal fluid (CSF) sodium concentrations.

Necropsy Findings

Cattle do not seem to develop the perivascular infiltration of eosinophils observed in swine. However, pathologic changes reported include cerebral edema, malacia of the cortical regions, and perivascular cuffing of mononuclear cells.

Treatment

Treatment of animals affected by salt poisoning remains a challenge. Even in a hospital situation where laboratory monitoring and precise fluid rate administration can be performed, the prognosis remains guarded. Treatment goals are the following: prevent ingestion of free water, progressively reduce the osmolarity in the CNS, and control cerebral edema and its consequences if problematic.

In neonatal calves suffering from salt poisoning/water deprivation, administration of hypertonic saline combined to regular feeding of milk (10% of their bodyweight per day) seems to give interesting results. No access to free water during the course of treatment is also important. After obtaining a first measurement of the plasma sodium concentration, a hypertonic saline solution is administered intravenously. The sodium concentration of the intravenous (IV) fluid solution should be equal to or even slightly greater than that of the plasma. The plasma electrolyte concentration is measured several times during the course of treatment (2 to 4 times per day). According to the measurements, the hypertonic solutions, as well as the rate of administration can be readjusted. The ultimate goal is to bring back the serum concentration to sodium to normal level over 2 to 4 days without the development of nervous signs. If nervous signs develop during the course of treatment (twitching, head-neck extension, or convulsions), mannitol should be used to control brain edema. Valium can be used to control the convulsions. Corticosteroids (dexamethasone, 0.4-0.8 mg/kg by slow IV injection given twice daily for 2-3 days) have been recommended in animals developing acute cerebral edema.[11]

Control

Control and prevention are aimed at reducing exposure to known risk factors, water deprivation being an important one.

LEAD POISONING

Definition and Etiology

Lead poisoning or plumbisms in ruminants cause acute encephalopathy. Cattle have a natural tendency to lick and/or ingest foreign materials. The fact that they may have access to such material predisposes them to the condition. In some geographic areas where pasturing is commonly used, access to areas where lead-containing chemicals materials are stored remain possible. The toxic doses vary and in general, as the dose increases, the severity of clinical signs increases and the time before apparition of signs decreases. Susceptibility is influenced by the age of the animal, the type of lead product, the stage of lactation, and possibly the diet.

Epidemiology

Reported sources of lead are used batteries and motor oil, lead-based paints, grease used for farm equipments, linoleum, and roofing materials. Access to pasture near a busy highway or an industrial zone may also be considered a potential source of lead.

Pathophysiology

Because ingestion is a common route of exposure, lead enters through the gastrointestinal tracts. Inhalation of lead particulate is also possible. Although lead may affect several organs, the clinical signs in ruminants are associated with encephalopathy and gastroenteritis. Degeneration of peripheral nerves associated with chronic lead exposure is rarely seen in cattle. A small percentage of the ingested lead is actually absorbed. Insoluble complexes are formed in the intestine and are excreted in the feces. Direct caustic effect of the lead salts on the intestinal mucosa causes diarrhea after an initial constipation episode. The lead absorbed combines with erythrocytes, resulting in a low concentration in the plasma.[12] As lead gets distributed to all body systems, the liver and kidneys accumulate a large amount of it and necrosis may occur. The nervous tissue suffers capillary damage and decreased blood supply, leading to edema.[12]

Clinical Signs

Acute, subacute, and chronic forms have been described and are associated with different clinical presentations. CNS derangement predominates in the acute form, but gastrointestinal signs may also be present (most often diarrhea). Neurologic signs include hyperesthesia and a period of excitement, muscular fasciculations, and twitching of the eyelids, ears, or jaw. Acute death without any clinical signs is possible. As the disease progresses, ataxia, cortical blindness, head-pressing, circling, opisthotonus, and convulsions develop.

In the subacute form associated with exposure to lower levels of lead in the diet, gastrointestinal signs are more often observed. Complete anorexia and severe diarrhea are present. Signs of colic may be seen. Severe depression, blindness, hyperesthesia, and twitching then develop. Although various theories exist as to the cellular effect of lead on the CNS, the exact cellular pathophysiology is unknown.

In the chronic form, considered uncommon in ruminants, clinical signs are less characteristic and more associated with poor performance. Normocytic, normochromic anemia and basophilic stippling have been described.

Clinical Pathology and Diagnosis

Clinical signs and a thorough investigation often lead to a presumptive diagnosis of lead poisoning; however, measurement of blood and tissue concentrations of lead is necessary to obtain a final diagnosis. Although tissue lead values are of great value, whole blood concentration can also be used on a living animal. Acceptable blood concentration may vary from one laboratory to another, but most laboratories consider any values above 0.35 ppm as abnormal. Chronic exposure to low levels of lead may not generate elevated blood lead concentrations. Tissues concentrations (liver and kidney) above 10 ppm are considered to be diagnostic of lead poisoning.

The hematologic changes associated with lead poisoning are subtle. Many animals have a completely normal complete blood count (CBC). In some cases the following have been observed: anisocytosis, poikilocytosis, polychromasia, hypochromia, Howel-Jolly bodies, metarubricytes, and basophilic stippling.[13,14]

Cerebrospinal fluid analysis may remain normal in acute cases or reveal a moderate elevated protein concentration and nucleated cells.

Other specific tests measure the metabolic effects of lead. For example, the determination of the level of activity of the enzyme delta aminolevulinic acid dehydratase (d-ALAD), which is inhibited by the presence of lead, can be used. This enzyme is necessary for the heme synthesis. As the activity of the enzyme decreases in the blood, the metabolite (d-ALA) concentration increases in the urine. One should contact the laboratory before sending a sample to verify if the test is available because it is not performed widely.

Necropsy Findings

The gross postmortem examination is of little value unless foreign material and/or odor are found in the rumen. The brain examination may reveal mild congestion of vessels of the cerebral cortex and edema, and cerebrocortical necrosis may create a yellow discoloration.

Histopathologic brain lesions include the following: petechial hemorrhages, endothelial swelling, edema, and cortical neuronal necrosis. Liver and kidney degeneration may be observed in some cases.

Treatment

Treatment goals in lead poisoning are removal of the lead from the digestive tract when considered appropriate, chelation therapy to help lead excretion, and adequate supportive care. Thiamine treatment has been studied and found to be effective.[15-17] According to experimental studies, appropriate dosage of thiamine for this purpose should be at least 2 mg/kg body weight. The nature of the protective effects of thiamine is unclear.

The potential source of lead must be identified to prevent further exposure. In the meantime, only access to safe feed must be allowed. This may mean restricting access to pasture until the source is identified.

Removal of lead from the digestive tract can be done by rumenotomy if judged appropriate for the situation. Magnesium sulfate laxatives form insoluble lead sulfides and may reduce further absorption.

Specific treatment requires administration of calcium disodium EDTA (ethylenediamine tetraacetic acid). IV administration of the solution may cause adverse effects (increase heart and respiratory rates and muscle tremors), but if done slowly it is considered safe. The daily dosage is approximately 60 to 100 mg/kg body weight divided in two, three, or four treatments. Several days may be necessary to obtain some response. Calcium disodium EDTA chelates lead from bone and not directly from soft tissue. However, as the equilibrium between soft tissue and bone occurs, soft tissue concentrations also decrease.

Supportive cares includes fluid therapy, maintaining the animal in a quiet environment, controlling convulsions if necessary, and providing extra bedding material and a safe stall because many animals are hyperactive.

CITRULLINEMIA

Bovine citrullinemia is an autosomal recessive fatal disorder. Affected newborns are normal at birth and develop clinical signs in the first few days of life. Death occurs shortly after the onset of clinical signs. Clinical signs include depression, head-pressing, tremors, compulsive walking, blindness, recumbency, opisthotonos convulsions, and death. Dysfunction of a urea cycle enzyme (arginosuccinate synthetase) is responsible for the clinical signs. Blood citrulline concentration is extremely elevated in both homozygotes and heterozygotes.

HYDROCEPHALUS AND HYDRANENCEPHALY OF CATTLE

David Francoz

Hydrocephalus is defined as an increase in the volume of CSF.[18] Hydrocephalus may be further categorized as normotensive or hypertensive.[18-20] Both types may be congenital or acquired.

Normotensive Hydrocephalus

Normotensive hydrocephalus occurs when CSF accumulates in the nervous system space not occupied by brain tissue.[18] In ruminants, normotensive hydrocephalus is mainly a congenital defect associated with cell growth or failure cellular destruction.[20] When the defect creates an abnormal cavity combined with CSF accumulation, the term *hydranencephaly* is used.[20,21] When the defect leads to cystic CSF-filled spaces, it is called *porencephaly*.[21] Hydranencephaly and porencephaly are most often associated with in utero viral infection. Viruses that have been implicated include Akabane virus, bovine viral diarrhea virus, border disease virus, Cache Valley virus, bluetongue virus, Aino virus, Kasba (Chuzan) virus, and Wesselsbron disease virus. Akabane virus belongs to the bunyavirus, in the Arboviridae family. The virus can infect cattle, sheep, and goats. It is reported in Africa, Japan, Israel, Korea, and Australia. Infection in adult animals is usually asymptomatic. Hydranencephaly and/or porencephaly associated with arthrogryposis have been reported in calves and lambs when they are exposed in utero between days 62 and 96 and days 30 and 36, respectively.[22,23] Similar defects have been reported in goat kids.[24] A brief description of CNS congenital defects of other viruses is presented in the cerebellar disorders section.

Acquired causes of normotensive hydrocephalus in ruminants include polioencephalomalacia.[18]

Hypertensive Hydrocephalus

Hypertensive hydrocephalus occurs when both CSF volume and pressure increases. It may result from flow obstruction, decreased absorption, or increased production of CSF.[18] Based on CNS pathologic lesions, other organs involved, and the affected breed, six different forms of congenital hypertensive hydrocephalus have been described in calves. Affected breeds include Hereford, Charolais, Ayrshire, Dexter, Holstein, Whitebred Shorthorn, and Jersey.[25-27] The conditions are thought to be hereditary.

Acquired hypertensive hydrocephalus can occur secondary to cerebral abscesses, lymphosarcoma, *Coenurus cerebralis* infestation, meningitis, or vitamin A deficiency.[20]

Clinical Signs and Diagnosis

In many cases, newborn animals are born dead or die shortly after birth. When they are born alive, clinical signs related to cerebral disorders are present. The animal is weak and depressed, and has a weak or absent suckle reflex. The neonates may have droopy ears and heads, head tremor, muscular fasciculations, blindness, ventrolateral strabismus, nystagmus, dysphonia, limb spasticity, hyperreflexia, recumbency, convulsions, and coma.[18,20] A domed skull may also be observed. In cases of hydranencephaly or porencephaly associated with viral infection, other malformation such as limbs deformities, brachygnathia, or ocular malformations may be present. The diagnosis is based on clinical signs and domed skull when present. Virus isolation, or antigen detection on fetal tissues or blood, and detection of antibodies in precolostral samples can be performed to include or exclude in utero viral infection.

No treatment is available at present.

References

1. Raisbeck MF: Is polioencephalomalacia associated with high-sulfate diets? *J Am Vet Med Assoc* 180:1303-1305, 1982.
2. Markson JM, Lewis G, Terlecki S et al: The effects of administering antimetabolites of thiamine to preruminant calves. The etiology of cerebrocortical necrosis, *Br Vet J* 128:488-498, 1972.
3. Morgan JT, Lawson GH: Thiaminase type 1-producing bacilli and ovine polioencephalomalacia, *Vet Rec* 95:361-363, 1974.
4. Gabbedy BJ, Richard RB: Polioencephalomalacia of sheep and cattle, *Aus Vet J* 53:36-38, 1977.
5. Evans WC, Evans A, Humphreys DJ et al: Induction of thiamine deficiency in sheep with lesions similar to those of cerebrocortical necrosis, *J Comp Pathol* 85:253-267, 1975.
6. MacPherson A, Moon FE, Voss RC: Biochemical aspects of cobalt deficiency in sheep with special reference to vitamin status and a possible involvement in the aetiology of cerebrocortical necrosis, *Br Vet J* 132:294-308, 1976.
7. Edwin EE, Markson LM, Shreeve J et al: Diagnostic aspects of cerebrocortical necrosis, *Vet Rec* 104:4-8, 1979.
8. Sandals WC: Acute salt poisoning in cattle, *Can Vet J* 19:136-137, 1978.
9. McCoy CP, Edwards WC: Sodium ion poisoning in livestock from oil wastes, *Bov Pract* 15:152-154, 1980.
10. Angelos SM, Smith BP, George LW et al: Treatment of hypernatremia in an acidotic neonatal calf, *J Am Vet Med Assoc* 214:1364-1367, 1999.
11. George LW: In Smith BP: *Large animal internal medicine*, ed 3, Philadelphia, 2002, Mosby, p 927.
12. Goldstein GW, Asbury AK, Diamond I: Pathogenesis of lead encephalopathy uptake of lead and reaction of brain capillaries, *Arch Neurol* 31:382-389, 1974.
13. Buck WB: Toxins and neurologic disease in cattle, *J Am Med Assoc* 166:222-226, 1975.
14. Georges JW, Duncan JR: The haematology of lead poisoning in man and animals, *Vet Clin Pathol* 8:23-30, 1979.
15. Gudmundson J: Lead poisoning in cattle, *Agric Pract* 14:43-47, 1993.
16. Bratton GR, Zmudski J, Kincaid N: Thiamine as treatment of lead poisoning in ruminants, *Mod Vet Pract* 62:441-446, 1981.
17. Bratton GR, Zmudzki J, Bell MC et al: Thiamine (vitamin B_1) effects on lead intoxication and deposition of lead in tissues: therapeutic potential, *Toxicol Appl Pharmacol* 59:164-172, 1981.
18. DeLahunta A: Cerebrospinal fluid and hydrocephalus. In DeLahunta A, editor: *Veterinary neuroanatomy and clinical neurology*, Philadelphia, 1983, Saunders, pp 30-52.
19. Greene HJ, Leipold HW, Huston K et al: Congenital defects in cattle, *Irish Vet J* 27:37-45, 1973.
20. Smith MO: Diseases of the nervous system. In Smith BP, editor: *Large animal internal medicine*, St Louis, 2002, Mosby, pp 873-1017.
21. Washburn KE, Streeter RN: Congenital defects of the ruminant nervous system, *Vet Clin North Am Food Anim Pract* 20:413-434. viii, 2004.
22. Kurogi H, Inaba Y, Takahashi E et al: Congenital abnormalities in newborn calves after inoculation of pregnant cows with Akabane virus, *Infect Immun* 17:338-343, 1977.
23. Parsonson IM, Della-Porta AJ, Snowdon WA et al: Congenital abnormalities in newborn lambs after infection of pregnant sheep with Akabane virus, *Infect Immun* 15:254-262, 1977.
24. Inaba Y, Kurogi H, Omori T et al: Akabane disease: epizootic abortion, premature birth, stillbirth and congenital arthrogryposis-hydranencephaly in cattle, sheep and goats caused by Akabane virus, *Aust Vet J* 51:784-785, 1975.
25. Baker M, Payne LC, Baker GN: The inheritance of hydrocephalus in cattle, *J Hered* 52:135-138, 1961.
26. Urman HK, Grace OD: Hereditary encephalomyopathy: a hydrocephalus syndrome in newborn calves, *Cornell Vet* 54:229-249, 1964.
27. Axthelm MK, Leipold HW, Howard D: Hereditary internal hydrocephalus, *Proc Am Assoc Vet Lab Diagn* 115-126, 1980.

CHAPTER 66

Central Nervous System Infection and Infestation

GILLES FECTEAU and LISLE W. GEORGE

MENINGITIS

Definition and Etiology

Meningitis, an inflammation of one or more of the three covering layers of the meninges (dura, arachnoid, and pia mater) in the central nervous system (CNS), may be classified by duration (acute or chronic); structures that are affected (meningitis, meningoencephalitis, or meningoventriculitis); location, (cerebral, cerebrospinal, or spinal); etiology (bacterial or viral); or histopathologic lesions (suppurative or nonsuppurative). The collective role of the meninges is to support, protect, and contribute to the irrigation of the nervous system. The dura mater is the most external layer and is mostly collagen, blood vessels, and neural terminations. The dura mater is the thicker and most resistant of the three meninges. The dura mater is adherent to the skull but is unattached to the vertebrae. The gaps between unattached meninges and the vertebral column form the epidural space. The pia arachnoid, which consists of the internal meningeal layer, is attached to the nervous tissue by fine trabeculae. The arachnoid surrounds a mass of capillaries to form the choroid plexus. Unlike the pia mater, the arachnoid does not follow all depressions of the nervous tissue.

The spaces that form between the arachnoid and the pia mater contain the cerebrospinal fluid (CSF), which is a clear fluid containing mainly water and electrolytes. The CSF protects and nourishes the CNS. The fluid is produced in several sites that include the lateral ventricles, choroid plexus, and pia arachnoid. The fluid is formed by the combined physiologic mechanisms of ultrafiltration and active transport. Reabsorption of CSF occurs at the arachnoid villi and at the dural reflections over the cranial and spinal nerves. The two most important clinically important cisternae are the cisterna magna and the lumbosacral cistern, both of which may be used to collect CSF on living animals.

Bacterial meningitis has been described in adult cattle but is most commonly seen in neonates.[1-4] Bacterial suppurative meningitis can also result from direct extension through the calvarium, as may occur with conditions that include otitis interna, sinusitis, and infected skull fractures or following bacteremia. The following section describes neonatal bacterial suppurative meningitis (NBSM).

Bacterial sepsis and NBSM are often linked. In human medicine, the frequency with which NBSM occurs in neonatal sepsis cases has decreased in recent years from 1 in 4 cases to 1 in 20 cases. In developed countries, the case fatality rate from NBSM is 3%, which is lower than the 25% to 30% rate that was reported 20 years ago.[5] Such statistics are not currently available in domestic animals, but a reported case fatality rate of 100%[6] indicates that the prognosis is poor in cattle. The reported prevalence of septic meningitis in necropsied calves has been as great as 43%.[7] However, the true prevalence of the disease in cattle remains to be studied.

Pathogenesis

Gram-negative bacteria, *Escherichia coli* in particular, are reported to be the most common meningeal pathogens in bovine neonates.[6,8-10] In sheep and goats, *E. coli*, *Pasteurella*, *Streptococcus*, *Staphylococcus pyogenes*, and *Arcanobacterium pyogenes* have been cultured from meningitis cases.[11,12] Some *E. coli* virulence factors may be of importance in the development of NBSM because the successful meningeal pathogen would have overcome sequential host defenses mechanisms to reach the CSF and to replicate.

E. coli that are found in meningitic calves are non-hemolytic, synthesize hydroxymate and colicin V, have expressed the 31a surface antigen, show antibody resistance, produce aerobactin, and are fimbriated.[13]

Before invading the meninges, the pathogen must colonize host mucosal epithelium. Bacterial omphalophlebitis or severe enteritis may lead to bacteremia without previous mucosal colonization.

The access of pathogens into the meninges is poorly understood. Specific mechanisms may include the development of a bacteremia in highly perfused dural venous system and choroid plexuses, adherence of S fimbriae of some strains of *E. coli* to macrophages, the phagocytosis of the pathogens by circulating monocytes, and endocytosis through the microvascular endothelial cells.[14] Environmental growth conditions that may influence the ability to invade brain microvascular endothelial cells (microaerophilic, pH, newborn bovine serum, magnesium, and iron) have been studied in vitro.[15]

Bacteria survive and proliferate in the poorly defended CSF. Complement is essentially nonexistent in CSF, which, when combined with low specific antibodies, leads to inadequate opsonization of meningeal pathogens. Despite an early influx of leukocytes into the CSF in bacterial meningitis, the host defense system remains suboptimal because opsonic activity is deficient.[16]

The sequelae of meningitis are associated with the release of cytokines and the direct effects of bacterial invasion.[16] Free bacterial endotoxins may thrombose the arachnoidal or subependymal veins. Thrombosis-related hemorrhagic infarction results in neural necrosis.[5] Inflammatory changes in the subarachnoid space may affect the choroid plexus, decreasing the absorption of fluid and potentially creating hypertensive hydrocephalus.

Risk Factors

Calves with failure of passive transfer (FPT) are at high risk for developing neonatal sepsis and subsequent bacterial meningitis.

Clinical Presentation

Calves suffering from NBSM lack a suckling reflex and appear lethargic. Previous treatment for undifferentiated diarrhea is common. According to two different studies, approximately 30% of critically ill neonatal calves are bacteremic.[17,18] Fever is usually present, unless some NSAI drugs have been administered or the animal is in an extremely cold environment. The calves have an extended head and neck. Attempts to flex or reposition the neck result in a tonic extension and thrashing of the limbs. Hyperesthesia is common. With time, a profound depression state develops and eventually the animal becomes comatose and nonresponsive, or it may develop tonic clonic seizures. Dysfunction of cranial nerve VI results in nystagmus and strabismus. Dysfunction of cranial nerve VII leads to facial palsy. Spinal reflexes are described to be exaggerated. Concurrent findings may include hypopyon, arthritis, omphalophlebitis, and diarrhea.

Diagnosis

The presumptive diagnosis of bacterial meningitis is based on demonstration of failure of passive transfer, presence of a septic focus such as omphalophlebitis or septic arthritis, and the clinical signs described earlier. However, the definitive diagnosis is based on an abnormal purulent exudate in the CSF analysis or on the presence of histopathologic lesions.

The CSF of meningitic patients contains large concentrations of degenerating neutrophils and high protein concentrations. The specimens may be grossly xanthochromic and are usually turbid. Some CSF specimens from meningitic patients clot if collected in tubes that are devoid of anticoagulant.

The offending bacteria may not be recoverable in all specimens of CSF. Lack of correlation between antemortem and postmortem culture results of lumbar CSF and cultures of tissues postmortem has been reported. Ferrouillet and colleagues[9] found in seven cases where premortem and postmortem culture results were available that there was no association between culture results in vivo and culture results at postmortem examination.[9] CSF specimens should be submitted for laboratory analysis within an hour of collection.[19] Whenever immediate analysis is impossible, a sedimentation procedure should be attempted to reduce artifactual lysis of white blood cells and reduction of glucose concentration. To perform a sedimentation assay, a 2-cm plastic cylinder is placed on a clean glass slide and filled with 1 ml of CSF. The CSF in the cylinder is allowed to sediment for 30 to 60 minutes. The supernatant is then removed, and the glass slide is stained. The interpretation can then be performed at a later time by qualified personnel.[2,20]

Microscopic examination of CSF is an important test for bacterial meningitis. Three different studies have examined CSF analysis in meningitic calves.[6,8,9] The three papers agreed that the number of nucleated cells and the protein concentration are markedly increased. The proportion of neutrophils may reach as high as 80%. The ratio of CSF to plasma glucose concentration is less than 1 in animals with bacterial meningitis because of bacterial metabolism of glucose in the CSF. Xanthochromia was frequent in one study and rarely seen in another. One author did not report this particular finding. Free or intracellular bacteria were observed in 45% of the specimens in Green's study.

The meningitic patient's hemogram usually reflects either a toxic degenerative left shift or a profound neutrophilia. Bacterial meningitis should be differentiated from other encephalopathies of neonates. The condition can appear to be similar to several particular congenital diseases and of acute diffuse cerebral edema due to salt toxicity.

Treatment

Treatment of bacterial meningitis is difficult. The mortality rate of meningitic calves ranges from 3% to 13% and has been reported to be as high as 100%.[5,6] Antimicrobials are the most important therapeutic modality for treatment of bacterial meningitis in calves. Selection of antimicrobial drugs should be based on sensitivity testing of isolates from the CSF. However, this is rarely possible in farm animals because isolation of the bacteria from the CSF may be difficult. In clinical settings, therapeutic delays that await bacteriologic results could increase the mortality rate in patients with fulminant bacterial meningitis.

The physicochemical properties (lipid solubility, molecular weight, protein binding, and ionization) and the pharmacokinetics of a drug influence its penetration through the blood-brain barrier (BBB). The CSF to blood concentration ratio is an indicator of the penetration of a drug into the CNS. These ratios are described for several antimicrobials used in human medicine and laboratory animals. However, in farm animals, very little is known on these numbers.[21] Another key factor to consider is the suboptimal immune response in the CSF (lack of complement and antibody), which implies that to be effective, an antibiotic needs to reach the minimal bactericidal concentrations (MBCs). The antibiotic concentrations in the CSF should be compared with the MBC value for the targeted pathogens rather than using the standard minimum inhibitory concentration (MIC). Drugs that diffuse into the CSF (e.g., aminoglycosides) may not always be the optimum because the CSF concentrations that are achieved only approximate the MBC.[21] On the other hand, the β-lactam antibiotics diffuse poorly through the

BBB but can reach multiples of MBC because larger doses can be used without risk of toxicity.[21] The expected ratios of CSF antibiotic concentrations to bacterial MICs (MBC would be better, but those numbers are not always available) are part of the equation. The data available on this matter are again lacking in farm animals. One study available in calves presents the pharmacokinetic of florfenicol. The maximum concentration of florfenicol achieved in the CSF after a single IV dose of 20 mg/kg was 4.67 ± 1.51 μg/ml. The concentration in the CSF remained above the MIC for *Histophilus somnus* for 20 hours.[22]

The optimal antimicrobial for the treatment of meningitis in ruminants should have a good spectrum against gram-negative and gram-positive pathogens. The availability, formulation, and approved use of the antimicrobial are also taken into consideration (residue, possible IV administration, cost of prolonged therapy). The actual selection is often reduced to third-generation cephalosporins (ceftiofur 5-10 mg/kg one to three times a day intramuscularly or IV), sodium ampicillin (10-20 mg/kg three times a day intravenously), fluoroquinolones (enrofloxacin 10 mg/kg IV once a day, subcutaneously), and trimethoprim-sulfonamide (5 mg/kg based on the trimethoprim two or three times a day IV). A combination of drugs could be used to broaden the spectrum. Such combinations could include ampicillin-ceftiofur or ampicillin-trimethoprim-sulfonamide. All antimicrobial regimens described earlier are empiric and derived from comparative medicine and clinical experience. Solid scientific evidence to corroborate those regimens in the treatment of bacterial meningitis in ruminants is not available at the moment. One should remember that the inflamed meninges increase the diffusion of drugs into the CSF and that as the animal improves, diffusion will decrease. Repair of the BBB leads to lower penetration of most antibiotics into the CSF. Less drug in CSF may be associated with an intratherapeutic relapse of clinical signs.

Intrathecal antibiotic treatment does not improve the prognosis in human medicine and is impractical for farm animal medicine.[5]

Duration of therapy is empiric—14 days appears to be the minimum in human medicine.[5,16] Antiinflammatory agents are indicated to improve the patient's attitude in general and also to control the secondary effects of sepsis. However, the choice between steroidal and nonsteroidal antiinflammatory agents remains empiric in farm animals. In human medicine, steroidal antiinflammatory agents are indicated in cases of meningitis associated with *Haemophilus influenzae*. In all other situations, the questions remain unanswered.[16]

General supportive measures are essential, and any concurrent disease must be treated adequately and aggressively because the continuous bacteremia may arise from another site (septic arthritis or omphalophlebitis).

Because failure of passive transfer could be a predisposing factor to septicemia, plasma transfusion seems to be of interest in the treatment. Convulsions should be treated appropriately. Diazepam (0.01-0.2 mg/kg), IV every 30 minutes should be administered until convulsions are controlled.

Nutritional support is most important. If the animals remain inappetant, they should either be given whole milk by tube or intravenous total parenteral nutrition, or both.

Prevention

Adequate volume of colostrum is essential for prevention of meningitis in neonates. Early recognition and prompt therapeutic intervention with prophylactic antimicrobials and intravenous administration of whole homologous plasma are also important for prevention of life-threatening meningitis. Reduction of the exposition to risk factors is important, so appropriate care to colostrum feeding is essential and early recognition and treatment of any bacterial diseases is also important.

THROMBOTIC MENINGOENCEPHALITIS ASSOCIATED WITH *HISTOPHILUS SOMNUS (HAEMOPHILUS SOMNUS)*

Etiology and Epidemiology

Histophilus somni (recently renamed, traditionally known as *Haemophilus somnus*) was first isolated from the nervous tissues of a calf that died of encephalitis. *H. somni* has traditionally been associated with a fatal septicemic condition of feedlot cattle often showing neurologic signs; however, it is now well recognized that the disease caused by *Histophilus* involves a number of organ systems including respiratory, bone, joint, mammary gland, genitals, heart, and eye.[23] *H. somni* is a gram-negative non–spore-forming coccobacillus.[24] Isolates from the genital tract (prepuce and vagina) and from septicemic animals differ with respect to serum sensitivity and presumably in antiphagocytic resistance.[25] The prevalence and case fatality rate of *H. somni* infection is high, but the occurrence of the clinical disease is relatively low. Feedlot cattle are more often affected than are pastured or dairy animals. Histophilosis has a worldwide distribution.

Pathogenesis

H. somni first colonizes the surface of a mucous membrane, proliferates locally, and eventually invades the host to cause bacteremia. Which mucous membranes (respiratory or genital) are most often infected are unclear. Interaction between endothelial cells and the bacteria results in collagen exposure to initiate thrombus formation. Thrombosis is seen in the brain, lungs, and heart of affected cattle.[26,27] A study that was performed in experimentally infected calves using the 43826 strain further elucidated the pathogenesis of the disease. In that study, Little[26] was capable of inducing a septicemic thrombotic meningoencephalitis in 60% to 70% of challenged calves. Clinical signs developed rapidly, and death occurred in less than 36 hours. Necrotic lesions were found in the vasculature of the challenged animals. Initiation of this process was associated with exposure of the underlying basement membrane.[28] Thrombosis developed after the coagulation cascade was initiated. The thrombotic lesion resulted in septicemia, which allowed the bacterium to embolize and then reach distant tissues, where they would cause the typical histologic lesions. These include small-vessel thrombosis and tissue necrosis, neutrophilic infiltration, and intracellular bacteria.

The serum antibody titer has not correlated to the outcome of challenge infection,[28] suggesting that humoral immunity does not provide complete protection against clinical disease.

Clinical Signs

In the nervous form of histophilosis, multiple animals are commonly affected and sudden death could be the first and only clinical sign. In other cases, respiratory disease may precede the neurologic signs (7-14 days earlier). When clinical signs develop, neurologic impairment is often severe. Common clinical signs include lateral recumbency, depression, closed to semiclosed eyelids, blindness, proprioceptive defects, cranial nerve deficits, and hyperreflexia. Animals in lateral recumbency may progress to opisthotonos and convulsions. Retinal hemorrhages have been described in affected cattle.[29]

Diagnosis

History and physical examination often lead to a presumptive diagnosis of *H. somni* meningo-encephalitis, but final diagnosis is often based on postmortem examination. CBC changes are nonspecific and reported to be consistent with gram-negative sepsis (leukopenia and neutropenia or neutrophilia with left shift).[4] CSF changes are reflective of bacterial infection combined with hemorrhage. The number of nucleated cells is increased (neutrophils), as well as protein concentration. Xanthochromia and increased number of red cells may also be present. One method recommended by some author to rapidly assess CSF globulin concentration is the Pandy reaction (saturated phenol). Mild to strong reaction are observed in cases of meningitis.[1,2]

The organism can be cultured from different body fluids if the animal had not been treated (blood, CSF, joint and pleural fluids).[30] Selective medium has been developed, and it is suitable to specifically request that *H. somni* is suspected to the laboratory.[31] Serology testing exists but does not seem to be routinely used to confirm diagnosis. Asymptomatic animals may show spontaneous seroconversion, so acute and convalescent sera are necessary to confirm the role of the organism in a particular case.

Necropsy findings related to the nervous forms are hemorrhagic infarcts in the brain and spinal cord. The lesions are most often multiple and of various sizes, some being visible macroscopically. Histologically, vasculitis, thrombosis, and neutrophils infiltrates are the signature of the disease.

Treatment

Treatment of affected animals should be attempted only if the animal is believed to be in the early stages of the disease. Animals that are standing and treated early in the disease process may recover. Animals that have delayed treatment usually die within 24 to 36 hours following the appearance of clinical signs. Because of the poor therapeutic responses in animals with advanced neurologic signs, emphasis should be directed toward early identification of affected penmates. *H. somni* is susceptible to most commonly used antimicrobials, and antibiotic penetration into the CSF is enhanced by the endothelial damage.[31] Parenteral oxytetracycline is the most commonly recommended treatment for commercial animals. Dosages of 10 mg/kg of a conventional formulation administered intravenously twice a day for at least 3 days or until clinical signs indicate improvement may be used. A dosage of 20 mg/kg of a long-acting formulation given intramuscularly every 48 hours for a maximum of three treatments may also be used. Following this regimen, procaine penicillin (22,000 U/kg) should be given intramuscularly until complete recovery.

Use of a nonsteroidal antiinflammatory is indicated to control pain, fever, and general inflammatory reaction. Supportive care that includes nutrition, good footing, heavy bedding, and correction of dehydration and electrolyte change is important.

Prevention and Control

When a case is suspected or confirmed, all other animals in contact should be monitored twice daily to detect new cases in the earliest stage. Observations every 6 to 8 hours for the following week have been recommended.[4,25] Mass medication on arrival into feedlots does not reduce the risk of mortality associated with *H somni*.[32] Vaccines that are effective against the neurologic disease are available in North America.[28] Field efficacy studies are difficult to perform given the sporadic and unpredictable appearance of the nervous form of the disease.

Mycoplasma Meningitis in Calf

A particular clinical entity has been described in newborn calves and associated with *Mycoplasma bovis* infection. Newborn calves (younger than a week of age) were presented with fever, depression, swollen joints, and in some cases nervous signs. Treatment was unrewarding, and most animals were euthanized. Although the clinical signs and necropsy findings related mainly to pneumonia and arthritis, fibrinous meningitis was found in some cases.[33]

BRAIN ABSCESS

Etiology and Pathogenesis

Brain abscessation is a relatively rare condition of cattle. Two different pathogeneses are postulated to be of importance: extension of a local suppurative sinusitis through the bone and hematogenous spread into the CNS. *A. pyogenes* is most frequently isolated from brain abscesses.

Clinical Signs

The clinical signs of brain abscess are progressive and asymmetric including vision loss in the contralateral eye, ipsilateral mydriasis, depression, mania, head pressing, coma circling, and head tilt. If the abscess is near the brainstem, other cranial nerve dysfunctions may be observed.

A single lesion can usually be localized by observing the clinical signs, but multiple lesions of various sizes create a confusing and conflicting clinical picture.

Diagnosis

The diagnosis of brain abscess is based on the combination of clinical signs, inflammatory changes in the complete blood count, and CSF having increased numbers of neutrophils and high concentrations of protein. These changes include hyperfibrinogenemia, hypergammaglobulinemia, and nonresponsive anemia. Contrast magnetic resonance imaging and electrodiagnostic techniques are useful but rarely performed because of costs and logistical concerns.[34,35] Most diagnoses of brain abscesses are made at postmortem examination.

Treatment

Rational treatment of a brain abscess would include long-term antibiotic therapy and supportive care. The prognosis is unknown because no retrospective data are available at the moment, but they must be considered to be grave.

PITUITARY ABSCESS

Etiology and Pathogenesis

Pituitary abscesses occur sporadically in ruminants. The bacteria isolated most often are *A. pyogenes*. The pathogenesis of the condition is still to be determined; however, it is routinely accepted that the extensive capillary bed known as *rete mirabile,* surrounding the pituitary gland, is important in the development of the disease. Multiple other explanations have been postulated and reviewed.[36]

Clinical Signs

The clinical presentation is often variable and somewhat chronic. Neurologic signs include depression, dysphagia, dropped jaw, blindness, bradycardia, and absence of pupillary light reflex.[37] Males from 2 to 5 years of age have the highest incidence of pituitary abscess, probably because of infected nose rings or because of their propensity to fight with their head. Cranial injury may fracture the calvarium, which eventually leads to infection. The insertion of nose rings in bulls has been associated with the development of pituitary abscess.

Diagnosis

The diagnosis of pituitary abscess is based on clinical signs, necropsy, and CSF analysis. The CSF may have increased protein concentrations and pleocytosis.

Treatment

Rational treatment would be based on long duration antibiotic therapy and supportive care. The prognosis of a pituitary abscess is grave.[37]

ENCEPHALITIC INFECTIOUS BOVINE RHINOTRACHEITIS VIRUS INFECTION

In some circumstances, infectious bovine rhinotracheitis virus (IBRV) infection causes CNS disease. It is reported to be highly fatal.[38-40] Calves are more susceptible than adults. After an upper respiratory viral growth, migration toward the CNS occurs (trigeminal nerve).[41] The clinical signs are those of a meningoencephalitis and include depression and/or excitement, head pressing, aimless circling, bellowing, salivation, bruxism, nystagmus, convulsions, and mild nasal and ocular discharge. Fever is usually present. Postmortem examination reveals the following changes in the neural tissue: perivascular cuffing with mononuclear cells, diffuse gliosis, and neuronal degeneration. A severe lymphocytic meningoencephalitis is present. No specific treatment is recommended. Supportive care and control of convulsions with Valium may be helpful.

PSEUDORABIES

Definition and Etiology

Pseudorabies is caused by a herpes virus. Most often a mild disease to asymptomatic disease in swine, it is highly fatal in cattle. The clinical signs are to some extent similar to rabies and justify the name, *pseudorabies.*

Epidemiology

Pseudorabies has a worldwide distribution. Infected pigs shed the virus in the nasal and pharyngeal secretions, and because of the proximity of the two species in some livestock operations, transmission of the virus from swine into ruminants may occur.[42,43] Ruminants are susceptible to pseudorabies infection after intradermal, subcutaneous, intranasal, or oral exposure to the virus. Following infection, the incubation period is between 2 and 7 days. Horses and human beings are resistant to pseudorabies virus infection.

Clinical Signs

Because of the relatively short incubation period of the pseudorabies virus, ruminants may die suddenly without premonitory signs.[42] In more slowly developing cases, intense pruritus that may be localized or generalized develops. Dermal abrasions, swelling, pruritus, and alopecia occur at the site of virus inoculation.[44] Fever is often present. Other clinical signs reported are bloating, ataxia, aggression or depression, salivation, excessive chewing of the tongue, pharyngeal/laryngeal dysfunction, dyspnea, and seizures. Most affected animals die shortly (within 2 days) after the onset of clinical signs.

Diagnosis

In ruminants, a tentative diagnosis is often based on clinical signs and history of possible contact with pigs. On postmortem, histologic examination reveals a nonsuppurative inflammation of the brain and spinal cord, with perivascular cuffing and focal necrosis. Virus isolation, immunohistochemistry, and polymerase chain reaction can be used to confirm the diagnosis. Serologic testing is most often used in pigs, since ruminants die rapidly and may not have detectable antibodies. Regional diagnostic laboratory should be contacted before submitting a sample.

Treatment and Prevention

There is no effective treatment, and prevention is targeted toward reducing the exposure of ruminants to swine.

RABIES

Etiology

Rabies is a fatal disease affecting ruminants worldwide except in some insular countries or areas applying strict quarantine measures (e.g., Australia, New Zealand, British Islands). It is caused by a Lyssavirus of the Rhabdoviridae family.

Epidemiology

The disease is endemic in Canada and the United States and many other countries. The disease is not present in livestock of Australia or New Zealand. Vector-specific serovars exist, and the predominant vectors vary regionally and include foxes, bats, raccoons, and skunks. Exposure to the virus is by contact with saliva from an infected animal. The virus may be present in the saliva of infected animals a few days before the development of clinical signs. However, transmission through aerosols and milk to offspring had been shown.

A seasonal variation exists, and the incidence increases in late summer to early fall. Homologous host serovar infections are frequently asymptomatic.

Pathophysiology

After the virus enters the body, there is initial local multiplication followed by migration of the virus through peripheral nerves into the CNS. Nasal epithelium and salivary glands become infected and begin shedding of the virus into the saliva. The incubation period of rabies is variable and is associated with the route of entry. Bites around the head and face have a shorter incubation time than do wounds on the extremities. The source of the virus, site of infection, size of inoculum, and geographic differences are all associated with the predominance of the furious or paralytic form of the disease. The disease is considered invariably fatal, and respiratory paralysis appears to be a common cause of death.

Clinical Signs

The clinical signs of rabies in ruminants are quite variable. Once the neurologic signs appear, the course of the disease is rapid (usually <3 days). Two clinical presentations exist: furious and dumb. During the course of the disease, clinical patterns in some animals may shift from the furious to the dumb forms within hours. Furious rabies produces behavioral changes that include rage, hyperexcitability, tonic clonic convulsions, vocalization, and sexual excitement. Dumb rabies presents with profound depression, ataxia, inappetence, distant stare, and possibly tenesmus. Animals may present with mild proprioceptive ataxia as the single clinical abnormality. Despite the presenting signs, the course of rabies is progressive until the animal dies. Ascending signs of paralysis are prominent in the paralytic form, so swaying of the hindquarters, knuckling, and flaccidity of the tail are observed. Excessive salivation is frequent and may be combined to a pharyngeal paralysis. Yawning movements and vocalization have been reported. Bladder paresis, reduced anal tone, and tenesmus are possible. Other clinical signs include a shifting lameness and an ataxia. The disease eventually causes the death of the animal with the last few moments sometimes difficult to witness. The animal may develop some hyperexcitability that, combined with the pharyngeal/laryngeal paralysis and excessive salivation, creates some upper airway obstruction by frothy material. Stridor caused by pharyngeal paralysis is evident. At this stage it may be dangerous to approach the animal.

Clinical Pathology and Diagnosis

On a living patient, laboratory procedures are performed to rule out other conditions or provide supportive care until a decision is made. The CSF may be normal or reveal increased protein and nucleated cell concentration. It is best to advise laboratory workers that a sample originates from a rabies-suspect animal. Final diagnosis is made by microscopic examination of CNS tissue. On regular histopathology slides, nonsuppurative encephalitis and Negri bodies are considered diagnostic. Fluorescent antibody tests and ELISA methods exist to confirm the diagnosis. All states require reporting of a rabies case along with a list of potentially exposed human beings. At that point assessments will be made regarding immunoprophylaxis of contact personnel, and quarantine and vaccination of herdmates.

Treatment

No treatment is recommended when clinical signs are evident and the level of confidence in the diagnosis considered adequate. On the other hand, early euthanasia of suspected animals is also not recommended, especially if humans have been exposed. To establish the final diagnosis, the disease must develop in the suspect animal. In Canada and the United States, the public health department should be notified and the approach of the situation discussed with public health officials. It is often best to observe the suspect animal and reduce the number of people involved in the care of the animal. State regulations relating to disposal of an exposed live animal may vary, but in California the following regulations have been drafted:

1. Slaughter for meat any animal that has been exposed for 7 days or less.
2. Quarantine unvaccinated, exposed animals for 6 months.
3. If the exposed animal is vaccinated, revaccinate it and quarantine for 45 days.

Prevention

In an endemic area, livestock may be vaccinated to reduce the risk of developing the disease. The vaccine used is an inactivated vaccine given to calves between 3 and 4 months of age and repeated annually.

NERVOUS COCCIDIOSIS

Definition and Etiology

Nervous coccidiosis is a clinical syndrome affecting young cattle that are associated with enteric infestations by *Eimeria* spp. The mortality rate of the disease is high and has been reported to be as great as 72%.[45]

Pathophysiology

Although the cause of the seizures and neurologic signs observed remains unexplained, the results of one study[46] suggest that electrolyte disturbances, vitamin A deficiency, thiamine deficiency, anemia, lead poisoning, uremia, *H. somni* infection, and hepatopathy were not involved in the pathogenesis. A soluble protein that has been found in the plasma of affected calves has been implicated in the neurotoxicity of *Eimeria bovis*.

Clinical Signs

No relation between the severity of enteric infestations and appearance of neurologic signs has been shown. Neurologic signs vary from minor muscular incoordination and twitching to continuous seizures. The seizures can also be intermittent and of variable frequency. Blindness and hyperexcitability have been reported in some cases. Convulsions tend to occur when the animal is manipulated.[47-49] Death may occur rapidly after the onset of clinical signs. Some animals survive 3 to 5 days, whereas others recover after 1 week.

Necropsy

No macroscopic lesions are observed in the CNS, and microscopic lesions are noncharacteristic.

Treatment and Prevention

Treatment goals include controlling the seizures, treatment of the coccidial infection, and provision of supportive care. The case fatality rate despite adequate treatment remains high in the nervous form of coccidiosis.

References

1. Rings DM: Bacterial meningitis and diseases caused by bacterial toxins, *Vet Clin North Am Food Anim Pract* 3:85-98, 1987.
2. Jamison JM, Prescott JF: Bacterial meningitis in large animals. *Comp Cont Educ Pract Vet* 9:F399, 1987.
3. Radostits OM, Gay CC, Blood DC et al: Diseases of the nervous system. In Radostits OM, Gay CC, Blood DC et al, editors: *Veterinary medicine: a textbook of the diseases of cattle, sheep, pigs, goats and horses*, London, 2000, Saunders, pp 501-549.
4. Smith MO, George LW: Diseases of the nervous system. In Smith BP, editor: *Large animal internal medicine*, St Louis, 2002, Mosby, pp 873-1018.
5. Philip AGS: Neonatal meningitis in the new millenium, *NeoReviews* 4:3:e73-e80, 2003.
6. Green SL, Smith LL: Meningitis in neonatal calves: 32 cases (1983-1990), *J Am Vet Med Assoc* 201:125-128, 1992.
7. Mosher AH, Helmboldt CF, Hayes KC: Coliform meningoencephalitis in young calves, *Am J Vet Res* 29:1483-1487, 1968.
8. Scott PR, Penny CD: A field study of meningoencephalitis in calves with particular reference to analysis of cerebrospinal fluid, *Vet Rec* 133:119-121, 1993.
9. Ferrouillet C, Fecteau G, Higgins R et al: Analysis of cerebrospinal fluid for diagnosis of nervous system diseases in cattle [French], *Le Point Vet* 29:783-788, 1998.
10. Cordy DR: Pathomorphology and pathogenesis of bacterial meningoventriculitis of neonatal ungulates, *Vet Pathol* 21:587-591, 1984.
11. Machen MR, Waldridge BM, Cebra C et al: Diseases of the neurologic system. In Pugh DG, editor: *Sheep and goat medicine*, Philadelphia, 2002, Saunders, pp 277-316.
12. Scott PR: Other nervous diseases. In Martin WB, Aitken ID, editors: *Diseases of sheep*, Oxford, England, 2000, Blackwell Science, pp 228-242.
13. Contrepois M, Ribot Y: Study of *Escherichia coli* isolated from bovine septicaemia cases. 1. With meningitis symptoms. 2. With an immunodepression syndrome and purpura haemorrhagica. [French], *Bulletin de L'Academie Veterinaire de France* 59:465-473, 1986.
14. Tunkel AR, Scheld WM: Acute meningitis. In Mandell GL, Bennet JE, Dolin R, editors: *Mandell: principles and practice of infectious diseases*, Philadelphia, 2000, Churchill Livingstone, pp 959-991.
15. Badger JL, Kim KS: Environmental growth conditions influence the ability of *Escherichia coli* K1 to invade brain microvascular endothelial cells and confer serum resistance, *Infect Immun* 66:5692-5697, 1998.
16. Polin RA, Harris MC: Neonatal bacterial meningitis, *Semin Neonatol* 6:157-172, 2001.
17. Lofstedt J, Dohoo IR, Duizer G: Model to predict septicemia in diarrheic calves, *J Vet Intern Med* 13:81-88, 1999.
18. Fecteau G, Metre DC, Pare J et al: Bacteriological culture of blood from critically ill neonatal calves, *Can Vet J* 38:95-100, 1997.
19. Brobst D, Bryan G: Cerebrospinal fluid. In Cowell RL, Tyler RD, editors: *Diagnostic cytology of the dog and cat*, Goleta, Calif, 1989, American Veterinary Publications, pp 141-149.
20. Ferrouillet C, Fecteau G, Lanevschi A: Cerebrospinal fluid sampling and analysis in cattle [French], *Le Point Vet* 29:777-782, 1998.
21. Lutsar I, Mccracken GH, Friedland IR: Antibiotic pharmacodynamics in cerebrospinal fluid [review], *Clin Infect Dis* 27:1117-1127, 1998.
22. de Craene BA, Deprez P, D'Haese E et al: Pharmacokinetics of florfenicol in cerebrospinal fluid and plasma of calves, *Antimicrob Agents Chemother* 41:1991-1995, 1997.
23. Harris FW, Janzen ED: The *Haemophilus somnus* disease complex (hemophilosis): a review, *Can Vet J* 30:816-822, 1989.
24. Radostits OM, Gay CC, Blood DC et al: Diseases caused by bacteria-III. In Radostits OM, Gay CC, Blood DC et al, editors: *Veterinary medicine: a textbook of cattle, sheep, pigs, goats and horses*, London, 2000, Saunders, pp 779-908.
25. Humphrey JD, Little PB, Barnum DA et al: Occurrence of *Haemophilus somnus* in bovine semen and in the prepuce of bulls and steers, *Can J Comp Med* 46:215-217, 1982.
26. Little PB: *Haemophilus somnus* complex: pathogenesis of the septicemic thrombotic meningoencephalitis, *Can Vet J* 27:94-96, 1986.

27. Momotani E, Yabuki Y, Miho H et al: Histopathological evaluation of disseminated intravascular coagulation in *Haemophilus somnus* infection in cattle, *J Comp Pathol* 95:15-23, 1985.
28. Stephens LR, Little PB, Humphrey JD et al: Vaccination of cattle against experimentally induced thromboembolic meningoencephalitis with a *Haemophilus somnus* bacterin, *Am J Vet Res* 43:1339-1342, 1982.
29. Dukes TW: The ocular lesions in thromboembolic meningoencephalitis (ITEME) of cattle, *Can Vet J* 12:180-182, 1971.
30. Nayar PSG, Ward GE, Saunders JR et al: Diagnostic procedures in experimental *Hemophilus somnus* infection in cattle, *Can Vet J* 18:159-163, 1977.
31. Humphrey JD: Haemophilus somnus: colonization of the bovine reproductive tract, strain variation and pathogenicity, *Dissert Abstr Int B* 43:3499-3500, 1983.
32. Vandonkersgoed J, Janzen ED, Potter AA et al: The occurrence of *Haemophilus-somnus* in feedlot calves and its control by postarrival prophylactic mass medication, *Can Vet J* 35:573-580, 1994.
33. Stipkovits L, Rady M, Glavits R: Mycoplasmal arthritis and meningitis in calves, *Acta Vet Hungarica* 41:73-88, 1993.
34. Tsuka T, Taura Y: Abscess of bovine brain stem diagnosed by contrast MRI examinations, *J Vet Med Sci* 61:425-427, 1999.
35. Strain GM, Claxton MS, Turnquist SE et al: Evoked potential and electroencephalographic assessment of central blindness due to brain abscesses in a steer, *Cornell Vet* 77:374-382, 1987.
36. Espersen G, Moller T: [A hypophysis-abscess-syndrome in cattle III. Pathogenesis (author's transl)]. [Danish], *Nordisk Vet* 27:627-632, 1975.
37. Perdrizet JA, Dinsmore P: Pituitary abscess syndrome, *Comp Cont Educ Pract Vet* 8:S311-S318, 1986.
38. Gardiner MR, Nairn ME, Sier AM: Viral meningoencephalitis of calves in western Australia, *Aust Vet J* 40:225-228, 1964.
39. Hill BD, Hill MW, Chung YS et al: Meningoencephalitis in calves due to bovine herpesvirus type 1 infection, *Aust Vet J* 61:242-243, 1984.
40. Carrillo BJ, Ambrogí A, Schudel AA et al: Meningoencephalitis caused by IBR virus in calves in Argentina, *Zentralbl Veterinarmed* 30:327-332, 1983.
41. Bagust TJ, Clark L: Pathogenesis of meningoencephalitis produced in calves by infectious bovine rhinotracheitis herpesvirus, *J Comp Pathol* 82:375-383, 1972.
42. Herweijer CH, De Jonge WK: De ziekte van Aujeszky bij de geit, *Tijdschr Diergeneeskd* 102:425-428, 1977.
43. Bitsch V: A study of outbreaks of Aujeszky's disease in cattle, *Acta Vet Scand* 16:420-433, 1975.
44. Dow C, McFerran JB: The pathology of Aujeszky's disease in cattle, *J Comp Pathol* 72:337-347, 1962.
45. Eness P, Owen W: Bovine coccidiosis survey results, Ames, Iowa, 1984, Iowa State University Newsletter.
46. Isler CM, Bellamy JEC, Wobeser GA: Labile neurotoxin in serum of calves with nervous coccidiosis, *Can J Vet Res* 51:253-260, 1987.
47. Nillo L: Bovine coccidiosis in Canada, *Can Vet J* 11:91-98, 1970.
48. Clayburg J: Neurological signs seen in coccidial infections, *Iowa State Vet* 2:85, 1970.

SECTION VII

Urinary System

Matt D. Miesner

CHAPTER 67

Urolithiasis

MEREDYTH L. JONES and MATT D. MIESNER

Obstructive urolithiasis is considered to be the most economically significant urinary tract disease of food animals, affecting primarily intact and castrated male ruminants, swine, and camelids.[1] Male small ruminants are particularly predisposed, whereas females are rarely clinically affected.

PATHOGENESIS

Uroliths are solid crystalline formations in the urine composed of organic matrix and organic and inorganic crystalloids.[2] Matrix, made up of sugars, proteins, and cells, results from urine super-saturation.[2] Factors affecting urine super-saturation include the rate of renal excretion of crystalloids, negative water balance, urine pH, and the presence or absence of crystallization inhibitors.[2] Metaplasia of uroepithelium, as a result of vitamin A deficiency, may contribute cells and protein for nuclear formation.[1,3] Suture, tissue debris, blood clots, or bacteria may also serve as nuclear components initiating urolith formation.[2] Infection, however, is considered to be a minor factor in urolith formation in ruminants. The formation of a nucleus is followed by deposition of inorganic minerals including magnesium, calcium, and phosphate onto the matrix.[1,3-6]

The anatomy of the distal urinary tract of male ruminants differs significantly from that of males of other species and contributes to the development of obstruction. It also increases treatment difficulty. The penis is sigmoid in arrangement,[7] with two major bends occurring between the urinary bladder and the distal glans penis. The distal flexure is a common site of urethral obstruction by uroliths.[1] The glans penis of the small ruminant also has a vermiform appendage, or urethral process, which is an extension of the urethra 2 to 4 cm beyond the distal end of the penis.[7] It has a narrowed diameter[7] compared with the more proximal portions of the urethra and also serves as a common location for obstruction.[1] The urethral diverticulum, an outpouching of the urethra at the level of the ischial arch,[7] complicates the treatment of affected animals. When a urinary catheter is passed into the urethra in a retrograde manner from the glans to access the urinary bladder, this diverticulum readily accepts the catheter,[7] rather than allowing the catheter to proceed into the urinary bladder.

Urolithiasis is a multifactorial disease with such inputs as diet, urine pH, and body water balance. Struvite (magnesium ammonium phosphate) and apatite (calcium phosphate) may be commonly seen in animals fed high-grain diets, whereas animals consuming legumes are predisposed to calcium carbonate uroliths. Silicate stones may be observed in animals grazing silicaceous plants and soils in the Western United States and Canada. Calcium oxalate stones may be associated with oxalate-containing plants.

A significant factor in the availability of urolith components and their binding ability is urine pH.[1,6,8] Struvite, apatite, and calcium carbonate uroliths are known to precipitate in alkaline urine.[2,4,5,8] Struvite crystallization occurs only at a pH range of 7.2 to 8.4, whereas apatite stones develop at a urine pH of 6.5 to 7.5.[9] Calcium carbonate stones also tend to form in alkaline urine, whereas pH may have little or no effect on silicate or calcium oxalate uroliths.

Total body water balance plays an important role in calculogenesis by its effects on urine volume and concentration. This may be seen in winter and during times of other systemic illness, when animals consume decreased volumes of water. A negative body water balance contributes to super-saturation, precipitation, and formation of residue of organic and inorganic crystalloids in urine.

Uroliths may obstruct urine flow anywhere from the renal pelvis to the distal urethra, although the most common sites of obstruction are at the distal sigmoid flexure or the vermiform appendage in sheep and goats. Obstruction at these sites may result in either rupture of the urethra or the urinary bladder.

CLINICAL SIGNS

Clinical signs depend on the degree of obstruction, location of obstruction, and duration of disease. Uroliths may not completely obstruct urine flow yet manifest as an incomplete or even intermittent obstruction resulting in periods of quiescence between active clinical signs of obstruction. Initial incomplete obstruction may become complete because of inflammation of damaged urethral mucosa.

Overt clinical signs of urinary obstruction may range from nonspecific inappetance and lethargy to overt colic. Restlessness, persistent straining, repetitive posturing to urinate, and vocalization are common. Swelling around the prepuce or bilateral ventral abdominal distension may be noted with rupture of the urethra or urinary bladder, respectively. Subcutaneous swelling or edema because of urine accumulation from urethral rupture should be differentiated from preputial infection or trauma.

Physical examination should include evaluation of the prepuce, which should normally be moist and devoid of crystals on the preputial hairs. Exteriorization of the penis should be performed in small ruminants when possible to allow examination of the urethral process and distal urethra. The distal sigmoid should be palpated for signs of swelling or sensitivity. Digital rectal palpation of the pelvic urethra in small ruminants and rectal examination in cattle should detect urethral pulsations and/or bladder distention. Urethral pulsations may also be visualized ventral to the anal sphincter. Abdominal palpation in small ruminants and percutaneous ultrasound of the abdomen can be used to detect bladder distention or free abdominal fluid. If free abdominal fluid is found, abdominocentesis may be performed to determine if it is consistent with urine.

Clinical pathology findings are related to the duration of obstruction and sequela such as uroabdomen and hydronephrosis. Elevations in blood urea nitrogen and creatinine and electrolyte derangements including hyponatremia, hypochloremia, and normal to low potassium may be noted, particularly in cases of urinary bladder rupture. Ruminants have the ability to more effectively manage uremia and maintain adequate phosphorus and potassium homeostasis through salivary secretions.[10] This often results in a longer period of time before the patient becomes clinically lethargic. Often the history of disease indicates that the animal had a period of undetermined lethargy days before urinary bladder rupture, appeared to recover, and is becoming lethargic again.

TREATMENT

Management of affected individuals consists of establishing a patent route of urine excretion, providing analgesia, correcting fluid deficits and electrolyte derangements, decreasing inflammation, and preventing infection.

The presence of the urethral diverticulum prevents passage of a urinary catheter retrograde from the urethral orifice to the urinary bladder. Retrograde catheterization or retropulsion of uroliths is not recommended to avoid further trauma or puncture of the urethra at the level of the diverticulum. Attempts at retropulsion of uroliths may result in overdistention of the urinary bladder as the stone is diverted into the diverticulum, allowing fluid to pass into the bladder, followed by the urolith falling back into the urethra and preventing the bladder from emptying. Occasionally, removal of the vermiform appendage in small ruminants establishes a patent urethra; however, inflammation in the proximal urethra from passage of the uroliths may still prevent normal urination. Uroliths tend to occur in multitudes in the urinary bladder, and 80% of animals initially relieved by amputation of the vermiform appendage will reobstruct with subsequent stone passage. Relief of urinary obstruction most often requires surgical intervention (see surgical management of urolithiasis).

Sedatives may be useful to facilitate treatment. Historically, acepromazine (0.05-0.1 mg/kg, IV or IM) has been used in the medical management of urolithiasis.[1,11,12] Unproven arguments for utilization of acepromazine have been to relax urethral tone through α-antagonistic effects on smooth muscle and relaxation of the retractor penis muscle. Benefits of acepromazine may also include suppressing the anxiety associated with the inability to urinate. Caution should be taken when using phenothiazine tranquilizers in patients who may already be hypotensive and hypothermic. Diazepam (0.1 mg/kg, slow IV) may also be used for urethral relaxation and as an anxiolytic. Xylazine (0.05-0.1 mg/kg, IV or IM) or other α-2 agonists may be used in attempt to restrain the patient for examination of the penis and have excellent analgesic properties in ruminants. Caution should be exercised when using xylazine before relief of the obstruction, as it promotes diuresis, as well as enhancing hypotension. Lumbosacral epidurals using 2% lidocaine (1 ml/7 kg) may be used in the place of sedation to relieve discomfort and aid in exteriorization of the penis in small ruminants.

Fluid therapy should be instituted as indicated by the clinical findings and economics of the case. After relief of the obstruction, diuresis is important to correct dehydration, reduce azotemia, and flush the urinary tract. For intravenous therapy, 0.9% NaCl is a good choice, although additional electrolyte and acid-base abnormalities should be considered.

Nonsteroidal antiinflammatory drugs should be administered to decrease inflammation and aid in the prevention of urethral stricture formation but should be used with caution until adequate renal perfusion is attained. Broad-spectrum antibiotic therapy should be instituted to prevent or treat infection resulting from devitalized or inflamed urinary tissues or cavitational accumulation of urine. β-Lactams (penicillins and cephalosporins) may be chosen because they have a good spectrum of activity and are excreted in the urine.

Once the obstruction is relieved, treatments to acidify the urine should be initiated in an effort to solubilize additional stones and sediment. Ammonium chloride at a dosage of 200 mg/kg may be orally administered initially and adjusted to attain a urine pH of 6 to 6.5. Care should be taken in dosing so that systemic overacidification does not occur.

PREVENTION

Because of the poor prognosis and expense associated with clinical cases of obstructive urolithiasis, as well as the herd or flock implications of the disease, considerable focus should be placed on prevention. The important role of metabolic byproducts and minerals in the pathophysiology causes diet to be the primary focus of disease prevention. Risk factors addressed in preventative strategies include high dietary phosphorus relative to calcium, high magnesium, low fiber content of rations, low urine output, and an alkaline urine pH. Additional factors including selective grazing and castration timing may be addressed.

An elevated level of phosphorus in the diet, with a calcium-to-phosphorus ratio less than 2:1 increases the excretion of phosphorus in the urine and provides an ion to bind to organic matrix.[1,4-6,13,14] Increasing the level of calcium in the diet markedly decreases the incidence of urolithiasis, probably because of competition with phosphorus for intestinal absorption and matrix binding.[14] Phosphorus should not comprise greater than 0.6% of the total ration,[8] and it is recommended that a 2.5:1 or 2:1 calcium-to-phosphorus ratio be achieved, by the use of calcium salts, if necessary.[1,6,13,14] Calcium oversupplementation should be avoided because increased calcium excretion in the urine may contribute to calcium-containing uroliths.[1] High phosphorus levels are present in grains, particularly sorghum, wheat, corn, milo, and oats.[1,5,13]

A reduction in phosphorus excretion into the urine is also desirable. Ruminants excrete phosphorus primarily by saliva, where it is then swallowed and removed from the body in the feces. Excessive dietary levels of phosphorus may saturate this salivary pathway, causing the excess to be excreted in the urine.[1,8] Urine phosphorus excretion is greater in animals fed pelleted rations as compared with meal-type rations,[10] because of a decrease in saliva production and therefore a pathway for excess phosphorus excretion. Increases in the roughage component of diets are important from this standpoint because they increase the amount of saliva that must be produced for proper mastication.[8]

Particularly in the case of struvite stones, but also with apatite stones, an increase in magnesium excretion into the urine is contributory to crystallization. It is recommended that magnesium not exceed 0.6% of the total ration of ruminants.[8] Magnesium is more available and absorbed more efficiently from concentrate rations than from roughage diets.[8]

Increasing water intake and urine volume is an important preventive measure for urolithiasis. Sources recommend the provision of adequate palatable water at desirable temperatures according to the ambient environment.[1,5,8,13] Ruminants demonstrate a reduction in water intake for grain feeding over roughage feeding.[8] Additionally, the feeding of intermittent meals may cause shunting of body water into the rumen because of increased osmotic pull from generated volatile fatty acids, resulting in a decrease in urine output. This has led to the recommendation that ruminants be fed ad libitum to maintain urine output.[1,8]

Increasing forage versus grain in the diet of animals at risk for urolithiasis has many benefits. Eating grain results in increased magnesium, phosphorus, and peptides in the urine.[1,13] Forage encourages saliva production for phosphorus excretion, potentially reduces magnesium uptake, reduces overall grain consumption, and increases water intake. Legumes and their hay should be avoided because they have high levels of calcium and are associated with calcium carbonate urolithiasis.

The role of urine pH in urolithiasis is well documented, and various sources recommend urine pH goals of 5.5 to 6.5, based on the solubilities of the common stone compositions. Because of an ability to alter acid-base balance and body water balance, salts have been widely used and recommended for the prevention of urolithiasis. Anionic salts containing primarily chlorides have been popular and used extensively because they reduce urine pH; increase urine output; and, ultimately, prevent urolithiasis.[1,5,6,8] Sodium chloride (1%-4%), calcium chloride (1%-2%), and ammonium chloride (0.5%-2%) have been traditionally added to as percentages of rations to increase water intake and produce acidic urine, with inconsistent results.

The traditional addition of these salts as a simple percentage of the diet without consideration for the components of the total ration may lead to inconsistent and unsuccessful maintenance of low urinary pH. The concept of DCAD states that with increased cations in the diet, alkalotic tendencies will occur. Conversely, increased anions in the diet have acidifying potential. Different commercial diets are commonly formulated using various commodities, and these commodities are interchanged regularly in feed preparation based on availability. If a feedstuff of a particular batch of feed is higher in cations or anionic salts are fed in conjunction with a high-potassium forage, the DCAD of the diet will be raised and urinary acidification may not occur, despite the addition of the standard dose of anions. This one-dose-fits-all method may be the major cause of sporadic urolith formation in animals being fed anionic salts. The use of DCAD balancing for goats and urolithiasis is mentioned as a recommendation in some sources,[1,5,15,16] and it is recommended that high cation-containing feedstuffs such as alfalfa and molasses should be avoided.[5] Few controlled studies for target DCAD levels currently exist, but a DCAD of 0 mEq/kg appears to achieve urine pH of intact and castrated goats of less than 6.5.[15,16] To accurately assess the efficacy of salts in the diet, whether DCAD balanced or not, owners should be encouraged to periodically assess urine pH at home.

Early castration is commonly thought to reduce the positive influence of testosterone on urethral diameter, as well as diminish normal preputial to penile attachments that are present in the neonate. Delaying castration in pet animals may serve to increase urethral diameter and the ability to examine the penis. Prophylactic removal of the vermiform appendage in young small ruminants may also serve to reduce the likelihood of obstruction.

Grazing of females on pastures that have high silica content of soil and plants is preferred to the grazing of males on these pastures. If males are to be grazed in these locations, water intake should be encouraged by maintaining desirable and accessible water sources and supplementation of anionic salts.

In summary, for prevention of urolithiasis, major efforts should be focused on reducing the grain and increasing the forage composition of the diet. A 2:1 calcium-to-potassium ratio should be attained, magnesium lowered to less than 0.6%, and anionic supplementation or DCAD balancing should be considered. Palatable, fresh water should be consistently available at temperatures that encourage consumption. Because urolithiasis is multifactorial, it is difficult to achieve consistent results from preventative strategies and can be frustrating for producers and veterinarians. With adherence to these goals, significant reductions in clinical cases can be achieved.

References

1. Van Metre DC, Divers TJ: Diseases of the renal system: urolithiasis. In Smith BP, editors: *Large animal internal medicine*, ed 3, St Louis, 2002, Mosby.
2. Osborne CA, Polzin DJ, Abdullahi SU et al: Struvite urolithiasis in animals and man: Formation, detection and dissolution, *Adv Vet Sci Comp Med* 29:1-45, 1985.
3. Packett LV, Coburn SP: Urine proteins in nutritionally induced ovine urolithiasis, *Am J Vet Res* 26:112-119, 1965.
4. Floyd JG Jr: Urolithiasis in food animals. In Howard JL, Smith RA, editors: *Current veterinary therapy 4: food animal practice*, Philadelphia, 1999, Saunders.
5. Pugh DG: Lower urinary tract problems. In Pugh DG, editor: *Sheep and goat medicine*, ed 1. Philadelphia, 2002, Saunders.
6. Jensen R, Mackey D: Urinary calculosis. In *Diseases of feedlot cattle*, ed 3, Philadelphia, 1979, Lea & Febiger.
7. Dyce KM, Sack WO, Wensing CJG: The pelvis and reproductive organs of male ruminants. In *Textbook of veterinary anatomy*, ed 3, Philadelphia, 2002, Saunders.
8. Hay L: Prevention and treatment of urolithiasis in sheep, *Vet Record Suppl In Pract* 12:87-91, 1990.
9. Elliot JS, Quaide WL, Sharp RF et al: Mineralogical studies of urine: the relationship of apatite, brushite and struvite to urinary pH, *J Urol* 80:269-271, 1958.
10. Sockett DC, Knight AP, Fettman MJ et al: Metabolic changes due to experimentally induced rupture of the bovine urinary bladder, *Cornell Vet* 76:198-212, 1986.
11. Oehme FW, Tillmann H: Diagnosis and treatment of ruminant urolithiasis, *J Am Vet Med Assoc* 147:1331-1339, 1965.
12. Van Metre DC, House JK, Smith BP et al: Obstructive urolithiasis: medical treatment and urethral surgery, *Compend Cont Educ* 18:317-328, 1996.
13. Kimberling CV: Diseases of the urinary system: calculosis. In *Jensen and Swift's diseases of sheep*, ed 3, Philadelphia, 1988, Lea & Febiger.
14. Hoar DW, Emerick RJ, Embry LB: Potassium, phosphorus and calcium interrelationships influencing feedlot performance and phosphatic urolithiasis in lambs, *J Anim Sci* 30:597-600, 1970.
15. Stratton-Phelps M, House JK: Effect of a commercial anion dietary supplement on acid-base balance, urine volume, and urinary ion excretion in male goats fed oat or grass hay diets, *Am J Vet Res* 65:1391-1397, 2004.
16. Jones M, Streeter RN: Dietary cation anion balancing for the reduction of urine pH in goats, *J Vet Intern Med* 19:412, 2005 (abstract).

CHAPTER 68

Urinary Tract Infection in Food Animals

MATT D. MIESNER

Urinary tract infection (UTI) in food animals, like other species, results most commonly from ascending infection of pathogenic bacteria normally inhabiting the genitourinary epithelium and gastrointestinal (GI) tract or residing in the environment. Infection may ascend proximal from the bladder to include unilateral or bilateral disease of the ureters and kidneys. Left-sided pyelonephritis is most commonly diagnosed clinically, although bilateral disease may be present. Hematogenous spread is reported much less frequently, but possible. Ascending infection may originate from the lower urinary tract, much more likely in females, and is often reported with a history of decreased frequency of urination and with postparturient diseases in cows. Dehydration may result in lower volumes of urine produced and stagnation of urine flow. Downer cows often urinate infrequently, if at all without assistance, and are in closer prolonged proximity to environmental contaminants. Other origins for ascending infection may be from an infected urachus in neonates or indwelling transabdominal cystostomy tubes or stoma postsurgery for urethral obstruction. Infection may also be introduced through urethral catheterization and obstetric manipulation. Inflammation within the urinary tract from trauma or urinary calculi increases the risk of an established UTI, although *Escherichia coli*, *Corynebacterium renale* (cattle), and *Eubacterium suis* (swine) can establish primary infections in normal mucosa.

The most commonly isolated organism from pyelonephritis cases in cattle is *E. coli*, followed closely by *C. renale*. *E. coli* would more commonly be considered in the environmental or opportunistic pathogen, whereas *C. renale* is commonly considered the agent of "infectious" pyelonephritis. Though both can normally reside subclinically in urogenital epithelium, poor environmental hygiene on farms increases the frequency of clinical disease. *C. renale* are continually disseminated into the environment from infected animals and may survive there for 2 months.[1] Other *Corynebacterium* species, coliforms, and *Arcanobacterium pyogenes* are also capable of causing disease. The ability to isolate *Corynebacterium* species, as well as *Eubacterium suis* (formerly *Corynebacterium*), from prepuces of bulls and boars (preputial diverticulum) makes venereal transmission possible.[2,3]

DIAGNOSIS

In cattle a history of illthrift, fever, and vague colic signs accompany a diagnosis of pyelonephritis. Careful questioning of the observant owner may also reveal a history of straining to urinate or pus in the urine. Often, cattle are diagnosed after a chronic course of disease. *E. suis* infections in swine may present as either a chronic disease or a short course of acute disease and death in less than a few days.

Physical examination of cattle with suspected pyelonephritis should include urinalysis for evidence of hematuria, leukouria, bacteriuria, and proteinuria. Isosthenuria with an alkaline pH is common. It is important to observe the complete urination period because debris may have settled to the ventral bladder wall and only be voided terminally in the urination process. Rectal examination should determine pain elicited on palpation of the kidneys (usually only the left can be palpated), which may feel enlarged, with decreased lobulations. The ureters can be located at approximately 11 and 1 o'clock anterior to the wings of the ilium and are retroperitoneal. Normal ureters are the size of a large pencil lead and can be "slipped" between the fingertips. Enlarged ureters can be palpated for enlargement and turgidity. The urinary bladder wall may feel thickened.

Ultrasonography of urinary soft tissues per rectum or kidneys per cutaneous in the paralumbar fossae provides a valuable diagnostic aid for determining the extent or severity of UTI. Ultrasound of the craniodorsal, right paralumbar fossa at the twelfth intercostal space is of particular benefit for determining pathology of the right kidney because palpation per rectum is limited. Findings may reveal dilated renal calices containing hyperechoic debris.[4]

TREATMENT

Antibiotic selection should be based on culture and sensitivity if available; however, penicillin is the most common initial treatment of choice. Overwhelming infection may result in a lack of therapeutic response despite bacterial susceptibility. Long-term antibiotic administration should be recommended, extending at least 4 weeks. Limited studies have suggested relapse rates of nearly 10% and overall mortality or culling rates of one third of clinical cases.[5] Medical treatment outcome depends largely on the duration and extent of infection.

Determining bilateral disease is important, and extent of renal function is more difficult to determine in ruminants. Measuring urine specific gravity and azotemia response to fluid therapy, as well as physical examination findings, should be combined to determine response to therapy. Nephrectomy may be an option for some individuals, and both kidneys can be carefully evaluated with palpation and ultrasound during the exploratory.

Promoting diuresis is an important adjunctive therapy in flushing the urinary tract. Intravenous fluids may be used initially or in severe cases. Oral fluids through tubing and encouraging water intake should be done. Providing salt and feeding ammonium chloride (maximum 200 mg/kg per day) will encourage water consumption. Ammonium chloride has the added benefit of urine acidification, which may prevent adhesion of some organisms.

References

1. Hayashi A, Yangawa R, Kida H: Survival of *Corynebacterium renale* and *Corynebacterium pilosum* and *Corynebacterium cystitidis* in soil, *Vet Microbiol* 10:381-386, 1985.
2. Pijoan C, Lastra A, Leman A: Isolation of *Corynebacterium suis* from the prepuce of boars, *J Am Vet Med Assoc* 183:428-429, 1983.
3. Tubbs RC: Cystitis, pyelonephritis, and miscellaneous diseases of swine. In Howard JL, Smith RA, editors: *Current veterinary therapy: food animal practice*, ed 4, Philadelphia, 1999, Saunders.
4. Hayashi H, Biller DS, Rings DM et al: Ultrasonographic diagnosis of pyelonephritis in a cow, *J Am Vet Med Assoc* 205:736-738, 1994.
5. Markusfeld O, Nahari N, Kessner D et al: Observations of bovine pyelonephritis in cattle, *Br Vet J* 145:573-579, 1989.

CHAPTER 69

Neonatal Urinary Disorders

RICHARD F. RANDLE

CONGENITAL DEFECTS

The occurrence of congenital anomalies associated with the urinary system in ruminant species is rare. Often, congenital defects are multiple and associated with more than one body system. A variety of urinary system defects have been recorded and include patent urachus, polycystic kidneys, renal oxalosis, hydronephrosis, renal dysgenesis, renal agenesis, hypospadias, and ectopic ureter.

Patent Urachus

At birth, the urachus should close rapidly in association with rupture of the umbilical cord. Situations that cause delayed or incomplete closure of the urachus can result in this condition. Congenital patent urachus in ruminants is rare; however, infections of other umbilical structures or the urachus itself may result in incomplete closure and lead to an acquired patent urachus after birth. Aggressive manipulation of the umbilical cord at parturition may predispose to an acquired patent urachus.

Patent urachus is most often diagnosed by direct visualization of urine dripping from the urachus or a persistently wet umbilical stump. Retrograde or intravenous contrast radiography may also be used as an aid in diagnosing a patent urachus.

The usual therapy is surgical removal of the entire urachus. The associated arteries and veins are typically ligated and removed as well. A common sequela of a patent urachus is cystitis secondary to ascending infections; therefore systemic antimicrobials are indicated. Conservative therapy may be considered and consists of medical management of infection and cauterization of the urachus with such agents as silver nitrate, iodine, or phenol. A potential problem exists with this therapy in that cauterization of the urachus at the umbilical stump may trap organisms higher up in the urachus and lead to infection and urachal abscessation, necessitating surgery later.

Polycystic Kidneys

The most commonly reported congenital defect seen in most species is polycystic kidneys. Typically the condition is unilateral, and no clinical signs appear because of compensation by the other kidney. If the defect is extensive and bilateral, the animal is usually stillborn or dies in the perinatal period. Frequently, other congenital anomalies are found in these animals.

Most often this condition is reported as a finding at necropsy. The affected kidney is enlarged and composed of either a few large cysts or numerous small cysts. A grossly enlarged kidney may be encountered on rectal examination in adult large ruminants. Ultrasonography may aid in the diagnosis of polycystic kidneys.

Renal Oxalosis

Renal oxalosis results from excessive deposition of calcium oxalate crystals in the glomeruli, tubules, and collecting ducts. This condition has been described in aborted fetuses and neonatal calves that have not been exposed to a known oxalate source. Calves with renal oxalosis have a frequent occurrence of cardiac and musculoskeletal defects such as arthrogryposis, osteopetrosis, and chondrodysplasia, which suggests a metabolic disorder involving glycine.

OMPHALITIS

Inflammation of the umbilical arteries, umbilical vein, urachus, or surrounding tissues is termed *omphalitis*. These structures combine to form the umbilicus, which represents the vestige of the fetal-maternal connection. The umbilical vein, which carries oxygenated blood from the placenta to the fetus via the liver and ductus venosus, becomes the round ligament of the liver. The two umbilical arteries, which carry waste materials from the fetus to the placenta, become the round ligaments of the bladder. The remnant of the urachus becomes incorporated into the apex of the bladder.

Pathogenesis

At parturition the umbilical arteries retract into the abdomen and close by smooth muscle contraction in response to the increased partial pressure of oxygen in the blood, and the umbilical vein and urachus remain outside the abdomen. The vein closes rapidly by smooth muscle contraction, and the urachus shrinks and dries within a few days.

Of the umbilical structures, the urachus is the most commonly infected in calves, with *Actinomyces pyogenes* being the most frequently identified organism involved. *Escherichia coli, Proteus, Enterococcus, Streptococcus*, and *Staphylococcus* species have also been identified as causative agents; therefore antimicrobial therapy should be based on culture results.

Clinical Signs

Clinical signs associated with omphalitis may be varied. Usually the animal has a history of purulent drainage from the umbilicus at 1 to 2 weeks of age. The umbilicus may be enlarged, firm, hot, and painful on palpation. In approximately 25% of the cases there is an associated umbilical hernia. The animals may have concurrent systemic infections such as bacteremia, septic arthritis, pneumonia, diarrhea, uveitis, or peritonitis. Some animals show no evidence of drainage or inflammation at the umbilicus but are febrile, appear depressed, and are tender in the abdomen on palpation. Other clinical signs include dysuria, pollakiuria, and cystitis as a result of direct communication between the urachus and the bladder or interference with filling and emptying of the bladder.

Diagnosis

Infections of the umbilicus are easily identified in the presence of a draining tract or enlarged umbilicus. For determining the extent of urachal involvement, a metal probe or radiopaque contrast material can be placed in the draining tract and radiographs taken. Radiographic findings include a cranioventrally positioned bladder and a radiopaque structure ventral to the bladder. Deep palpation above the umbilicus with the animal either standing or in lateral recumbency may reveal an abdominal mass or painful areas. Ultrasonography may also be used as an aid in determining involvement of the various umbilical structures. Omphalitis should be considered in neonates with a normal-appearing umbilicus but that are unthrifty or have a fever of unknown origin.

Treatment

The treatment of choice is exploratory laparotomy and surgical excision of the abscesses. Urachal infections extending into the bladder require excision of the apex of the bladder and ligation of the umbilical arteries. In the absence of systemic involvement, the prognosis is good and recovery is usually uneventful.

Prevention

The control of umbilical infections centers on good sanitation and hygiene at parturition. The use of astringents and disinfectants on the umbilicus at birth is widely practiced, but there is limited evidence that this is of significant benefit.

Recommended Readings

Baxter GM: Umbilical masses in calves: diagnosis, treatment, and complications, *Compend Contin Educ* 11:505-513, 1989.

Dennis SM: Urogenital defects in sheep, *Vet Rec* 105:344-347, 1979.

Fetcher A: Renal disease in cattle. Part I. Causative agents, *Compend Contin Educ* 7(suppl):701-708, 1985.

Smith BP: *Large animal internal medicine*, St Louis, 1990, Mosby, pp 370-372.

Trent AM, Smith DE: Surgical management of umbilical masses with associated umbilical cord remnant infections in calves, *J Am Vet Med Assoc* 185:1531-1534, 1984.

CHAPTER 70

Ulcerative Posthitis

MEREDYTH L. JONES

Ulcerative posthitis, also known as *enzootic balanoposthitis, pizzle rot,* and *sheath rot,* is an infectious disease of the external genitalia of primarily male small ruminants and, occasionally, cattle. The etiologic agent is *Corynebacterium renale,* a normal inhabitant of the skin and external genitalia of small ruminants.

RISK FACTORS

Risk factors for infection include high-protein diets, thick fiber, wet conditions, and venereal exposure from infected animals. *C. renale* proliferates on genital mucosa in the presence of urea, which increases in concentration in the urine of animals fed high protein, legume pasture, and non-protein-nitrogen (NPN) diets. It then acts to hydrolyze urea to ammonia, resulting in necrosis of the surrounding tissue. Merino and Angora animals have an increased incidence due to dense fiber coats, and adults are more commonly affected than youngstock. Symptomatic or asymptomatic carriers may spread large numbers of the bacteria venereally.

CLINICAL SIGNS

Clinical signs associated with ulcerative posthitis in rams, bucks, and wethers include moist ulcers and thin, brown, malodorous scabs at the mucocutaneous junction of the prepuce. The infection may become internalized, with diffuse swelling of the prepuce, and necrotic tissue and exudate are present. Eventually, fibrinous or fibrous adhesions may form between the penis and prepuce and stenosis of the preputial orifice may occur. The lesions are quite painful and lead to dysuria, vocalization during urination, a stilted gait, and possibly chronic weight loss. In does and ewes, ulcerative lesions of the perineum and vulva occur with vulvar swelling. Dysuria may result in cases where infection and inflammation involve the urethral orifice, and longstanding cases may result in fibrosis and contracture of the vulva.

DIAGNOSIS

Diagnosis of this condition is usually based on lesion characteristics and dietary information. Histopathology or culture of the organism provides definitive diagnosis; however, herpesvirus and *Actinobacillus seminis* have also been reported to cause ulcerative posthitis lesions. Differential diagnoses for the clinical presentation of ulcerative posthitis include obstructive urolithiasis, preputial trauma, ulcerative dermatosis (sheep poxvirus), and contagious ecthyma (Orf). Serum chemistry may reveal an increased blood urea nitrogen, creatinine, and potassium if urinary outflow is obstructed.

TREATMENT

Medical treatment involves reducing the protein or NPN levels in diet to less than 16%, which may alone effect a cure with no further treatment in mild cases. Shearing fiber away from the external genitalia to allow airflow and irrigation of the sheath and application of nonirritating antiseptic/antibiotic solutions are useful. Iodine solutions should be avoided due to their encouragement of adhesions and production of granulation tissue. Systemic use of penicillin or oxytetracycline should be initiated in internalized cases and continued until lesions are dry and inflammation is reduced. Surgical management may involve lesion débridement or, as a salvage procedure, 2- to 4-cm incisions may be made through the ventral skin into the prepuce to allow drainage and lavage. In attempt to retain animals for breeding, one can perform preputial resection to allow urine flow and prevent adhesions. Sedation with xylazine should be avoided in cases of suspected urinary obstruction due to acute increases in urine volume. After treatment, patients should be monitored closely to ensure patency of the urinary tract.

PREVENTION

Control and prevention of ulcerative posthitis should involve isolation of affected individuals and a reduction in dietary protein to less than 16%. Supplementation with grass hay may limit intake of high-protein feeds and legume pastures. Shearing animals at times of high-protein intake, the inclusion of the urinary acidifier ammonium chloride, or chlortetracycline added to the feed may reduce disease incidence. The fiber of affected animals should be burned. The bacterium is environmentally resistant in exudate.

PROGNOSIS

The prognosis for recovery depends largely on the severity of signs when treatment is initiated. Without a reduction in dietary protein, it is unlikely that any treatment or preventative regimen will be successful. If the disease is recognized before fibrosis, there may be a good prognosis for a full recovery with appropriate medical and dietary management. Potential sequelae in males include loss of breeding soundness because of adhesion of penis to prepuce, scarring of the preputial orifice, urethritis, and urethral obstruction. In females there may be urine scalding and loss of breeding soundness caused by impaired vulvar conformation. Fibrosis of the vulva may be severe enough to cause dystocia.

Recommended Readings

Belknap EB, Pugh DG: Diseases of the urinary system: ulcerative posthitis. In Pugh DG, editor: *Sheep and goat medicine*, Philadelphia, 2002, Saunders.

Brook AH, Southcott WH, Stacy BD: Etiology of ovine posthitis: relationship between urine and a causal organism, *Aust Vet J* 42:9, 1966.

Grewal AS, Wells R: Vulvovaginitis of goats due to a herpesvirus, *Aust Vet J* 63:79, 1986.

Horner GW, Hunter R, Day AM: An outbreak of vulvovaginitis in goats caused by a caprine herpesvirus, *N Z Vet J* 30:150, 1982.

Loste A, Ramos JJ, Garcia L et al: High prevalence of ulcerative posthitis in Rasa Aragonesa rams associated with a legume-rich diet, *J Vet Med Assoc* 52:176, 2005.

McMillian KR, Southcott WH: Aetiological factors in ovine posthitis, *Aust Vet J* 49:405, 1973.

Mickelsen WD, Meman MA: Infertility and diseases of the reproductive organs of bucks: posthitis. In Youngquist RS, editor: *Current therapy in large animal theriogenology*, Philadelphia, 1997, Saunders.

Shelton M, Livingston CW: Posthitis in Angora wethers, *J Am Vet Med Assoc* 167:154, 1975.

Southcott WH: Epidemiology and control of ovine posthitis and vulvitis, *Aust Vet J* 41:225, 1965.

Southcott WH: Etiology of ovine posthitis: description of a causal organism, *Aust Vet J* 41:193, 1965.

Tarigan S, Webb RF, Kirkland D: Caprine herpesvirus from balanoposthitis, *Aust Vet J* 64:321, 1987.

Uzal FA, Woods L, Stillian M et al: Abortion and ulcerative posthitis associated with caprine herpesvirus-1 infection in goats in California, *J Vet Diagn Invest* 16:478, 2004.

Van Metre DC, Divers TJ: Ulcerative posthitis and vulvitis. In Smith BP, editor: *Large animal internal medicine*, ed 3, St Louis, 2002, Mosby.

CHAPTER 71

Bovine Enzootic Hematuria

MATT D. MIESNER

Prolonged ingestion of bracken fern by cattle and sheep is associated with a syndrome of chronic/intermittent hematuria and neoplasia of the urinary bladder. Growing evidence suggests that urinary bladder neoplasia is enhanced with concomitant bovine papillomavirus-2 (BPV-2) infection in cattle via synergistic effects of chromosomal aberrations and clastogenesis.[1-3] Neoplastic lesions do occur in chronic enzootic hematuria (CEH) cases without evidence of BPV-2 DNA.[2] Enzootic hematuria is the milder form of bracken fern toxicosis. Ingestion of large amounts (animal's body weight/1-3 months) of bracken fern results in acute bracken toxicosis and presents as acute systemic hemorrhage, fever, and pancytopenia because of thrombocytopenic coagulopathy, septicemia, and bone marrow suppression.[4,5]

Typically multiple animals are affected with CEH and initially show clinical signs of marked hematuria and anemia with a history of consuming bracken fern (*Pteridium aquilinum*) on pasture or in hay. Hematuria may be persistent or intermittent, with or without blood clots, but prolongation of the disease results in blood loss anemia and associated clinical signs. Clinical signs of stranguria may be present due to cystitis, and urethral obstruction with clotted blood can occur. Rectal examination and ultrasound may reveal a thickened bladder wall and/or intramural masses protruding into the lumen.

Urine sedimentation from a freshly voided sample should be performed to differentiate hematuria (intact red blood cells) from pigmenturia. Urinalysis will also reveal proteinuria and, occasionally, mild pyuria, although secondary cystitis pyelonephritis may occur. Primary urinary tract infections such as cystitis/pyelonephritis manifest as marked pyuria and bacteriuria without gross evidence of hematuria. In the early to mid stages of the disease, a marked monocytosis has been suggested as being of some diagnostic value as an early hematologic marker.[6]

Preventing consumption of bracken fern is the only treatment and preventive measure to be taken. Resolution of hematuria can occur if tumors have not yet formed.

References

1. Stocco dos Santos RC, Lindsey CJ et al: Bovine papillomavirus transmission and chromosomal aberrations: an experimental model, *J Gen Virol* 79:2127-2135, 1998.
2. Lioi MB, Barbieri R, Borzacchiello G et al: Chromosome aberrations in cattle with chronic enzootic haematuria, *J Comp Pathol* 131:233-236, 2004.
3. Wosiacki SR, Claus MP, Alfieri AF et al: Bovine papillomavirus type 2 detection in the urinary bladder of cattle with chronic enzootic hematuria, *Mem Inst Oswaldo Cruz* 101:635-638, 2006.
4. Osweiler GD: Bracken fern toxicity. In Osweiler GD, editor: *The national veterinary medical series: toxicology*, Media, Pa, 1996, Williams & Wilkins.
5. Humphreys DJ: In *Veterinary toxicology*, ed 3, London, 1988, Bailiere Tindall.
6. Perez-Alenza MD, Blanco J, Sardon D et al: Clinico-pathological findings in cattle exposed to chronic bracken fern toxicity, *N Z Vet J* 54:185-192, 2006.

Recommended Readings

Radostits OM, Gay CC, Blood DC et al: Diseases caused by major phytotoxins; bovine enzootic hematuria. In Radostits OM, Blood DC, Gay CC et al, editors: *Veterinary medicine*, ed 9, London, 2000, Saunders.
Van Metre DC, Divers TJ: Diseases of the renal system: enzootic hematuria. In Smith BP, editor: *Large animal internal medicine*, ed 3, St Louis, 2002, Mosby.

CHAPTER 72

Surgery of the Urinary Tract

JENNIFER IVANY EWOLDT

URETHRAL EXTENSION

Urethroplasty is a useful technique for treatment of urine pooling (urovagina or vesicovaginal reflux) in the cranial vaginal cavity. Cows that experience urine pooling often fail to conceive because of metritis and vaginitis induced by the presence of urine.[1-6] Urine pooling may be visualized by vaginal speculum or noted during vaginal palpation. Urovagina may be due to trauma (lacerations or dystocia). The condition can also be anatomic in nature, most common in cows having an abnormal, cranially sloping vulva. The condition is aggravated by age and multiple parities because the uterus and cervix advance cranially into the abdominal cavity after supporting ligaments are stretched.[1,4]

Before performing urethral extension surgery, a complete reproductive examination should be performed to rule out any other causes of infertility. Cervical tears, cystic ovaries, and periuterine scar tissue can be identified in this manner, and the expense of surgery can be avoided if they are present.

Following the diagnosis of urine pooling, urethral extension (urethroplasty) may be attempted to resolve the problem. The cow is prepared for surgery by placing her in standing stocks with her tail elevated and tied. A caudal epidural is performed using lidocaine, xylazine, mepivacaine, or a combination of these. The rectum is evacuated and packed with a sterile tampon of gauze. The vulva and surrounding hair are washed well, and the vaginal cavity is flushed with a dilute disinfectant solution. Any remaining vaginal fluid (urine or disinfectant) should be evacuated before starting surgery. Stay sutures, towel clamps, or a self-retaining Balfour retractor are used to pull open the vulvar lips to expose the surgical field. Long-handled instruments and good lighting (such as a headlamp) are vitally important to ease the procedure. If desired, a large-diameter Foley catheter (28 French [Fr]) may be placed in the urethra to divert urine and provide a scaffold for repair.

Urethroplasty in cows is performed using a modification of the technique described by Brown and colleagues[7] for mares. To initiate the procedure, the transverse fold is grasped with forceps and retracted caudally. Approximately 1 cm cranial to the urethral orifice, the fold is split in a transverse orientation to create two layers (dorsal and ventral). The incision is then extended caudally along the lateroventral walls of the vaginal vault (3 o'clock and 9 o'clock) at the level of the transverse fold, creating a U-shaped incision with the base at the transverse fold. Incisions end approximately 2 cm cranial to the mucocutaneous junction of the vulva edges.[1-6] Dorsal and ventral flaps are created by careful undermining of the tissue until the ventral flaps can be pulled together without tension, creating a tube on the ventral floor of the vaginal vault. Lack of tension is essential to the success of this procedure, so more undermining of tissue is better than less.[4] The size of the newly created urethral extension depends on the size of flaps created. A large-diameter extension is preferable to prevent stress on the urethroplasty during urination and reduce postoperative urethral obstruction by swelling.

Following creation of tension-free flaps, closure can begin. Closure begins at the cranial aspect of the U-shaped incision. Closure is performed using 2-0 monofilament absorbable suture material in a continuous pattern, inverting the edges into the newly created urethral lumen. A horizontal mattress, vertical mattress, or Lembert pattern is ideal for this purpose. The incision can be closed in the Y-shaped pattern as described by Brown and colleagues[7] or simply sutured side to side with no Y at the proximal aspect. It is recommended that before continuing far along the ventral flap, the closure of the dorsal flaps be initiated at the cranial aspect of the incision, in a manner similar to the closure of the ventral flaps. In this manner the surgeon continues to suture caudally in two layers at the same time, closing each layer separately (Fig. 72-1). The dorsal flaps are sutured to evert the edges into the vaginal vault. Some surgeons prefer to perform a three-layer closure, suturing the submucosal tissues between dorsal and ventral flaps in a simple continuous pattern to provide strength to the repair. The Foley catheter may be left in place for 72 hours or removed at the surgeon's discretion. Routine antiinflammatory and antibiotic treatment is continued for 7 days following surgery.

The most critical point in the repair is at the proximal aspect of the suture line, where dehiscence and fistula formation are common.[1,3,4] Fistula formation in this area is the most common complication following urethroplasty in mares and cows.[3] Special attention should be paid to this area when suturing. Other major complications are insufficient length of the urethroplasty, allowing urine reflux, and insufficient diameter of the urethroplasty, causing difficulty in urination and stress on the suture line, sometimes leading to fistula formation. The repair should be rechecked in 2 to 3 weeks, and breeding by artificial insemination may begin following the first heat cycle after surgery (usually 4-6 weeks after surgery).[4] Breeding by natural methods will endanger the repair and is not recommended. Revision of a failed urethroplasty

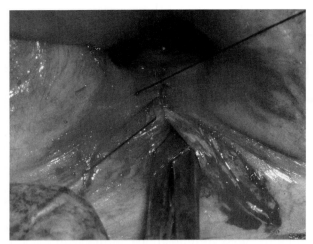

Fig 72-1 Urethral extension in progress showing two layers of suture being placed concurrently. (Courtesy Bruce L. Hull, DVM.)

procedure (other than fistulation) is not recommended because scar tissue will limit the mobility of tissues and the success of repair.[3]

A modification of the previously mentioned method has been described in mares in which no dorsal flap is sutured, leaving instead exposed submucosal tissue to heal by second intention.[8] This method has been reported to be successful in cows.[1] Another modification involved use of horizontal mattress sutures to pull vaginal mucosa in folds from either side of the vault over the top of a Foley catheter, without the creation of a U-shaped incision. The edges were then trimmed to create fresh edges, which were sutured together. This technique was successful in the report and may provide a simpler technique than the urethral tube technique. Monin[9,10] described an alternative procedure in horses in which the transverse fold is caudally retracted and sutured in place to deflect urine caudally. I have no experience with this technique in cows, but reports indicate that it is not effective in cows.[1]

CYSTOTOMY/BLADDER REPAIR

Urinary bladder rupture is most common secondary to urolithiasis and therefore occurs most often in males.[11-13] Bladder rupture can occur, however, in cattle of all ages. Bladder rupture can occur during or following dystocia because of direct trauma or focal pressure necrosis.[12-16] Bladder rupture or leakage can also occur in conjunction with patent urachus or urachal remnants.[17] Leakage can occur following cystotomy, partial cystectomy, cystocentesis, or transcutaneous bladder catheterization. Leakage can also occur through microscopic holes caused by prolonged overdistension.[18] The most common location of bladder rupture is in dispute in cattle. In horses, dorsocranial ruptures are most common.[19] In cattle, however, there is a lack of consensus on the most likely location.[11,14,16,17]

Metabolic consequences of bladder rupture or leakage have been well described elsewhere. Diagnosis is usually by clinical signs of intra-abdominal fluid accumulation,

abdominocentesis, or serum biochemistry. Following diagnosis, the choice for medical versus surgical correction must be made based on the cause, value of the animal, and knowledge of success rates for different procedures.

Experts disagree regarding the ability of dorsal bladder ruptures to spontaneously heal if provided with bladder drainage using a Foley catheter (size 12-20 in an adult cow).[11,12] Care must be taken to place the catheter within the intact bladder and not through the rupture into the abdominal cavity. Some anecdotal success has been reported with this technique, but many bladders eventually require surgical closure to restore complete patency. Also controversial is the strength of spontaneous healing of bladder ruptures in comparison with surgical closure.

Ventral bladder ruptures require surgical repair via general anesthesia.[11,12] Depending on the size of the animal, the approach can be made by ventral midline, caudal flank, or ventrolateral incisions, although the ventral midline approach gives the best visualization.[11] Accessibility of the bladder is often an issue, especially in adult cattle. Grasping the bladder and fatiguing it by traction may be necessary to bring it closer to the incision. Repair of bladder ruptures through standing caudal flank approaches have also been reported, with varying success dependent on location of the tear. Much of the suturing in standing approaches is performed blindly within the abdominal cavity because of the caudal location of the bladder and the interference of intra-abdominal organs with visibility.

Following the approach to the bladder, the tear in the bladder wall is located, débrided, and closed in two layers using 2-0 or 0 monofilament absorbable suture material. Inclusion of mucosa in the first layer of closure does not seem to cause problems with incisional healing. Care should be taken to leave as little suture material as possible exposed to the bladder lumen to prevent foci for urolith formation and premature degradation of suture material by urine. The extremely alkaline nature of ruminant urine can speed degradation of polyglycolic acid and poliglecaprone suture material, making it less than ideal for bladder repair. Polydioxanone is a superior choice for bladder repair. The second layer of closure should invert the bladder edges (Cushing, Lembert, mattress patterns). Following repair, the bladder should be distended with sterile saline to ensure secure closure of the incision and look for further sources of leakage.

Recently, there has been much interest in laparoscopic repair of bladder ruptures, especially in foals.[20,21] Laparoscopic repair avoids the complications of open abdominal surgery in neonatal animals and can provide superior visualization of the bladder in the caudal abdomen. Closure of the bladder may be performed in one or two layers using endoscopic suturing devices. Results thus far have been encouraging, but repair has been reported in neonatal or very young animals only.

Cystotomy may also be performed for removal of uroliths from the bladder.[18] In these cases, surgeon's preference determines if the incision will be made in the dorsal or ventral surface of the bladder. For gravitational reasons, the dorsal surface may be best for healing but the ventral surface is most accessible. Stay sutures are useful in controlling the bladder for cystotomy and should be placed

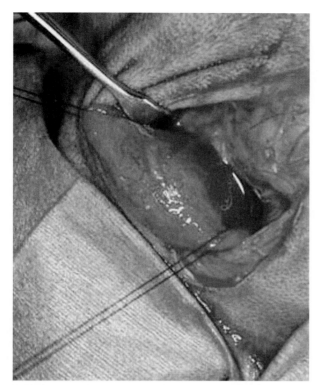

Fig 72-2   Stay sutures holding bladder in position for surgery. (Courtesy Kimberly A May, DVM, MS, DACVS.)

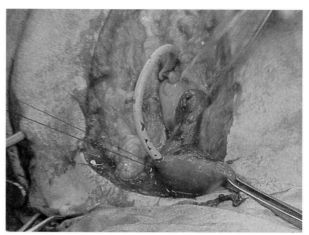

Fig 72-3   Placement of Foley catheter for tube cystostomy. The catheter enters the abdomen through the body wall *(left)* and enters the bladder through a stab incision. The Foley cuff has not yet been inflated. Sutured cystotomy incision for removal of uroliths is evident on bladder surface.

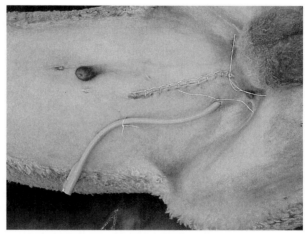

Fig 72-4   Completed tube cystostomy showing locations of abdominal incision and tube placement, with stay sutures stabilizing Foley catheter.

before performing the cystotomy incision (Fig. 72-2). Cystotomy should be performed in a manner to avoid major blood vessels in the bladder wall. Closure is in two layers, as previously described for bladder rupture.

Partial cystectomy has been described following bladder rupture, trauma, prolapse, devitalization, and as treatment for patent urachus/omphalitis.[12] A large portion of the bladder wall can be resected without undue effects, as long as the trigone and ureteral insertions are not involved. Resection should be performed in healthy tissue and is closed in two layers as previously described.

UROLITHIASIS CORRECTION

Surgical treatment of urolithiasis in ruminants has traditionally been limited to short-term salvage procedures in feedlot animals destined for early slaughter. These methods often involved resection of the penis and experienced numerous complications, most commonly stricture formation at the site of entry into the urethra. Success rates varied and were dependent on the duration of obstruction before surgery; condition of the animal and urethral tissue at the time of treatment; concurrent urethral rupture; and location of the urolith itself. Most techniques were, therefore, not useful in breeding animals or in animals kept as pets.

More recently, an increase in the number of small ruminants kept as pets has led to the development of several other techniques for resolution of urolithiasis. The intent is to develop a procedure that does not form a stricture rapidly and that does not end the breeding ability of intact males. Research has led to ways to replace ruptured urethral

tissue to salvage animals that would otherwise be doomed to slaughter or euthanasia. The perceived value of these animals as pets also provides the opportunity to perform procedures that would not be cost effective in feedlot animals.

Surgical tube cystostomy provides an excellent method of treating urolithiasis and has been applied to both cattle and small ruminants.[22-24] In this technique the patient is anesthetized in dorsal recumbency, and the bladder approached via a paramedian incision. A cystotomy is performed to remove any uroliths present and perform normograde flushing of the urethra if desired. A Foley catheter (12 to 24 Fr) is then passed through a stab incision in the body wall of the inguinal region, placed into the bladder through a stab incision, and sutured into place with the cuff inflated (Fig. 72-3). Following closure of the celiotomy incision, extra catheter is secured with sutures or bandages to the abdominal wall (Fig. 72-4).

The catheter is allowed to drain freely for several days, after which time it is periodically occluded with a clamp to test for normograde urine flow through the urethra. Once normograde flow is established, the catheter cuff is deflated and the catheter is removed. In two separate reports, urine flow was reestablished in a mean of 11.5 and 11 days.[22,23] Success of this procedure was 76% to 90% in the short term and 86% in the long term.[22,23] Success rates have been shown to be dependent on several factors. Sheep, animals with serum potassium level greater than 5.2 mEq/L at admission, the presence of fluid in the abdomen at admission, and previous urethral process amputation have all been shown to be associated with poorer survival.[23] In a separate study, increased blood urea nitrogen and respiratory rate were associated with poorer survival.[25] The major drawback of surgical tube cystostomy is the cost associated with the procedure because animals must be hospitalized during the waiting period before catheter occlusion. Repeat obstruction and premature tube removal have not been major problems following tube cystostomy.[23] Tube cystostomy has been used to restore breeding function in intact males, avoiding the loss of breeding function previously described.[26]

In addition to its use in small ruminants, tube cystostomy is useful in other species as well. I have experience with the technique in llamas, alpacas, whitetail deer, and a camel and anecdotal evidence of its use in potbellied pigs. Success rates vary widely in these alternative species, but the technique is the same.

To reduce the costs associated with the tube cystostomy procedure, a *percutaneous tube cystostomy* technique has been developed for placement of the cystostomy tube.[27] This technique was successful in the initial description, but subsequent reports indicated that it is 5.6 times more likely to require a second procedure to replace the tube following premature tube loss.[25] If successful, percutaneous tube cystostomy is managed similarly to the surgically placed tubes, in that the tube is periodically occluded after a waiting period of approximately 7 days and removed once urination is reestablished.

Urinary bladder marsupialization in small ruminants has been moderately successful in restoring urination.[28,29] It does, however, eliminate urinary continence and may, as a result, be unacceptable to some pet owners. In this technique the apex of the bladder is marsupialized to the ventral body wall at midline during a midline celiotomy, creating a stoma that allows for free drainage of urine from the bladder (Fig. 72-5). Major complications involved include bladder mucosal prolapse through the stoma, urine scald on the ventrum of the animal, and ascending urinary tract infections through the marsupialization site.[28,29] The marsupialization stoma formed a stricture in 3 of 25 goats.[28,29] Success rates were 66% and 94% in two separate studies.[28,29] Hospitalization was significantly shorter than tube cystostomy (mean of 4 vs. 14 days), which may reduce the cost associated with the procedure.

Prepubic urethrostomy has been described in a sheep and a goat for relief of obstructive urolithiasis.[30] In the report described, prepubic urethrostomy was used for relief of urinary obstruction following perineal urethrostomy stricture formation. The technique used is similar to that performed in dogs and cats. In dorsal recumbency

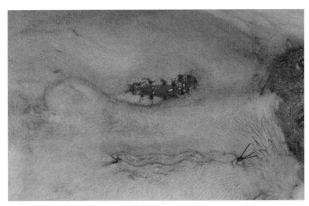

Fig 72-5 Completed bladder marsupialization surgery demonstrating placement of stoma and abdominal incision. (Courtesy Kimberly A May, DVM, MS, DACVS.)

the pubic bone of the pelvis was approached, all attached muscles elevated and reflected, and the pubic bone transected with an oscillating bone saw. The urethra was then mobilized from its caudal location by blunt dissection and brought through the ventral midline incision. The pubic bones were reapposed with orthopedic wire, and all elevated muscles reapposed. The urethra was then positioned near the caudal abdomen and carefully reapposed to the skin edges. Both animals described were able to void normally after the procedure, but recurrent cystitis and further stricture formation were complications. Because of its proximal location in the urethra and the difficulty of the procedure, this technique should be reserved for revision of previously performed techniques for stricture.

Laser lithotripsy has recently been investigated as a technique for dissolution of uroliths in ruminants.[31,32] A chromium-thulium-holmium:yttrium-aluminum-garnet (Ho:YAG) laser was successfully used to rupture a urethral calculus when placed via an ischial urethrotomy in a steer.[31] In a separate study, a Ho:YAG laser was successfully used to fracture uroliths in three goats and two potbellied pigs.[32] The use of lithotripsy depends on the presence of a urethra sufficiently large for passage of the laser in an endoscope and the location of uroliths in the distal urethra. Lithotripsy, however, presents a viable option for removal of uroliths in the future, and further investigation is warranted. Advantages include reduced cost and rapid discharge from the hospital.

Buccal mucosal grafting has recently been described for the reversal of a perineal urethrostomy in a goat.[33] In this case the urethra was reconstructed using a strip of tissue from the buccal mucosa following unsuccessful revision of the urethrostomy site. Buccal mucosa proved to be an excellent tissue for this procedure, and healing was excellent, with good long-term survival.

Vesicular irrigation with hemiacidrin was used in conjunction with percutaneous tube cystostomy to restore urinary function in a goat.[27] The authors concluded that irrigation resulted in rapid dissolution of calcium phosphate uroliths without the need for celiotomy and cystotomy. Vesicular irrigation could be combined with surgical or percutaneous tube cystostomy and perhaps also with other techniques to dissolve uroliths in situ. The efficacy

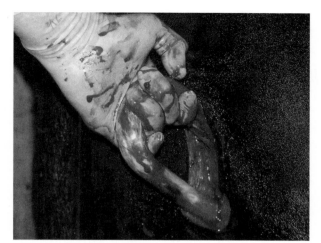

Fig 72-6 Perineal urethrostomy in a steer. The penis has been mobilized and brought to the incision with good mobility, allowing for a tension-free fixation. (Courtesy Bruce L Hull, DVM, MS.)

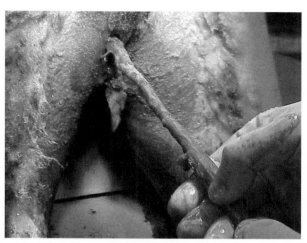

Fig 72-7 Perineal urethrostomy (penile amputation) in a lamb. The penis has been freed from its preputial attachments and is ready for fixation and amputation.

of this technique on different types of uroliths is not known.

Cystotomy with urolith removal combined with normograde and retrograde urethral flushing was successful in restoring urinary function in seven of eight small ruminants with obstructive urolithiasis.[34] The authors concluded that this technique was more successful than perineal urethrostomy in restoring urinary function. However, at the time of their study, further techniques such as tube cystostomy, urinary bladder marsupialization, and laser lithotripsy had not been described.

Perineal urethrostomy has long been the mainstay of urolithiasis treatment in ruminants. It is considered a salvage technique in most cases, though some animals have survived for long periods of time after surgery. With this technique, a permanent opening is made in the urethra through which the animal voids urine. Perineal urethrostomy does not guarantee urethral patency because an animal can still obstruct proximal to the stoma. As a result, the urethrostomy stoma should be placed as distally as possible to allow for repeat surgery more proximally. The most common complication of urethrostomy is stricture of the stoma, which may occur rapidly (weeks to months) after surgery.[35]

The penis is approached via a midline incision in a standing animal under epidural anesthesia. The ideal location for the incision is just caudal to the scrotum because this location is usually proximal to the obstruction but sufficiently distal to provide penile mobility and the opportunity for more proximal urethrostomy in the future. The retractor penis muscles are located and traced to the penis itself within the thick tunica albuginea. The retractor muscles can be transected or left in place at the discretion of the surgeon, though transection of the muscles helps reduce any tension that may result in breakdown of the stoma site. The penis is dissected free of the surrounding tissues and mobilized to the incision site (Fig. 72-6). A tension-free position of the penis is required to prevent breakdown of the urethrostomy. The penis is stabilized at the incision with horizontal mattress

stay sutures of large monofilament, nonabsorbable suture material passing through the lateral aspects of the fibrous tunica albuginea and then through the skin. Once stabilized, the urethra on the dorsal aspect of the penis (under the bulbospongiosus muscle) is then opened with a single longitudinal incision. Small-gauge (0 to 2-0), nonabsorbable monofilament suture material is used to appose skin edges and urethral edges, creating a stoma.

Perineal urethrostomy can also be performed at a location much more proximal, even as high as the level of the ischium. At this location the stoma thus created may allow catheterization of the bladder for relief of bladder distension. The proximal location is much more likely to experience urine scald on the perineal region and does not allow for a secondary procedure to relieve any further urinary obstruction. The technique is similar to that described for the distal urethrostomy.

Penile amputation (penectomy) is similar to the technique described for perineal urethrostomy; however, the penis is transected and may be completely removed rather than creating a stoma in the penis. This is a simpler procedure than the perineal urethrostomy but has the disadvantage of increased stricture rate and speed. It is strictly a salvage procedure. The approach to the penis is identical to that described for the perineal urethrostomy; however, once the penis is identified and mobilized to the incision, the retractor penis muscles are transected. The penis itself is brought to the incision and sufficiently mobilized so that the transection can be performed several inches below the ventral aspect of the skin incision to allow for tension-free positioning of the penis (Fig. 72-7). The distal penis may be excised completely, in which case the dorsal vessels of the penis are ligated immediately proximal to the transection site. The distal penis may also be left in place, in which case the dorsal vessels are carefully separated from the dorsal aspect of the tunica albuginea and protected from damage during the penile transection.

Following sharp transection of the penis at the desired location, mattress sutures of heavy, nonabsorbable monofilament suture material are placed at the lateral aspects to secure the penis to the skin edges (Fig. 72-8). Care must

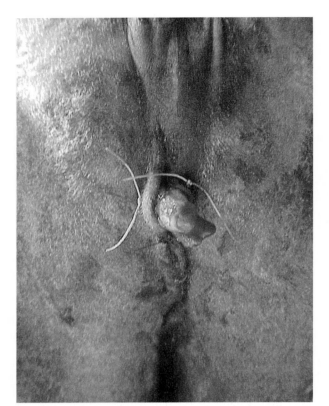

Fig 72-8   Perineal urethrostomy in a lamb showing suture placement and final appearance of penis. Note the dorsally placed urethra visible in this photo.

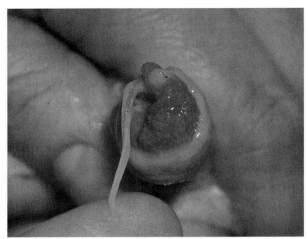

Fig 72-9   Normal urethral process in a ram. The lumen of the process is extremely narrow and prone to obstruction with uroliths. (Courtesy Michael Rings, DVM, MS.)

be taken to avoid penetrating or ligating the urethra with these mattress sutures. The penis should be positioned such that the stump projects approximately 1 inch from the incision and is oriented such that the urine will flow caudoventrally. Once the penis is secure, the urethra may be spatulated to create a larger opening or left unspatulated. If hemorrhage is severe from the exposed corpus spongiosum and cavernosum, the cut edge of the penis may be closed with interrupted sutures of small monofilament suture.

Urethrotomy can be performed over the urolith itself or adjacent to the urolith in healthier tissue. The urolith must be located in an area that can be reached easily, determined by catheterization or palpation. Following incision at the urolith, it is removed with forceps or is crushed to allow the pieces to pass. An alternative technique involves retropulsion of a urolith from the distal urethra to an ischial urethrotomy, where it can be removed. Ischial urethrotomy also allows for placement of a long urethral catheter to act as a stent for a ruptured urethra. Urethral stricture formation is a common side effect of urethrotomy, but the simplicity of the procedure makes it popular, especially in breeding animals in which the penis must remain intact.[35] The urethrotomy incision may be allowed to heal without suturing because suturing may increase the likelihood of stricture formation. Some surgeons, however, recommend suture closure of the urethrotomy as soon as possible to prevent stricture formation.

Urethral process amputation in small ruminants is the simplest procedure for relief of obstructive urolithiasis (Fig. 72-9). The uroliths must be present in the process itself or in the distal penile urethra to pass. Examination of the urethral process should be performed in every animal with urolithiasis, and often the process is removed as a precautionary measure. The procedure is performed quickly with scissors or scalpel and is easiest with the animal restrained in a sitting position on its rump. Unfortunately, urethral process amputation usually results in reobstruction within a short period of time because there are more uroliths further proximal in the urethra. Approximately half of the animals treated with amputation will have urine flow restored.[34] Amputation can be performed as an adjunct therapy for other procedures. Amputation of the urethral process is only possible in ruminants that have reached the age of puberty, at which time the prepuce separates from the penis and allows access to the distal penis.

Unlike other animals, ruminants, swine, camelids, and cervids cannot be catheterized to relieve obstructive urolithiasis because their urethra has a diverticulum in the region of the ischial portion of the urethra.[36,37] This diverticulum results in the redirection of any catheter into the diverticulum, rather than into the bladder itself. Only with special precurved catheters has bladder catheterization been possible.[37] Catheterization and retrograde flushing are therefore not useful in ruminants for resolution of obstructive urolithiasis and may result in urethral rupture if too much force is used.

References

1. Fubini SL: Surgery of the vagina. In Fubini SL, Ducharme NG, editors: *Farm animal surgery*, St Louis, 2004, Saunders.
2. Hooper RN, Taylor TS: Urinary surgery, *Vet Clin North Am Food Anim Pract* 11:95-121, 1995.
3. Madison JB: Surgery of the urinary tract. In Wolfe DF, Moll HD, editors: *Large animal urogenital surgery*, ed 2, Baltimore, 1999, Williams & Wilkins.

4. St-Jean G, Hull BL, Robertson JT et al: Urethral extension for correction of urovagina in cattle: a review of 14 cases, *Vet Surg* 17:258-262, 1988.

5. Wolfe DF, Baird AN: Female urogenital surgery in cattle, *Vet Clin North Am Food Anim Pract* 9:369-388, 1993.

6. Gilbert RO, Wilson DG, Levine SA et al: Surgical management of urovagina and associated infertility in a cow, *J Am Vet Med Assoc* 194:931-932, 1989.

7. Brown MP, Colahan PT, Hawkins DL: Urethral extension for treatment of urine pooling in mares, *J Am Vet Med Assoc* 173:1005-1007, 1978.

8. Mckinnon AO, Belden JO: A urethral extension technique to correct urine pooling (vesicovaginal reflux) in mares, *J Am Vet Med Assoc* 192:647-650, 1988.

9. Monin T, *Vaginoplasty: a surgical treatment for urine pooling in the horse.* Proceedings 18th Annual Meeting American Association Equine Practice, Atlanta, 1973, pp 99-102.

10. Turner AS, McIlwraith CW: Urethroplasty by caudal relocation of the transverse fold. In Turner AS, McIlwraith CW, editors: *Techniques in large animal surgery*, ed 2, Philadelphia, 1989, Lea & Febiger.

11. Fubini SL: Surgery of the urinary bladder and ureters. In Fubini SL, Ducharme NG, editors: *Farm animal surgery*, St Louis, 2004, Saunders.

12. Baird AN: Surgery of the urinary bladder. In Wolfe DF, Moll HD, editors: *Large animal urogenital surgery*, ed 2, Baltimore, 1999, Williams & Wilkins.

13. Dart AJ, Dart CM, Hodgson DR: Surgical management of a ruptured bladder secondary to urethral obstruction in an alpaca, *Aust Vet J* 75:793-795, 1997.

14. Carr EA, Schott HC, Barrington GM et al: Ruptured urinary bladder after dystocia in a cow, *J Am Vet Med Assoc* 202:631-632, 1993.

15. Roussel AJ, Ward DS: Ruptured urinary bladder in a heifer, *J Am Vet Med Assoc* 186:1310-1311, 1985.

16. Smith JA, Divers TJ, Lamp TM: Ruptured urinary bladder in a post-parturient cow, *Cornell Vet* 73:3-12, 1983.

17. Hooper RN, Taylor TS: Urinary surgery, *Vet Clin North Am Food Anim Pract* 11:95-121, 1995.

18. Ewoldt JM, Anderson DE, Miesner MD et al: Short- and long-term outcome and factors predicting survival after surgical tube cystostomy for treatment of obstructive urolithiasis in small ruminants, *Vet Surg* 35:417-422, 2006.

19. Madigan JE: Diagnosing and treating the foal with bladder rupture, *Vet Med* 82:1048-1052, 1987.

20. Bouré LP, Kerr CL, Pearce SG et al: Comparison of two laparoscopic suture patterns for repair of experimentally ruptured urinary bladders in normal neonatal calves, *Vet Surg* 34:47-54, 2005.

21. Bouré LP, Foster RA, Palmer M et al: Use of an endoscopic suturing device for laparoscopic resection of the apex of the bladder and umbilical structures in normal neonatal calves, *Vet Surg* 30:319-326, 2001.

22. Rakestraw PC, Fubini SL, Gilbert RO et al: Tube cystostomy for treatment of obstructive urolithiasis in small ruminants, *Vet Surg* 24:498-505, 1995.

23. Ewoldt JM, Anderson DE, Miesner MD et al: Short- and long-term outcome and factors predicting survival following surgical tube cystostomy for treatment of obstructive urolithiasis in small ruminants, *Vet Surg* 35:417-422, 2006.

24. Hastings DH: Retention catheters for treatment of steers with ruptured bladders, *J Am Vet Med Assoc* 147:1329-1330, 1965.

25. Fortier LA, Gregg AJ, Erb HN et al: Caprine obstructive urolithiasis: requirement for second surgical intervention and mortality after percutaneous tube cystostomy, surgical tube cystostomy, or urinary bladder marsupialization, *Vet Surg* 33:661-667, 2004.

26. Todhunter P, Baird AN, Wolfe DF: Erection failure as a sequela to obstructive urolithiasis in a male goat, *J Am Vet Med Assoc* 209:650-652, 1996.

27. Streeter RN, Washburn KE, McCauley CT: Percutaneous tube cystostomy and vesicular irrigation for treatment of obstructive urolithiasis in a goat, *J Am Vet Med Assoc* 221:546-549, 2002.

28. May KA, Moll HD, Wallace LM et al: Urinary bladder marsupialization for treatment of obstructive urolithiasis in male goats, *Vet Surg* 27:583-588, 1998.

29. May KA, Moll HD, Duncan RB et al: Experimental evaluation of urinary bladder marsupialization in male goats, *Vet Surg* 31:251-258, 2002.

30. Stone WC, Bjorling DE, Trostle SS et al: Prepubic urethrostomy for relief of urethral obstruction in a sheep and a goat, *J Am Vet Med Assoc* 210:939-941, 1997.

31. Streeter RN, Washburn KE, Higbee RG et al: Laser lithotripsy of a urethral calculus via ischial urethrotomy in a steer, *J Am Vet Med Assoc* 219:640-643, 2001.

32. Halland SK, House JK, George LW: Urethroscopy and laser lithotripsy for the diagnosis and treatment of obstructive urolithiasis in goats and pot-bellied pigs, *J Am Vet Med Assoc* 220:1831-1834, 2002.

33. Gill MS, Sod GA: Buccal mucosal graft urethroplasty for reversal of a perineal urethrostomy in a goat wether, *Vet Surg* 33:382-385, 2004.

34. Haven ML, Bowman KF, Engelbert TA et al: Surgical management of urolithiasis in small ruminants, *Cornell Vet* 83:47-55, 1993.

35. Van Metre D: Urolithiasis. In Fubini SL, Ducharme NG, editors: *Farm animal surgery*, St Louis, 2004, Saunders.

36. Garrett PD: Urethral recess in male goats, sheep, cattle, and swine, *J Am Vet Med Assoc* 220:1831-1834, 1987.

37. Palmer JL, Dykes NL, Love K et al: Contrast radiography of the lower urinary tract in the management of obstructive urolithiasis in small ruminants and swine, *Vet Radiol Ultrasound* 39:175-180, 2002.

Genital Surgery—Male

Dwight Wolfe

CHAPTER 73

Diagnosis and Management of Juvenile Anomalies of the Penis and Prepuce

DWIGHT WOLFE and SOREN P. RODNING

PREMATURE SEPARATION OF THE PENIS AND PREPUCE

Prepubertal bulls are incapable of penile extension due to the lack of a sigmoid flexure and because the epithelium of the free portion of the penis is attached to the epithelium of the prepuce at birth. The sigmoid flexure develops before puberty under androgenic stimulation, and the epithelial attachment between the penis and prepuce begins separating at about 1 month of age and continues caudally until completely separated by 8 to 11 months of age, thus allowing normal penile extension. Mounting behavior is normal for peripubertal bulls, and occasionally the penile and preputial epithelium separates prematurely in young bulls as a result of these early attempts to extend the penis. The condition is usually self-limiting and goes unnoticed, but sufficient hemorrhage may create a noticeable swelling within the sheath. The hematoma typically resolves with time and does not require therapy, but occasionally an abscess forms that creates adhesions between the damaged penile and preputial epithelium, leading to permanent phimosis. Therapy for the calf includes separation from the herd to eliminate mounting behavior, irrigation of the preputial cavity with a 3% povidone-iodine and saline solution, and systemic antibiotics.

PERSISTENT FRENULUM

The penile frenulum is a thin band of connective tissue on the ventrum of the penis that extends from the prepuce to near the tip of the free portion of the penis (Fig. 73-1). The frenulum normally ruptures during separation of the preputial and penile epithelium. If the frenulum fails to rupture, a bull can still extend the penis but has a marked ventral bending of the free portion of the penis on erection. A persistent frenulum is usually first noticed when the bull begins to masturbate or attempt breeding or when he undergoes his first breeding soundness evaluation. The persistent frenulum may be narrow or broad based and contains one or more blood vessels.

Repair of a persistent frenulum is accomplished with the bull restrained in a squeeze chute or on a tilt-table. Manually extend the penis and place a towel clamp under the dorsal apical ligament to maintain penile extension. Clean the penis with a preoperative scrub, and infiltrate

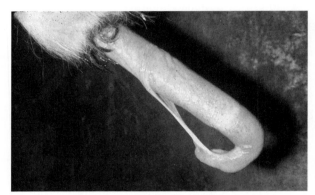

Fig 73-1 Ventral bending of bull penis caused by persistent frenulum.

both ends of the frenulum with 1 to 2 ml of 2% lidocaine hydrochloride. If the distal attachment of the frenulum is near the urethral orifice, place a 10-French (Fr) male dog catheter in the urethra to avoid incising the urethra. Because the frenulum often contains a large vein, ligate each end of the frenulum with No 0 or 1 chromic gut and excise the frenulum (Fig. 73-2). Application of a topical antibiotic ointment is optional. The bull should be ready for breeding service after 2 to 4 weeks of sexual rest. Cattle producers should be advised, however, that persistent penile frenulum is considered a heritable condition. Therefore all male offspring produced from a bull with a repaired persistent frenulum should be castrated.

CONGENITAL SHORT PENIS

Another developmental anomaly is a congenitally short or underdeveloped penis. Typically the circumference of the penis is near normal, but the penis is too short to allow intromission. Although the condition may be suspected on physical examination or part of a routine breeding soundness examination, a test mating is advised to confirm the diagnosis. Even with a test mating, however, caution should be exercised when diagnosing an underdeveloped penis.

Young bulls occasionally become overstimulated and as a result do not completely relax their retractor penis muscles, thereby limiting penile extension. The limited

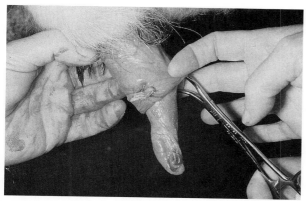

Fig 73-2 Bull penis after ligation and excision of persistent frenulum.

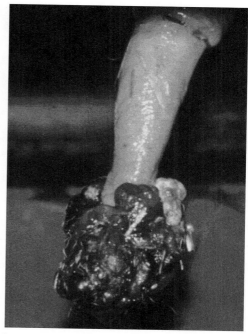

Fig 73-3 Fibropapilloma near the glans penis of a bull.

penile extension mimics a congenitally short penis. Such bulls develop adequate erections, however, so observing the sheath during attempted mating should allow determination of whether the sigmoid flexure fails to straighten. Additionally, with the bull restrained in a livestock chute and the penis relaxed, palpate the sigmoid area to confirm that fibrosis from a previous penile hematoma does not prevent the sigmoid from straightening. Also rule out the possibility that penile extension is limited by adhesions between the peripenile elastic tissue and skin of the sheath. Overly conditioned young bulls with adequate penile size may also fail to achieve intromission because of their large abdomens.

PENILE FIBROPAPILLOMA

Penile fibropapillomas, or penile warts, are common in pens of young bulls and are caused by the bovine papilloma virus. Often these young bulls exhibit homosexual behavior and mount their penmates, causing penile abrasions. The papilloma virus enters the penile skin via these abrasions and causes neoplastic growth of fibroblasts. If one bull in a pen has penile warts, often several of his penmates will have them also. The lesions do not metastasize and are not locally invasive. The warts typically occur on the free portion of the penis, most commonly near the glans penis (Fig. 73-3), and only rarely do they occur on the prepuce. Bulls frequently have a single pedunculated wart, but occasionally several growths are present. Generally, bulls with penile fibropapillomas do not have warts on other body parts. Other neoplasias of the bull penis are rare.

Fibropapillomas most commonly occur in bulls between 1 and 3 years of age. The first clinical sign is often scant hemorrhage from the preputial orifice following coitus, and sometimes affected bulls are reluctant to breed. The warts are also frequently first noticed during routine breeding soundness examination and are either palpated as a mass in the sheath or seen on extension of the penis. Occasionally, large warts may result in paraphimosis or phimosis.

Penile fibropapillomas are easily removed with the bull restrained in a squeeze chute or on a tilt-table. Manually extend the penis and place a towel clamp under the apical ligament proximal to the lesion to maintain penile extension. Clean the penis with a preoperative scrub, and administer local anesthesia via 5 to 10 ml of 2% lidocaine hydrochloride injected subcutaneously on the dorsum of the penis to block the dorsal penile nerves. Rescrub the operative field and place a gauze or Penrose drain tourniquet proximal to the lesion. Because of the proximity of the urethra, it is often advisable to place a 10-Fr male dog catheter into the urethra to aid in identification of this structure during sharp dissection of the papilloma. Inadvertently incising the urethra can lead to urethral fistula formation.

Remove the growth by dissecting its pedunculated base with a scalpel. Larger growths are more manageable by first debulking the lesion with a scalpel to allow clear identification of the pedunculated stalk. Ligate any small vessels and close the skin with No 0 chromic gut. Topical antibiotics are optional, and the bull should be ready for breeding service after 2 to 4 weeks of sexual rest. Recurrence of penile warts is common, however, and bulls should therefore be reexamined before resuming breeding service. Penile warts are most likely to recur when the bull is in an active state of the disease. Commercial and autogenous wart vaccines may decrease the incidence of recurrence.

PENILE HAIR RINGS

Another problem in young bulls is penile hair rings resulting from the previously described homosexual activity of young bulls. Body hair from the bull being ridden accumulates on the penis of the aggressor and results in a ring of hair just proximal to the glans penis (Fig. 73-4). Bulls may also accumulate hair in the same location from their own preputial orifice during masturbation. The hair ring may cause pressure necrosis of the urethra with a resulting

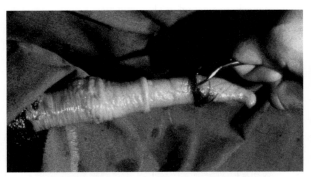

Fig 73-4   Hair ring proximal to the glans penis of a bull.

Recommended Readings

Ashdown RR: Adherence between the free end of the bovine penis and its sheath, *J Anat* 94:198, 1960.

Ashdown RR: Persistence of the penile frenulum in young bulls, *Vet Rec* 74:1464, 1962.

Carroll KJ, Aanes WA, Ball L: Persistent penile frenulum in bulls, *J Am Vet Med Assoc* 144:747, 1964.

Roberts SJ: Infertility in male animals. In Roberts SJ, editor: *Veterinary obstetrics and genital diseases (theriogenology)*, ed 3, Woodstock, Vt, 1986, Edwards Bros.

Wolfe DF: Surgical procedures of the reproductive system of the bull. In Morrow DA, editor: *Current therapy in theriogenology*, ed 2, Philadelphia, 1986, Saunders.

Wolfe DF, Beckett SD, Carson RL: Acquired conditions of the penis and prepuce. In Wolfe DF, Moll HD, editors: *Large animal urogenital surgery*, ed 2, Baltimore, 1998, Williams & Wilkins.

Wolfe DF, Carson RL: Juvenile anomalies of the penis and prepuce. In Wolfe DF, Moll HD, editors: *Large animal urogenital surgery*, ed 2, Baltimore, 1998, Williams & Wilkins.

urethral fistula. If the condition goes unnoticed for too long, avascular necrosis can result in damage to the dorsal nerves of the penis or sloughing of the glans penis. However, if extensive damage has not already occurred, the hair ring is simply removed and an emollient antibiotic ointment applied. Urethral fistulas require surgical repair before breeding can resume.

CHAPTER 74

Diagnosis and Management of Penile Deviations

DWIGHT WOLFE and SOREN P. RODNING

Penile deviations occasionally cause copulation failure in bulls, but they are rare in other domestic ruminants. Penile deviations, in descending order of occurrence, are classified as either spiral (corkscrew), ventral, or S-shaped. Bulls affected with penile deviations typically had one or more successful breeding seasons before copulation failure, but there is usually no known history of previous traumatic penile injury. Affected bulls are usually between 2.5 and 5 years of age.

SPIRAL DEVIATION

Two potential explanations exist for the development of spiral deviations. The first involves malfunction of the apical ligament, whereas the second is based on a more current understanding of erectile physiology. The

apical ligament is a thick collagen band arising from the dorsum of the tunica albuginea about 2.5-cm proximal to the distal end of the prepuce and inserting back into the tunica albuginea near the distal end of the corpus cavernosum penis (CCP). The apical ligament helps maintain the shape of the penis during erection. Historically, spiral deviations were considered the result of a short apical ligament that slipped off to the left side of the penis at peak erection just before intromission. More recently, based on a better understanding of erectile pressures and ejaculation, spiral deviations have been associated with the high maximum pressures within the CCP that occur during ejaculation. In fact, the penis of many normal bulls likely develops a spiral orientation in a cow's vagina during ejaculation. Therefore a possible explanation for a spiral deviation is that a bull whose penis spirals before

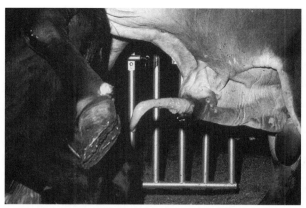

Fig 74-1 Intromission failure secondary to spiral deviation.

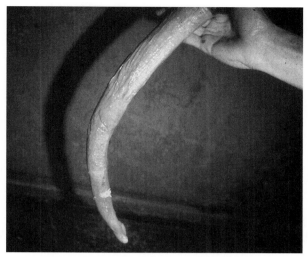

Fig 74-2 Ventral penile deviation originating proximal to the free portion of the penis.

intromission reaches this maximum CCP pressure prematurely. Although the cause of spiral deviations remains uncertain, both apical ligament malfunction and altered penile pressure may contribute in some cases.

An important consideration when diagnosing spiral deviations is that the distal portion of a bull's penis frequently spirals during electroejaculation and masturbation. A spiral deviation should therefore be diagnosed only after observing natural mating (Fig. 74-1). Several test matings are sometimes necessary because the deviation often occurs intermittently, especially during the early stages of the condition. Diagnosis is also difficult in *Bos indicus* bulls because the deviation may occur before penile extension. In such cases the deviation remains hidden in the bull's pendulous sheath and excessive prepuce. Careful observation of the test breeding including palpation and manual retraction of the prepuce may be necessary to differentiate from erection or extension failure.

VENTRAL DEVIATION

Ventral penile deviations are less common than spiral deviations, and their etiology is uncertain. Ventral deviations may occur as a result of altered architecture of the tunica albuginea of the penis or apical ligament and altered blood flow through the ventral portion of the CCP, both of which probably result from chronic traumatic injury. Ventral deviations present as long, gradual curvatures of the erect penis, with the curvature frequently originating proximal to the junction of the sheath and prepuce (Fig. 74-2). The deviation becomes more apparent as the bull's erection increases. Ventral deviations can be diagnosed during electroejaculation, but observation during natural breeding is recommended, especially for less dramatic cases.

S-SHAPED DEVIATION

The S-shaped deviation is the least common type of penile deviation and typically occurs in bulls older than 4 years old as a result of apical ligament malfunction. The S-shaped curvature results from either a normal penis with a short apical ligament or an excessively long penis with

a normal apical ligament. A short apical ligament may result from trauma with resultant contracture of the ligament. In either case, the apical ligament does not allow the penis to fully straighten during erection. No effective therapy exists for this type of penile deviation, but the bull could be used for artificial insemination if the deviation prevents copulation.

REPAIR OF SPIRAL AND VENTRAL PENILE DEVIATIONS

Repair of spiral deviations is much more successful than repair of ventral deviations. In fact, repair of ventral deviations is only recommended when the deviation is limited to the free portion of the penis. Spiral and ventral deviations are both repaired with a fascia lata graft. Autogenous grafts are preferred, but homologous grafts preserved in 70% ethyl alcohol are satisfactory. The narrow strip of fascia lata is sutured between the apical ligament and the tunica albuginea of the penis. The graft serves as a fibroblast lattice that homogenizes with adjacent structures to strengthen and stabilize the apical ligament on the dorsum of the penis. Complete reorganization requires about 90 days, but, if successful, adequate healing usually occurs by 60 days to allow natural breeding.

Fascia Lata Graft Technique

Fast the bull for 24 to 48 hours before general anesthesia. Place the bull in right lateral recumbency and aseptically prepare two operative sites. First, clip and scrub a 20-cm wide × 40-cm long area dorsal to the left patella and extending toward the tuber coxae. Next, clip the hair around the preputial orifice, manually extend the penis, and then place towel forceps under the distal portion of the apical ligament to aid with penile extension (Fig. 74-3). Scrub the penis and prepuce and allow them to return to the sheath while the fascia lata graft is harvested, but leave the towel forceps in place to assist penile extension once the fascia lata harvest is complete.

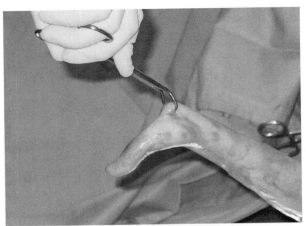

Fig 74-3   Towel forceps placed underneath apical ligament to aid in penile extension.

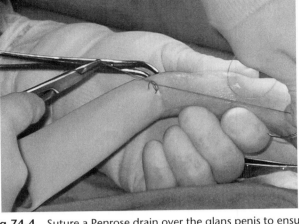

Fig 74-4   Suture a Penrose drain over the glans penis to ensure urine drains away from the incision.

Harvest the fascia lata graft via a 20-cm incision proximal to the patella. The incision should begin about 10 cm dorsal to the anterior border of the patella and extend toward the tuber coxae. The incision must continue through the superficial fascia to expose the thicker layer of deep fascia. Excise a 2-cm wide × 15-cm long section of the deep fascia lata and place in warm saline while closing the incision. Close the fascia lata with No 1 polyglycolic acid suture in a bootlace pattern. Secure closure is imperative to prevent any muscle herniation that could result in severe lameness. Suture the subcutaneous tissue with No. 1 chromic gut, and close the skin with nonabsorbable 0.6-mm synthetic suture in a continuous interlocking pattern. Prepare the fascia lata graft by removing any loose connective tissue and fat and then replace it in warm saline.

Extend the penis and have an assistant maintain penile extension for the remainder of the operation. Place a 2.5-cm Penrose drain around the penis and prepuce as a tourniquet. Beginning just caudal to the glans penis, make a 20-cm skin incision along the dorsum of the penis. Continue the incision through the loose fascial layers in the free portion of the penis and through the thin elastic layers in the preputial portion to expose the apical ligament. Incise the entire length of the apical ligament through its thickest portion along the dorsum of the penis. Reflect both edges laterally to expose the tunica albuginea of the penis and create a bed for the fascia lata graft. Be careful to avoid the two large veins that drain the corpus spongiosum penis because these veins are located deep to the apical ligament on the right ventral aspect of the penis.

Place the fascia lata graft between the apical ligament and tunica albuginea as far proximally as possible. Using No 0 polyglycolic acid suture, place four simple interrupted sutures through the proximal border of the fascia lata graft and into the tunica albuginea. Do not penetrate the entire thickness of the tunica albuginea into the corpus cavernosum penis because this could result in vascular shunt formation and erection failure. Continue placing interrupted sutures along the lateral border of the

graft at 2-cm intervals while stretching the fascia lata in both directions. Trim the graft to fit at the distal end, and then suture it under mild tension with three interrupted sutures. Finish suturing the graft with simple interrupted sutures at 0.5-cm intervals. Remove the tourniquet and check for hemorrhage. Once hemostasis is complete, reappose the edges of the apical ligament over the fascia lata graft with No 1 polyglycolic acid suture in a simple interrupted pattern that engages the fascia lata.

Suture the elastic tissue with No 3-0 chromic gut in a closely spaced simple continuous pattern, and then close the skin with a simple interrupted suture pattern using No 0 chromic gut. Suture a 2.5-cm Penrose drain over the glans penis to ensure urine egress from the incision (Fig. 74-4), and apply antibacterial ointment to the incision. Finally, remove the towel forceps and allow the penis to retract.

Postoperative care includes systemic antibiotics and 60 days sexual rest. Remove the penile skin sutures 10 days postoperatively, but do not remove the thigh skin sutures for 3 weeks to reduce the risk of muscle herniation. Bulls should undergo a breeding soundness examination before the next breeding season.

Recommended Readings

Ashdown RR, Smith JA: The anatomy of the corpus cavernosum penis of the bull and its relationship to spiral deviation of the penis, *J Anat* 104:153, 1969.

Ashdown RR, Pearson H: The functional significance of the dorsal apical ligament of the bovine penis, *Res Vet Sci* 12:183, 1971.

Ashdown RR, Coombs MA: Experimental studies on "corkscrew penis" in the bull, *Vet Rec* 93:30, 1973.

Carson RL, Hudson RS: Diseases of the penis and prepuce. In Howard JL, editor: *Current veterinary therapy 3: food animal practice*, Philadelphia, 1993, Saunders.

Hanselka DV: Bovine penile deviations: a review, *Southwest Vet* 3:265, 1973.

Roberts SJ: Infertility in male animals. In Roberts SJ, editor: *Veterinary obstetrics and genital diseases (theriogenology)*, ed 3, Woodstock, Vt, 1986, Edwards Bros.

Seidel GE, Foote FH: Motion picture analysis of ejaculation in the bull, *J Reprod Fertil* 20:313, 1969.

Walker DF: Deviations of the bovine penis, *J Am Vet Med Assoc* 147:677, 1964.

Walker DF, Young SL: *The fascia late implant technique for correcting bovine penile deviations.* Proceedings of the Annual Meeting of the Society for Theriogenology, 1979.

Walker DF: Surgery of the penis. In Walker DF, Vaughan JT, editors: *Bovine and equine urogenital surgery*, Philadelphia, 1980, Lea & Febiger.

Wolfe DF, Beckett SD, Carson RL: Acquired conditions of the penis and prepuce. In Wolfe DF, Moll HD, editors: *Large animal urogenital surgery*, ed 2, Baltimore, 1998, Williams & Wilkins.

Wolfe DF, Hudson RS, Walker DF: Common penile and preputial problems of bulls, *Comp Cont Ed* 5:447, 1983.

CHAPTER 75

Diagnosis and Management of Injuries to the Penis and Prepuce of Bulls

HERRIS S. MAXWELL and MISTY A. EDMONDSON

Injuries to the penis and prepuce occasionally occur in breeding bulls. The type and extent of injury and the time from injury to recognition and intervention are critical in determining appropriate therapy and prognosis for return to breeding soundness. To make a definitive diagnosis, a veterinarian must be familiar with the regional anatomy and etiology of preputial and penile injuries. Knowledge of therapeutic options and prognosis, coupled with economic constraints and the expectations of the owner, guide case management.

PREPUTIAL INJURIES

Clear breed predilections to preputial injury exist in that the pendulous sheath, excessively long prepuce, and large preputial orifice in *Bos indicus* breeds of bulls and their crosses increase the risk for laceration of the prepuce and subsequent preputial prolapse when compared with *Bos taurus* breeds (Fig. 75-1).

During intromission, the excess prepuce of *Bos indicus* bulls is forced caudally and may form a collar or doughnut at the preputial orifice. During the ejaculatory lunge this collar may be trapped between the abdomen of the bull and the bony pelvis of the cow, with subsequent contusion of the tissues on the ventral aspect of the prepuce. Occasionally the preputial skin ruptures in response to compressive forces generated during the ejaculatory lunge, leading to a preputial laceration. This rupture of the preputial skin predictably occurs on the ventral aspect of the prepuce along a longitudinal axis but assumes a transverse orientation as the penis and prepuce are retracted into the preputial cavity (Fig. 75-2). Edema quickly develops in the traumatized skin and elastic tissues of the prepuce, resulting in preputial prolapse. As the laceration assumes a transverse orientation, the effective length of the skin of the ventral portion of the prepuce decreases, resulting in a characteristic appearance of the prolapsed tissues that is sometimes likened to an elephant's trunk (Fig. 75-3). If the bull continues to attempt to breed, repeated trauma worsens the condition.

In contrast to the *Bos indicus* breeds, *Bos taurus* bulls can usually completely retract the damaged prepuce into the preputial cavity following injury. Consequently, the laceration of the prepuce may go unnoticed until cellulitis, abscessation, or stenosis occurs.

When the prepuce prolapses in response to injury, the increased size and weight of the edematous tissues create a vicious cycle, which may worsen the condition and lead to prolapse of additional lengths of prepuce. The presence of the retractor prepuce muscle may modify this cycle to some extent. In naturally polled bulls, which lack a functional retractor prepuce muscle, the progression of preputial prolapse may be more rapid and severe than in nonpolled bulls. Conversely, the ability of nonpolled

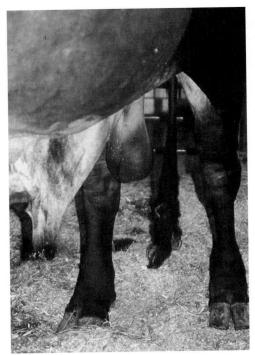

Fig 75-1 *Bos indicus* bull with excessive preputial skin, which is likely to "bunch up" during intromission.

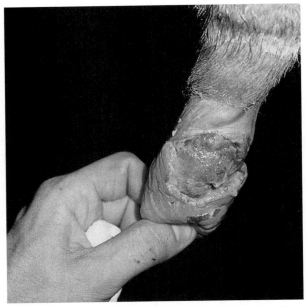

Fig 75-2 Laceration on ventral aspect of the prepuce of a *Bos indicus* bull. Note that original longitudinal laceration is healing with a transverse orientation.

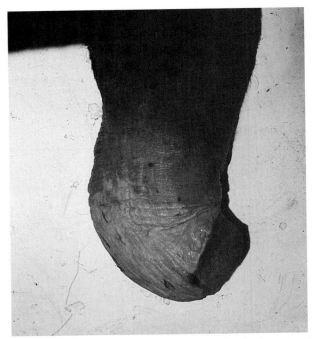

Fig 75-3 Prolapsed prepuce with a typical "elephant trunk" appearance.

bulls to actively retract the prepuce may help minimize preputial edema following trauma.

Some bulls with poor conformation of the prepuce and sheath may appear to spontaneously prolapse. In reality the preputial prolapse is the result of impaired lymphatic drainage of the prepuce induced by repeated trauma during natural service or secondary to posthitis.

When edema in the traumatized tissues impairs the bull's ability to retract the prolapsed prepuce into the preputial cavity, additional trauma or mutilation combined with desiccation of the exposed tissues may lead to extension of the laceration, wound sepsis, and necrosis of tissues. Cellulitis and abscessation may accompany bacterial contamination of the initial laceration or of the wounds that develop secondarily in the exposed preputial tissues. In adverse climatic conditions, frostbite of exposed tissues is a concern.

A classification scheme for preputial injuries that uses the severity of the injury to estimate the prognosis for return to fertility is presented in Table 75-1. Examples of the various classifications are shown in Figs. 75-4 to 75-7. The length and depth of laceration and the extent of damage to the peripenile elastic tissues are the factors most critical in determining the prognosis.

If surgical repair is indicated, the preputial tissue remaining following resection must be at least 1.5 times the length of the free portion of the penis to allow adequate preputial and penile extension at the time of breeding. Additionally, the peripenile tissues must be free of scar tissue that could interfere with the free extension and retraction of the penis and prepuce.

MEDICAL MANAGEMENT OF PREPUTIAL PROLAPSE

Proper care of all categories of preputial prolapse requires cleansing the damaged tissues, support bandaging to reduce edema and prevent secondary injury, and application of emollient antiseptic or antibacterial ointments. One commonly used topical treatment consists of 2 g of tetracycline powder and 60 ml of Scarlet oil mixed into 500 g of anhydrous lanolin.

Table 75-1

Classification of Preputial Prolapses

Category I	Simple preputial prolapse with slight to moderate edema
	Responds well to either surgical or conservative treatment
	Prognosis for return to service: good (see Fig. 75-4)
Category II	Prolapsed prepuce with moderate to severe edema
	May have superficial lacerations or slight necrosis, but no evidence of fibrosis
	Surgery usual course of therapy
	Prognosis for return to service: good to guarded (see Fig. 75-5)
Category III	Prolapsed prepuce with severe edema and deep lacerations, moderate necrosis, and slight fibrosis
	Surgery indicated
	Prognosis for return to service: guarded (see Fig. 75-6)
Category IV	Prolapsed prepuce exposed for a prolonged time, severe edema, deep lacerations, deep necrosis, fibrosis, and often abscessation
	Surgery or salvage by slaughter only options
	Prognosis for return to service: guarded to poor (see Fig. 75-7)

After the damaged tissues are cleaned with surgical scrub and emollient ointment is applied, cover the prolapsed prepuce with a clean 5-cm orthopedic stockinette (Fig. 75-8). Prepare a length of latex tubing, 6.35 mm in diameter or larger, and place it in the preputial cavity for urine drainage (Fig. 75-9). Apply an elastic tape bandage snugly, beginning at the distal end of the prepuce and advancing proximally so that the tape can be anchored on the haired skin of the sheath, being careful to avoid direct contact of the tape with the preputial epithelium (Fig. 75-10). The bandage may be left in place for up to 3 days but should be changed more frequently if it becomes excessively soiled.

A support sling designed to lift the sheath close to the body may be useful in reducing preputial edema. Fashion the sling from burlap, heavy netting, or other loosely woven material and suspend it under the bull's abdomen with bungee cords or strips of inner tubing placed across the bull's back. Adjust the sling so that it supports the weight of the prepuce (Fig. 75-11).

Once the initial edema has resolved, most Category I and II prolapses can be reverted into the preputial cavity and held in place by elastic tape, using a piece of latex

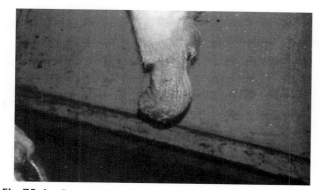

Fig 75-4 Category I prolapsed prepuce; there is slight to moderate edema, no laceration, necrosis, or fibrosis.

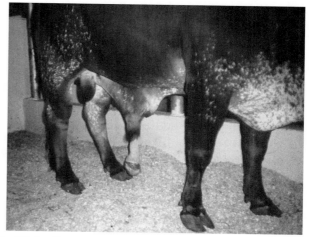

Fig 75-6 Category III preputial prolapse; there is deep laceration and slight fibrosis of the elastic tissue.

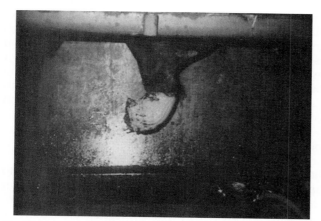

Fig 75-5 Category II preputial prolapse; there is moderate edema and superficial laceration of the skin of the prepuce.

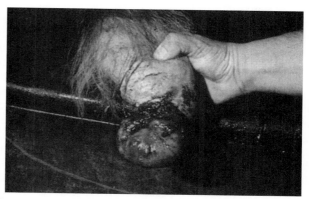

Fig 75-7 Category IV preputial prolapse; there is severe edema and laceration with deep necrosis of the elastic tissue.

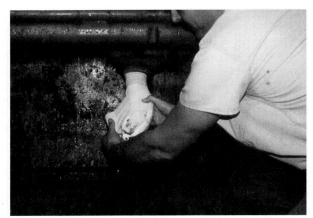

Fig 75-8 Place orthopedic stockinette to protect the exposed prepuce from irritation, and allow placement of a pressure bandage made from adhesive tape.

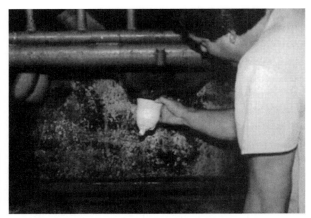

Fig 75-10 Snugly wrap the stockinette with elastic tape, and anchor the tape to the hair of the sheath proximally and to the urine drainage tube distally.

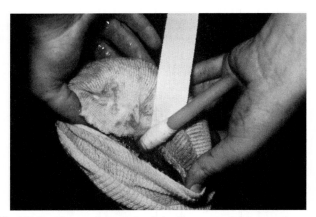

Fig 75-9 Place a latex tube into the preputial lumen to carry urine away from the damaged tissues. The tube should extend 2 to 3 cm proximal to the top of the preputial bandage.

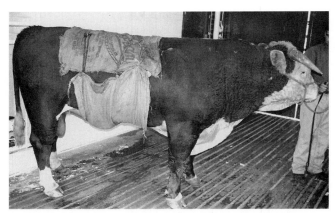

Fig 75-11 To elevate the sheath and help reduce edema, fashion a support sling from burlap or other open mesh material.

tubing placed in the preputial lumen for urine drainage (Fig. 75-12). Avoid placement of a purse-string suture to retain the prepuce because its use is associated with abscess formation and stenosis of the preputial orifice. Retention of a reduced prepuce with a purse-string suture may be considered in bulls destined for immediate salvage at slaughter.

Bulls with Category I or II preputial prolapse treated with a series of bandage changes and supportive therapy are often able to return to service without surgery. In such cases the redundant prepuce that initiated the first incident is still present and may be hypertrophied or stretched to such an extent that recurrence is extremely likely. These bulls should be allowed a minimum of 30 days' sexual rest followed by thorough examination of the damaged tissues before returning to breeding. When surgery is chosen, the prepuce must be conditioned before surgery by the methods described for medical management of nonsurgical cases.

Category III and IV prolapses often have a fibrotic area on the ventral aspect of the prepuce where a previous laceration healed transversely. In Category III and

IV preputial prolapse there are areas of superficial and possibly deep necrosis of tissues, and these tissues may slough following the first few bandage changes. Healthy granulation tissue must cover these areas and any skin lacerations before the prepuce is reversed into the preputial cavity and before surgery. Two to 6 weeks of bandaging and support may be required before this granulation is complete. To expedite the healing process, spray water as a massage (hydrotherapy) and apply antiseptics and osmotic soaks to the prolapsed tissues. Observe the bandage frequently to ensure that it does not roll down and compromise circulation in the damaged tissues.

Bos taurus bulls typically retract the prepuce into the preputial cavity following injury. Because wound drainage is compromised, these bulls may benefit from systemic antibiotics. A pressure bandage to reduce edema is difficult to apply, and the risk of retropreputial abscess is greater than in *Bos indicus* bulls. Complications may be reduced by irrigating the preputial cavity with antiseptic solutions and by hydrotherapy of the sheath over the area where the swelling is most evident. Enforce sexual rest for at least 60 days after the swelling subsides. During convalescence, advise owners to observe the area for any recurrent swelling, which could indicate abscess formation. Because the original longitudinally oriented laceration heals in a transverse plane, impaired extension of the penis is likely. Before returning the bull to service, extend the penis and evaluate the prepuce for stenosis or restriction caused by scar formation.

Do not suture acute lacerations of the prepuce. The peripenile elastic tissue is invariably contaminated by bacteria, and suturing the wound will impede drainage and increase the likelihood of abscess formation. Medical management as previously described, until granulation is complete, is the indicated treatment.

AVULSION OF THE PREPUCE

Occasionally, bulls avulse the prepuce from its attachment to the free portion of the penis. This injury is most common in bulls that serve an artificial vagina (AV) while

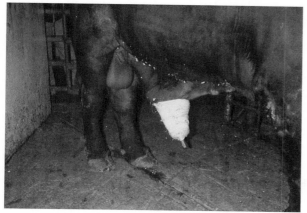

Fig 75-12 Once the prolapsed prepuce can be reduced, hold it in the preputial cavity with elastic tape around the haired portion of the preputial orifice. Note the continued use of the urine tube.

being collected for artificial insemination but rarely may occur during natural service. When the injury occurs while serving the AV, the prepuce adheres to the latex liner of the AV, and during the ejaculatory thrust, the preputial attachment to the penis separates. In contrast to other preputial lacerations, this injury is relatively free of bacterial contamination and should be sutured immediately. Excellent healing occurs following primary wound closure. Attempts to repair avulsion injuries that have undergone delayed healing involve undermining the prepuce, sliding the freed edge to its normal position, and anastomosis to the penis with absorbable suture (Fig. 75-13).

SURGICAL MANAGEMENT OF PREPUTIAL INJURIES

Circumcision

The surgical technique most likely to restore a bull's ability to successfully service cows is resection and anastomosis of the prepuce. Commonly called *circumcision,* this procedure requires full extension of the penis and prepuce, which may necessitate incision of stenotic areas of the prepuce. Although general anesthesia greatly assists the procedure, regional analgesia using an internal pudendal nerve block is sometimes employed.

Following surgical preparation, place a 2.5-cm Penrose drain as a tourniquet around the extended penis at the level of the preputial orifice to achieve a relatively bloodless surgical field. Use the length of the free portion of the penis as a guide for the maximal amount of preputial tissue that may be removed. At a minimum, the remaining prepuce should be 1.5 times the length of the free portion of the penis. Two times the length of the free portion of the penis is preferred (Fig. 75-14). If the prepuce is shortened excessively, the bull will be unable to completely extend the penis, and, conversely,

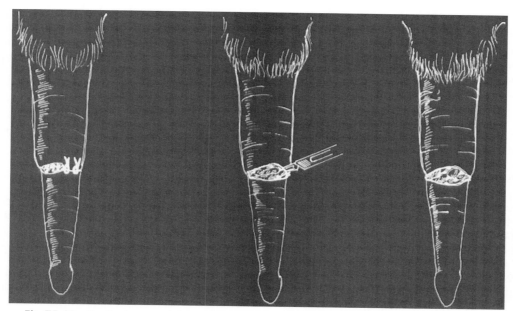

Fig 75-13 Reattachment of the prepuce to the free portion of the penis following avulsion.

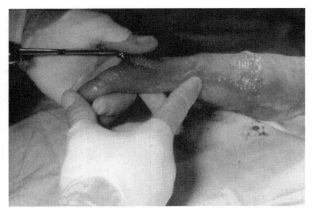

Fig 75-14   Measure the length of the free portion of the prepuce, and ensure that the remaining prepuce is at least one and a half times that length.

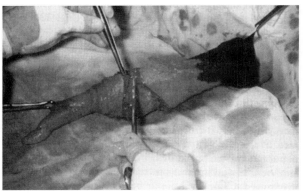

Fig 75-16   Use a simple continuous suture for closure of the peripenile elastic tissue.

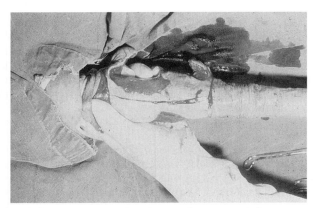

Fig 75-15   To remove the damaged portion of the prepuce, make circumferential incisions proximal and distal to the damaged preputial tissues and connect these incisions with a single longitudinal incision. Carefully dissect under the fibrotic tissues, being careful to preserve as much normal tissue as possible.

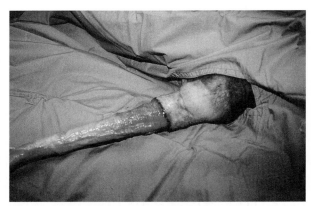

Fig 75-17   Use No 0 chromic gut to close the preputial skin. Align the skin edges closely to ensure first intention healing.

if the prepuce is not shortened sufficiently, recurrence of the prolapse may occur when the bull resumes breeding. Identify the tissues to be excised and make circumferential skin incisions proximal and distal to these tissues. Connect these two incisions with a longitudinal incision (Fig. 75-15).

Use sharp and blunt dissection of the elastic layers beneath the preputial skin to remove the fibrotic tissues, taking care to dissect to the depth adequate to undermine all abnormal tissues while preserving as much normal tissue as possible.

Following removal of the excessive preputial skin and scar tissues, identify all vessels within the elastic tissue and ensure hemostasis by ligature or electrocautery. Remove the tourniquet and ligate or cauterize any remaining vessels to ensure complete hemostasis. Close the subcutaneous elastic tissue with No 2-0 chromic gut in a simple interrupted pattern or, alternately, in a simple continuous pattern tied at each quadrant of the preputial circumference (Fig. 75-16).

Close the skin in a similar fashion, and suture a 2.5-cm Penrose drain over the tip of the penis to drain urine away from the surgical site (Fig. 75-17). Following suturing, place the penis and prepuce back into the preputial cavity and insert a firm, flexible rubber tube of a diameter sufficient to fill the preputial cavity into the lumen of the prepuce. Place elastic tape on the haired distal portion of the sheath to create a bandage that applies pressure to the area opposite the incision site (Fig. 75-18).

Remove the bandage in 3 days, and remove the Penrose drain and sutures in 10 days. Ensure sexual rest for a minimum of 60 days postsurgery. Extend the penis and evaluate for preputial strictures before returning the bull to service.

Amputation of the Prepuce

Prophylactic amputation of the prepuce is occasionally performed in young bulls of the *Bos indicus* breeds to lessen the likelihood of preputial laceration when the bull begins breeding. The procedure can also be used to remove the mass of prolapsed tissue in bulls with grade III or IV preputial prolapse that are expected to be salvaged for slaughter. The procedure is sometimes erroneously referred to as "reefing," a term that means infolding or tucking tissues rather than amputation.

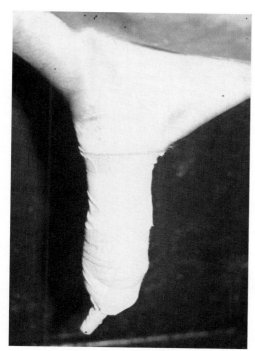

Fig 75-18   After returning the penis and prepuce to the preputial cavity, place a flexible plastic tube in the preputial cavity to serve as a stent, suture a Penrose drain over the tip of the penis, and apply a pressure bandage.

The chief advantage of amputation is that the procedure is simpler and more quickly performed than circumcision. The major disadvantage is a higher incidence of preputial stenosis following wound contracture due to the removal of more elastic tissues and the less precise apposition of skin edges than occurs with circumcision.

Amputation of the prepuce may be performed with the bull standing in a chute or restrained in lateral recumbency on a tilt-table. Achieve anesthesia by subcutaneous infiltration of a local anesthetic into the area of the sheath just proximal to the preputial orifice. Make an incision into the prolapsed prepuce, and extend it into the lumen of the preputial cavity. Initially incise only one third of the circumference of the prepuce. Ligate bleeders and appose the internal and external layers of preputial skin with No 0 chromic gut using a simple continuous pattern. Repeat this procedure for each remaining one third of the prepuce so that the entire prolapsed portion is removed and the sutures are anchored in three places. Suture a Penrose drain over the end of the penis as described for circumcision, and revert the prepuce into the preputial cavity. Place an elastic bandage as described for circumcision to maintain pressure on the incision. Leave the bandage in place for 3 days. Remove the Penrose drain in 10 days.

An alternate to preputial amputation that may be considered when surgical facilities are limited or when the economic value of the bull prohibits expensive surgical treatment is amputation of the prepuce using a plastic ring and a special suture pattern to assist hemostasis. This procedure may also be considered in bulls with grade III or grade IV preputial prolapse when the goal is to reduce the mass of prolapsed tissues before submitting the bulls to slaughter.

The goal of this procedure is to place a ring of ligating sutures through holes in a plastic ring in a manner that completely ligates the prepuce and its associated vessels. Nonabsorbable suture, 0.6 mm in diameter, is used in a special suture pattern, dubbed the "booger suture" by Dr. Don Walker and Dr. Robert Hudson.

Amputation with a plastic ring is not suitable for bulls that have considerable edema and fibrosis of the prepuce adjacent to the preputial orifice, making preoperative evaluation and conditioning of the preputial prolapse necessary in the selection of surgical candidates.

Although technically less challenging than circumcision, amputation of the prepuce with a plastic ring has inherent disadvantages. The amputation occurs with the prepuce in the prolapsed position, making it impossible to determine if the length of remaining prepuce will be sufficient to allow normal extension of the prepuce and penis. The procedure also has a predictably high incidence of postsurgical preputial stenosis as a result of the less precise alignment of the preputial tissues.

Although cleanliness in the procedure is important, absolute asepsis is not required because of the limited exposure of the tissues and placement of sutures before amputation of pathologic tissue. This procedure results in only minimal hemorrhage.

Before surgery, prepare the amputation ring using a ⅛-inch drill or similar device to place 10 to 15 holes around the circumference near the middle of a 7.5-cm long section of flexible polyvinyl tubing that is 3 to 5 cm in diameter.

Restrain the bull and clip the hair around the preputial orifice. Thoroughly scrub the area with surgical soap and infiltrate the subcutaneous tissues around the preputial orifice with a local anesthetic. Place the previously prepared polyvinyl tubing into the preputial cavity and position it so that the ring of holes aligns with the area selected as the site of the amputation. If the opening at the end of the prolapsed prepuce is constricted, the flexible tubing may be compressed as it is inserted and allowed to spring back to its original diameter within the preputial cavity.

Begin the suture pattern by passing a 10-cm, half-curved, cutting-edge suture needle into the lumen of the prepuce, through the first hole of the polyvinyl ring, and through the prolapsed prepuce to the outside. Pull the tail of the suture through the tissue, and then remove the needle. Create a loop of suture between the previously placed suture and the suture cassette. Thread the loop onto the suture needle and introduce the needle through the next hole in the ring to pass the double strand of suture through the plastic ring and preputial tissues (Fig. 75-19). Remove the needle from the double strand of suture and cut the suture in the middle of the loop. Tie the tail of suture introduced with the first bite as snugly as possible to the strand that is continuous with that tail. The free end of the double strand then becomes the tail for the second suture. Repeat the pattern until the entire circumference of the prepuce is ligated. When complete,

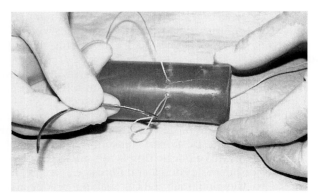

Fig 75-19　The polyvinyl ring used for amputation of the prepuce with a plastic ring.

the pattern ligates 100% of the prolapsed preputial tissues. Amputate the damaged prepuce 0.5 cm distal to the suture line, leaving the plastic ring in place. Extend the penis through the plastic ring and suture a 2.5-cm Penrose drain over the tip of the penis to divert urine past the suture line. Allow the penis to retract, and push the plastic ring into the preputial cavity. Place an elastic bandage, or alternately a purse-string suture, to hold the ring in place. Trim the Penrose drain to an appropriate length.

Irrigate the preputial cavity daily with a nonirritating antibacterial or antiseptic solution, and leave the bandage or purse-string suture in place for 1 week. Two weeks following the procedure, grasp the ring with a pair of forceps and apply traction to extract the ring. The ligating sutures and a ring of necrotic tissue distal to the sutures will accompany the ring as it is removed. Maintain the Penrose drain for an additional 3 days, and continue the preputial flushes as indicated. As with other procedures, a minimum of 60 days' sexual rest is required. The bull's ability to extend the penis should be verified before returning to service.

Preputial Reconstruction by Scar Revision

When scar revision is indicated, the scar tissue is removed and the laceration reoriented to its original longitudinal plane with sutures (Fig. 75-20, *A*). If sutures in the prepuce were to be tightened with the penis in an extended state, tension on the elastic layers would prevent reversion of the prepuce. To avoid this problem, align the cut edges of the preputial skin with a loosely placed bootlace suture pattern, leaving the untied suture ends aligned toward the sheath. Revert the prepuce into the preputial cavity and tighten the sutures from outside the preputial orifice to appose the skin edges (Fig. 75-20, *B*). This orients the sutured wound in a longitudinal plane and allows primary healing to occur (Fig. 75-20, *C*). The likelihood of stenosis is reduced because minimal elastic tissue or preputial skin is removed.

Suture a Penrose drain over the end of the penis to divert urine from the suture line and leave in place for 10 days. Maintain the bull on prophylactic antibiotic therapy.

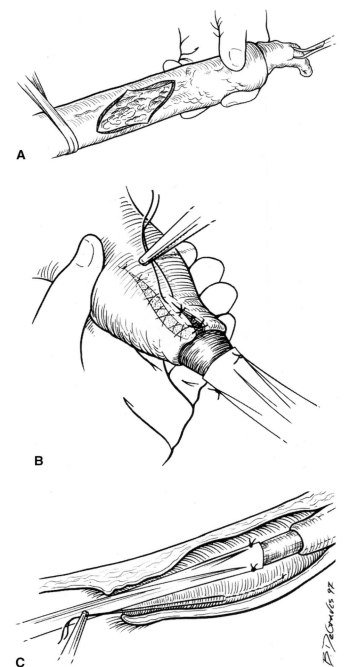

Fig 75-20　Preputial scar revision. **A,** Excise scar and extend prepuce to orient wound with the long axis of the penis, and loosely place a bootlace suture such that the free ends of the suture are located toward the preputial orifice. **B,** Gently return the penis and prepuce to the preputial cavity before tightening the bootlace suture. **C,** Align the wound edges by tightening the suture from outside the prepuce.

Following scar revision the penis is not generally freely capable of extension for 60 to 120 days. Do not forcefully extend the penis during the convalescent period. Most bulls begin to masturbate within a few weeks of the surgery and will stretch the contracted tissues without causing permanent damage.

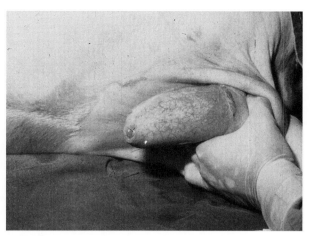

Fig 75-21   Retropreputial abscess.

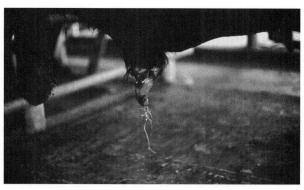

Fig 75-22   Circular stenosis of the prepuce. Note that the opening is barely large enough for urine drainage.

COMPLICATIONS OF PREPUTIAL INJURY

Retropreputial Abscess

Formation of a retropreputial abscess may occur following preputial laceration. This condition occurs more commonly in bulls of *Bos taurus* breeds than in *Bos indicus*–influenced breeds. As previously noted, *Bos taurus* breeds usually do not prolapse the prepuce following laceration, being more likely to retract the contaminated wound into the preputial cavity. In addition to cellulitis and phlegmon, bacterial contamination may result in formation of an abscess at the site of the laceration. The affected area may extend from the preputial orifice to the scrotum or may be confined to a small, well-circumscribed area along the cranial portion of the sheath. The swelling associated with preputial lacerations or abscess can generally be differentiated from that due to penile hematoma by the differences in location and by the lack of symmetry generally associated with the preputial injury (Fig. 75-21).

Appropriate surgical drainage of retropreputial abscesses is difficult but may be attempted. The drainage must be established through the original preputial laceration and into the preputial cavity, not through the external skin of the sheath. Attempts to drain the abscess to the outside invariably results in bacterial seeding of the peripenile elastic tissues and likely result in adhesion formation. Systemic antibiotics and hydrotherapy should be used following establishment of drainage. Because of the high probability that adhesions within the elastic layers of the prepuce or between the elastic layers and the skin will adversely affect normal penile extension, the prognosis for return to breeding soundness for bulls with retropreputial abscesses is always poor.

Phimosis

Stenosis of the preputial cavity resulting from scar contraction may follow preputial injury or surgery. This stenosis may be severe enough to result in phimosis, the inability to extend the penis. Other causes of phimosis may include a congenitally short penis or penile deviation, which are discussed elsewhere.

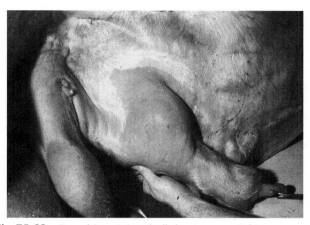

Fig 75-23   Paraphimosis in a bull due to preputial trauma.

Preputial stenosis severe enough to prevent penile extension may occur in two forms. A circular stenosis (Fig. 75-22) develops when scar tissue encircles the prepuce and can follow amputation of the prepuce or be due to frostbite or other trauma. The second form of preputial stenosis occurs when a longitudinally oriented preputial laceration heals in a transverse plane as previously described. Either form of stenosis may be surgically corrected.

If there is sufficient length of preputial skin, a circular stenosis may be incised to allow penile extension and preputial resection and anastomosis performed. Similarly, with transverse healing of a longitudinal wound, the penis can usually be partially extended. If the prepuce is sufficiently long, the scar can be removed by resection and preputial anastomosis. Where the length of healthy prepuce is limiting, reconstruction by scar revision is necessary.

Paraphimosis

The inability to retract the penis into the preputial cavity is known as *paraphimosis*. The most common cause of paraphimosis is preputial trauma in *Bos taurus* bulls. Edema formation subsequent to preputial contusion or laceration prevents the penis from being withdrawn into the sheath (Fig. 75-23). In rare instances, bulls with balanoposthitis caused by herpes virus infection extend the inflamed penis, which then becomes edematous, preventing penile retraction. Regardless of cause, the exposed tissues of the penis and prepuce become dehydrated and the superficial layers of skin may become necrotic and slough.

Treatment for paraphimosis consists of topical application of emollient ointments or creams and application of an orthopedic stockinette to protect the exposed penis and prepuce from environmental contamination and further dehydration. Hydrotherapy may also be beneficial. Treat daily until the bull is able to retract the penis into the preputial cavity, and continue infusing the antibacterial emollient ointment into the prepuce for an additional 7 to 10 days. At least 30 days' sexual rest should be provided before returning the bull to breeding.

Prognosis for return to breeding soundness depends on the cause of the paraphimosis and the extent of damage to the penile and preputial tissues. Bulls with paraphimosis resulting from herpes viral infections have a good prognosis unless there is deep necrosis of the peripenile tissues. Bulls with paraphimosis secondary to preputial laceration have a fair to guarded prognosis, depending on the extent of the damage from the primary injury.

PENILE INJURIES

Deviations of the penis and treatment of penile fibropapillomas are covered elsewhere in this text. Traumatic injuries of the penis also occur in breeding bulls, and as with preputial injuries, recognition and assessment of the injury by the veterinarian are required to determine proper treatment and establish a prognosis.

Penile Hematoma

Although any injury that results in the accumulation of a blood clot within the tissues surrounding the penis could be called a *hematoma of the penis,* in the bull the term *hematoma of the penis* refers to a specific condition in which a peripenile blood clot forms from blood that escapes from the erectile tissues of the corpus cavernosum penis following rupture of the tunica albuginea. This injury occurs most commonly in bulls used in natural service.

Normal erection pressure in the corpus cavernosum penis of the bull may exceed 14,000 mm Hg. The creation and maintenance of this pressure is due to the transient existence of a closed, fluid-filled system in which the venous outflow of the corpus cavernosum penis is occluded and additional pressure is applied to the system by contraction of the ischiocavernosus muscles over the crua of the penis. The tunica albuginea surrounds the erectile tissue of the corpus cavernosum penis. The penis becomes erect as the retractor penis muscles relax and the sigmoid flexure extends in response to the generated pressure. Normally the tunica albuginea easily contains these high pressures. However, if sudden angulation of the erect penis is induced when a heifer or cow collapses during intromission or if the breeding lunge accidentally forces the penis against the escutcheon rather than into vagina, the internal pressure of the penis dramatically increases and the tunica albuginea may rupture in response to extraordinary pressures. Rupture of the tunic

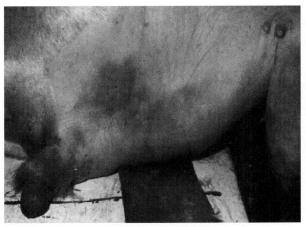

Fig 75-24 Discoloration or bruising of the skin over the site of the hematoma.

predictably occurs on the dorsum of the penis at the level of the distal sigmoid flexure, opposite the insertion of the retractor penis muscles. The typically transverse tear of the tunic is from 2 to 7 cm in length.

Following rupture of the tunica albuginea, externally visible subcutaneous swelling develops as a result of the blood that escapes from the corpus cavernosum penis. Although only 250 ml of blood is required for penile erection in the bull, several liters of blood may accumulate around the penis if the bull makes additional attempts to breed following the injury.

Diagnosis of penile hematoma is not difficult and is based on history and physical findings. Owners frequently become aware of the condition when they notice a prolapsed prepuce, which often occurs secondary to the swelling and blood accumulation in the peripenile elastic tissues. The preputial prolapse often appears congested and may be bluish or dark red and edematous. Immediately anterior to the scrotum, a symmetrical swelling can be detected by visual observation and palpation. This swelling may completely surround the penis or be located only over the dorsum of the penis. Because of the high pressures at the time of rupture, the skin over the hematoma site may be discolored for the first few days following injury (Fig. 75-24). The initially fluctuant clot begins to organize as fibrous tissue replaces blood. By day 10 postinjury, the swelling will have become quite firm.

Hematoma of the penis must be differentiated from other conditions including retropreputial abscess, preputial laceration with or without abscessation, or posthitis. Retropreputial abscesses are generally located distal to the usual site of a penile hematoma, lack symmetry, and may be warm to the touch. Avoid percutaneous needle aspiration as a means of differentiation because this procedure may create a tract of infection into the elastic tissues, which could lead to adhesions and prevent penile extension.

Treatment

More than 50% of bulls with rupture of the tunica albuginea undergo spontaneous recovery if given 90 days' sexual rest. Because of the likelihood of abscessation,

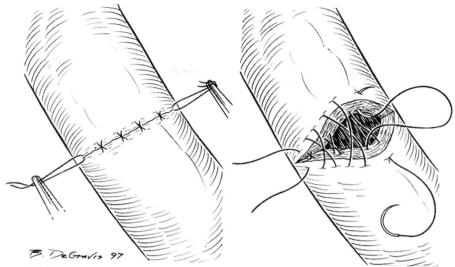

Fig 75-25   Tighten the bootlace suture in the tunica albuginea from both ends.

prophylactic parenteral antibiotics are recommended for 10 days as part of conservative therapy.

Surgical removal of the clotted blood in the hematoma coupled with repair of the rent in the tunica albuginea is felt to reduce the occurrence of complications that can follow this injury and may increase the recovery rate to 80%. Although surgical repair can be accomplished with an internal pudendal nerve block and local infiltration, general anesthesia offers many advantages and greatly facilitates the procedure.

Because fibrous organization of the hematoma makes exteriorization of the penis difficult, surgery should be performed as soon after the injury as possible, preferably from day 3 to day 7 following injury. Surgery is not recommended after day 10 because the clot will have become well organized.

Following a 48-hour fast, induce general anesthesia with the bull in right lateral recumbency. Secure the left rear leg in flexed abduction to improve access to the surgical site, and prepare the skin over the hematoma for aseptic surgery.

Make a 20-cm skin incision over the site of the hematoma, anterior and parallel to the rudimentary teats. Carefully deepen the incision through the subcutaneous tissues and into the elastic tissues until the hematoma is encountered. Ligate any subcutaneous vessels encountered, and when hemostasis is achieved, incise the connective tissue over the hematoma and remove clotted blood. Remove large fragments of clot manually and smaller clots by irrigating the cavity with warm saline.

Following removal of the clotted blood, exteriorize the penis and the surrounding elastic tissues through the incision and locate the paired retractor penis muscles near the distal sigmoid flexure. Identify the urethral groove on the ventral aspect of the penis, and make a longitudinal incision through the elastic tissues over the lateral aspect of the penis to expose the tunica albuginea. Bluntly dissect the elastic layers and elevate the tissues dorsally to reveal the rent in the tunica albuginea. Approaching the rent in this manner rather than directly

lessens the possibility of injury to the dorsal vessels and nerves of the penis.

After identifying the edges of the rent, remove a small wedge of tissue to establish healthy wound edges. Remove only the minimal amount of tissue necessary to freshen the wound margins because excessive tissue removal may result in interference with extension of the penis at the level of the distal sigmoid flexure. Appose the edges of the rent with No 1 polyglycolic acid suture in a bootlace pattern (Fig. 75-25). Appose the elastic layers over the lateral side of the penis and close with 3-0 chromic gut in the superficial layers. Return the penis to its normal position. Flush with saline and close the subcutaneous tissues and skin in a routine manner.

Postoperatively, administer systemic antibiotics and monitor the wound. A seroma commonly occurs and subsides over the next 10 days. As with conservative therapy, ensure sexual rest for 60 days following surgery.

A number of complications may occur following hematoma of the penis in the bull. Recurrence in subsequent breeding seasons is not uncommon. Contamination of the hematoma site from hematogenous bacterial spread or surgical sepsis can lead to functional disruption of the peripenile elastic tissues, adhesions, and abscessation. Loss of sensation to the penis may occur coincident with the initial injury if the dorsal penile nerves are damaged by the explosive forces accompanying the rupture. Penile desensitization may also be delayed until the bull returns to service if the dorsal penile nerves become entrapped in the fibrous tissue that replaces the hematoma and are injured by stretching or tearing as the penis becomes erect. Although bulls with penile analgesia are incapable of servicing cows successfully, semen may be collected by electroejaculation and used for artificial insemination.

Erectile failure may develop following penile hematoma. Although the erectile failure may be the result of bacterial infection or thrombus formation of the cavernous spaces of the corpus cavernosum penis, the most common cause of erectile failure following penile hematoma is the formation of vascular shunts between the corpus cavernosum penis and the peripenile vasculature. The formation of shunts allows blood to escape from the corpus cavernosum penis and, as a result, sufficient erectile pressure is not achieved. These vascular shunts may be demonstrated by injecting contrast media into the corpus cavernosum penis while taking serial radiographs. Surgical repair of the posthematoma shunt can be accomplished by wedge resection of the tunica albuginea and closure similar to the technique described for hematoma repair.

Recommended Readings

Ashdown RR, Pearson H: Anatomical and experimental studies on eversion of the sheath and protrusion of the penis in the bull, *Res Vet Sci* 15:13, 1973.

Bellenger CR: A comparison of certain parameters of the penis and prepuce in various breeds of beef cattle, *Res Vet Sci* 12:299, 1971.

Carson RL, Hudson RS: Diseases of the penis and prepuce. In Howard JL, editor: *Current veterinary therapy: food animal practice*, ed 3, Philadelphia, 1993, Saunders.

Cardwell WH: The surgical correction of the preputial and penile disorders of the bull, *Southwestern Vet* Summer:270, 1961.

Dawson LJ, Rice LE, Morgan GL: Management of the preputial prolapse in the bull fact sheet, *Soc Therio Bull*, 1989.

Long SE, Hignett PG: Preputial eversion in the bull, *Vet Rec* 86:161, 1970.

Madill JW: Amputation of the sheath in Brahma or Brahma crossbred bulls, *Auburn Vet* Fall:25, 1958.

Memon MA, Dawson LJ, Usenik EA et al: Preputial injuries in beef bulls, *J Am Vet Med Assoc* 193:484, 1988.

Musser JM, St-Jean G, Vestweber JG et al: Penile hematoma in bulls: 60 cases (1979-1990), *J Am Vet Med Assoc* 201:1416, 1992.

Walker DF, Vaughan JT: *Bovine and equine urogenital surgery*, Philadelphia, 1980, Lea & Febiger.

Wolfe DF, Hudson RS, Walker DF: Common penile and preputial problems of bulls, *Comp Cont Ed* 5:447, 1983.

CHAPTER 76

Diagnosis and Management of Inguinal Hernia in Bulls

DWIGHT WOLFE and SOREN P. RODNING

The three most common types of bovine inguinal hernias are acquired indirect hernias in mature bulls, acquired direct hernias in mature bulls, and congenital hernias in neonatal bulls. The direct/indirect classification of hernias refers to whether or not the abdominal viscera exits the abdomen through a normal body opening, in this case the inguinal ring. Direct hernias are the result of disruption of normal anatomy, whereas indirect hernias occur through dilated, but otherwise normal, inguinal rings. The two acquired inguinal hernias in mature bulls are not considered heritable, and therefore repair focuses on maintaining breeding soundness. Occasionally, however, acquired inguinal hernia repair requires unilateral castration to preserve the contralateral testicle. Congenital hernias are considered heritable, and therefore bilateral castration is recommended.

INDIRECT INGUINAL HERNIA

An indirect inguinal hernia presents as a chronic, nonemergency condition. A cattle producer often notices a characteristic hourglass-shaped scrotum that may appear intermittently as viscera moves in and out of the vaginal tunics in the scrotal neck. More than 90% of indirect inguinal hernias occur through the left inguinal ring because of the weight of the rumen and because mature cattle prefer to rest in right sternal recumbency with their left rear leg abducted. This recumbent position tends to stretch the left inguinal ring, allowing viscera to exit the abdominal cavity, and most bulls do not develop clinical signs of gastrointestinal obstruction.

On physical examination, rectal palpation of the inguinal rings reveals dilation of the ring with viscera often herniated through the affected ring. Occasionally the herniated viscera is reducible via rectal palpation. The remaining physical examination is usually normal, with the notable exception that an indirect inguinal hernia can negatively affect a bull's semen quality through interference with normal testicular thermoregulation.

A bull with an indirect inguinal hernia often has a history of having been overconditioned at some point in his life, and overconditioned bulls tend to have enlarged inguinal fat pads that are an accumulation of retroperitoneal fat protruding through the inguinal ring (Fig. 76-1). The enlarged inguinal fat pad dilates the inguinal ring and when a bull loses excessive body condition the fat pad shrinks, but the inguinal ring remains dilated and more prone to inguinal herniation.

DIRECT INGUINAL HERNIA

Direct inguinal hernias in men occur through the body wall near the inguinal rings, but a bull's abdominal tunic is too strong to allow herniation and most often the more delicate peritoneum near the inguinal ring tears if stressed sufficiently. Significant increases in intra-abdominal pressure often result from bulls fighting or attempting to jump a fence. If the bull hangs on the fence and the fence does not break, intra-abdominal pressure may increase sufficiently to tear the peritoneum. A tear in the peritoneum near the inguinal ring allows viscera to herniate retroperitoneally through the inguinal ring and into the neck of the scrotum, resulting in a direct inguinal hernia. No right- or left-sided predilection for direct inguinal hernias exists.

Direct inguinal hernias are emergencies. Regardless of the cause, intestinal incarceration is common and results in both intestinal obstruction and vascular compromise. Clinical presentation may vary depending on the duration of the condition, but bulls often show signs of obstructive or ischemic bowel disease. The characteristic hourglass shape associated with indirect inguinal hernias is not seen with direct inguinal hernias. Instead, the inguinal area and scrotum are significantly swollen as a result of the incarcerated bowel. Bulls may present with signs of colic, abdominal distention, and systemic shock. Most bulls will not survive beyond a few days without operative intervention.

REPAIR OF INDIRECT INGUINAL HERNIAS

Indirect inguinal hernias are not considered heritable, and therefore repair focuses on salvaging both testicles to return the bull to breeding soundness. Repair of an indirect inguinal hernia is an elective procedure, so proper timing is a consideration. The optimal time to perform the operation is predicated on the breeding status and semen quality of the bull. Both the hernia and the postoperative swelling may or may not negatively affect semen quality by disruption of normal testicular thermoregulation. Also, regardless of the effects on semen quality, bulls will need several weeks of sexual rest to allow for postoperative healing. Indirect inguinal hernia repair is accomplished via a standing flank approach or an inguinal approach, the latter requiring lateral recumbency and

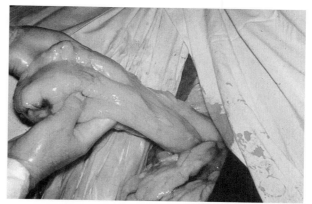

Fig 76-1 Inguinal fat pad.

general anesthesia. Both approaches are performed ipsilateral to the hernia.

Standing Flank Approach for Repair of Indirect Inguinal Hernias

Adequately restrain the bull in a livestock chute. After the ipsilateral paralumbar fossa is clipped, scrubbed, anesthetized, and prepared for aseptic surgery, enter the abdominal cavity via routine laparotomy. Palpate the affected inguinal ring and apply traction to the herniated intestine to reduce the hernia. Close the inguinal ring with blindly placed simple interrupted or simple continuous sutures, being careful not to occlude any of the large blood vessels in the inguinal ring.

A standing flank laparotomy for repair of indirect inguinal hernias is advantageous because of the ease of animal positioning, simple anesthesia, and applicability as a field procedure. However, there are two common conditions associated with indirect inguinal hernias that may interfere with repair via a standing flank approach. Because of the chronicity of many indirect inguinal hernias, the herniated viscera is often adhered to the parietal vaginal tunic of the spermatic cord, thus preventing reduction of the hernia. Also, remnants of the inguinal fat pad, which may have been one of the predisposing factors, can remain prolapsed through the inguinal ring and interfere with appropriate closure.

Inguinal Approach for Repair of Indirect Inguinal Hernias

An inguinal approach for repair of indirect inguinal hernias requires lateral recumbency and general anesthesia. After a 24- to 48-hour fast, induce general anesthesia and place the bull in lateral recumbency on the side opposite the hernia. Next, elevate the upper rear leg to expose the affected inguinal area and then clip and aseptically prepare the operative field.

Begin the operation with a 20-cm vertical skin incision over the inguinal ring, and continue the incision through the subcutaneous tissue and tunica dartos to expose the spermatic cord (Fig. 76-2). First mobilize the spermatic cord by blunt dissection, and then extend the dissection to expose the inguinal ring. The inguinal ring is identified

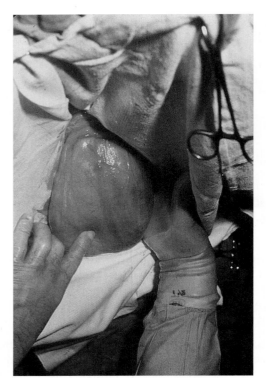

Fig 76-2 Enlarged spermatic cord containing herniated intestine.

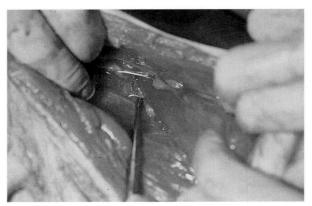

Fig 76-3 Two sutures placed from the edge of the internal abdominal oblique muscle superficial and deep to the spermatic cord.

by its predominantly longitudinal orientation with cranial and caudal endpoints, and the medial and lateral edges of the inguinal ring consist of the thick abdominal tunic. After the spermatic cord is isolated and the inguinal ring identified, incise the parietal vaginal tunic to evaluate the herniated viscera for adhesions. The jejunum or jejuno-ileum is the most common portion of the intestinal tract found in inguinal hernias. If no adhesions are present, replace the viscera and close the inguinal ring before suturing the incision in the parietal vaginal tunic.

If adhesions are present between the herniated viscera and the parietal peritoneum containing the spermatic cord, place one or more ligatures around the adhesions before sharp dissection. Blunt separation of adhesions without ligatures may damage the bowel or cause unnecessary hemorrhage. Any hemorrhage into the scrotum may alter thermoregulation of the testicle through the formation of a hematoma and/or subsequent testicular adhesions to the scrotum. After separating any adhesions, reduce the herniated viscera and explore the inguinal ring for the presence of an inguinal fat pad. If present, the retroperitoneal fat pad appears as a pedunculated mass protruding through the inguinal ring cranial to the spermatic cord (see Fig. 76-1). Bluntly dissect around the fat pad to allow secure ligation, and then amputate the pad as close to the inguinal ring as possible. Ensure complete hemostasis of the fat pad before closure of the inguinal ring.

Close the dilated inguinal ring in multiple layers with nonabsorbable, 0.6-mm synthetic suture on a tapered needle. First, insert the needle through the medial edge of the external ring approximately 2 cm from the caudal apex of the ring. Pass the suture deep to the spermatic

cord, through the caudal border of the internal abdominal oblique muscle, and back under the spermatic cord to exit adjacent to the first suture bite. Place a second suture in a similar manner through the lateral edge of the inguinal ring and external to the spermatic cord at least 3 cm away from the first suture in the edge of the internal abdominal oblique muscle (Fig. 76-3). Simultaneously tighten both sutures while avoiding excessive pressure on the spermatic cord. Next, close the external border of the inguinal ring with an overlapping (vest-over-pants) pattern beginning at the cranial border of the ring where a natural overlap is present. Tighten this layer enough to allow two fingers between the spermatic cord and the closed inguinal ring. A tighter closure causes excessive postoperative edema, whereas a looser closure may not prevent recurrence of the hernia. Finally, place a simple continuous suture to secure the lateral and medial edges of the ring. Again, be careful to avoid compromising the spermatic cord and vessels exiting the inguinal ring.

After verifying that no viscera remains herniated, close the incision in the parietal vaginal tunic of the spermatic cord in a simple continuous pattern with absorbable suture. Next, close the inguinal area and subcutaneous tissues in a simple continuous pattern with absorbable suture while attempting to minimize any dead space. Close the skin in a continuous pattern with nonabsorbable suture.

Postoperative care includes systemic antibiotics to prevent infection and diuretics as needed to manage edema. Slow, forced exercise often assists with resolution of minor edema, whereas hydrotherapy is beneficial with more extensive postoperative swelling. Remove the skin sutures in 14 days.

REPAIR OF DIRECT INGUINAL HERNIAS

Repair of direct inguinal hernias is identical to the repair of indirect inguinal hernias, except for several complicating factors associated with direct inguinal hernias that should be considered. Initially, the bull is often metabolically compromised due to intestinal obstruction leading to greater risks associated with general anesthesia. Appropriate supportive care including intravenous fluid therapy is therefore necessary to ensure patient survival both during and after the operation. Also, the herniated viscera may be nonviable due to incarceration and is often nonreducible because of adhesions resulting from excessive fibrin production secondary to trauma and ischemia. Reducing the herniated viscera will then require dissecting the adhesions and may actually require enlarging the hernial ring. A flank laparotomy may also be necessary to provide traction on the herniated viscera and to assist resection of any nonviable bowel. Because direct inguinal hernias are traumatically induced, the potential for recurrence following repair is less than that associated with indirect hernias. Other than treatment for metabolic aberrations, repair and aftercare for a direct inguinal hernia are essentially identical to that required for repair of an indirect inguinal hernia. Castration may be necessary if sufficient necrosis or trauma has occurred to testicular or spermatic cord tissues.

REPAIR OF CONGENITAL INGUINAL HERNIAS

Congenital inguinal hernias are present at birth either unilaterally or bilaterally, with no right- or left-sided predisposition for unilateral hernias. Because congenital inguinal hernias are considered heritable, all calves affected by this condition should be castrated bilaterally. Depending on the size of the calf, the surgeon may prefer manual restraint in dorsal recumbency with local anesthesia, heavy sedation, or general anesthesia.

Begin the hernial repair with a skin incision over the scrotum, and bluntly dissect the testicle and spermatic cord free from surrounding tissues. Because there is no inflammatory response associated with congenital inguinal hernias, the herniated viscera is easily reduced by twisting the testicle within the vaginal tunic, forcing the viscera back into the abdominal cavity (Fig. 76-4).

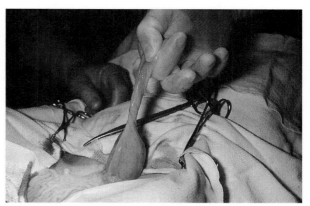

Fig 76-4 Twist the testicle to force intestines out of the vaginal tunic and back into the abdominal cavity.

Ligate the spermatic cord before excision of the testicle, and then close the inguinal ring in one layer with either a continuous vest-over-pants or simple continuous pattern with No 1 or No 2 absorbable suture. After repairing a unilateral congenital inguinal hernia, castrate the remaining testicle and leave the scrotal incision open to drain and heal by second intention.

Recommended Readings

Noordsey JL: *Food animal surgery*, ed 3, Trenton, NJ, 1994, VLS Books.

Riddell MG: Developmental anomalies of the scrotum and testes. In Wolfe DF, Moll HD, editors: *Large animal urogenital surgery*, ed 2, Baltimore, 1998, Williams & Wilkins.

Roberts SJ: *Veterinary obstetrics and genital diseases (theriogenology)*, ed 3, Woodstock, Vt, 1986, Roberts.

Walker DF: Genital surgery in the bull. In Morrow DA, editor: *Current therapy in theriogenology*, Philadelphia, 1980, Saunders.

CHAPTER 77

Diagnosis and Management of Conditions of the Scrotum and Testes

DWIGHT WOLFE and ROBYN WILBORN

ABNORMALITIES OF THE SCROTUM

The veterinarian should be thoroughly familiar with normal anatomic structures of the scrotum and testes to accurately determine diagnosis and prognosis for fertility. Diagnosis of scrotal or testicular pathology requires visual examination, as well as palpation of the scrotum and its contents. Visual examination and palpation should include evaluation for size, shape, symmetry, swelling, or skin conditions such as scars or dermatitis.

Because of its location and pendulous nature, the scrotum is susceptible to environmental injury such as frostbite during the winter, as well as photosensitization and sunburn in bulls lacking scrotal skin pigment. Fungal or bacterial dermatitis may also affect the skin of the scrotum in bulls and should be included on the list of differential diagnoses.

Abnormalities of the scrotum can potentially be severe enough to alter thermoregulatory mechanisms and lead to testicular degeneration. The scrotal neck is an important location for temperature control because of the presence of the pampiniform plexus. Conditions that alter thermoregulation in this area include excessive fat accumulation and, rarely, mastitis of supernumerary teats. Inflammatory responses such as scrotal edema alter insulation by increasing the thickness of the scrotal wall, thereby altering testicular cooling. Scars following injury, dermatitis, or frostbite may cause elevation of the testicles within the scrotum, thereby altering thermoregulation (Fig. 77-1). Scrotal examination and considerations for the ram and buck are similar to the bull. Species-specific conditions are discussed in more detail in the following section.

DIFFERENTIATION AND MANAGEMENT OF SCROTAL SWELLINGS

Scrotal enlargement may be unilateral or bilateral and can be caused by a variety of conditions. Using both visual and palpable information to determine the source of the swelling and make a definitive diagnosis is important. Scrotal enlargement may be caused by swelling of the scrotal wall, testis, or epididymis or most commonly by the presence of fluid within the vaginal cavity.

Swelling of the wall of the scrotum, usually because of edema, typically occurs as an inflammatory response. This enlargement can usually be differentiated from other

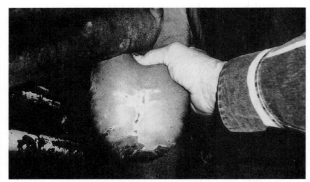

Fig 77-1 Frostbite affecting distal portion of scrotum. Scarring following injuries such as this can cause elevation of the testicles, thereby altering thermoregulation.

causes by palpation of the thickened scrotal skin and the presence of pitting edema and may be confirmed by ultrasound (Fig. 77-2).

Testicular swelling is uncommon due to the tough, fibrous nature of the tunica albuginea. However, orchitis may affect one or both testes. On examination, a size disparity of more than 25% is considered abnormal. In the bull, orchitis is usually caused by hematogenous spread of bacteria during a systemic infection. In rare cases, however, orchitis may be due to puncture wounds to the scrotum. Severity may range from mild and subclinical to suppurative and severe. Although rare, testicular rupture may occur and is diagnosed by its amorphous, clot-like consistency on palpation and ultrasound (Fig 77-3). Orchitis in the ram is a fairly common occurrence and is usually caused by trauma or an extension of infectious epididymitis.

Epididymitis is more common than orchitis and may be diagnosed by thorough examination of the testes and scrotal contents. In the bull, this condition is commonly unilateral and may present as a swollen, painful epididymal tail in the acute phase of the disease. Chronic epididymitis usually results in epididymal tails that are small and firm, and infertility is often caused by their eventual obstruction. *Actinomyces pyogenes* and *Brucella abortus* have been implicated in this condition in the bovine. Epididymitis is more common in the ram than any other domestic species and is considered to be due to *Brucella*

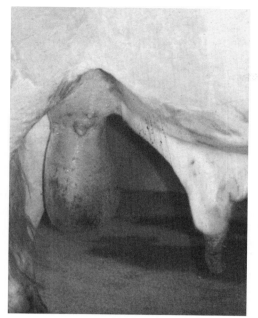

Fig 77-2   Generalized scrotal edema.

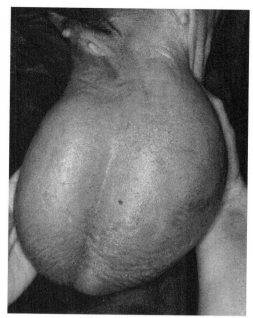

Fig 77-4   Unilateral scrotal edema.

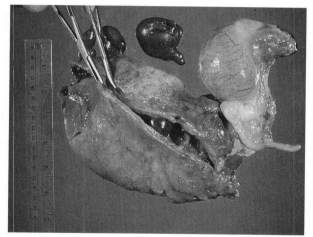

Fig 77-3   Ruptured testicle shown next to normal testicle. This may be diagnosed on physical examination by its clotlike, characteristic palpation.

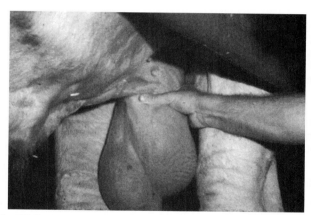

Fig 77-5   Unrestricted movement of testicle within scrotum.

ovis until otherwise confirmed. *B. ovis* is not discussed in detail in this text but should be the primary differential for epididymitis in older rams. The effects of acute and chronic epididymitis in rams are similar to the bovine, also resulting in obstruction and infertility. In cases of bovine or ovine epididymitis, treatment procedures are generally ineffective and affected animals are usually culled.

Accumulation of fluid within the vaginal cavity is the most common cause of scrotal enlargement in the bull and may be due to periorchitis, hydrocele, or hematocele. The presence of fluid is usually unilateral and is discernible by palpation of the testis (Fig. 77-4). Character of the fluid may be thin and easily displaced by palpation, or it may be thickened such as purulent material or clotted blood. Ultrasonographic examination should be helpful

in confirming the nature of the fluid present. With fluid accumulation, fibrous adhesions may form between the testis or epididymis and parietal vaginal tunic, which may be detected as the testis is moved within the vaginal cavity (Fig. 77-5). Periorchitis is most commonly due to infection, whereas hematocele and hydrocele are usually a result of trauma.

Valuable animals with orchitis or periorchitis may be able to resume breeding soundness with unilateral castration. Although these conditions are not emergencies, prognosis improves if surgery is performed early in the disease process. The longer the normal testis is subjected to the heat generated by inflammation, the more likely that testicle will undergo irreversible testicular degeneration. Depending on the degree of degeneration already present, most males will return to fertility following surgery. Compensatory hypertrophy can be expected in the normal testis, allowing the animal to produce up to 75% of normal sperm capacity. Owners should be advised that restrictions may be necessary following surgery. Although he may be productive in a herd situation, a unilaterally castrated male cannot pass a standardized breeding soundness evaluation and is therefore ineligible for certain shows or sales.

Rarely, male ruminants present for evaluation of the presence of a single scrotal testis. The following conditions should be considered in these animals: true cryptorchidism, ectopic testis, complete aplasia of the testis and epididymis, or previous unilateral castration. In ruminants ectopic testes are more likely to be encountered than retained testes because true cryptorchidism is rare. In cases of testicular ectopia, the testis becomes misguided after passing through the inguinal canal and is often found positioned alongside the penis several centimeters cranial to the scrotum. Remove the misdirected testis by making a skin incision over the testis followed by blunt dissection. Use an emasculator or ligatures for hemostasis, and leave the surgical wound to heal by second intention.

ROUTINE CASTRATION—BOVINE

In the United States, cattle are most often castrated without anesthesia, but use of anesthesia is at the surgeon's and owner's discretion. The procedure should be performed at an early age, and every effort should be made to minimize discomfort and stress by completing the procedure quickly and efficiently. Depending on the owner's wishes and the surgeon's preference, local anesthesia, heavy sedation, or general anesthesia may be used.

Most calves can be adequately restrained for castration using a squeeze chute and a firm tail hold. Calves younger than 4 weeks of age are usually restrained in lateral recumbency. These forms of restraint will apply to both the surgical and nonsurgical techniques discussed here.

Surgical Techniques

The most common type of castration involves surgical removal of the testes and can be accomplished using either of two different approaches: vertical scrotal incision using a Newberry knife or incision and removal of the distal scrotum altogether. Using the Newberry knife, grasp the distal scrotum firmly and pull it away from the body. Position the Newberry knife just distal to both testes through both lateral walls and the median septum. Pull quickly through the distal aspect of the scrotum, thereby exposing both testes, which are easily grasped by the surgeon. Apply traction to the testis with one hand while using the other hand to bluntly separate the spermatic cord from fascia to allow for better exposure. As soon as possible, grasp the cord just proximal to the pampiniform plexus and continue traction and stripping of the cord until the cremaster muscle and vasculature have been ruptured and the testis is released. Repeat this procedure with the opposite testicle. The incision with the Newberry knife creates a cranial and caudal flap of skin, allowing for adequate postsurgical drainage.

The second surgical approach involves complete removal of the distal one third or one half of the scrotum. Grasp the distal scrotum and pull away from the body

as with the first approach. Using a scalpel blade, make a quick horizontal incision to excise the distal one third of the scrotum just below the testes, thereby exposing both testes. Use traction to remove the testes as described earlier. This approach produces a relatively small postsurgical scrotal opening and is not recommended for calves weighing more than 300 lb because of the potential for inadequate postsurgical drainage.

Surgical methods using an open technique are recommended for older, larger bulls. These methods include incision of the vaginal tunic, allowing for direct traction on the testis, and subsequent removal of the tunics to eliminate hydrocele formation following surgery. Emasculators or ligatures may prevent excessive hemorrhage. Adequate restraint for these animals is usually more challenging and may require the use of a tilt-table with head and leg restraints.

Nonsurgical Techniques

Rather than removal of the testes, these techniques create ischemia with subsequent atrophy of the testes. Band emasculation continues to be the most common method of nonsurgical castration. Following restraint as described earlier, grasp both testes and force them distally in the scrotum. Place an elastrator band, presoaked in antiseptic, around the neck of the scrotum using elastrator pliers. Exercise caution to ensure that both testes are entrapped in the banded scrotum with no bowel loops included. For larger calves, commercial tools that use latex tubing secured with a clip in the same fashion as the bands are available. Using either product, the scrotum and testes usually slough within 3 weeks. Tetanus prophylaxis is mandatory and should be administered at the time of banding.

A second type of bloodless castration uses the Burdizzo emasculatome. Isolate the spermatic cord laterally in the neck of the scrotum and crush it with the emasculatome. Repeat this procedure on the opposite side, being careful to stagger the crushing sites to preserve blood supply to the scrotum. The testes will atrophy but not slough with this technique compared with the bands. As with banding, care should be taken to avoid entrapment of extraneous tissues and tetanus prophylaxis should be administered.

ROUTINE CASTRATION OF OVINE AND CAPRINE

Small ruminants may be castrated using any of the techniques discussed earlier for cattle, but surgical removal is considered by most to be superior. Regardless of the method, castration in these species is best accomplished before the animal reaches 4 weeks of age and is preferably done in the first week of life. In young animals, castration is accomplished with only physical restraint and is most often performed using elastrator bands or surgical castration via removal of the distal scrotum as described earlier. Tetanus prophylaxis is essential in these species, particularly when using elastrator bands. If young animals have not received vaccinations by the time of castration, tetanus antitoxin should be given on the day of surgery (150-250 units). If surgical removal is elected in young animals, pressure should be applied to the inguinal ring while using traction to remove the testis. This helps to prevent herniation via stretching of the inguinal ring during castration.

For older, larger rams or bucks, administer anesthesia before castration to reduce animal stress and risk of hypotensive shock. Administration of a sedative and local anesthetic is usually adequate and greatly minimizes stress and discomfort to the ram or buck. Mature animals should then be castrated using the surgical methods discussed earlier for the older bovine, and the surgeon should also use an emasculator or ligatures to reduce hemorrhage. Administer tetanus toxoid booster to adult rams and bucks of known vaccination history at the time of castration. If history is unknown, administer 500 to 750 units of tetanus antitoxin at the time of surgery.

Older rams and bucks may be castrated using the Burdizzo emasculatome. The procedure is identical to that discussed previously for the bovine. Many surgeons and owners now consider this technique to be inhumane, and therefore this method has decreased in popularity.

UNILATERAL CASTRATION

Implications for unilateral castration have been discussed previously and include unilateral orchitis, periorchitis, traumatic injury, and, occasionally, neoplasia. For this procedure, fast the animal for at least 24 hours and restrain him in right lateral recumbency. Induce either general anesthesia or a combination of heavy sedation and local anesthesia of the scrotum. Clip and prepare the entire scrotum for aseptic surgery.

Make a vertical skin incision approximately the length of the testicle on the lateral aspect of the scrotum, preserving the parietal vaginal tunic. Manipulate the affected testis by blunt dissection to separate the parietal vaginal tunic from the surrounding scrotal fascia. Make a shorter vertical incision through the parietal tunic of sufficient length to remove the testis, and exteriorize the testicle and spermatic cord.

Identify the spermatic vessels and ductus deferens proximal to the pampiniform plexus, doubly ligate using No 0 chromic gut, and then transect these structures between the ligatures. Ligate and transect the cremaster muscle distal to the remaining cord. Transect the parietal vaginal tunic distal to the stump of the spermatic cord, and close using No 0 chromic gut in an inverting pattern such as the Connell.

Excise excessive scrotal skin to decrease dead space before closure. Appose the tunica dartos with a simple continuous pattern using No 0 chromic gut, and close the scrotal skin using a simple continuous or interlocking pattern with the surgeon's suture of choice.

Administer an antibiotic just before surgery and continue for at least 5 days postoperatively. Examine the incision daily for excessive swelling or discharge and, if necessary, remove skin sutures 10 to 14 days following surgery. The patient should be encouraged to exercise to minimize postoperative scrotal swelling.

Unilateral castration is also a viable option for small ruminants. Implications and surgical procedures are the same as those discussed here for the bovine.

Recommended Readings

Baird AN, Wolfe DF: Castration of the normal male. In Wolfe DF, Moll HD, editors: *Large animal urogenital surgery*, ed 2, Baltimore, 1998, Williams & Wilkins.

Pugh DG: *Sheep and goat medicine*, Philadelphia, 2002, Saunders.

Radhakrishnan J: Testicular developmental anomalies. In Knobil E, Neil JD, editors: *Encyclopedia of reproduction*, vol 4, New York, 1998, Academic Press.

Riddell MG: Developmental anomalies of the scrotum and testes. In Wolfe DF, Moll HD, editors: *Large animal urogenital surgery*, ed 2, Baltimore, 1998, Williams & Wilkins.

Wolfe DF: Unilateral castration for acquired conditions of the scrotum. In Wolfe DF, Moll HD, editors: *Large animal urogenital surgery*, ed 2, Baltimore, 1998, Williams & Wilkins.

Youngquist RS: *Current therapy in large animal theriogenology*, Philadelphia, 1997, Saunders.

CHAPTER 78

Preparation of Teaser Bulls, Rams, and Bucks

DWIGHT WOLFE, ROBERT H. WHITLOCK, and BRIAN K. WHITLOCK

Detection of estrus is often a problem in breeding programs using artificial insemination. Observation of animals for estrus detection is time consuming, and frequently many animals displaying signs of behavioral estrus go undetected. Estrus-detector animals can improve estrus detection if they are used properly and supplement visual observations. Therefore surgically or hormonally altered males are often used to assist with estrus detection. Such animals have the potential to increase the sexual activity in the herd. The more animals sexually active at one time, the more mounting will occur for each animal in estrus. Additionally, precocious stimulation of puberty by male contact is well recognized in swine and may occur in heifers. Male presence also stimulates postpartum estrous activity in gilts, cows, and ewes. Therefore the addition of males that are incapable of breeding to the herd may shorten time to rebreeding.

The optimum technique for teaser preparation should be a simple procedure that alters the male in a humane manner. The altered male should heal and be ready for service in a minimum amount of time following surgery. Regardless of the technique used, certain objectives should be satisfied for the altered male to be a safe and effective aid to the estrus detection program. First, the male should be healthy, display obvious male characteristics, and have good libido. Because teasers are usually used to improve estrus detection efficiency for artificial insemination and will therefore have frequent human contact, teasers with aggressive temperaments should not be used. If the proposed teaser is a new herd addition, he should be free of contagious diseases, vaccinated according to the program in use for the breeding herd, and quarantined for a minimum of 30 days before introduction to the herd. Well-developed postpubertal males are usually preferred to older, larger mature breeding animals that may injure females during mounting activity. Additionally, many breeders prefer the teaser to be a breed of different color than the female herd.

Next, the selected surgical method of teaser preparation should render the bull incapable of intromission without causing discomfort. This objective is essential for successful artificial insemination programs in cattle. Intromission causes microbial contamination of the vagina, thereby risking transmission of venereal or nonspecific pathogens. In cattle that are inseminated by intrauterine techniques, the insemination pipette may carry microorganisms into the cervix or uterus, with negative effects on fertility. In species such as sheep and goats in which semen is deposited in the cranial vagina, this prevention of intromission is less critical. Prevention of intromission should be accomplished in a manner that does not make copulation attempts uncomfortable for the male, consequently reducing libido or discouraging estrus-seeking activity.

PREVENTING INTROMISSION

Numerous surgical techniques are available to prevent intromission by estrus-detector males. Intromission is prevented in one of three ways: by translocation of the penis, by adhesion of the penis in the retracted position, or by preventing erection. Procedures to prevent intromission include but are not limited to penile translocation, preputial obstruction, artificial corpus cavernosal thrombosis, penectomy, and penile fixation. Each procedure has its advantages and disadvantages in terms of cost, reliability, potential postsurgical complications, and technical ease.

Penile Translocation

Penile translocation consists of relocation of the penis and preputial orifice to just above the fold of the left flank, rendering the bull incapable of gaining intromission while maintaining libido and the ability to achieve erection and extension. This procedure is best performed well in advance of the breeding season on yearling bulls. Unfortunately, this technique requires the bull to be restrained in right lateral recumbency under heavy sedation or general anesthesia. Clip and prepare the skin of the caudal ventral abdomen from the preputial orifice to the scrotum and from the lower left flank to the right side of midline for aseptic surgery. Some surgeons prefer to leave the long preputial hairs to aid urine egress from the postoperative surgery site.

First, excise a 7-cm circle of skin and underlying cutaneous trunci muscle above the fold of the left flank so that the lower opening is a few centimeters above the flank fold (Fig. 78-1). After hemostasis is attained, cover the excision with a moist, sterile, surgical sponge and proceed with the next phase of dissection.

Place an identifying suture in the skin at the ventral aspect of the preputial orifice to serve as a reference to prevent twisting of the prepuce during translocation and orientation into the new opening in the flank. Make a circumferential skin incision 3 to 5 cm caudal to the preputial orifice. Begin a longitudinal skin incision along the

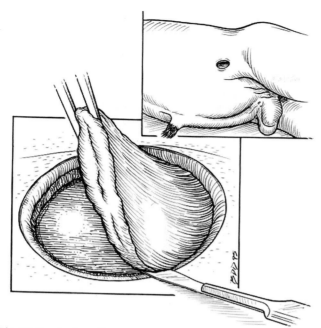

Fig 78-1 Excise a 7-cm circle of skin and underlying cutaneous trunci muscle above the left flank fold.

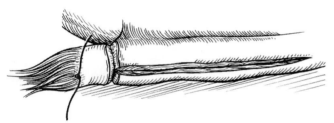

Fig 78-2 Circumferential incision through the skin of the sheath 5 cm caudal to the preputial orifice. Note the longitudinal skin incision on the ventral midline of the sheath from the circumferential incision and the single reference suture placed on the ventrum of the preputial orifice.

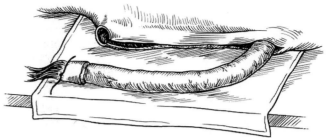

Fig 78-3 Schematic of the penis and prepuce dissected from the sheath and abdominal wall.

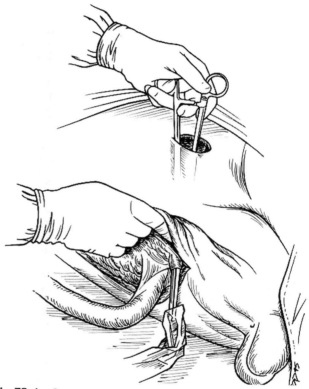

Fig 78-4 Grasp a moistened, sterile, obstetrical sleeve with Knowle's forceps, and pull through the undermined area to exit the flank incision.

ventral midline of the sheath at the circumscribing incision, and extend caudally 25 to 40 cm (Fig. 78-2). Deepen the incisions by blunt dissection to free the penis, prepuce, and surrounding elastic tissue from the abdominal wall, taking care to avoid large vessels and preserve the blood supply to the prepuce and penis (Fig. 78-3).

Pass a long pair of blunt forceps such as Knowle's cervical forceps through the circular flank incision deep to the cutaneous trunci muscle, and bluntly dissect a tunnel to the ventral midline incision. The tunnel should be sufficiently wide to allow relocation of the penis and prepuce without constraint. To avoid contaminating the tunnel with debris, with the Knowle's forceps pull a sterile, disposable, obstetrical sleeve with the hand portion removed through the undermined area (Fig. 78-4). Reintroduce the Knowle's forceps through the circular incision and into the plastic sleeve, grasp the skin of the preputial orifice with the forceps, and with gentle traction pull the preputial orifice through the circular incision while avoiding

torsion (Fig. 78-5). Remove the sleeve through the flank incision.

Align the reference suture in the preputial orifice with the ventral aspect of the circular flank incision. Appose the cutaneous trunci muscle to the subcutaneous tissue of the preputial orifice with No 1 absorbable suture using a simple interrupted pattern at each quadrant and then around the remaining periphery of the opening (Fig. 78-6, *A* and *B*). Appose the skin of the preputial orifice to the skin of the flank with interrupted, nonabsorbable, monofilament suture. Close the ventral midline incision with nonabsorbable suture in a simple continuous or continuous interlocking pattern, making no attempt to reduce dead space. Do not close the circular preputial incision at the end of the sheath to allow for wound drainage (Fig. 78-7).

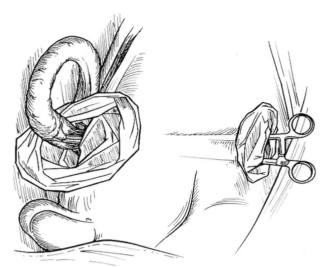

Fig 78-5 Introduce the Knowle's forceps through the sterile obstetrical sleeve with the fingers removed, and grasp the preputial orifice.

Five days of prophylactic antibiotics are indicated in addition to petroleum jelly around the preputial orifice for 3 to 4 days to reduce potential urine scald. Remove skin sutures in 14 days, and the bull should be ready for service 1 month postoperatively.

Preputial Pouch Technique

The preputial pouch technique prevents intromission by closure of the preputial orifice, which forms a blind pouch that prevents extension of the penis while allowing for urine drainage through the formation of a fistula or stoma on the ventrum of the sheath. Perform this procedure with the bull in lateral recumbency under local anesthesia with or without sedation. This technique results in excellent estrus detector bulls that maintain libido for several years and experience no pain during attempted coitus. Unfortunately, debris such as urinary calculi can accumulate in the pouch, which requires periodic lavage with a mild antiseptic. Because of the potential for urine pooling, this technique is not considered appropriate for bulls that possess a pendulous sheath. The finished size of the preputial fistula is critical. If it is too large, the penis may extend through the opening and permit intromission. If it is too small, urine drainage may be compromised.

With the bull restrained in lateral recumbency, clip and prepare the preputial orifice and the cranial aspect of the sheath for aseptic surgery. Infiltrate a local anesthetic agent into the preputial orifice and at the fistula site. To avoid postoperative urine irritation of the suture lines, extend the penis and insert the glans into the lumen of a Penrose drain. Next, suture the drain in place with three to five interrupted absorbable sutures, taking care to avoid the urethra and ventral groove. After the penis is returned to the sheath, insert sponge forceps 7 to 10 cm into the preputial cavity. Direct the tip of the forceps away from the body wall, forming a stent over which to make a 2 × 3 cm, longitudinally oriented, elliptical incision through the skin, subcutaneous tissues, and preputial epithelium.

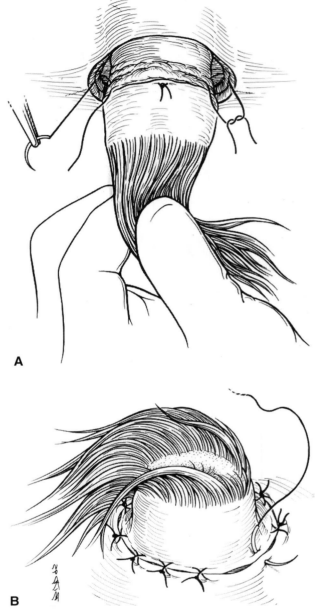

A

B

Fig 78-6 **A,** Place interrupted sutures at each quadrant to appose the subcutaneous tissue of the preputial orifice with the cutaneous trunci muscle. **B,** Interrupted sutures apposing the skin of the preputial orifice with the skin of the flank incision.

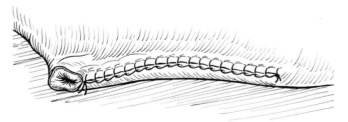

Fig 78-7 Continuous, interlocking closure of ventral midline incision in the sheath.

Appose the internal epithelium of the prepuce to the skin of the sheath with a monofilament, nonabsorbable suture material in a simple interrupted pattern, and then exteriorize the Penrose drain through the fistula.

The final step of this procedure is closure of the preputial orifice. Place Backus towel clamps at the cranial and caudal limits of the preputial orifice and have an assistant stretch the orifice taut. Excise a half-centimeter ring of tissue at the junction of the haired sheath and the non-haired prepuce, which results in separating the preputial skin into an inner and outer edge with an interposed connective tissue layer. Close the preputial epithelium and the subcutaneous tissue individually with simple, continuous patterns of absorbable material. Appose the skin edges with interrupted or continuous nonabsorbable sutures.

After the effects of sedation have ended and the penis is fully retracted, shorten the Penrose drain to allow 10 to 15 cm exposed through the fistula. Systemic antibiotics are recommended for 3 to 5 days. Two weeks following surgery, remove the Penrose drain and skin sutures. Observe 30 to 45 days of sexual rest before using the bull for estrus detection.

Artificial Corpus Cavernosal Thrombosis

The purpose of this technique, performed by injecting soft acrylic in the corpus cavernosum penis (CCP) at the proximal sigmoid flexure, is to create an artificial thrombus that causes erection failure and prevents intromission. This relatively quick procedure is most easily performed in the standing patient, and animals so altered by this technique tend to maintain libido and remain useful for several breeding seasons. Inadvertent injection of acrylic into the corpus spongiosum penis (CSP) or urethra should be carefully avoided.

With the animal restrained standing in a chute, achieve caudal epidural anesthesia. Clip and prepare the perineal area, from just below the anus to the base of the scrotum, for aseptic surgery. Make a vertical 15-cm midline skin incision that ends 10 cm dorsal to the base of the scrotum. Sharply dissect the underlying thick subcutaneous fascia, followed by blunt dissection of the elastic layers surrounding the penis. Dissect between the retractor penis muscles and identify the sigmoid flexure by palpation. Free the entire sigmoid flexure from the associated elastic tissues by blunt dissection, and exteriorize it through the incision. Identify the urethral groove on the ventral aspect of the penis and the attachment of the retractor penis muscles at the distal sigmoid flexure. The site of injection is approximately 15 cm proximal to this point at the proximal sigmoid flexure. This site is chosen to prevent straightening of the sigmoid caused by the erection failure resulting from the artificial thrombus.

Insert a 14-gauge, 1.5-inch needle through the tunica albuginea at a slight dorsal angle into the lateral aspect of the CCP. This insertion route minimizes the potential for an injection into the CSP or urethra. Make a trial injection using 5 to 20 ml of saline to ensure free flow of material into the CCP. If the needle is positioned correctly, the test injection requires little pressure and palpation of the penis during injection detects filling of the CCP. Once the test injection indicates an appropriate needle position, remove the syringe while leaving the needle in place. Mix a thin solution of soft acrylic and place 6 to 10 ml in a 20-ml disposable syringe. Inject the acrylic into the CCP through the previously placed needle. The acrylic should inject easily and filling of the CCP can be detected by palpation.

When the bull mounts a cow in heat, the nonerect penis can still be extended because of reflex relaxation of the retractor penis muscles. To prevent this, place nonabsorbable fixation sutures into both lateral aspects of the CCP through the tunica albuginea at the distal sigmoid flexure to the tough subcutaneous fascia in that area. When tightening the sutures, do not pull the sigmoid flexure into a position that might compromise the bull's ability to urinate. Close the skin with an interrupted or continuous suture pattern of nonabsorbable material. Observe the bull immediately after the procedure to ensure that he can urinate and during the first use as an estrus detector to guarantee erection failure. Remove sutures in 2 weeks, but use bulls to detect estrus as early as 3 to 5 days after surgery.

Penectomy

Penile amputation is another surgical technique for teaser bull preparation. The advantages of this procedure are that it can be performed on standing animals and there is no chance of intromission following penile amputation. A disadvantage is that many teaser bulls prepared by this technique lose their libido within one breeding season.

Surgery is most easily performed with the bull restrained in a squeeze chute. Administer epidural anesthesia and prepare an area on the posterior midline from the perineum to the scrotum for aseptic surgery. Make a 10-cm vertical midline skin incision midway between the anus and base of the scrotum. Deepen the incision through the dense subcutaneous fascia, and identify the paired retractor penis muscles (Fig. 78-8). Continue the dissection deep between the retractor muscles and free the penis from its surrounding tissues.

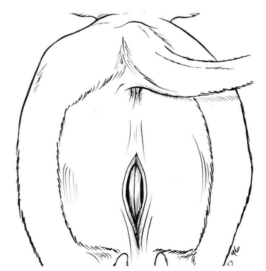

Fig 78-8   Make a 10-cm vertical incision on the middle beginning 5 cm below the anus.

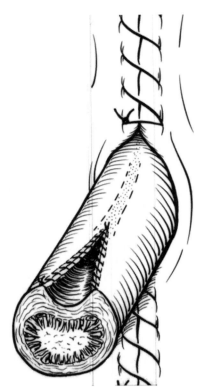

Fig 78-9   The urethral mucosa is sutured with a closely spaced, simple, continuous suture to help reduce hemorrhage from corpus spongiosum penis. Close the skin incision above and below the penile stump with a continuous suture pattern.

Grasp the penis firmly, and apply traction caudally and dorsally to bluntly dissect the penis from the surrounding tissue and exteriorize it through the incision. After the penis is exteriorized, ligate and transect the retractor penis muscles as far proximally as possible. Ligate the dorsal vessels of the penis proximal to the point of amputation. Transect the penis 5 cm distal to the dorsal apex of the skin incision and generously spatulate the urethra with scissors to the incision apex. Hemorrhage from the cavernous tissue may occur in bulls when erection is stimulated. Wedge excision of the end of the stump with suture closure will minimize hemorrhage in bulls.

Suture the penile stump to the skin using nonabsorbable monofilament suture material. Place the suture through the skin and body of the penis, and exit the skin on the opposite side of the incision. Place the second limb of the suture through the skin and under the penis, and exit in the skin on the original side of the incision and ties. This suture prevents the penile stump from retracting into the incision. Using No 2-0 chromic gut, place closely spaced simple continuous sutures around the incision in the urethral mucosa to reduce hemorrhage from the CSP during urination (Fig. 78-9).

Hemorrhage from the CSP may still be a problem in bulls during urination. Insert a 15-cm length of 1-cm diameter latex tubing into the urethra, and fix it in place with a single suture through the tubing and penile stump. This tubing serves as a stent to compress the CSP and

reduce hemorrhage in the early postoperative period. Observe the bull frequently to ensure that he is able to urinate freely. Administer systemic antibiotics and local wound care for 5 days and remove the tubing from the urethra in 7 to 10 days. The bull should have a minimum of 6 weeks' rest before entering the breeding herd to ensure adequate healing.

Penis Tie-Down

The penis tie-down technique results in a permanent adhesion of the penis to the ventral body, preventing extension of the penis and intromission, and is a relatively quick and simple procedure to perform. Failure of the procedure or urethral penetration may occur if the sutures are not placed properly. To guarantee sterility in the event of procedure failure, perform an epididymectomy or vasectomy. Many teaser bulls prepared by this technique lose their libido within 1.5 years of the surgery.

Place the bull in right lateral recumbency and clip and prepare the ventral abdomen, from the preputial orifice to the base of the scrotum for aseptic surgery. Infiltrate local anesthetic subcutaneously 2 cm lateral and parallel to the penis halfway between the preputial orifice and the base of the scrotum. Make a skin incision in this same plane and continue it through the connective tissue until the penis is located. Identify the urethral groove on the ventral aspect of the penis to avoid this area during suturing the penis to the body wall. Bluntly dissect to the abdominal tunic and the tunic albuginea of the penis 15 cm distal to the distal sigmoid flexure. Débride these two surfaces with dry surgical sponges, and then appose them with four to six simple interrupted sutures of slowly absorbed or nonabsorbable suture material placed through the dorsal one third of the penis and into the linea alba. Close the deep and superficial subcutaneous tissues with simple continuous layers of absorbable suture. Close the skin incision with a continuous interlocking pattern of nonabsorbable suture material. Prophylactic antibiotics are optional following this procedure. Bulls prepared for estrus detection with this technique should be isolated for 30 to 45 days, at which time they can be placed into use.

PREVENTION OF EJACULATION OF SPERM

The last objective of teaser male preparation is to render the estrus detector incapable of ejaculating live spermatozoa. This objective is necessary to ensure that the animal is incapable of fertilization in the unlikely event that surgical alteration to prevent intromission fails or the altered bull learns to achieve intromission. The most reliable methods of accomplishing this objective without causing undue discomfort are epididymectomy or vasectomy. When performed correctly, either technique is satisfactory. Epididymectomy is easier and quicker to perform and is less likely to fail when compared with vasectomy.

Epididymectomy

Bilateral caudal epididymectomy is recommended to sterilize bulls, rams, and bucks used as teasers for estrus detection. With the animal adequately restrained, clip

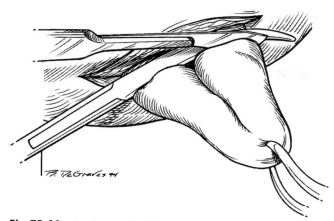

Fig 78-10 Apply crushing hemostatic forceps across the tail of the epididymis and excise.

and prepare the skin of the distal one third of the scrotum for aseptic surgery. Force both testes to the bottom of the scrotum, and infiltrate local anesthetic into the scrotal skin over the epididymal tail and into the epididymis. Grasp the neck of the scrotum to force the testes to the bottom of the scrotum, and make a 2.5-cm skin incision directly over the most prominent bulge of the cauda epididymis. Deepen the incision through the scrotal fascia and tunica vaginalis parietalis, and apply pressure to the neck of the scrotum until the cauda epididymis protrudes through the incision. Grasp the epididymis with towel forceps, and apply sufficient traction to exteriorize the entire cauda epididymis. Apply crushing hemostatic forceps across the vas deferens and the most proximal part of the cauda epididymis. Although unnecessary, it is preferable to ligate above both forceps with a No 0 absorbable suture material. Remove the tail of the epididymis by excising the tissue between the forceps with a scalpel (Fig. 78-10). If the tunica albuginea is inadvertently incised, suture it with absorbable suture material to achieve adequate hemostasis. Remove the hemostats, and examine the excised tissue to verify that the entire cauda epididymis was removed. Leave the wound open to enable healing of the incision by second intention within 3 weeks. Postsurgical antibiotics are not routinely used, although tetanus prophylaxis is recommended when this procedure is performed on rams or bucks. The teaser animal should not be used for heat detection for approximately 3 weeks to ensure complete sterility.

Vasectomy

Vasectomy is performed at the neck of the scrotum. With the animal restrained in lateral recumbency, clip and prep the neck of the scrotum for aseptic surgery and infiltrate local anesthetic into the skin and spermatic cord on the posterior aspect of the scrotum just above each testicle. Make a 2- to 4-cm incision through the skin and tunica dartos of the scrotal wall to expose the spermatic cord within the tunica vaginalis. Once the spermatic cord has been isolated and freed from the surrounding tissue, place

a hemostat under the cord and elevate the cord through the skin incision. Avoiding the cremaster muscle, make a 2.5-cm incision through the tunica vaginalis to expose the contents of the spermatic cord. Take care to avoid incising the underlying pampiniform plexus.

The ductus deferens is readily identified by palpation as a cordlike, firm structure approximately 2 to 3 mm in diameter alone in a fold of tunica vaginalis. Also, identify the testicular artery, vein, and nerve located in a common fold to ensure that these structures are not damaged during the surgical procedure. Once the ductus deferens is identified, place two encircling ligatures approximately 3 to 5 cm apart using No 0 chromic gut. Excise the ductus and tunica vaginalis between the ligatures, and close the incision in routine fashion. As with epididymectomy, teaser animals should not be used for heat detection for a minimum of 3 weeks after vasectomy to ensure sterility.

Researchers have reported different results on the seminal characteristics, structure and function of the testes, and libido of bucks and rams subjected to vasectomy. Current research reports full sterility in the buck 1 week after vasectomy because no motile spermatozoa have been found beyond this point. However, the vasectomized male should have 2 to 3 weeks of sexual rest before being used as an estrus detector. Vasectomy does not alter plasma testosterone concentration in the buck, although unfortunately libido of vasectomized bucks may decline as a consequence of orchitis or sperm granuloma at the tail of the epididymis.

Recommended Readings

Arkins S, Thompson LH, Giles JR et al: Bilateral removal of the cauda epididymides in the neonatal pig as a technique for creating teaser boars, *J Anim Sci* 67:15, 1989.

Batista M, Prats N, Calero P et al: Semen characteristics and plasma levels of testosterone after bilateral vasectomy in bucks, *Reprod Dom Anim* 37:375, 2002.

Brooks PH, Cole DJA: The effect of the presence of a boar on the attainment of puberty in gilts, *J Reprod Fertil* 23:435, 1970.

Gill MS: Surgical techniques for preparation of teaser bulls, *Vet Clin North Am Food Anim Pract* 11:123, 1995.

Morgan G: Surgical correction of abnormalities of the reproductive organs of bulls and preparation of teaser animals. In Youngquist RS, editor: *Current therapy in large animal theriogenology*, Philadelphia, 1997, Saunders.

Riddell MG: Prevention of intromission by estrus-detector males. In Wolfe DF, Moll HD, editors: *Large animal urogenital surgery*, ed 2, Baltimore, 1998, William & Wilkins.

Walker DF: Surgery of the penis. In Walker DF, Vaughan JT, editors: *Bovine and equine urogenital surgery*, Philadelphia, 1980, Lea & Febiger.

Wolfe DF: Surgical preparation of estrus-detector males. In Wolfe DF, Moll HD, editors: *Large animal urogenital surgery*, ed 2, Baltimore, 1998, William & Wilkins.

Wolfe DF: Surgical procedures of the reproductive system of the bull. In Morrow DA, editor: *Current therapy in theriogenology*, Philadelphia, 1986, Saunders.

Wolfe DF, Baird A: Philosophy of teaser male preparation, section II, B, 3. In Dzuik P, Wheeler M, editors: *Handbook of methods for study of reproductive physiology in domestic animals*, Champaign-Urbana, 1991, University of Illinois.

SECTION IX

Genital Surgery—Female

David E. Anderson

CHAPTER 79

Bovine Cesarean Sections: Risk Factors and Outcomes

KENNETH D. NEWMAN

The cesarean section (C-section) is probably one of the oldest surgical procedures both in human and veterinary medicine. In veterinary medicine, geography tends to influence the frequency, ease, and success of this procedure. Dairy practices tend to perform fewer C-sections year round and usually do them on the farm. In comparison, C-sections in beef practice are numerous and heavily concentrated during the late winter and early spring. Furthermore, adverse weather conditions associated with beef calving practices require appropriate in-clinic or farm facilities for performing C-sections. Nevertheless, the basic goals of performing a C-section remain independent of geography: preservation of both the cow and her calf, as well as the future reproductive efficiency of the cow.

This chapter briefly reviews the salient points of C-sections. Risk factors and complications that affect outcome from published literature and Ohio State University (OSU) data are covered next. Included as outcomes are reproductive efficiency and milk production. Finally, an example of the worst possible case scenario, dealing with an emphysematous fetus, is provided.

INDICATIONS

Both maternal and fetal indications warrant performing a C-section. Maternal indicators include immature heifers, pelvic deformities, failure of cervical dilation, uncorrectable uterine torsion, uterine tear, hydrops, and prepartum paralysis.[1] Beef breeds that have double muscling (hypertrophied semitendinosus and semimembranosus muscles) such as Charolais, Limousine, and Belgian Blue breeds[2,3] by definition often require C-sections. The risk factors in dairy cattle for C-sections are increased by heifers' age younger than 2 years (odds ratio [OR] 3.09 compared with multiparous cows), long gestation period, preceding long interval from first service to conception, long dry period, double-muscled (OR 10.85) or Piedmont sire (odds ratio 4.26), and previous C-section calving (OR 18.89 compared with those having a previous normal calving).[4]

Fetal indicators include both normal and pathologic fetal conditions. Normal fetal conditions consist of absolute fetal oversize (relative to a normal maternal pelvis size) and malposition. A high-value calf such as an embryo transfer may also be an indication for a C-section. Pathologic fetal conditions include fetal anasarca, schistosomus reflexus, hydrocephalus, cojoined twins, mummification, and prolonged gestation.[1] Under certain conditions an emphysematous fetus can best be removed by

C-section: a tightly contracted uterus, little uterine fluid present, incompletely dilated cervix, or a friable uterus. A fetotomy under these conditions is probably not ideal.[1]

APPROACH

Once the decision has been made to perform a C-section, the next step is to determine the approach. Depending on the practice area, there may be few options available. Restraint (appropriately based on the breed), space, light, help available, location, and the veterinarian's experience and confidence[1] are issues that must be considered, in conjunction with the underlying reason for performing the C-section because this can determine the surgical approach.[1,5]

In general, the two main options are whether to do a C-section on a standing or recumbent animal. In an ideal setting, standing C-sections are selected when there is little concern of uterine contents (i.e., live calf or recently dead calf vs. an emphysematous fetus). Dairy cows often require a mere halter, whereas most beef cows require an appropriate chute to protect the veterinarian, client, and cow. If no chute is available, a recumbent approach using sedation and tying the legs forward and back works. If there is concern that the cow may not remain standing for the C-section, then it may easier to start with her already down rather than having her fall down during surgery. The recumbent approach allows the best exposure and exteriorization of the uterus, thus reducing the opportunity to contaminate the abdominal cavity.[5]

Though the standing flank approach may be done from either the left or right, it is more commonly done from the left.[1,5,6] Based on coded C-sections retrieved from the OSU Medical Record, 102 cesareans were performed between 1998 and 2002; the left approach was used 83% of the time compared with 2% on the right.[7] The overall percentage of left approaches done at OSU is likely lower compared with private practice due to case bias. The left approach almost always avoids the small intestines. Purists may consider a right approach when the pregnancy is in the right horn. In practice, there is usually not enough help to retain the small intestines within the abdominal cavity during surgery. A vertical incision approximately 40 cm in length is made in the paralumbar fossa. Alternatively, the left oblique in standing cows has been described.[8] An incision is started 10 cm cranial and 8 to 10 cm ventral to the cranial aspect of the tuber coxae. The incision is extended cranioventrally at a 45-degree angle, ending 3 cm caudal to the last rib.

The apex of the uterine horn is more readily accessible, therefore facilitating manipulation and exteriorization of the uterus. This incision is larger and extends more cranial-ventrally compared with the traditional vertical incision. Some surgeons find this technique useful to remove large calves or when the uterine contents are contaminated. Furthermore, the transversus and internal muscle layers are incised parallel to the muscle fibers. The abdominal viscera apply tension to these muscles, thus facilitating their apposition during closure.

The recumbent approach can be midline or over the pregnant horn using ether a paramedian or low-flank approach.[5] The midline was used 13% of the time compared with the low right (2%) approach.[7] The main advantage of the recumbent approaches is the ability to exteriorize the uterus and therefore avoid contaminating the abdomen. Compared with the paralumbar approach, the ventral approach can assist the removal of an oversized fetus. A large incision is required to exteriorize the uterus because the linea alba is not too flexible. In comparison, the paramedian and low flank oblique approaches are more pliable and require smaller incisions to exteriorize the uterus but require more layers of closure. Furthermore, the ventral midline approach can be used to exteriorize either horn, whereas the paramedian and low oblique approaches need to be over the pregnant horn.

ANESTHESIA

Periodically sedation is required, especially on nervous heifers when the primary method restraint is a halter. Xylazine HCl is the most widely used drug to provide sedation in bovine practice. An unfortunate side effect of xylazine HCl is that it increases uterine tone, thus making manipulation and exteriorization of the gravid uterus more difficult.[9,10] In addition, a more recent study using endoscopy demonstrated that xylazine altered laryngeal and pharyngeal anatomy and impaired sensation in adult dairy cattle.[11] This impairment increases the risk of aspiration if the cow is positioned in either lateral or dorsal recumbency. Furthermore, xylazine can also induce ataxia—an undesirable effect while doing a standing C-section. In the author's experience, acepromazine maleate (0.03 mg/kg) and butorphanol tartrate (0.02 mg/kg) administered intravenously provided adequate sedation (unless the cow was not already in a high state of excitement), without ataxia or increasing uterine tone.

The approach determines which technique is used for local anesthesia. These techniques for local anesthesia using 2% lidocaine HCl are well documented in the literature.[12-14] The most common techniques are the proximal and distal paravertebral, inverted L, and line blocks. Proximal paravertebral blocks work for all standing surgeries and all breeds, whereas distal paravertebral blocks are more difficult to perform on well-conditioned beef cattle. The technique used tends to reflect the surgeons' preference. These techniques can be used for standing approaches. For the recumbent approaches, sedation using with xylazine HCl (0.03-0.05 mg/kg) intravenously[15] is required in addition to a local block.

The proximal paravertebral block can be technically more challenging, requiring more restraint, a long needle

(minimum 20-gauge, 10-15 cm long), and the smallest dose of local anesthetic.[12-14] The distal block requires less skill and can be performed using an 18-gauge, 1½-inch needle. This block works well provided the local anesthetic injections are fanned above and below the cranial edge of the transverse processes.

A caudal epidural anesthesia, which desensitizes the caudal nerve roots as they emerge from the dura, is often indicated if either the calf or obstetrical manipulation has initiated strong abdominal contractions (Ferguson's reflex). An 18-gauge, 1½-inch needle and 2% lidocaine HCl (0.2-0.4 mg/kg) are required.[12-14] As the name implies, a caudal epidural should not affect motor control of the hind limbs. The onset of a properly placed epidural is usually within minutes.

A xylazine caudal anesthesia epidural has been described in the literature.[16-18] A dose of 0.05- to 0.07-mg/kg body weight diluted to a 5- to 7.5-ml volume with 0.9% NaCl has been used. Volumes of 10 ml and greater have led to excessive systemic effects. The advantage of this technique is the sedation achieved in addition to the paralumbar analgesia for at least 2 hours[17] by a single epidural administration. The disadvantages of this technique are that cows develop a mild ataxia 80% of the time (but remain standing), onset of paralumbar analgesia of 30 minutes on average, and analgesia (requiring additional local analgesia) 17.2% of the time.[18] Therefore this technique may not be the most efficient in field situations. Other systemic effects of the xylazine with this technique have been observed in healthy cows: heart rate, respiratory rate, ruminal contraction rate, arterial blood pressure, PAO_2, PVC, and total solids were significantly ($P<0.05$) decreased, whereas $PACO_2$, base excess, and bicarbonate concentrations were significantly ($P<0.05$) increased.[17] This study cautions that the use of the xylazine epidural should be restricted to healthy cows. Despite it shortcomings, this technique can be used in conjunction with local techniques to enhance sedation and analgesia in uncooperative patients. In practice, part of the 0.9% NaCl volume can be substituted in part with 2% lidocaine HCl for a more complete caudal epidural anesthesia.[14]

When performing local anesthesia with small ruminants, or even small heifers, one should remain aware of the toxic dose of lidocaine HCl (>5 mg/kg).[12] The clinical signs of systemic toxicity predominantly involve the central nervous system (drowsiness, convulsions, respiratory depression) and can include cardiovascular collapse leading to death.[12-14] For practical purposes, the volume of 2% lidocaine HCl required to elicit systemic toxicity works out to 0.2 ml/kg or 9 ml/45 kg.

General anesthesia may be administered for recumbent approaches. A general anesthetic ensures minimal patient movement during the surgical procedure and a speedy recovery. Ruminants typically lie quietly in sternal recumbency until they have sufficiently recovered to stand steadily. In field situations, sedation (typically xylazine) in conjunction with either a high epidural (dose) or local anesthetic can be used for these approaches. The disadvantages of these anesthetic protocols include inopportune patient movements during surgery and the prolonged effects of the high epidural.

SURGICAL TECHNIQUE

Details of the surgical techniques for performing a C-section are well described in the literature.[1,12,19] After identifying the uterus, the portion of the uterus containing a leg (preferably the rear) is pulled up into the abdominal incision. Usually it is the greater curvature of the uterus that can be exteriorized. An incision is made along the greater curvature of the uterus, which tends to avoid the majority of blood vessels and caruncles. Ideally, there should be no spillage of uterine contents into the abdomen. Once both legs are exteriorized (and sometimes the head if dealing with a posterior presentation), clean (or sterile) calving chains can be placed on the calf's legs to assist removing the calf from the uterus. While the calf is being removed, the uterus needs to be held in place to prevent spillage of uterine contents into the abdomen. In addition, the umbilical cord should be stretched and ruptured in a controlled fashion by holding it adjacent to the abdominal wall. Normal retraction and contraction of the umbilical arteries may be impaired by surgical excision of the umbilical cord. A large incision is required to safely remove the fetus from the uterus and through the abdominal wall. A small uterine incision increases the risk of tearing the uterus. A small abdominal incision increases the level of difficulty in removing the fetus and the risk of subcutaneous emphysema formation. After the calf is removed, the uterus should be fully exteriorized. If the placenta readily detaches from the caruncles, it should be removed. Otherwise, trim the portion that is hanging outside the uterus. Ensure there is not a twin calf before closing the uterine incision. If the calf is alive, one layer of closure using No 2 chromic catgut is usually sufficient. Two-layer closure is required if the calf is dead or contaminated uterine fluids are present. Changing to fresh surgical gloves once the uterus is closed potentially reduces abdominal contamination.

Abdominal walls usually require two to three layers of closure. The peritoneum and transversus are usually closed in one layer. When the first layer is almost closed, have an assistant (usually the client) push the opposite abdominal wall to push out the extra air inside the abdominal cavity. The internal and external obliques are closed together in a second layer. Typically No 2 or 3 chromic gut is used in a simple continuous pattern to close the muscle layers. To reduce dead space and potential seroma formation, the layers can be periodically tacked down to the preceding layer. The skin can be closed using either a continuous ford interlocking, simple interrupted cruciate, or simple interrupted sutures using No 3 polymerized caprolactam (Vetafil, Braunamid). If the ford interlocking pattern is used, the current recommendation is to place a couple of simple interrupted sutures at the base of the incision. If necessary, these sutures could be cut to assist drainage.

In cases of uncorrected uterine torsions, experts debate whether the uterus should be detorsed before or after removal of the calf. If the calf is removed first, the incision tends to be in the horn opposite the body wall incision, which is proposed to make suturing the uterine incision more difficult. Interestingly, in cases when there is no uterine torsion and the calf's hind legs are located in the opposite horn from the incision, the only way to exteriorize the uterus is by iatrogenically inducing a uterine torsion. Therefore this supposed debate should not even be an issue.

CALF MANAGEMENT

Once removed from the uterus, the calf should be rigorously dried off and the navel dipped in 7.5% iodine. In cases of prolonged dystocias, additional support may be required. Briefly, warmth, oxygen (either mask or endotracheal tube), naloxone, flunixin meglumine, and lactated Ringer's solution can be administered to support fetal anoxia and metabolic acidosis. As part of good calf management practices, colostrum should be given in a reasonable, timely matter and an injection of selenium administered. In instances when the cow will be transported home immediately after surgery, attention should be given to the environmental temperature and the trailer should be partitioned to keep the cow and calf separated. The proximal local anesthetic block can induce a mild to severe ataxia in the cow for up to several hours after surgery.

POSTOPERATIVE CARE

The use, type, and frequency of antibiotics vary on a case-by-case basis. The most commonly used antibiotics are either penicillin G procaine (22,000 U/kg IM q24h for 3-5 days), oxytetracycline (20 mg/kg IV, IM, or SQ q1-3 days), or ceftiofur (1 to 2 mg/kg IV, IM, or SQ q12-24 hr for 3-5 days). The appropriate milk and meat withdrawals need to be followed. In cases of future breeding animals, flunixin meglumine (1 mg/kg IV, IM q12h for 2 days) is used in an effort to reduce abdominal adhesion formation. Typically, stitches are removed in 3 weeks. A breeding soundness examination is recommended to evaluate uterine health and abdominal adhesions between 4 and 6 weeks after surgery in order to maximize reproductive efficiency.

COMPLICATIONS

Dehghani and Ferguson[20] described preoperative, operative, postoperative, and long-term complications.[20] These authors summarized the potential complications of C-sections in a flow chart format shown in Fig. 79-1.

One study observed that 30% of the cows had poor appetite, fever, metritis, or diarrhea after surgery.[21] At OSU, 56.4% of the cows had complications either during or after surgery.[7] This higher figure likely reflects case bias. Because most C-sections at OSU are done on an outpatient basis, this figure may be much higher.

Case Selection

An easily overlooked point is case selection. C-sections can sometimes be a self-fulfilling prophecy for both clients and veterinarians alike.[22] When a C-section is considered an option of last resort, a negative outcome (losing both the cow and calf) is more likely. A bad experience in turn fuels the desire to further avoid this surgical procedure in

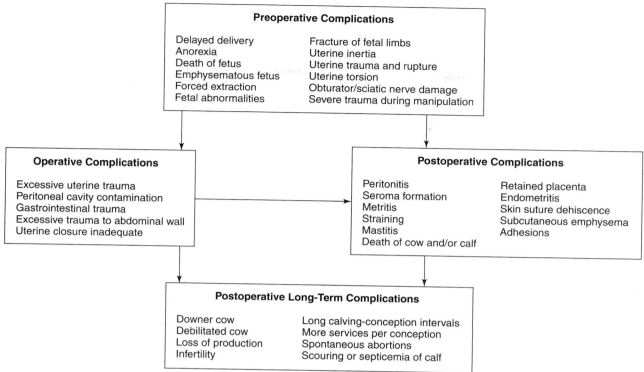

Fig 79-1   Complications.

the future. Alternatively, when a C-section is NOT considered an option of last resort, the procedure is much more rewarding because the outcomes tend to be more positive. Furthermore, clients tend to be more agreeable to C-sections provided their previous experiences have been positive. The ideal case is an animal that has been in labor briefly, and the decision to perform a C-section is made quickly without prolonged obstetrical manipulation by either the client or attending veterinarian. A survey conducted in Ireland revealed that 12.7 minutes was the average (range 0-60 minutes) time spent trying to deliver a calf before deciding on surgery.[6] Rapid clinical assessment was associated with improved success in another practitioner survey.[22] Excessive manipulations by the owner and veterinarian alike were associated with higher postoperative complications.

In general, if the client or veterinarian is unable to hand pull both the legs and head into the birth canal, the decision to perform a C-section should be immediate. The pelvic canal should have sufficient room for both the calf's head and legs and a person's arm to sweep around the calf's shoulders and safely extract the fetus through the birth canal.

Exteriorizing the Uterus

A bovine C-section is considered a clean-contaminated procedure at best. The belief is that exteriorizing the uterus and avoiding abdominal contamination are likely most important when dealing with a dead calf and/or extensive obstetrical manipulations (by either the client or veterinarian). One study[23] of 1000 C-sections found the most important complication was exteriorizing the uterus (20.8% difficult, 5.8% impossible), but the more experienced surgeons appeared to have less difficulty. Unfortunately, this study did not determine whether there was an association among calf viability, exteriorizing the uterus, and cow outcome. Based on the retrospective study of OSU cases,[7] the uterus is not exteriorized 24% of the time. Lack of surgeon experience likely accounts for the bulk of this percentage. The OR of a cow surviving with an exteriorized uterus is estimated to be 7.86 times the odds of a cow surviving with a uterus that was not exteriorized (95% confidence interval [CI]: 2.24-27.44). This result confirms that exteriorizing the uterus does, in fact, positively contribute toward cow survival.

Calf viability, exteriorizing the uterus, and cow survival were the next factors addressed. The survival odds of a cow that had a live calf removed without exteriorizing the uterus were estimated to be 0.17 times the odds of a cow that had a dead calf removed without exteriorizing the uterus (95% CI: 0.12-0.26).[7] This result was unexpected and likely due to the small sample size. Of the original 102 cases, several records are missing information regarding calf viability and whether the uterus was exteriorized. The survival odds of a cow that had a live calf removed by exteriorizing the uterus were estimated to be 1.16 times the odds of a cow that had a dead calf removed by exteriorizing the uterus (95% CI: 0.18-7.51). This suggests that exteriorizing the uterus is important for the removal of a dead calf. The OR seems rather small and, again, is probably affected by the small sample size.

According to three European practitioner surveys, uterine relaxants at the time of surgery are used frequently

(50%-100%).[6,21,22] When the uterus has contracted down tightly on the fetus, it is difficult to either correct malpresentations or exteriorize the uterus during a C-section. Historically, clenbuterol and isoxsuprine have been available to bovine practitioners as aids in obstetrical manipulation.[24,25] Currently, these drugs are not permitted for use in food animals. Over the past few years there has been some discussion on the American Association of Bovine Practitioners-List concerning the use of epinephrine as a tocolytic agent. Because isoxsuprine is a sympathomimetic with structural similarities to epinephrine,[24] it would make pharmacologic sense that epinephrine may have inherent tocolytic properties. The best way to delay parturition in heifers by several hours is to relocate them to a calving pen. The release of endogenous epinephrine is thought to be responsible for this inhibition. An empiric dose of 10 ml of 1:1000 epinephrine, diluted in isotonic fluid, and administered IV 10 minutes preoperatively appears to relax the uterus quite well clinically, making it much easier to grasp hold of a leg to pull up into the incision. Occasionally the relaxed myometrium makes the uterine wall thin, which makes closing the uterine incision more challenging. A small tapered needle is required to avoid full-thickness bites, and the stitches need to be placed much more closely together to ensure proper closure. The use of uterine relaxants may be a confounding variable not accounted for in the European studies.

Uterine Tears

Dawson and Murray[22] reported that tearing the uterus during surgery accounted for 6.8% of complications in their Cheshire, England, practice, which contrasts with a rate of 8.8% at OSU.[7] Only cows with uterine tears and emphysematous feti at the time of surgery were euthanized. No difference was observed in cow survival with uterine tears and whether the calf was alive or dead at the time of surgery. Unfortunately, the impact of uterine tears on adhesion formation and reproductive efficiency is not known.

Mortality

Cows become recumbent during surgery (14.8%)[22] compared with 2.9% at OSU.[7] Cattle are more likely to become recumbent if difficulty was encountered trying to exteriorize the uterus. Pain, thought to be caused by traction on the broad ligament, is believed to be the cause. Cattle that remain standing during the procedure have a better chance of survival, with a reported 91% survival rate for the cows and a 95% survival rate for the calves.[21] Another study reported a 94% cow survival rate and that 100% of the calves alive at the start of surgery survived.[22] These numbers appear comparable with OSU, where 90.1% of the cows and 100% of the calves alive at the time of surgery were released from the hospital after C-section. Fifty-seven percent of the calves were dead before surgery.

A retrospective study that looked at 159 dairy cow C-sections found a strong correlation between cow survival and calf viability at the time of surgery.[26] Cow survival decreased from 86% with a live calf, to 79% with a dead calf, to 33% with an emphysematous fetus. At OSU the odds of a cow that had a live calf at surgery surviving were estimated to be 1.88 times the odds of a cow that had a dead calf at surgery surviving (95% CI: 0.66-5.21).[7]

Surgery time greater than 1 hour reduced the dam survival rate from 96% to 86%.[23]

Unfortunately, surgery time is often not recorded in the literature or at OSU (unless a general anesthetic is administered). However, it is generally accepted that increased surgical time is a key factor in surgical morbidity and mortality. The most common complications associated with maternal death are peritonitis, toxemia, metritis, uterine rupture, and fatty liver.[7,20] Reportedly rare (0.5%), infection by *Clostridium chauvoei* at a site distant to the surgery site can result in sudden death of the cow within 24 hours of surgery.[27]

Peritonitis

One European practitioner survey[6] in 1993 (381 respondents, representing an estimated 60,195 deliveries/year, and 10,457 cesareans) reported that the leading causes of mortality associated with C-sections were peritonitis (70.3%) and shock (18.1%). Interestingly, 5% of the respondents did not routinely disinfect the surgical site.

Spillage of uterine contents during surgery is not always necessary to cause peritonitis. A compromised uterine wall can occur, even before surgery.[20] Peritonitis can be caused by either exogenous (through the abdominal incision) or endogenous bacterial flora.[28] Exogenous bacteria are considered minor. Fetal fluids can become contaminated by obligate, anaerobic vaginal bacterial flora, especially after rupturing the amniotic sac or extensive obstetrical manipulations. Bacteria can be cultured from uterine fluids before amniotic sac rupture; however, their numbers increase significantly after the sac ruptures. During hysterotomy, uterine fluids are heavily contaminated 83% of the time by a polymicrobial population. Therefore it is appropriate to consider the C-section a clean-contaminated procedure, thus warranting the use of antibiotics, preferably before surgery. The use, dose, and frequency of antibiotics at OSU appeared to vary greatly among cases. Traditionally, the appropriate antibiotic selection is directed toward the anticipated bacteria of the postpartum uterus. Fifty percent of cows that had a normal calving on two hygienically contrasting farms were positive on uterine culture: *Arcanobacterium pyogenes* (formerly known as *Actinomyces pyogenes*) was the most common isolate, followed by *Escherichia coli, Fusobacterium nucleatum, Proteus mirabilis,* and *Bacteroides melanogenicicus.*[29] Enterobacteriaceae, *Clostridium,* and *Actinomyces* spp. have been cultured from peritonitis and incisional infections.[23] This study also observed that despite the apparent bacterial contamination, the incidence of peritonitis was relatively low (10.5%).

Clinical signs of peritonitis are expected to occur 3 to 4 days after surgery.[1,9] Though the peritonitis incidence rate at OSU is 7.8%,[7] the majority of cases are outpatients and therefore this rate is likely not accurate. However, based on the information available, the odds of peritonitis developing when the uterus is not exteriorized are estimated to be 2.04 times the odds of peritonitis developing when the uterus is exteriorized (95% CI: 0.61-6.82).

Retained Fetal Membranes

In Dawson and Murray's[22] experience, the authors found that the placenta was removed easily during surgery in 14.2% of C-section cases and that stillborn calves were present in 72.7% of the cases in which the placenta could be easily removed. Interestingly, postoperative complications were higher in these cases compared with those that expelled the placenta in 24 hours. The occurrence of retained fetal membranes was between 35% and 40.8% in a study by Cattell and Dobson and Bouchard.[21,26] Both rates are accepted as being significantly higher compared with unassisted calvings. In contrast, Barkema and colleagues[30] observed that C-sections reduced the occurrence of retained fetal membranes (relative risk = 0.49) but were unable to explain the difference.

In cases when the placenta was not removed during surgery, Frazer[27] administered oxytocin on days 2 and 3 postcalving at 20 USP q3hr and then increased both the dose and frequency of oxytocin to 30 USP q2hr on day 4. The half-life of oxytocin is 3 to 5 minutes in humans and 22 minutes in goats.[31] Small doses administered frequently are recommended rather than high doses administered less frequently. High doses appear to cause tetanic-like spasms, which can last between 6 and 10 minutes.[27] The ideal productive uterine response to oxytocin is tubalocervical.

Adhesions

An imbalance between fibrin formation and fibrinolysis is thought to result in adhesion formation. Adhesions can be either beneficial or detrimental. Furthermore, the presence of abdominal adhesions is not always clinically relevant. Detrimental effects of adhesions can be both partial and complete intestinal obstruction, pain, and infertility. Halsted's principles of surgery have been viewed as the mainstay of adhesion prevention: minimal and atraumatic tissue handling, meticulous hemostasis, preservation of adequate blood supply, strict asepsis, no tension on tissues, careful approximation of tissues, and obliteration of dead space.[32,33] One study that looked at the complications associated with standing C-sections observed a significant difference between surgeons and adhesion formation.[28]

The significance of adhesions is determined by their degree and location. Detrimental adhesions in the bovine abdomen following C-section are primarily associated with elements of the reproductive tract: the ovary, infundibulum, oviduct, and uterus in decreasing order are the most critical elements with respect to future fertility. Uterine adhesions were found in 9.4% of cattle at the time of surgery and in 31% of cattle that had had a previous C-section.[23] Older studies observed uterine adhesions between 20% and 60%.[28] Adhesions were not noted in the surgery reports of the OSU cases.

Continuous inverting patterns that do not take full-thickness bites such as the Lembert, Cushing, Guard, Utrecht, or reverse Utrecht are preferred because these patterns provide an excellent seal and the uterus heals by serosal-to-serosal contact. One should ensure adequate infolding of the serosal surfaces or leakage of uterine contents into the abdomen will occur. According to two European practitioner surveys,[6,21] the Lembert pattern was most commonly used (73%-88.2%) compared with the Cushing (5.8%) or Utrecht (6%) pattern, using either chromic gut (87.2%) or plain catgut (10.6%). A third European study used the Lembert pattern exclusively.[22] No differences between the Lembert and Utrecht suture patterns and adhesion formation were noted.[28] Instead, this study revealed a dramatic difference between surgeons and adhesion formation. This illustrates the basic principle of good surgical technical skill and how this can affect adhesion formation. The Lembert pattern requires more suture material, has more suture material exposed, and takes more time to complete. Unfortunately, none of these studies compared surgery time. At OSU the Cushing pattern was used the most, followed by the Utrecht pattern. The Lembert pattern was used the least.

Once the uterus is closed, blood clots and debris from the serosal surface of the uterus must be removed. The ovarian bursa should be closely examined because blood clots can lodge there, cause adhesions, and adversely affect future fertility. Gauze squares used to help remove blood clots should be avoided because the gauze will remove the thin mesothelial layer on the serosal surface of the uterus, which can result in adhesion formation and therefore adversely affect fertility. Sterile physiological saline (usually 2 L) is sufficient to rinse off the uterus. After rinsing, the uterus is replaced inside the abdomen. Lavage of the abdominal cavity may be required to remove blood clots and debris.

Suture type has been the subject of great debate with regard to adhesion formation. Synthetic material has significant advantages over biologic material. Polyglactin 910 has the advantages of uniform material quality; being less readily damaged by surgical instruments; superior handling qualities (less stiff, knot tying, less fraying); and a mild inflammatory reaction compared with plain catgut. One study demonstrated there was no advantage using polyglactin 910 compared with plain catgut.[34] Currently, it is not known whether polyglactin 910 induces less scar formation within the myometrium, which could positively affect future fertility. The disadvantages of polyglactin 910 are increased drag (because it is braided) and cost. Suture material exposure, rather than type of suture material, especially knots, is thought to be the most significant cause of adhesions, especially along the uterine incision.

Researchers have experimented with other modalities in an effort to reduce adhesion formation. Abdominal lavage during and after surgery using lactated Ringer's solution has been used in horses to reduce adhesion formation.[35] The removal of inflammatory products and cytokines are believed to be the mechanism by which adhesion formation was reduced. Unfortunately in the bovine, the greater omentum sheet makes abdominal lavage after surgery ineffective. However, abdominal lavage during surgery after the uterine incision is closed to remove blood clots is probably beneficial.

Flunixin meglumine administered intravenously for 72 hours after surgery (in addition to potassium penicillin and gentamycin) reduced adhesion formation in a foal intestinal ischemia model.[36] The suggested mechanism of action has been the reduction of flunixin-mediated endotoxemia. Endotoxemia increases tPA inhibitor-1, which reduces fibrinolytic activity. Therefore flunixin meglumine may prevent inhibition of tPA and assist fibrinolysis.

Heparin has long been used as an antiadhesion drug in abdominal surgery. Heparin increases the activity of antithrombin III, which reduces the amount of thrombin that is available to convert fibrinogen to fibrin. Reports concerning the efficacy and side effects of heparin in reducing adhesion formation are conflicting.[37] In women, abdominal lavage using heparin (5000 U/L) with Ringer's solution did not reduce adhesion scores.[38] In contrast, intraperitoneal heparin administration has been effective in reducing adhesion formation in laboratory models.[35] In foals, a high dose of heparin administered subcutaneously for 3 days was not effective in reducing adhesion formation compared with flunixin meglumine, antibiotics, and DMSO.[36] In contrast, heparin administered initially intravenously (40 USP/kg) during surgery and subcutaneously (40 USP/kg q12hr for 2 days) significantly reduced adhesion formation.[37] Therefore the dose and route of heparin administration may be factors associated with its efficacy in preventing adhesions.

Sodium carboxymethylcellulose (SCMC) has been used as a protective lubricant agent for viscera, used most commonly during equine colic surgery. The proposed mechanisms by which SCMC prevents adhesion formation have been hydroflotation of the abdominal viscera, prevention of serosal surfaces from coming into contact with one another, and/or minimizing serosal damage during intestinal manipulation. A 1% SCMC solution has been used successfully intraoperatively[39] and after celiotomy closure[40] in reducing adhesion formation. Delayed healing after equine jejunal resection and anastomosis[41] and incision complications[39] have not been observed. Though SCMC precipitate is detectable in both equine and bovine serum 15 minutes after intraperitoneal administration, no clinical complications were observed in a study by Burkhard and colleagues.[42] Because of the gravitational effect in quadrupeds, SCMC may not elicit much of a protective effect on the reproductive tract because it hangs above the abdominal organs. However, a 1% SCMC solution reduced adhesion formation after uterine trauma in ewes.[43] Traditionally, large volumes of SCMC (1-2 L/horse) have been used. However, this volume in the horse's abdomen would seem insufficient to provide a hydroflotation effect. Therefore the mechanism by which SCMC prevents adhesion formation is likely local surface activity.[43] In a laparoscopic ewe uterine trauma model, traumatic forceps were used to create a 1.5 cm × 5 cm long area of serosal trauma and bleeding along the left uterine horn.[43] A low dose (30 ml) of SCMC applied directly to the traumatized serosal area prevented adhesion formation. Extrapolating this amount to the bovine hysterotomy, a volume of 150 ml would probably be required to adequately cover the uterine incision. The use of SCMC before hysterotomy would make exteriorizing the uterus difficult. In addition, healing of the uterine incision may be impaired because it heals by serosal-to-serosal contact. Once the uterine incision is closed, a low dose of 1% SCMC applied to the uterus after abdominal lavage may be beneficial in reducing detrimental adhesion formation.

I have used an abdominal lavage and a combination of flunixin meglumine (1 mg/kg), heparin (20 U/kg), and potassium penicillin (22,000 U/kg) mixed in 500 ml of 0.9% sodium chloride irrigation solution and instilled into the abdomen is sometimes used as an aid to reduce adhesion formation.[44] Based on the current knowledge, instilling flunixin meglumine, heparin, and potassium penicillin G into the abdomen during surgery is strictly empiric.[44] Postoperatively, flunixin meglumine is administered (1 mg/kg q12 IV, IM) for 2 to 3 days in an effort to reduce adhesion formation. Some scientific merit of flunixin meglumine (1 mg/kg IV) before surgery, abdominal lavage, applying 1% CSMC on the uterine incision, and using both flunixin meglumine (1 mg/kg q12h for 2 days) and heparin (20 USP/kg q12h for 3 days) after surgery may exist.[35]

Incisions

The disadvantages of the recumbent approaches are the increased risks of intraoperative hemorrhage, postoperative seroma formation, and incisional herniations. The overall surgical time is also increased. Standing cesareans typically required 1 hour to complete, whereas a minimum of 2 hours are required for the recumbent approaches. More time is required for preparation, suturing, and recovery. One article suggested the paramedian approach to be superior to the ventral approach[5] because the presence of increased vascularity and muscle tissues was thought to enhance healing. Furthermore, this paper suggested that this enhanced healing reduces the incidence of incisional herniation, although healing likely occurs faster compared with the linea alba.

The advantage of the midline approach is that the linea alba provides a stronger holding layer compared with either the paramedian or low oblique approaches. The thin facial layers, with interposed muscle layers, likely cause the lateral approaches to herniate. Furthermore, fewer layers of closure compared with the paramedian and low oblique approaches reduce surgery time.

Reports of paralumbar incisional complications in the literature are scarce: two practitioner surveys reported infections between 1.3% and 8.2%[21,22] and dehiscence of 3.8%.[22] At OSU the reported incidence is 5.9%. Because most C-sections are handled as outpatients, this incidence rate is likely not accurate. One study did report an incisional infection rate of 15%[3] caused by *Actinobacillus lignieresii*. The veterinarian apparently spread this infection by either poor aseptic technique or inadequately sterilized equipment. Subcutaneous emphysema has been reported between 0% and 41%.[9,21,22] Subcutaneous emphysema could be avoided by closing the peritoneum along with the transversus and thus sealing the abdomen. Unfortunately, these numbers are fraught with confounding variables. Differences in surgical site preparation, local anesthetic technique, incision length, difficulty removing the calf through the incision, time of surgery, and the use, type, and duration of postoperative antibiotics make it difficult to make clear inferences. Applying pressure to the opposite abdominal wall to expel intra-abdominal air during closure of the first layer has also been suggested as a means to reduce subcutaneous emphysema.[20]

The incidence and predisposing factors of incisional hernias in the horse have been reported.[45] The linea alba was closed with a simple interrupted suture with one of the following: chromic gut, 2 polydioxanone, or 2 polyglactin 910. Polydioxanone retains 70% of its tensile strength after 14 days, 50% after 28 days, 25% after 42 days, and 0% after 90 days. Polyglactin 910 retains 75% of its tensile strength after 14 days, 50% after 21 days, 8% after 28 days, and 0% after 35 days. No difference in incision complications (infection, hernia formation) was observed between polydioxanone and polyglactin 910. Chromic gut had a significantly higher hernia complication rate; however, the small sample size ($n=4$) may be subject to bias. Suture pattern and skin staples likely reduced the overall incisional complication rates of this study in sharp contrast with previous studies. Using the near-far-far-near pattern for abdominal closure has been associated with an increased incisional drainage in horses.[46] In another study, 97% of incisional hernias were preceded by either infection or edema.[45]

Recent research[47] in the healing of the normal equine linea alba had some interesting results. Simple interrupted cruciate sutures using No 2 lactomer taking 15-mm bites were used to close the linea alba. Lactomer retains 80% of its tensile strength at 14 days and 30% after 21 days. The tensile strength of the linea was weakest at 2 weeks compared with the control (nonincised) linea alba. No statistical significant difference in tensile strength was observed at 4, 8, and 16 weeks after surgery. However, no practical significance in tensile strength was observed at 8 and 16 weeks after surgery. Interestingly, the incised linea alba samples were significantly stronger compared with the controls at 24 weeks. The incised linea alba samples at 2 weeks were characterized primarily by granulation tissue—at 4 weeks unbundled, immature collagen fibers were present. At 8, 16, and 24 weeks bundles of mature collagen were present.

The principles of the previously mentioned findings can probably be extrapolated to the bovine linea alba. Traditionally, chromic catgut, polyglactin 910, polydioxanone, and occasionally polyglycolic acid are used to close the linea alba. Polyglycolic acid retains 65% of its tensile strength after 14 days, 35% after 21 days, and 5% after 28 days; is completely hydrolyzed between 100 and 120 days; and has poor knot security. Based on the previously mentioned studies looking at healing and suture type, it may make more sense to select a suture material that retains its tensile strength closer to 8 weeks such as either polydioxanone or polyglyconate. Polyglyconate retains 80% of its tensile strength after 7 days, 75% after 14 days, 65% after 21 days, 50% after 28 days, and 25% after 42 days and is completely hydrolyzed between 180 and 200 days. The disadvantage of polyglyconate is difficulty in tying knots under tension.

Reproductive Economics of Cesarean Section

Good practice management for future breeding cows should include observing for estrus 21 to 28 days after surgery. If estrus is not detected, an injection of prostaglandin F2a (25 mg dinoprost tromethamine IM) between days 21 and 28 and repeated 14 days later will improve reproductive efficiency.[48] If endometritis is suspected, the cow should be short cycled using prostaglandin F2a to eliminate the infection. A breeding soundness examination is recommended 4 to 6 weeks postsurgery to evaluate for adhesions, ovarian activity, and uterine health. If the owner elects to breed back the cow within 6 to 8 weeks after surgery, artificial insemination (using a bull known for calving ease) is recommended because the abdominal incision has not reached maximum strength. Alternatively, natural breeding can be started 8 weeks after surgery.

C-sections in dairy cattle did not change the interval to first service or subsequent gestation length in a study by Noakes and colleagues.[29] The calving to first service was 81 ± 29 in dairy cattle.[21] Studies have demonstrated that cows having C-sections had an increase in services per conception and days open.[1,20] The number of services per conception was 2.1 ± 1.4 for dairy cows and 1.2 ± 0.4 for beef cows.[21] The calving to conception interval was 110 ± 43 days in dairy cows and 99 ± 18 days in beef cattle. No difference occurred in the rate of abortion between cesarean and normal deliveries.[29] The overall pregnancy rate in dairy and beef cows that had had C-sections has been demonstrated to be 72% and 91%, respectively.[21] These rates appear reasonable for routine cases. The lower pregnancy rates in the dairy cattle could be attributable to confounding variables. The reproductive reasons for culling can be easily influenced by nonreproductive reasons such as lameness. Therefore it is possible the apparent culling for reproductive reasons is an overestimation of the true rate. Furthermore, it is generally accepted that beef cows likely tolerate surgery better with better outcomes because they are usually in better body condition and have significantly lower metabolic demands compared with high-producing dairy cows. In beef cows, infertility increased as the level of calving assistance was required, especially when a C-section was performed.[49] The effect of body condition was not considered in this study and may have been confounding variable in the pregnancy rates. Poorly and overly conditioned cows are well known to have difficulty getting pregnant.

The effect of a C-section on milk production is difficult to elucidate because of numerous confounding variables. Accurate information in beef cows is not available. In dairy cattle, milk production/lactation following a C-section is thought to be reduced by 80 to 1500 L when compared with their previous lactation.[21] When the effects of herd, year, parity, calving season, and abortion were corrected, cows that had a C-section were less likely to reach 100 days in milk (DIM) and produced on average 79.9 kg less milk in the first 100 DIM compared with controls.[29] A second study confirmed that the entire milk reduction occurred during the first 100 DIM.[50] No difference was observed in groups between 100 DIM and 240 DIM.[29]

In the Netherlands, dairy cattle are frequently crossbred to beef sires. A risk-benefit economic study considered the extra income received by Dutch dairies compared with the increased costs associated with C-sections. Based on the extra return from crossbred calve sales, the OR would have to increase to 26 before being economically unjustifiable in Dutch dairies.[49] The overall risk of being culled is higher for cows with C-sections compared with controls.[2]

Emphysematous Fetus

A retrospective study[26] found that dairy cows ($n = 16$) had a 33% rate of survival if they had an emphysematous fetus at the time of surgery. Between 1985 and 1989, 159 cows were referred to the veterinary hospital for C-section. Of the 16 cows with emphysematous feti, 6 survived and were released from the hospital. A ventral midline approach was used to remove these calves. These results are neither surprising nor encouraging for either the client or surgeon.

The experience at OSU has been dramatically different. Unfortunately, relatively few C-sections have been coded in the OSU medical record computer system. Between April 12, 1998 and July 12, 1998, 11 cows were admitted to OSU with emphysematous feti. A local block and ventral midline approach was used. Nine cows were released. Two cows were euthanized during surgery because the uterus had already ruptured. Since August 2002, nine cows (three dairy, six beef) have had a ventral midline C-section under a general anesthetic to remove emphysematous feti. All cows survived surgery and were released from the hospital. Unfortunately, the earlier study made no comment other than the approach regarding preoperative, intraoperative, or postoperative factors, which could significantly influence survival rates. It would be interesting to know more in order to explain the differences in survival.

Typically these cows are toxic, pyrexic, hypotensive, and in shock. A minimum database composed of a packed cell volume (PCV) and total protein (TP) is collected. Fluid therapy is initiated, usually at shock rates (80 ml/kg/hr),[14] using either Ringer's solution or 0.9% NaCl. Oxytetracycline (200 mg/ml, 20 mg/kg q24 IV) and flunixin meglumine (50 mg/ml, 1 mg/kg q12 IV) are administered preoperatively. Once the cardiovascular system is sufficiently stabilized, the cow is induced, intubated, and maintained on gas anesthetic. The anesthetic protocol varies according to the individual anesthetists' preferences.

Fluids are continued during the surgery. Blood gas is taken every hour of surgery, and abnormalities are identified and addressed if possible. The uterus must be exteriorized as much as possible to prevent contamination of the abdominal cavity. The cow is positioned in right lateral recumbency, with the upper hind leg tied up and back, which assists exteriorizing of the uterus, and allowing it to somewhat hang down. Lately, a Mayo Stand Cover has been used to envelop the exteriorized uterine horn, placing the ends of the cover as deep as possible within the abdominal cavity. The cover effectively isolates the uterus from the abdominal cavity and surgical field. The end of the cover is cut open to reveal the exteriorized uterine horn. The surgical instruments required for the hysterotomy are partitioned on the table. To ensure proper aseptic technique, "clean" instruments are used to close the body wall.

The uterus is incised, the fetus is removed, and the uterus is closed in two inverting layers by a simple, continuous Cushing pattern using No 2 chromic catgut. Chromic gut loses 50% of its tensile strength after 14 days and is absorbed by phagocytosis. Premature absorption occurs in infected environments and highly vascularized tissues. Because the uterus is both highly vascularized and contaminated after the emphysematous calf is removed, there may be some merit in selecting another suture type such as polycaprone 25. This suture type retains 70% of its tensile strength after 7 days, 40% after 14 days, and 0% after 28 days, which is when the uterus should be fully healed and involuted. After the uterus is extensively lavaged to remove blood clots and contaminated fluids, the cover is removed. Changing to clean gloves and, if necessary, clean gowns likely reduces abdominal contamination. Contaminated instruments are kept separate on the surgery table.

The clean instruments are then used to close the linea alba, subcutaneous tissue, and skin. The linea alba is closed using No 2 polyglactin 910 in a simple cruciate pattern. Research done in horses demonstrated that chromic gut suture had a higher incision dehiscence, compared with either polyglactin 910 or polyglycolic acid.[45] After 21 days polyglactin 910 has no detectable strength. Because the risk of incisional herniation is greater compared with paralumbar approaches, there may some merit in selecting a suture material that retains its tensile strength longer such as polydioxanone or polyglyconate.

The subcutaneous layer is closed using No 2 polyglactin 910 in a simple continuous pattern. Careful attention in closing the dead space associated with the subcutaneous layer will prevent significant seroma formation postoperatively. The skin is closed using No 3 vetafil (Braunamid) in a continuous ford interlocking pattern. A few simple interrupted sutures are placed at the cranial portion of the incision because this will be the most dependent portion of the incision once the cow is standing. If necessary, these sutures can be cut to assist drainage. The cow is recovered either in the stall on tan bark or in the induction/recovery stall if the halter is broken.

Postoperatively, the cow is kept on fluids usually for 24 hours at a maintenance rate (2 ml/kg/hr).[14] Antibiotics are continued for a minimum of 3 to 7 days. Anti-inflammatories are continued q12h for several days and then reduced to q24h. Typically, the number of days hospitalized ranges from 3 to 7. In addition to the routine C-section take-home instructions, daily monitoring of lethargy, appetite, manure production, and the incision is recommended. Skin stitches are removed after 3 weeks. The cow is kept separated in a pen for 4 weeks. A breeding soundness examination is strongly recommended 4 to 6 weeks after surgery to evaluate for adhesions and uterine health. Artificial insemination is recommended if breeding is less than 2 months after surgery.

Reproductive Economics of Emphysematous Fetus

The cost of a replacement animal can range from $500 for a commercial-grade, nonpregnant heifer to $1200 to $1500 for a commercial-grade, pregnant cow. A purebred pregnant cow can cost several thousand dollars, depending on the breed, conformation, and genetic value. Cow survival represents only a portion of a successful outcome of surgery. The future reproductive efficiency of the cow is equally important. Reasonably good information is available in the literature concerning rebreeding rates in both dairy and beef cattle after routine C-section. Unfortunately, this is not the case with emphysematous feti. The earlier study did not stratify which cows were bred back successfully.[26] Not enough time has elapsed to determine reproductive efficiency on the cows seen at OSU since last July. The most accurate technique of determining these rates would be pregnancy checks. The reality is that this information will be collected the following year when these cows calve (or fail to calve) again.

CONCLUSIONS

A number of risk factors adversely affect outcome. Case selection, surgical time, calf viability at the time of surgery, and exteriorizing the uterus can affect outcome. Reducing excessive adhesion formation, which can adversely affect reproductive efficiency, is equally important. Gentle tissue handling, good surgical technique, appropriate suture pattern with adequate serosal infolding, abdominal lavage, and preoperative and postoperative antiinflammatories can minimize adhesions. The intravenous administration of heparin preoperatively, SCMC applied to the uterine incision, and postoperative subcutaneous heparin may be additional adjuncts in reducing adhesions.

When dealing with emphysematous fetus, aggressive fluid therapy to stabilize the cow's cardiovascular system is likely the critical determining factor of cow survival. Antiinflammatories; high doses of intravenous antibiotics; and using a ventral midline approach, which permits adequate uterine exteriorization and therefore reduces abdominal contamination, are also likely key elements that contribute to the high survival rates of cows with emphysematous feti at OSU.

References

1. Campbell ME, Fubini SL: Indications and surgical approaches for cesarean section in cattle, *Compend Contin Ed* 12:285-291, 1990.
2. Walker DF, Vaughan JT: *Bovine and equine urogenital surgery*, Philadelphia, 1980, Lea & Febiger, pp 85-98.
3. deKruif A, Mitjen P, Haesebrouck F et al: Actinobacillosis in bovine caesarean sections, *Vet Rec* 414-415, 1992.
4. Barkema HW, Schukken YH, Guard CL et al: Cesarean section in dairy cattle: a study of risk factors, *Theriogenology* 37:489-506, 1992.
5. Noorsdy JL: Selection of an incision site for cesarean section in the cow, *Vet Med [Small Anim Clin]* 74:530-537, 1979.
6. Vaughan L, Mulville P: A survey of bovine caesarean sections in Ireland, *Irish Vet J* 48:411-415, 1995.
7. Newman KD: *Bovine caesarean sections: Ohio State University clinical cases 1998-2003.* Unpublished data, 2003.
8. Parish SM, Tyler JW, Ginsky JV: Left oblique celiotomy approach for cesarean section in standing cows, *J Am Vet Med Assoc* 207:751-752, 1995.
9. Sloss V, Duffy JH: Elective caesarean operation in Hereford cattle, *Aust Vet J* 53:420-424, 1977.
10. LeBlanc MM, Hubbell JAE, Smith HC: The effects of xylaxine hydrochloride on uterine pressure in the cow, *Theriogenology* 21:681-690, 1984.
11. Anderson DE, Gaughan EM, DeBowes RM et al: Affects of chemical restraint on the endoscopic appearance of laryngeal and pharyngeal anatomy and sensation in adult cattle, *Am J Vet Res* 55:1196-1200, 1994.

12. Turner SA, McIlwraith CW: *Techniques in large animal surgery*, Philadelphia, 1989, Lea & Febiger, pp 225-228, 277-283.
13. Thurmon JC, Tranquilli WJ, Benson GJ: *Lumb and Jones' veterinary anesthesia*, ed 3, Baltimore, 1996, Lippincott Williams & Wilkins, 486-496.
14. Muir WW, Hubbell JAE, Skarda RT et al: *Handbook of veterinary anesthesia*, ed 3, St Louis, 2000, Mosby, pp 57-71.
15. Knight AP: Xylazine, *J Am Vet Med Assoc* 176:454, 1980.
16. Zuagg JL, Nussbaum M: Epidural injection of xylazine: a new option for surgical analgesia of the bovine abdomen and udder, *Vet Med* 1043-1046, 1990.
17. St-Jean G, Skarda RT, Muir WW et al: Caudal epidural analgesia induced by xylazine administration in cows, *Am J Vet Res* 8:1232-1236, 1990.
18. Caulkett N, Cribb PH, Duke D: Xylazine epidural analgesia for cesarean section in cattle, *Can Vet J* 34:674-676, 1993.
19. Frazer GS, Perkins NR: Cesarean section, *Vet Clin North Am Food Anim Pract* 11:19-35, 1995.
20. Dehghani SN, Ferguson JG: Cesarean section in cattle: complications, *Comp Contin Educ Vet Prac* 4:s387-s392, 1982.
21. Cattell JH, Dobson H: A survey of caesarean operations on cattle in general veterinary practice, *Vet Rec* 127:395-399, 1990.
22. Dawson JC, Murray R: Caesarean sections in cattle attended by a practice in Cheshire, *Vet Rec* 131:525-527, 1992.
23. Hoeben D, Mijten P, de Kruif A: Factors influencing complications during caesarean section on the standing cow, *Vet Quart* 19:88-92, 1997.
24. Menard L: Tocolytic drugs for use in veterinary obstetrics, *Can Vet J* 25:389-393, 1984.
25. Menard LD, Diaz CS: The use of clenbuterol for the management of large animal dystocias: surgical corrections in the cow and ewe, *Can Vet J* 28:585-590, 1987.
26. Bouchard E, Daignault D, Belanger D et al: Césarienne chez la vache laitière: 159 cas, *Can Vet J* 35:70-774, 1994.
27. Frazer GS: Hormonal therapy in the postpartum cow—days 1 to 10—fact or fiction, *AABP Proceed* 109-130, 2001.
28. Mijten P, van den Bogaard AE, Hazen MJ, de Kruif A: Bacterial contamination of fetal fluids at the time of cesarean section in the cow, *Theriogenology* 48:513-521, 1997.
29. Noakes DE, Wallace L, Smith GR: Bacterial flora of uterus of cows after calving on two hygienically contrasting farms, *Vet Record* 128:440-442, 1991.
30. Barkema HW, Schukken YH, Guard CL et al: Fertility, production and culling following cesarean section in dairy cattle, *Theriogenology* 38:589-599, 1992.
31. Plumb DC: *Veterinary drug book*, ed 2, Ames, Iowa, 1995, Iowa State University Press, p 515.
32. Slatter D: *Textbook of small animal surgery*, ed 2, Philadelphia, 1985, Saunders, p 42.
33. Southwood LL, Baxter GM: Current concepts in management of abdominal adhesions, *Vet Clin North Am Equine Pract* 13:415-435, 1997.
34. Mijten P, de Kruif A, Van der Weyden GC et al: Comparison of catgut and polyglactin 910 for uterine sutures during bovine caesarean section, *Vet Rec* 140:458-459, 1978.
35. Hague BA, Honnas CM, Berridge BR et al: Evaluation of postoperative peritoneal lavage in standing horses for prevention of experimentally induced abdominal adhesions, *Vet Surg* 27:122-126, 1998.
36. Sullins KE, White NA, Lundin CS et al: Treatment of ischemia induced peritoneal adhesions in foals, *Vet Surg* 20:348, 1991 (abstract).
37. Parker JE, Fubini SL, Car BD et al: Prevention of intra-abdominal adhesions in ponies by low-dose heparin therapy, *Vet Surg* 16:424-431, 1987.
38. Jansen RP: Failure of peritoneal irrigation with heparin during pelvic operations upon women to reduce adhesions, *Surg Gynecol Obstet* 166:154-160, 1988.

39. Mueller PO, Hunt RJ, Allen D et al: Intraperitoneal use of sodium carboxymethylcellulose in horses undergoing exploratory celiotomy, *Vet Surg* 24:112-117, 1995.

40. Moll HD, Wolfe DF, Schumacher J et al: Evaluation of sodium carboxymethylcellulose for prevention of experimentally induced abdominal adhesions in ponies, *Am J Vet Res* 52:88-91, 1991.

41. Mueller PO, Harmon BG, Hay WP et al: Effect of a carboxycellulose and a hyaluronate-carboxycellulose membrane on healing of intestinal anastomoses in horses, *Am J Vet Res* 61:369-374, 2000.

42. Burkhard MJ, Baxter G, Thrall MA: Blood precipitate associated with intra-abdominal carboxycellulose administration, *Vet Clin Pathol* 25:114-117, 1996.

43. Ivany JM: *Evaluation of sodium carboxymethylcellulose and a novel carbohydrate polymer gel for the prevention of adhesions using a sheep laparoscopic uterine trauma model*, Ohio State University, 2002 (master's thesis).

44. Anderson DE: *Surgical management and decision in problem birthing* (website): www.vet.ohio-state.edu/docs/ClinSci/bovine/repro/cset.html. Accessed December 30, 2007.

45. Gibson KT, Curtis CR, Turner SA: Incisional hernias in the horse: incidence and predisposing factors, *Vet Surg* 18:360-366, 1989.

46. Kobluk C, Ducharme N, Lumsden J et al: Factors affecting incisional complication rates associated with colic surgery in horses: 78 cases (1983-1985), *J Am Vet Med Assoc* 195:639-642, 1989.

47. Chism PN, Latimer FG, Patton CS et al: Tissue strength and wound morphology of the equine linea alba after ventral median celiotomy, *Vet Surg* 29:145-151, 2000.

48. Luchsinger JH, Boucher JF: Postpartum use of Lutalyse/Dinolytic sterile solution in problem cows, *AABP Proc* 2001, p 184.

49. Ducrot C, Cimarosti I, Bugnard F et al: Calving effect on French beef-cow fertility, *Prev Vet Med* 19:126-136, 1994.

50. Rougoor CW, Dijkhuizen AA, Barkema HW et al: The economics of caesarean section in dairy cattle, *Prev Vet Med* 19:27-37, 1994.

CHAPTER 80

Vaginal and Uterine Prolapse

MATT D. MIESNER and DAVID E. ANDERSON

Vaginal and uterine prolapse are common problems in cattle, occasional problems in sheep, but more rarely seen in goats. When vaginal prolapse is seen in goats, these occur more frequently in dairy breeds. Acute vaginal prolapse may be seen prepartum or postpartum. Animals suffering prepartum vaginal prolapse should be selected for culling after weaning the current offspring. Dietary factors implicated in vaginal prolapse include poor-quality forage, hypocalcemia, high-estrogenic-content foodstuffs such as legumes and soybean meal, and overcrowding. Individual animal risk factors include obesity, chronic coughing, chronic straining to urinate or defecate, and excessively short tail docking in sheep. Vaginal prolapse may be described using a grade scale of I to IV (Table 80-1; Figs. 80-1 to 80-4). In this grading scale, vaginal prolapse severity and extent of damage are used to assess treatment options.

ACUTE VAGINAL PROLAPSE

A plethora of techniques have been described for treatment of acute vaginal prolapse including Buhner's suture, boot lace sutures, paravaginal stents, Caslik's suture, rope slings or harnesses in sheep, and indwelling vaginal retainers in sheep (Figs. 80-5 to 80-9). Indwelling retainers and rope slings are purported to have the advantage that kids and lambs may be able to birth around or through the device. However, dystocia is a concern whenever these devices are left in place. Ideally, rope slings or retainers should be removed within a few days of expected parturition. Alternatively, parturition may be induced to allow a shorter interval for close observation or for elective C-section. In small ruminants, suture techniques have a higher risk of tearing through the perineal tissues. When necessary, I have chosen 6- to 12-mm diameter rubber stents to place under mattress sutures. I place three to five vertical or horizontal mattress sutures over a stent that is positioned perpendicular (for vertical mattress) or parallel (for horizontal mattress) to the vulva (Fig. 80-10). All of these techniques are used to maintain the position of the vagina cranial to the vulva and ideally within the vaginal vault. Vaginal vault retention requires replacement of the function of the vestibular sphincter muscles. Thus the sutures must be placed along the hair-nonhaired margin of the vulva such that the depth of the suture will mimic the effect of the vestibular sphincter muscle. Placement of

Table 80-1

Clinical Grading Scale for Vaginal Prolapse in Cattle

Grade	Description	Relevance	Treatment
I	Intermittent prolapse of vagina; most common when lying down	Likely to progress to grade II if not treated	Use temporary retaining suture Cull after calving or perform permanent fixation technique if embryo donor cow
II	Continuous prolapse of vagina ± urinary bladder retroflexed	Urinary bladder involvement (common) can obstruct urination or cause persistent straining	Use temporary retaining suture Cull after calving or perform permanent fixation technique if embryo flush cow
III	Continuous prolapse of vagina, urinary bladder, and cervix (external os visible)	Can cause compromise to urine outflow and ureters Should be treated quickly to prevent life-threatening injury	Perform permanent fixation technique if embryo flush cow Induce parturition or perform elective C-section if commercial cow
IV	Grade II or III with trauma, infection, and/or necrosis of vaginal wall a. Subacute such that replacement into vaginal vault is possible b. Chronic with fibrosis such that the vagina cannot be replaced	Grade IVa: repair laceration, débride wounds, treat infection, and replace into vaginal vault Grade IVb: requires elective C-section or vaginal resection	Perform permanent fixation technique if embryo flush cow Induce parturition or perform elective C-section if commercial cow

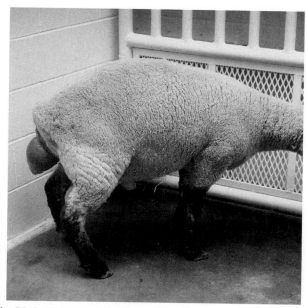

Fig 80-1 Prepartum vaginal prolapse in a ewe.

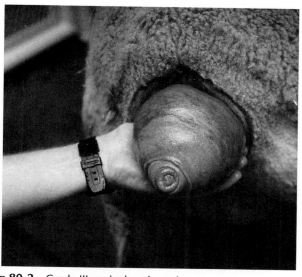

Fig 80-2 Grade III vaginal prolapse in a ewe.

the sutures too superficially will result in insufficient support of the vaginal tissues and thus persistent or recurrent straining. Persistent straining and recurrent prolapse will result in tearing of the vulva (Fig. 80-11).

Buhner's sutures should be placed using a Buhner needle inserted through a 1-cm incision made approximately at the level of the ischium (4-cm width proximal to the ventral commissure of the vulva) and exiting a 1-cm incision made on midline of the perineum 4-cm dorsal to the dorsal commissure of the vulva. The needle is inserted first, and then ¼-inch (6.4-mm) width umbilical tape is inserted in the end of the needle and the suture is pulled back through as the needle is removed. The procedure is repeated on the contralateral side with the needle exiting the same proximal midline perineal incision.

CHRONIC VAGINAL PROLAPSE

Although Buhner's suture and other methods of fixation give temporary relief from vaginal prolapse, chronic vaginal prolapse requires more invasive techniques to stabilize the vagina (Fig. 80-12). The Johnson button and Minchev suture techniques are appropriate for vaginal prolapse associated with excessive redundancy of the dorsal vaginal wall. These techniques are traumatic and may result in tearing of the vagina into the abdomen because of chronic straining after surgery. They may cause damage to the sciatic nerve or internal pudendal artery if these structures are not avoided. In these techniques an indwelling needle (Johnson button) or umbilical tape suture (Minchev) is placed from the dorsolateral vaginal wall through the sacrotuberous ligament and through the gluteal musculature (Figs. 80-13 to 80-16). In the case of the Johnson button, large, flat disks are attached to each

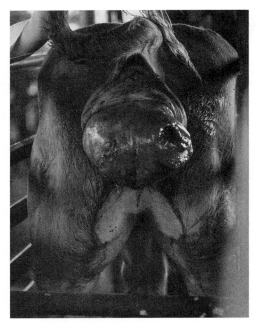

Fig 80-3   Grade III vaginal prolapse in a cow.

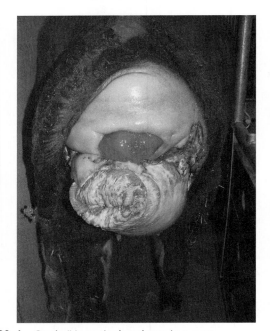

Fig 80-4   Grade IVa vaginal prolapse in a cow.

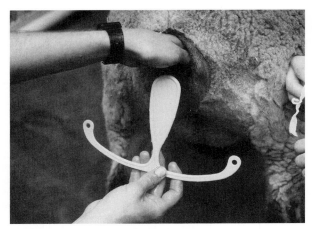

Fig 80-5   Vaginal retainer for sheep.

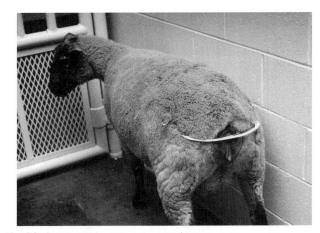

Fig 80-6   Vaginal retainer inserted into a ewe.

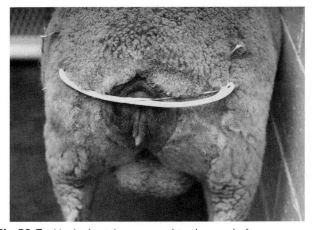

Fig 80-7   Vaginal retainer secured to the wool of a ewe.

end to secure the device. With the Minchev suture, rolls of gauze sponges are attached to each end to secure the device (Fig. 80-17). These are left in place for 2 to 6 weeks to allow formation of extensive fibrous adhesions, which serve as anchors for the vaginal shelf.

Cervicopexy is appropriate for vaginal prolapse associated with excessive redundancy of the ventral vaginal wall. Cervicopexy can be performed transvaginally or via flank laparotomy. Flank laparotomy offers the best approach for anatomic and permanent fixation because the cervix can be more accurately anchored without interference with the bladder, the suture can be placed without compromise of the cervical lumen, and the suture is permanently placed with little risk of infection. However, cows having chronic vaginal prolapse are often obese and excessive abdominal fat increases the difficulty of this procedure dramatically. Transvaginal cervicopexy offers the easiest and least invasive surgical approach and is amenable to field conditions. Two sutures of No 3 vetafil are placed through the cervix (being careful not to penetrate the lumen of the cervix) and are anchored to the prepubic tendon (being careful not to entrap

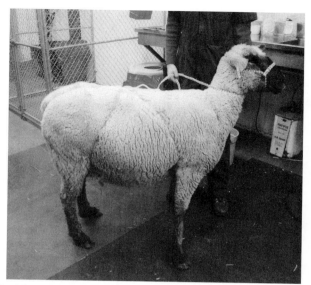

Fig 80-8 A rope harness for prolapse retention in sheep.

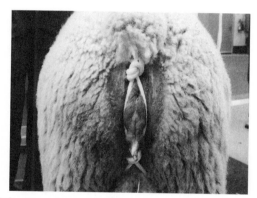

Fig 80-9 Rope harness applied to a ewe with vaginal pro-lapse.

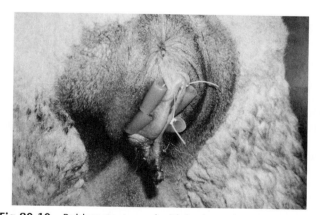

Fig 80-10 Rubber stents used with horizontal suture retention of vaginal prolapse.

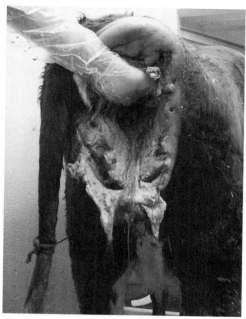

Fig 80-11 Severe vulvar and perineal injury caused by excessive straining after prolapse retention using Buhner's suture.

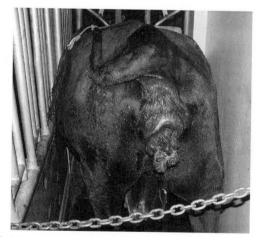

Fig 80-12 Type IV vaginal prolapse in a cow.

the bladder, urethra, or intestines). Disadvantages of cervicopexy include increased risk of entrapment of the urethra, increased risk of sepsis of the abdomen or cervix, increased risk of compromise of the lumen of the cervix, and suboptimal anatomic positioning.

Vaginoplasty and vaginal resection are effective in the elimination of vaginal prolapse and may be used for either dorsal or ventral wall prolapse, but this procedure prevents the animal from being used in natural service or going through normal parturition. This technique is done with the animal standing with epidural anesthesia. A triangular segment of the dorsal lateral vaginal wall is resected on both sides with the triangles based on dorsal midline (Figs. 80-18 and 80-19). Next, the sides are sutured closed together. The vaginal wall resection should only leave enough room for embryo flushing equipment to be passed through the vagina. Vaginal resection can be performed in chronic vaginal prolapse when vaginal redundancy is circumferential such that a complete segment of the vaginal can be removed. Vaginal resection is performed much like rectal amputation. A vaginal speculum is placed into the lumen of the prolapsed vagina, and then cross-fixation

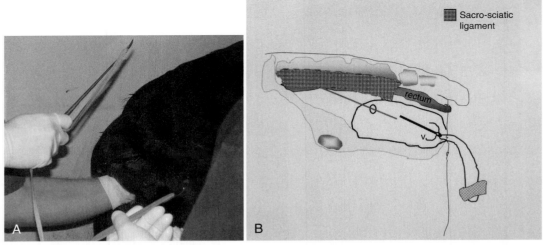

Fig 80-13   A, Umbilical tape in Buhner needle before insertion for modified Minchev vagino-pexy. **B,** Diagram showing intended path of needle for placement of the umbilical tape during placement of modified Minchev vaginopexy. v, Vaginal vault.

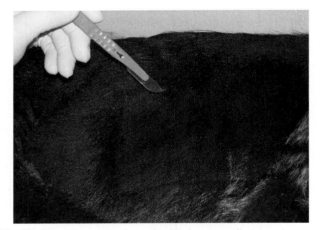

Fig 80-14   Gluteal site for exit of Buhner needle in vaginopexy (tail head to left).

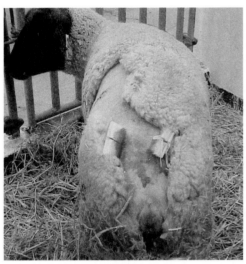

Fig 80-16   Gauze padding secured to end of umbilical tape placed in modified Minchev vaginopexy.

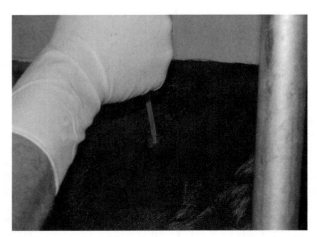

Fig 80-15   Umbilical tape being drawn through the gluteal site for modified Minchev vaginopexy suture.

pins are placed through the vaginal prolapse and tube to stabilize the segment for surgery (Figs. 80-20 to 80-22). The injured portion of the vaginal prolapse is resected, and an end-to-end anastomosis performed using No 1 or 2 polyglycolic acid in interrupted suture pattern. Complications of vaginal resection include stricture, dehiscence, hemorrhage, abscess, and reoccurrence of prolapse.

After surgery, the animal should be rested for 30 days after surgery before insemination or breeding activity is resumed. We only recommend treatment of chronic vaginal prolapse when there is a history of chronic hormonal manipulation. Other vaginal prolapses have a high concern for heritability and these animals should be culled. If the animal is to be made a pet, ovariohysterectomy is recommended. Complications of surgical treatments for vaginal prolapse include recurrence, dehiscence, hemorrhage, abscess, damage to vital structures (urethra, sciatic nerve, pudendal artery), and peritonitis.

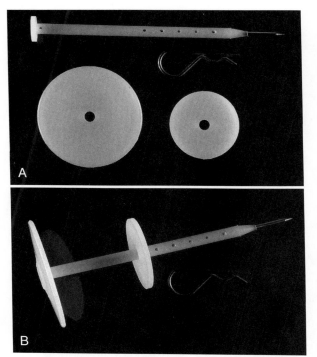

Fig 80-17   **A,** Disassembled Johnson button device used for dorsal and lateral stabilization of dorsal vaginal shelf for vaginopexy. **B,** Assembled Johnson button device used for dorsal and lateral stabilization of dorsal vaginal shelf for vaginopexy.

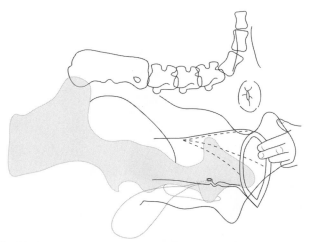

Fig 80-18   Diagram of incisions at dorsal midline and lateral aspects of vaginal vault in vaginoplasty.

Long-term prognosis for vaginal prolapse is limited because of culling.

UTERINE PROLAPSE

Uterine prolapse in cows is a historic topic, well discussed in scientific veterinary literature and texts, argued at legendary proportion between practitioners, and even referenced in western poetry. The condition occurs sporadically, is easily recognized, and is sometimes not easily repaired. Replacing, repairing, and removing the uterus is discussed in this chapter along with helpful techniques and potential

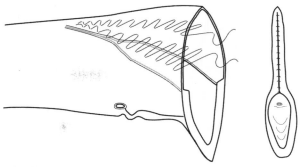

Fig 80-19   Suture placement in closure of vaginoplasty technique for permanent reduction of vaginal prolapse.

complications. Occasionally the veterinarian encounters situations where manual eversion (iatrogenic prolapse) of the uterus is helpful, particularly for efficiently repairing the traumatized uterus in the field. Therefore a technique for iatrogenic prolapse is discussed as well.

Spontaneous uterine prolapse in cows is an occasionally encountered postparturient complication requiring immediate attention. It almost always happens within 12 to 24 hours after calving. Occasionally, occurrence is delayed until days after calving and complicated by partial cervical involution (closure), creating added difficulty in replacing the uterus. Cervical involution may necessitate and combination of laparotomy in addition to external reduction. Midgestation prolapse of the nongravid uterine horn, with successful management and maintaining a viable pregnancy, has been reported.

Uterine prolapse occurs sporadically, with dairy cattle appearing to be more frequently represented than beef cattle. Decreased myometrial tone is a logical predisposing mechanism for occurrence, leading to the proposed risk factors of hypocalcemia, as well as dystocia, causing myometrial fatigue and trauma. Manual extraction of the calf and retained fetal membranes may initiate uterine eversion of the gravid horn(s) followed by complete uterine prolapse after delivery. Uterine prolapse should be regarded as an emergency condition, for one to assist replacement before accumulation of excessive edema, contamination, mucosal trauma, and cervical closure occurs. In addition, client communication to restrict movement should be stressed to decrease the chance of uterine artery rupture or avulsion from the internal iliac leading to fatal hemorrhage. Without timely intervention, the prognosis for life is grave.

Unlike vaginal prolapse, heritability and/or additive individual susceptibility with subsequent pregnancies is not apparent with uterine prolapse. Prognosis for surviva depends on timely intervention, parity, calf viability, an lack of secondary metabolic or musculoskeletal disease. 1-year study from a large dairy practice in California su gested an incidence of less than 0.1% (200/220,000 co and a 2-week postincident survival of 72.4%. A retros tive questionnaire regarding 90 cases of uterine prol and two matched case control herdmates per farm, o 3-year period in the United Kingdom, found only on prolapsed a second time. In the same study, surviva was approximately 80% with the 20% mortality res from shock (evisceration), blood loss, refractory

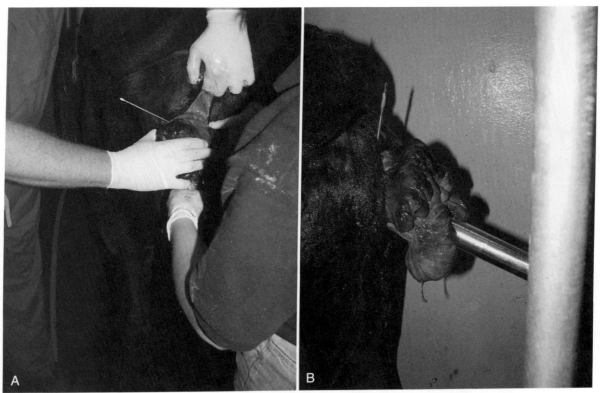

Fig 80-20   A, Grade IVb vaginal prolapse being prepared for vaginectomy by placement of transfixing pin using a 3.2-mm diameter stainless steel pin. **B,** Placement of a disposable vaginal speculum as a luminal stent for placement of transfixing pins and sutures.

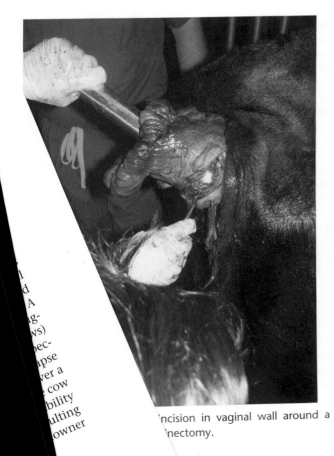

...ncision in vaginal wall around a ...nectomy.

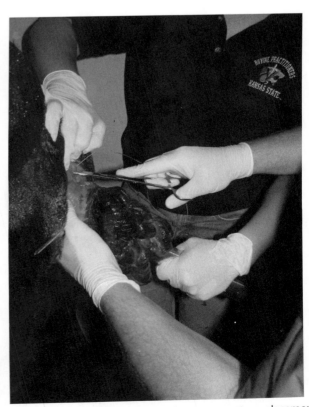

Fig 80-22   Overlapping horizontal mattress suture placement for vaginectomy.

cow syndrome, and humane euthanasia. Jubb and colleagues suggested a 73.5% (50/68) survival rate with only one cow having a history of a previous uterine prolapse. A longer calving-to-conception interval varied between studies, an additional 10 to 50 days longer. Prognosis for life and future fertility is expected to be good with timely veterinary intervention and recognition and treatment of secondary complications. In most instances the decision to treat should be cost effective for the producer.

Replacing the Prolapsed Uterus

Prolapse of the uterus is a diagnosis of observation and physical examination. A large, reddened heavy mass of everted uterus is dramatically visualized, thus exposing placentomes and possibly attached fetal membranes (Fig. 80-23). Treatment should begin with restraining and evaluating the patient for the presence of metabolic and/or musculoskeletal disease and treated as indicated. Animal restraint and cleansing of the exposed endometrium, preferably with hypertonic solutions, should be emphasized as priority treatment. Various rope casting restraint methods are described to maintain recumbency and can be applied. In retractable animals chemical restraint may be indicated. Caudal epidural anesthetics prevent straining and assist replacement of the uterus and, at higher volumes, provide a method of restraint through posterior muscle paralysis. Often, the urethra is positioned in the prolapse such that urination is prevented. By lifting the uterus and allowing urination, additional cow comfort and reduced straining are achieved. This is also a good time to rule out bladder prolapse as an additional complication. It should also be noted that the bladder, and even intestinal viscera, can be contained within the prolapsed uterus. Bladder retroflexion may persist once the uterus is replaced and results in continued straining by the cow. Ultrasonic evaluation of the pelvic canal for urinary bladder retroflexion should be performed with persistent straining. When bladder retroversion is present, placement of an indwelling catheter (e.g., Foley catheter) will help maintain normal bladder position until healing has occurred.

Topically applying osmotic agents such as salts and/or sugar has proved beneficial to begin reducing and preventing the edema, which rapidly accumulates within the prolapsed tissue. These products are known to amplify endometrial trauma. Manual massage during replacement, using ointment with lubrication and emollient properties, is an effective alternative. Attempt to keep the uterus elevated off the ground while cleaning to prevent ongoing contamination. Laundry baskets, kennel grates, and a plethora of fenestrated supportive/containment devices have been used to replace uterine prolapse reduction. We prefer a ceramic, coated, adjustable cooking grill grate (20 × 30 inches) when assistance is unavailable. The grate is easily supported between the cranial thighs/hip of the practitioner and the caudal thighs of the sternal recumbent or standing cow, allowing both hands to be used to work. Evaluate the surface of the exposed endometrium for tearing and perforations and repair at this time, if possible. Alternatively, if repair is not possible, as in the case of severe necrosis or circumferential lacerations, amputation of the uterus should be considered (see later). Protecting the exposed uterus from further trauma and environmental contamination should be performed by wrapping the uterus in plastic or dampened cloth under compression. Confining the uterus in a wrapped plastic or porous fabric bag aids in control of the uterus during replacement and prevent handling-induced trauma to the friable mucosa. If a compression wrap is applied, do so in a manner that allows sequential removal of portions of the wrap as the uterus is replaced from the base (near vagina) to the apex of the prolapse. Additionally, to reduce handling trauma, as well as keep hands warm during cold weather, mittens can be worn while kneading and massaging the uterus during replacement (Fig. 80-24). Begin reducing the prolapse at the base and continue to the apex. Evaluate for complete reduction, and passively infuse warm fluid into the uterus to completely reduce the inverted uterine horns. Failure to achieve complete reduction of the prolapse can result in continued straining and uterine necrosis. Remove excess infused fluid by siphoning it out of the uterus after infusion. Administer oxytocin (20-40 IU, IM) to enhance uterine involution.

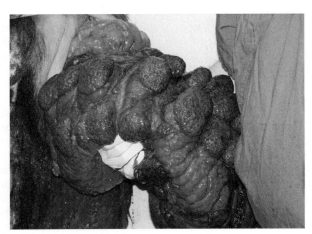

Fig 80-23 Prolapsed uterus in a cow.

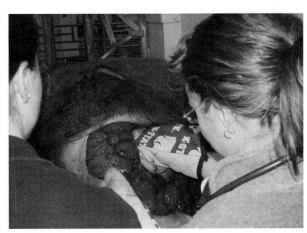

Fig 80-24 Use of oven mitts to massage uterus and thus reduce risk of iatrogenic injury.

Full-thickness lacerations should be repaired when visualized. It is often suggested that repair can be foregone if lacerations are less than 2 to 3 inches and dorsal (most common), as the defect will close sufficiently with oxytocin therapy and uterine involution. The statement is often implied when tears are noted after live-calf extraction and without uterine prolapse or complications. We strongly encourage client communication about the risks associated with not repairing uterine lacerations when diagnosed. With a prolapsed uterus, repair is easy to perform with a simple continuous pattern of No 2 or 3 catgut suture. With wide, radiating areas of devitalized or traumatized tissue from the free edges of the laceration, vertical mattress sutures should aid in minimal tension apposition and result in an inverting pattern of the uterus when replaced. Repair should be performed whenever possible because postpartum metritis caused by gross contamination and additional trauma has occurred.

Positioning of the cow can assist replacement. An efficient means of positioning is with the cow in sternal recumbency and "frog legged" (stifles down, pelvic limbs stretch out behind the cow) (Fig. 80-25). This position can put the cow at risk for coxofemoral luxation. When available in the field, hip lifters can also help support the tuber coxae or even allow some ventral support of the quadriceps draped over a bale of straw. When replacing the prolapse in the standing animal, a support device (see earlier) should be used. Allowing the cow to stand as soon as possible is best. Application of vaginal retention sutures (see vaginal prolapse section) are at the discretion of the individual but are often unnecessary. Vaginal retention sutures may stimulate additional straining by the cow.

Amputation of the Prolapsed Uterus

Occasionally, extensive calving or environmental trauma has occurred, necessitating a complete ovario-hysterectomy to attempt salvage of the cow for slaughter. Another indication may be when significant delay in treatment has occurred, allowing time for cervical involution to occur

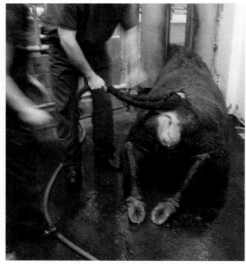

Fig 80-25   Position of cow with "tipped pelvis" to ease reduction of uterine prolapse.

and preventing reduction of the prolapsed uterus. When deciding on amputation, it is important to remember that the uterine broad ligaments and reproductive tract vasculature are contained within the prolapse and abdominal viscera and urinary bladder may also be enclosed. The near uterine wall should be incised carefully and the inner prolapse evaluated for contained viscera and vasculature. Viscera should be repelled into the abdomen. Visualize and ligate large uterine arteries and veins with large (No 3) moistened and doubled catgut suture or umbilical tape.

Differing techniques for removing the uterus have been described. The surgeon may elect to ligate each entire half of the uterus with two complete hemicircumferential or transfixing sutures using umbilical tape, amputate the uterus distal to the sutures, and replace stump into the pelvic canal. A second technique would be to place a series of overlapping interrupted crushing sutures with catgut for hemostasis of the cut surface, followed by a continuous appositional suture pattern to close the lumen. The latter technique is more time consuming but provides more accurate hemostasis and reconstruction. Another described technique is to circumferentially ligate the prolapsed uterus tightly near the vulva with either surgical tubing or broad suture (umbilical tape) and allow the uterus to slough distal to the suture. The uterus should slough within a week to 10 days.

Iatrogenic Uterine Prolapse

Forced extraction of calves and dystocia can result in uterine tears for various reasons. Laparotomy exposure and "blind" one-handed suturing techniques through vaginal access are described elsewhere. One technique for attempting repair of uterine rupture is by manually exteriorizing the uterus to gain visual access of the traumatized area. The cervix must be adequately relaxed for the procedure to be successful, thus limited to within the first few hours (maximum <12 hours) after calving. The cow should be adequately restrained, and surgical instruments and suture material including a uterine support device (see earlier) or clean plastic drape to support the uterus should be available. The repair should be performed as quickly as possible to prevent accumulation of excessive edema. Because most uterine tears are dorsal and just cranial to the cervix, complete uterine prolapse may not be necessary.

Beta$_2$-adrenergic agonist drugs (betamimetics) have historically been used in veterinary medicine to relax the uterus (tocolysis) for procedures such as assisting fetal manipulation during assisted vaginal delivery, as well as providing more complete exteriorization of the uterus during C-section. Examples of these drugs are clenbuterol, isoxsuprine, ritodrine, and epinephrine. Of these pharmaceuticals, only epinephrine is permitted for use in food-producing animals in the United States. A Canadian study indicated successful tocolysis with ritodrine. We are unaware of the availability, cost, or legal limitations with the use of ritodrine in the United States. Personal experience and communication is limited to the use of epinephrine for tocolysis. Epinephrine does have inherent side effects associated with betamimetics such as altering blood pressure, increasing heart rate and myocardial work, and inducing irreversible fatal cardiac arrhythmia. Use as a tocolytic should be weighed on a case-by-case basis and other options considered.

Most commonly, an intravenous dose of 10 ml of 1:1000 epinephrine is used. A dilution with 250 ml of sterile saline administered as a constant rate infusion over 10 minutes has been described. A bolus IV administration with 10 ml of 1:1000 epinephrine diluted in 50 ml of sterile saline has also been successful without adverse effects in our experience. A uterine caruncle, fold of endometrium, or placenta is grasped and steady traction applied to evert the uterus. The surgeon should be patient and not overzealous with traction. As progress is made, the surgeon can advance the grip cranial toward the apex of the uterine horn until the uterus is exteriorized. Difficulty in this procedure arises when the weight of the uterus prevents exposure. It is more successfully done before caudal epidural anesthesia, allowing the cow to aid expulsion through abdominal press. The defect is then repaired and the uterus replaced within the abdomen.

Recommended Readings for Vaginal Prolapse

Mobini S, Heath AM, Pugh DG: Theriogenology of sheep and goats. In Pugh DG, editor: *Sheep and goat medicine*, St Louis, 2002, Saunders, pp 129-186.

Wolfe DF, Carson RL: Surgery of the vestibule, vagina, and cervix: cattle, sheep, and goats. In Wolfe DF, Moll HD, editors: *Large animal urogenital surgery*, Baltimore, 1999, Williams & Wilkins, pp 397-411.

Recommended Readings for Uterine Prolapse

Abdullahi US, Kumi-Diaka J: Prolapse of the nongravid horn in a cow with a seven-month pregnancy: a case report, *Theriogenology* 26:353-356, 1986.

Boileau M, Babkine M, Desrochers A: Effet de la ritodrine sur le myomètre lors de manipulations obstètricales chez la vache, *Med Vet Q* 31:191, 2001.

Carson RL, Wolfe DW: Surgery of the uterus; uterine prolapse. In Wolfe DF, Moll HD, editors: *Large animal urogenital surgery*, Baltimore, 1999, Williams & Wilkins, pp 421-424.

Fubini SL: Surgery of the uterus. In Fubini SL, Ducharme NG, editors: *Farm animal surgery*, Philadelphia, 2004, Saunders, pp 382-390.

Garcia-Seco E, Gill MS, Paccamonti DL: Theriogenology question of the month. Laparotomy to assist replacement of the uterus, *J Am Vet Med Assoc* 219:443-444, 2001.

Gardner IA, Reynolds JP, Risco CA et al: Patterns of uterine prolapse in dairy cows and treatment, *J Am Vet Med Assoc* 197:1021-1024, 1990.

Hopper RM: Surgical correction of abnormalities of genital organs of cows: management of uterine prolapse. In Youngquist RS, Threlfall WR, editors: *Current therapy in large animal theriogenology*, ed 2, Philadelphia, 2007, Saunders, pp 470-471.

Jubb TF, Malmo J, Brightling P et al: Survival and fertility after uterine prolapse in dairy cows, *Aust Vet J* 67:22-24, 1990.

Murphy AM, Dobson H: Predisposition, subsequent fertility, and mortality of cows with uterine prolapse, *Vet Rec* 151:733-735, 2002.

Newman KD, Anderson DE: Cesarean section in cows, *Vet Clin North Am Food Anim Pract* 21:91, 2005.

Roberts SJ: Injuries and diseases of the puperal period, *Vet Obstet Genital Dis (Theriogenology)*.

Youngquist RS: Bovine uterine prolapse, *Theriogenology Handbook* B-3(2/89).

CHAPTER 81

Umbilical Surgery in Calves

D. MICHAEL RINGS and DAVID E. ANDERSON

A variety of publications have addressed the development of neonatal bovine physiology and umbilical changes in the early postpartum period.[1-9] Normal anatomic (embryonic) structures are the urachus, paired umbilical arteries, umbilical vein (paired externally), and external umbilicus. After rupture of the umbilical cord at birth, the urachus, arteries, and umbilical vein normally retract into the abdomen, thus protecting them from environmental contamination. C-sections have a much greater risk of umbilical infection because of clamping or ligation of the umbilical cord, thus preventing normal retraction of the umbilical structures. Several publications have addressed the association of umbilical abnormalities with calf morbidity and mortality.[10-14]

ANATOMY

The umbilicus is a remnant of the fetal-maternal connection. At birth the structure consists of the paired umbilical arteries, a single umbilical vein, and the urachus. Before birth, the umbilical vein serves as the source of oxygenated blood to the fetus via the liver and ductus venosus/portal vein. The paired umbilical arteries are branches of the internal iliac artery and carry waste materials and unoxygenated blood to the placenta. The urachus is the connection from the fetal bladder to the allantoic sac. Following a normal delivery, the smooth muscle that surrounds the umbilicus contracts in response to the stretching of the cord at parturition. Separation of the umbilical cord allows the umbilical arteries and urachus to retract into the abdomen, where they close by smooth muscle contraction.[15] The umbilical vein and remnants of the amniotic membrane remain outside the body wall but rapidly collapse in association with smooth muscle contraction; therefore the umbilicus shrinks and shrivels. The umbilical stalk normally dries and thins out by 3 to 4 days postdelivery. The scabbed over and desiccated umbilical stalk should be totally eliminated by 3 to 4 weeks of age.[16]

As the animal matures, the umbilical vein undergoes fibrosis and becomes the round ligament of the liver suspended in the falciform ligament. The umbilical arteries collapse and become the lateral ligaments of the urinary bladder. The body wall normally closes completely around the umbilical structures within a few days, but occasionally, small openings in the linea alba (<1.2 cm) are palpable for a few months. These most often close spontaneously.

DISEASES

Umbilical abnormalities have been extensively described in the literature and can be divided into three categories: umbilical infection, umbilical hernia, and umbilical hernia with infection.[17-41]

Umbilical Hernias

Among the most common congenital defects in cattle are umbilical hernias, which are seen in all breeds and have been postulated to be related to heritable factors or in association with inflammation of the umbilicus.[42,43] However, many umbilical hernias are secondary to umbilical sepsis. Most owners are willing to "tolerate" umbilical hernias as a side effect of genetic pressures for high lactation production or growth rates (the same may be said to be true for cystic ovaries, poor conformation, dystocia, etc.). Because the issue is clouded, most veterinarians perform herniorrhaphy as a service without extensive discussions about heritability. Hernias are made up of the hernia sac and peritoneum and may contain peritoneal fluid and viscera. Depending on the size of the hernial ring, omentum, the abomasums, intestines, or a combination of these may be inside the sac. Longstanding hernias are more likely to develop adhesions between the abdominal structures and the everted peritoneum. Strangulations occasionally occur,[3] but the greater omentum tends to slide into the hernial sac first, preventing other abdominal viscera from falling in. Large hernias, although more susceptible to external trauma (via scraping the ventrum against the ground) and resulting skin abrasions and superficial infection, seldom cause strangulation. Small hernia rings (<2 cm) rarely cause strangulation because of insufficient room in the body wall opening for more than omentum. Simple umbilical hernias are nonpainful to the affected individual. The

most common viscera involved in umbilical hernias in cattle is the abomasum with or without omentum. Hernias may be small at birth and enlarge with age. These should be differentiated from umbilical sepsis. Simple (or uncomplicated) hernias are easily reducible. Complicated hernias (incarcerated viscera usually without strangulation or concurrent infection of umbilical structures) cannot be completely reduced. Rarely, the viscera may become locally devitalized and rupture to the outside, resulting in an enterocutaneous fistula. Our subjective clinical experience working with cloned dairy calves over the past 2 years suggests that cloned calves may have a greater likelihood of umbilical hernia/infection and that there may be a difference in the holding strength of collagen in the ventral abdominal wall of clones.

Umbilical Infections

Five anatomic types of umbilical infections exist. Most infections are caused by *Actinomyces pyogenes*. *Escherichia coli* is the second most commonly isolated bacteria and is the most likely to cause systemic infection and septic polyarthritis. The risk of septicemia is closely associated with ingestion of colostrum. The quantity of immunoglobulin transferred has been correlated with morbidity, mortality, and performance in calves (Table 81-1). Urachal sepsis is the most common structure infected. *Omphalophlebitis* is infection/inflammation of the umbilical vein and is the second most commonly infected structure. *Omphaloarteritis* refers to infection/inflammation of the umbilical arteries and is the least commonly infected (but this does not mean rare!). *Umbilical abscess* refers to the external umbilicus and is an umbilical mass that is nonreducible. *Navel Ill* refers to septicemia and possibly hematogenous septic polyarthritis ("Joint Ill"). Any of these umbilical infections may lead to this eventually.

Umbilical abscesses can result from inflammation of any of the umbilical structures and, in fact, may be iatrogenic. The practice of dipping navels in strong iodine solutions (i.e., 7%) may create such a degree of inflammation and necrosis that organisms may more easily penetrate the stalk, or the sealing of the umbilical vessels is so complete that minor infections may not be permitted to drain to the outside.[44] Abscessation of these components, singly or in combination, can be totally external to the body wall, both external and internal, or totally internalized. Large external abscesses such as pendulous hernias are susceptible to skin abrasions. Drainage from the umbilical stalk, although confirmation of abscess formation, does not identify which of the umbilical structures is involved. In addition to the presence of drainage from the umbilical stalk, calves affected with omphalitis often suffer from poor performance and recurring fevers and are prone to develop bacteremias/septicemias that may result in joint infections and meningitis. Because the infection can be totally internalized, the umbilicus should be palpated carefully for the presence of increased sensitivity around the navel. Young calves that show signs of abdominal pain, stand with an arched back (urination posture), or show poor performance should have the navel area closely evaluated before excluding "navel ill" as a diagnosis. Stranguria and pollakiuria (passage of

Table 81-1

Correlation Between Quantity of Transferred Immunoglobulin and Calf Morbidity, Mortality, and Performance

Variable	Odds Ratio for Development of "Variable" in Calves with Inadequate IgG (<800 mg/dl)	Odds Ratio for Development of "Variable" in Calves with Inadequate Plasma Protein (<4.8 g/dl)
Preweaning mortality	5.4	
Neonatal morbidity	6.4	
Preweaning morbidity	3.2	
Morbidity		3
Respiratory tract morbidity		3.1
Weaning weight	16-kg lower weaning weight	
Respiratory disease	0.04-kg loss in daily rate of gain	

Modified from Wittum TE, Perino LJ: Am J Vet Res 56:1149-1154, 1995.

small quantities of urine with increased frequency) are most often associated with inflammation or abscessation of the urachus. This inflammation results in a firm fibrous band forming between the tip of the bladder and the body wall that prevents the bladder from voiding totally.

Umbilical Infection with Hernia

Umbilical infection may result in weakening of the adjacent abdominal wall and cause an acquired umbilical hernia (or sepsis and hernia may simply occur concurrently). These are usually partially reducible. Umbilical hernias may be treated using various techniques. Small hernias may respond to digital irritation of the hernia ring one to two times daily until closed. "Hernia belts" to maintain reduction of the hernia for a period of time may be successful in small (<4-cm diameter) hernias. Larger hernias may be treated using hernia clamps or surgical closure. Hernia clamps should be reserved for hernias less than 5 cm diameter. Be absolutely sure that no viscera are adhered to the interior of the sac and no internal umbilical structures are infected. Also, administer a tetanus toxoid vaccine. Surgical closure may be accomplished by inverting the hernia sac, scarifying the hernia ring, and suturing the edges of the ring/sac closed. You must be absolutely sure that no internal umbilical structures are infected and that you do not puncture any viscera with the needle.

SONOGRAPHIC FINDINGS

The surgeon, ideally, should know what structures are involved in any umbilical mass before repair, especially with umbilical masses that are not reducible. Because of the limitations of physical examination including external palpation, sonographic examination of the ventral abdomen is advisable for patients with potentially internalized abscesses.[45] Either a sector scan or linear array probe of 3.5 to 7.5 mHz provides sufficient depth of field to view the umbilical structures adequately.[46] The abdomen must be clipped to give sufficient contact to accurately image the structures. The area from the sternum to the udder should be imaged to evaluate involvement of the umbilical vein (cranially) or the umbilical arteries or urachus (posteriorly). Abdominal scanning is best performed on the standing animal. This allows the weight of the abdominal viscera to push potentially involved structures close to the abdominal wall. Imaging should start at the umbilicus, with the operator scanning from side to side to view what resides within the protruding mass. The use of a standoff pad may aid the operator in better visualizing the contents of pendulous structures. Abscesses appear as granular, echoic, amorphous material within a defined cavity, often surrounded by a dark space, indicating fluid. The operator should visualize the abdominal wall and scan from front to back and side to side to look for openings through the abdominal body wall above the umbilical mass. In instances of urachal abscesses and omphaloarteritis, the bladder may be held down close (within 4 inches) to the umbilical stalk and imaged as a fluid-filled sac with a cord running from the apex of the bladder to the umbilicus. The paired umbilical arteries should atrophy and can be seen only sporadically after 1 week of age. In the normal calf the arteries are found caudal to the apex of the bladder. Dilation of the vessel's lumen supports a diagnosis of umbilical artery abscessation.[46]

PREOPERATIVE PREPARATIONS

Accurate assessment of involved structures allows the surgeon to select the most appropriate type of anesthesia to be used. With urachal, umbilical vein, or umbilical artery abscesses, the intricacy of the surgical dissection likely consumes more time than is routinely provided by simple injectable anesthetic agents. Inhaled anesthetic agents provide greater freedom to the surgeon by providing better patient control for longer periods. Simple umbilical hernias can usually be repaired by an experienced surgeon with either injectable anesthetics or tranquilization and infiltration around the surgical site with a local anesthetic agent (lidocaine, procaine). In all cases, because repair is an elective procedure, the patient should be held off feed for at least 24 hours to minimize the risk of regurgitation and aspiration and bloat. Withholding water before surgery is not recommended. Preoperative antibiotic administration may be helpful in decreasing postoperative incisional abscesses.[47] *Arcanobacterium pyogenes* is frequently isolated from umbilical infections, and antibiotics with the appropriate sensitivity should be selected.[48,49]

SURGICAL PROCEDURES FOR REPAIR OF UMBILICAL HERNIAS

Open herniorrhaphy is the treatment of choice for umbilical hernias. This technique ensures that the hernia is removed and permanently closed, no infected umbilical structures are closed within the abdomen, recurrence of the hernia is minimal, and no viscera are entrapped. You must be sure to remove the hernia ring. This part of the abdominal wall is abnormal and should not be used to anchor sutures.

The ventral abdomen is clipped generously and scrubbed from the sternum to the pubis, and from the left subcutaneous abdominal vein (caudal superficial epigastric vein) to the right subcutaneous abdominal vein. An elliptical incision is made through the skin equal to twice the length of the base of the hernia. The incision should be centered on the hernia sac but kept close to it as the sac passes laterally. This should prevent excessive skin removal that may pose a problem at closure. Conversely, excess skin at closure results in a dependent, pendulous area, leading to possible seroma formation and, perhaps, abscessation. Hemorrhage is controlled, and the connective tissue around the base of the hernial ring is freed from the sac using blunt dissection. This can be accomplished readily using Metzenbaum scissors, placing the tips into the tissue and opening the ends, thereby spreading the tissues apart. Dissection by this method appears to minimize hemorrhage as compared with sharp dissection. This should free the hernia sac and the overlying skin. A 1-inch incision parallel to and on either side of the hernia base is made into the abdomen by elevating the sac and dissecting through the abdominal wall and peritoneum. It is important to enter the abdomen laterally to minimize the risk of hitting abscessing structures that may lie cranially (the umbilical vein) or caudally (the urachus and umbilical arteries). The umbilical area is explored digitally from the peritoneal side to determine involvement of additional structures. If it is determined that no abscesses are present, the incision can be carried around the base of the hernia sac. This should totally free the sac from all structures, but omentum commonly adheres to the base of the hernia and must be loosened or resected so that the sac can be discarded. Any hemorrhage around the incision is controlled, and the surgeon prepares to close the body wall.

Several approaches are used to close the hernial opening including the vest-over-pants method (modified Mayo), vertical mattress, and appositional closure. Vest-over-pants is a descriptive method of depicting how one lateral wall is pulled over the opposite wall. The area around the resected ring should be freed of connective tissues for 1.2 cm so that the linea alba or fascia of the rectus abdominis muscle is exposed. The overlapping or leading edge of the body wall is then tacked down to the exposed fibrous surface so that an adhesion of 0.6 cm or greater width and running the length of the incision may form. A subcutaneous suture pattern is recommended to eliminate dead space between the skin and subcutaneous tissues, where blood and serum tend to accumulate. Remember, this will be the dependent area of the abdomen, so elimination of potential pockets helps prevent likely complications from arising in the postoperative period. Vest-over-pants sutures have been shown to be significantly weaker than appositional closure and result in poorer healing. This technique is no longer advocated based in inferior results compared with appositional closure of the abdominal wall.

The preferred method of closure is to suture the edges into direct apposition. The edges of the hernia ring should be freshened to create a new bed for healing. Simple interrupted sutures or a simple continuous pattern can be used in hernias that close with minimal tension. The use of interrupted, tension-absorbing suture patterns such as the near-far, far-near, and vertical mattress can be used to close fairly large defects.

When prior hernia surgery fails to hold or the defect is too large to allow proper apposition, the use of prosthetic meshes to bridge the defect should be considered. With ventral or ventrolateral body wall defects (other than umbilical hernias and especially in adult animals), the tissue surrounding the hole may not retain sufficient strength to hold sutures under tension and the used of mesh must be considered. Ideally, mesh should maintain its strength over an extended time, become incorporated into the surrounding tissues, and not stimulate adhesions of the viscera to the implant.[50,51] Mesh serves as a template for ingrowth of fibrous tissue across the defect. A number of materials, both natural and manmade, have been investigated including pericardial sac, nylon mosquito screen, polypropylene mesh, Teflon, polytetrafluoroethylene mesh, polyglactin 910 mesh, stainless steel mesh, Dacron-reinforced silicone rubber, and preserved human dura.[47,50,52-56] No single mesh totally fulfills the ideal. Many materials have been found to elicit a strong foreign body response and be extruded from the implantation site, often with evisceration. Others lack holding power over time (absorbable meshes such as polyglactin 910) and allow reherniation.

Prosthetic material should be implanted only into wounds devoid of infection. Because all meshes tend to induce inflammatory reaction at the margins, the presence of an existing infection would hasten the breakdown of suture (and perhaps the mesh) and cause failure. A number of methods of mesh implantation are described: Nelson[57] mentions placement of mesh between the peritoneum and the internal muscle fascia. In this method the hernia sac is dissected from the surrounding overlying tissues but not removed; rather, the sac (hernia sac) is infolded/invaginated into the abdomen and the peritoneum is carefully dissected free from the internal fascia of the rectus abdominis muscle around the ring to allow placement of the mesh across the defect without exposing the viscera to direct contact with the mesh. This method should prevent the adhesion of viscera against the mesh but is time consuming to perform because of the more delicate dissection required for mesh placement. We personally have found it easier to open and remove the hernia sac and place the implant directly against the peritoneal surface. Fortunately, in cattle, the greater omentum serves as a formidable barrier in preventing direct contact between the intestine and the mesh. If adhesions form, they should therefore not involve the intestine and should cause little or no problem for the patient.

The size of the implant should be only slightly larger than the defect; one reference cites the mesh being 2 to 3 cm greater than the diameter of the hernia/defect.[56] When mesh is sutured in place, it should draw the edges of the rim close together and be sufficiently tight that no wrinkles in the mesh are present. One entire side of the mesh may be sutured fast to the ring before preplacing sutures along the opposite margin. Both monofilament absorbable and nonabsorbable suture material can be used to hold the mesh in place. Chromic gut suture has been used, but it lacks the long-term holding power and is less satisfactory than synthetic sutures. Sutures placed into the mesh should be at least 6 mm (0.25 inches) from its edge to prevent unraveling of the mesh as tension is applied. At the discretion of the surgeon, a second layer of mesh can be placed over the external muscular fascia to improve the holding power of the area. The subcutaneous tissues should be closed tightly to prevent edema pockets and to lessen the opportunity for bacterial invasion.

UMBILICAL ARTERY ABSCESSES AND URACHAL ABSCESSES

Umbilical infections may be treated medically or surgically. If medical treatment has not resolved or significantly improved the umbilical infection within 5 days, then surgery is probably indicated. If the calf is overtly sick, the umbilicus should probably be removed as soon as the calf is stabilized. The antibiotic of choice for umbilical infections is penicillin because of the spectrum against *A. pyogenes*, *Actinomyces* sp., and anaerobic organisms. Surgical treatment of umbilical infection involves removal of the umbilicus and all infected structures:

Urachus → resection of the apex of the bladder
Omphaloarteritis → omphalectomy and artery resection
Omphalophlebitis: Stops before liver → omphalectomy with vein resection
Enters liver → umbilical vein marsupialization

The incidence of omphaloarteritis in calves is open to discussion. One author reported it to be among the least commonly infected umbilical structures, whereas another[58] believes it to be frequently involved in navel infections. The distinction between umbilical artery and urachal abscesses is often difficult and of little consequence because of the similar course these structures take toward the bladder. The paired arteries that run from the umbilicus posteriorly to the internal iliac artery course alongside the urinary bladder. Ascending infections of the arteries often incorporate omentum, and the adjacent inflammation may lead to adhesions of the bladder wall to the arteries. Infections of the urachus are also common. Patent urachus, with the flow of urine from the umbilical stump, is seen more commonly in horses than in cattle, but urachal abscesses that restrict bladder emptying frequently or that seem uncomfortable during urination should be examined specifically with a urachal abscess in mind (see section on sonographic findings). Sonographic evidence of involvement of the bladder should cause the surgeon to consider inhalation anesthesia for the superior time this method provides. In addition, the surgical preparation area should be much larger than that normally required for a simple hernia. The entire ventral abdomen back to the mammary gland should be surgically prepared because the total length of the incision cannot always be anticipated before the abdomen is opened. If draining openings are present in the umbilical stalk, these should

be flushed thoroughly (with a weak povidone-iodine solution) and the openings oversown before the final surgical preparation.

A normal elliptical incision is made around the umbilical stalk and the tissues are dissected down to the abdominal wall. As with a hernia, the abdomen is entered lateral to the stalk, a finger is inserted through this opening, and the posterior aspect of the abdomen is explored digitally. A thickened stalk will be felt running toward the pubis. Differentiation of an urachal abscess from an umbilical artery abscess is of little consequence because both run in the same direction. Once the involved structures have been evaluated by digital palpation, the abdominal incision may be extended posteriorly along the linea alba. Abscessed umbilical arteries should be followed until the enlarged portion decreases to a fibrous stalk (usually lateral to the bladder). The stalk should then be double-ligated and transected between the ligatures. The stump should be inspected for drainage before being released into the abdomen.

Urachal abscesses and umbilical arteritis tend to cause more adhesions of the omentum around the inflamed stalk than are usually seen with umbilical vein infections. The surgeon should free this connective tissue from the fibrous stalk(s) carefully to prevent accidentally puncturing the abscess. Quite often, the capsule of a urachal abscess involves the wall of the apex of the bladder or, less frequently, communicates and drains directly into the bladder. The incision through the linea alba must be sufficiently long to allow the best possible exteriorization of the bladder and mass, or purulent material may spill into the abdomen. Resecting the bladder is usually quicker and easier than dissecting the urachus from the bladder wall. Normal urine is a sterile fluid and small-volume spillage into the abdomen should cause no real concern to the surgeon. The mass is removed from the site before closure of the bladder. When suturing the bladder, care is taken to avoid penetration of the mucosa to prevent wicking of urine and early degradation of the suture material. A Lembert or Cushing's pattern works well in the bladder wall. All rents in the omentum created during removal of the abscess should be closed to prevent intestine from adhering to the body wall at the incision site. With potentially infected incision lines, it is best to close the abdomen with as many layers as possible to minimize the risk of early suture breakdown.

UMBILICAL VEIN ABSCESSES

Umbilical vein marsupialization has been described as a one-step or two-step procedure. In the one-step procedure, a ventral midline celiotomy is performed and the infected umbilical vein isolated. The umbilicus is excised and the umbilical vein sutured closed. A sterile glove may be placed over the stump to prevent abdominal contamination. Next, the umbilical vein is marsupialized through a separate 2- to 4-cm incision in a right paramedian location as close to the liver as possible to minimize the length of vein to provide drainage. The vein is sutured to the abdominal wall and skin. The celiotomy incision is closed. As the vein infection resolves, granulation tissue contraction closes the defect in the rectus abdominis muscle such that no hernia forms at the incision site. In the two-step procedure a ventral midline celiotomy is performed and the infected umbilical vein isolated (first step). The umbilicus is moved as far cranially in the incision as possible and the umbilical vein sutured to the cranial aspect of the wound. The vein is sutured to the linea alba and skin. The celiotomy incision is closed. As the vein infection resolves, a defect in the linea alba remains as a small hernia. This hernia is closed at a second surgery to repair the small defect (second step).

The surgical approach for the umbilical vein abscesses is similar to that for an umbilical hernia. The elliptical incision around the umbilical stalk is made as already described and the dissection carried down to the linea. Once the peritoneum has been punctured (lateral to the mass), digital exploration should identify the enlarged vein coursing cranially toward the liver. The incision is extended cranially so that a greater portion of the vein is accessible. In many instances the abscess or enlargement of the vein ends before entering the liver. In these instances the vein is freed from the surrounding tissue by a combination of blunt and sharp dissection, and transfixion sutures are placed through the vein anteriorly to any enlargement. The vein is then severed between the sutures, and the end of the stump to be left in the abdomen is examined for evidence of exudates. If the end is free of infection, the incision can be closed like a simple hernia.

The surgeon occasionally recognizes infection extending into the liver or sufficiently close to the liver's parenchyma that total resection is not achievable. Partial hepatic resection of a single liver abscess can be attempted,[59] but marsupialization of the vein is a more easily accomplished technique to achieve proper drainage of the abscess.[48,60] Two methods have been described: the first involves translocation of the infected, but resected, umbilical vein to a new incision site created lateral to the original incision. A 2- to 3-cm skin incision is made in the right paramedian area, adjacent to the site where the vein enters the liver. A sponge forceps is poked into the abdomen at the new incision site, and the free end of the resected umbilical vein stalk is grasped and pulled back through the incision and sutured snugly to the skin. At least 1 cm of vein should extend beyond the skin margin so that as the vein dries and retracts, the infected stump is not pulled back into the abdomen. The transfixion ligature is then removed to allow drainage. The opening can be lavaged (using a soft, flexible catheter) to remove exudate from the lumen. The biggest drawback to this approach is the potential to carry infection cranially as the umbilical vein is relocated to the new incision site. This risk is minimized by enclosing the tissue in a sterile receptacle (e.g., sterile surgery glove) during transit through the abdomen and passage through the abdominal wall.

The second method described involves carrying the entire infected stalk as far cranially as possible and suturing the vein into the primary incision.[60] This method better limits the risk of spreading infection because the stalk need not be opened until it has been sutured in place. The stalk is severed as in the first method, and the postoperative care is the same. One drawback of this approach is that the infected stalk is left in the primary incision.

Should infection from the stalk invade the incision line, the chance of dehiscence greatly increases. Calves treated in this fashion may require a second surgery to repair the defect left by the marsupialized umbilical vein stalk. This two-step technique is no longer advocated because of the inferior healing results compared with the one-step method and the need for a second surgery to repair the incisional hernia.

Postoperatively, the incision site can be supported by an abdominal wrap. A commercial elastic bandage that allows a large area to be covered and can be reused is available.

References

1. Staller GS, Tulleners EP, Reef VB et al: Concordance of ultrasonographic and physical findings in cattle with an umbilical mass or suspected to have infection of the umbilical cord remnants: 32 cases (1987-1989), *J Am Vet Med Assoc* 206:77-82, 1995.
2. Lischer CJ, Iselin U, Steiner A: Ultrasonographic diagnosis of urachal cyst in three calves, *J Am Vet Med Assoc* 204: 1801-1804, 1995.
3. Watson E, Mahaffey MB, Crowell W et al: Ultrasonography of the umbilical structures in clinically normal calves, *Am J Vet Res* 55:773-780, 1994.
4. Kasari TR: Physiologic mechanisms of adaptation in the fetal calf at birth, *Vet Clin North Am Food Anim Pract* 10:127-136, 1994.
5. Anderson DE, Cornwell D, Anderson LS et al: Comparative analyses of peritoneal fluid from calves and adult cattle, *Am J Vet Res* 56:973-976, 1995.
6. Lischer CJ, Steiner A: Ultrasonography of the umbilicus in calves. Part 2: Ultrasonography, diagnosis and treatment of umbilical diseases, *Schweiz Arch Tierheilkd* 136:227-241, 1994.
7. Lischer CJ, Steiner A: Ultrasonography of umbilical structures in calves. Part I: Ultrasonographic description of umbilical involution in clinically healthy calves, *Schweiz Arch Tierheilkd* 135:221-230, 1993.
8. Steiner A, Fluckiger M, Oertle C et al: Urachal disorders in calves: clinical and sonographic findings, therapy and prognosis, *Schweiz Arch Tierheilkd* 132:187-195, 1990.
9. Flock M: Ultrasonic diagnosis of inflammation of the umbilical cord structures, persistent urachus and umbilical hernia in calves, *Berl Munch Tierarztl Wochenschr* 116:2-11, 2003.
10. Donovan GA, Dohoo IR, Montgomery DM et al: Calf and disease factors affecting growth in female Holstein calves in Florida, USA, *Prev Vet Med* 33:1-10, 1998.
11. Virtala AM, Mechor GD, Gröhn YT, Erb HN: Morbidity from nonrespiratory diseases and mortality in dairy heifers during the first three months of life, *J Am Vet Med Assoc* 208:2043-2046. 1996.
12. Virtala AM, Mechor GD, Grohn YT et al: The effect of calfhood diseases on growth of female dairy calves during the first 3 months of life in New York State, *J Dairy Sci* 79:1040-1049, 1996.
13. Muniz RA, Anziani OS, Ordonez J et al: Efficacy of doramectin in the protection of neonatal calves and post-parturient cows against field strikes of, *Cochliomyia hominivorax*, *Vet Parasitol* 58:155-161, 1995.
14. Curtis PE: A knackery survey of calf disease, *Vet Rec* 86: 454-456, 1970.
15. Norden DM, deLahunta A: Umbilical venous system. In *The embryology of domestic animals*, Baltimore, 1985, Williams & Wilkins, pp 220, 259.

16. Stober M: Procedure for clinical examination. In Rosenberger G, editor: *Clinical examination of cattle*, Philadelphia, 1979, Saunders.

17. Boure L, Foster RA, Palmer M et al: Use of an endoscopic suturing device for laparoscopic resection of the apex of the bladder and umbilical structures in normal neonatal calves, *Vet Surg* 30:319-326, 2001.

18. Lopez MJ, Markel MD: Umbilical artery marsupialization in a calf, *Can Vet J* 37:170-171, 1996.

19. Lewis CA, Constable PD, Huhn JC et al: Sedation with xylazine and lumbosacral epidural administration of lidocaine and xylazine for umbilical surgery in calves, *J Am Vet Med Assoc* 214:89-95, 1999.

20. Rings DM: Umbilical hernias, umbilical abscesses, and urachal fistulas. Surgical considerations, *Vet Clin North Am Food Anim Pract* 11:137-148, 1995.

21. Kumper H: New therapy for acute abomasal tympany in calves, *Tierarztl Prax* 22:25-27, 1994.

22. Baxter GM, Zamos DT, Mueller PO: Uroperitoneum attributable to ruptured urachus in a yearling bull, *J Am Vet Med Assoc* 200:517-520, 1992.

23. Mee JF: Navel ill, *Vet Rec* 126:341, 1990.

24. Shearer AG: Internal navel abscesses in calves, *Vet Rec* 118:480-481, 1986.

25. Hylton WE, Trent AM: Congenital urethral obstruction, uroperitoneum, and omphalitis in a calf, *J Am Vet Med Assoc* 190:433-434, 1987.

26. Brodrick TW: Internal navel abscesses, *Vet Rec* 118:620, 1986.

27. Mbassa G: Diffuse gangrene of the hindlimb associated with umbilicus infection in a calf, *Vet Rec* 116:662, 1985.

28. Clemente CH: Drainage: a possible treatment method in ascending umbilical abscess in calves, *Tierarztl Prax* 13:159-161, 1985.

29. Trent AM, Smith DF: Surgical management of umbilical masses with associated umbilical cord remnant infections in calves, *J Am Vet Med Assoc* 185:1531-1534, 1984.

30. Fubini SL, Smith DF: Umbilical hernia with abomasal-umbilical fistula in a calf, *J Am Vet Med Assoc* 184:1510-1511, 1984.

31. Rotimi VO, Duerden BI: The development of the bacterial flora in normal neonates, *J Med Microbiol* 14:51-62, 1981.

32. Dirksen G, Hofmann W: Experiences with surgical treatment of ascending umbilical infections in calf, *Tierarztl Prax* 4:177-184, 1976.

33. Esiutin AV, Girin VA: Prevention and treatment of omphalitis in calves, *Veterinariia* Oct:90-2, 1975.

34. Mesaric M, Modic T: Strangulation of the small intestine in a cow by a persistent urachal remnant, *Vet Rec* 153:688-689, 2003.

35. Starost MF: Haemophilus somnus isolated from a urachal abscess in a calf, *Vet Pathol* 38:547-548, 2001.

36. Hassel DM, Tyler JW, Tucker RL et al: Clinical vignette: urachal abscess and cystitis in a calf, *J Vet Intern Med* 9:286-288, 1995.

37. Hooper RN, Taylor TS: Urinary surgery, *Vet Clin North Am Food Anim Pract* 11:95-121, 1995.

38. Rijkenhuizen AB, Sickmann HG: Incarcerated umbilical hernia with enterocutaneous fistula in a calf, *Tijdschr Diergeneeskd* 120:8-10, 1995.

39. Hunt RJ, Allen D Jr: Treatment of patent urachus associated with a congenital imperforate urethra in a calf, *Cornell Vet* 79:157-160, 1989.

40. Trent AM, Smith DF: Pollakiuria due to urachal abscesses in two heifers, *J Am Vet Med Assoc* 184:984-986, 1984.

41. Smart ME, Ferguson JG, Vaillancourt D: Sequela to a urachal abscess in a Hereford heifer (a case report), *Vet Med Small Anim Clin* 73:1557-1558, 1978.

42. Muller W, Schlegel F, Haase H et al: Congenital umbilical hernia in the calf (Zum angeborenen Nabelbruch beim Kalb), *Monatschefte fur Veterinarmedizin* 43:161-163, 1988.

43. Trent AM: Surgical management of umbilical masses in calves, *Bovine Pract* 22:170-173, 1987.

44. Baxter GM: Umbilical masses in calves: diagnosis, treatment and complications, *Compend Contin Educ Pract Vet* 11:505-513, 1989.

45. Taguchi K, Ishida O, Suzuki T et al: Surgical management of umbilical infection in calves, *J Jap Vet Med Assoc* 43:793-797, 1990.

46. Lischer CJ, Steiner A: Ultrasonography of umbilical structures in calves. Part 1: Ultrasonographic description of umbilical involution in clinically healthy calves, *Schweiz Arch Tierheilk* 135:221-230, 1993.

47. Klein WR, Firth EC: Infection rates in clean surgical procedures with and without prophylactic antibiotics, *Vet Rec* 123:542-543, 1988.

48. Smith DF: Clinical assessment and surgical management of umbilical masses in calves, *Bovine Pract* 20:82-84, 1985.

49. Steiner A, Fluckiger M, Oertle C et al: Urachuserkeankungen beim Kalb: Klinische und Sonographische befunde Sowie Therapie und Prognose, *Schweiz Arch Tierheilk* 132:187-195, 1990.

50. Jenkins SD, Klamer TW, Parteka JJ et al: A comparison of prosthetic materials used to repair abdominal wall defects, *Surgery* 94:392-398, 1983.

51. Santora TA, Roslyn JJ: Incisional hernia, *Surg Clin North Am* 73:557-570, 1993.

52. Becker M, Kaegi B, Waxenberger M: Bovines Perikard Eine Bioprothese fur den Verschluss von Bauchdeckendefekten beim Kalk, *Schweiz Arch Tierheil* 127:379-383, 1985.

53. Sen TB, Paul MK: Further studies on the use of nylon mosquito net mesh in hernioplasty in bovine, *Indian J Animal Health* 28:65-66, 1989.

54. Hylton WE, Rousseauz CG: Intestinal strangulation associated with omphaloarteritis in a calf, *J Am Vet Med Assoc* 186:1099, 1985.

55. Lamb JP, Vitale T, Kaminski DL: Comparative evaluation of synthetic meshes used for abdominal wall replacement, *Surgery* 93:643-648, 1983.

56. Kanade MG, Kumar R, Kumar A: Mechanical evaluation of healing of abdominal defects repaired by stainless steel, nylon, and cotton mesh in bovine, *Indian Vet J* 67:47-50, 1990.

57. Nelson DR: The abdominal wall. In Oehme FW, editor: *Textbook of large animal surgery*, Baltimore, 1988, Williams & Wilkins, pp 383-398.

58. Hull BL: Personal communication, 1994.

59. Parker JE, Gaughan EM: Partial hepatic resection for the treatment of a single liver abscess in a dairy heifer, *Vet Surg* 17:87-89, 1988.

60. Steiner A, Lischer CJ, Oertle C: Marsupialization of umbilical vein abscesses with involvement of the liver in 13 calves, *Vet Surg* 22:184-189, 1993.

CHAPTER 82

Diagnosis and Management of Teat Injury

SYLVAIN NICHOLS

Teat injuries are common in dairy cattle and, compared with other frequently occurring diseases, these injuries often result in premature culling of affected cows.[1,2] High milk production and udder conformation of modern cows are likely the main contributing factors to this problem. From calving to the peak of lactation, the enlarged udder exposes the teats to various traumas. Most are self-inflicted when the cow tries to get up. The risk of teat trauma is increased by improper housing of animals; small pens and overcrowded barns predispose teats to injuries. To maintain milk production at its highest level, the cows need to have a healthy udder. Teat surgery can be performed to suture teat lacerations, restore normal milk flow, and keep the normal anatomic shape of the udder.

The clinical manifestations of teat lesions are variable but can be defined in two categories: external (uncovered) (Fig. 82-1) and internal (covered) (Fig. 82-2) lesions. Laceration of the teat wall with or without milk leakage from the wound is classified as an external lesion. This type of lesion requires early surgery to achieve good results.[3] Internal lesions are more common and are defined as swelling and fibrosis of the teat cistern or the papillary duct. Cows with internal lesions become increasingly difficult to milk and are more susceptible to mastitis. Depending on the location of the lesion, a thelotomy or theloscopy may have to be performed to restore normal milk flow. Successful teat surgery requires atraumatic tissue handling, appropriate hemostasis, and reconstruction of the tissue incised or traumatized. If those principles are not followed, fibrosis of the teat, dehiscence of the incision, fistula formation, and mastitis will result, compromising milk production of the quarter and limiting survival of the cow in the herd.

This chapter reviews and presents new diagnostic tools available to practitioners to evaluate teat injury and milk flow disturbance. Following the evaluation section, each type of injury is presented and classified. Surgical and medical principles to approach each problem are presented. Finally, a prognosis for each condition is given to help practitioners in the decision process of culling the animal, doing on-farm surgery, or referring the case to a specialized hospital.

TEAT EVALUATION

Evaluation of cows having teat injury must be thorough including visual examination, palpation, California Mastitis Test (CMT), ultrasonography, microbial culture, and milk outflow evaluation. A complete history should be obtained from the farmer before examination of the cow to detect any herd problems (housing, conformation or vacuum problems) that could be contributing to teat injuries. The examination begins with visual examination of the udder looking for asymmetry, laceration, and swollen or empty teats. This is followed by palpation of the gland and teat, and signs of inflammation should be noticed. Based on clinical findings and CMT, milk samples of affected glands are submitted for bacterial culture. Milk

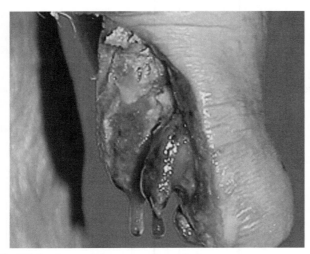

Fig 82-1 External (uncovered) teat lesion.

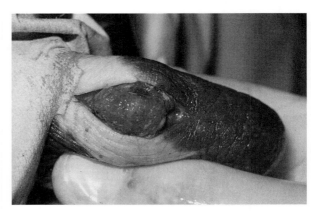

Fig 82-2 Thelotomy incision exposing a large teat spider. This type of lesion is classified as an internal (covered) lesion.

outflow is evaluated while doing the CMT. Palpation and milking should be done cautiously if the teat is lacerated. By rolling the teat between the fingers, a mass or a swollen area can be localized. The palpation is followed by introduction of a teat probe into the streak canal and teat cistern to determine patency of the canal. Care must be taken with streak canal traumas not to further damage the mucosa by the introduction of the probe. By rotating the probe around the teat mucosa, a focal defect (fibrosis or teat spider) can be localized.

The length of the streak canal can be evaluated with a special graduated probe (Dr. Fritz LLC, Louisville, Ky.) (Fig. 82-3). An increased length of the canal could be indicative of distal end injury. In a study done by Geishauser,[4] many false positives were found when the diagnosis of distal teat injury was based only on the measurement of the streak canal length. Normal streak canal averaged 8 mm in length.[3,4]

Ultrasonography has been used to evaluate milk outflow problems in recent years.[5,6] A 5- to 10-MHz linear probe is used to visualize the streak canal, teat cistern, and gland cistern. The longitudinal view allows an overview of the teat with specific relation among the annular ring, teat cistern, and teat end. It is used specifically to evaluate the distal end of the teat (Fig. 82-4). The transverse view may be more useful to localize specific lesions like a mass within the cistern or fibrosis of the annular ring area. The contralateral teat, if normal, can be used as a control. When a cow is evaluated for outflow problems, it is important to evaluate the dimension of the gland cistern with sonography before surgery. After calving, a large gland cistern filled with homogeneous hyperechoic fluid compatible with milk should be visualized. The diameter of the cistern should be compared with the contralateral quarter. Without ultrasound, it can be difficult to evaluate the quarter for presence of milk. With palpation, the edema present after calving may give the false impression of an engorged quarter. If no milk is detected by ultrasound in the gland cistern, surgery will be unrewarding.

Before the use of ultrasonography, contrast and double-contrast radiography were commonly used techniques to assess milk outflow problems.[3,7] Filling capacity of the teat and glandular cisterns, as well as anatomic disorders, can be evaluated. The double-contrast technique helps to detect irregularities around the rosette of Furstenberg or within the teat cistern. The correlation between the radiologic findings and surgical findings for distal teat lesions is around 63%.[8] Contrast radiography can be useful to localize a proximal lesion or evaluate the dimension of an accessory gland. Radiographic techniques are less useful for teat lesions located in the mid to proximal teat cistern and are no more sensitive than other imaging techniques for distal teat injuries.[3] Udder conformation and teat position (hind vs. rear quarter) are factors complicating radiographic evaluation. The technique consists of aseptic infusion of a contrast product (50% diatrizoate sodium solution) in the affected teat. If a double-contrast study is performed, a teat clamp is placed at the teat-gland junction before the injection of the contrast product. The product is drained from the teat and the teat is inflated with air before the radiograph is taken. The cassette is placed in between the quarters to avoid superimposition of the teats.

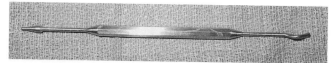

Fig 82-3 Teat probe (Dr. Fritz, Louisville, Ky.) used to measure the length of the streak canal. A 3-mm scale is present at both ends of the probe.

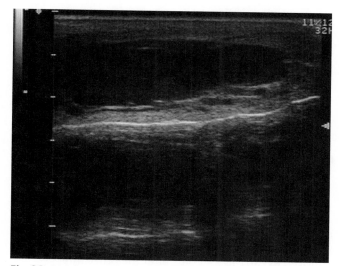

Fig 82-4 Ultrasound evaluation of the teat (longitudinal view).

In the past decade, teat endoscopy (theloscopy) has been developed.[9-11] This procedure allows direct visualization of lesions located at the distal aspect of the teat cistern. It can be used for diagnostic purposes or to treat specific lesions. The theloscope can be introduced from the streak canal for axial and proximal evaluation (Fig. 82-5) of the teat or from the lateral wall for lateral and distal evaluation of the teat (Fig. 82-6). In slaughtered cows, 70% of all teat injuries were located around the Furstenberg area or the streak canal (50% of the case had inversion of the streak canal in the gland cistern).[9] Theloscopy can be done with the cow in a standing position or in lateral recumbency with light sedation and local infiltration of anesthetic solution. A specially designed teat clamp (Dr. Fritz LLC, Louisville, Ky.), a Doyen forceps, or an elastrator band is applied proximal at the teat-gland interface. A teat cannula is inserted to allow lavage of the teat cistern. Lavage is performed with sterile saline until the solution becomes clear. A blunt trocar and its theloscopic sheath are inserted through the streak canal. With a narrow streak canal, it may be necessary to enlarge the canal using Hug's lancet knife. The trocar is replaced by the theloscope and the teat is inflated with air. The proximal and mid portions of the teat are evaluated (see Fig. 82-5). Evaluation of the distal teat is performed by introduction of a sharp trocar through the streak canal and the lateral wall of the teat. The theloscopic sheet is slid over the end of the trocar and the trocar is replaced by the theloscope. The teat is inflated with air and the theloscope is directed downward to visualize the rosette of Furstenberg (see Fig. 82-6). After evaluation,

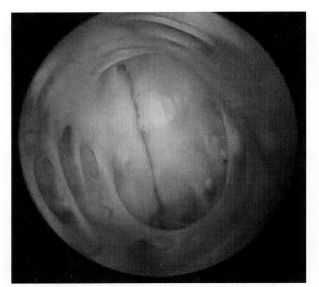

Fig 82-5   Axial theloscopy. The theloscope is entered from the streak canal and is looking at the proximal aspect of the teat cistern.

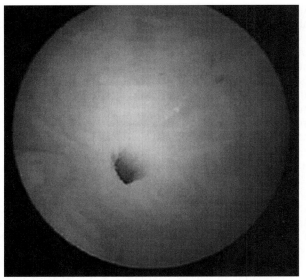

Fig 82-6   Lateral theloscopy. The theloscope is inserted from the lateral wall of the teat and is looking at the distal aspect of the teat (rosette of Furstenberg).

the lateral port is closed with a single cruciate stitch and a bandage is applied around the teat. The stitch can be removed as early as 24 hours after the procedure.

TEAT INJURY AND SURGERY

External (a.k.a. Uncovered) Lesions

Teat injuries can be divided in two categories: external or "uncovered" lesions and internal or "covered" lesions. The uncovered lesions include lacerations with an external wound visible on the teat (see Fig. 82-1). The lacerations are divided in subcategories that are important to consider before posing a prognosis. A laceration can be classified as being partial thickness (skin to submucosa) or full thickness (skin to mucosa with milk leaking out of the incision). With full-thickness lesions, the defense mechanisms of the teat against mastitis are compromised and the cow has a higher risk of developing mastitis. Prompt surgical reconstruction of the injured tissue is necessary to protect the quarter against environmental pathogens.[12] In teats with incomplete lacerations (when the integrity of the teat cistern has not been compromised), surgical intervention may not be necessary. In that situation, secondary healing by medical management of the wound can be sufficient. However, contraction of the tissue during healing can change the alignment of the teat creating problems during machine milking. With show cows, reconstructive surgery of the teat is necessary to obtain cosmetic outcome.

Lacerations can also be categorized as acute or chronic (>12 hours old). Surgical intervention on the teat is best performed during the first 12 hours following the injury. Later, swelling of the teat can be too severe to permit adequate reconstruction of the tissue. These injuries benefit from medical therapy (hydrotherapy and nonsteroidal anti-inflammatory drugs [NSAIDs]) before attempting primary closure of the defect (delayed first-intention healing).

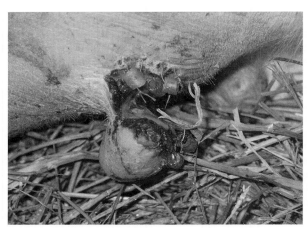

Fig 82-7   Dehisced transverse laceration that was fixed using rubber tubing as a stent between mattress sutures.

Finally, lacerations can be classified according to configuration and location on the teat. Because of the orientation of the teat's vasculature, a transverse laceration (Fig. 82-7) is regarded as having a poorer prognosis compared with a longitudinal laceration. Many blood vessels are transected by a transverse laceration, and this could lead to sloughing of the injured tissue or avascular necrosis of the distal end of the teat. Distal injuries involving the streak canal are also regarded as having a poor prognosis. Reconstruction of the streak canal is difficult and can cause partial or complete milk flow obstruction. Distal injuries may also lead to avascular necrosis of the distal end of the teat.

Surgery on a teat to repair a laceration is considered a contaminated procedure. The surgery is best performed under sedation (xylazine 0.05 mg/kg IV) and local anesthesia[13] (lidocaine 2% as a ring block, V block, or local intravenous perfusion) with the patient standing or in lateral or dorsal recumbency depending on the orientation, severity, and localization of the wound. After adequate surgical preparation, the wound is carefully débrided and lavaged. Care should be taken to reconstruct the mucosa and submucosa. Wounds with irregular edges should be sutured with a simple interrupted suture pattern. With a linear configuration, a simple continuous pattern produces the best results. Synthetic, absorbable monofilament suture of size 3.0 or 4.0 mounted on a swedged-on atraumatic needle should be used. Teat incisions are expected to heal during a period of 21 days.[14] A recent in vitro study demonstrated an increased degradation rate of poliglecaprone 25 (Monocryl, Ethicon, Inc., Cincinnati) and polyglycolic acid (Dexon II, Ethicon, Inc., Cincinnati) after incubation in milk and bacteria-contaminated milk.[15] Poliglecaprone lost all tensile strength within 14 days and polyglycolic acid lost all tensile strength within 21 days after incubation. According to this study, polydioxanone (PDS II, Ethicon, Inc., Cincinnati) was the ideal suture to use in the face of milk degradation because it retained tensile properties for more than 21 days. The subcutaneous layer should be closed in a simple continuous pattern with 4.0 synthetic, absorbable suture material. The skin should be carefully apposed with 2.0 synthetic, nonabsorbable monofilament suture material using a simple interrupted pattern. Care should be taken to leave the skin sutures slightly loose because swelling is expected at the surgery site. When severe postoperative edema is suspected (transverse and/or chronic laceration), mattress suture and stent (see Fig. 82-7) can be used to decrease the risk of wound dehiscence. The wound is protected with a teat bandage and the quarter is treated appropriately for mastitis.

NSAIDs (flunixin meglumine 1 mg/kg IV, sid for 3 days) and antimicrobials (procaine penicillin 22,000 IU/kg IM bid for 3 days) should be given postoperatively. Depending on the severity of the lesion, the milking machine may or may not be used at the following milking. A larger teat cup is recommended if a machine milking is used. Hand milking should be avoided because it is associated with wound dehiscence. The skin sutures are removed 9 days after the surgery. If the sutures are left in place longer, excessive fibrosis and suture tract infection will occur.[3] Complications following surgical reconstruction of a teat laceration are wound dehiscence (see Fig. 82-7), fistula formation, mural abscess, teat cistern fibrosis, and mastitis. If a fistula is formed, surgery can be performed later to close the teat cistern.

Different suture patterns have been tested (Gambee, continuous two layers, and separated two layers). However, the best healing was achieved by using the three-layer technique described earlier.[16] Tissue adhesives have also been used with some success in teat surgery.[14,17] When used in combination with sutures between layers, severe inflammation was created. The adhesive needs to slough out of the tissue at some point during the healing to avoid prolonged or excessive foreign body reaction. Failure of reconstruction with tissue adhesive is usually catastrophic and results in complete dehiscence of the incision.

In cases of catastrophic distal injury, teat reconstruction by supernumerary teat auto-transplantation has been described.[18] After complete transection of the injured teat,

a nearby supernumerary teat was partially transected, leaving a portion of the skin and muscular layer intact. The proximal mucosa of the injured teat was sutured to the distal mucosa of the supernumerary teat with 4.0 polyglactin 910 (Vicryl, Ethicon, Inc.) with a simple continuous pattern. The submucosa/muscular layers were sutured with 4.0 polyglactin 910 in a simple continuous pattern except for the attached portion. The teat was bandaged for 14 days with a teat cannula left in the teat cistern. At day 14, the attached portion was gradually incised. Approximately one third of the portion was incised every 2 days to avoid necrosis of the transplanted end. On day 18, when the transplantation was completed, the donor site was closed.

Internal (Covered) Lesions

The second type of teat injury is the internal or "covered" lesion, defined as a partial or total obstruction of milk flow at any level of the mammary gland without loss of the skin integrity. Ducharme (1987) described five types of covered teat injuries requiring extensive surgery.[8] At that time, distal teat injuries were not included in his classification. Distal teat injuries are discussed later in this section.

Type I Lesions

The first type of teat lesion is a focal teat cistern obstruction involving less than 30% of the mucosal surface of the cistern.[8] This type of obstruction is also termed a *teat spider*.[19] The specific lesions referred to as teat spiders are defined as a mass (scar tissue or neoplasia) protruding from the mucosal surface into the teat cistern. The mass can be transmural or pedunculated. In the last case, it is often possible to remove the mass through the streak canal with the help of alligator forceps. When the mass is transmural, curetting the mass from the streak canal has been attempted. Poor success rates were obtained with this technique because the specialized vascularization of the teat resulted in transmural bleeding at the surgical site and the exposed submucosa was expected to cause excessive scar tissue formation, leading to the teat cistern becoming obstructed again. Better success was obtained in Ducharme's study when a thelotomy and primary closure of the mucosa were performed after resection of the mass. One month after surgical removal of the obstruction, 77% of the cows were still milking. Today, theloscopy can be used in selective cases to remove small lesions precisely without extensive surgical incision.[20,21]

Type II Lesions

The second type of teat lesion is a diffuse teat cistern obstruction involving more than 30% of the teat cistern mucosa (see Fig. 82-2).[8] A surgical approach similar to the one described for type I lesions is necessary to remove the obstructive tissue. Because of the large size of the lesion, primary closure of the teat mucosa is frequently not possible. In those cases, a teat implant will be necessary to keep the teat functional. Implant properties and types are discussed later in this section. In Ducharme's study, 75% of the cows were milking 1 month following surgery for a type II obstruction. Clinicians often classify type I and type II lesions as similar lesions and refer to both as "teat spiders." These lesions are most often caused by external trauma creating bruising at the level of the mucosa with secondary submucosal hemorrhage leading to excessive granulation tissue formation.

Type III Lesions

The third type of teat lesion is a membranous or fibrous structure separating the gland cistern from the teat cistern.[8] This obstruction can be congenital or acquired. Cows that are affected by ongoing mastitis at the time of dry-off at the end of a lactation period may develop this type of lesion. These lesions become apparent when the cow "freshens" again (e.g., starts lactating after parturition). When a thin membranous-like structure forms at the level of the annular ring, a sharp, pointed bistoury can be introduced through a thelotomy incision to create a large X-shaped incision in the membrane. Care must be taken to avoid cutting into the annular ring in order to avoid hemorrhage and hematoma formation. Active milking is necessary to prevent reobstruction. However, a fibrous structure (≥5 mm in thickness) forms more commonly than membranous structures. In this situation, resection of the fibrous structure via a thelotomy incision and implantation of a silicone implant will be necessary to avoid recurrence of the obstruction (Fig. 82-8). In Ducharme's study, 37% of the cows with a proximal obstruction at the level of the annular ring were still milking a month after the surgery.

Type IV Lesions

The fourth type of teat lesion is a stenosis, or obliteration of the gland and teat cistern.[8] This category includes the syndrome called *congenital obstruction of the teat cistern* (Fig. 82-9). The etiology of this condition is uncertain, but it has been speculated that mastitis secondary to suckling by another calf at a young age could be the predisposing factor.[3] Surgery in these cases is rarely rewarding. Presence of some normal mucosa at the distal and proximal aspect of the teat is necessary to achieve a successful surgical outcome. If little milk is obtained from the gland after removal of the scar tissue, the prognosis is poor to grave. The use of an implant is necessary in affected cows to preserve the patency of the canal during the healing phase. In Ducharme's study, 30% of the cows with a type IV lesion were still milking a month after the surgery.

Type V Lesions

The fifth type of teat lesion is a teat fistula, or webbed teat. In the case of a fistula, an elliptic incision is made around the opening on the longitudinal plane of the teat. The soft tissue and the mucosa are dissected and resected. The teat mucosa is then closed. A webbed teat is a supernumerary teat attached to the side of the teat. It may be visible as a swelling or an opening (like a fistula) on the side of the teat. In this case it is important to assess the milk production of the supernumerary teat. This can be achieved by cannulating the accessory teat or by using positive contrast radiography to evaluate the dimension of the accessory quarter. For this reason, it is better to evaluate and treat webbed teat when the animal is in lactation. If the production is minimal, the webbed teat is resected like a fistula. If the accessory gland produces a significant amount of milk, the supernumerary teat cistern can be

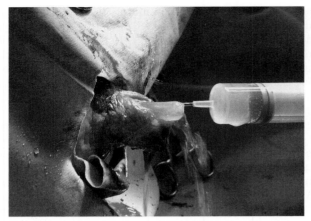

Fig 82-8 Insertion of a silicone implant in a teat with fibrosis at the teat cistern and gland cistern junction (type III lesion).

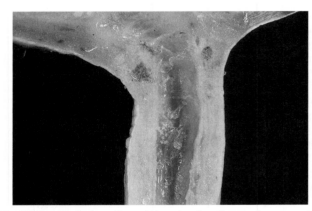

Fig 82-9 Sagittal section of the gland and teat of a cow with congenital atresia of both cisterns. Performing surgery in this case will be unrewarding because no milk is produced by the quarter.

anastomosed to the primary teat canal.[22] Milk culture should be performed before anastomosing the supernumerary teat cistern to the main cistern. In Ducharme's study, 83% of the cows were milking 1 month following surgery for type V lesions.

Distal Teat Injury

Lesions involving the streak canal or rosette of Furstenberg are frequently found. In an abattoir study, the prevalence of lesions of the distal teat was approximately 70% among culled dairy cows slaughtered for milk outflow problems.[9] These types of injury can be secondary to trauma, improper cannulation techniques, or repeated cannulation of the teat. Frequently, no lesion can be palpated at the time of examination of the teat. The farmer will report an increased milking time for that quarter. The cow is then qualified as a slow or "hard milker." Lesions at this level will predispose the cow to mastitis. The most frequent lesions seen are fibrosis of the Furstenberg rosette (Fig. 82-10), partial disruption of the streak canal, or complete disruption and inversion of the streak canal

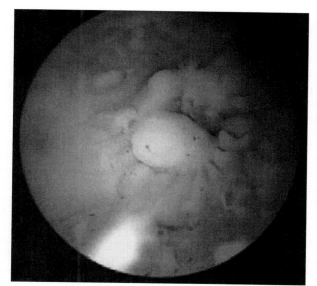

Fig 82-10 Fibrosis around the rosette of Furstenberg (most frequent lesion found in cow culled for reason related to the udder).

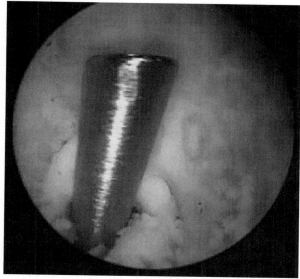

Fig 82-11 Theloscopic triangulation. The theloscope was entered from the lateral wall, and the Eisenhut stenosis remover was entered from the streak canal to remove the obstruction involving the rosette of Furstenberg.

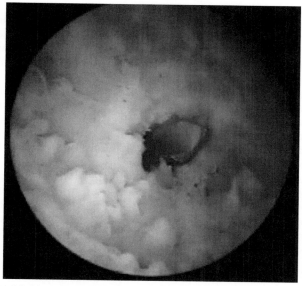

Fig 82-12 Rosette of Furstenberg after theloscopic removal of the obstruction.

into the teat cistern.[23] In 1987 Ducharme did not include this type of lesion in his classification because management of those obstructions did not require invasive (e.g., thelotomy) surgery. At present, most of those injuries are still managed blindly, using a curette and specialized knives. Recently, theloscopic examination and treatment of these lesions has allowed for specific surgery with direct viewing of the surgeon, resulting in improved outcome in lactating dairy cows.

In the acute phase of the injury, medical therapy ($2 \times 3 = 2$ periods of 3 days of rest) should be used before theloscopic evaluation and surgery. The milking should be stopped, and a natural teat insert (slow dissolving wax implant) (Keratelin, Dr. Fritz LLC, Louisville, Ky.) should be introduced in the streak canal for 3 days. After the third day, the quarter is milked with a teat cannula. Another insert is then introduced in the streak canal for another 3 days. On day 6 of treatment, the teat flow is evaluated. If the quarter is still hard to milk, theloscopic evaluation and surgery should be considered.

In the late 1980s, Tulleners described for the first time in North America the use of endoscopy to evaluate covered teat injury.[24] He used a 4-mm arthroscope inserted through a 5-mm self-locking sleeve to evaluate the teat and gland cistern from the streak canal. The technique was quick and easy to perform, but more than 50% of the cows developed mastitis and had lesions affecting the streak canal following the endoscopic evaluation. The technique was abandoned until new instrumentations (2-mm theloscope, Dr. Fritz LLC, Louisville, Ky.) were developed in the mid 1990s. At this time, theloscopy was not only a diagnostic tool but also a minimally invasive surgical tool to treat distal teat injuries.[9-11] When the theloscope is inserted through the lateral wall of the teat, distal teat lesions can be visualized and removed by an instrument entered from the streak canal (Figs. 82-11 and 82-12). This procedure, termed *theloscopic*

triangulation, allows accurate removal of the obstructive tissue and complete evaluation of the teat cistern. When the procedure is finished, the lateral port is closed with a single interrupted suture (2.0 monofilament, nonabsorbable suture material). The suture can be removed as early as 24 hours after the surgery. Milk from the quarter is passively drained using a cannula and mammary antibiotics are infused into the quarter to prevent or treat mastitis. A natural teat insert is introduced through the streak canal and the teat is bandaged to avoid losing the insert.[25] For surgical interventions performed around the streak canal or rosette of Furstenberg, a 3×3 (3 periods of 3 days without milking the affected quarter) convalescence treatment should be done to allow healing of the streak canal. The treated teat is milked with a cannula every 3 days for 9 days. Between milking, a natural teat insert is left in place. If mastitis is present, the quarter will have to be milked more often, but only with a teat cannula. No milking with the machine is allowed before day 9. This protocol is important in the success of the technique.[3] Without appropriate rest, the streak canal will heal with excessive granulation tissue that may lead to reobstruction of the quarter. If only diagnostic theloscopy is performed, milking with the machine can be resumed at the following milking.

A specialized theloscope has been designed to remove distal teat lesions in a procedure called *theloresectoscopy*.[20] The theloresectoscope consists of a wire snare, connected to an electrosurgical unit for monopolar cutting, mounted on an endoscope. The major advantage of using this technique over the standard theloscopic triangulation is that a cautery excision causes less bleeding than a sharp resection.[3] Better hemostasis is thought to decrease the chance of reobstruction and adhesion formation at the surgery site. The theloresectoscope allows the manipulator to perform the procedure without any extra help (theloscopic triangulation necessitates an assistant to hold the scope during removal of the lesion from the streak canal).[11] However, theloresectoscopy is more difficult to perform and the unit is more expensive. Improper setup on the cautery unit can damage the teat. Also, smoke created when working from the streak canal rapidly obstructs the surgical view and venting is necessary to provide a clear view. Finally, it is difficult to clean the wire snare without breaking the fine copper filament.

A retrospective study evaluating the short-term and long-term prognosis of theloscopic surgery versus thelotomy for treatment of distal teat obstructions showed that on the fourth milking, the milk flow improved significantly for the theloscopic group.[26] Fewer postoperative manipulations (cutting the sphincter end) were necessary in the theloscopic group. The hospitalization time and convalescence time were also shorter for the theloscopic group. However, no differences were found for the long-term prognosis or the frequency of mastitis between both groups.

One retrospective study showed that teats with a distal milk flow obstruction produced approximately 24% of the milk produced by the contralateral teat.[23] One month after removal of the obstruction by theloscopic triangulation, milk production of the affected quarter had increased to 73% of the contralateral teat. Six months after the procedure, milk production had increased to 82% of the contralateral quarter. The somatic cell count (SCC) of teats with a distal outflow obstruction was, on average, 2.9 million cells/ml before the theloscopic surgery, 725,000 cells/ml 1 month after the surgery, and 426,000 cells/ml 6 months after the surgery. In 67% of the cases, a pathogen was isolated before the surgery. In 69% and 61% of the cases a pathogen was isolated 1 month and 6 months after the surgery, respectively. These numbers show that mastitis is often associated with distal milk flow obstruction. However, surgical intervention with the help of theloscopy can significantly decrease the SCC of the affected quarter.

A retrospective study of 52 cases treated with theloresectoscopy showed that teats with sinusitis (erythema and proliferation of the mucosa) at the time of the procedure had higher SCC throughout the entire lactation and were more at risk of developing mastitis than teats without sinusitis.[27] Sinusitis is often created by excessive cannulation of the teat or blind resection of the tissue. Of the 52 cases, 15 milk cultures grew a single or double pathogen before the surgery. Those cows were 4.95 times more at risk of being culled before the end of their lactation because of mastitis. Cows with a 2+ or 3+ California Mastitis Test (CMT) before the surgery had a higher SCC than negative or 1+ cows throughout the lactation. Twenty cows out of 52 were culled before the end of their lactation. Of those 20, 13 were culled because of a problem in the affected quarter (mastitis or reobstruction). Of the cows still in production or culled for a reason not related to the udder, 24 (60%) had milk flow and milk production comparable with the contralateral quarter.

TEAT IMPLANTS

In teats with lesions involving more than 30% of the mucosa, it can be difficult to appose the edges of the mucosa together. When lesions are located in the proximal teat causing obstruction, reestablishment of a connection between the gland cistern and teat cistern is difficult without reobstruction. In these situations an implant is required to keep the teat functional. Several types of implants have been developed and used to promote healing of the mucosa and keep the cistern functional. In 1987 Ducharme reported the use of silicone implants after removal of defects of variable sizes and locations in 27 teats.[28] The diameter of the tube varies according to the size of the teat (average 11-mm tube). The implant should be long enough to extend into the gland cistern. A long tube is more susceptible to break. The free portion within the gland cistern should be fenestrated. Care should be taken in the placement of the fenestration holes to avoid weakening of the tube. The distal end must be rounded to avoid trauma to the rosette of Furstenberg. The implant is sutured in the mid teat cistern with nonabsorbable material. One month after surgery, 60% of the teats carrying an implant were still functional. At 1 year, 41% were successfully able to be milked. Eighteen percent of the implants encountered technical problems throughout the process. The silicone prosthesis broke in two cases. A longer prosthesis was necessary in two other cases. In one cow, the prosthesis became loose and needed to be removed and replaced. Finally, one implant was extruded from the incision when dehiscence of the incision occurred.

In 1988 Nassef and colleagues[29] created an artificial model of a teat defect. The model attempted to stimulate mucosal proliferation and silicone teat implants were used to keep the teat cistern open. The implants were constructed of a silicone tube coated with Dacron (12 teats) or Teflon (6 teats). Both implants stimulated a certain degree of mucosal metaplasia, but only the Teflon strips became anchored by fibrotic invasion, decreasing the chance of dislodging of the implant. Several complications were associated with the procedure. Mastitis (16 cases), migration of the implant (3 cases), and milk fistula (1 case) were the most common.

In 1989 Bristol published a case report using a buccal mucosal graft to repair an extensive teat injury.[30] He used a silicone implant to apply pressure on the graft postoperatively. However, the silicone tube had to be removed 27 days after implantation because the tube migrated into the gland cistern. In this case a successful outcome was observed for at least 2 years after the surgery. The owner reported decreased milk production in the affected quarter, but the production was sufficient to justify retention of the cow in the herd.

In 1990 Trent and colleagues used a buccal mucosal graft (12 teats) in a model of teat mucosal lesions.[31] Without any support, the graft collapsed and the teat cistern became obstructed within 6 weeks after the surgery. When a silicone tube was used as a stent to maintain pressure on the graft, 11 teats out of 12 remained patent for 12 weeks after the surgery. Ten of those 11 teats had marked narrowing (>80%) of the teat cistern. This narrowing, caused by increased fibrous tissue at the graft site, was associated with increased milking times. Other postoperative complications included mastitis (six cases) and tube migration.

In 1999 Metzger and colleagues[32,33] used a reinforced polytetrafluoroethylene vascular graft (nine teats) to correct teat flow obstructions in a model of teat trauma. Ninety days after the implantation, all of the grafts had collapsed. After collapse, all of the cows had an increased milking time from the affected quarter. At the lactation following the surgery, all of the teats had become obstructed. Other complications were mastitis (five cases), graft migration (seven cases), and ingrowth of obstructive tissue (all cases). They concluded that the early milking with the machine (15 days after the surgery) was one of the reasons for the collapse of the graft.

In 2001 Molaei and colleagues[34] used a vestibular mucosal graft (eight teats). He found that the thickness of the graft had a better correlation with the thickness of the teat mucosa removed compared with the buccal mucosa used by Trent and Bristol. Instead of using a silicone tube to support the graft, they used an external teat cannula for 10 days. In this study only one of eight teats became obstructed 125 days after the surgery. In our judgment, the narrowing of the cistern seemed to be less than the narrowing reported after buccal mucosal graft.

At this time, silicone implants are the implants most frequently used in teat surgery. The search for new implants with better long-term prognosis and minimal complications is still on-going.

References

1. Beaudeau F, Ducrocq V, Fourichon C et al: Effect of disease on length of productive life of French Holstein dairy cows assessed by survival analysis, *J Dairy Sci* 78:103, 1995.
2. Michigan Dairy Herd Improvement Association: *Animal summary*, Lansing, 1981, Michigan DHIA.
3. Couture Y, Mulon PY: Procedures and surgeries of the teat, *Vet Clin North Am Food Anim Pract* 21:173, 2005.
4. Geishauser T, Querengässer K: Investigations on teat canal length in teats with milk flow disturbances, *J Dairy Sci* 83:2000, 1976.
5. Franz S, Hofmann-Parisot M, Baumgartner W et al: Ultrasonography of the teat canal in cows and sheep, *Vet Rec* 149:109, 2001.
6. Trostle SS, O'Brien RT: Ultrasonography of the bovine mammary gland, *Comp Cont Educ Pract Vet* 20:564, 1998.
7. McDonald JS: Radiographic method for anatomic study of the teat canal: observations on 22 lactating dairy cows, *Am J Vet Res* 29:1315, 1968.
8. Ducharme NG, Arighi M, Horney D et al: Invasive teat surgery in dairy cattle. I. Long-term follow-up and complications, *Can Vet J* 28:757, 1987.
9. Geishauser T, Querengässer K: Using teat endoscopy (theloscopy) to diagnose and treat milk flow disorders in cows, *Bov Pract* 35:156, 2001.
10. Hirsbrunner G, Steiner A: Use of a theloscopic triangulation technique for endoscopic treatment of teat obstructions in cows, *J Am Vet Med Assoc* 214:1668, 1999.
11. Seeh C, Hospes R: Experiences with a theloresectoscope compared with conventional teat endoscopy in diagnosis and therapy of covered teat lesions, *Tierarztl Prax* 26:110, 1998.
12. Trent AM: Teat surgery, *Agri Pract* 14:6, 1993.
13. Steiner A, Von Rotz A: The most important local anesthesia in cattle: a review, *Schweiz Arch Tierheilkd* 145:262, 2003.
14. Makady FM, Whitmore HL, Nelson DR et al: Effect of tissue adhesives and suture patterns on experimentally induced teat lacerations in lactating dairy cattle, *J Am Vet Med Assoc* 198:1932, 1991.
15. Nichols S, Anderson DE: Breaking strength and elasticity of synthetic absorbable suture materials incubated in phosphate-buffered saline solution, milk, and milk contaminated with *Streptococcus agalactiae*, *Am J Vet Res* 68:441-445, 2007.
16. Ghamsari SM, Taguchi K, Abe N et al: Effect of different suture patterns on wound healing of the teat in dairy cattle, *J Vet Med Sci* 57:819, 1995.
17. Grymer J, Watson GL, Coy CH et al: Healing of experimentally induced wounds of mammary papilla (teat) of the cow: comparison of closure with tissue adhesive versus nonsutured wounds, *Am J Vet Res* 45:1979, 1984.
18. Saifzadeh S, Ardebili FF, Hobbenaghi R et al: Teat tip reconstruction by supernumerary teat autotransplantation in cattle, *Vet Surg* 34:366, 2005.
19. Hull BL: Teat and udder surgery, *Vet Clin North Am Food Anim Pract* 11:1, 1995.
20. John H, Sicher D, Ousterla JB et al: Video-assisted theloscopic electroincision of a high teat stenosis, *Schweiz Arch Tierheilkd* 140:282, 1998.
21. John H, Hassig M, Gobet D et al: A new operative method to treat high teat stenosis in dairy cows, *Br J Urol* 82:906, 1998.
22. Schimt KA, Arighi M, Dobson H: Postoperative evaluation of the surgical treatment of accessory teat and gland cistern complexes in dairy cows, *Can Vet J* 34:25, 1994.
23. Geishauser T, Querengässer K, Querengässer J: Teat endoscopy (theloscopy) for diagnosis and therapy of milk flow disorders in dairy cows, *Vet Clin North Am Food Anim Pract* 21:205, 2005.
24. Tulleners E, Hamir A: Effects of teat cistern mural biopsy and teatoscopy stab versus longitudinal incision with or without tube implant on incisional healing in lactating dairy cattle, *Am J Vet Res* 51:1257, 1990.
25. Querengässer J, Geishauser T, Querengässer K et al: Comparative evaluation of SIMPL silicone implants and NIT natural teat inserts to keep the teat canal patent after the surgery, *J Dairy Sci* 85:1732, 2002.
26. Hirsbrunner G, Eicher R, Meylan M et al: Comparison of thelotomy and theloscopic triangulation for the treatment of distal teat obstructions in dairy cows: a retrospective study (1994-1998), *Vet Rec* 148:803, 2001.

27. Bleul UT, Schwantag SC, Bachofner C et al: Milk flow and udder health in cows after treatment of covered teat injuries via theloresectoscopy: 52 cases (2000-2002), *J Am Vet Med Assoc* 226:1119, 2005.

28. Ducharme NG, Arighi M, Horney D et al: Invasive teat surgery in dairy cattle II. Long-term follow-up and complications, *Can Vet J* 28:763, 1987.

29. Nassef MT, Coy CH, Watson GL: Method to create and maintain the patency of the bovine mammary papilla, *Am J Vet Res* 49:1131, 1988.

30. Bristol DG: Treatment of teat obstruction in a cow by transfer of oral mucosa and temporary implantation of an intraluminal tube, *J Am Vet Med Assoc* 195:492, 1989.

31. Trent AM, Smith DF, Cooley AJ et al: Use of mucosal grafts and temporary tube implants for treatment of teat sinus mucosal injuries, *Am J Vet Res* 51:666, 1990.

32. Metzger L, Hirsbrunner G, Waldvogel A et al: Permanent implantation of a reinforced polytetrafluoroethylene vascular graft for treatment of artificial defects of the teat cistern mucosa in cows, *Am J Vet Res* 60:56, 1999.

33. Hirsbrunner G, Metzger L, Steiner A: Implantation of a reinforced polytetrafluoroethylene vascular graft for treatment of obstructions of the teat and mammary gland cisternae in cattle, *J Am Vet Med Assoc* 212:1432, 1998.

34. Molaei MM, Oloumi MM, Maleki M et al: Experimental reconstruction of teat mucosa by vestibular graft in cows. A histopathologic and radiographic study, *J Vet Med* 49:379, 2002.

CHAPTER 83

Laparoscopy in Large Animal Surgery

KENNETH D. NEWMAN

The development of laparoscopy as another tool in the surgeon's toolbox paralleled the advances in imaging over the past century. The first report of laparoscopy in veterinary medicine was in a dog in 1902. An oblique lens developed in 1929 was the second development in laparoscopy. Not until the technologic explosion during the latter half of the twenty-first century did laparoscopy begin to steadily evolve: the invention of fiberoptics, computer chips, video cassette recorders, and the miniaturizing of said technology. Today, digital cameras and recording devices offer unparalleled video quality and storage capabilities.

Laparoscopy was first being used as a diagnostic tool in horses in the 1970s. In the 1990s laparoscopy evolved from a strictly diagnostic tool to become an extension of the surgeon's surgical tools. The development of arthroscopy and its widespread clinical application in equine surgery was likely responsible in part for the evolution of laparoscopy as a therapeutic tool. In addition, the advancement of the surgeon's skills, surgical techniques, and our understanding of what laparoscopy has to offer has led to the continued development of specialized laparoscopic instruments. Not until 2002 was the first textbook on equine diagnostic and surgical laparoscopy published.[1] The use of hand-assisted laparoscopy surgery (HALS) has become a useful and acceptable technique in laparoscopic surgery. The advantages of this technique include lowered learning curve, minimal intraoperative blood loss, significantly decreased surgical time, minimal postoperative pain, and shorter hospitalization.[2,3] The intraoperative advantages include tactile sensation to assist dissection, rapid blunt-finger dissection, hand retraction, easier suturing, and access for immediate hemostasis if required.[3,4]

The advantages of laparoscopy include minimal invasiveness; ability to visualize and perform surgical operations in areas not readily accessible; minimizing surgical and anesthetic time; fewer postoperative surgical complications; reduced postoperative recuperative time; and, in some instances, the option of performing procedures on standing but sedate patients that are at high risk for complications of anesthesia.

As with any technique, laparoscopy has a number of disadvantages. The capital costs for equipment and consumables can be expensive. Limited training is available for veterinary surgeons. Increased anesthetic and surgical times are likely during the initial learning curve. These times could possibly be longer compared with traditional surgical approaches. General anesthesia requires positive pressure ventilation and close monitoring of blood gas values to correct alterations caused by body position and CO_2 insufflation. Finally, the equipment traditionally used in large animal surgery was designed primarily for use in humans.

Laparoscopy is not the panacea of surgical techniques—to use it as such would be a disservice to our patients and clients and a discredit to fellow veterinary surgeons and the veterinary profession itself. After critically evaluating patient and disease issues, laparoscopy should be offered and applied in strategic clinical cases as a safe and efficient alternative to traditional laparotomy.

ANATOMY

The laparoscopic anatomy of the abdomen in several large animal species has been well described in the literature. The equine adult abdomen both in standing[5] and dorsally recumbent[6] positions has been documented. Significant structures that could be visualized from the left paralumbar fossa in the standing horse include hepatic duct; left lateral and quadrate liver lobes; stomach; spleen; left kidney and its association with the nephrosplenic ligament; segments of the jejunum, descending colon, and ascending colon; left side of both the male and female reproductive tracts; urinary bladder; vaginal ring; and mesorchium.[5] Relevant structures that could be visualized from the right paralumbar fossa in the standing horse include portions of the common hepatic duct; the left lateral, quadrate, and right liver lobes; caudate process of the liver; stomach; duodenum; right dorsal colon, epiploic foramen; omental bursa, right kidney; base of the cecum; segments of the jejunum, descending colon, and ascending colon; urinary bladder, right portion of the male and female reproductive tracts; and rectum.[5]

Significant structures in the caudal region of the abdomen in dorsally recumbent adult horses that can be visualized include urinary bladder; mesorchium, ductus deferens; left and right vaginal rings; insertion of the prepubic tendon; segments of the jejunum and descending colon; pelvic flexure of the ascending colon; body of the cecum; and the cecocolic fold.[6] Relevant structures in the cranial region of the abdomen in dorsally recumbent horses that can be visualized include the ventral surface of the diaphragm; falciform and round ligaments of the liver; ventral portion of the left lateral, left medial, quadrate, and right lateral lobes of the liver; spleen; right and left ventral colons; sternal flexure of the ascending colon; apex of the cecum; and stomach.[6]

In comparison with adult horses, the laparoscopic abdominal anatomy of foals in dorsal recumbency includes umbilical structures, urinary bladder, male and female reproductive tracts, the inguinal area, the liver, and various segments of the intestinal tract.[7] These authors indicated they could not identify either the duodenum or ileum but did observe a greater quantity of loops of small intestine in foals between 1 and 12 days of age. The umbilical structures were observed in all foals 45 days of age or younger.

The laparoscopic anatomy in camelids has been described.[8,9] The left paralumbar approach was used with the llamas positioned in right lateral recumbency.[8] Significant structures visualized from this approach are the first forestomach (C1), spleen, diaphragm, left kidney, loops of small intestines, and left inguinal ring. The relevant structures identified from the right paralumbar approach (llama positioned in left lateral recumbency) are the first and third forestomachs (C1 and C3); liver; right kidney; small intestine, including segments of the duodenum and jejunum; proximal aspect of the spiral colon; urinary bladder; and right inguinal ring.[8] Ventral midline laparoscopy permitted adequate visualization of relevant viscera, including the ventral aspect of C1, C3, liver, spleen, diaphragm, and small intestine. The ileum was identified by locating the antimesenteric artery. The proximal loop of the ascending colon and the spiral colon were also identified.[8]

Laparoscopic anatomy of the bovine abdomen was first described in 1993.[10] The left paralumbar fossa typically provides excellent visualization of the left cranial abdomen, including the diaphragm, spleen, rumen, left kidney, and small intestine. Occasionally the pancreas, spiral colon, and bladder can be adequately visualized. In contrast, laparoscopy of the bovine abdomen from the cranioventral midline laparoscopy provides visualization of the cranioventral abdomen, including the diaphragm, rumen, reticulum, abomasum, pylorus, spleen, and sometimes the left liver lobe.

TECHNIQUE

Standing laparoscopy can be done under sedation and local infiltration of the muscle and subcutaneous layers using 2% lidocaine hydrochloride at each laparoscopic site.[5] Laparoscopic insertion consisted of a 33-cm, 30-degree laparoscope for peritoneal puncture. This permits visualization of the peritoneum before entry into the abdomen, compared with the smooth serosal surface of the viscera after peritoneal penetration. Furthermore, intra-abdominal pressure (−3 to −5 mm Hg) could be recorded on the lapoflator.[5] After confirmation of correct laparoscopic placement and pneumoperitoneum established during the peritoneal puncture, the cannula could be advanced along the laparoscope or additional laparoscopic portals could be placed and the abdomen can be insufflated with carbon dioxide. These investigators believe that their technique reduced the likelihood of accidental visceral puncture.[5]

Ventral laparoscopy in the horse requires general anesthesia and intermittent positive pressure once pneumoperitoneum is established.[6] In addition, varying degrees of head-up and head-down positions were required to adequately visualize the abdomen. In foals, a 10-degree Trendelenburg position was sufficient to provide visualization of the caudal abdomen by clearing the pelvic inlet of intestinal loops.[7] Laparoscopy in camelids is more easily performed under general anesthesia, regardless of the approach.[8,9] In one report, a standing approach under sedation was used while a bilateral ovariectomy was performed.[11] However, this approach was challenging because one llama had a tendency to lean on the sidebars.

Hand-assisted laparoscopy (HAL) is a modification of the laparoscopic technique. A hand is used intra-abdominally to assist with laparoscopic manipulations.

COMPLICATIONS

The most common complications in humans include hypercapnia, decreased cardiac output, gas emboli, emphysema, bowel perforation, hemorrhage, and coagulation injury associated with operative laparoscopy.[12]

Animal position, rather than intra-abdominal carbon dioxide or abdominal pressure, significantly affected mean, diastolic, and systolic blood pressures in the dorsally recumbent horses.[6] These pressures were greatest during the head-up, followed by the horizontal position, and least during the head-down position.

Blood gas values varied in anesthetized, dorsally recumbent horses that underwent laparoscopy.[6] PaO_2 was significantly ($p > 0.003$) lower during the head-down position, whereas there was no effect during either the horizontal or head-up positions. $PaCo_2$ was lower for the horizontal than the head-down position. The pH was greater that during the horizontal than the head-down position. Furthermore, the pH was higher ($p = 0.05$) before than after CO_2 administration.

In dorsally recumbent horses anesthetized using halothane, PaO_2 and ph of arterial blood, tidal volume, and systemic vascular resistance decreased during abdominal insufflation and laparoscopy surgery.[13] Furthermore, mean arterial pressure, right atrial pressure, cardiac and stroke indices, $PaCO_2$, and end-tidal respiratory gases increased significantly. Interestingly, only the systemic vascular resistance returned to preinsufflation levels after deflation. These authors concluded that perioperative complications could arise because of hypercapnia, acidosis, and the apparent increased cardiac work that occur with CO_2 pneumoperitoneum. Close anesthetic monitoring, as well as correcting blood gas alterations and instituting supportive cardiovascular therapy during laparoscopy surgery, should reduce these potential complications.

In standing, sedate, adult horses, pneumoperitoneum with CO_2 at 15 mm Hg had no significant effect on cardiopulmonary function during laparoscopy.[14] No significant differences in blood gas values, complete blood cell count, or serum biochemical values were observed. In contrast, a mild inflammatory response was noted. These authors concluded that laparoscopic surgery can be safely performed in healthy, sedated, standing adult horses without any adverse affects on the hemodynamic or cardiopulmonary function.

In anesthetized foals, hypercarbia and respiratory acidosis developed during peritoneal insufflation with CO_2.[7] These blood gas alterations were easily corrected by adjusting ventilation using a positive-pressure ventilator.

Blood gas values remained within the normal range in anesthetized llamas that underwent laparoscopy.[9] A more detailed study observed that insufflation of CO_2 and changing body position had minor and transient effects on cardiopulmonary functions.[15] Significant decreases in systolic and mean arterial pressures and $PaCO_2$, and increased pH were observed when the position of the llamas changed from right lateral to dorsal recumbency. Interestingly, the mean arterial pressures were significantly lower when the llamas were placed in either dorsal or left lateral recumbency compared with right lateral recumbency. The authors suggest that compression of the great vessels both in the thorax and abdomen may be responsible. Bicarbonate values were unaffected by position but were lower than preinduction values.

Localized emphysema developed at the laparoscopy site in one mare,[5] likely because of a large peritoneal tear and manipulation of the laparoscopic cannula through a large amount of retroperitoneal fat and thick body wall. Compared with the days and weeks for air emphysema to resolve, carbon dioxide emphysema completely resolved within 12 hours. The same situation occurred in llamas and resolved over 48 hours.[8,11] In addition, mild to moderate edema developed postoperatively at the ventral midline laparoscopy site and resolved without further complications in one llama.[8]

Some abdominal discomfort was observed in one foal postoperatively.[7] Abdominal discomfort has been noted in adult horses[16] and is thought to be caused by the formation of carbonic acid, which is a by-product of the combination of carbon dioxide and abdominal fluids.[16] Passively deflating the abdomen of all possible carbon dioxide at the end of the laparoscopic procedure may eliminate this complication.

In one report, a horse was accidentally injured during placement of the laparoscopy portals.[17] Damage to the vessels increased surgical time, subcutaneous hematoma formation, and hemoperitoneum. In foals, these vessels can be easily avoided by transilluminating the body wall with the laparoscope before trocar insertions.[18]

Laparoscopy can be performed in cows with few adverse effects.[10] Significant differences were not observed with CBC, serum biochemical, and peritoneal fluid variables before and 72 hours after laparoscopy. However, in llamas the mean white blood cell count peaked (23,500 cells/μL) 24 hours after laparoscopy.[8]

INDICATIONS

Urinary Bladder

The literature contains one report regarding laparoscopic repair of a ruptured bladder in a stallion.[19] Though not a common condition in adult horses, it was likely iatrogenic as a result of the initial endoscopic examination of the bladder. This stallion had a history of a septic urachus as a foal, and possibly the resulting scar and damage to the bladder formed an area of weakness. When nonsurgical management of the case failed, the stallion was anesthetized and placed in dorsal recumbency, with his head down. A 4-cm tear near the apex of the bladder was visualized. The tear margins were grasped using two 5-mm Babcock forceps. Necrotic tissue along the tear margin was débrided using 17-mm curved spoon scissors. The defect was closed in two layers: full-thickness, simple, continuous pattern using No 0 polyglycolic acid suture with a laparoscopic autosuture device and laparoscopic needle holder oversewn with a Cushing pattern using No 0 polyglycolic acid. The stallion was discharged 5 days postoperatively and was free of clinical signs 2 years later.

Ruptured bladders are more common in foals, specifically males during birth. Consequently, laparoscopic techniques have been developed to repair ruptured bladder in foals. After anesthetizing the foal, it is placed in dorsal recumbency with the head down. The first report used a gastrointestinal linear stapler device to repair a 2-cm tear near the apex.[20] The necrotic margins along the tear were resected and removed through an instrument portal. Unfortunately, the foal developed stranguria 10 months after surgery. A urolith was removed endoscopically from the penile urethra: Endoscopic examination of the bladder revealed an ulcerated area in the area of the staple line. The authors suggested that the staples in the lumen of the bladder may have served as a nidus for urinary calculi formation. A more recent experimental study used seven normal neonatal calves as a model to develop a laparoscopic technique using an endoscopic suturing device for resection of the bladder apex and the associated umbilical structures.[21] The bladder apex was resected using a staggered row of vascular clips. The bladder apex was resected, and the cut edge of the bladder was closed with an endoscopic suturing device: first using full-thickness, simple, continuous suture of either No 2-0 or 0 glycoside lactide copolymer suture and over-sewn using similar suture material in a Lembert pattern. No postoperative surgical complications were observed. More recently, this investigator successfully applied these techniques in clinical cases of ruptured urinary bladders in foals.[18]

Laparoscopy has been used successfully to resect umbilical structures in foals. The first report in the literature used a hand-assisted technique in 11 foals.[22] The umbilical vein, umbilical arteries, and ventral and lateral ligaments of the bladder were laparoscopically ligated using endoscopic ligating clips. An elliptical incision was made around the umbilicus, thus permitting exteriorizing of the umbilical remnants and the apex of the bladder. The bladder was resected, and the umbilical remnants removed. The end of the bladder was closed using No 3-0 polyglactin 910 in a full-thickness, simple, interrupted pattern, which was then oversewn using a Lembert pattern. More recently, the technique of laparoscopically resecting the apex of the bladder has been described.[18] These authors have further modified their technique by closing the bladder as a single layer using the endostitch laparoscopic suturing device and full-thickness, simple, continuous suture pattern without surgical complications.[23] No significant difference occurred in mean bladder bursting strength between one- and two-layer closure. One-layer closure required significantly less time to complete. Interestingly, the histologic examination revealed that one-layer closure was superior compared with two-layer closure. Differences in tissue at a ruptured site versus the model suggest that further work is required before the one-layer laparoscopic closure is recommended in clinical cases.

Hernias

Nonstrangulating hernias have been repaired by a laparoscopic technique. A bilateral scrotal hernia reduced itself when a 4-week-old Percheron was placed in dorsal recumbency. Laparoscopy revealed that both vaginal rings were 4 cm long. Laparoscopic grasping forceps and an atraumatic right-angle forcep were used to retract both testes into the abdomen. A bipolar electrocautery unit was used to cauterize the tail of the epididymis and transected it with scissors. The mesenteric portion of the mesorchium was cauterized, and No 0 polydioxanone ligature (endoloop ligature) was used for ligation. The stalk was transected (the testes were later retrieved during a celiotomy to remove enlarged umbilical remnants). Both

vaginal rings were closed using a stapling instrument. A second 4-week-old Percheron that presented for a unilateral scrotal hernia had a similar laparoscopy surgery, but this time the testes were removed using a 16-mm cannula, thereby avoiding a celiotomy. Both foals recovered uneventfully from surgery. The advantage laparoscopy provided in these cases was the ability to visualize the incarcerated bowel.

A testis-sparing laparoscopic herniorrhaphy procedure in stallions has been described. Two stallions had surgery done in dorsal recumbency, in the head-down position.[24] A peritoneal flap was dissected cranial and ventral to the inguinal ring. A polypropylene mesh was placed over the inguinal ring, and the peritoneum was drawn over the mesh and stapled in place. These two stallions recovered uneventfully, resumed breeding activity, and completed two breeding seasons without recurrence of herniation. This technique is limited to when the hernia can be reducible by reduction per rectum before surgery or by celiotomy and when the vasculature of both the bowel and testis has not been compromised. Nine stallions had surgery done standing through the paralumbar fossa.[25] A coiled polypropylene mesh was inserted and fixed in the inguinal canal. A combination of either laparoscopic or rectal reexamination revealed obliteration of the inguinal ring 2 to 4 weeks postsurgery. Sperm quality control 4 months after surgery revealed no changes.

Male Reproductive Tract

Laparoscopic cryptorchid castration has been described in the dorsally recumbent horse under a general anesthetic[26,27] and in the standing, sedated horse.[27-29] In the dorsally recumbent horse, the head was pointed down to assist visualization of the caudal abdomen. A ligating loop technique[26] or endo-gastrointestinal anastomosis (GIA)[30] can be used to ligate the testicular vessels. However, routine clinical use of the endo-GIA for cryptorchidectomy is cost prohibitive. The testis can be removed through an enlarged portal, using Semms forceps.[26] This technique is ideal in cases of bilateral cryptorchids, which would require two inguinal incisions. In these two studies, more than 56 horses have successfully had laparoscopic cryptorchidectomies. The dorsal approach may be preferable to use in young horses untrained to stand comfortably in stocks. The standing approach on the same side as the retained testis was used for 22 horses.[27-29] Local anesthetic was injected into the intra-abdominal testis before laparoscopic manipulations, unless a caudal epidural anesthesia was performed. The testis was either ligated within the abdomen using No 0-polydioxanone (endoloop)[29] or withdrawn from the abdomen through a laparoscopic portal and then emasculated or ligated.[28] It is possible to explore both sides of the abdomen through a single paralumbar approach: either by lifting the descending colon and rectum with instruments or inserting an arm into the rectum and by perforating the mesocolon. Though the perforation in the mesocolon was small at 1 cm, to reduce the risk of incarcerating a segment of bowel, the veterinarians closed this perforation with staples. It was possible to transect the spermatic cords on both sides if either long instruments were used or the horse was thin. No postoperative surgical complications were observed.

Electrosurgical instrumentation as the sole means of hemostasis of the equine mesorchium has been described[31] as a safe, reliable, efficient alternative technique for hemostasis. A laparoscopic cryptorchidectomy in camelids has been briefly described.[31,32] This procedure has been performed successfully in calves, lambs, pigs, alpacas, and llamas (D.E. Anderson, unpublished data).

Laparoscopy has been used to castrate ponies and juvenile horses.[33] In this study the testis was either retracted into the abdomen by enlarging the vaginal ring using scissors and then ligating the mesorchium and removing the resected testis through an enlarged laparoscopy portal or ligated by vascular cauterization and left in situ. Though no complications were observed in this study, these authors recommend further experience with this approach before use in mature stallions. In a later clinical case,[34] instead of avascular necrosis of testicular tissue, revascularization occurred, which resulted in testosterone production and stallionlike behavior. It is thought that testicular tissue survived as a result of peritesticular angiogenesis before testicular necrosis was complete.

Intra-abdominal vasectomy in camelids has been used successfully without impairing libido or male sexual behavior for many years.[35] Vasectomized males are useful to induce ovulation in females or detect sexually receptive females. This technique might be an interesting alternative to teaser bull preparation.

Laparoscopic intra-abdominal ligation of the testicular artery for postcastration hemorrhage after routine orchidectomy has been described.[36,37] This has been performed in the dorsally recumbent horse under a general anesthetic[36] and in the standing horse using a paralumbar approach.[37] These approaches may provide alternative solutions when complications such as swelling in the inguinal area and previous failure to identify the testicular stump through the previous scrotal incision have occurred.

Female Reproductive Tract

Laparoscopic ovariectomy in the mare has been thoroughly described in the literature: a bilateral paralumbar fossae approach in the standing sedated mare[38,39] or a ventral abdominal approach in the dorsally recumbent mare under general anesthetic.[40] In both approaches the ovaries were removed through a single, enlarged laparoscopy portal. Ligation of the ovarian pedicle can be accomplished using endoloop sutures,[38] a modified Roeder knot and modified Camber's urinary catheter,[39] Kleppinger bipolar electrocoagulation[41] device, LigaSure bipolar vessel sealing device,[42] Harmonic Scapel,[43] and an 800-μm neodynmium:yttrium (Nd:YAG) aluminum garnet attached to a 100-W Nd:YAG laser.[44] Complications associated with these techniques include incomplete hemostasis of the ovarian pedicle,[39] transient inappetence,[39] pyrexia,[39,44] and incisional infection.[39] Most postoperative complications were considered minor.

The ventral approach has been described for efficient and safe ovariectomy for foals and adults,[40] as well as the removal of granulose cell tumors in two horses.[45]

Abdominal pain was observed in the immediate postoperative period in three mules and one horse.[40] Fluid was removed from the granulosa cell tumor using a 14-gauge, 12-cm needle placed through the body wall to reduce the volume and wall tension of the affected ovary. The granulosa cell tumor was placed inside a sterile plastic bag; a small incision through the body wall was required to remove the tumor. Enclosing the tumor may prevent neoplastic tissue or fluids from spilling into the abdomen.[45] However, this technique required a hand to be placed within the abdomen to open the bag. Interestingly, these investigators also chose not to insufflate the abdomen; instead, a hand was used to retract the abdominal wall through the celiotomy site, through which the tumor was removed. This eliminated the detrimental cardiovascular and acid-base abnormalities associated with pneumoperitoneum.

One report concerns removal of granulose cell tumors in 10 standing mares.[46] A hand-assisted technique was used to assist manipulation of the ovary, and a stapling device (TA-90) was used to provide hemostasis. The authors felt the increased incisional complications were associated with trauma to the incision edges during removal of the ovary.

Laparoscopic ovariectomy has been described in camelids: a standing approach through the left paralumbar fossa[11] and a caudal ventral midline approach under general anesthetic.[47] No intraoperative or postoperative complications were observed in either study. Laparoscopic and hand-assisted laparoscopic techniques have been used for ovariohysterectomy, ovariectomy, uterine masses and neoplasia, and ovarian neoplasia (D.E. Anderson unpublished data).

A hand-assisted ovariohysterectomy has recently been described.[48] A hand access port (Omniport) was placed to maintain the abdomen insufflated during the procedure. A combination of a stapling device (Endo GIA II), an ultrasonically activated instrument (Harmonic Scalpel), and endoscopic clips (Endo Clip II) were used for ligation and hemostasis of the ovarian pedicles and the broad ligament. The ovaries and uterus were exteriorized through a celiotomy site, and the body of the uterus was resected using No 1-0 polydioxanone in a Parker-Kerr pattern. This technique was first developed in two mares in a nonsurvival procedure. Four mares recovered uneventfully, one was euthanized at recovery for bilateral femur fractures, and another mare developed pleuropneumonia postoperatively. No postoperative surgical complications were observed at postmortem in the surviving mares. The hand-assisted laparoscopic technique is a safer and more efficient alternative to conventional ovariohysterectomy, which is more technically demanding, invasive, and associated with high morbidity.

Kidneys

Recently a hand-assisted laparoscopic technique for left nephrectomy in standing horses has been described.[49] Special care must be taken to identify and ligate all the accessory branches of the renal artery. One horse was euthanized before incisional closure because of arterial hemorrhage from a transected accessory branch of the renal artery that had not been ligated. This technique provides an alternative to rib resection or a dorsal paralumbar incision.

Laparoscopic ablation of the renosplenic space in standing horses has been described[50] and may be useful in preventing recurrent incarceration of the ascending or descending colon in this space. Closure of the space was accomplished by apposing the dorsomedial splenic capsule to the dorsal portion of the renosplenic ligament using No 1 polyglactin 910 in a continuous pattern. No intraoperative or postoperative surgical complications were observed. Laparoscopic reexamination 3 weeks after closure of the renosplenic space revealed a smooth connecting fibrous-like tissue between the dorsal splenic capsule and the dorsal portion of the renosplenic ligament. In addition to pleasure-type horses, this technique could likely be used in performance-type horses in which colopexy is contraindicated. Long-term evaluation of laparoscopic ablation of the renosplenic space is still required before this technique can be recommended for clinical use.

A serial renal biopsy technique has been described in the bovine.[51] This is a much safer and more efficient alternative technique compared with the keyhole and laparotomy techniques for renal biopsy. No complications including disturbance to renal function after surgery were observed.

Adhesiolysis

Intra-abdominal adhesions that form after colic surgery are usually broken down through a repeat laparotomy. Reformation and new adhesions are a common complication associated with repeated laparotomies. In humans, laparoscopy is the preferred approach for the diagnosis and treatment of abdominal adhesions.[52] Furthermore, laparoscopy results in a decrease in new adhesion formation, but not in reformation.[53,54] Laparoscopy was used in a sedated, standing, 18-month-old Standardbred filly to access intra-abdominal adhesions in the dorsal portion of the abdominal cavity.[55] The approach was through the right paralumbar area. Fibrinous adhesions were observed among the base of the cecum, right uterine horn, and pelvic flexure. Using both a 10-mm laparoscopic Babcock and a 10-mm atraumatic, laparoscopic Kelly forceps, the adhesions between the viscera were broken. The filly recovered from surgery uneventfully and 11 months later was racing. These authors concluded that laparoscopy may be an option in the surgical treatment of localized intra-abdominal adhesions.

A 14-year-old Arabian mare developed signs of colic 7 days after a traditional laparotomy for a unilateral ovariectomy to remove a granulose cell tumor.[56] Suspecting adhesions, the veterinarian reanesthetized the horse, placed her in dorsal recumbency (head down), and performed an exploratory laparoscopy. Two well-vascularized adhesions were visualized between the small intestine and the paramedian incisions from the first surgery: 10-cm and 6-cm segments of small intestine were adhered to the cranial and caudal aspects, respectively. The adhesions were broken down using the combination of a blunt cherry dissector, 10-mm laparoscopic Metzenbaum scissors, and 10-mm curved laparoscopic Kelly forceps. Adhesiolysis was further aided by gentle transrectal traction of the adhered small intestine. The horse recovered without further complications and remained incident free 12 months later.

Laparoscopic adhesiolysis was used successfully in experimentally induced adhesions in pony foals.[57] This procedure was done during the early maturation stage of adhesion formation, 10 days after laparotomy and serosal abrasions were created. At postmortem, thin adhesions between the omentum and laparoscopic portals were observed in five of eight foals. The clinical importance of these adhesions is unknown; therefore the clinical use of this technique in foals is not recommended. Laparoscopic adhesiolysis has been performed to resolve uterine, ovarian, and intestinal adhesions in cattle and alpacas (D.E. Anderson, S. Nichols, unpublished data).

Colopexy

Laparoscopic colopexy in six horses has been described.[58] Placed in dorsal recumbency under a general anesthetic, the lateral taenia of the left ventral colon was laparoscopically sutured to the body wall just left of the midline, using 2-monofilament nylon in a continuous pattern. No surgical complications were observed. Postmortem examination 90 days after surgery revealed a firm, fibrous adhesion of the colon to the abdominal tunic. Histologic examination revealed a mature fibrous tissue with no evidence of inflammation.

Rectal and Colonic Tears

Brugmans and Deegen[59] described a laparoscopic surgical technique for repair of rectal and colonic tears in 2001. This technique needs further investigation to determine whether it can be used in clinical cases. Laparoscopic examination of rectal tears in cows has been accomplished to aid in treatment decisions and establish prognosis (D.E. Anderson, unpublished data).

Splenectomy

Laparoscopic splenectomy has been successfully performed in steers and heifers up to 250 kg for creation of research animals (D.E. Anderson, unpublished data).

References

1. Fischer AT: *Equine diagnostic and surgical laparoscopy,* Philadelphia, 2002, Saunders, p 290.
2. Bemelman WA, van Doorn RC, de Wit LT et al: Hand-assisted laparoscopic donor nephrectomy. Ascending the learning curve, *Surg Endosc* 15:442-444, 2001.
3. Rehman J, Landman J, Andreoni C et al: Laparoscopic bilateral hand assisted nephrectomy for autosomal dominant polycystic kidney disease: initial experience, *J Urol* 166:42-47, 2001.
4. Sosa R, Seiba M, Shichman S: Hand-assisted laparoscopic surgery, *Semin Laparosc Surg* 7:185-194, 2000.
5. Galuppo LD, Snyder JR, Pascoe JR: Laparoscopic anatomy of the equine abdomen, *Am J Vet Res* 56:518-531, 1995.
6. Galuppo LD, Snyder JR, Pascoe JR et al: Laparoscopic anatomy of the abdomen in dorsally recumbent horses, *Am J Vet Res* 57:923-931, 1996.

7. Boure L, Marcoux M, Laverty S: Laparoscopic abdominal anatomy of foals positioned in dorsal recumbency, *Vet Surg* 26:1-6, 1997.

8. Anderson DE, Gaughan EM, Baird AN et al: Laparoscopic surgical approach and anatomy of the abdomen in llamas, *J Am Vet Med Assoc* 208:111-116, 1996.

9. Yarbrough TB, Snyder JR, Harmon FA: Laparoscopic anatomy of the llama abdomen, *Vet Surg* 24:244-249, 1995.

10. Anderson DE, Gaughan EM, St-Jean G: Normal laparoscopic anatomy of the bovine abdomen, *Am J Vet Res* 54:1170-1176, 1993.

11. King MR, Hendrickson DA, Southwood LL et al: Laparoscopic ovariectomy in two standing llamas, *J Am Vet Med Assoc* 213:523-525, 1998.

12. Nord HJ: Complications of laparoscopy, *Endoscopy* 24:693-700, 1992.

13. Donaldson LL, Trostle SS, White NA: Cardiopulmonary changes associated with abdominal insufflation of carbon dioxide in mechanically ventilated, dorsally recumbent, halothane anaesthetised horses, *Equine Vet J* 30:144-151, 1998.

14. Latimer FG, Eades SC, Pettifer G et al: Cardiopulmonary, blood and peritoneal fluid alterations associated with abdominal insufflation of carbon dioxide in standing horses, *Equine Vet J* 35:283-290, 2003.

15. Lin HC, Baird AN, Pugh DG et al: Effects of carbon dioxide insufflation combined with changes in body position on blood gas and acid-base status in anesthetized llamas *(Llama glama)*, *Vet Surg* 26:444-450, 1997.

16. Fischer AT Jr, Lloyd KC, Carlson GP et al: Diagnostic laparoscopy in the horse, *J Am Vet Med Assoc* 189:289-292, 1986.

17. Ragle CA, Southwood LL, Schneider RK: Injury to abdominal wall vessels during laparoscopy in three horses, *J Am Vet Med Assoc* 212:87-89, 1998.

18. Boure L: Laparoscopic surgical techniques in foals, *Am Coll Vet Surg 2003 Proc.*

19. Walesby HA, Ragle CA, Booth LC: Laparoscopic repair of ruptured urinary bladder in a stallion, *J Am Vet Med Assoc* 221:(1715), 1737-1741, 2002.

20. Edwards RB III, Ducharme NG, Hackett RP: Laparoscopic repair of a bladder rupture in a foal, *Vet Surg* 24:60-63, 1995.

21. Boure L, Foster RA, Palmer M et al: Use of an endoscopic suturing device for laparoscopic resection of the apex of the bladder and umbilical structures in normal neonatal calves, *Vet Surg* 30:319-326, 2001.

22. Fischer AT Jr: Laparoscopically assisted resection of umbilical structures in foals, *J Am Vet Med Assoc* 214:1791-1792, 1813-1816, 1999.

23. Boure L, Kerr C, Pierce SO et al: Comparison of two laparoscopic suture patterns for the repair of experimentally ruptured bladders in normal neonatal calves, *Am Coll Vet Surg 2003 Proc.*

24. Fischer AT Jr, Vachon AM, Klein SR: Laparoscopic inguinal herniorrhaphy in two stallions, *J Am Vet Med Assoc* 207:1599-1601, 1995.

25. Marien T: Standing laparoscopic herniorrhaphy in stallions using cylindrical polypropylene mesh prosthesis, *Equine Vet J* 33:91-96, 2001.

26. Ragle CA, Southwood LL, Howlett MR: Ventral abdominal approach for laparoscopic cryptorchidectomy in horses, *Vet Surg* 27:138-142, 1998.

27. Fischer AT Jr, Vachon AM: Laparoscopic cryptorchidectomy in horses, *J Am Vet Med Assoc* 201:1705-1708, 1992.

28. Davis EW: Laparoscopic cryptorchidectomy in standing horses, *Vet Surg* 26:326-331, 1997.

29. Hendrickson DA, Wilson DG: Laparoscopic cryptorchid castration in standing horses, *Vet Surg* 26:335-339, 1997.

30. Fischer AT, Vachon AM: Laparoscopic intra-abdominal ligation and removal of cryptorchid testes in horses, *Equine Vet J* 30:105-108, 1998.

31. Fowler ME: *Medicine and surgery of South American camelids: llama, alpaca, vicuna, guanaco,* Ames, Iowa, 1998, Iowa State University Press, p 137.

32. Wilson DG: *Surgery of the genitalia of llamas.* In Youngquist RS, editor: *Current therapy in large animal theriogenology,* Philadelphia, 1997, Saunders, p 840.

33. Wilson DG, Hendrickson DA, Cooley AJ et al: Laparoscopic methods for castration of equids, *J Am Vet Med Assoc* 209:112-114, 1996.

34. Bergeron JA, Hendrickson DA, McCue PM: Viability of an inguinal testis after laparoscopic cauterization and transection of its blood supply, *J Am Vet Med Assoc* 213:1280, 1303-1304, 1998.

35. Bravo PW, Sumar J: Evaluation of intra-abdominal vasectomy in llamas and alpacas, *J Am Vet Med Assoc* 199:1164-1166, 1991.

36. Trumble TN, Ingle-Fehr J, Hendrickson DA: Laparoscopic intra-abdominal ligation of the testicular artery following castration in a horse, *J Am Vet Med Assoc* 216:1569, 1596-1598, 2000.

37. Waguespack R, Belknap J, Williams A: Laparoscopic management of postcastration haemorrhage in a horse, *Equine Vet J* 33:510-513, 2001.

38. Boure L, Marcoux M, Laverty S: Paralumbar fossa laparoscopic ovariectomy in horses with use of Endoloop ligatures, *Vet Surg* 26:478-483, 1997.

39. Hanson CA, Galuppo LD: Bilateral laparoscopic ovariectomy in standing mares: 22 cases, *Vet Surg* 28:106-112, 1999.

40. Ragle CA, Schneider RK: Ventral abdominal approach for laparoscopic ovariectomy in horses, *Vet Surg* 24:492-497, 1995.

41. Rodgerson DH, Belknap JK, Wilson DA: Laparoscopic ovariectomy using sequential electrocoagulation and sharp transection of the equine mesovarium, *Vet Surg* 30:572-579, 2001.

42. Hand R, Rakestraw P, Taylor T: Evaluation of a vessel-sealing device for use in laparoscopic ovariectomy in mares, *Vet Surg* 31:240-244, 2002.

43. Dusterdieck KF, Pleasant RS, Lanz OI et al: Evaluation of the harmonic scalpel for laparoscopic bilateral ovariectomy in standing horses, *Vet Surg* 32:242-250, 2003.

44. Palmer SE: Standing laparoscopic laser technique for ovariectomy in five mares, *J Am Vet Med Assoc* 203:279-283, 1993.

45. Ragle CA, Southwood LL, Hopper SA et al: Laparoscopic ovariectomy in two horses with granulosa cell tumors, *J Am Vet Med Assoc* 209:1121-1124, 1996.

46. Rodgerson DH, Brown MP, Watt BC et al: Hand-assisted laparoscopic technique for removal of ovarian tumors in standing mares, *J Am Vet Med Assoc* 220:1475, 1503-1507, 2002.

47. Rodgerson DH, Baird AN, Lin HC et al: Ventral abdominal approach for laparoscopic ovariectomy in llamas, *Vet Surg* 27:331-336, 1998.

48. Delling U, Pleasant RS, Lanz OI: Hand assisted laparoscopic ovariohysterectomy in the mare, *Am Coll Vet Surg 2003 Proc* (abstract).

49. Keoughan CG, Rodgerson DH, Brown MP: Hand-assisted laparoscopic left nephrectomy in standing horses, *Vet Surg* 32:206-212, 2003.

50. Marien T, Adriaenssen A, Hoeck FV et al: Laparoscopic closure of the renosplenic space in standing horses, *Vet Surg* 30:559-563, 2001.

51. Naoi M, Kokue E, Takahashi Y et al: Laparoscopic-assisted serial biopsy of the bovine kidney, *Am J Vet Res* 46:699-702, 1985.

52. Hershlag A, Diamond MP, DeCherney AH: Adhesiolysis, *Clin Obstet Gynecol* 34:395-402, 1991.

53. La Morte AI, Diamond MP: Adhesion formation after laparoscopy, *Prog Clin Biol Res* 381:51-58, 1993.

54. Operative Laparoscopy Study Group: Postoperative adhesion development after operative laparoscopy: evaluation at early second-look procedure, *Fertil Steril* 55:700-704, 1991.

55. Boure L, Marcoux M, Lavoie JP et al: Use of laparoscopic equipment to divide abdominal adhesions in a filly, *J Am Vet Med Assoc* 212:845-847, 1998.

56. Bleyaert HF, Brown MP, Bonenclark G et al: Laparoscopic adhesiolysis in a horse, *Vet Surg* 26:492-496, 1997.

57. Boure LP, Pearce SG, CL Kerr et al: Evaluation of laparoscopic adhesiolysis for the treatment of experimentally induced adhesions in pony foals, *Am J Vet Res* 63:289-294, 2002.

58. Trostle SS, White NA, Donaldson L et al: Laparoscopic colopexy in horses, *Vet Surg* 27:56-63, 1998.

59. Brugmans F, Deegen E: Laparoscopic surgical technique for repair of rectal and colonic tears in horses: an experimental study, *Vet Surg* 30:409-416, 2001.

Recommended Readings

Hanrath M, Rodgerson DH: Laparoscopic cryptorchidectomy using electrosurgical instrumentation in standing horses, *Vet Surg* 31:117-124, 2002.

Janowitz H: [Laparoscopic reposition and fixation of the left displaced abomasum in cattle], *Tierarztl Prax Ausg G Grosstiere Nutztiere* 26:308-313, 1998.

Kehler W, Stark M: [*Laparoscopic repositioning and fixation of the left-displaced abomasum: anatomic assessment of the development of the fixation in the abdominal cavity in the following six months*], XXII World Buiatrics Congress 2002 (abstract).

Seeger T, Kumper H, Doll K: [*Surgical treatment of left displaced abomasum: results of laparoscopic reposition with abomasopexy (Janowitz-method) compared to right flank laparotomy with omentopexy (Dirken-mentod)*], XXII World Buiatrics Congress 2002, 2003 (abstract).

van Leeuwen E, Janowitz H, Willemen MA: [Laparoscopic positioning and attachment of stomach displacement to the left in the cow], *Tijdschr Diergeneeskd* 125:391-392, 2000.

van Leeuwen E, Muller K: [*Laparoscopic treatment of the left displaced abomasum in cattle and results of 108 cases treated under field conditions*], XXII World Buiatrics Congress 2002, (abstract).

SECTION X

Ophthalmic Examination Techniques

Harriet J. Davidson

CHAPTER 84

Ophthalmic Examination Techniques for Production Animals

HARRIET J. DAVIDSON

An ophthalmic examination is necessary when animals are suffering from obvious ocular problems, but it may be a diagnostic aid for general health abnormalities. The extra information gained from the ophthalmic examination may support the need for further systemic testing. Animals with neurologic disease in particular may benefit because of the number of cranial nerves involved in normal ocular health. To complete a successful ophthalmic examination, the practitioner must have the proper equipment, an appropriate facility for examination, and knowledge of normal ocular anatomy.

The purpose of this section is to review the common ophthalmic examination techniques, with adaptations that may be used by the production animal veterinarian. Covering all ophthalmic examination techniques or providing an in-depth description of anatomy is beyond the scope of this chapter. Practitioners are referred to the bibliography for further information.

HISTORY

Before making a trip or immediately on arrival at the farm or ranch, an ophthalmic history should be completed. Because of the nature of production medicine, information should be gathered about individual animals, herd problems, and general management techniques. Questions such as, "What are the symptoms?" and "What is the duration?" seem straightforward but can be complicated depending on how closely the animals are monitored. It may be helpful to ask the manager to describe what he or she has observed and when. Asking how often the animals are viewed and in what manner may also help in determining the length of time for the problem. In many cases the animal may be evaluated from a distance, and close observation of both eyes may have been impractical. Asking which animals are affected should be combined with questions on the location and times that the animals are affected. Variations in the likelihood of certain diseases affecting different ages of animals exist. Changes in pastures, locations, or activities may result in problems in different age groups or types of animals. Questions regarding what has been changed with the general management of the animals should include changes on diets, treatments, and vaccine protocols, as well as new animals brought into

the herd. Questions regarding what treatments have been used on the animals for the current condition may help in diagnosis of the problem, as well as prevent repetition of treatments that have not worked. Questions should be asked in an open and nonjudgmental manner to elicit the greatest amount of information and improve the success of future treatments.

INSTRUMENTS AND SUPPLIES

The items listed in Box 84-1 are my recommendations for materials used in performing a complete ophthalmic examination. It may be helpful to have these items packed into a carry box, or tackle box, to assist on-site examination. Ophthalmic instruments can be delicate and require gentle handling; careful packing of the instruments helps prevent on-site damage. A preprinted ophthalmic examination sheet may help remind the practitioner of the best order to complete each task and prevent the omission of procedures. The examination form should allow for the drawing of pictures of ocular lesions. Detailed descriptions, including measurement of lesions or pictures, aid in monitoring the progression or resolution of the disease. The use of each instrument is discussed in the following section involving detailed ocular examination.

EXAMINATION AREA AND RESTRAINT TECHNIQUES

Area

Examination should begin with a general inspection of the animals and farm or ranch site. This includes a general physical inspection of the animals to determine clinical signs of respiratory diseases, malnutrition, or unthriftiness. These conditions may be related to ocular problems. It may be helpful to evaluate the area for housing conditions such as the degree of shade, dust conditions, and fly control efforts because these factors may also be related to ocular lesions.

Ophthalmic examination is best completed in a dark, quiet environment. This may be a stall or shed. In many cases the animal chute is outside, which does not allow for a dark environment. Although it seems cumbersome, it may be helpful to temporarily drape a tarp or blanket

Box 84-1

Instruments and Supplies Recommended for Ophthalmic Examination

Instruments
Ophthalmic/otic diagnostic set with fiberoptic Finoff transilluminator (No. 41100), direct ophthalmoscope (No. 11720), and otoscope (No. 20260) interchangeable heads with a 3.5-V rechargeable nickel-cadmium battery (Welch Allyn, Skaneateles, Wash.)
Panoptic ophthalmoscope
20-D (5×) veterinary viewing lens (Welch Allyn)
Magnifying head loupe (Donegan Optical Company Inc., Kansas City, Mo.)
Dressing forceps with rounded, serrated tips (or a curved Kelly hemostat)

Supplies
Eye wash, normal saline, or lactated Ringer's solution
Fluorescein-impregnated paper strips (Fluor-I-Strips, Ayerst Laboratories, New York)
Schirmer tear test strips (Schering-Plough Animal Health, Kenilworth, N.J.)
Culturette II (Becton-Dickinson, Franklin Lakes, N.J.)
Cotton-tipped applicators
Roll cotton or cotton balls
3½-Fr tomcat catheter, polyethylene (Sovereign)
20-, 22-gauge Teflon intravenous catheters (Angiocath, Becton-Dickinson)
No. 15 Bard-Parker scalpel blade
Tropicamide, 1% (Mydriacyl, Alcon, Fort Worth, Texas)
Proparacaine, 0.5% (Ophthetic, Allergan, Irvine, Calif.)
Lidocaine, 1% or 2% (Butler, Columbus, Ohio)

around the animal's head and examiner to darken the environment and allow better examination of intraocular structures.

The type of restraint for a close and detailed ophthalmic examination depends on the species, type, and demeanor of the animal. A stanchion, chute, or crate and a halter, nose lead, and/or snare are frequently required. Position of the head substantially alters the position of the eye. Pulling the head up tends to cause the eye to roll ventrally. Animals in lateral recumbency also tend to roll the eye ventrally. This deviation of the eye makes it difficult to examine the ventral half of the globe or have access to examine the posterior segment. Pulling the head laterally may expose more of the medial aspect of the globe in the eye away from the direction that the head/neck is bent.

In most production animals, chemical restraint for the ophthalmic examination is not necessary. However, it may be necessary in extremely fractious animals. Xylazine may be used to adequately restrain most food animals, but drug withdrawal times and the risk of apnea, bradycardia, and recumbency following sedation should always be considered. Additionally, xylazine alters the palpebral, corneal, menace, and dazzle reflexes and may cause enophthalmos and third eyelid protrusion, which may hinder a complete ophthalmic examination.

Nerve Blocks

Local nerve blocks may help overcome blepharospasm that may be seen with painful ocular conditions. The simplest nerve block involves injection of lidocaine around the palpebral branch of the auriculopalpebral nerve (cranial nerve VII). This local block gives partial eyelid akinesia but offers no analgesia and does not affect retraction of the globe or third eyelid movement. In most ruminants the nerve can be palpated subcutaneously as it courses along the zygomatic arch midway between the base of the ear and lateral canthus. The nerve can be difficult to palpate in heavy fleshed animals (beef cattle and bulls) and swine. Local infiltration about the nerve (1-5 ml of 1% injectable lidocaine) followed by vigorous massage of the area will usually negate the animal's ability to forcibly close the lids.

Topical anesthesia of the cornea, conjunctiva, and third eyelid may be achieved with commercially available topical anesthetic. For minor procedures (conjunctival scrapings or superficial biopsies), several applications of 0.2 ml of a topical anesthetic at approximately 5-minute intervals or placement of a cotton tip applicator that has been soaked in ophthalmic anesthetic on the area in question provides adequate anesthesia. More extensive procedures (third eyelid excision, deep eyelid resection, or enucleation) require regional anesthetic blocks.

Unlike the adequately described regional nerve blocks for the lids and adnexa in the horse, species and animal-to-animal variation makes it impossible to describe the exact location of the distribution of the zygomatic, lacrimal, infraorbital, and frontal nerves (sensory branches to the lids and adnexa) in production animals. For palpebral and third eyelid surgery, local infiltration (line blocks) of injectable anesthetic with a small-gauge needle (23-25 gauge) usually provides adequate anesthesia. The Peterson eye block, which allows for placement of local anesthetic behind the globe to provide anesthesia of the orbit and the structures cranial to the orbit, can cause inadvertent injection of anesthetic into the subdural space, with resultant death from apnea and cardiac arrest, and I do not recommend using it. A four-point nerve block involving the use of a bent 18-gauge spinal needle to deliver retrobulbar anesthetic (the needle is passed through the skin and walked along the orbital bone to a site behind the globe; injections are made at four sites: dorsal, ventral, lateral canthus, and medial canthus) should be used to anesthetize the orbit for extensive surgical procedures (e.g., enucleation or orbital exenteration). The amount of anesthetic agent per site depends on the size of the animal (2-6 ml per site for sheep and goats to 10-15 ml per site for adult cattle).

VISION AND OPHTHALMIC REFLEXES

Vision should be accessed before restraint of the animal. This may be accomplished by observing the animal in its normal environment; in some cases visual deficits are obvious. However, because of the herd mentality of most production animals, those being studied may need to be separated from the herd to observe them moving alone. A maze or obstacle course can be made using buckets, hay bales, and other objects. Importantly, the objects must not have hard or sharp edges that may injure the animal. Equally important is ensuring that the animal can be caught again without injuring itself or personnel. If unilateral blindness is suspected, alternately patching the eyes with gauze or cloth taped over the eye may help with the diagnosis. Animals may use their other senses more aggressively when they are blind. They may carry the head lower with ear position more forward and active. Animals with acute vision loss frequently keep their eyes open wider than normal and ears more erect. Animals that cannot see and have recently been separated from their companions may be more easily frightened and can be dangerous.

The animal must be restrained for examination of ophthalmic reflexes. The pupillary light reflex (PLR), menace response, dazzle reflex, and vision are described in greater detail in the section on neurogenic vision loss. In short, the pupillary light reflex tests the following pathway: retina→optic nerve (II)→optic chiasm→optic tract→Edinger-Westphal nucleus of the brain→midbrain →parasympathetic fibers of the oculomotor (III) nerve and the iris structure. Initially note the size of the pupils in both the light and dark environment. Note the size of the pupils relative to each other, as well as in normal animals. Stressed animals may have large pupils that are slow to respond. Patience and a bright light aids the response. Using a bright, finely focused light held approximately 3 to 6 inches from the eye, the direct reflex is accessed by observing that eye for pupillary constriction. The consensual, or indirect, reflex is evaluated by quickly moving the light to the opposite eye and evaluating its size. A normal response is to find the opposite pupil constricted. The menace reflex tests the retina→optic nerve (II)→optic chiasm→optic tract→visual cortex→facial nerve (VII). The dazzle reflex is similar, but it tests the subcortical area of the brain. This reflex is elicited by rapidly moving an object into the animal's visual field and observing it for a blink. The examiner must be careful not to touch the eye or surrounding face physically or with air currents because this may elicit a palpebral or corneal reflex. The menace reflex can be overridden in some animals and is not present in neonates. The dazzle reflex is elicited by shining a bright light into the eye from a close distance and observing the animal for a blink or retraction of the eye. The palpebral reflexes can be elicited by lightly touching the medial or lateral canthus and observing the animal's blink. The corneal reflex is tested by lightly touching the cornea with finger, cotton tip applicator, or small section of soft cloth. The normal responses are blinking and retraction of the globe. These reflexes test the palpebral nerve or corneal nerve→trigeminal nerve→brainstem→facial nerve. Twisting the head from side to side or up and down causes a nystagmus, with the fast phase of the nystagmus being in the direction of head movement. This tests the function of the extraocular muscles and their corresponding innervation: oculomotor (III), trochlear (IV), and abduces (VI).

EXAMINATION OF THE EYE AND ADNEXA

The face should be evaluated for symmetry of the eyelids, ears, and lip position. Abnormalities may be indicative of neurologic abnormalities involving the vestibular system or facial nerve. The lids should be examined to ensure there is no entropion (inward turn of the eyelid) or ectropion (outward turn of the eyelid). Digital retropulsion with the flat surface of the fingers through closed eyelids helps to access any space-occupying lesions within the orbit. Keeping the superior lid slightly open with digital pressure applied through the lid retropulses the globe and allows the third eyelid to be passively moved across the surface of the eye, allowing examination of the palpebral surface. Retropulsion of the globe should not be done in cases of suspected corneal ulceration because this may inadvertently rupture the globe.

Schirmer Tear Test

A Schirmer tear test (STT) is used to measure aqueous tear production. Although this test is rarely necessary in production animal medicine, it should be completed if low tear production is suspected. Clinical signs of low tear production include mucoid discharge; dull, lusterless cornea; and chronic conjunctivitis. An STT should be performed before placing any substances into the eye, or at least 15 minutes following, because fluid in the conjunctival sac alters the results. The test is completed by bending the STT strip at the notched mark, placing it in the lower conjunctival sac, and holding it gently in place for 30 seconds or 1 minute. The result is the millimeter of wetting of the strip in that time period. Normal values for cattle are 24 mm/30 sec; values for other animals have not been reported.

Fluorescein Stain

Fluorescein stain is used to test for corneal ulceration. Several possible methods of applying the fluorescein are available. One method is to moisten the fluorescein strip and touch the strip to the bulbar surface of the eye. A second method is to mix the fluorescein in eye wash or topical anesthetic solution in a 1-ml syringe. The needle is then broken from the hub and the solution is sprayed on the corneal surface. This must be performed carefully because the hub of the needle can still damage the cornea of it is poked directly onto the ocular surface. It is also not recommended to store this suspension for more than a few hours because it may become contaminated. (If large volumes of liquid ophthalmic fluorescein are necessary, the sterile solution can be purchased.) Using either method, washing of the excess stain may not be required because of the high rate of normal tearing in most production animals. Excess stain may be picked up by mucus strands and misinterpreted as a positive ulcer. This can be prevented by washing the ocular surface with eye wash or saline or manually blinking the eyelids. The stain can be viewed with a normal light source or a cobalt blue filter, which aids in fluorescence; a positive stain is green. To access the depth of the ulcer, the cornea can be viewed from the side.

Intraocular Pressure Measurement

Intraocular pressure (IOP) is rarely measured in production animal medicine. However, measurements may aid in the diagnosis of uveitis (a lower than normal IOP) and glaucoma (a higher than normal IOP). A Tonopen uses applanation to measure the IOP. The Tono-vet measures IOP by rebound. Using either instrument, it may be helpful, although not required, to apply topical anesthetic to the eye before measurement. Each of these instruments is handheld and easily used in animals. The instrument reports the IOP in mm Hg. The average IOP reported in cattle is between 16 and 28 mm Hg. This value is rather standard across species and may be extrapolated to be considered normal in other production animal species.

Anterior Segment Examination

Close examination of the eye generally requires the eyelids to be physically opened. This is accomplished by placing the side of the thumb or forefinger directly along the lid margin, rolling or pressing the eyelid against the orbital rim, either dorsally or ventrally. The closer the finger is placed to the eyelid margin, the easier it is to open. If the eye is painful, the resulting blepharospasm will make opening the lids extremely difficult. In these cases a nerve blocks may aid in examination and treatment (see end of this section). In many large animals the pupil is large enough to allow for fairly good examination of the lens and fundus. However, dilation of the pupil allows easier and more extensive examination. Pupillary dilation is most efficiently accomplished with the administration of tropicamide ophthalmic solution.

Examination of ocular structures for opacities may begin by viewing the eye from an arm's distance away and aiming a bright, finely focused light into the animal's eye (like sighting down a gun barrel). This causes light to be reflected back at the examiner as retroillumination. Opacities of structures within the eye appear as dark foci, or shadows, against the bright fundic reflex. Detailed examination of the anterior segment (lids, third eyelid, conjunctiva, sclera, cornea, iris, pupil, and anterior lens) is best done with a bright, well-focused light source such as a transilluminator with a Finoff tip, an otoscope head, or a bright penlight. Using a magnification loupe or glasses allows the examiner to focus on small, delicate lesions. The surfaces of the eye and adnexa should be viewed from the front, as well as the side, with illumination both from the front and the side. Evaluation from the side allows for assessment of depth of corneal ulcers or localization of opacities to the cornea, anterior chamber, or lens. An additional method to localize an opacity is to use the slit beam from a direct ophthalmoscope shown into the eye, while the eye is examined from a different angle using some form of magnification. As a linear focal light beam passes through the eye, light is refracted and reflected along the cornea, anterior lens capsule, and posterior lens capsule. The first two beams (cornea and anterior lens capsule) appear convex (bow outward) when viewed from the side, and the third beam (posterior lens capsule) appears concave (bows inward). As the light is swept slowly back and forth across the eye, the reflected light moves across the opacity. Additionally, the direct ophthalmoscope may be used to focus on intraocular structures. The cornea is generally in focus at a setting of +20 D, the anterior lens and iris at +10 to +12 D, and the posterior lens at +7 to +9 D.

Fundic Examination

The ocular fundus can be examined with many things, including the naked eye and a bright light source, direct ophthalmoscope, panoptic ophthalmoscope, or indirect ophthalmoscope. The examiner places his or her eye approximately 2 to 5 cm from the animal's eye and then shines a light into the eye. This can be an otoscope with the objective lens flipped out of the line of sight or another form of bright, well-focused light. The direct ophthalmoscope is also used from a distance of 2 to 5 cm at a setting of −2 to +2 D. These two methods allow direct viewing of the fundus, but only a small area is seen, so it is difficult to view the periphery of the fundus and may be dangerous if the animal bangs its head into the examiner. The panoptic ophthalmoscope allows for a larger area of the fundus to be examined. Although the instrument is held approximately 4 cm from the animal's eye, the unit is slightly larger than the ophthalmoscope, so the examiner is slightly farther from the animal. Indirect ophthalmoscopy requires a bright, well-focused light source and a condensing lens, generally 15, 20, or 25 D. At approximately an arm's distance from the animal the light is shown into the eye, creating a fundic reflex. The lens is held in the opposite hand and placed in the line of light, perpendicular to the line of light, approximately 2 to 6 cm from the animal's eye. This creates a virtual image; the image is upside down and backward. The magnification is much less than with direct ophthalmoscopy, but the periphery of the fundus is readily visible and the examiner is less likely to be hit by the animal's head. A variation in the appearance of the normal fundus exists, depending on the species. The bovine, ovine, and caprine fundus is holangiotic (there are arteries and veins extending the entire portion of the fundus). In these species the optic nerve is oval in shape and white, pink, or gray, depending on the degree of myelination. The dorsal portion of the fundus contains the tapetum, which is generally blue, green, yellow, or orange, depending on the coat color of the animal.

Lacrimal Duct Flush

Animals that have epiphora (excessive tearing) with no obvious cause may benefit from flushing of the lacrimal duct either as a diagnostic test or a treatment to remove debris. In most ruminants the eyelid puncta are on the inner lid margin approximately 5 to 10 mm from the medial canthus, on the upper and lower eyelids. Swine have only one punctum on the upper eyelid. A topical ophthalmic anesthetic is placed on the ocular surface to prevent the animal from feeling the procedure. Normograde flushing of the duct may be accomplished by sliding a small cannula into the puncta and flushing fluid into the cannula. The cannula may be a lacrimal cannula made for this purpose or a 3½-French (Fr), open-ended polyethylene tomcat catheter or 26-22–gauge Teflon intravenous catheter with the stylet removed. The cannula is inserted approximately 5 to 10 mm. Occluding the opposite duct with digital pressure prevents reflux of fluid. Generally 5 ml of fluid such as eyewash, sterile saline, or lactated Ringer's solution is adequate to flush the duct. More fluid may be necessary to therapeutically remove debris. Gentle pressure is used on the syringe. Because the duct is small, fluid does not travel rapidly to the end. If resistance is met while flushing, pulsing the injection may aid in dislodging an obstruction. Fluid should be seen exiting the nose. Fluorescein stain may be mixed with the flush solution to allow for easier identification of substance in the nasal vestibule. However, stain can be messy when the animal snorts or shakes its head. Retrograde flushing of the nasolacrimal duct may be achieved by catheterizing the nasal punctum with a red rubber 3- or 5-Fr canine urinary catheter or 3½-Fr closed or open-ended polyethylene tomcat catheter. In the cow the nasal punctum is laterally positioned under the alar cartilage; in sheep and goats, it is on the medial surface of the alar fold, just off the floor of the nasal vestibule. The puncta may be visually identified by pulling the alar cartilage laterally and shining a light into the nasal vestibule. The puncta may be cannulated while viewing them or, more easily, through blind insertion following visual identification. Fluid flushed into the cannula will exit the eyelid puncta. In swine the nasal vestibule is usually too small to allow observation or catheterization of the nasal punctum.

Third Eyelid Examination

Examining behind the third eyelid requires a palpebral nerve block and/or topical ophthalmic anesthetic. A non-toothed, serrated dressing forceps or a hemostat may be used to gently grasp the third eyelid margin and evert the nictitans to allow examination. The hemostat should not be locked or the tissue grasped too firmly with the dressing forceps because the topical anesthetic does not alleviate the deep pain that occurs when too much pressure is applied to these structures. A cotton tip applicator may also be used to slide between the third eyelid and the cornea and then push the third eyelid up and out to allow examination underneath. A bright light source should be used to illuminate the pocket that is formed behind the third eyelid. Digital palpation may be used to identify any foreign objects that may be deep within the pocket.

Sample Collection

Scrapings of the external ocular surface may be evaluated microscopically to diagnose infection or neoplasia. To obtain adequate cells for evaluation, a palpebral nerve block and topical anesthetic are first administered. With the flat handle end of a scalpel blade, the surface of the lesion is repeatedly scraped gently in the same direction until a pellet of cellular material clings to the blade. This material is gently blotted onto a slide and stained with Diff-Quik or Wright's stain (for cellular morphology) or with Gram stain (for bacterial identification).

Recommended Readings

Barnett KC: *Color atlas of veterinary ophthalmology*, St Louis, 1996, Mosby.

Gelatt KN: Ophthalmic examination and diagnostic procedures. In Gelatt KN, editor: *Veterinary ophthalmology*, ed 2, Philadelphia, 1991, Lea & Febiger, pp 195-236.

Severin GA: Examination of the eye. In *Severin's veterinary ophthalmology notes*, ed 3, Fort Collins, Colo, 1996, DesignPointe Communications, pp 1-62.

Whitley RD, Moore CP: Ocular diagnostic and therapeutic techniques in food animals, *Vet Clin North Am Large Anim Pract* 6:553-575, 1984.

CHAPTER 85

Selected Eye Diseases of Cattle

HARRIET J. DAVIDSON and J. PHILLIP PICKETT

Infectious bovine keratoconjunctivitis (IBK), or "pink-eye"; ocular squamous cell carcinoma; and orbital lymphosarcoma are the most common eye diseases production animal practitioners diagnose and treat. These three entities are responsible for the majority of ocular-based economic losses for cattle producers. However, many ocular disorders can cause pain and blindness in the animal, with subsequent economic loss for the producer. This section covers IBK, as well as other ocular disorders. Squamous cell carcinoma and lymphosarcoma are covered under the ocular neoplasia section. Except for systemic diseases in which the ocular signs are a minor component of the overall disease entity, specific therapy and potential preventive measures are discussed. In the case of systemic diseases with ophthalmic manifestations, although supportive ocular therapy may be described, the practitioner is referred to other sections within this text for specific therapy.

ORBIT/GLOBE DISORDERS

Congenital anophthalmia (total absence of the eye) and congenital microphthalmia (a small, usually nonfunctional eye) are occasionally found in cattle. If the condition is unilateral, clinical signs may include a serous, mucous, or purulent ocular discharge; secondary entropion; or simply the appearance of a small or absent globe in the socket. Bilaterally afflicted animals are usually blind. Any disorder (physical, toxic, or infectious) that can cause in utero maldevelopment could cause microphthalmia. Bovine viral diarrhea (BVD)/mucosal disease infection between days 75 and 150 of gestation can cause cataract formation, retinal and optic nerve degeneration/dysphasia, nystagmus, and microphthalmos, as well as central nervous system disease.

Genetic anophthalmia/microphthalmia is seen in several breeds of cattle. The ocular disease may be seen alone, or there may be multiple congenital anomalies associated with the eye disease. In Herefords, inherited microphthalmia has been described in association with muscular dystrophy and hydrocephalus. Microphthalmia and other ocular defects have been associated with hydrocephalus in Shorthorn cattle. Inherited microphthalmia in Jerseys, Guernseys, and Holsteins may be seen in conjunction with cardiac malformations (high ventricular septal defects), as well as skeletal abnormalities (vertebral defects of the lumbar and/or sacral vertebrae, wrytail, or total absence of a tail). Because the inheritance of these disorders appears to be autosomal recessive, rebreeding the carrier sire and dam together is not recommended and culling of apparent carriers may be in order.

Phthisis bulbi (an acquired shrunken eye) is normally secondary to injury such as a perforated wound, ruptured corneal ulcer, or severe uveitis. These eyes are blind and may be ugly in appearance but generally are not painful and require no treatment. Secondary entropion or kerato-conjunctivitis, which can be painful, may occur because of loss of normal globe eyelid conformation. In these cases enucleation is the only option.

Congenital megaloglobus (enlarged eye) secondary to glaucoma is seen in Holsteins in association with malformation of the anterior chamber and lens. Calves with unilateral disease may have one enlarged, blind, nonpainful eye or may have secondary exposure keratitis, corneal ulceration, and pain. Bilaterally afflicted animals are blind. If painful, the globe should be enucleated. Acquired glaucoma in cattle is uncommon and usually secondary to corneal perforation following IBK or traumatic or infectious uveitis. Treatment recommendations are the same as for congenital glaucoma.

Esotropia, also known as convergent strabismus or "crossed eyes," with or without exophthalmos may be congenital or acquired. In Holsteins, Jerseys, Shorthorns, Ayrshires, and Brown Swiss, strabismus is occasionally seen at birth. A motor deficiency of the extraocular muscles (lateral rectus and retractor bulbi) innervated by the abducens nerve (VI) causes a nonpainful, non–vision-threatening disorder that appears to be autosomal recessive in inheritance. In the Jersey breed, a recessively inherited, progressive convergent strabismus has also been described and is first noted at 6 to 12 months of age. Exotropia, or divergent strabismus, may be seen in cattle and is usually associated with hydrocephalus. Congenital nystagmus has been described in Holsteins (and other breeds) and is seen as a pendular, constant horizontal nystagmus that seems to cause no vision deficit. The disorder is familial, but the mode of inheritance is unknown. Acquired strabismus and/or nystagmus may be seen in cattle as a result of neurologic disorders such as polioencephalomalacia, listeriosis, thromboembolic meningoencephalitis, toxic phenomena, and other nonspecific disorders of the brainstem and cerebellum. These systemic diseases are generally accompanied by other neurologic conditions and require specific therapy.

Exophthalmos (normal size globe protruding outward from the socket) may be due to retrobulbar neoplasia, orbital cellulitis, or periorbital sinusitis. Orbital cellulitis is generally acute and frequently accompanied by a swelling of the lids and conjunctiva and third eyelid protrusion. Fever, anorexia, and depression are usually present with orbital cellulitis, which is not usually the case with orbital lymphosarcoma unless the tumor involves multiple body systems. Puncture wounds through the lids or conjunctiva, maxillary molar root abscess, and migration of herbaceous material from the mouth into the orbital space are causes of orbital cellulitis. Differentiation of orbital cellulitis from orbital neoplasia may be accomplished by aspiration and cytologic evaluation of material from behind the eye. Neutrophils, macrophages, bacterial organisms or foreign material generally suggest orbital cellulitis. Lymphosarcoma is the more likely diagnosis when the cell types are predominately lymphocytes, lymphoblasts, and/or neoplastic cells. Periorbital sinusitis usually involves a more chronic, progressive distortion of the bony periocular tissue. Maxillary or frontal sinusitis is usually due to infection secondary to dehorning or trauma resulting in fractures. Infectious agents such as *Actinomyces pyogenes*, *A. bovis*, and *Pasteurella* spp. are common with periorbital sinusitis. Treatment of orbital cellulitis involves protection of the eye. A temporary tarsorrhaphy or frequent lubrication with ophthalmic ointment may be necessary if the animal cannot blink. A warm, moist compress may be used to reduce swelling, along with analgesics (aspirin, phenylbutazone, flunixin meglumine) and systemic antibiotic therapy. If a tract from a foreign body can be found, it should be probed and drainage should be attempted. Unresponsive orbital cellulitis with extensive ocular damage and a blind eye may necessitate orbital exenteration and placement of drains. Treatment of periorbital sinusitis may involve trephination of the sinus to establish drainage, curettage, and broad-spectrum antibiotic therapy.

EYELID/THIRD EYELID/NASOLACRIMAL SYSTEM DISORDERS

The two most common congenital disorders of the adnexa are a dermoid and a supernumerary opening of the nasolacrimal duct. A dermoid is aberrant skin; diagnosis and treatment are covered under cornea/conjunctiva in this section. Accessory opening to the nasolacrimal duct appears as a hairless, depigmented opening on the face inferior to the medial canthus. Tear staining and minor facial dermatitis may occur as a result of this deformity. Treatment requires surgical intervention to reform or close the irregular duct. Because the clinical problem is not severe, treatment is generally not warranted. Brown Swiss and Holsteins seem to be afflicted most commonly.

Acquired lagophthalmos (inability to close the eyelids) may be a result of nerve damage or secondary to exophthalmos. Lagophthalmos may result in drying of the corneal surface and ulceration. Nerve damage may be a result of trauma to the facial nerve caused by a severe blow to the head or as the animal attempts to pull its head from the stanchion. Central nervous system disorders such as polioencephalomalacia or listeriosis may also result in lagophthalmos. Symptomatic therapy includes application of topical ophthalmic ointment or temporary tarsorrhaphy to protect the cornea while waiting to see whether the nerve paralysis resolves.

Acute eyelid edema and conjunctival chemosis may be seen as a result of allergic reactions to antibiotics, intravenous fluids, blood transfusions, or, rarely, vaccines. This allergic phenomenon is usually bilateral and may be seen in conjunction with urticaria, skin wheals, generalized facial swelling, and other mucocutaneous junction swelling. Systemic antihistamines, corticosteroids, and/or epinephrine along with cold compresses are recommended, as well as attempts to identify the offending agent and avoidance of future exposure. Sunburn of the eyelids may occur in white-faced animals. It may also occur secondary to photosensitization following phenothiazine administration or the ingestion of toxic plants. Conjunctival necrosis and severe corneal edema, particularly ventrally, may occasionally be present as a result of photosensitization. Supportive care includes providing shade for afflicted animals and topical application of antibiotic ointment to the lids, conjunctiva, and cornea to prevent secondary bacterial infection.

Treatment of traumatic eyelid lacerations depends on the severity of the lesion. Minor lid lacerations may heal following cleansing and the application of antibiotic ointment. If the eyelid is damaged such that lid closure and protection of the globe cannot be achieved, gentle, judicious débridement of necrotic tissue followed by multiple-layer surgical closure of the wound is indicated. A palpebral nerve block and local anesthesia help assist meticulous placement of two layers of sutures, one deep in the eyelid musculature with absorbable suture while making sure that no suture can come in contact with the corneal surface and another in the external skin.

Ocular squamous cell carcinoma is the most common neoplasm involving the lids, the third eyelid, or the globe itself in cattle. The second most common eyelid mass is fibropapilloma or warts. These virally induced growths are typically seen in the young and are mostly self-limiting. Large warts may be successfully removed by debulking and cryosurgery with liquid nitrogen.

Occlusion of the nasolacrimal duct is clinically seen as epiphora (excess tearing) or a mucoid ocular discharge in animals with minimal other signs of conjunctival or corneal disease. Lack of passage of fluorescein dye through the nasolacrimal system is diagnostic. Inflammatory debris, food particles, weed seeds, and parasites (*Thelazia* spp.) may occlude the nasolacrimal duct. Treatment involves flushing the nasolacrimal duct and removal of the inciting cause.

Keratoconjunctivitis sicca (KCS) caused by a lack of aqueous tear production is rarely seen in cattle, but it can be seen after the ingestion of locoweed (*Oxytropis* and *Astragalus*). Supportive therapy includes frequent application of ophthalmic ointment or artificial tears to protect the cornea. A partial or total temporary tarsorrhaphy will also protect the globe and decrease drying of the corneal surface. This form of KCS may be transient or permanent. If normal tear production does not return within a reasonable period of time, the animal should be culled from the herd, preferably before it develops severe keratitis. Topical ophthalmic cyclosporine (0.2%-2%) and tacrolimus (0.02%-0.03%) applied twice daily have been shown to improve natural tearing. These medications may be considered for treatment of KCS in pets but are not logistically possible for production animals.

CONJUNCTIVAL AND CORNEAL DISORDERS

Conjunctival Disorders

The appearance of the conjunctiva may be useful in diagnosing systemic disease. Icterus may first be seen on the bulbar conjunctiva; conjunctival hemorrhage may indicate thrombocytopenia, warfarin toxicity, and/or septicemic states and pallor may indicate anemia. Subconjunctival hemorrhage in newborns is commonly seen following birth trauma and usually resolves without therapy. Bovine viral diarrhea infection in adult cattle occasionally causes mild conjunctivitis. Conjunctivitis may also be due to exposure to ocular irritants such as ammonia fumes, dust and feed material, plant awns and seeds, and disinfectants. History, physical examination, and complete ophthalmic examination helps to rule out some of these other disorders.

Infestation of the conjunctival fornices (recesses around the third eyelid) and the nasolacrimal ducts with the nematode *Thelazia*, several species of which are called "eye worms," usually causes little or no surface ocular disease, but keratoconjunctivitis may occur with heavy infestations. The diagnosis is based on identifying the 1- to 2-cm-long worms in the tears, examination under the lids or behind the third eyelid, or from nasolacrimal duct flushing. Treatment in severe cases involves the use of oral levamisole or fenbendazole, topical application of ivermectin formulated into an eye drop (2 μg/ml), or physically picking the worms out after application of topical ophthalmic anesthetic. Systemic ivermectin at recommended doses is not consistently effective against conjunctival *Thelazia*. Reinfection is likely if measures are not taken to eradicate face flies, the biologic vector.

Corneal or conjunctival dermoid may occur as a congenital anomaly. This appears as keratonized or hairy skin on the corneal or conjunctival surface. These are seen more commonly in the dorsal and lateral aspects of the eye at the limbus. The eye should be examined to determine if the hairs are rubbing on the ocular surface, resulting in chronic keratitis or conjunctivitis. If this is the case, surgical excision of the dermoid is the best method of therapy. Best surgical results are achieved with the animal under general anesthesia or heavy sedation to prevent inadvertent movement of the eye. The dermoid is completely resected using a scalpel with a No 15 blade or 6400 beaver blade. Postoperative topical antibiotic should be applied three times daily until the surgically induced ulcer has healed. A bilateral, congenital, recessively inherited corneal endothelial dystrophy is seen in Holsteins. Clinically this appears as a nonpainful, diffuse corneal edema that can be severe enough to cause blindness. No effective treatment for this condition is available. Animals afflicted with either of the disorders should not be used for breeding purposes.

Ulcers and Keratitis

Topical application of toxic substances in the form of insecticides, disinfectants, and chemicals may cause corneal ulcers and stromal necrosis. Chlorhexidine is a common disinfectant used in dairies. When accidentally sprayed on the corneal surface, it can result in serious ocular injury. Anhydrous ammonia used as a fertilizer and as a silage additive is equally toxic to the corneal surface. Immediate therapy for any toxic substance on the ocular surface is copious lavage with water followed by symptomatic therapy. Systemic antiinflammatory medications decrease the concurrent uveitis that may develop with corneal ulcers. Topical ophthalmic antibiotic steroid combinations may be helpful in some cases of chemically induced ulceration, although they may not be physically practical. Additionally, systemic injections of antibiotics may aid in prevention of secondary bacterial corneal infections.

Photosensitization secondary to toxic plant or phenothiazine ingestion may cause severe corneal edema and has been described earlier in this article. Severe long-term vitamin A deficiency may cause corneal edema along with retinal and optic nerve disease.

Trauma to the ocular surface is a common cause of corneal ulceration. Hay and straw, weeds and grasses, conjunctival foreign bodies, restraint devices, and even switching tails may disrupt the corneal epithelium. Exposure keratitis caused by an inability to blink because of exophthalmos or facial nerve paralysis may result in ulcers found in a central position on the cornea. The clinical appearance of an ulcer may begin with epiphora and blepharospasm; close examination may reveal corneal opacity caused by edema and miosis. Superficial abrasions frequently heal without medical intervention. Secondary bacterial infection may occur and result in more serious corneal ulceration. Infected ulcers have a white to yellow appearance in the surrounding cornea. White may be a result of corneal edema, which is a normal response to injury. The yellow color may be a result of inflammatory cells. Superficial blood vessels may extend from the limbus to the ulcer. These vessels are a normal response to injury and aid in the healing process. The ulcer is confirmed with a positive uptake of fluorescein stain. Treatment depends on the use and type of the animal. Infected ulcers are best treated by application of broad-spectrum topical ophthalmic antibiotics four or more times daily. If the ulcer fails to improve within 2 to 4 days, a culture of the ulcer may be necessary to determine the organism present. Ophthalmic atropine may be applied once or twice daily to dilate the pupil, decrease the ciliary muscle spasm that results in pain, and help stabilize the blood aqueous barrier that results in secondary uveitis. Systemic nonsteroidal antiinflammatory drugs (NSAIDs) may also help relieve the secondary uveitis. The vast majority of ulcers heal with medical therapy. Surgical corrective options are generally not an option for production animals but may be considered in animals that are kept as pets. These include such options as conjunctival or corneal grafting procedures. These are delicate procedures that can be accomplished by a veterinary ophthalmologist. Again, these are not necessary for the majority of cases and only possible on an individual basis.

Infectious Bovine Keratoconjunctivitis

Infectious bovine keratoconjunctivitis (IBK), also known as *pink eye complex* and *infectious ophthalmia*, is characterized by blepharospasm, conjunctivitis, lacrimation, and varying degrees of corneal opacity and ulceration. The diagnosis is made by either identification of the Moraxella organism or when multiple animals within the herd are affected with the same clinical symptoms and no other cause has been identified (see earlier).

Moraxella bovis with multiple serovars is the most commonly recognized cause of IBK. *M. bovis* exists in both a piliated and nonpiliated form. It is the piliated form that causes the clinical disease. The organism has within its genetic makeup the ability to shift between the piliated and nonpiliated forms, but what is not known are the factors that cause the organism to shift. Several strains of the organism have been isolated worldwide; these strains generally fall into seven serotypes. These serotypes have enough genetic variation that immunity to one does not always provide immunity to another serotype. *M. bovis* has been shown to have enzymatic properties that result in corneal epithelial destruction. Other organisms that may cause conjunctivitis of cattle, either alone or in conjunction with *M. bovis,* include *Moraxella ovis* (previously *Branhamella ovis*), *Mycoplasma* spp., and *Neisseria* spp. Infection with infectious bovine rhinotracheitis (IBR) or other organisms may increase the severity of infection with *M. bovis.* Dry, dusty environmental conditions; shipping stress; bright sunlight; and irritants such as pollens, grasses, and flies tend to predispose or exacerbate the disease. Flies *(Musca autumnalis)* also serve as vectors. Hereford cattle are more susceptible to IBK than other breeds. Although degree of pigmentation surrounding the eye may be partly responsible for this susceptibility, it does not account for all of it. *Bos indicus* breeds are more resistant to infection when compared with *Bos taurus* breeds. In all breeds, young animals are affected most frequently, but animals of any age are susceptible.

The initial clinical signs are photophobia, blepharospasm, and epiphora; later, the ocular discharge may become mucopurulent. Conjunctivitis, with or without varying degrees of corneal edema (white appearance to cornea), is always present. Appetite may be depressed due to ocular discomfort or decreased vision that results in an inability to locate food. The clinical course varies from a few days to several weeks unless complicated by other diseases. The disease is generally acute and tends to spread rapidly. One or both eyes may be affected. Lesions vary in severity from small ulcers in the center of the cornea, but occasionally near the limbus, which are often preceded by cloudiness of the central cornea. Initially, the cornea around the lesion is clear, but within a few hours a faint haze appears and subsequently becomes denser. Opacity of the cornea may be a result of edema, which is a part of the inflammatory process or leukocyte infiltration that indicates severe infection. Lesions may regress in the early stages or continue to progress. In severe cases the entire cornea may be opaque and the animal is blind. Blood vessels may invade the cornea from the limbus and move toward the ulcer at an approximate rate of 1 mm per day. Continued active ulceration may result in rupture of the cornea. The primary differential diagnosis is IBR, which causes severe conjunctivitis and edema of the cornea near the corneoscleral junction, but corneal ulceration is uncommon.

M. bovis is susceptible to a variety of antibiotics that may vary in different geographic locations because of serovar differences. If there is no response to initial therapy, bacterial culture and susceptibility testing is advised because of possible infection with other organisms. Ampicillin (50 mg/ml) or penicillin (300,000 units/ml) can be injected subconjunctivally; best results are obtained with injection into the bulbar conjunctiva. Oxytetracycline has historically been considered the drug of choice for systemic therapy because it is concentrated in corneal tissue. However, it should not be injected subconjunctivally because it causes tissue necrosis. Two injections (20 mg/kg, SC) of a long-acting oxytetracycline formulation (200 mg/ml) at 72-hr intervals are an effective treatment. Sulfonamides (e.g., sulfadiazine and sulfamethazine) may also be effective when administered systemically because most of them pass readily into the tear film. Florfenicol (20 mg/kg, IM, 2 doses or 40 mg/kg, SC, 1 dose) tilmicosin (10 mg/kg, IM, 1 dose) and tulathromycin (2.5 mg/kg SC) may also be used systemically. Ceftiofur crystalline-free acid 6.6 mg/kg injected into the posterior aspect of the pinna has been shown to be effective in an experimental setting. Systemic therapy can be augmented with topical ophthalmic applications, subconjunctival injection of antibiotic, or both. Topical applications of ophthalmic preparations should be applied at least four times daily to be maximally effective and are therefore neither cost effective nor practical. Effective antibiotics for topical ophthalmic use include triple antibiotic combinations, gentamicin, and a combination oxytetracycline/polymyxin B ointment.

Covering the eye may provide shade and prevent exposure to flies, thereby decreasing spread of the organism. A temporary eye patch glued to the hair surrounding the eye is an inexpensive and easily applied treatment. The patch must allow for airflow to the ocular structures and should not be allowed to be constantly wet because this may lead to further bacterial contamination. A third-eyelid flap and partial tarsorrhaphy are other forms of covering the eye. No data exist to suggest that these therapies are any better than an eye patch at healing an ulcer. Animals that have painful uveitis secondary to ulceration may benefit from topical ophthalmic application of 1% atropine ointment one to three times daily. Doing this prevents painful ciliary body spasms and reduces the likelihood of posterior synechia that can occur with miosis. Because of mydriasis caused by atropine, treated animals should be provided with shade. Systemic NSAIDs may be used to provide relief from the secondary uveitis.

Good management practices are necessary to reduce or prevent spread of infection. Separation of affected from nonaffected animals is beneficial when possible. Temporary isolation of animals newly introduced to the herd may be helpful because some of these animals may be asymptotic carriers. Ultraviolet radiation from sunlight may enhance disease, so affected animals should be provided with shade. Dust bags or insecticide tags can be used to reduce the number of face flies, which may help decrease spread of the disease. *M. bovis* bacterins are available and can be administered before the beginning of fly season; however, the efficacy of these bacterins is controversial. Autogenous bacterins have not been shown to provide adequate immunity in field trials. Current bacterins based on surface proteins do not produce consistent immunity for all serovars. Commercially produced vaccines contain several serovars in an attempt to improve immune coverage. They can be protective in the face of certain outbreaks, but they are not consistently reliable. Future vaccines may be more protective because they are based on immunity to the enzymatic action of the organism. Concurrent IBR infection may predispose cattle to infection with *M. bovis;* thus vaccination of herds against IBR may reduce outbreaks of *M. bovis.* However, cattle should not be vaccinated during an outbreak with *M. bovis.*

ANTERIOR UVEAL DISORDERS

The uvea is the vascular portion of the eye and is made up of the iris, ciliary body, and choroid. Commonly used terminology includes anterior uvea for the iris and ciliary body and posterior uvea for the choroid. Because the uvea is highly vascular, it has the capacity to become inflamed after local or systemic stimuli. Congenital defects and malformations, with or without a hereditary predisposition, are rare in cattle and usually important only for recognition purposes so that these animals are not used for breeding. Aniridia (total absence of an iris); iris hypoplasia; persistent pupillary membranes (iris strands bridging across the iris, from the iris to the cornea, or from the iris to the lens); previously described anterior segment dysplasia with glaucoma and megaloglobus; and heterochromia iridis (depigmented or multicolored iris tissue) are commonly occurring congenital/hereditary uveal defects that have been described in food animals.

Inflammation is the most common and most important uveal disease. Commonly used terms are iritis (inflamed iris), cyclitis (inflamed ciliary body), iridocyclitis or anterior uveitis (inflammation of the iris and ciliary body), chorioretinitis (inflammation of the choroid and adjacent retina), endophthalmitis (inflammation of the uvea and intraocular chambers), and panophthalmitis (inflammation of the internal and external ocular structures and adjacent adnexa and orbit). Common clinical signs of uveitis may include blindness, photophobia, blepharospasm, tearing, episcleral and conjunctival vascular injection, and corneal edema. The anterior chamber may be cloudy as a result of aqueous flare (elevated protein levels), hypopyon (white cells), hyphema (blood), or fibrin. The iris may be swollen and irregular on the surface with increased vascularization and a miotic pupil. Uveitis initially causes a soft eye, but chronic uveitis can cause obstruction of aqueous humor outflow with secondary glaucoma. Measurement of the intraocular pressure aids in diagnosis. Chronic uveitis can lead to poor lens nutrition and cataract formation.

Because most cases of uveitis are due to an underlying systemic disease, a thorough physical examination and workup are indicated. Appropriate treatment of the underlying disease is the most important part of a treatment strategy for uveitis. Symptomatic ocular therapy may include topical application of 1% atropine ophthalmic ointment one to three times daily to achieve mydriasis and negate painful ciliary spasm. If the cornea is nonulcerated, topical steroids (dexamethasone or prednisolone)

two to four times daily or bulbar subconjunctival corticosteroids (betamethasone acetate or dexamethasone) will help relieve the anterior uveitis and should have no systemic immunosuppression. Systemic NSAIDs may also be used to reduce ocular inflammation and pain.

Blunt trauma to the globe may produce traumatic anterior uveitis. This is usually, but not always, unilateral and hyphema or subconjunctival hemorrhage is often present. Symptomatic therapy as described earlier is indicated. Anterior uveitis secondary to surface eye disease (pinkeye complex) is usually mild in comparison to uveitis caused by systemic disease (except for a perforated eye and secondary endophthalmitis). Treatment of the surface eye disease and systemic NSAIDs usually resolves this form of anterior uveitis. Neonatal septicemias caused by navel ill, scours, and pneumonia may cause anterior uveitis in calves. *Escherichia coli, Corynebacterium, Klebsiella, Listeria, Salmonella, Staphylococcus,* and *Streptococcus* spp. are common etiologic agents. Comatose calves with anterior uveitis often have meningoencephalitis, so the presence of anterior uveitis is an important negative prognostic sign. In adult cattle, anterior uveitis is most commonly seen secondary to systemic infection such as metritis, mastitis, peritonitis, and reticulopericarditis.

Tuberculosis may be a cause of granulomatous anterior uveitis and should be ruled out as an underlying disease because of its public health significance. Clinical signs of malignant catarrhal fever in the acute form include bilateral mucoid to mucopurulent ocular discharge with severe episcleral and conjunctival injection; initial peripheral corneal edema and neovascularization that eventually become complete; hypopyon; and meiosis. Blindness can result from this initial anterior uveitis or from the subsequent panophthalmitis. Listeriosis in young cattle being fed silage may result in anterior uveitis, as well as posterior uveitis and neurologic disease.

LENS

Disorders of the lens are uncommonly reported in food animals, possibly because unless noticeable vision loss is observed, the lenses are not examined. The lenses are seldom evaluated with full pupillary dilation, adequate instrumentation, or appropriate light conditions, and as a result subtle changes go unnoticed and cattle usually do not live long enough for senile lens changes to develop. A cataract, opacity of the lens, is the most commonly seen lens change. The cataract is most often a congenital anomaly, but it may be acquired.

Congenital cataracts may be due to inheritance or in utero infection or any toxic, traumatic, or other metabolic disorder that affects development of the eye and/or lens. Generally, evaluating a single calf and determining the cause of the cataract are not possible. If cataracts are found in other age-matched calves from different genetic lines within a herd, a toxic or infectious disease may be the cause. When calves of common genetic lines are repeatedly afflicted, inheritance should be suspected. Unless inheritance can be definitively ruled out, bull calves with congenital cataracts should be rejected for use as studs. In the Jersey, Hereford, Holstein, and Shorthorn breeds, autosomal recessive inheritance of cataracts has been described. In the Jersey breed, congenital cataracts with other anomalies such as lens luxation and microphakia, with or without megaloglobus, have been described. In Hereford and Holstein cattle, a form of congenital cataract that becomes totally mature at 4 to 11 months of age has been noted. Other ocular anomalies may or may not be associated with these cataracts. In Shorthorns a congenital cataract that may also be seen in conjunction with microphthalmos, hydrocephalus, cerebellar hypoplasia, and myopathy has been described. Affected cattle should be culled from the herd. Infection in utero between days 75 and 150 of gestation with BVD virus can cause congenital cortical cataracts in conjunction with microphthalmos, retinal dysplasia, cerebellar hypoplasia, and brachygnathism. If minimally afflicted, some of these calves may be visual enough to be raised for production purposes.

Anterior uveitis may cause degenerative changes leading to secondary cataract formation. Young animals with neonatal septicemias, animals with severe IBK, animals with trauma to the globe, and adults with systemic disease and secondary uveitis may have posterior synechia (adhesion of the iris to the lens capsule), inflammatory debris on the lens capsule, and cataract formation that may lead to vision loss. For this reason, all animals with uveitis should have supportive, symptomatic treatment of the eye in conjunction with definitive systemic treatment for the underlying primary disease.

The degree of cataract formation is variable, so the degree of vision is variable. If animals are kept within a herd, they generally are able to find food and water but are generally lower in the herd order. Isolated animals should be kept in small enclosures to ensure they have access to food and water. Cataracts are not painful, but the leakage of lens proteins may result in a secondary uveitis. The long-term productivity of blind cattle is poor; the best recommendation is to cull them from the herd. Cataract surgery is a physical possibility but not a practical treatment. The procedure requires delicate instrumentation, magnification, and special equipment to perform adequately. It is cost prohibitive for cattle production, but it could be considered in the occasional pet with cataracts.

DISORDERS OF THE FUNDUS

Fundic disorders may be grouped into congenital, degenerative, and inflammatory diseases. Congenital disorders may be due to inheritance, in utero infection, or deficiencies that lead to abnormal ocular development. In calves the hyaloid vessels, in the embryonic vascular stalk that runs from the optic nerve to the lens, may contain blood, and thin, white strands from the optic nerve to the back of the lens may be seen in adult animals. The persistent hyaloid remnant emanating from the optic nerve is called Bergmeister's papilla. Coloboma of the optic nerve and peripapillary choroid are seen in the Hereford and Charolais breeds. Inherited colobomas are typically seen at the 6 o'clock position and are bilateral. Vitamin A deficiency in cows may cause in utero optic nerve hypoplasia and retinal degeneration. In utero infection with BVD virus at 75 to 150 days of gestation causes multifocal areas

of chorioretinal scarring/dysplasia as a result of virally induced necrosis of the developing retina. Total generalized retinal degeneration leading to total blindness may be seen in some calves. Neonatal septicemias may cause multifocal or generalized chorioretinitis, as well as anterior uveitis. Animals that survive may have multifocal chorioretinal scars.

Degenerative disorders can be caused by nutritional deficiencies or ingestion of toxic substances that cause retinal or optic nerve death. Ingestion of the male fern *Dryopteris filix-mas* may cause acute papilledema and end-stage changes that can be seen as generalized retinal atrophy. Locoweed toxicity may result in KCS and generalized retinal degeneration along with other central nervous system disorders.

Inflammatory diseases of the fundus are often due to infections involving the vascular choroid and retina. Many inflammatory diseases of the fundus also involve the anterior uvea. Vision loss may not be noticeable unless bilateral, end-stage chorioretinal disease is present. Clinical signs of active chorioretinal disease include subretinal exudate or hemorrhages that appear as a poorly delineated, dull discoloration of the tapetal and nontapetal zones. Gray exudates are more easily seen when perivascular in location or when in the nontapetal zone than when the tapetal zone is involved. Total separation of the retina from the underlying retinal pigment epithelium and choroid is seen as retinal detachment (a thin, gray "veil" protruding forward from the back of the eye like a "sail in the wind"). Inactive chorioretinal lesions are typically well demarcated, depigmented areas in the nontapetal fundus and shiny, hyperreflective areas (sometimes surrounding hyperpigmented foci) in the tapetal zone. Active optic neuritis appears as swelling of the optic nerve with indistinct exudates, edema, and/or hemorrhage seen within the nerve head or immediately adjacent to it. Optic nerve atrophy is manifested as a pale, shrunken, sometimes avascular nerve head.

Thromboembolic meningoencephalitis caused by *Haemophilus somnus* infection in young cattle usually does not cause anterior uveitis, but characteristics of chorioretinal and perivascular exudates ("cotton-wool" spots) and multifocal retinal hemorrhage are often seen. Multifocal scars may be seen if the animal survives. Listeriosis usually causes anterior uveitis, but it can cause multifocal areas of chorioretinitis as well. Other diseases that can cause retinal hemorrhage, chorioretinitis, retinal detachment, and/or optic neuritis are malignant catarrhal fever, tuberculosis, and toxoplasmosis. Polioencephalomalacia secondary to thiamine deficiency occasionally causes papilledema, as well as other neurologic signs.

Recommended Readings

George LW, Borrowman AJ, Angelos JA: Effectiveness of a cytolysin-enriched vaccine for protection of cattle against infectious bovine keratoconjunctivitis, *Am J Vet Res* 66:136, 2005.

Lavach JD: *Large animal ophthalmology*, St Louis, 1990, Mosby-Year Book.

Leipold HW: Congenital ocular defects in food-producing animals, *Vet Clin North Am Large Anim Pract* 6:577, 1984.

Moore CP, Miller RB: Infectious and parasitic diseases of cattle. In Howard JL, editor: *Current veterinary therapy: food animal practice,* ed 3, Philadelphia, 1993, Saunders.

Rebhun WC: *Diseases of dairy cattle,* Baltimore, 1995, Williams & Wilkins.

Rebhun WC: Ocular manifestations of systemic diseases in cattle, *Vet Clin North Am Large Anim Pract* 6:623, 1984.

Snowder GD, VanVleck LD, Cundiff LV et al: Genetic and environmental factors associated with incidence of infectious bovine keratoconjunctivitis in preweaned beef calves, *J Anim Sci* 83:507, 2005.

Whittaker CJ, Gelatt KN, Wilkie DA: Food animal ophthalmology. In Gelatt KN, editor: *Veterinary ophthalmology,* ed 2, Philadelphia, 1991, Lea & Febiger.

CHAPTER 86

Selected Eye Diseases of Sheep and Goats

HARRIET J. DAVIDSON and J. PHILLIP PICKETT

Sheep and goats are uncommonly examined for primary ocular disease and few systemic diseases have ocular lesions as part of the clinical presentation. Because of the behavior of small ruminants and management techniques, the eyes are rarely closely examined. For these reasons data on ocular diseases and treatment in small ruminants are scarce.

The anatomy of sheep and goat eyes is similar. The eyelids are pliable and thin, although sheep have slightly thinner skin than goats, and the lids fit tightly to the globe. Both lids have cilia; superior lid cilia are longer than on the inferior lid. The lacrimal puncta are located approximately 5 mm from the medial canthus superiorly and inferiorly. The third eyelid is in the medial canthus and moves passively in the superior lateral direction. The third eyelid contains lymphatic nodules within and beneath the conjunctiva. The cornea is generally oval in the horizontal plane, with a slightly broader medial aspect. The limbus is frequently pigmented. The iris ranges in color from yellow to brown with variations in color and a slightly folded appearance. The pupil is generally oval when contracted, being broader medially and more round in shape when dilated. The corpora nigra is prominent and placed forward on the pupil margin. The fundus has a tapetum that may vary in color from yellow to orange to green to blue. The optic nerve is oval with a pinkish white color. Generally, four main blood vessels radiate in each quadrant.

ORBIT/GLOBE DISORDERS

Inherited microphthalmos is seen in conjunction with multiple ocular anomalies in British, Dutch, and German Trexel sheep. The mode of inheritance appears to be autosomal recessive. Ingestion of the insect chemical sterilant apholate by pregnant ewes can cause congenital microphthalmos and other ocular anomalies, as well as malformation of periorbital bones. Chronic ingestion of plants containing high levels of selenium (>3 ppm) by pregnant ewes can also cause microphthalmos, ocular cysts, and other ocular malformations. Overzealous selenium supplementation to pregnant ewes by herdsmen can have the same effect.

Consumption of the plant *Veratrum californicum* ("skunk cabbage"), most common in the high mountain pastures of western North America, by ewes and does can cause cyclopia (presence of one central eye) in lambs and kids. Other facial skeletal malformations frequently referred to as "monkey face" and absence of the pituitary gland and other brain malformations can also be seen. The plant must be ingested on day 14 of gestation to result in this facial/ocular malformation. Consumption of the plant later in gestation normally results in embryonic death. Cyclopia has been seen in the eastern United States and Canada in areas where *V. californicum* does not grow. The etiology of the facial/ocular malformation in these areas is unknown.

Glaucoma and megaloglobus are rare in sheep and goats and are usually secondary to ocular puncture wounds or severe uveitis. Enucleation is recommended when the enlarged globe has exposure keratitis or is painful. Orbital cellulitis occurs rarely in sheep and goats. Causes include puncture wounds, migration of foreign plant material from the mouth to the orbit, and, rarely, caseous lymphadenitis (*Corynebacterium pseudotuberculosis*).

EYELID/THIRD EYELID

Congenital Anomalies

Dermoids are uncommon, but they may occasionally be identified. These have not been shown to be genetic in small ruminants. A dermoid is a section of skin either with or without hair in an incorrect location. The most frequently identified location is the superior or lateral limbal region. This skin may contain hairs that rub on the conjunctival or corneal surface, causing chronic irritation. Clinical signs are swelling of the conjunctiva, corneal opacities, ulcers, and an ocular discharge. If these signs occur, the dermoid should be surgically removed. Entropion is the most common congenital eyelid disorder in sheep. Afflicted lambs usually have inrolling of the lower lid, which causes irritant keratoconjunctivitis with pain, ocular discharge, and potential blindness from corneal perforation or scarring. The disorder has a hereditary predisposition but may be augmented by factors such as windy or dusty environmental conditions. Immediate therapy is aimed at reducing the frictional irritation and protecting the cornea. Having the shepherd frequently manually roll the lids out in conjunction with the application of lubricant antibiotic ointment may be too labor intensive for a large flock. Temporary eversion of the lid margin with skin clips (Michel clips), skin staples, or vertical mattress sutures or injection of penicillin (1-2 ml) into the lid to evert the lid margin may break the cycle of irritation. Most animals will do well with a single temporary eversion technique, but some animals may require a Hotz-Celsus procedure to remove eyelid skin and permanently repair the defect. This should only be done in older animals (4-6 months or older) when temporary techniques have failed. This is a relatively simple method of making an incision 3 to 5 mm from and parallel with the eyelid margin. A second curvilinear incision is made beginning and ending at the same place as the first incision, outlining a crescent-shaped area of skin. This crescent-shaped area of skin is sharply dissected using scissors. The deep subcutaneous fat is also removed. The wound is closed with simple interrupted sutures in the skin. Sutures should be removed in approximately 10 days. Entropion afflicted animals should not be bred, and sires and dams producing multiple afflicted offspring should be culled.

Blepharitis

Numerous infectious and parasitic diseases of the skin may cause blepharitis in sheep. The viral infections that cause cutaneous ecthyma and sheep pox, ulcerative dermatosis, and blue tongue may cause exudative skin lesions about the eyelids. *Dermatophilus congolensis, Actinobacillus lignieresii,* and *Trichophyton verrucosum* infections can cause exudative, scablike eyelid lesions. *Clostridium novyi* infection ("big head") can cause eyelid and facial edema. Sarcoptic and demodectic mange, as well as keds, lice, and ticks, can cause blepharitis along with facial dermatitis. Ocular therapy for these disorders is supportive (the eyelids should be kept cleansed and the cornea protected with ophthalmic ointment), and precautions should be taken to prevent the spread of these infections to other animals and/or humans.

As with cattle, photosensitization and keratoconjunctivitis sicca (KCS) can occur in sheep and goats secondary to the ingestion of toxic substances. St. John's wort, buckwheat, and spineless horsebrush are common plants that contain these toxins. Locoweed ingestion causes KCS and palpebral nerve paralysis, which can in turn cause severe exposure keratoconjunctivitis.

Although biopsy of the third eyelid is one method used in detection of scrapie, there are no ophthalmic lesions associated with the disease. Samples may be collected by restraining the sheep, placing a topical ophthalmic anesthetic on the surface of the eye and eyelids, and grasping the third eyelid and rolling it outward, exposing the bulbar conjunctiva. Scissors are used to snip the biopsy sample. No treatment is necessary post sample collection.

CONJUNCTIVAL AND CORNEAL DISORDERS

In sheep, infection with *Chlamydophila pecorum* (*Chlamydia psittaci* is the former taxonomic name) and *Moraxella ovis* (*Branhamella ovis* is the former taxonomic name) is most common. *Mycoplasma* spp. and other aerobic bacteria, notably *Neisseria ovis*, may also cause conjunctivitis. In goats, mycoplasmal infections are most common, although aerobic bacteria have also been isolated. Although much of the syndrome in young goats is caused by *Mycoplasma agalactiae*, it may also be caused by *Mycoplasma conjunctivae*. For sheep and goats, in which chlamydophilal and mycoplasmal infections are most likely, topical ophthalmic tetracycline, oxytetracycline/polymyxin B, or erythromycin ointments are the treatments of choice. These preparations should be applied 3 to 4 times daily. When topical therapy is not practical, an injection of long-acting oxytetracycline (10-20 mg/kg, IM) or the addition of oxytetracycline to the feed (80 mg/head/day) may be beneficial. In sheep and goats, concurrent polyarthritis may be present. In goats, mammary gland and uterine infection may also occur simultaneously with keratoconjunctivitis. Disease rarely advances beyond a mild corneal opacity, with the occasional accompanying ulcer and conjunctivitis. Relapse may occur at any stage of recovery, but late lesions are not as severe as initial lesions.

Thelazia californiensis infection is widespread in North America, but clinical disease is uncommon. Conjunctival or nasolacrimal duct involvement with the nasal botfly *Oestrus ovis* may cause irritant conjunctivitis and epiphora. Systemic organophosphate anthelmintics and ivermectin are effective in killing the parasite. Treatment is best performed in the fall when the larvae are small. Manual extraction of the larvae from the conjunctival cul-de-sacs and flushing the nasolacrimal ducts may also be useful in severe cases.

The filarid nematode *Elaeophora schneideri* afflicts sheep, deer, and elk in the high mountain regions of western North America. The disease is sometimes called "sore head" or clear-eyed blindness. Adult worms live in the carotid and internal maxillary arteries, but microfilaria can lodge in the capillary beds of the face and orbit and produce an immunologic reaction with facial swelling, alopecia, encrustations, conjunctival swelling, and corneal ulcerations. Diagnosis using skin biopsy is difficult and best confirmed at necropsy and evaluation of the carotid or internal maxillary arteries. Therapy may include oral piperazine (50 mg/kg-220 mg/kg once daily) or diethylcarbamazine (100 mg/kg). The efficacy of ivermectin therapy is unknown.

ANTERIOR UVEAL DISORDERS

Clinical signs of inflammation of the uvea, or uveitis, include aqueous flare (hazy opacity to the anterior chamber), hypopyon (white cells in the anterior chamber), swollen irregular iris, misshapen pupil, cataracts, chorioretinitis, and optic neuritis. Uveitis may be caused by septicemia. *Mycoplasma agalactiae* infection is most common, but neonatal septicemias caused by coliforms, *Staphylococcus* spp., and *Streptococcus* spp. have been reported. Listeriosis in 4- to 6-month-old feedlot lambs being fed silage may cause anterior uveitis similar to that seen in calves. *E. schneideri* infection in sheep may cause uveitis in conjunction with the previously described lesions of the lids and conjunctiva. Toxoplasmosis is an uncommon cause of anterior uveitis and chorioretinitis in sheep, goats, and cattle. Treatment is primarily directed at the systemic disease. Medical therapy may include application of topical ophthalmic steroids such as dexamethasone or prednisolone two to six times daily depending on the severity of the ophthalmic lesions and the use of the animal. Atropine ophthalmic ointment may be applied one to three times daily to control ciliary spasms, which are painful and help to stabilize the blood aqueous barrier. These medications should be decreased in frequency or discontinued as the clinical symptoms improve.

LENS

A cataract is any opacity of the lens. Inherited cataracts have been described in New Zealand Romney sheep. Cataracts have been reported as sequelae to uveitis secondary to *E. schneideri* infestation or *M. agalactiae* infection. Cataracts in general are rarely identified in small ruminants. No medical therapy is available to restore the lens to its normal clarity. Cataract surgery is a possibility but is generally cost prohibitive for production animals. Pet animals that have lost vision from cataracts may benefit from referral to a veterinary ophthalmologist for possible surgery.

FUNDUS

Bluetongue virus exposure during the first half of gestation (either as a viral infection or as a vaccination with modified live virus vaccine) may cause in utero necrosis of the developing retina with subsequent postpartum signs of multifocal retinal dysplasia, vision impairment, and cerebellar hypoplasia and hydrocephalus.

Neonatal septicemias, listeriosis, and toxoplasmosis may cause chorioretinitis. *E. schneideri* infestation may cause chorioretinitis and optic neuritis during acute disease and chorioretinal scars, optic nerve atrophy, and blindness as sequelae to the acute disease. Scrapie virus has been reported to cause a retinopathy that accompanies the neurologic disease. Multifocal, oval, raised "blisterlike" lesions less than 1 disk diameter in size scattered throughout the tapetal fundus have been described.

Chronic bracken fern (*Pteridium aquilinum*) ingestion causes "bright blindness" in sheep. After many months of grazing, progressive, generalized retinal degeneration results in blindness. In western Australia ingestion of "blind grass" (*Stypandra imbricata*) causes a similar retinal atrophy in sheep. Chronic ingestion of locoweed causes retinal atrophy in sheep, the same as in cattle. Hexachlorophene (used in countries outside the United States to treat liver flukes) can cause acute optic nerve–head edema within 24 hours of ingestion of a toxic dose, with subsequent generalized retinal atrophy, optic nerve atrophy, and blindness.

Recommended Readings

Moore CP, Wallace LM: Selected eye diseases of sheep and goats. In Howard JL, editor: *Current veterinary therapy: food animal practice*, ed 3, Philadelphia, 1993, Saunders.

O'Rourke KI, Duncan JV, Logan JR et al: Active surveillance for scrapie by third eyelid biopsy and genetic susceptibility testing of flocks of sheep in Wyoming, *Clin Diagn Lab Immunol* 9:996, 2002.

Prince JH, Diesem CD, Eglitis I: *Anatomy and histology of the eye and orbit in domestic animals*, Springfield, Ill, 1960, Charles C. Thomas.

Smith MC, Sherman DM: *Goat medicine*, Philadelphia, 1994, Lea & Febiger.

Webb AI, Bayenes RE, Craigmill AL et al: Drugs approved for small ruminants, *J Am Vet Med Assoc* 224:520, 2004.

CHAPTER 87

Ophthalmology of South American Camelids: Llamas, Alpacas, Guanacos, and Vicuñas

JULIET R. GIONFRIDDO and DEBORAH S. FRIEDMAN

South American camelids have become companion animals of importance to veterinary practice. Llamas and alpacas have considerable economic value in the United States, and in South America these animals are necessary for food, wool, transportation, and fuel. The ocular anatomy of the South American camelid differs greatly from that of other domestic species.

ANATOMY AND PHYSIOLOGY

The large and prominent eyes of camelids are only slightly smaller than equine and bovine eyes despite their considerably smaller body size. They are framed with long lashes and three pairs of vibrissae. The eyelids are tightly adherent to the globe, which makes examination of the conjunctival fornices difficult. Unlike in other domestic animals, no meibomian gland duct openings are present on the eyelid margin. In the camel, a closely related species, meibomian glands are also absent but are replaced by sebaceous glands on the lacrimal caruncle.[1] This is probably the case in the llama as well.

Magnification is helpful in observation of the nasolacrimal puncta, which are 4 to 6 mm inside the medial canthus. The tear drainage system starts with dorsal and ventral canaliculi, which join to form a lacrimal sac. The nasolacrimal duct extends from the lacrimal sac through the lacrimal and maxillary bones and then traverses the nasal cavity. The nasal opening of the nasolacrimal duct is 1.5 to 2 cm proximal to the nares and laterally placed as in sheep and goats. In the adult llama, the duct is 11 to 15 cm long and 2 to 4 mm in diameter.[2]

The prominent appearance of the llama eye is enhanced by the lack of visible sclera within the palpebral fissure. Often the conjunctiva overlying any exposed sclera is pigmented so that no white is evident. The limbus has a dark brown pigment band 2 to 3 mm wide.

The elaborate structure of the iris is a striking feature of the llama eye (Fig. 87-1). On the dorsal and ventral margins of the pupil, the posterior pigment epithelium of the iris is proliferated and folded vertically. This pupillary ruff is analogous to the corpora nigra of horses but is significantly larger and consists of folded layers rather than globular masses. Iris pigmentation is usually various shades of brown and occasionally blue. Persistent pupillary membranes are common, especially near the pupillary margin. Neonatal llamas occasionally have thin, gray fibrinous strands spanning one or two folds of the pupillary ruff.

The fundus of camelids lacks a tapetum.[1,3-5] However, it may appear highly reflective because of a prominent Bruch membrane that has been identified histologically.[5] Ophthalmoscopic examination shows the fundus to be either red and brown or blue and brown. The red coloration is due to choroidal vessels being visible through a nonpigmented retinal pigment epithelium.

A study of 29 alpacas demonstrated a relationship among coat color, iris color, and retinal pigmentation.[6] Animals with light coat colors had various combinations of gray, blue, and brown irides and reduced pigmentation of the fundus. Those with dark coat colors had brown irides and pigmented fundi.[6]

The optic disc and retinal vasculature are similar to those of the bovine. A large Bergmeister papilla (hyaloid remnant) may protrude from the disc, and three to five pairs of large retinal vessels emerge from its periphery. Two pairs of vessels leave the optic disc horizontally and are usually accompanied by myelin, which extends several disc diameters peripherally into the fundus (Fig. 87-2).

The bony orbit of the llama, like that of the horse and ox, is complete and made up of the frontal, lacrimal, zygomatic, maxillary, palatine, temporal, and sphenoid bones. A large notch located dorsally in the frontal bone is

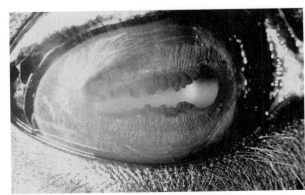

Fig 87-1 Llama iris showing the distinctive pupillary ruff, which represents a protrusion and folding of the posterior pigment epithelium of the iris.

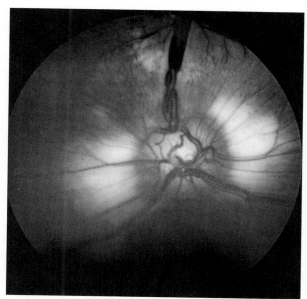

Fig 87-2 Fundus of a llama. Note the large retinal blood vessels and the myelin from the optic disc, which is extending out into the fundus.

palpable in living animals. Rostral to the medial aspect of the orbit is a 2-cm-diameter opening into the nasal cavity. This opening is probably associated with a scent gland.

EXAMINATION

A complete evaluation of the camelid eye is important as part of a routine physical examination and when ophthalmic disease is suspected. In addition, the eyes of all sick camelids should be examined because many systemic diseases have ophthalmic manifestations.[7]

Ocular examination is optimally undertaken with the llama restrained in stocks. Chemical sedation (butorphanol, 0.02 to 0.04 mg/kg) is occasionally necessary to control head movement.[7] Liquids such as tropicamide, topical anesthetic, and fluorescein may be applied to the eye with a "squirt gun" made from a 3-ml syringe and a needle broken at the hub.

A complete ocular examination should include an external eye and anterior segment examination under magnification, reflex responses, a Schirmer tear test, measurements of intraocular pressure, and funduscopy. The menace reflex for testing vision may be elicited by a sudden hand movement across the visual axis. The llama should blink or jump back. Direct and indirect pupillary light reflexes are slow, and movement of the iris is minimal. The mean Schirmer tear test value is 19 mm/minute in a nonanesthetized eye.[8] Fluorescein dye is applied to the eye to help detect corneal ulcers and for the diagnosis of tear drainage problems. Intraocular pressure is most easily measured with an applanation tonometer and averages 14 mm Hg. One application (about 0.25 ml) of 1% tropicamide causes mydriasis within 20 to 45 minutes.

Dacryocystorhinography may be used for detailed examination of the nasolacrimal drainage system. For this procedure, 5 ml of a sodium and meglumine diatrizoate mixture are injected into the dorsal lacrimal punctum and lateral and dorsoventral radiographs are then taken.[9]

CAMELID OCULAR DISEASE

Limited information is available concerning the types and frequencies of ocular disease in camelids. Gelatt and colleagues[6] reported on routine ophthalmic examinations of 29 healthy alpacas in South America. In this report, 38% of the alpacas had at least one ocular problem including conjunctivitis, corneal scars, posterior synechiae, cataracts, a subluxated lens, vitreous opacities, and an optic disc coloboma. Most were thought to be secondary to trauma, but some may have been hereditary.[6] A recent retrospective study of the Veterinary Medical Database (VMDB) for a 13-year period found that at least one ocular problem was diagnosed in 6% (194 of 3243) of the llamas seen at veterinary teaching hospitals.[10] Trauma was also considered the primary cause in many of these cases.

Cornea

Corneal disease is the most common ocular abnormality in llamas. Forty-one percent of the llamas with ocular disease reported to the VMDB had corneal disease, and more than half of these were ulcers.[10] Most of them were of unknown cause but were probably traumatic in origin. There is no evidence that llamas or other camelids have primary corneal invasion by bacteria such as *Moraxella bovis*, the main cause of infectious bovine keratoconjunctivitis.[6,7,10] Other trauma-associated corneal diseases in llamas include corneal lacerations, foreign bodies, and stromal abscesses.[8,10] Corneal trauma may be seen in recumbent llamas because of anesthesia, tick paralysis, meningeal worms, or illnesses secondary to a lack of passive transfer.[8,10]

Treatment of corneal ulcers, lacerations, and infection in camelids is similar to that in other species.[11] Because bacterial pathogens are often present on the normal camelid eye, topical broad-spectrum antibiotics should be used in all cases of corneal ulcers or lacerations.[8] Corneal lacerations may be sutured directly with small-gauge (6-0–8-0), absorbable suture material. Deep ulcers in llamas often heal well under the protection of conjunctival grafts as in other species.

Other corneal diseases include dystrophies, degenerations, dermoids, and edema.[10,12,13] Bilateral corneal edema was reported in a guanaco and her offspring.[14] The corneal endothelium of camelids appears to be highly sensitive and, if irritated, becomes ineffective in removing excess water from the corneal stroma. Severe corneal edema develops readily after intraocular surgery and corneal trauma.

Conjunctiva

Diseases of the conjunctiva were reported in 19 llamas (10% of the llamas with ocular disease) in a study of the VMDB.[10] Most of these cases were conjunctivitis "due to unknown cause," but there were several conjunctival infections.[10] Numerous bacteria have been isolated from llamas with conjunctivitis.[15] These were suspected to be the primary cause of the disease, although they may have been secondary invaders. *Staphylococcus aureus* was isolated from the inflamed conjunctiva of a llama with keratoconjunctivitis.[16] Clinical signs of bacterial conjunctivitis include hyperemia, serous or mucopurulent ocular discharge, and blepharospasm.

Microbiologic culture (both bacterial and fungal) and sensitivity testing are recommended in most cases of conjunctivitis and keratoconjunctivitis. Most bacterial infections respond well to appropriate topical antibacterial therapy.

Other causes of infectious conjunctivitis include chlamydiae[13] and parasites. *Thelazia californiensis,* a nematode, has been found in the conjunctival sac of many species including llamas.[17] The pathology of *Thelazia* in llamas ranges from mild conjunctivitis[17] to severe ulcerative keratitis.[8] The initial signs of infection are usually those of nonspecific conjunctivitis. If corneal ulcers are present, however, there may be purulent discharge and photophobia. The nematode is transmitted among animals by face flies, and *Thelazia* may be seen on the surface of the eye or beneath the third eyelid.[17] Treatment consists of mechanical removal following topical anesthesia or instillation of diethylcarbamazine or ivermectin drops into the conjunctival sac to kill the parasite.[17] Many types of flies feed on llama lacrimal secretions and cause conjunctival irritation. Consequently, fly control is important for minimizing this form of conjunctivitis.

Noninfectious conjunctival abnormalities include trauma, foreign bodies, dermoids, and congenital cysts.[8,10,18] Large conjunctival wounds should be sutured with small-gauge, absorbable suture material. Small wounds usually heal with medical therapy alone. Congenital cysts have been reported infrequently in crias (neonatal llamas).[19] Schuh and colleagues[18] reported a cystlike structure on the bulbar conjunctiva of a cria. Aspiration of this structure yielded a clear fluid. Because the same eye had other defects, the cyst was thought to be part of a general ocular maldevelopment.[18] A conjunctival cyst, without other ocular lesions, was reported by Johnson.[19] After drainage of the cyst failed to permanently resolve the problem, surgical excision proved curative.

Eyelids and Nasolacrimal System

In the VMDB study only 13 llamas (7%) were reported to have eyelid diseases.[10] Blepharitis was the most common eyelid problem, and several of these llamas had concurrent dermatitis. Blepharitis caused by bacterial infection has been seen and often occurs in conjunction with bacterial conjunctivitis.[13]

Eyelid lacerations in llamas were uncommon in the VMDB study; they were seen in only two animals.[10] Eyelid lacerations can be serious in llamas because of the potential for secondary corneal damage from exposure. Therefore all full-thickness eyelid lacerations should be sutured.

Nasolacrimal duct disorders seem to be relatively common in camelids. Congenital nasolacrimal duct/punctal atresia was recorded in five crias in the VMDB.[10] Four llamas examined by Severin[13] had congenital punctal atresia. The puncta were successfully opened with

a procedure similar to that used in horses.[20] Sapienza and colleagues[9] described a case of severe epiphora caused by bilateral atresia of the nasolacrimal ducts in a cria. The palpebral puncta were patent and the congenital obstruction was at the nasal opening of the duct. Surgical opening of the obstruction was successful.

Lens

Cataracts are the most common abnormalities of the camelid lens. They were reported in 20 animals (10%) in the VMDB.[10] Mature, hypermature, and immature cataracts have been reported.[6,8,13,14,21,22] In a South American herd of 29 alpacas, Gelatt and coworkers[6] saw 1 animal with apparently normal vision but with nuclear cataracts. Whether small, immature cataracts in camelids progress to maturity or whether they are inherited is unknown.[14,17,21,22] Some cataracts in camelids severely impair vision.[14,21,23] Attempts at cataract removal have had poor outcomes. In a report of cataract surgery in a llama, lens extraction was followed by severe corneal edema, ulcerative keratitis, and phthisis bulbi.[23] Recently, the use of phacoemulsification and viscoelastics for cataract extraction has greatly improved the success rate in dogs. Yet these new techniques do not seem to have improved the success rate for cataract surgery in camelids. Veterinary ophthalmologists report severe, intractable corneal edema in most camelids that have undergone cataract surgery, no matter what surgical techniques are used or which medications are used perioperatively.[15]

Although infrequently seen, other lens diseases in llamas include luxated lenses, traumatic lens rupture, and lens colobomas. A lens coloboma was seen temporally in the left lens of a female guanaco and was associated with nuclear and perinuclear cataracts and corneal edema.[14] A hereditary cause for the defects was suspected.

Uvea

Uveitis (anterior and posterior combined) was the second most commonly diagnosed ocular problem in llamas in the VMDB.[10] Thirty-five llamas (18%) had uveitis. Most were recorded as having "endophthalmitis uveitis" or were "due to unknown cause." Trauma was also a frequent cause of uveitis. Anterior uveitis has been seen in septicemic neonates and crias with juvenile llama immunodeficiency syndrome.[10,19] Uveitis may also be secondary to deep ulcerative keratitis, trauma, and infectious disease such as equine herpesvirus type 1 (EHV-1).[10,24]

Posterior Segment: Retina, Optic Nerve

Diseases of the posterior segment are relatively common in camelids. In the VMDB, 11 animals (6%) were reported to have retinal lesions[10] including retinitis, retinal detachment, retinal dystrophy, and retinal degeneration. Optic nerve disease was reported in two llamas: One had optic nerve hypoplasia and the other had a coloboma.[10]

Congenital defects of the retina, choroid, and optic nerve of camelids have been reported.[6-8,18] These defects may be confined to a single structure or, more often, may involve multiple structures. During histopathologic examination of the eyes of neonatal llamas, Dubielzig saw multiple ocular defects including peripapillary colobomas, retinal dysplasia, retinal detachment, and vitreous fibrosis and ossification.[5] A large optic disc coloboma was observed in a young llama during routine ocular examination.[3] Schuh and colleagues[18] described a llama with a large coloboma near the optic disc. Although colobomas are known to be hereditary in cattle,[20] their heritability has not been established in camelids. In general, however, camelids with congenital posterior segment defects should not be bred.[7]

Two infectious diseases have been reported to cause posterior segment disease in camelids: EHV-1 and disseminated aspergillosis, with EHV-1 being the more widely seen. Camelids acquire EHV-1 by contact with members of the family Equidae. Rebhun and associates[24] reported that members of a mixed herd of camelids became blind after exposure to infected zebras. Neurologic signs including head tilt, nystagmus, and paralysis developed in four alpacas. Ophthalmoscopy showed vitritis, retinitis, and optic neuritis. Histopathologic examination of the eyes of two animals showed retinal and subretinal hemorrhage, vasculitis, subretinal exudate, and retinal detachment. Two alpacas also had hypopyon and iritis. All attempted treatments failed to restore vision to any animal. Histologic identification of eosinophilic inclusions in the brain and measurement of high EHV-1 antibody titers in the serum confirmed EHV-1 as the cause.

In 1989 a similar outbreak occurred in a herd of llamas in Illinois.[3] Twenty-eight llamas were exposed to zebras with rhinitis. In 10 to 17 days, neurologic signs including blindness, deafness, head tilt, and circling developed in most of the llamas. Ophthalmic examination showed severe anterior uveitis and chorioretinitis. Equine herpesvirus type 1 was confirmed as the cause of this outbreak.

The extreme pathogenicity of EHV-1 in llamas was shown when three llamas were experimentally infected intranasally with EHV-1.[25] Two of the llamas exhibited severe neurologic signs including blindness, staggering, head tremors, and depression. Histopathologic assessment showed severe neuronal changes in the brain and optic nerve. Isolation of EHV-1 was successful in only one (the most clinically ill) of the three infected animals, which suggests that it may be difficult to isolate the virus from infected animals.

Paulsen and colleagues[26] described a llama with chorioretinitis, optic neuritis, and encephalitis. Serologic tests failed to implicate EHV-1, and no intranuclear inclusion bodies were seen histopathologically. The similarity of this animal to the chronically affected alpacas described by Rebhun and coworkers[24] suggests that this may have been a case of chronic EHV-1 in which the virus was not identified.

No effective treatment or method of prevention of EHV-1 infection in camelids is known. Vaccination of llamas for EHV-1 with the equine vaccine has been attempted, but its efficacy has not been evaluated.

Aspergillosis was implicated as a cause of neurologic disease and chorioretinitis in a wild-caught, zoo-housed alpaca.[27] On necropsy, *Aspergillus* was identified in the lung and eye. The fungus was thought to have spread from the lungs to the eye hematogenously.

Toxoplasmosis, a known cause of chorioretinitis in dogs and cats, may also cause blindness in camelids. During an investigation of causes of late-term abortions in llamas, a serologic survey showed an extremely high antibody titer for *Toxoplasma* in a nonaborting blind llama.[19] The llama had lesions of chronic panophthalmitis. Tinsley described a 15-year-old llama with signs of bilateral uveitis.[28] Vitreous humor was collected from one eye at hospital admission and 1 month later. Vitreous toxoplasmosis antibody titers showed a marked rise, although serum antibody titers were negative. These results suggested that an ocular *Toxoplasma gondii* infection may have caused the uveitis.

Miscellaneous Diseases

Although rare, glaucoma has been seen in camelids; two cases were reported in the VMDB.[10] Severin[13] observed increased intraocular pressure in two llamas with normal-appearing eyes. No known reports of secondary glaucoma in camelids exist. Barrie and associates[14] used gonioscopy to examine the drainage angle of a guanaco with corneal edema and normal intraocular pressure. They found the drainage angle to be closed and spanned by uveal tissue. The prevalence of goniodysgenesis and subsequent glaucoma is unknown. Routine tonometry and gonioscopy on diseased and healthy eyes may show a higher prevalence of glaucoma than has been reported.

Visual deficits are being diagnosed with increasing frequency in camelids. Eleven blind neonatal crias with apparently normal fundi were seen at Colorado State University Veterinary Teaching Hospital.[13] Vision gradually returned to all crias; no cause was found. Congenital nystagmus and amblyopia have also been diagnosed in crias.[13] Reports of permanent blindness with no apparent ocular defects or diseases in adult llamas are numerous.[15] These cases may be due to sudden retinal degeneration or a brain disorder. In some cases, electroretinograms and/or visual evoked potentials can be generated in camelids to test the visual pathways and explore the cause of the blindness.

Neoplasia

Ocular and periocular neoplasia seems to be rare in llamas. In 14 years only two cases of neoplasia were reported to the VMDB.[10] One was an intraocular medulloepithelioma, and the other was an unspecified corneal tumor. No cases of squamous cell carcinoma were reported. This is particularly interesting inasmuch as almost 50% of the cases in the VMDB were from Colorado State University, which serves a region having a relatively high elevation.[10] The increased exposure to ultraviolet light at high altitudes is a predisposing factor to squamous cell carcinoma in cattle and horses.[29] The low tumor incidence in llamas may reflect an adaptation of camelids to exposure to ultraviolet light.

Much remains to be learned about llama eyes. The results of research into the etiology of various ocular diseases, especially the mode of inheritance of suspected hereditary problems (such as cataracts and colobomas), have practical value for veterinary practitioners advising llama owners about breeding programs and treating camelids with ocular disease.

References

1. Duke-Elder S: *System of ophthalmology, vol 1, the eye in evolution*, St Louis, 1959, CV Mosby.
2. Sapienza JS, Isaza R, Johnson RD et al: Anatomic and radiographic study of the lacrimal apparatus of llamas, *Am J Vet Res* 53:1007, 1992.
3. Friedman DS: Unpublished data, 1989.
4. Rahi AHS, Sheikh H, Morgan G: Histology of the camel eye, *Acta Anat* 106:345, 1980.
5. Dubielzig RR: Personal communication, 1990, 1997.
6. Gelatt KN, Otzen Martinic GB, Flaneig JL et al: Results of ophthalmic examinations of 29 alpacas, *J Am Vet Med Assoc* 206:1204, 1995.
7. Gionfriddo JR: Ophthalmology, *Vet Clin North Am Food Anim Pract* 16:371-382, 1994.
8. Gionfriddo JR, Friedman DS: Ophthalmology of South American camelids: llamas, alpacas, guanacos, and vicuñas. In Howard JL, editor: *Current veterinary therapy: food animal practice*, ed 3. Philadelphia, 1993, Saunders.
9. Sapienza JS, Isaza R, Brooks DE et al: Atresia of the nasolacrimal duct in a llama, *Vet Comp Ophthalmol* 6:6, 1996.
10. Gionfriddo JR, Gionfriddo JP, Krohne SG: Ocular diseases of llamas: 194 cases (1980-1993), *J Am Vet Med Assoc* 210:1784, 1997.
11. Severin GA: *Severin's veterinary ophthalmology notes*, ed 3, Fort Collins, Colo, 1996, DesignPointe Communications.
12. Severin GA: Personal communication, 1993.
13. Severin GA: Unpublished data, 1993.
14. Barrie KP, Jacobson E, Peiffer RL Jr: Unilateral cataract with lens coloboma and bilateral corneal edema in a guanaco, *J Am Vet Med Assoc* 173:1251, 1978.
15. Gionfriddo JR: Unpublished data, 1990.
16. Brightman AH, McLaughlin SA, Brumley B: Keratoconjunctivitis in a llama, *Vet Med Small Anim Clin* 76:1776, 1981.
17. Fowler ME: *Medicine and surgery of South American camelids*, Ames, Iowa, 1989, Iowa State University Press.
18. Schuh JCL, Ferguson JG, Fischer MA: Congenital coloboma in a llama, *Can Vet J* 32:432, 1991.
19. Johnson LW: Personal communication, 1983.
20. Lavach JD: *Large animal ophthalmology*, St Louis, 1990, Mosby.
21. Donaldson LL, Holland M, Koch SA: Atracurium as an adjunct to halothane-oxygen anesthesia in a llama undergoing intraocular surgery, *Vet Surg* 21:76, 1992.
22. Boer M, Schoon HA: Untersuchungen zu erblich bedingten Augen- und ZNS-Verdanderungen in einer Zuchtgruppe von Vikunjas *(Lama vicugna)* im Zoologischen Garten Hanover, *Verhandlungsbericht des Internationalen Symposiums über die Erkanungen der Zootier* 26:159, 1984.
23. Ingram KA, Sigler RL: *Cataract removal in a young llama.* Proceedings of the annual meeting of the American Association of Zoo Veterinarians, Tampa, Fla, 1993.
24. Rebhun WC, Jenkins, Riis RC et al: An epizootic of blindness and encephalitis associated with a herpes virus indistinguishable from equine herpesvirus I in a herd of alpacas and llamas, *J Am Vet Med Assoc* 192:953, 1988.
25. House JA, Gregg DA, Lubroth J et al: Experimental equine herpesvirus-1 infection in llamas *(Lama glama)*, *J Vet Diagn Invest* 3:137, 1991.
26. Paulsen ME, Young S, Smith JA et al: Bilateral chorioretinitis, centripetal optic neuritis, and encephalitis in a llama, *J Am Vet Med Assoc* 194:1305, 1989.
27. Pickett JP, Moore CP, Beehler BA et al: Bilateral chorioretinitis secondary to disseminated aspergillosis in an alpaca, *J Am Vet Med Assoc* 187:1241, 1985.
28. Tinsley D: Unpublished data, 1996.
29. Dugan SJ, Roberts SM, Curtis CR et al: Prognostic factors and survival of horses with ocular/adnexal squamous cell carcinoma: 147 cases (1978-1988), *J Am Vet Med Assoc* 198:298, 1991.

CHAPTER 88

Selected Eye Diseases of Swine

HARRIET J. DAVIDSON

Swine are frequently used as ophthalmic research animals, but they are rarely examined or treated for primary ocular disease because of the nature of production management. Ocular lesions may be seen in conjunction with other systemic diseases, toxins, or genetic abnormalities. Ocular diseases may be of primary importance in pet pigs. Ophthalmologic examination of a pig is difficult at best. They may require restraint with a snare or squeeze chute and muzzle. Some animals may be examined if they are stroked to calm them and only gentle manipulations are made of the eyes. Pig eyelids are thick because of a layer of subcutaneous fat, and the extraocular muscles are strong. Cilia exist along the superior lid with a single lacrimal puncta in the medial aspect, but no cilia or puncta are found in the inferior lid. The corneal appearance is slightly horizontal in shape. The pupil is round to oval in shape. Iris color is generally brown, although this can vary with breed. The fundus does not have a tapetum and is generally a reddish brown color with blood vessels radiating outward from an oval-shaped optic nerve.

ORBIT/GLOBE DISORDERS

Congenital microphthalmos, thought to be inherited, has been seen in Yorkshire pigs. One study reported the most common congenital malformations were cyclopia, anophthalmia, and microphthalmia. Although these malformations may occur, they are not treatable, with affected animals being culled early. In sows fed a vitamin A–deficient diet, especially during the first month of gestation, microphthalmos and, rarely, megaloglobus were seen in conjunction with other developmental ocular anomalies.

EYELID

Entropion

Vietnamese pot-bellied pigs may have eyelid abnormalities that require surgical intervention. One problem is a large fat pad on the forehead that pushes the eyelids down, resulting in functional blindness. Other problems are keratitis, conjunctivitis, and corneal ulcers caused by entropion. Determining whether the eyelids are actually touching the corneal surface is an important factor in what type of procedure is necessary for correction. Weight loss is generally helpful in prevention and/or treatment. However, these animals are generally pets and management can be difficult. Temporary eyelid eversion combined with weight loss may prevent the animal from requiring a permanent surgical correction. Temporary eyelid

tacking is accomplished by placing mattress sutures from the eyelid margin to the skin, exposing the conjunctival surface. The sutures are left in place for approximately 1 to 2 weeks. Skin staples can be used, but pig skin does not allow for easy placement and care must be given to ensure the staple does not rub on the corneal surface.

Surgical correction for this condition is directed at two areas, the first being elevation of the heavy brow, for which there are two different types of surgery. One method is a brow sling procedure. This involves placement of two slings, one medial and one lateral for each eye. The sling suture should be a heavy, nonabsorbable material, preferably on a straight needle. The suture is placed subdermally through a series of small incisions made between the top of the head and the eyelid margin. A set of four incisions is made for each sling, beginning with two 5-mm incisions along the eyelid margin, one 5-mm incision at the orbital rim, and one 5-mm incision several centimeters dorsal to the orbital rim. The middle incision is to allow for placement and manipulation of the long suture that ultimately needs to run from the top of the animal's head to the eyelid margin. The needle is inserted into the most dorsal incision and passed subdermally to the middle incision, where it exits the skin. The needle is then passed back into the middle incision and again passed subdermally to one eyelid incision, where it exits. The needle is again inserted into the same incision and then passed horizontally to the adjacent eyelid incision, where it exits. The needle again enters the same incision it just exited but now passes to the incision at the dorsal rim. The needle exits and is again passed back into the same incision and back out the original incision. The second sling is placed in the same manner before tying a knot in the first sling. The two sutures are tightened slowly; this pulls the skin upward like a window shade. The individual sutures are then tied and the small skin incisions closed with simple interrupted skin sutures. The same procedure is then completed on the opposite eye. A different form of correction for the heavy fat pad involves dissecting away the subcutaneous periocular fat. This is done by making an incision in the cleavage line of the ventral aspect of the forehead fat pad extending from the tragus rostromedially toward the lateral canthus, above the superior eyelid, extending to the midline of the animal's nose. A second incision is made on the opposite side, joining the first incision at the midline. The skin is then sharply incised, elevating the forehead skin to expose the hard fat underneath. Slices of the subdermal fat are excised until the hair follicles are visible under the skin, being careful not to transect major muscles or nerves underneath. The skin is then laid back down, redundant skin is removed, and the incision is closed with simple interrupted sutures. Sources for more specific surgical description are listed in the Recommended Readings section. The second area of concern is everting the eyelids if they are turned inward and are rubbing on the corneal surface. This is a relatively simple method of making an incision 3 to 5 mm from and parallel with the eyelid margin. A second curvilinear incision is made beginning and ending at the same place as the first incision, outlining a crescent-shaped area of skin. This crescent-shaped area of skin is sharply dissected using scissors. The deep subcutaneous fat is also removed. The wound is closed with simple interrupted sutures in the skin. Sutures should be removed in approximately 10 days. Some animals may benefit from application of topical ophthalmic artificial tears to provide a layer of protection to the cornea if the eyelids cannot be adequately rolled out.

Blepharitis

Historically, phenothiazine toxicity in pigs may cause photosensitization phenomena just as in cattle, sheep, and goats. The treatment is to provide shade for the animals and application of ophthalmic antibiotic ointment to the surrounding lids. Swinepox may cause pox lesions of the lids, third eyelids, and conjunctiva similar to those seen elsewhere on the body. *Escherichia coli* infections (edema disease and endotoxemia) in pigs may cause severe eyelid edema, conjunctival chemosis and inflammation, and even exophthalmos as part of the clinical disease. Treatment is aimed at the primary disease.

CONJUNCTIVAL AND CORNEAL DISORDERS

The microbial population of the ocular surface is most frequently α-hemolytic *Streptococcus* spp., *Staphylococcus epidermidis*, and *Staphylococcus* spp. Sows have a higher level of organism growth compared with feeder pigs, although bacteria are found in all ages of animals. Chlamydial organisms have been identified in all age groups of pigs but are most prevalent in feeder pigs when compared with sows.

Dust, pollen, and noxious fumes may cause conjunctivitis or keratoconjunctivitis. In swine with conjunctivitis and keratoconjunctivitis, the most frequently implicated infectious organisms are *Mycoplasma* and *Chlamydia* spp. It is unknown the exact role these two organisms play in the disease process, whether they are the primary source of disease or secondary invaders. In general conjunctivitis may spread through a herd but is self-limiting, with no long-lasting effects. In a herd operation ophthalmic treatment may not be possible and may not be necessary as long as no other clinical symptoms are found. Management practices may need to be evaluated to ensure environmental factors are not the source of the ocular irritation.

Systemic diseases may present with concurrent ocular lesions. Pseudorabies may have severe clinical symptoms along with ocular discharge and blindness. The ocular form of pseudorabies itself is usually a mild, self-limiting keratoconjunctivitis. Hog cholera may have an early clinical presentation of profuse conjunctivitis and a mucoid to purulent ocular discharge. In most cases the animals progress to other clinical symptoms.

ANTERIOR UVEAL DISORDERS

Anterior uveitis and chorioretinitis are uncommonly diagnosed in pigs, but they may occur with systemic diseases such as hog cholera, Glasser's disease *(Haemophilus somnus* infection in young piglets), and septicemia secondary to erysipelas.

LENS

Cataracts in pigs are uncommon. Starvation and riboflavin deficiency have been described as causing incomplete cataracts. The feed additive Hygromycin B can cause cataracts in adult sows. Toxins from feeds should be considered a possible cause agent if several animals develop cataracts at the same time. In Vietnamese pot-bellied pigs, juvenile cataracts are seen with an age of onset of 1 to 4 years. This type of cataract may be inherited. Uveitis can cause cataracts in pigs just like in sheep, goats, and cattle.

FUNDUS

Optic nerve colobomas (holes or pits) have been reported as a presumed inherited defect in miniature pigs. The lesions are typically bilateral and located at the 6 o'clock position. Listeriosis, tuberculosis, toxoplasmosis, and Glasser's disease may cause multifocal areas of chorioretinitis in swine. Arsanilic acid toxicity can cause optic nerve atrophy in swine.

Recommended Readings

Andrea CR, George LW: Surgical correction of periocular fat pad hypertrophy in pot-bellied pigs, *Vet Surg* 28:311-314, 1999.

Davidson HJ, Rogers DP, Yeary TJ et al: Conjunctival microbial flora of clinically normal pigs, *Am J Vet Res* 55:7; 949-951, 1994.

Prince JH, Diesem CD, Eglitis I et al: *Anatomy and histology of the eye and orbit in domestic animals*, Springfield, Ill, 1960, Charles C Thomas.

Willis AM, Martin CL, Stiles J et al: Brow suspension for treatment of ptosis and entropion in dogs with redundant facial skin folds, *J Am Vet Med Assoc* 214:4; 660-662, 1999.

Vestre WA: Porcine ophthalmology, *Vet Clin North Am Large Anim Pract* 6:667-676, 1984.

CHAPTER 89

Food Animal Ocular Neoplasia

CARMEN M.H. COLITZ and ELLEN B. BELKNAP

The development of neoplasia, benign or malignant, is a multistep process that involves mutations in different genes. These mutations may be caused by spontaneous mutations, the environment, toxins, and viruses. The malignant phenotype is attained when growth of the tumor harms the host because of tissue invasion and metastasis to other sites. Regardless of the initiating cause, cancer is a genetic disease.

Neoplastic disease affecting the eye and periocular structures in cattle results in considerable economic losses every year. Ocular squamous cell carcinoma (OSCC) and orbital lymphosarcoma are the most common tumors affecting cattle. Numerous other neoplasia have been reported to occur in cattle, but little is known about their pathophysiology and subsequent treatment because of the limited number of cases.

OCULAR SQUAMOUS CELL CARCINOMA

Bovine OSCC, also referred to as "cancer eye," is the most economically important neoplasm of cattle. Over the past 50 years, numerous studies have investigated the prevalence of disease in certain breeds, in breeds with certain periocular pigmentation, and in cattle exposed to a number of risk factors.[1-3] The future of this disease's understanding and treatment will no doubt turn toward a genetic cause.

Bovine OSCC is a disease of high morbidity that results in early culling and carcass condemnation at slaughter (Box 89-1). Approximately 12.5% of all carcass condemnations in the United States occur because of OSCC.[4] One study showed the association between solar ultraviolet (UV) radiation and the occurrence of OSCC. As radiation levels increased, the average ages of affected cattle decreased. Also important was the presence of periocular pigmentation, which both lessened the susceptibility to lesion development and lessened the probability of its development.[5] Squamous cell carcinoma does develop in animals with periocular pigmentation, but less often than in nonpigmented animals. In another study, preneoplastic periocular squamous cell carcinoma developed in 75% of the Hereford cattle exposed to solar UV radiation for 16 weeks.[2] Animals living at lower latitudes are exposed to higher intensities of solar UV light and are more prone to the development of OSCC than those at higher latitudes.[2] Therefore the amount and intensity of exposure to solar UV light are probably the most important risk factors for the development of OSCC, especially in cattle with lightly pigmented periocular structures.

The peak age of incidence of OSCC in cattle is between 7 and 9 years, and OSCC is practically unheard of in cattle younger than 4 years.[1,6] These data support the environmental component of the disease (i.e., solar UV light) inasmuch as a purely genetic disease would probably be manifested in the younger age group. No difference in incidence between males and females exists. Females seem to be affected more often than males, but this is probably because cows are used for breeding purposes and milk production and are therefore allowed to age. Males are usually slaughtered at a younger age.[4]

Hereford cattle are the most represented of breeds in which OSCC develops. Herefords also outnumber all other breeds of range cattle and cattle at slaughter, so these statistics must be interpreted with care.[3] Ocular squamous cell carcinoma has also been reported in Hereford crossbreeds and Brahman, Charolais, and dairy breeds.[7]

Factors believed to play a role in the development of squamous cell carcinoma include viruses, nutrition,

---

Box 89-1

Federal Guidelines for Carcass Condemnation

1. Any animal whose eye has been obscured or destroyed by neoplastic tissue and which is infected, suppurative, and necrotic, usually accompanied by a foul odor, or any animal that is cachectic will be condemned.
2. Carcasses with an affected eye or orbit will be condemned if the following occur:
   a. Extensive infection, suppuration, and necrosis are affecting the osseous structures of the head.
   b. Metastasis has occurred from the eye to any lymph node (including the parotid lymph node), internal organ, or any other structure.
   c. Cachexia is present to any extent.
3. If the carcass is not affected other than the eye, it may be passed for human food after removal and condemnation of the head and tongue.
4. Any individual organ or affected part of a carcass with a neoplasm will be condemned. The entire carcass will be condemned if there is evidence of metastasis or if the size, position, or nature of the neoplasm has adversely affected the general condition of the animal.
5. Any animal affected with bovine lymphoma will be condemned.

Modified from *Code of Federal Regulations*, Title 9, Chapter 3, parts 309.6, 311.11, and 311.12 (1-1-90 edition).

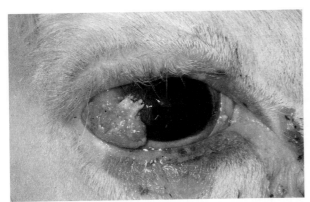

Fig 89-1   Bovine eye affected with squamous cell carcinoma. Note the large, proliferative mass originating from the lateral limbus and the small, plaquelike lesion on the leading edge of the nictitans.

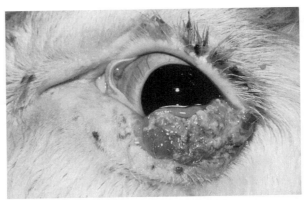

Fig 89-2   Bovine orbit affected by squamous cell carcinoma. Note the large, proliferative, necrotic mass of the ventral lid and the red, raised lesion on the bulbar aspect of the nictitans.

periocular pigmentation, and solar UV light. As already mentioned, UV light in combination with a lack of periocular pigmentation increases the chances for mutations that can lead to the development of OSCC. The lateral limbus is affected most often (66%) (Fig. 89-1), followed by the nasal limbus, nictitans, lacrimal caruncle, and medial canthus.[1,8,9]

Pathophysiology

Initially, sun-damaged, nonkeratinized, stratified squamous epithelial cells of the cornea or conjunctiva become hyperplastic plaques. Plaques may regress spontaneously, progress to a papilloma, or advance to a noninvasive carcinoma (carcinoma in situ); finally, noninvasive carcinoma may develop into an invasive carcinoma.[9] Noninvasive carcinoma usually remains confined to the epithelium but infrequently can be invasive.[10] Invasive carcinoma varies in clinical appearance with the degree of differentiation, extent of neovascularization, amount of secondary inflammation, and duration.[10] Necrosis, hemorrhage, ulceration, and inflammatory cell invasion characterize an invasive carcinoma.[1] It is not uncommon for these lesions to grow large enough to protrude and cause difficulty in closing the eyelids (Fig. 89-2). Carcinomas affecting the nictitans consume the structure but usually do not invade the cartilage.[1] Carcinomas that affect the cornea are usually noninvasive.[11] Early lesions in the skin of the eyelid appear as hyperkeratotic plaques or keratoacanthomas and usually occur at mucocutaneous junctions at or near the hairline.[1,11] These lesions usually regress but infrequently progress into a papilloma or invasive carcinoma.[4]

Tumors of the eyelid, nictitating membrane, and conjunctival fornix metastasize more readily than those at the limbus and cornea.[12] Metastases from OSCC pass through lymph nodes in the head and neck before arriving at the thoracic duct and venous circulation to affect the heart, lungs, pleura, liver, kidney, and neighboring lymph nodes.[13]

Diagnosis

The diagnosis of OSCC is often made by gross appearance, although cytologic and histopathologic examination confirms the diagnosis. Cytologically, benign lesions have anucleated superficial squamous cells and vesicular nuclei with coarse chromatin clumping in deeper cells.[8,11] Lesions of OSCC are typically characterized by enlarged hyperchromatic nuclei with large clumps of chromatin and prominent nucleoli.[8,9] In 90% of the cases there is agreement between the cytologic diagnosis and the histologic diagnosis.[14] If regional lymph nodes are enlarged, fine-needle aspiration and/or biopsy is indicated. Overexpression of p53 protein has been reported in bovine OSCC by immunohistochemistry, indicating a possible role of this protein in the pathogenesis of OSCC.[15,16] The index of cells immunopositive for Ki67, a marker for cell proliferation, has also been reported to show significant correlation with histologic patterns regarding degree of tumor differentiation.[17]

Treatment

Numerous modalities are available for the treatment of OSCC, but one should first consider the practicality of treatment. That is, the extent of the disease, as well as the intended use of the animal and its value, should be assessed before investing time and money. If OSCC has invaded the bony orbit or parotid lymph node, the animal should be sent to slaughter because the cost of treatment and probability of its recurrence often preclude any attempt to treat the animal.[14] The smaller the lesion, the better the chance for successful treatment; the bigger the lesion, usually the more expensive the treatment with a lower chance for remission. Smaller lesions are usually more superficial and more amenable to the available treatment options, but larger lesions usually need more than one type of treatment modality.[18]

Complete surgical excision is the treatment of choice for OSCC, although it has been shown that additional lesions may develop within 2 years of surgery.[19] Small lesions with well-defined margins are easily excised and may then be treated with adjunctive cryosurgery or hyperthermia.[18] Lesions involving the nictitans may require amputation of the structure. More extensive lesions or multiple lesions may require either enucleation or exenteration.

Another common treatment modality is cryosurgery. Cryosurgery involves selectively destroying tissue with a cryogen, usually liquid nitrogen. Nitrous oxide is not usually used because it does not attain as suitable a temperature as liquid nitrogen. A double freeze-thaw protocol involves freezing the lesion to between −25° and −40° C, allowing it to thaw slowly, and repeating the cycle; this is the most useful method. When used in lesions smaller than 2.5 cm in diameter, cryosurgery has been shown to have a 97% cure rate.[20] Lesions greater than 5 cm in diameter did not respond well to cryosurgery and had high rates of recurrence. Cryosurgery can also be used in conjunction with surgical excision to destroy the remaining neoplastic cells not removed by excision. Recognizing the extent of the disease is important because even extensive excision and cryosurgery cannot help invasive and metastatic OSCC.[21] Cryosurgery is an easy, rapid, relatively inexpensive procedure that provides analgesia, requires little postoperative care, causes minimal adverse side effects, and can be repeated.[20]

Radiation therapy can also be used to treat OSCC, either alone or in conjunction with surgical excision, depending on the size of the lesion. This modality is usually reserved for extremely valuable animals because of the expense, the need for a radiologist to handle the radioactive isotopes, and public health concerns.[14,22]

Radiofrequency current hyperthermia involves heating the tumor tissue above normal body temperature (42°-45° C). Tumor cells are more susceptible to heat damage than are normal cells, so the tumor cells are selectively killed.[8] Heat normally penetrates only 3 to 4 mm into tissues and covers an area of 1 cm^2; therefore larger tumors need to be surgically debulked before hyperthermia can be used effectively.[9,18] It is recommended that the instrument be applied 3 to 4 mm beyond the tumor margin. A handheld radiofrequency device is available commercially (Thermoprobe, Hach Co, Loveland, Colo.) and consists of electrodes on a surface probe that can heat tissues to 50° C when placed on a lesion for 30 seconds. This increase in temperature results in necrosis of both neoplastic and normal cells and sloughing of the treated tissue.[9] Successful treatment with hyperthermia in small, localized lesions is approximately 90%, and if the tumor should recur, the procedure can be repeated.[15]

Immunotherapy is a treatment option that attempts to stimulate the host's immune system against the tumor. Various antigens including allogeneic or freeze-dried saline phenol extract of squamous cell carcinoma and emulsified cell walls of *Mycobacterium bovis* (cell walls of the Calmette-Guérin bacillus) have been used in an attempt to initiate active immunity against the tumor. Other agents that have been used to stimulate immunity include levamisole and H$_2$-receptor blockers. Immunotherapy is ineffective in the treatment of cancer, probably because tumor cells are capable of evading the immune system either by downregulation of major histocompatibility antigens or tumor-specific immunosuppression.

Herd Management

Careful and proper herd management practices will substantially reduce the economic losses from OSCC. Animals older than 2 years of age should be examined for ocular lesions two to three times per year when they are rounded up for routine examination. If suspicious lesions are found, they should be treated immediately by surgical excision, cryotherapy, radiofrequency hyperthermia, and/or immunotherapy.[9,14] Large, noninvasive lesions of the globe or adnexa may require orbital exenteration or culling, depending on the productivity of the animal and market prices. Cattle with invasive and/or metastatic OSCC should be shipped to slaughter immediately.[14] Lines of cattle highly susceptible to OSCC should be culled or bred for pigmented periocular structures, which will decrease the incidence of the disease. Choosing breeds of cattle (Charolais, Angus, and Brahman) that are less predisposed to OSCC will also decrease economic losses.[7]

BOVINE LYMPHOSARCOMA

Enzootic bovine lymphosarcoma is an insidious systemic disease of the reticuloendothelial system that has ocular manifestations. It is responsible for most of the economic losses in dairy cattle and is the most common orbital neoplasia affecting dairy cattle.[8] Clinically, progressive unilateral or bilateral exophthalmos results from a retrobulbar neoplastic infiltrate that usually affects the caudal periorbital tissues.[11] More cases (13%) have bilateral involvement than unilateral (9%).[23] Extraocular muscles are often infiltrated by tumor cells. The globe itself is not usually involved.[8] As the disease progresses, exposure keratitis and eventual proptosis occur. The initial complaint may be an acute onset of exophthalmos, although the orbital involvement has probably been present for some time. Subtle signs of exophthalmos are difficult to assess, especially because dairy cattle naturally have slightly exophthalmic eyes. Physical examination usually reveals other systemic abnormalities.[24] Less than 2% of cattle infected with bovine leukemia virus (BLV) develop enzootic bovine lymphosarcoma.[25]

The methods most often used to detect bovine leukemia virus infection are the agar gel immunodiffusion test (AGID) and the enzyme-linked immunosorbent assay (ELISA), both of which are directed at detecting antibodies to the viral envelope glycoprotein, gp51.[26] Two negative tests 2 to 3 months apart are necessary to consider cattle BLV free because seroconversion occurs 3 weeks to 3 months postinfection. Most ELISA tests for BLV correlate well with specificity of AGID tests yet have greater sensitivity when used for pooled sera or milk samples as herd screening tests.[26-28] A definitive diagnosis of enzootic bovine lymphosarcoma requires histologic or cytologic examination (Fig. 89-3) of affected lymph nodes, organs, or body fluid.

Treatment is not attempted in systemically affected cattle because there is no curative therapy. Cattle will probably be condemned if sent to slaughter. Exenteration of involved eyes provides palliative treatment in cows in late gestation until calving or until embryos or ova are obtained.[11]

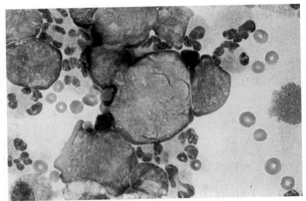

Fig 89-3   Photomicrograph of a cytologic specimen aspirated from the retrobulbar area of a bovine orbit. Note the large, immature lymphocytes with a high nuclear-to-cytoplasmic ratio and fine chromatin in the nuclei, typical of bovine lymphoma.

References

1. Russell WO, Wynne ES, Loquvam GS et al: Studies on bovine ocular squamous carcinoma ("cancer eye"): I. Pathological anatomy and historical review, *Cancer* 9:1, 1956.
2. Kopecky KE, Pugh GW, Hughes DE et al: Biological effect of ultraviolet radiation on cattle: bovine ocular squamous cell carcinoma, *Am J Vet Res* 40:1783, 1979.
3. Russell WC, Brinks JS, Kainer RA: Incidence and heritability of ocular squamous cell tumors in Hereford cattle, *J Anim Sci* 43:1156, 1976.
4. Heeney JL, Valli VEO: Bovine ocular squamous cell carcinoma: an epidemiological perspective, *Can J Comp Med* 49:21, 1985.
5. Anderson DE, Skinner PE: Studies on bovine ocular squamous cell carcinoma ("cancer eye"): XI. Effects of sunlight, *J Anim Sci* 20:474, 1961.
6. Blackwell RL, Anderson DE, Knox JH: Age incidence and heritability of cancer eye in Hereford cattle, *J Anim Sci* 15:943, 1956.
7. Bailey CM, Hanks DR, Hanks MA: Circumocular pigmentation and incidence of ocular squamous cell tumors in *Bos taurus* and *Bos indicus* × *Bos taurus* cattle, *J Am Vet Med Assoc* 196:1605, 1990.
8. Moore CM: Diseases of the eye. In Smith BP, editor: *Large animal internal medicine*, St Louis, 2002, Mosby.
9. Gilger BC, Whitley RD, McLaughlin SA: Bovine ocular squamous cell carcinoma: a review, *Vet Ann* 31:73, 1991.
10. Spencer WH: Conjunctiva. In Spencer WH, editor: *Ophthalmic pathology*, Philadelphia, 1996, Saunders.
11. Whittaker CJG, Gelatt KN, Wilkie DA: Food animal ophthalmology. In Gelatt KN, editor: *Veterinary ophthalmology*, ed 3, Philadelphia, 1999, Lippincott Williams & Wilkins.
12. Kircher CH, Garner FM, Robinson FR: Tumors of the eye and adnexa, *Bull WHO* 50:135, 1974.
13. Moulton JE: *Tumors in domestic animals*, Los Angeles, 1961, University of California Press.
14. Kainer RA: Current concepts in the treatment of bovine ocular squamous cell tumors, *Vet Clin North Am Large Anim Pract* 6:609, 1984.
15. Sironi G, Riccaboni P, Mertel L et al: p53 Protein expression in conjunctival squamous cell carcinomas of domestic animals, *Vet Ophthal* 2:227, 1999.
16. Teifke JP, Lohr CV: Immunohistochemical detection of p53 overexpression in paraffin wax-embedded squamous cell carcinomas of cattle, horses, cats and dogs, *J Comp Pathol* 114:205, 1996.
17. Carvalho T, Vala H, Pinto C et al: Immunohistochemical studies of epithelial cell proliferation and p53 mutation in bovine ocular squamous cell carcinoma, *Vet Pathol* 42:66, 2005.
18. Roberts SM, Kainer R: Food animal ocular neoplasia. In Howard JL, editor: *Current veterinary therapy: food animal practice*, ed 3, Philadelphia, 1993, Saunders.
19. Lavach JD: Ocular neoplasia. In Lavach JD, editor: *Large animal ophthalmology*, St Louis, 1990, Mosby.
20. Farris HE, Fraunfelder FT: Cryosurgical treatment of ocular squamous cell carcinoma of cattle, *J Am Vet Med Assoc* 168:213, 1976.
21. Farris HE: Cryosurgical treatment of bovine ocular squamous cell carcinoma, *Vet Clin North Am Large Anim Pract* 2:861, 1980.
22. Banks WC: Radioactive gold in the treatment of ocular squamous cell carcinoma of cattle, *J Am Vet Med Assoc* 163:745, 1973.
23. Radostits OM, Gay CC, Blood DC et al: *Veterinary medicine*, ed 9, London, 2000, Saunders.
24. Malatestinic A: Bilateral exophthalmos in a Holstein cow with lymphosarcoma, *Can Vet J* 44:664, 2003.
25. Thurmond MC: Retrospective study of four years of carcass condemnation rates for malignant lymphoma in California dairy cows, *Am J Vet Res* 46:1387, 1985.
26. Simard C, Richardson S, Dixon P et al: Enzyme-linked immunosorbent assay for the diagnosis of bovine leukosis: comparison with the agar gel immunodiffusion test approved by the Canadian Food Inspection Agency, *Can J Vet Res* 64:101, 2000.
27. Monti GE, Frankena K, Engel B et al: Evaluation of a new antibody-based enzyme-linked immunosorbent assay for the detection of bovine leukemia virus infection in dairy cattle, *J Vet Diagn Invest* 17:451, 2005.
28. Nguyen VK, Maes RF: Evaluation of an enzyme-linked immunosorbent assay for detection of antibodies to bovine leukemia virus in serum and milk, *J Clin Micro* 31:979, 1993.

CHAPTER 90

Neurogenic Vision Loss

PAUL E. MILLER

Differentiation among the causes of neurogenic vision loss in food animals is often frustrating because many of these entities have a similar range of clinical presentations and it is difficult, if not impossible, to accurately assess the visual capability of obtunded animals. The purpose of this chapter is to consider the common causes of neurogenic vision loss in food animals and to discuss methods of distinguishing these disorders from each other from an ophthalmic standpoint. The reader is referred to previous editions of this text, as well as the many textbooks on neurology that review the basic science and neuro-circuitry of these disorders.

EXAMINATION

Normal Vision

Any attempt to determine the nature and extent of vision loss first requires an understanding of the normal visual abilities of that species. Unfortunately, this knowledge is relatively limited in domestic ruminants. Their large eyes probably give them a visual acuity (e.g., the ability to see the details of an object separately and unblurred) in the 20/45 to 20/50 range. This is superior to that of dogs and cats and means that they can differentiate the details in an object from 20 feet away that the normal human could do at 45 to 50 feet. The lateral placement of their eyes also gives them a larger, virtually 360-degree visual field of view, with blind spots only anteroventral to the nose and the width of the head posteriorly.

Visual clues are more important to cattle than auditory clues in acquiring feed, and calves have been demonstrated to have a hierarchical attraction for certain colors with green being preferred over white (incandescent), which is preferred to red. Studies have led to a general consensus that cattle have imperfect, although useful, color vision. It appears that they can readily distinguish longer light wavelengths such as red, orange, and yellow from gray but have more difficulty in differentiating short wavelength colors (green, blue, violet) from gray. It has also been suggested that anatomic differences in the density and biochemical composition of the cone photoreceptors among different cattle breeds may result in breed-related differences in color perception. Pigs also appear to have useful color vision and can differentiate many colors on behavioral testing.

Assessment of Vision

Most clinical tests of animal vision are crude and only able to discern gross deficiencies in visual function bordering on total vision loss. Therefore the first indication

of vision loss in a herd or flock is often aberrant, visually oriented behavior or an increase in self-inflicted injuries resulting from falling into gutters or bumping into objects. More detailed investigation of the visual capabilities of an individual animal usually begins with the assessment of a menace response in which the open hand is rapidly moved parallel to, and across, the animal's visual field. Care should be exercised to avoid disturbing the vibrissae or periocular hairs, which may initiate a blink response via touch receptors rather than the visual pathway. If the animal lacks a menace response, the ability to blink should be verified by gently tapping with a finger on the skin of the medial canthal region. This stimulation can also be used in uncooperative or somewhat obtunded animals to amplify the response to a subsequent menacing gesture. Because the menace response is a learned response, it may be slow or absent in naive, normal neonatal animals for the first several weeks of life. It should be remembered, however, that a menace response often is retained in the presence of a visual acuity of 20/1000 or poorer and that it is not particularly reliable for determining the presence or absence of *partial* visual field deficits. Tossing cotton balls across the animal's visual field or maze testing (with or without a pink-eye patch over one eye) may also provide crude estimates of an animal's visual capabilities.

In addition to the menace response, the pupillary light reflex (PLR), swinging flashlight test, and dazzle response should also be assessed, although the presence of these reflexes does not guarantee that vision is normal. Pupillary contraction in response to bright light in large animals is relatively slow compared with most carnivores, making a bright halogen light source and darkened quarters for examination nearly essential for the accurate evaluation of this reflex. Both the direct and consensual pupillary light reflexes should be assessed to adequately localize the lesion(s). A swinging flashlight test may also aid in localizing unilateral lesions by verifying that the deficit is not at the level of cranial nerve III or the iris sphincter muscle. In this test a bright light source is shone into one eye for several seconds and then immediately shifted to the other eye, and then back and forth between the two eyes. Severe unilateral lesions of the retina or optic nerve result in an eye in which the pupil constricts when the contralateral eye is stimulated, but in pupillary dilation when the affected eye is illuminated. The dazzle reflex is a subcortical response to bright light and is determined by quickly shining a bright light into a dark, adapted eye. A positive response is manifested as blinking or withdrawal of the head in response to light. Visual animals have a positive dazzle reflex, which may also occur in animals with cerebral cortical disease because the reflex is mediated subcortically.

Once the status of the pertinent neurologic reflexes has been determined, careful examination of the ocular media is warranted. I prefer to begin by standing approximately arm's distance from the eye and looking at the tapetal reflex through a direct ophthalmoscope set at "0" diopters. This technique screens for opacities in the ocular media located between the examiner and the tapetum. Small corneal scars, cataracts, or vitreal debris appear as black spots obtunding the tapetal reflex. If the animal is observed directly head-on so that the tapetal reflex from both eyes is seen simultaneously, it may also be used to screen for anisocoria. If the tapetal reflex cannot be readily obtained, it is likely that the cause of vision loss is not neurologic but related to an abnormality of the globe itself. Once the eye is examined at a distance, the clinician then moves to within a few centimeters of the animal and views the fundus and optic nerve head with the ophthalmoscope still set at "0" diopters. Alternatively, a 20-diopter, indirect ophthalmoscope hand-lens (20-diopter veterinary viewing lens, Welch Allyn, Skaneateles Falls, N.Y.) and a focal bright light source may be used to view the retina and nerve head. The latter is especially useful in animals with horns or dispositions such that it would be unsafe to approach them closely.

This rapid screening approach allows the clinician to determine whether neurogenic vision loss is present and to further subdivide vision loss into two groups: those with and those without a discernible PLR. Although imperfect, the presence or absence of a PLR is often the most reliable clinical parameter because of the difficulty in thoroughly evaluating the visual status of neonatal or obtunded animals. The absence of a PLR in a blind eye that is not inflamed suggests a lesion of the optic nerve/chiasm. Such eyes also typically fail to exhibit dazzle reflexes (or a menace response) and may or may not have abnormalities of the optic disc discernible on ophthalmoscopy. An intact PLR in a blind eye that otherwise appears normal is typical of lesions of the higher visual pathway. Although these eyes lack a menace response, they may or may not exhibit a positive dazzle reflex. The fundus examination should be within normal limits. The following is an attempt to use the PLR as a method of differentiating the most common neurogenic causes of vision loss in food animals—with the realization that in some circumstances overlap in presentation in a small percentage of animals may occur.

DISORDERS WITH AN ABSENT PUPILLARY LIGHT REFLEX

Vitamin A Deficiency

Calves born to dams that were vitamin A deficient during gestation may be congenitally blind and exhibit bilateral optic nerve atrophy. Affected animals may also be uncoordinated and have thickened carpal joints and hydrocephalus. Acquired vitamin A deficiency most frequently occurs in young (younger than 2 years of age), rapidly growing, feedlot steers that are nongrazing and consuming diets high in concentrate with low-quality roughage for a prolonged period of time (>200 days).

Heifers appear to be more resistant even if eating the same diet. The development of clinical signs varies with the animal's age, its liver stores of vitamin A, and the duration/severity of the deficiency. Five to 18 months of a deficient diet are usually required before clinical signs become readily apparent, although affected animals are often in poorer condition than normal. Early clinical signs include night blindness (usually not recognized until some animals in the herd are completely blind) and papilledema, which results from both increased cerebrospinal fluid (CSF) pressure and bony compression of the optic nerve by a stenotic optic canal. Papilledema occurs before complete vision loss and alterations in the PLR and initially appears as a bilateral, occasionally asymmetric, subtle blurring of the optic disc margins. As the deficiency progresses the disc may become two to three times normal size and markedly protrudes into the vitreous, suggesting the extent of papilledema may indicate the duration of the deficiency. Later in the course of the disease the retinal vasculature may become congested and torturous, and peripapillary hemorrhages and retinal detachment may occur. The nontapetal region is often focally depigmented, and in advanced stages the optic nerve head becomes atrophic. Some animals may have tonic/clonic seizures, exophthalmia, nystagmus, strabismus, and, uncommonly, corneal edema and conjunctivitis.

Diagnosis is based on clinical signs and determination of vitamin A levels in the serum or liver. Serum levels less than 25 µg/dl and liver values less than 2 µg/g of liver tissue are considered diagnostic. Initial treatment for cattle consists of parenteral vitamin A (440 IU/kg), and long-term control can be achieved by repeated IM injections of 3000 to 6000 IU/kg of vitamin A every 60 days. Alternatively, long-term control may be achieved by addition of exogenous stabilized vitamin A to the ration or by permitting access to leafy, freshly cured hay; green pasture; or 0.5 to 2 kg of alfalfa meal daily. Night-blind animals typically respond well to treatment, but those with marked retinal degeneration and optic canal stenosis with secondary optic neuropathy should not be expected to regain useful vision.

Orbital Diseases

Inflammatory diseases of the orbit may secondarily involve the optic nerve and cause vision loss (usually unilateral) in individual animals. Unilateral exophthalmia ranging from only a mild resistance to retropulsion of the globe to overt proptosis is almost always present, and many animals also exhibit periorbital or temporomandibular joint pain (manifested as pain on opening the mouth), anorexia, fever, eyelid swelling, and chemosis. Common causes include periocular puncture wounds, actinobacillosis, plant or other foreign material migrating into the orbit from the oral cavity, and extension of frontal or maxillary sinusitis into the orbit. Diagnosis is based on clinical signs and examination of an aspirate/biopsy of retrobulbar tissues. An elevated white blood cell count and skull radiograph/orbital ultrasound study may be supportive. Untreated, orbital cellulitis is potentially fatal and management should consist of ensuring adequate hydration, removing any foreign material from the orbit, establishing drainage, hot packing the affected area, and systemic/topical antibiotics. The cornea must be protected with either topical antibiotic ointments, a temporary tarsorrhaphy, or third eyelid flap until the exophthalmia resolves. In some circumstances exenteration of the orbit is required.

Ocular squamous cell carcinoma and lymphosarcoma are the most common orbital neoplasms that can induce neurologic vision loss via secondary optic nerve involvement. In contrast to inflammatory orbital disease, orbital tumors usually present as a nonpainful, slowly progressive exophthalmia or as an externally apparent mass invading the orbit.

Arsanilic Acid

Phenylarsonic derivatives such as arsanilic acid and roxarsone ("3-nitro") have been used as feed additives in the swine industry in the past, both as growth promoters and, at higher levels, as therapeutic agents for swine dysentery. Acute symptoms after exposure to high levels of an organic arsenical may occur within 4 to 6 days and include blindness, head tremors, incoordination, euphoria, ataxia, paraparesis, and paraplegia, but affected animals typically continue to eat and drink. Lower, but still excessive, levels of arsanilic acid such as those used for treating swine dysentery may take weeks or months to induce clinical signs and may cause only partial or complete vision loss and possibly paresis. Fundus examination may reveal optic nerve atrophy, supporting the diagnosis. Confirmation of the diagnosis may be difficult because the gross postmortem examination is often unremarkable, and the only characteristic histologic feature is demyelination and necrosis of the optic nerves, optic tracts, and some peripheral nerves. Because of rapid excretion, tissue or blood levels of arsenic are rarely diagnostic and feed levels are more indicative of the true level of exposure. Treatment consists of complete withdrawal of any arsenic-containing compound. The prognosis is fairly good in all but the severely affected, although permanent vision loss or neurologic damage may persist and recovery may require 2 to 4 weeks.

Plant Toxicities

In England, ingestion of the rhizomes of male fern (*Dryopteris filix-mas*) by cattle has been associated with permanent or, more frequently, transient blindness. Blindness may be the primary presenting sign, although drowsiness, weakness, malaise, and constipation also occur. Retinal ganglion cells and optic nerve fibers are destroyed, and on ophthalmoscopy, variable amounts of papilledema and peripapillary hemorrhages are observed initially (thus necessitating differentiation from hypovitaminosis A). In advanced cases, optic nerve head atrophy and retinal vascular attenuation are noted. A similar syndrome has been reported in Australia in sheep and goats after ingestion of *Stypandra imbricata* ("blind grass") and the spring flowering phase of *Stypandra glauca* ("nodding blue lily").

DISORDERS WITH AN INTACT PUPILLARY LIGHT REFLEX

Polioencephalomalacia

Polioencephalomalacia (PEM) is most common in young feedlot cattle and weaned calves 6 to 12 months old receiving a low-fiber, high-concentrate ration. Lambs and kids are typically 2 to 6 months old. Early in the course of the disease affected animals may be anorectic, hypersalivate, appear blind, walk with the head erect or in circles, show incoordination, and become detached from the rest of the herd or flock. Diarrhea, hyperesthesia, muscle tremors, and head pressing may also be present. Vision loss is central in origin and may be accompanied by dorsomedial strabismus secondary to trochlear nerve dysfunction, variable nystagmus, and head tilt. Dorsomedial strabismus, however, is not diagnostic for PEM by itself. Papilledema and an impaired PLR secondary to increased intracranial pressure has been reported but is uncommon. In some cases, intense miosis may make interpretation of the PLR difficult. In the latter stages the animal becomes recumbent and develops tonic/clonic seizures.

A tentative diagnosis of PEM is made by observing blindness, muscle tremors, and opisthotonos in cattle 4 to 18 months of age that are being fed high-concentrate rations and by assessing response to therapy. Thiamine (10 mg/kg IV or IM) every 6 hours for the first day usually results in significant improvement in 24 hours (often within 6-8 hours). Therapy should continue every 6 to 12 hours for 2 more days and recovery may take as long as a week. Euthanasia should be considered in patients not responding to treatment within 3 days. Proper hydration needs to be ensured and seizures may be controlled with a barbiturate or diazepam. Mannitol (1-2 g/kg of a 20% solution IV), DMSO (1-2 g/kg of a 40% solution IV), or dexamethasone (1-2 mg/kg IV) may be useful in reducing cerebral edema. PEM resulting from high-sulphur diets such as barley malt sprouts, corn byproducts, molasses-based supplements, or *Brassica oleracea* ingestion may not respond to thiamine supplementation, and patients with cortical necrosis may not regain vision. Consideration should also be given to supplementation of high-concentrate diets with thiamine (3-10 mg/kg of feed) or allowing access to pasture or good-quality green hay.

Lead Poisoning

Lead is ubiquitous in the environment and although the risks of ingestion of lead based paint are well recognized, there are numerous other sources of lead such as grease, used crankcase oil from engines burning leaded fuels, discarded lead-acid batteries, plumbing materials, and possibly other sources discarded into rural trash piles. Central vision loss may affect up to 50% of cattle with lead poisoning. Fixed and dilated pupils, however, have been occasionally reported. Most cattle will exhibit other symptoms such as muscle twitching, hyperirritability, depression, convulsions, ataxia, circling, bruxism, excessive salivation, tucked abdomen, anorexia, or diarrhea. Diagnosis is based on clinical signs; history or circumstantial evidence of lead poisoning; and excessive lead levels in blood, feces, liver, kidney, or rumen contents. Whole blood lead levels in excess of 0.35 ppm in cattle and probably other ruminants are significant. Unlike listeriosis and thrombotic meningoencephalitis (TEM), lead toxicity typically lacks a fever, does not have elevated protein or white blood cells on a CSF tap, and is unresponsive to antibiotic therapy. In contrast to PEM, it frequently affects cattle younger than 6 months and older than 18 months of age. In general, treatment is by eliminating the source of lead, inhibiting further absorption (i.e., using gastroprotectants or surgically removing large objects from the gastrointestinal tract), and chelation of the lead in bone with calcium versenate (CaEDTA) (66 mg/kg/day slow IV) in divided doses two to three times daily and continued for 3 to 5 days. If additional treatment is indicated (usually multiple courses are required because calcium versenate does not remove soft tissue lead), rest for 2 days to allow for lead redistribution and renal recovery, and follow with another 5-day treatment period. Thiamine hydrochloride alone (250-1000 mg SQ or IM daily) may be beneficial in the treatment of lead toxicity, although a combination of thiamine hydrochloride (25 mg/kg SQ q12h) and 110 mg Ca-EDTA/kg IV 6 hours apart twice daily was more effective in one study. Chelation therapy should be continued despite the apparent lack of clinical improvement because lead first mobilizes from tightly bound tissue depots.

Thrombotic Meningoencephalitis

Although less common than in the past, the neurologic form of septicemia secondary to *Hemophilus somnus* may cause high fevers, unilateral or bilateral blindness, strabismus, nystagmus, anorexia, staggering, paralysis, tonic/clonic seizures, opisthotonus, and partial paralysis of multiple cranial nerves in any bovine, but especially calves and feedlot cattle 1 to 12 months of age. Death may occur in a few hours to days. Although vision loss is typically central in origin, approximately 50% of patients have fundus lesions consistent with septicemia, which can be a useful aid in diagnosis. Visualization of the fundus may be difficult if strabismus and miosis secondary to anterior uveitis are also present, but retinal hemorrhages (secondary to thrombosis of retinal vessels) and small, sometimes coalescing white "cotton-wool" spots with indistinct borders are seen ophthalmoscopically. Focal areas of retinal detachment and mild papilledema may also be seen. Chronic cases may show only chorioretinal scarring. In contrast to PEM, often there is fever, multifocal cranial nerve deficits, leukocytosis on CSF tap, and a history of respiratory infection in the group. Therapy consists of fluid support and anticonvulsant agents if necessary; systemic nonsteroidal antiinflammatory drugs; and systemic oxytetracycline, ampicillin, penicillin, ceftiofur, or florfenicol. If the animal is still ambulatory, the prognosis is fair to good with intensive therapy. Bacterins are of questionable economic benefit in preventing the relatively sporadic neurologic form of the disease, although they may be useful in other forms of the disease.

Water Deprivation Sodium Ion Toxicosis

Water deprivation sodium ion toxicosis (salt toxicity) occurs primarily in swine but may also be seen in ruminants consuming a high concentration of sodium with limited access to water. It also occurs in cattle when thirsty animals are given access to saline water or allowed free access to a salt supplement after a period of salt restriction. Generally, as long as water intake is adequate, relatively large intakes of sodium (up to 13% salt) can be tolerated in the diet. Limited water intake may occur as a result of neglect, malfunction of automatic waterers, freezing of water sources, overcrowding, placing the animals in unfamiliar environments, and unpalatable water from the addition of drugs or minerals. Clinical signs are associated with central nervous system edema, and in the initial stages increased thirst, pruritus and constipation may be noted. In the later stages (1-5 days), vision loss is associated with other neurologic signs such as deafness, circling or running movements, aimless wandering, altered consciousness, walking backward, sialorrhea, and seizures. Seizures in pigs are characterized by sitting on the rear quarters, jerking the head backward and upward, and falling over in a tonic-clonic seizure and opisthotonus. Cattle may exhibit gastrointestinal symptoms, blindness, convulsions, and often characteristically drag their rear feet or even walk on the dorsal surface of the fetlock. Diagnosis is based on a history of limited water intake (which may be difficult to elicit), clinical signs, the finding of serum sodium levels above 160 mEq/L and cerebral cortex tissue sodium concentrations above 1800 ppm. An increase of 5 mEq or greater in sodium levels in the CSF versus the serum is also supportive of the diagnosis, especially if water-deprived animals are allowed access to water immediately before an examination. Additionally, in pigs a characteristic eosinophilic meningoencephalitis is present histologically early in the course of the disease. Treatment is nonspecific and directed at slowly restoring CNS and serum sodium and water values to normal levels, either by giving small amounts of fresh water frequently (up to 0.5% of body weight every 60 minutes) or appropriate intravenous fluid support. Approximately 50% of affected animals die regardless of treatment, but those who recover do so within 4 to 5 days.

Listeriosis

Listeria monocytogenes may produce a bacterial encephalitis or meningoencephalitis in adult sheep and sometimes cattle, which occasionally results in blindness. Ophthalmic clinical signs vary but may include amaurosis, facial paralysis, optic neuritis (with an obtunded PLR), and secondary endophthalmitis. Hypopyon is common, and a unilateral uveitis in the absence of systemic signs may occur. Listeriosis is more commonly manifested as a vestibular syndrome with head tilt, circling, and ataxia or as a medial strabismus with head pressing, unilateral facial paralysis, dysphagia, limb paresis, and depression. It can be distinguished from PEM by the presence of fever, asymmetric cranial nerve deficits, and mononuclear leukocytosis on CSF tap. Cultures of CSF fluid may be useful diagnostically. Treatment with penicillin (22,000-44,000 IU/kg, IV q6h or IM q12h) and oxytetracycline (20 mg/kg IV once a day or 10 mg/kg IV q12h) may be effective, although some strains may exhibit in vitro resistance to these compounds. Other authors have advocated using ampicillin, amoxicillin, or gentamicin, but aminoglycosides are subject to a voluntary ban in North America. Animals exhibiting a weak or absent menace response, recumbency, or excitement have a poorer prognosis for recovery than those showing other signs of the disease.

Miscellaneous

Virtually any cause of encephalitis or meningitis is capable of presenting in select circumstances as blindness. Infrequent but potential causes include hydrocephalus, brain tumors, bacterial meningitis, brain abscesses, nervous coccidiosis, *Sarcocystis* infection, *Neospora* spp. infection, the encephalitic form of infectious bovine rhinotracheitis, pseudorabies, rabies, ammoniated forage toxicosis, ethylene glycol ingestion, nitrofurazone toxicosis, neuronal ceroid lipofuscinosis, and intracarotid drug injection. Vision loss has also been described in sheep with scrapie, *Parelaphostrongylus tenuis* (meningeal worm), the intermediate stages of *Taenia multiceps (Coenurus cerebralis),*

inherited ceroid-lipofuscinosis, and following overdosage with closantel. In the latter disorder the retina was also degenerate and there was a severe optic neuropathy.

Recommended Readings

Collins BK: Neuro-ophthalmology in food animals. In Howard JL, Smith R, editors: *Current veterinary therapy food animal*, ed 4, Philadelphia, 1999, Saunders.

Constable PD: Ruminant neurologic diseases, *Vet Clin North Am Food Anim Pract* 20:185, 2004.

Dey S, Swarup D, Kalicharan et al: Treatment of lead toxicity in calves, *Vet Hum Toxicol* 37:230, 1995.

Gould DH: Update on sulfur-related polioencephalomalacia, *Vet Clin North Am Food Anim Pract* 16:481, 2000.

Kul O, Karahan S, Basalan M et al: Polioencephalomalacia in cattle: a consequence of prolonged feeding of barley malt sprouts, *J Vet Med A Physiol Pathol Clin Med* 53:123, 2006.

Mayhew IG: *Large animal neurology*, Philadelphia, 1989, Lea & Febiger.

Plumless K: *Clinical veterinary toxicology*, St Louis, 2004 Mosby.

Schweizer G, Ehrensperger F, Torgerson PR et al: Clinical findings and treatment of 94 cattle presumptively diagnosed with listeriosis, *Vet Rec* 158:588, 2006.

Smith BP: *Large animal internal medicine*, ed 2, St Louis, 1996, Mosby.

CHAPTER 91

Ophthalmic Therapeutics

HARRIET J. DAVIDSON

Treatment plans for ophthalmic diseases in production animals are complicated because of the multiple factors of animal use and temperament along with the financial and physical ability of the owner or manager. The treatment plan is further complicated by the limited number of drugs approved for use in food animals, particularly for ophthalmic diseases. Ophthalmic examination of the affected animal or selected animals within the herd helps in determination and documentation of the diagnosis. Documentation of the diagnosis may be helpful when considering the use of extra-label drugs. In general, treatment is initiated after a tentative diagnosis and should be altered based on response to treatment or diagnostic test results. Selection of medications should be based on the location, type, and severity of disease, as well as the potential use of the animal. The route of drug administration may be dictated by the type of animal, as

well as financial and physical constraints. The frequency of administration is determined by the individual drug(s) and route of administration. Although the vast majority of production animals are considered commodities, a number of animals are considered pets or show animals. Individual animals may be treated by local and aggressive administration of ophthalmic drugs to achieve improved results over mass systemic treatment needed for herds or flocks.

ROUTES OF DRUG ADMINISTRATION

The most practical routes of administration include the topical ophthalmic, subconjunctival, and parenteral routes. Retrobulbar injection is used for surgical intervention and not as a therapeutic method. The route of administration is important when attempting to establish therapeutic drug levels in ocular tissues. Factors to consider when selecting the route of administration include the type of disease, ability of a given drug to achieve a therapeutic level in affected tissue, number and type of animals requiring treatment, physical constraints of the operation, and financial commitment for the owner or manager. Many drugs administered systemically do not establish therapeutic levels in ocular tissues, so effective treatment requires topical or subconjunctival administration. Drug penetration into specific ocular tissues is impeded by the blood-aqueous barrier and the corneal structure. The blood-aqueous barrier is similar to the blood-brain barrier; this barrier is lowered when inflammation is present. The cornea prevents drug penetration because of the combination of lipophilic hydrophobic epithelium and lipophobic hydrophilic stroma. This barrier prevents invasion of organisms and toxins but hinders drug delivery. To overcome this barrier, topical drug application must be frequent to achieve therapeutic levels within the cornea or anterior chamber.

Topical Ophthalmic Application

The normal corneal anatomy along with constant washing from the tear film prohibits high levels of drug penetration. Manufactured ophthalmic medications attempt to overcome this obstacle by adding wetting agents to the drug preparation; altering the drug tonicity, pH, particle size, or concentration; or incorporating lipophilic derivatives of parent drugs. Drugs are better able to penetrate the cornea when an ulcer is present, as a result of the loss of the epithelial layer. Common drug vehicles include solutions, suspensions, ointments, and contact lenses. Solutions and suspensions are difficult to administer to production animals without the use of physical restraint. The contact time for these medications is generally short, and only a small percentage of the medication (1%-10%) is absorbed by the corneal stroma or anterior segment of the eye. Surface contact time and subsequent drug absorption are greater for solutions with increased viscosity. Ointments have a longer surface contact time and are not lost as readily, so the frequency of administration is slightly reduced, but the drug may be bound slightly higher and have lower levels of true corneal penetration depending on the drug. Because of head position, administration of an ointment is easier than administration of a solution or suspension but careful control of the amount of ointment used is not always possible, so material may be wasted. Ophthalmic ointments do not generally cause delay in corneal wound healing. Drugs that drain through the nasolacrimal system can be absorbed systemically; they may have undesired side effects. Soft contact lenses are not specifically made for production animal eyes, but devices manufactured for horses may fit. Soft contact lenses or dehydrated collagen shields can be presoaked in a drug solution to promote the accumulation of drug in the device. The lenses act as a reservoir that releases the drug over several days. Corneal edema from tissue hypoxia has been reported with the use of poorly fitted contact lenses in cattle. Contact lenses are generally not cost effective for large groups of animals, but they may be considered for individuals. Conjunctival or scleral implants are also infrequently used in

production animals due to the cost. Drugs manufactured in a powder form are not recommended for application to the eye because they are extremely irritating and have low drug bioavailability. In the future it may be possible to implant subconjunctival inserts that will allow for longer drug delivery.

Subconjunctival Injection

Subconjunctival injection of drugs may be used to achieve high local concentrations in anterior ocular tissues. An auriculopalpebral nerve block may be used in some animals to assist the injection, but it is not generally required. Topical ophthalmic anesthetic applied to the eye before injection provides comfort to the animal by decreasing its sensation of the needle; this in turn may help decrease the animal's eye and head movements and make the injection easier. The head should be restrained with a halter to avoid unintentional intraocular penetration. A maximum volume of 1 ml in large eyes and 0.5 ml in small eyes is injected under the bulbar conjunctiva over the dorsolateral surface approximately 5 mm posterior to the limbus. This is easily accomplished with a 25-gauge needle and 1-ml syringe. The needle is inserted bevel up, with a finger on the plugger ready to inject as soon as the conjunctiva has been penetrated. The fluid is injected slowly to ensure proper placement of the needle. A small bleb should be seen to form. Drug should not be injected in the superior lid or third eyelid because these do not allow for maximal drug delivery to the eye. Subconjunctival injection is recommended for drugs with low solubility and poor corneal penetration. Drugs injected subconjunctivally may bypass the corneal epithelial barrier and enter the corneal stroma or sclera directly, or they may escape back through the conjunctival injection site onto the ocular surface and be absorbed by the cornea. Unless repository forms of the drug are available, drug concentration and activity are not sustained and repeated subconjunctival injections may be necessary to establish therapeutic levels of drug in ocular tissue. These repeated subconjunctival injections may result in the formation of small granuloma complexes along the bulbar surface. These should not be misdiagnosed as other forms of ocular disease. Drugs given as a subconjunctival injection should be considered a form of systemic therapy; the same extralabel drug rules should be followed for safe treatment. In cattle subconjunctival injections are most frequently used as the initial treatment for infectious bovine keratoconjunctivitis (IBK).

Systemic Administration

Frequent application of ophthalmic medications or subconjunctival injections may be impractical in many production operations. Treatment by systemic administration may be feasible, but not all drugs administered systemically will achieve therapeutic ophthalmic levels. The relative distribution of drug administered by the systemic routes to ocular tissue is determined by the inherent drug properties, intended ocular tissue, stability of the blood-aqueous barrier, and removal of drug by metabolic pathways. The oral or parenteral routes of administration are better for diseases of the eyelids, orbit, and sclera than for diseases of the vitreous, retina, or choroid due to difficulty in penetration of these tissues. Inflammation of intraocular tissue frequently compromises the blood-ocular barriers and increases the ability of drugs to penetrate. Parenteral injections generally need to be repeated depending on the severity of the ocular disease and the drug being used. Oral administration with bolus-type medication is generally not cost effective. The medications may be poorly absorbed by the gastrointestinal tract; be degraded rapidly by the rumen; or require frequent administration, making labor costs too high. Feed additives are a cost-effective method of drug delivery; however, calculation of appropriate dosage may require feeding separate rations. The most common parenterally administered drug for ophthalmic disease is oxytetracycline, used in the treatment of IBK. Fortunately oxytetracycline is known to establish therapeutic levels in conjunctiva, cornea, and the tear film.

SPECIFIC THERAPY

The most commonly treated ophthalmic diseases in production animals affect the conjunctiva, cornea, and uveal tract, with the common processes being infectious or inflammatory. In conjunctival diseases the clinical appearance for both processes is similar. A cytology sample may be helpful in determining which process is involved. A swab for culture, immunofluorescent antibody (IFA) test, or polymerase chain reaction (PCR) test may determine the infective organism.

Few systemic or ophthalmic medications are approved for treatment of ocular diseases in production animals in the United States. Drugs not specifically approved for ocular disease or unapproved for use in a species may be used following extra-label guidelines (see the Pharmacology and Therapeutics section later in this book).

Antibiotic Drugs

Antibiotic selection should be based on susceptibility of the organism; however, this is not possible in many situations and documentation is not required in all cases. Once a tentative diagnosis has been achieved, historical response to treatment or published information regarding the likely causative organism and general susceptibility may be used. Antibiotic administration may be in the form of intramuscular (IM), subcutaneous (SC), or subconjunctival injection or oral or topical ophthalmic. Oxytetracycline is approved in the United States for treatment of IBK. It is most successful when used at a dosage of 20 mg/kg given SC or IM as a long-lasting formulation and given twice, 72 hours apart. Oxytetracycline is not used subconjunctivally due to severe ocular irritation. Oral administration of tetracyclines is 22 mg/kg once daily for approximately 5 days. Other systemic antibiotics that may be effective in treatment of IBK or other ocular infections include florfenicol 20 mg/kg IM or 40 mg/kg SC as a single dosage, single dosage of tulathromycin 2.5 mg/kg SC, and ceftiofur crystalline-free acid 6.6 mg/kg injected into the posterior

aspect of the pinna. Drugs that have been administered subconjunctivally include gentamicin (50 mg/ml) and procaine penicillin (300,000 units/ml). Currently, several topical ophthalmic ointment preparations are available, although all are manufactured for human use. These ointments include ciprofloxacin, erythromycin, gentamicin, sulfacetamide, tobramycin, and combinations of bacitracin-neomycin-polymyxin B or polymyxin B-trimethoprim.

Mydriatic/Cycloplegic Drugs

Tropicamide and atropine are parasympatholytic ophthalmic medications that cause pupillary dilation. Tropicamide is used diagnostically because it has a rapid onset and short duration. Atropine is most frequently used in the treatment of uveitis, either as the primary problem or secondary to corneal ulceration. The induced mydriasis decreases the likelihood of posterior synechia; the paralysis of the ciliary muscle relieves the pain from cyclitis. Atropine may help stabilize the blood-aqueous barrier, which decreases uveitis. Ophthalmic 1% tropicamide solution (1-2 drops or 0.2 ml) is sprayed on the ocular surface to achieve maximum pupillary dilation for complete lens and funduscopic examination. Ophthalmic 1% atropine solution (1-2 drops or 0.2 ml) or ointment (¼-½ inch) may be used one to three times daily depending on the severity of the ocular disease.

Steroid and Nonsteroidal Antiinflammatory Drugs

Steroids and nonsteroidal antiinflammatory drugs (NSAIDs) are used to control inflammation in the conjunctiva, cornea, and uvea. They are also used to decrease pigmentation of the corneal surface, which is an uncommon problem in production animals. Topically applied steroids have been shown to slow the rate of epithelialization in healing ulcers. Subconjunctival administration of steroids should be used cautiously with ulcerative keratitis because it may potentate infection. Ocular immunity may be suppressed following steroid administration, which may contribute to microbial overgrowth if appropriate antibiotic treatment is not concurrent with therapy. For these reasons steroids are generally contraindicated in the treatment of most corneal ulcers. However, the most common historical use of subconjunctival steroids is to reduce the inflammation associated with IBK. The secondary degeneration that results from neutrophil infiltration into the cornea may be reduced with steroid administration. In one study of IBK in heifers comparing no treatment, subconjunctival procaine penicillin G, and procaine penicillin G plus dexamethasone once daily for 3 days, there was no significant difference in the three groups. However, this study used the palpebral conjunctiva for deposition of the drug rather than the bulbar conjunctiva, which is the better mode of therapy. The decision to use steroids in therapy should be made based on the severity of the concurrent inflammation, the likelihood that the infective process has been controlled, and the cosmetic results necessary for the animal.

NSAIDs may be administered systemically or topically to treat inflammatory ocular diseases in food animals. These medications may decrease the pain associated with disease. Aspirin has been used orally (100 mg/kg PO bid for cattle and 10 mg/kg tid for swine) to treat uveitis. The frequent dosage necessary makes this drug difficult to use clinically. Phenylbutazone, ketoprofen, and flunixin meglumine may be used to treat ocular inflammation; however, residue and milk withholding guidelines and extra-label drug use regulations should be followed (see the Pharmacology and Therapeutics section later in this book). Phenylbutazone may be administered IV or per os (cattle 10 mg/kg loading dose, followed by 5 mg/kg every 2 days, swine 4 mg/kg once daily) to treat inflammatory ocular disease. Ketoprofen has been used IV or IM (cattle 2-4 mg/kg once daily). Flunixin meglumine (1.1-2.2 mg/kg IV slowly) may be administered once daily for a total of 3 days. No topical ophthalmic NSAIDs are commercially available in an ointment form. Solutions of diclofenac, flurbiprofen, and ketorolac are commercially available. Although these drugs can be compounded into an ophthalmic form, the frequency with which they should be used (two to four times daily), the cost, and the unknown residue times make them difficult to use in production animal medicine. They may be considered in pets or show animals to decrease inflammation, minimize corneal scarring, and improve the clinical appearance of the cornea and conjunctiva.

Cyclosporine and tacrolimus are T-cell modulating agents that have been used in small-animal ophthalmology to increase an animal's natural tearing ability and decrease corneal inflammation. These medications come in both ointments and solutions. Cyclosporine (0.2%-2%) or tacrolimus (0.02%-0.03%) is used twice daily in small animals. These medications should not be used in production animals that may enter the human food supply, because of unknown withdrawal times. They may be considered for pets.

Recommended Readings

Allen LJ, George LW, Willits NH: Effect of penicillin or penicillin and dexamethasone in cattle with infectious bovine keratoconjunctivitis, *J Am Vet Med Assoc* 206:1200, 1995.

Angelos JA, Dueger EL, George LW et al: Efficacy of florfenicol for treatment of naturally occurring infectious bovine keratoconjunctivitis, *J Am Vet Med Assoc* 216:1,62, 2000.

Dueger EL, George LW, Angelos JA et al: Efficacy of a long-acting formulation of ceftiofur crystalline-free acid of the treatment of naturally occurring infectious bovine keratoconjunctivitis, *Am J Vet Res* 65:1185, 2004.

Shryock TR, White DW, Werner CS: Antimicrobial susceptibility of *Moraxella bovis, Vet Microbiol* 61:305, 1997.

CHAPTER 92

Ocular Surgery: Enucleation in Cattle

KARA SCHULZ

Enucleation of the bovine eye is one of the most common ocular surgical procedures in cattle and is used to palliate and cure a wide variety of diseases. Much of the surgical protocol remains unchanged from previous publications, although perioperative management varies from veterinarian to veterinarian. Effective perioperative management of the patient allows for efficient removal of the diseased eye, decrease patient distress and discomfort, and decrease the risk of complications.

INDICATIONS FOR ENUCLEATION

Indications for enucleation include invasive ocular neoplasia, severe perforating ocular trauma, uncontrollable endophthalmitis or panophthalmitis, and severe exophthalmos leading to exposure keratitis.[1,2] Some of the more common disease entities encountered include ocular squamous cell carcinoma, retrobulbar lymphosarcoma, perforating ulcers, congenital defects, and abscessation or infection of the periorbital tissues resulting from trauma or foreign bodies.

PERIOPERATIVE MANAGEMENT

Restraint

Most adult bovine enucleations are performed using standing restraint. This yields the benefits of time and cost efficiency without the associated risks of general anesthesia. Adequate restraint in the form of a chute or stanchion is essential, as is sturdy restraint of the head.

Sedation

The demeanor of the animal determines the degree of sedation required. Most animals, with proper restraint and adequate local anesthesia, need little to no sedation. As with any standing surgery, the need for sedation must be balanced with the risk of recumbency during the procedure. Pregnancy status and general health of the animal determine the type of sedation or tranquilization used.[3-4]

Surgical Preparation

A wide margin surrounding the eye should be clipped and aseptically prepared for surgery using an appropriate antiseptic agent such as povidone iodine scrub.

Local Anesthesia

The most common regional anesthetic blocks performed include the Peterson nerve block and the four-point retrobulbar nerve block. The nerve blocks are described in several textbooks.[1-10] Reasons for choosing one block over the other should include the surgeon's comfort and skill at performing the blocks, the disease process present, and the knowledge of the risks associated with each block. Although the Peterson eye block is considered more technically challenging, it is associated with less risk of trauma to the orbit with regard to penetration of the globe, hemorrhage, and damage to the optic nerve. However, neurologic signs and cardiopulmonary arrest can occur if lidocaine is injected into the optic nerve meninges or nasal turbinates. The four-point block is technically less challenging to perform and appears to yield better anesthesia of the periocular tissues as supported by clinical experience, as well as published work by Pearce and colleagues.[9] Although there is risk of intrameningeal injection, clinical experience has shown it to be less of an issue than with the Peterson nerve block.

Auriculopalpebral Nerve Block
To allow for general ease, an auriculopalpebral nerve block can be placed to reduce upper eyelid movement before performing a Peterson or retrobulbar block. The auriculopalpebral nerve can be palpated as it crosses the zygomatic arch, roughly 5 to 6 cm behind the supraorbital process. Three to 5 ml of 2% lidocaine are deposited subcutaneously on the dorsal aspect of the zygomatic arch at this location.

Peterson Nerve Block
After performing a small local skin block over the intended site of puncture, a 14-gauge needle used as a cannula is placed caudal to the junction of the supraorbital process and zygomatic arch and is introduced through the skin. An 18-gauge, 3- to 4-inch needle is then introduced through the guide needle and directed in a horizontal and slightly proximal direction until the coronoid process is encountered. The needle is then walked off the rostral aspect of the coronoid process and advanced in a ventromedial direction along the caudal aspect of the orbit until the needle encounters the bony plate encasing the foramen orbitorotundum. Once the needle is advanced to the foramen, it is advised that the needle be drawn back a few millimeters to

reduce the risk of intrameningeal injection. After aspirating to ensure the needle is not in the internal maxillary artery, 10 to 15 ml of lidocaine (2%) are deposited, with an additional 5 ml of lidocaine deposited as the needle is slowly withdrawn. Mydriasis indicates a successful block.

Four-Point Retrobulbar Nerve Block

An 18-gauge, 3- to 4-inch needle is introduced through the skin on the dorsal, lateral, ventral, and medial aspects of the eye, at 12, 3, 6, and 9 o'clock, respectively. Introduction of the needle through the conjunctiva should be avoided to reduce the occurrence of ocular contamination. The needle is directed behind the globe using the bony orbit as a guide. When the needle is introduced into the retrobulbar sheath, the eye moves slightly with a tug of the needle. After this location is reached and aspiration is performed to ensure that the needle is not in a vessel, 5 to 10 ml of lidocaine (2%) are deposited at each site. Mydriasis indicates a successful block.

Ring Block

Additional local anesthesia of the eyelids is recommended because the Peterson and retrobulbar blocks typically result in incomplete analgesia of the eyelids. As a ring block, 5 to 10 ml of lidocaine (2%) are infiltrated subcutaneously 2.5 cm from the eyelid margins.

Lidocaine Toxicity

Particular care should be taken in young calves not to exceed the toxic dose of lidocaine (10 mg/kg). This calculates out to a maximum of 1 ml of 2% lidocaine per 5 kg of body weight, or roughly 2 ml per 10 lb of body weight. Dilution of 2% lidocaine in saline can assist distribution when restricted amounts are necessary.

SURGICAL PROCEDURE

The degree of invasiveness and infectious nature of the diseased globe determine the required surgical procedure. Classification of the enucleation procedure can be grouped into one of the following categories as described in the major ophthalmologic textbooks.* Evisceration entails the removal of ocular contents with retention of the globe.

The globe, conjunctiva, and nictitating membrane are removed in enucleation (Fig. 92-1). Removal of all the periocular contents, including the muscle and associated structures, is defined as extirpation or exenteration, the latter typically involving periosteal removal. In cattle the enucleation procedure is generally extended into an extirpation or exenteration procedure to allow for complete excision of diseased tissues.

ENUCLEATION

A transpalpebral ablation technique is used to remove the eye. The upper and lower eyelids are sutured closed. Alternatively, eyelids can be closed using multiple towel clamps. A circumferential skin incision is made approximately 1 cm from the edges of the eyelids. Using a combination of

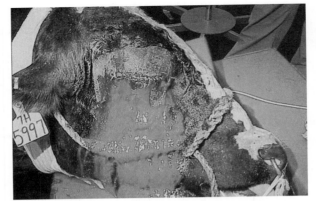

Fig 92-1 Immediate postoperative appearance of hemorrhage after enucleation and suture closure.

blunt and sharp dissection, Mayo scissors are used to dissect through the orbicularis oculi muscle, fascia, and subcutaneous tissue surrounding the eye. The interior of the bony orbit is used as a guide. The medial and lateral canthal ligaments are sharply transected to allow access to the caudal aspect of the orbit. Because a large vessel is associated with the medial canthus, transaction of the medial canthal ligaments is best left until necessary. Aggressive excision of orbital tissue is necessary in most cases of eye removal. The retrobulbar musculature and the optic nerve sheath should be transected as far caudally as feasible. A vascular clamp can aid in hemostasis while additional excision of remaining orbital tissue is undertaken. In cases in which neoplastic infiltration of the bony orbit has occurred, affected areas of ocular periosteum should be thoroughly excised. An orbitotomy may be necessary to remove affected areas of orbital bone; however, radical resection of orbital bone and associated lymph nodes is an extensive procedure not recommended except for extremely valuable animals in a referral setting.[11]

The skin incision can be closed in a variety of patterns with a nonabsorbable suture such as No 2 or 3 nylon. Common patterns include the Ford interlocking, cruciate, or simple continuous. An interrupted suture should be placed in the medial canthal portion of the skin closure to allow for facilitation of drainage if necessary.

If a cosmetic result is desired, a "trampoline" suture can be employed to reduce the hollow appearance of the orbit. However, it is not recommended when there is periorbital infection or neoplasia present. The periosteum on the inner dorsal and ventral rim of the orbit is grasped using a cruciate or simple interrupted pattern with No 2 or 3 nylon or equivalent nonabsorbable suture. The sutures are tightened to allow for support of the overlying ocular skin. The skin is subsequently sutured using a Ford interlocking, cruciate, or simple continuous pattern and No 2 or 3 nylon suture. The skin sutures are removed routinely in 14 to 21 days, leaving the underlying trampoline sutures in place as a permanent support.

ANTIINFLAMMATORY/ANALGESIC THERAPY

The disease process and degree of invasiveness determine the degree of antiinflammatory therapy required. Flunixin meglumine (1 mg/kg IV) at the time of surgical excision is usually adequate for general enucleation procedures, but further antiinflammatory management may be warranted depending on the disease process and extent of excision.

ANTIBIOTIC THERAPY

Because of the typical field conditions present during enucleation procedures, broad-spectrum systemic antibiotic therapy is indicated. The disease process dictates the duration of antibiotic therapy. Although there have been no publications regarding the placement of intraorbital suspensions or boluses, general observation cautions against the use of any material that may act as a future nidus of infection or cause inflammation or exacerbation of pain caused by caustic or chemical effects. Systemic antibiotics combined with general surgical asepsis are likely to be the most efficacious therapeutic option.

POSTOPERATIVE CARE

The animal should be kept in a confined area for several days after surgery to allow for appropriate hemostasis to occur. Daily observation of the surgical site and assessment of general well-being is recommended until suture removal (Fig. 92-2). Sutures should be removed in 14 to 21 days to allow for complete healing of the skin.

POSTOPERATIVE COMPLICATIONS

Postoperative complications can include simple incisional infection, orbital infections, dehiscence of the suture, significant infections of the periorbital tissue, or progression of neoplasia into bone or regional lymph nodes. Cattle often demonstrate pruritus after surgery, which can lead to incisional dehiscence because of head rubbing. If purulent drainage is noted during the course of healing, the medial interrupted suture may be removed and the cavity flushed with a dilute disinfectant solution daily until resolution of the orbital infection. Antibiotic therapy is recommended if systemic signs of infection are noted.

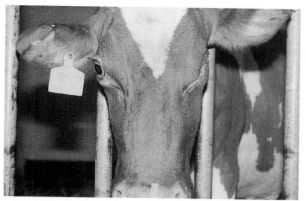

Fig 92-2   Typical appearance of orbit several months after enucleation.

References

1. Bistner S et al: Diseases of the orbit. In *Atlas of veterinary ophthalmic surgery*, Philadelphia, 1977, Saunders, 265-277.
2. Slatter D: Orbit. In *Fundamentals of veterinary ophthalmology*, ed 3, Philadelphia, 2001, Saunders, pp 516-531.
3. Irby NL: Surgical diseases of the eye in farm animals. In *Farm animal surgery*, St Louis, 2004, Saunders, pp 429-459.
4. Ivany JM: Farm animal anesthesia. In *Farm animal surgery*, St Louis, 2004, Saunders, pp 97-112.
5. Brooks DE: Orbit. In *Equine surgery*, ed 2, Philadelphia, 1999, Saunders, pp 497-514.
6. Muir MW: Local anesthesia in ruminants and pigs. In *Handbook of veterinary anesthesia*, ed 4, St Louis, 2005, Mosby, pp 72-99.
7. Rubin LF: Large animal ophthalmic surgery. In *The practice of large animal surgery*, Philadelphia, 1984, Saunders, pp 1151-1201.
8. Turner AS et al: Miscellaneous bovine surgical techniques. In *Techniques in large animal surgery*, ed 2, Philadelphia, 1989, Lea & Febiger, pp 337-340.
9. Pearce SG et al: Comparison of the retrobulbar and Peterson nerve block techniques via magnetic resonance imaging in bovine cadavers, *J Am Vet Med Assoc* 223:852-855, 2003.
10. Welker B: Ocular surgery, *Vet Clin North Am Food Anim Pract* 11:149-157, 2005.
11. Klein WR et al: Radical surgery of bovine ocular squamous cell carcinoma (cancer eye): complications and results, *Vet Surg* 13:236-242, 1984.

SECTION XI

Pharmacology and Therapeutics

Virginia R. Fajt

CHAPTER 93

Ethical Responsibilities of Bovine Veterinarians in Selecting, Prescribing, and Using Therapeutic Drugs

M. GATZ RIDDELL, JR.

The selection and use of therapeutic agents in veterinary medicine utilizes many of the diagnostic and critical thinking skills developed during the educational process and refined by previous case experience. Part of the "art of veterinary medicine" is being able to combine the skills of diagnosis; the knowledge of pharmacology and therapeutics; an understanding of contraindications and specific patient considerations (renal failure, geriatrics, breed predisposition); and effective communication skills into a successful outcome for a patient. With sufficient knowledge-base acquisition, conscientiously updated by continuing education of some type, as well as adequate diagnostic and therapeutic experience, treatment decisions can be made with a significant level of confidence. Fewer black and white decision-making challenges occur when issues of medical ethics arise. Pharmaceutical sourcing options and channels of acquisition can make for challenging ethical decisions for all veterinarians, but the food animal veterinarian has one overarching concern that has little, if any, applicability to companion animal or equine medicine. Human food safety concerns override all other considerations in the selection, prescription, and use of therapeutic drugs in food animal medicine.

VETERINARIAN-CLIENT-PATIENT RELATIONSHIP

The veterinarian-client-patient relationship (VCPR) concept (Box 93-1) provides the basis for the appropriate use of prescription drugs and was an integral component in the development, passage, and regulation writing for the Animal Medicinal Drug Use Clarification Act (AMDUCA) of 1994.[1] Before AMDUCA, extralabel use of drugs in veterinary medicine was illegal and was only allowed under a policy of regulatory discretion. The VCPR is critical in maintaining the trust of the regulatory agencies and the consuming public. The medical, pharmacologic, and food safety knowledge that the veterinary profession furnishes through the VCPR allows pharmaceutics to be used in food-producing animals including extralabel uses where

indicated and justified, while maintaining the high expectations of the consuming public for food safety.

The VCPR is defined in the Code of Federal Regulations.[2] The relationship is defined in terms of veterinarian availability for follow-up, knowledge of management practices, and owner acceptance of veterinary input rather than number of visits per year or month. This broad definition was considered appropriate because of the diversity found in the types of food animal practices and veterinary services offered from emergency work to consultation to employment by agricultural operations and corporations. Unfortunately, this broad definition has been misused through misinterpretation solely for the purpose of sales and distribution of products as an income stream. Exploitation of the VCPR for economic reasons not only reduces the credibility of the profession but also places pharmaceutic agents in untrained hands without adequate professional input to ensure human food safety.

Box 93-1

Veterinarian-Client-Patient Relationship as Defined by the Animal Medicinal Drug Use Clarification Act of 1994

1. A veterinarian has assumed the responsibility for making medical judgments regarding the health of (an) animal(s) and the need for medical treatment, and the client (the owner of the animal or animals or other caretaker) has agreed to follow the instructions of the veterinarian;
2. There is sufficient knowledge of the animal(s) by the veterinarian to initiate at least a general or preliminary diagnosis of the medical condition of the animal(s); and
3. The practicing veterinarian is readily available for follow-up in case of adverse reactions or failure of the regimen of therapy. Such a relationship can exist only when the veterinarian has recently seen and is personally acquainted with the keeping and care of the animal(s) by virtue of examination of the animal(s), and/or by medically appropriate and timely visits to the premises where the animal(s) are kept.

ANTIMICROBIAL SUSCEPTIBILITY

Antimicrobial use leads to selection for antimicrobial resistance or reduced susceptibility in bacteria. This occurs because of the adaptability of bacteria. The areas of concern are the target animal pathogens and commensal organisms, some of which are potentially zoonotic organisms transmissible to humans as food-borne pathogens. Antimicrobial prudent use guidelines[3] developed for cattle are designed to minimize the impact by designing programs to reduce unsubstantiated antimicrobial usage and maximize therapeutic effectiveness.

The debate on the role that antimicrobial therapy in food animals plays in human medicine will continue (see Chapter 98). The current prohibition on the extralabel use of fluoroquinolones and glycopeptides in food animals is one example of the veterinary profession's obligation to self-educate and self-police. Through the approval of several fluoroquinolone antibiotics, the Center for Veterinary Medicine has allowed the profession the opportunity to use another class of antibiotics proven to be effective for bovine respiratory disease. The caveat associated with the approval of the fluoroquinolones is that they cannot be used in an extralabel manner in food-producing animals. Practitioners have become familiar with the AMDUCA regulations and the additional requirements for extralabel drug use (ELDU) of U.S. Food and Drug Administration (FDA)-approved products. The current prohibition on ELDU of fluoroquinolones is more difficult to grasp and even more challenging to explain to nonprofessionals such as producers and their suppliers. However, compliance with this mandate is essential to maintaining the profession's credibility in the eyes of the regulatory agencies. Lack of VCPR-based professional oversight for any reason or claims of ignorance of the prohibition subvert the process and damage the image of the profession in the eyes of the regulatory agencies and, ultimately, the consuming public.

COMPOUNDED DRUGS

The subject of drug compounding is complicated. The profession of veterinary medicine has been involved with compounding at many levels, particularly in the 1970s and 1980s. Therapeutic needs for which there are no approved products and that require some form of compounding are encountered in veterinary medicine. The food animal practitioner is held to a higher standard than the rest of the profession because of the involvement with production of food for human consumption. This limits the potential for compounding in food animal practice to either the compounding of FDA-approved drugs or the compounding of a short list of antidote drugs as outlined in an FDA Compliance Policy Guideline (CPG)—Compounding of Drugs for Use in Animals (http://www.fda.gov/ora/compliance_ref/cpg/cpgvet/cpg608-400.html).[4]

Using compounded products produced from raw active ingredients, whether made in the practice environment or purchased from a compounding pharmacy, is a violation of federal law. Certain forms of compounding may be allowed by CPG 608.400.[4] This type of CPG provides for regulatory discretion for specific needs when there is little

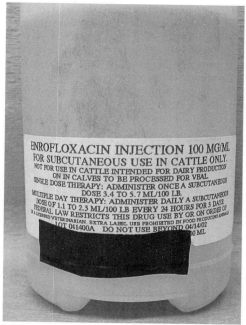

Fig 93-1 Bottle of illegally compounded enrofloxacin seized from compounding pharmacy.

potential harm to the target animal or human food safety. However, use of these types of products in food-producing animals raises concerns on multiple fronts. Bulk pharmaceutic ingredients (bulk products) that do not bear a certificate of analysis from a scientifically recognized authority on quality and purity or that have been produced in a facility not subject to FDA Good Manufacturing Practices inspections should not be administered to food-producing animals (Fig. 93-1). Even with quality assurance information for the bulk products, a lack of pharmacokinetic data and hence accurate withdrawal information exists on the finished product. The potential for both inadvertent and malicious adulteration of the human food supply exists. The specific risks include but are not limited to inaccurate drug concentrations resulting in treatment failures or residues, toxins, potentially infectious endemic agents, and foreign animal disease. Veterinarians engaged in food animal practice to any degree cannot accept this type of liability and the profession cannot risk the potential damage to its credibility. Veterinarians should avoid using or prescribing products from unknown or suspicious sources.

DECISIONS IN SOURCING AND DELIVERY OF PHARMACEUTICS

Veterinarians and their clients are presented with a variety of options for sourcing therapeutic drugs. A long-standing source, pharmaceutical sales as profit centers in veterinary practices, has been affected by a diminished sales trend because of the development of alternative distribution methods. Internet pharmacies, catalog sales, and route trucks are commonplace. Producers are aware of these sources and the potential cost savings and may either request a prescription from a local or consulting veterinarian, purchase the products through channels that claim to meet the requirements of a VCPR but provide little if any on-farm resources, or purchase them directly from the source with no pretense of a VCPR. Of these three potential scenarios, only the first (prescription from a veterinarian with a VCPR as defined by federal regulations[2]) creates a situation that provides the producer access to the level of veterinary advice and information that promotes prudent drug use and optimally protects the human food supply.

Practice models continually change, and the transition from being the source of the products to providing the prescription that allows the producer to purchase elsewhere is not always easy for the practitioner involved. The American Veterinary Medical Association Principles of Veterinary Medical Ethics states that if a prescription therapeutic drug is considered medically indicated and the owner requests a prescription to obtain the product from a source other than a veterinarian's practice, the veterinarian should honor the client's request. The practitioner is faced with the loss of one source of income and the need to generate another, while retaining the responsibility to educate and inform the client to ensure appropriate drug use and human food safeguards. Producers and others involved in the food animal industries cannot be expected to understand the intricacies and implications of ELDU, the differences between FDA-approved drugs (both pioneer and generic) and compounded drugs, or the subject of reimportation of drugs, particularly where they apply to food animals and withdrawal recommendations that are consistent with a safe food supply. Practice models can be changed and the profession must remain engaged at the farm level because both prescription drug approval and extralabel use are predicated on the involvement of a licensed veterinarian.

RESOURCES AVAILABLE TO THE FOOD ANIMAL PRACTITIONER

The food animal practitioner needs to use resources outside the traditional scientific journals and textbooks. The FDA-CVM website (http://www.fda.gov/cvm) offers current updates and regulatory items that affect food animal medicine, as well as other aspects of veterinary medicine. This site provides specific information relative to the list of drugs prohibited for extralabel use in food-producing animals. Concerning the enforcement arm of the agency, this site and an agency service referred to as *CVM Updates* provide information on recent regulatory actions against both producers and veterinarians. The *FDA Green Book* for veterinary drugs (http://www.fda.gov/cvm/greenbook. html) provides current information on both pioneer (New Animal Drug Application [NADA] numbers) and generic (Abbreviated New Animal Drug Application [ANADA] numbers) products, which helps the practicing veterinarian differentiate between approved drugs and illegally compounded products. FDA-approved drug withdrawal times apply to label use of the product and should be relied on. Extralabel use shifts the burden of information for withdrawal recommendations to the veterinarian

involved in the VCPR allowing the extralabel use. The Food Animal Residue Avoidance Database (FARAD, http:// www.farad.org/) is a readily accessible, easily navigated source of current information on which to base withdrawal recommendations. The Veterinary Antimicrobial Decision Support database is a science-based tool to aid in developing and adapting treatment protocols with antimicrobial drugs (VADS, http://www.vads.org). This effort is supported by grants from numerous allied species organizations and the FDA and is focused on providing tools to maximize treatment effectiveness and minimize risk to human food safety.

PRACTICE CHALLENGES—PHILOSOPHY

The complexity of the issues facing the food animal practitioner is compounded by the economic demands on the food animal producer and a lack of regulatory support on certain critical issues. These issues include but are not limited to nontraditional drug-marketing channels, ELDU outside of a VCPR, and the availability of illegally compounded products. The lack of regulatory support results from either limited resources for enforcement or poorly defined roles on the part of licensing boards, both veterinary and pharmacy. This may result in the veterinarian being seen as an enforcer while providing informed opinions on the legality and appropriateness of product acquisition and use. Within the profession of veterinary medicine, these issues are best self-policed within our ranks rather than regulated by state and federal agencies and boards.

Consultants without a veterinary degree and producers often challenge the role and even the need for veterinary input in treatment decisions made on animal agriculture operations. However, the FDA has entrusted the distribution of prescription drugs and the extralabel use of all drugs to the oversight of the veterinary profession. Without this level of veterinary input and involvement, many of the currently available prescription drugs would not be on the market and all extralabel use would be a violation of federal law. Of vital importance is that the industries, profession, and regulatory agencies continue a cooperative relationship to maximize successful animal treatment and maintain the integrity of the human food supply. The consumer, the ultimate client of both food animal practitioners and the producers, expects and demands no less.

References

1. Animal Medicinal Drug Use Clarification Act of 1994, Pub L No 103-396.
2. *Code of Federal Regulations*, 21 CFR 530.3(i), 1996.
3. American Association of Bovine Practitioners: *Prudent Drug Use Guidelines, AABP Policy and Procedure Manual*, Auburn, Ala, 1999, AABP.
4. U.S. Department of Health and Human Services, Food and Drug Administration, Office of Regulatory Affairs, Center for Veterinary Medicine, 2003.

CHAPTER 94

Ethical Responsibilities of Small Ruminant Veterinarians in Selecting and Using Therapeutics

JOAN S. BOWEN and JOE SNYDER

SMALL RUMINANTS ARE FOOD ANIMALS

Small ruminant veterinarians face more complex decisions than those working with more traditional food animal species when it comes to responsible and ethical use of pharmaceutics and therapeutic drugs. Few drugs are licensed or labeled for use in sheep, goats, camelids, or farmed cervids. However, small ruminant producers can easily purchase over-the-counter (OTC) drugs available for other species and use these freely, often without veterinary consultation. Because of unregulated access and lack of veterinary input, small ruminant producers often lack adequate information regarding dosage, frequency and route of administration, duration of therapy, and withdrawal time of pharmaceutics in animals before use of products for human consumption. Also, producers may not be receptive to decisions that prevent the use of certain drugs because of regulatory or ethical issues. Other small ruminant owners consider their sheep, goat, camelid, or cervid to be a pet rather than a food animal and expect veterinary care and use of therapeutics like that provided by a small animal or equine hospital. Because therapeutic guidelines are not readily available to small ruminant producers, veterinarians must exercise a leadership role in the judicious and ethical use of pharmaceuticals in small ruminants.

Many small ruminant producers begin as hobbyists whose herds outgrow family use of the milk, fiber, or meat produced. Some enter commercial production, while others sell products at farmers' markets or through advertising at local feed stores or food cooperatives. Many producers do not have a livestock production background and are unaware of potential problems with drug residues in meat and milk. Small ruminant producers often purchase medications from lay outlets and make diagnostic and treatment decisions without veterinary input. In the search for quick diagnosis and fast remedy, long-term disease control through improved management practices is often overlooked.

Good management practices prevent major disease outbreaks and lower the incidence of drug residue problems by decreasing the need for pharmaceutical use. Reviewing management practices is an integral part of a quality assurance program for small ruminant veterinarians and their clients. When the veterinarian and producer work together in this assessment on the farm, one of the criteria for a veterinary-client-patient-relationship (VCPR) is satisfied. The review should include but is not limited to nutrition, parasite prevention, vaccine protocols, stress reduction, and biosecurity. Good management practices not only prevent disease and the ethical dilemmas associated with treating it but also have the potential to increase profit by lowering expenses for pharmaceutics.

The distinction between "food animal" and "companion animal" is often blurred when trying to categorize small ruminants. Many small ruminant owners develop as much emotional attachment to their livestock as others with dogs or cats. Some small ruminants, especially camelids, are considered valuable breeding stock that would never grace a dining room table. In the eyes of regulatory agencies such as the U.S. Food and Drug Administration and the Food Safety and Inspection Service, all sheep, goats, and farmed cervids are considered food animals under all circumstances. At this time, classification of camelids as companion animals or food animals is less clear. In some areas of the United States, camelids are entering the food chain and should be treated as food animals. To the best of our knowledge, regulatory agencies currently regard camelids in the same manner as they consider horses, species that are so unlikely to enter the food chain as to require little regulatory effort. This issue presents a dilemma for veterinarians working with small ruminants, especially camelids. Do we take a "proactive" stance and treat these species as food animals, or should they be treated more like companion animals until forced to do otherwise? Camelid veterinarians should be aware of the local pattern for disposal of camelids in terms of entry into the human food chain. Although each veterinarian has to address this issue when treating small ruminants, the decision of whether a particular small ruminant is a pet or food animal needs to be examined seriously and thoughtfully. When there is any question as to the status of a particular small ruminant, the attending veterinarian should err on the side of caution and follow the established guidelines for use of drugs in food animals. *Neither the small ruminant producer nor the veterinarian should endanger the food chain or the integrity of the veterinary profession by treating small ruminants inappropriately.*

At what point should the veterinarian consider reporting illegal or unethical drug use to a legal authority? At this time we are unaware of any regulatory agencies that are actively enforcing Animal Medicinal Drug Use Clarification Act of 1994 (AMDUCA) rules in small ruminants. However, ethical veterinarians should consider to whom, when, and if they should report veterinarians or producers who are mishandling drugs or using drugs in a manner that would yield violative drug residues.

EXTRALABEL DRUG USE

Few drugs are licensed or labeled for use in small ruminants. AMDUCA was passed to establish guidelines under which approved animal drugs and certain human drugs could be used in a manner other than labeled. Extralabel drug use (ELDU) is the use or intended use of a drug in a manner that is not in accordance with its approved labeling. This includes, but is not limited to, use in species not listed in the labeling; use for indications (disease or other conditions) not listed on the labeling; use at dosage levels, frequencies, or route of administration other than those stated on the labeling; and deviation from the approved, labeled withdrawal time based on these different uses. The full text of AMDUCA and specific updates may be found at www.fda.gov/cvm/amducatoc.htm. AMDUCA addresses three key issues: (1) drugs must be prescribed by a veterinarian within an established VCPR, (2) no violative drug residues should be detected in animals or animal products used for human consumption, and (3) ELDU should comply with all regulations.

The required valid VCPR has three components (see Box 93-1 in Chapter 93 for a complete description). The herd veterinarian must assume responsibility for making medical judgments regarding the health of the animals and the need for medical treatment, and the small ruminant producer must agree to follow the instructions of the veterinarian. Also, the veterinarian must have sufficient knowledge of the animals to initiate a general or preliminary diagnosis of the medical condition of the small ruminants. The veterinarian must have visited the farm and examined the animals in question and must be personally acquainted with the management of the animals. Lastly, the veterinarian must be readily available for follow-up consultation in case of adverse reactions or failure of therapy.

The AMDUCA also provides specific guidelines that govern ELDU. ELDU is permitted only by or under the supervision of a veterinarian in a valid VCPR. ELDU is allowed only for FDA-approved animal and human drugs and is for therapeutic purposes only when an animal's health is suffering or threatened. Drugs used for production purposes may not be used in an extralabel manner. The rules apply to dosage-form drugs and drugs administered in water, whereas ELDU in feed is prohibited. ELDU is not permitted if it results in a violative food residue or any residue that may present a risk to public health. Lastly, FDA maintains the right to prohibit certain drugs from extralabel use.

Currently, 10 drugs are banned from use in food animals and no circumstances permit use of any of these drugs in small ruminants that are intended for food production.

This list includes chloramphenicol, clenbuterol, diethylstilbestrol, dimetridazole, dipyrone, ipronidazole, other nitroimidazoles, fluoroquinolones, glycopeptide antibiotics, and nitrofurans. Phenylbutazone is restricted from use in lactating dairy cattle older than 20 months of age, so it should probably not be used in lactating sheep or goats either. One formulation of enrofloxacin, a fluoroquinolone antibiotic, has received restricted FDA approval for treatment of respiratory disease complex in cattle because of concern about selection for antimicrobial resistance in food-borne pathogens. Development of antibiotic resistance by pathogenic microorganisms is of growing concern to both the medical community and the consuming public. We do not debate either the wisdom of public policy on this subject or the accuracy of the data that has led to it. It is our responsibility as public health officials to uphold both the letter and the spirit of that policy even if we may disagree with some aspects of it. Small ruminant veterinarians often lack clear guidelines because of the absence of label suggestions for drug use in these species. In those situations, veterinarians must make ethically sound decisions based on both the available scientific knowledge and the outlines of responsibility mandated by public policy. The FDA will not tolerate any extralabel use of enrofloxacin, so it should not be used in any sheep, goat, camelid, or farmed cervid.

Although not specifically banned by AMDUCA or any other regulation, the American Association of Small Ruminant Practitioners concurs with the recommendation of the American Association of Bovine Practitioners and the American Veterinary Medical Association prohibiting the use of gentamicin in food animals because of the inability to establish a withdrawal time for this drug.

Small ruminant veterinarians and producers should examine the requirements for extralabel drug use carefully. Low price is not on the list of reasons that a drug may be used in an extralabel manner when there is an approved drug that is available and effective. Also, ELDU is not allowed for purely production purposes such as use of growth implants or low-level feeding of antibiotics to improve growth rate. No provision is in the ELDU rules for compounding of drugs for use in food animal species. No drugs are currently approved for estrus cycle manipulation in small ruminant species, and it is unclear to what extent drugs may be legally used to manipulate or time reproduction. No rule is available as to whether use of prostaglandin to terminate an untimely pregnancy would be considered therapeutic or for production purposes. Manipulating reproductive cycles to achieve out-of-season or year-round breeding in sheep or goats would also be questionable. Guidelines to answer these questions have not been published, but our responsibility to protect the food supply should be the foremost guide in making decisions about drug use. This involves not only protecting the public from consumption of any amount of potentially toxic or harmful substance but also in protecting the *perception* of a safe food supply. Every small ruminant, except possibly for some camelids, should be considered a food-producing animal when making decisions regarding therapeutic use of pharmaceutics. *Too many incidents of presumptive pet animals entering the food supply when the owner's circumstances changed abruptly and unexpectedly have occurred.*

When drugs are used in an extralabel manner, the veterinarian must determine reasonable and adequate withdrawal times in order to prevent drug residues in products used for human consumption. The Food Animal Residue Avoidance Databank (FARAD, www.farad.org) uses data from many sources to assist veterinarians in selecting adequate withdrawal times for extralabel use (see Chapter 96 for further discussion of FARAD). Occasionally the practitioner must extrapolate from withdrawal periods for related species, in which case a generous allowance for potential variance is recommended. Many drugs are labeled and licensed for use in small ruminants in other countries, and those label restrictions and recommendations can be accessed via the Internet. However, veterinarians should remember that other countries may have established tolerances for drugs for which there is zero tolerance in the United States.

DAIRY SHEEP AND GOATS

Of special concern are the use of drugs in sheep or goats producing milk or dairy products for human consumption. Many producers have access to OTC drugs and may use them without realizing that the drugs could produce residues in the milk. Small-scale sheep or goat dairy producers may not be subject to the regulatory agency monitoring for drug residues required of large-scale commercial producers. It is incumbent on the small ruminant veterinarian to educate clients about the importance of residue avoidance.

CERVIDS

Veterinarians working with farmed cervids should also be aware of drug residue issues associated with the collection of velvet antler. Veterinarians or cervid producers administer local anesthetics around the base of the antler in preparation for surgical removal of velvet antler, and this may lead to anesthetic residues in the velvet. Velvet antler is consumed orally by humans for a variety of reasons and farmed cervid producers should be educated about drug residue avoidance.

RESPONSIBLE USE OF PARASITICIDES

Another area of drug use in which veterinarians face complicated ethical decisions is the use of anthelmintics. Multi-drug-resistant parasites, most notably gastrointestinal nematodes such as *Haemonchus* species, have become increasingly more common and are a real threat to the future of small ruminant production in many areas. Resistant parasites develop independently with overly aggressive or inappropriate anthelmintic use and spread through shipments of animals infested with resistant strains. Veterinarians must be vigilant to check both the development and spread of parasite resistance. In this case, it is not a concern for human health but concern for the well-being of the animals and future of the industry that is deemed important. Producers are driven by the need for profit from this year's crop or production and may not deem it economically reasonable to make changes in parasite control that will result in significantly lower profits today for the sake of preventing a problem that may occur in the future. Corporate sales pitches and the network of shared producer information can make the veterinarian's educational task even more difficult. Nevertheless, veterinarians must persist in making the case for wise and discriminate use of anthelmintics in small ruminants. See Chaper 97 for further discussion of parasite resistance to anthelmintics.

HELPING PRODUCERS MAKE TREAMENT DECISIONS

Small ruminant veterinarians have the responsibility to inform producers about a variety of treatment options and management practices and can assist the producer in making ethical choices for the specific situation. Circumstances may arise when it would be more prudent to consider humane slaughter or euthanasia rather than medical treatment or surgery. This decision must be made before initiating treatment with drugs that may preclude slaughter for many days or weeks. Commercial producers may need to be educated about effective and profitable procedures that can save an animal such as fracture repair or cesarean section. Those owners with a deep attachment to their animals may need help understanding that extensive medical or surgical intervention may not be in the best interest of a severely ill or injured small ruminant.

PAIN MANAGEMENT

Appropriate use of analgesics and anesthetics for control of pain and suffering in small ruminants presents another ethical challenge. Without veterinary intervention, commercial producers may not recognize the economic benefits of pain management for routine procedures such as dehorning, tail docking, or castration. The consuming public is increasingly demanding assurance that their meat, milk, and fiber products are produced with minimum pain and suffering. Small ruminant veterinarians should practice good pain management to decrease pain and suffering during all medical treatment or surgical procedures.

Pain management drugs commonly used in other species are not labeled or licensed for use in small ruminants, so the AMDUCA extralabel drug restrictions must be followed. The small ruminant veterinarian is responsible for educating both himself or herself and the client about the potential toxicity of pain control agents in these species. Drugs with narrow margins of safety or potential human abuse should not be dispensed to producers. Many pain relief medications are controlled substances that require accurate records of their use. The extra care involved in using controlled substances should not discourage veterinarians from using them when circumstances indicate their use.

RESPONSIBILITY TO PRODUCERS AND THE PUBLIC

Many small ruminants are seen by veterinarians whose primary practice is with companion animals or horses. Because of limited course time in veterinary school, many such practitioners may have limited experience and knowledge with the idiosyncrasies of medicating these species, as well as the responsibilities of treating food-producing animals. Those veterinarians who find themselves involved in small ruminant medicine on any level have an obligation to educate themselves about small ruminant diseases and pharmacology. Membership and participation in organizations such as the American Association of Small Ruminant Practitioners (AASRP) provides an important educational resource for veterinarians.

Veterinarians, by virtue of their profession, are often the first to observe operations in which substandard care is provided to small ruminants. They are also frequently the first person a concerned citizen contacts in raising a concern about animals suffering from less than adequate care. Veterinarians prepared with the knowledge of good management practices can mediate the conflicting concerns of the small ruminant producer and consuming public. Small ruminant veterinarians serve an important educational role in assisting sheep, goat, camelid, and farmed cervid producers in improving their management practices to decrease unnecessary use of pharmaceuticals, preventing drug residues in foods produced for human consumption, and selecting and using therapeutic drugs in a judicious manner.

CHAPTER 95

Practical Pharmacokinetics for the Food Animal Practitioner

RONETTE GEHRING

Assuming that an appropriate drug has been selected for the treatment of a disease, successful pharmacotherapy depends on selecting an appropriate dosing regimen to ensure that effective concentrations of the drug are achieved and maintained at the site of action without causing toxicity. Rarely can a drug be administered directly at the site of action. Rather, most drugs move from a site of administration to the site of action, while simultaneously being distributed throughout the rest of the body including the organs of elimination (most notably the kidney and liver). Questions that need to be answered to determine a dosage regimen are: By which route should the drug be administered? How much of the drug should be administered? How often should the drug be administered? And for how long should the drug be administered?

Pharmacokinetics is the study of drug disposition and how drug concentrations change in the body over time following administration. Measurements of drug concentrations are usually taken from blood, a practical and convenient site for sampling, as well as the vehicle that receives the drug from site of administration and carries it to the site of action and organs of elimination. A successful dosing regimen can therefore be defined as one that achieves and maintains blood, plasma, or serum concentrations that are associated with therapeutic success without producing unacceptable toxicity (often referred to as the "therapeutic window").

The observed data, typically measurements of drug concentrations in blood, plasma, or serum with samples taken at different time points following administration, are summarized and described using mathematic equations. These equations can then be used to predict plasma concentrations for different doses and, depending on the complexity of the model, could also be used to account for changes in disposition due to factors such as species, age, or disease. Clinical pharmacokinetics is the application of these mathematic models in the rational design of dosing regimens to achieve target plasma concentrations. In food animals, an additional consideration is avoiding drug residues in edible tissues, which are potentially harmful to the consumer.

PHYSIOLOGIC CONCEPTS

Following the administration of a drug formulation to an animal, the blood and tissue concentrations change over time as a result of three processes: absorption, distribution, and elimination (Fig. 95-1). These processes occur simultaneously, with each dominating at a different time following administration. Initially, absorption dominates, adding drug to the body and resulting in rising drug concentrations in the blood and other tissues. Later, distribution and elimination dominate, with both of these removing the drug from the systemic circulation,

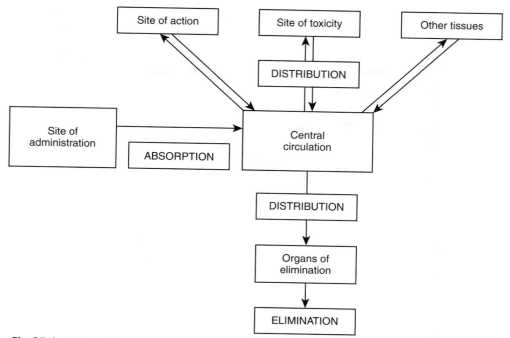

Fig 95-1   Schematic representation of pharmacokinetic processes responsible for changing plasma drug concentrations.

resulting in decreasing blood concentrations and ultimately subsiding effect(s).

Absorption, distribution, and elimination require that drug molecules be transported across a series of membranes and spaces. In addition, elimination may require that the drug is metabolized. Differences in the rates of these processes result in variations in the time-concentration profiles observed for different drugs and animals. The membranes through which drugs must be transported are composed of lipophilic cellular membranes; aqueous interstitial spaces; and in some membranes (e.g., capillary endothelia, intestinal epithelia), narrow aqueous-filled channels between cells. Most drugs pass through these membranes by simple diffusion from areas of higher concentration to areas of lower concentration. The rate of drug penetration is therefore determined by the magnitude of the concentration difference across the membrane, the surface area of the membrane, and the ease with which the drug can penetrate through the membrane. The latter is quantitatively expressed as permeability, which is affected by the molecular size, lipophilicity, and charge of the drug. Active and passive carrier-mediated transport processes may be involved for some drugs, resulting in the rate of transport approaching a maximum value at high concentrations (Fig. 95-2). Because saturation of active transport processes is uncommon at concentrations typically used for treatment, this phenomenon is not considered further in this chapter.

PHARMACOKINETIC PARAMETERS AND DOSING REGIMENS

A *parameter* can be defined as a quantifiable characteristic of a system that is used as input for a predictive model. In pharmacokinetic modeling, parameters are quantitative

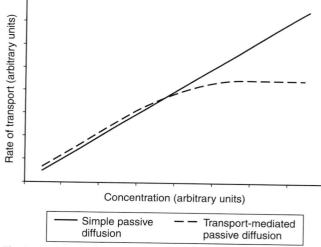

Fig 95-2   Relationship between concentration and rate of transport for drugs transported by simple passive diffusion and transport-mediated processes.

estimates of the rate and extent of distribution, elimination, and absorption, which are used to predict plasma drug concentrations for specific doses of a drug in individuals or groups of animals. These pharmacokinetic parameters are estimated by fitting a pharmacokinetic model to observed data, and they are then used to construct dosing regimens that will achieve a specified target plasma concentration. The target concentration may be the minimum inhibitory concentration (MIC) for an antimicrobial drug or a concentration that has been associated with the desired therapeutic effect.

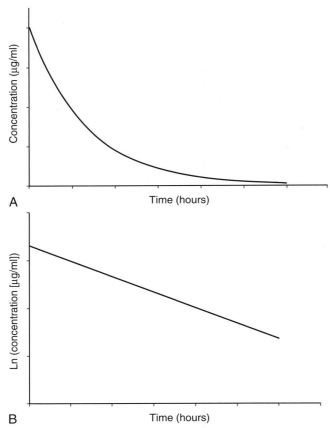

Fig 95-3 Typical time-concentration profile of a drug best described using a one-compartment model on a linear (**A**) and a semilogarithmic (**B**) scale.

Single Intravenous Dose

Rapid intravenous administration ensures that the entire dose enters the general circulation and that effective concentrations are achieved quickly. Typical drugs that are administered by this route include those for the management of acute pain, anesthesia, and severe bacterial infections. It is also the route that should be used to investigate the disposition of a drug (distribution and elimination) because the time-concentration curve is not confounded by variations in the rate and extent of absorption.

A graphic representation of the time-concentration data for a hypothetical drug following intravenous administration is shown in Fig. 95-3. Notice that the relationship between the x (time) and y (concentration) variables becomes linear if the y-axis is transformed to a logarithmic scale. Also, notice that the concentration declines over time at a constant rate (Fig. 95-3, *B*). The data can therefore be described using a simple monoexponential mathematic equation that is conventionally referred to as a *one-compartment pharmacokinetic model*. At this point, it is important to point out that the plasma concentrations of many drugs decline in a biexponential or multiexponential manner, requiring that additional term(s) are added to the mathematic equation to adequately describe the time-concentration data. Suffice it to mention that the pharmacokinetic parameters discussed in this chapter can also be calculated for these

drugs, but that it is computationally more complex to do so because the processes of distribution and elimination need to be distinguished from each other. In this chapter, we concentrate on one-compartment models.

Drugs that can be described using a one-compartment model typically equilibrate rapidly between the blood and tissues. This makes it possible to describe their disposition as the drug being injected into a single compartment of uniform liquid with the dose distributing instantaneously and homogenously throughout this compartment and the drug being eliminated from the compartment immediately after injection.

The two parameters that are necessary to describe the time-concentration curve of a drug following intravenous administration using a one-compartment model are *apparent volume of distribution* (V_d) and *elimination rate constant* (k_{el}). The relationship between these parameters and plasma concentrations is given in Equation 1.

Equation 1

$$C(t) = D \times e^{-k_{el}t}$$

Where: D = dose

Apparent Volume of Distribution

The volume of distribution (V_d; units: volume/body-weight) is the volume of fluid into which the total amount of drug in the body must be dissolved to account for the concentration that is measured in the plasma following equilibration. For a drug that has been administered by the intravenous route and can be described using a one-compartment model, the amount of drug in the body at the time of injection (time = 0) is the dose and, because distribution is essentially instantaneous, equilibration can also be considered to be complete at this time. Equation 2a can therefore be used to calculate V_d. Conversely, if the V_d of a drug is known, the equation can be rearranged to calculate the dose required to obtain a target plasma concentration (Equation 2b).

Therefore

Equation 2a

$$V_d = \frac{D}{C_p(0)}$$

Equation 2b

$$D = C_p(0) \times V_d$$

Where: $C_p(0)$ = concentration of drug in plasma at time = 0
D = dose

Because it is not practical to measure $C_p(0)$, its value is usually determined by back-extrapolation of the time-concentration curve to the y-axis.

Although the value of the V_d does not have a true physiologic meaning (hence the designation *apparent*), it can be related to the different fluid and tissue volumes of the body, thus giving an indication of the extent of distribution of a drug (Fig. 95-4). Notice that the dose required to achieve a specific plasma concentration is directly proportional to the V_d and that any increase or decrease

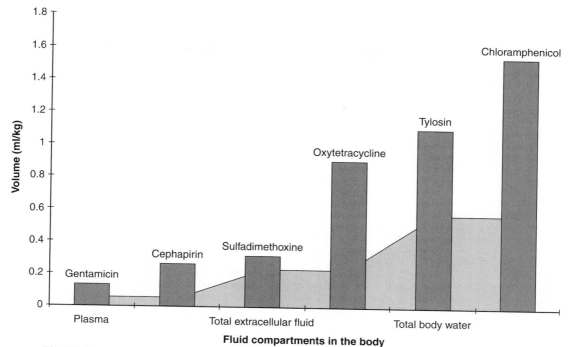

Fig 95-4 Typical values of apparent volumes of distribution (V_d) for selected drugs in cattle compared with the volumes of fluid spaces in the body.

in the value of this parameter will require that the dose is adjusted accordingly to maintain efficacy or prevent toxicity, respectively. Numerous factors could affect the value of V_d including species, age, obesity, pregnancy, and disease conditions (e.g., ascites).

Elimination Rate Constant

In a one-compartment model, the rate of elimination of a drug is characterized by the slope of the time-concentration curve (Fig. 95-5). This pharmacokinetic parameter, also known as the *elimination rate constant* (k_{el}; units: time^{-1}), is essentially a proportionality constant that relates the rate of elimination of a drug to the amount of drug in the body (Equation 3).

Equation 3

$$Rate\ of\ elimination = A \times k_{el}$$

Where: A = Amount of drug in the body
This means that the steeper the slope of the time-concentration curve, the larger the value of k_{el} and the faster the rate of elimination of a drug. Practically, if two drugs are administered at the same dose, the plasma concentrations of the drug with the higher k_{el} value will deplete to ineffective levels faster than those of the drug with the lower k_{el} value (see Fig. 95-5).

The plasma half-life ($T_{1/2}$; units: time) is a parameter that is derived from k_{el} (Equation 4) and is defined as the time required for plasma drug concentrations to decrease by half.

The value of $T_{1/2}$ is often conceptually easier to relate to reality and the time needed for drug concentrations to deplete to ineffective levels. It is also important to

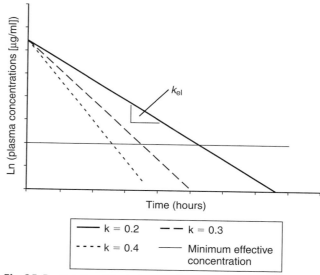

Fig 95-5 Relationship between the value of k_{el} and the rate of depletion of plasma concentrations to ineffective levels.

remember that, although one may be tempted to increase the dose to prolong the activity of a drug that has a fast rate of elimination, this will only extend the duration of action by $T_{1/2}$ for each doubling of the dose (Fig. 95-6).

Equation 4

$$T_{1/2} = \frac{\ln 2}{k_{el}}$$

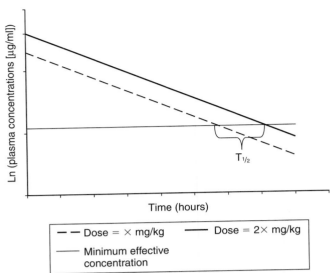

Table **95-1**

Percentage of Steady-State Concentrations Reached as a Function of Elapsed Time in Terms of Half-Lives

Time in Half-Lives	Percentage of Steady-State Concentrations Reached
1	50
2	75
3	88
4	94
5	97
6	98
7	99

Fig 95-6 Plasma time-concentration profile of a hypothetical drug following single intravenous administration to illustrate that doubling the dose extends the duration of action by one half-life ($T_{1/2}$).

Clearance

Clearance (Cl; units: volume/bodyweight/time) is the pharmacokinetic parameter that quantifies drug elimination without identifying the mechanism or process. It characterizes the rate of elimination of a drug by relating it to plasma concentrations (Equation 5). Conceptually, Cl represents the volume of plasma cleared of drug per unit time, which can be related to physiologic processes such as glomerular filtration rate and hepatic blood flow.

Equation 5

$$Rate\ of\ elimination = C_p \times Cl$$

Where: C_p = Plasma drug concentration
Because the amount of drug in the body, and hence plasma drug concentrations, is continually changing, the value of Cl is not determined directly from time-concentration data, but rather it is calculated based on its relationship with the two other pharmacokinetic parameters, k_{el} and V_d (Equation 6b).

Equation 6a

$$Rate\ of\ elimination = A \times k_{el} = \frac{A}{V_d} \times Cl$$

Equation 6b

$$\therefore\ Cl = k_{el} \times V_d$$

Where: A = Amount of drug in the body
Notice that the value of k_{el}, and hence the rate of decline of plasma drug concentrations, is dependent on the value of both Cl and V_d (Equation 7).

Constant Rate Intravenous Infusions

Drugs that are generally administered as constant rate intravenous infusions are those for which it is important that constant plasma concentrations are maintained

throughout the treatment period. Examples would include anesthetic drugs and drugs used to treat cardiac arrhythmias. The two questions that need to be answered when considering an intravenous infusion are (1) At what rate must the drug be administered to achieve target plasma concentrations? and (2) How long will it take to reach target concentrations?

The former question is easily answered if the desired concentration at steady state (C_{ss}) and Cl are known. Because the aim of the infusion is to replace the drug at the same rate at which it is being eliminated from the body, Equation 8 can be used to calculate the rate of infusion (R_0; units: amount/time).

Equation 7

$$R_0 = C_{ss} \times Cl$$

Where: C_{ss} = desired steady state concentration
The time taken to reach C_{ss} is dependent on the value of the $T_{1/2}$ of the drug (Table 95-1). Once C_{ss} has been reached, plasma concentrations remain steady as the amount of drug eliminated from the body is matched by the amount of drug that is replaced by the infusion. A bolus dose (D_{bolus}) should be administered if target concentrations need to be reached quickly or if a drug has a long $T_{1/2}$ (Equation 8).

Equation 8

$$D_{bolus} = C_{ss} \times V_d$$

Where: C_{ss} = desired steady state concentration

Multiple-Dose Regimens

Despite the advantages of a constant rate infusion, this method of administration requires intensive patient management and is often impractical in food-producing animals. More commonly, if effective concentrations must be maintained for longer than are achievable with a single dose, drugs will be administered as multiple discrete doses. In this way, an average effective plasma concentration can be maintained, although it will fluctuate between dosing intervals. The magnitude of these fluctuations depends on the relationship between the dosing interval (τ) and

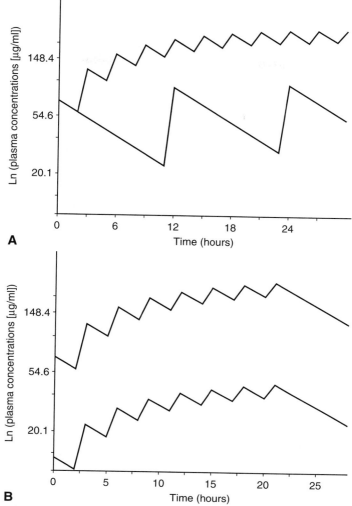

Fig 95-7   Plasma time-concentration profile following multiple intravenous administrations to illustrate that either decreasing the dosing interval **(A)** or increasing the dose **(B)** will increase the average plasma concentrations.

the rate of elimination of the drug (k_{el}) (Equation 9) (Fig. 95-7, *A*). Products for food-producing animals are often formulated for extended-release, which prolongs their elimination (decreases the value of k_{el}), making it possible for dosing intervals to be extended without causing unacceptably large fluctuations in plasma concentrations.

Equation 9

$$\ln \frac{C_{max}}{C_{min}} = \tau \times k_{el}$$

Where: C_{max} = Maximum plasma concentration
$\quad\quad\quad C_{min}$ = Minimum plasma concentration

The average concentration (C_{avg}) is a function of the administered dose (*D*), V_d, and the ratio $T_{1/2}/\tau$ (Equation 10a) (see Fig. 95-7) and can be manipulated by either changing the dose (*D*) or the dosing interval (*τ*).

Equation 10a

$$C_{avg} = \frac{D}{V_d} \times \frac{(1.44) \times T_{1/2}}{\tau}$$

For food-producing animals, because of the inconvenience of handling the animals, longer dosing intervals are generally preferred. The dosing interval (and hence the value of *τ*) is therefore often extended to as long as possible within the constraints of acceptable fluctuations in plasma concentrations and the values of C_{max} required to prevent toxicity and the values of C_{min} required to ensure efficacy. If *τ* has been calculated using Equation 10, the dose required to achieve the target average plasma concentration can be calculated by rearranging Equation 10 (Equation 10b).

Equation 10b

$$D = C_{avg} \times V_d \times \frac{(0.693) \times \tau}{T_{1/2}}$$

Once again, it will take approximately 5 $T_{1/2}$s to reach this target concentration and a loading dose (Equation 2b) should be administered if target concentrations need to be achieved earlier.

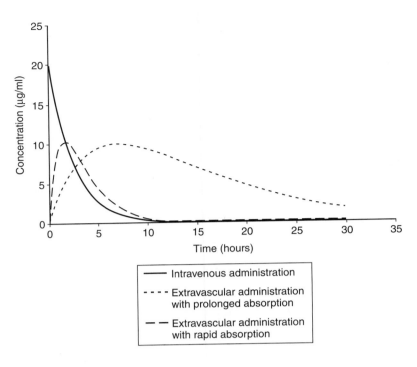

Fig 95-8 Plasma time-concentration profiles of different formulations of the same drug to illustrate the effect of differences in absorption rate.

Extravascular Administration

Drugs are most frequently administered extravascularly (e.g., intramuscularly or subcutaneously), which means that absorption is a prerequisite for activity. Plasma concentrations are dependent on the rate and extent of this process, which can be affected by many factors including the site of administration and drug formulation. If absorption is rapid, as is the case for some solutions that are administered intramuscularly, the rate of elimination will not be affected and the time-concentration profile will be similar to the intravenous route except for a brief absorption period. In contrast, if the drug has been formulated to delay absorption, peak concentrations will be lower and will occur later. In some cases the rate of elimination may be determined by the rate of absorption (flip-flop kinetics), therefore extending the duration of action of the drug (Fig. 95-8).

Extravascular administration may result in some of the dose not being absorbed into the central circulation. Bioavailability *(F)* is the measure of the extent of absorption and can be defined as the percentage of a dose that is absorbed and reaches the site of action. It is calculated by comparing the area under the time-concentration curves *(AUC)* for the extravascular *(ev)* and intravenous *(iv)* routes (Equation 11).

Equation 11

$$F = \frac{AUC_{ev} \times D_{iv} \times \left(T_{\frac{1}{2}}\right)_{iv}}{AUC_{iv} \times D_{ev} \times \left(T_{\frac{1}{2}}\right)_{ev}}$$

Bioavailabilities of greater than 100% are sometimes reported in the literature, which is conceptually impossible. Numerous factors could lead to such a result including experimental errors and deficiencies in the analytic

technique used to generate the data. Most importantly, if the rate of elimination is prolonged due to flip-flop kinetics, this must be accounted for in the bioavailability calculation (see Equation 11). Low bioavailability is compensated for by increasing the dose, but it should be remembered that low bioavailability is often associated with high variability and this may result in toxicity or inefficacy in some individuals.

WITHDRAWAL TIMES

An additional consideration for designing dosing regimens in food-producing animals is that illegal drug residues, which may be harmful to the consumer, must be avoided in the edible tissues. All drugs approved for use in food-producing animals have a withdrawal time included in the label, which is the time that must elapse from the administration of the last dose until the edible tissues can be harvested for human consumption. These withdrawal times are determined experimentally. The drug is administered to healthy animals, groups of which are then slaughtered at sequential time intervals to allow samples of their edible tissues to be taken. These samples are analyzed for drug concentrations and the withdrawal time is calculated using a statistical method to determine the time, rounded to the next whole day, at which the upper bound of the marker residue tissue concentration (representing 99% of the population with 95% confidence) is below the established safe concentration in the target tissue. Additional studies measuring the concentrations in the milk must be performed if a drug is to be approved in dairy cattle.

These label withdrawal times only apply if the drug is administered according to label directions, which would include the dose, dosing interval, route of administration, and indication. Veterinarians are legally allowed to use

Table **95-2**

General Approach to Estimating Extended Withdrawal Times Following the Extralabel Use of Drugs in Food-Producing Animals

Scenario	Possible Approach to Estimating an Extended Withdrawal Time	Caveats and Considerations
Drug approved in a food-producing species is administered at a higher-than-label dose to the same species	Extend the label withdrawal time by one tissue elimination half-life for each doubling of the dose.	An accurate estimate of the tissue elimination half-life is required. Invalid if any circumstances exist that may prolong absorption (e.g., large amounts are administered at a single injection site). Invalid if any circumstances exist that may prolong elimination (e.g., severe illness, saturation of elimination processes at higher doses).
Drug approved in a food-producing species is administered to an animal in which a prolonged tissue half-life is anticipated	Extend the label withdrawal time by a factor that is the ratio of the prolonged half-life to the half-life in the approved species.	An accurate estimate of the tissue elimination half-lives is required. When extrapolating between different species it should be remembered that differences in metabolism could lead to accumulation in different tissues or the production of an unknown toxic metabolite.
Administered drug is not approved in any food-producing species	Wait 10 half-lives (to allow 99.9% of the drug to be eliminated).	The safe concentration in the target tissue is unknown and any detectable residues will be considered violative. The target tissue elimination half-life is unknown and will not necessarily be the same as the plasma half-life.

drugs in an extralabel manner but must ensure that this does not result in violative tissue residues. A list of "rules of thumb" that can be used to estimate an appropriately extended withdrawal time following extralabel use is given in Table 95-2. Importantly, there are several caveats to the use of any of these rules. In the United States, the Food Animal Residue Avoidance Databank (FARAD) serves as a resource of information regarding the avoidance of violative residues following extralabel use of drugs in food-producing animals, and practitioners are strongly advised to make use of this service if they have any doubts regarding the potential for extralabel drug use to result in violative residues (see Chapter 96 for further discussion of FARAD).

Recommended Readings

Riviere JE: *Comparative pharmacokinetics: principles, techniques and applications*, ed 2, Ames, Iowa, 2003, Blackwell Publishing.

Toutain PL, Bousquet-Melou A: Plasma clearance, *J Vet Pharmacol Ther* 27:415-425, 2004.

Toutain PL, Bousquet-Melou A: Plasma terminal half-life, *J Vet Pharmacol Ther* 27:427-439, 2004.

Toutain PL, Bousquet-Melou A: Volumes of distribution, *J Vet Pharmacol Ther* 27:441-453, 2004.

Toutain PL, Bousquet-Melou A: Bioavailability and its assessment, *J Vet Pharmacol Ther* 27:455-466, 2004.

CHAPTER 96

FARAD and Related Drug Regulations

GEOFFREY SMITH

The Food Animal Residue Avoidance Databank (FARAD) is a drug and chemical database that can be used by veterinarians to obtain drug residue information. The ultimate goal of this U.S. Department of Agriculture (USDA)-sponsored program is to use regulatory and pharmacokinetic data to provide food animal practitioners with drug withdrawal information so that residues are minimal in meat and milk products, thereby reducing the public health risk associated with contaminated food. FARAD provides the following information via its Internet website (http://www.farad.org) or by telephone/e-mail consultation: (1) approved food animal drugs and their approved dose, route(s) of administration, and indications; (2) approved withdrawal times; (3) approved tolerances (United States) and foreign maximum residue levels (MRLs); and (4) information regarding various drug tests for milk residues. FARAD has been in existence since 1982 as part of the USDA's national residue avoidance program, which was designed to help producers and veterinarians prevent food residues by education rather than regulation. Congress more permanently authorized the FARAD program in the Agricultural Research, Extension, and Education Reauthorization Act of 1998 (Public Law 105-185, Title 6, Subtitle A, Section 604).

AMDUCA

Under the Animal Medicinal Drug Use Clarification Act of 1994 (AMDUCA), veterinarians are legally allowed to use drugs in food-producing animals in an extralabel manner, provided that certain conditions have been satisfied. Requirements for extralabel drug use (ELDU) are that (1) ELDU be conducted under the supervision of a licensed veterinarian, (2) ELDU is allowed only for FDA-approved animal and human drugs, (3) a valid veterinarian-client relationship exists, and (4) ELDU must be for therapeutic purposes only (not to improve production). Except for minor species (i.e., goats, sheep), the use of extralabel drugs in feed is prohibited and the FDA also has a list of drugs prohibited from ELDU in food-producing animals. Box 96-1 contains a complete list of prohibited drugs (current as of April 2007). It should be emphasized that any use of a drug from this list in any manner other than what is specifically approved on the label would be considered illegal. Drugs on this list that are approved (i.e., fluoroquinolones in beef cattle) must be used exactly according to label directions and would be limited to the specific age and type of animal the drug is approved for, the approved drug dose and duration of therapy, and approved indication for treatment.

Extralabel drug use is not permitted if it might result in a violative food residue or any residue that may present a risk to public health. Therefore the establishment of an appropriate withdrawal time for meat, milk, or eggs following ELDU is essential and represents the primary function of FARAD. The withdrawal time required following ELDU is a function of the dose of drug administered, the tolerance level in the edible product, and the rate at which the drug is depleted from the body.[1]

Box 96-1

Drugs Prohibited by AMDUCA* for Use in Food-Producing Animals

Diethylstilbestrol (DES)
Chloramphenicol
Nitroimidazoles (including dimetridazole, metronidazole, and ipronidazole)
Sulfonamide use in adult dairy cattle†
Clenbuterol
Fluoroquinolones (e.g., enrofloxacin, danofloxacin)
Glycopeptides (vancomycin)
Nitrofurans (including nitrofurazone and furazolidone; topical use prohibited as well)
Phenylbutazone use in adult dairy cattle‡
Adamantine (amantadine and rimantadine) and neuraminidase inhibitor (oseltamivir and zanamivir) classes of drugs that are approved for treating or preventing influenza A are prohibited in poultry (including chickens, turkeys, and ducks)
Dipyrone‡

*Animal Medicinal Drug Use Clarification Act of 1994.
†Lactating (adult) dairy cattle are defined by FDA as dairy cattle 20 months of age or older *regardless of whether they are milking or dry*. Currently the only sulfonamide available for use in dairy cattle older than 20 months of age is sulfadimethoxine (SDM). In adult dairy cattle this drug may only be used per the label. Administering higher doses or sustained release SDM products is prohibited.
‡Because dipyrone-containing products are not available for either humans or animals, they are not typically included on lists of extralabel prohibitions published by the Center for Veterinary Medicine. Old stockpiles of the drug, however, do occasionally surface. Any use of dipyrone in food animals remains a violation of the Food Drug and Cosmetic Act.
Aside from this AMDUCA list, regulations related to the Pasteurized Milk Ordinance (PMO) prohibit the presence of dimethyl sulfoxide (DMSO) and colloidal silver on dairies.

TOLERANCE LEVELS

According to AMDUCA, "establishing a safe level or tolerance is a priori for establishing an extended withdrawal time or interval for extralabel drug use."[2] The tolerance is defined as the safe level above which there may be adverse health effects if humans were to consume animal-derived products containing drugs above that level. Risk assessment groups derive tolerance levels (or minimal risk levels, as they are referred to outside the United States) for different drugs based on a number of factors. The first step in quantitative risk assessment requires some indication of the toxicity of the chemical, which involves identification of the no observable effect level (NOEL) or the no observable adverse effect level (NOAEL). The NOEL is based on dose-response studies and pharmacologic or toxicologic end points.[3] Although human toxicology data are ideal for calculating NOELs, data from laboratory animals are often used to determine the lowest dose that can be given and cause no adverse effects across all organ systems following a chronic exposure.

With an accurate NOEL value, an acceptable daily intake (ADI) can be determined. This is defined as a dose or concentration of drug that humans can be exposed to during a lifetime without experiencing adverse effects. The ADI is calculated by dividing the NOEL by safety factors that are used to compensate for interspecies extrapolation and intraspecies variability and to cover uncertainties caused by a diverse population of consumers. Finally, the likely intake of drug residues is considered to ensure that consumers would not exceed the ADI for a specific drug residue. Among several indices of daily intake of residues is the estimated maximum daily intake (EMDI), which is based on a "heavy meat consumption" diet and food consumption values derived from national food consumption surveys.[3]

If a specific drug or chemical has a tolerance level, generally accurate information about withdrawal times following ELDU drug use can be determined providing there are sufficient pharmacokinetic data available. If a tolerance level is not available in the United States, often FARAD will consider MRLs that have been set for the European Union. However, in the absence of a specific tolerance or "safe" level, a violative residue following ELDU is defined as any detectable concentration, regardless of the level detected. Therefore a drug residue would mean any concentration that could be detected in meat, milk, or eggs with current analytic methods. As a result, drugs or chemicals without established tolerances or MRLs generally have substantially longer withdrawal intervals compared with approved drugs because the levels in edible tissues must be essentially undetectable.

USING FARAD

FARAD is operated jointly by North Carolina State University, the University of California-Davis, and the University of Florida and can be contacted by toll-free access (1-888-873-2723) and/or via e-mail at farad@ncsu.edu or usfarad@gmail.com. The FARAD regional offices are staffed by specialists in pharmacokinetics and will work to provide veterinarians with specific information regarding their particular extralabel dosage conditions. When contacting FARAD, the following information is necessary to ensure an accurate response: (1) name of drug including the specific formulation and/or brand name, (2) dose of the drug (including frequency and duration of administration), (3) route of drug administration, and (4) species in which drug was administered.

FARAD personnel analyze the data on a case-by-case basis and provide withdrawal recommendations according to the specific features of each case. The vast majority of withdrawal information given to veterinarians comes from the FARAD database, which contains more than 5000 scientific articles with data on residues, pharmacokinetics, and the fate of chemicals in food animal species. The database also contains data from foreign approval of drugs (primarily Europe), freedom of information summaries on approved drugs, as well as proprietary data from private companies. The extensive database contains sufficient information to answer 90% to 95% of all calls that come into the center. For the rest of these calls, which usually involve unusual drugs or unusual chemical exposures, other methods can be used to determine an approximate withdrawal period.

One FARAD tool is known as the *extrapolated withdrawal-interval estimator* (EWE) *algorithm*. This patented method consists of a series of pharmacokinetic algorithms that first normalize the label dosage conditions to the extralabel scenario, then extract tissue depletion data from the approved label information, and finally estimate a withdrawal interval for the extralabel dosage regimen.[4] Pharmacokinetic data can also be extrapolated from other species when necessary to come up with an approximate withdrawal interval.

Another tool FARAD uses to estimate withdrawal intervals is called the half-life multiplier. This is based on the concept that the drug half-life does not change with different doses, which is probably the case for most drugs administered at therapeutic levels. Under this assumption, the withdrawal period would need to be increased by one half-life of the drug for each doubling in dose. This would be equivalent to the time required for the concentration of the residue to deplete to the same concentration as it would following the administration at the approved dose.[5] When an accurate estimate of elimination half-life is not available, it can be estimated on the basis of the approved withdrawal time, which is a direct reflection of the number of tissue elimination half-lives required for the concentration of the residue to reach tolerance levels. The process of estimating the number of drug half-lives contained within an approved withdrawal time is referred to as the *half-life multiplier* and is sometimes used to estimate withdrawal intervals on drugs when appropriate pharmacokinetic data are not available.

A relatively novel approach is the use of physiologically based pharmacokinetic (PBPK) models to describe and predict the kinetics of drugs or chemicals based on physiologic mechanisms by linking physiologic tissue blocks together via a communal plasma compartment.[6] These models have been used in human medicine to predict therapeutic doses for drugs during the development phase and now are being applied to veterinary drugs to predict withdrawal intervals for populations of animals.

OTHER FARAD RESOURCES

In addition to the regional offices, FARAD also maintains the newly updated Veterinarian's Guide to Residue Avoidance Management (VetGRAM). This program will assist access to a variety of therapeutic information including approved drugs, active ingredients, labeled indications, and specific withdrawal times. This database is accessible through the FARAD website found at www.farad.org. Members of FARAD also regularly contribute publications to the Journal of the American Veterinary Medical Association (JAVMA) under the heading "FARAD Digest." These articles appear several times per year and cover a number of topics related to ELDU including the pharmacokinetics and withdrawal intervals for drugs in food animal species. The "FARAD Digest" articles are meant to serve as reference resources for food animal practitioners, but the withdrawal information included in these manuscripts is always subject to change in the advent of new pharmacokinetic data and/or new regulatory guidelines from the FDA. FARAD has also compiled its pharmacokinetic database into a single published compendium.[7]

A final point of emphasis is that although FARAD is partly funded by the USDA and frequently collaborates with the FDA Center for Veterinary Medicine (CVM), FARAD is not obligated or under any contract to relay specific case-sensitive information from our clients (veterinarians) to these or other state/federal regulatory agencies or cooperatives. This confidentiality encourages open communication between FARAD and food animal practitioners, which promotes residue avoidance by education rather than by regulation.

References

1. Riviere JE: Pharmacologic principles of residue avoidance for veterinary practitioners, *J Am Vet Med Assoc* 198:809, 1991.
2. Baynes RE, Martín-Jiménez T, Craigmill AL et al: Estimating provisional acceptable residues for extralabel drug use in livestock, *Reg Toxicol Pharmacol* 29:287, 1999.
3. Gehring R, Baynes RE, Riviere JE: Application of risk assessment and management principles to the extralabel use of drugs in food-producing animals, *J Vet Pharmacol Therap* 29:5, 2006.
4. Martín-Jiménez T, Baynes RE, Craigmill A et al: Extrapolated withdrawal-interval estimator (EWE) algorithm: a quantitative approach to establishing extralabel withdrawal times, *Reg Toxicol Pharmacol* 36:131, 2002.
5. Gehring R, Baynes RE, Craigmill A et al: Feasibility of using half-life multipliers to estimate extended withdrawal intervals following the extralabel use of drugs in food-producing animals, *J Food Prot* 67:555, 2004.
6. Buur JL, Baynes RE, Craigmill AL et al: Development of a physiologic-based pharmacokinetic model for estimating sulfamethazine concentrations in swine and application to prediction of violative residues in edible tissues, *Am J Vet Res* 66:1696, 2005.
7. Craigmill AL, Riviere JE, Webb AI: *Tabulation of FARAD comparative and veterinary pharmacokinetic data*, Ames, Iowa, 2006, Blackwell.

CHAPTER 97

Anthelmintic Treatment in the Era of Resistance

RAY M. KAPLAN

Beginning with phenothiazine in the 1950s, followed by the benzimidazoles in the 1960s, the imidazothiazole/tetrahydropyrimidines in the 1970s, and the avermectins/milbemycins (AMs) in the 1980s, a new class of anthelmintics was introduced into the marketplace each decade. This arsenal of highly effective and relatively inexpensive drugs led to recommendations for parasite control that were based almost solely on the frequent use of anthelmintics, the goals of which were to maximize livestock health, productivity, and profitability. Though this approach was highly successful for a number of decades, it is now viewed as shortsighted and unsustainable. Two major factors have led to this change of mindset: (1) No new class of anthelmintics has been introduced into the marketplace in more than 25 years; and (2) the prevalence and distribution of multiple-drug–resistant parasites has increased dramatically. Consequently, the traditional paradigm of control based on relatively frequent treatment is threatened and new approaches are required.

Anthelmintics can no longer be thought of as an inexpensive management tool to be used as needed to maximize animal productivity. Instead, anthelmintics must be thought of as extremely valuable and limited resources that should be used prudently. In response to this changing paradigm of anthelmintic use, new recommendations for parasite control are being advocated. The basis of this new approach, commonly referred to as "smart drenching," is to use the knowledge we have about the parasite, animal, and drugs to develop strategies that maximize the effectiveness of treatments while also decreasing the development of drug resistance. Due to the complexities of instituting such a program, successful implementation is only possible with the help and active involvement of veterinarians and other animal health professionals. Additionally, innovative schemes using novel and sustainable approaches must be integrated into more traditional programs. A number of novel, nonchemical technologies will become increasingly important in gastrointestinal nematode (GIN) control programs both in the short- and long-term future. However, all of these novel approaches are less effective than anthelmintics (before emergence of drug-resistant parasites). Therefore as novel, nonchemical control modalities become available and widely applied, anthelmintics will still be required when control fails. Unless veterinarians take an active and leading role in the education of livestock owners and help to implement these new approaches to parasite control, there may be no effective anthelmintics remaining when that time comes.

The problem of resistance is by far the most severe in parasites of small ruminants, and it is in these animals where the most dramatic changes in how nematode control is practiced must be made. Multiple-drug resistance in parasites of small ruminants is the norm throughout much of the world, and there are increasing numbers of farms where resistance to all available drugs is being reported. But what about in parasites of cattle? The seriousness of resistance in cattle parasites is unmistakable in some areas of the world; a recent study in New Zealand reported that ivermectin resistance was evident on 92% of farms, and resistance to both ivermectin and albendazole was evident on 74% of farms. However, the general consensus in most areas of the world is that resistance in parasites of cattle is not yet an important problem. Despite this, most evidence suggests the problem is likely considerably worse than is generally recognized and will continue to worsen in the future. Because no studies have been performed investigating the prevalence of resistance in cattle parasites in most countries, it is difficult to know if the current levels of resistance in cattle nematodes warrant recommendations for major changes in how control is practiced. But based on the worldwide crisis of parasite control that is developing in small ruminants, it seems reasonable to assume that the problem in cattle should not be ignored.

Important GIN parasite genera of sheep, goats, and cattle include *Haemonchus, Trichostrongylus, Teladorsagia, Ostertagia, Cooperia, Oesophagostomum, Trichuris, Strongyloides,* and *Bunostomum.* Although all of these parasites have pathogenic potential, only a limited number of species are considered extremely important in terms of health and economic impact. In sheep and goats the highly pathogenic blood-sucking parasite *Haemonchus contortus* is by far the most prevalent and important in the warm, wet areas of the world including the United States. *Trichostrongylus colubriformis* is usually the second

most prevalent and noteworthy parasite and should not be ignored, but it rarely trumps *H. contortus* in importance where both species are prevalent. *Teladorsagia circumcincta* is commonly found in cooler climates and also has significant pathogenic potential. Multiple-drug resistance is extremely common in all three of these species and, depending on the country or area of the world, one or more of these species will predominate in importance. In cattle, *Ostertagia* is usually considered the most pathogenic and important species but resistance is still only rarely reported in this parasite. In contrast, *Cooperia* spp. have been gaining in importance because ivermectin resistance is most commonly diagnosed in these species.

ANTHELMINTICS USED IN RUMINANTS

Three primary classes of anthelmintics are available for use in treatment of helminth infections in ruminants: (1) benzimidazoles (BZs); (2) imidazothiazoles/tetrahydropyrimidines (I/Ts), also referred to as *membrane depolarizers;* and (3) AMs (also referred to as *macrocyclic lactones* and *macrolide endectocides*). All three of these major anthelmintic classes are broad-spectrum nematocides, but effectiveness against other groups of parasites varies widely (see Tables 97-1 and 97-2 for a list of drugs, recommended doses, and indications). Livestock are typically infected with multiple species of helminth parasites that differ somewhat in their susceptibilities to the different anthelmintic drugs, but most of the commonly used drugs are effective against the most economically important species. This is important because some species of parasites are much more pathogenic than others and are therefore much more important to target with treatment.

Benzimidazoles

Benzimidazoles are broad-spectrum nematocides with some drugs also having activity against tapeworms and flukes. Fenbendazole is also effective against the protozoan parasite *Giardia.* Many BZs kill larval stages of nematodes, as well as the adults, but usually larval efficacy is lower than for adults. In some cases increasing the dose and/or duration of treatment (e.g., treat for multiple days) increases efficacy, particularly against larval stages. BZs are safe; the toxic dose is 10 to 100 times the therapeutic dose depending on the drug, so they can be used safely in debilitated animals. BZs must be administered orally but are available in numerous formulations such as feed premix, bolus, drench, paste, mineral/protein block, and pellets. Albendazole is teratogenic in mice, but little evidence of teratogenicity exists in ruminants. Nevertheless, there is a label warning to not use albendazole in cows and sheep during the first 45 and 30 days of gestation, respectively. The prevalence of resistance to BZ drugs is extremely high in GIN parasites of small ruminants; however, in GIN of cattle, reports of resistance are uncommon. This may be largely due to the fact that BZs are typically used much less frequently in cattle than the AM drugs. BZ drugs are nonpersistent and rapidly metabolized; however, a rumen reservoir and gut recycling leads to prolonged gut levels of BZs in ruminants (but still of short duration, <24 hours).

Table 97-1

Commonly Used Anthelmintics in Sheep and Goats

Drug	Class	Approved for Sheep, Goats	Dosage (mg/kg)	How Supplied	Prevalence of Resistance*	Meat WDT	Milk WDT For Goats	Remarks
Ivermectin	AM	Yes / No	Sheep 0.2 Goats 0.4	Sheep oral drench	High	Sheep 11 days Goats 14 days†	8 days†	Cattle injectable formulation not recommended
Doramectin	AM	No / No	Sheep 0.2 Goats 0.4	Injectable	High	ND	NE	Not recommended because long residual activity promotes resistance
Moxidectin	AM	Yes / No	Sheep 0.2 Goats 0.2	Sheep oral drench Cattle injectable	Low to moderate	Sheep 14 days Goats 30 days†	NE	Use oral drench in sheep Use cattle injectable in meat goats (if using sheep oral drench dose = 0.4 mg/kg) Kills ivermectin-resistant *Haemonchus* Minimize use to preserve efficacy
Levamisole	I/T	Yes / No	Sheep 8 Goats 12	Soluble drench powder	Low to moderate	Sheep 3 days Goats 4 days†	NE	Toxic side effects = salivation, restlessness, muscle fasciculations Recommend weighing goats before treatment
Morantel	I/T	No / Yes	10	Feed premix	Moderate	30 days	0 days	Approved for use in lactating goats Surveys for prevalence of resistance have not been performed
Fenbendazole	BZ	No[a] / Yes	Sheep 5 Goats 5[b]	Paste Suspension Feed block Mineral pellets	High	Goats 6 days[c] (for suspension only)	4 days[c] (for suspension only)	[a]Approved in bighorn sheep [b]Label dose is 5 mg/kg but 10 mg/kg is recommended for goats [c]Listed WDT are for the 5 mg/kg dose. At 10 mg/kg, WDT should be extended to 7 days for meat and 5 days for milk†
Albendazole	BZ	Yes / No	Sheep 7.5 Goats 15-20	Paste Suspension	High	Sheep 7 days Goats 9 days†	7 days†	Do not use within 30 days of conception Effective against *Moniezia* tapeworms

Information in this table regarding extra-label dosages and withdrawal times is based on the best available data at the time of submission for publication. However, no guarantees can be made as to the future accuracy of this information because the data used to calculate withdrawal intervals are continuously updated and these may affect future recommendations. Please note that the withdrawal interval recommendations listed in this table are intended for veterinary use only, are only for use within a valid veterinary-client-patient relationship, and the prescribing veterinarian is ultimately responsible for potential residues resulting from extra-label drug use. Non-veterinarians should always consult with their veterinarian before using any drug in an extra-label manner.

*In the southern United States. Prevalence of resistance has not been established elsewhere.

†Based on the Food Animal Residue Avoidance Databank recommendations.

AM, Avermectin/milbemycin (macrocyclic lactone); BZ, benzimidazole; I/T, imidazothiazole/tetrahydropyrimidine; NE, milk WDT has not been established in goats; product should not be used in lactating dairy goats; ND, meat withdrawal time has not been established. To be safe it is suggested to double cattle WDT; WDT, withdrawal time.

Table 97-2

Commonly Used Anthelmintics in Cattle

Drug	Class	Spectrum	Dosage (mg/kg)	How Supplied	Meat Withdrawal	Approved for Use in Dairy Cattle	Remarks
Clorsulon	Other	F	7	Drench	8 days	No	
Ivermectin	AM	D,T,H,E	0.2	Injectable	49 days	No	Avermectin
			0.5	Pour-on	48 days		
Eprinomectin	AM	D,T,H,E	0.5	Pour-on	None	Yes, no milk withdrawal	Avermectin
Doramectin	AM	D,T,H,E	0.2	Injectable	35 days	No	Avermectin
			0.5	Pour-on			
Moxidectin	AM	D,T,H,E	0.5	Pour-on	None	Yes, no milk withdrawal	Milbemycin
Levamisole	I/T	T,D	6	Oral (powder, bolus)	48 hr	No	Toxic side effects = salivation, restlessness, and muscle fasciculations
			8	Injectable	7 days		
			10	Pour-on	9 days		
Morantel	I/T	T	10	Feed premix	14 days	Yes, no milk withdrawal	
Fenbendazole	BZ	T,D,C	5	Paste/Suspension	8 days	Yes, no milk withdrawal for paste/suspension	10 mg/kg for *Trichuris*, *Moniezia*, arrested *Ostertagia* larvae
				Protein feed block	16 days		
				Mineral, Pellets	13 days		
Oxfendazole	BZ	T,D,C	4.5	Suspension	7 days	No	
Albendazole	BZ	T,D,C,F	10	Paste/Suspension	27 days	No	Do not use within 45 days of conception

AM, Avermectin/milbemycin; *BZ*, benzimidazole; *C*, cestodes (*Moniezia* tapeworm); *D*, *Dictyocaulus viviparous* (lungworm); *E*, ectoparasites (lice, mange mites, horn flies); *F*, *Fasciola hepatica*; *H*, *Hypoderma* spp. (grubs); *I/T*, imidazothiazole/tetrahydropyrimidine; *T*, trichostrongylid/strongylid nematodes.

Membrane Depolarizers

This drug class is composed of two chemically unrelated groups having similar mechanisms of action. These drugs act as cholinergic (nicotinic) agonists causing paralysis of worms. Levamisole (imidazothiazole) is a broad-spectrum nematocide but has no effect on any other groups of parasites. Similar to BZs, this drug is short acting but may have added benefits as an immune stimulator by potentiating T cells and stimulating phagocytosis in monocytes. Safety can be an issue with levamisole; toxicity appears at three to five times the therapeutic dose. Overdose of levamisole resembles organophosphate poisoning, with transient ataxia, salivation/muzzle foaming, and muscle fasciculations as common symptoms. Levamisole also may potentiate organophosphates, causing signs of toxicity, especially in Brahman cattle. Because of this, it is best to not use levamisole in debilitated animals, but levamisole is considered safe in pregnant ruminants so long as it is dosed appropriately. In hot climates, levamisole should be used carefully in sheep during the summer because subclinical dehydration at the time of treatment could lead to toxicity. Morantel (tetrahydropyrimidines) is a broad-spectrum nematocide that is approved for use in lactating animals. In contrast to levamisole, morantel is safe and gentle with no contraindications for debility, pregnancy, or age. Presently, morantel is available only as feed premix, making accurate dosing a little more challenging.

Avermectins/Milbemycins (Macrocyclic Lactones, Macrolide Endectocides)

AMs are derivatives of naturally occurring antibiotic-like compounds secreted by soil-dwelling bacteria of the genus *Streptomyces*, presumably as a defense against bacteria-feeding soil nematodes. Drugs in this group are broad spectrum, being effective against most nematode and arthropod parasites. AMs have excellent efficacy (>99%) against both adult and larval stages of most trichostrongyle parasites including arrested (hypobiotic) larvae and also have excellent efficacy against most ectoparasites and fly larvae (myiasis). Moxidectin (milbemycin group) tends to be more potent against nematodes than the avermectins; however, drugs in the avermectin group are more potent against arthropod parasites than is moxidectin. AMs are highly lipophilic and provide residual activity against reinfection of many parasites for periods of time that vary depending on the worm species and the particular drug. Though commonly administered as pour-ons with a dose of 0.5 mg/kg, the bioavailability is superior when administered orally or by injection at a dose of 0.2 mg/kg. Of importance is the fact that a considerable percentage of the pour-on dose is ingested and absorbed orally as a consequence of cattle licking behavior. This is one of several reasons why pour-ons do not work as well in other ruminant species. Little metabolism of AM drugs occurs—most of the drug is excreted unchanged in the feces.

Ivermectin versus Moxidectin

Ivermectin and moxidectin are closely related drugs belonging to the AM class of anthelmintics. It is generally recognized that resistance to one drug in an anthelmintic class confers resistance to all of them, a phenomena referred to as *side resistance*. However, differences in potency of different drugs within a particular class can result in this side resistance being overwhelmed, so it appears that two drugs within a class differ in some important way. This is frequently seen with moxidectin because this drug is considerably more potent than the avermectins against many species of parasitic nematodes. Though precise mechanisms are not well understood, and some minor differences almost certainly exist, most published data suggest that ivermectin and moxidectin have similar mechanisms of action and resistance. Researchers do not know what is required to make the jump from ivermectin to moxidectin resistance, or how rapidly this process can occur, but recent data suggests that it can occur relatively quickly.

ANTHELMINTIC THERAPY IN SMALL RUMINANTS (see Table 97-1)

Most of the anthelmintics available for use in cattle are also labeled for use in sheep and should be administered according to label directions. In contrast, only four drugs are approved for use in goats: morantel tartrate, thiabendazole (TBZ), fenbendazole (FBZ), and phenothiazine, and TBZ is no longer marketed. This list is further limited in usefulness because drug resistance to benzimidazoles (TBZ, FBZ, and related compounds) and phenothiazine is common. Consequently, extralabel use of drugs is an important issue that must be considered when treating goats with anthelmintics. Additionally, because of the high prevalence of multiple-drug resistance, no general recommendations can be made regarding optimal drug choice. (See Table 97-1 and Anthelmintic Resistance later for guidance.)

All anthelmintics should be given orally to sheep and goats except for moxidectin in meat goats. Moxidectin has a superior pharmacokinetic profile in goats when administered by subcutaneous injection as compared with oral administration; therefore the cattle injectable product should be used. Pour-on anthelmintics are poorly absorbed in small ruminants and have a low bioavailability, so they should never be used unless specifically for ectoparasites. As a general rule, goats metabolize anthelmintic drugs much more rapidly than other livestock and require a higher dosage to achieve proper efficacy. A rule of thumb is that goats should be given a dose 1.5 to 2 times higher than for sheep or cattle. A 1.5× dose is recommended for levamisole because a 2× dose is approaching a level that could be toxic. For all other drugs it is recommended that a 2× dose be given to goats, except for moxidectin, which should be administered by subcutaneous injection using the label cattle dose.

Dairy goats present a more difficult problem in drug selection. Only morantel is approved for use in dairy goats and this drug has no milk withdrawal when used according to label instructions. FBZ can be used at 5mg/kg with a 4-day milk withdrawal or at the suggested 10mg/kg

dose with a 5-day milk withdrawal. But resistance to FBZ is highly prevalent, so this drug must be used with caution. No studies on prevalence of resistance to morantel have been conducted, but based on what we know about resistance to levamisole, it can be assumed that it will not work well on many farms. The Food Animal Residue Avoidance Databank (FARAD) has recommended a 1-day milk withdrawal for pour-on moxidectin, but this route of administration cannot be recommended due to poor absorption and bioavailability together with long persistence. Other drugs that can be used in an extralabel manner include albendazole and ivermectin, but these have milk withdrawal times of 7 and 8 days, respectively (as recommended by FARAD).

Anthelmintic Resistance

Resistance to anthelmintic drugs is reaching alarming levels in GIN parasites of small ruminants, and in the United States the biggest problem is with *H. contortus*. Resistance is reported to all available drugs, multiple-drug resistance is common, and resistance to all available anthelmintics is being diagnosed with increasing frequency. The prevalence of resistance has only been investigated in the southern United States, so it is not known what the prevalence of resistance is in other regions. It is possible that the problem is not as severe in the north and west as in the south, but the limited data available suggest the problem is not limited by geography. Resistance to ivermectin and the benzimidazole drugs is highly prevalent and these drugs should no longer be relied on unless first proven effective. Resistance to levamisole and moxidectin is less prevalent but still common enough to warrant concern, particularly if there is a history of regular use of these drugs on the farm. From a clinical standpoint it is important to appreciate that the prevalence of resistance only tells you what you can expect across many farms; it tells you nothing about which drug(s) are effective on any particular farm. Therefore it is not possible to make medically sound recommendations regarding drug choice for an individual farm without first doing a test to determine whether resistant worms are present there and, if present, to which drugs and at what levels. Given this reality, resistance testing should be performed on every farm as a standard component of herd health management every 2 to 3 years. This can be done in one of two ways: (1) by performing a fecal egg count reduction test (FECRT) or (2) by performing an in vitro larval development assay (LDA). The FECRT is presently the most definitive means of determining whether resistance is present on a particular property, but this test is labor intensive and expensive to perform. An alternative to the FECRT is the LDA (DrenchRite), but this test is not suited for in-clinic use and can only realistically be performed in a parasitology diagnostic laboratory.* A DrenchRite test can detect and measure resistance to benzimidazole drugs, levamisole, ivermectin, and moxidectin, all from a single pooled fecal sample.

---

*The DrenchRite LDA is available as a diagnostic service in the laboratory of Dr.Ray Kaplan. Contact Sue Howell at showell@vet.uga.edu for more information.

Fecal Egg Count Reduction Test

Guidelines for FECRT in sheep are published by the World Association for the Advancement of Veterinary Parasitology (WAAVP), and it is recommended that these be followed in principle. Briefly, animals that have not been treated with anthelmintic within the past 8 weeks are divided into groups of 10 to 15 and treated with anthelmintic or left untreated to serve as controls. If enough animals are present on the farm, multiple drugs can be tested simultaneously, but a control group of equal size must always be included. Fewer than 10 animals per group can be tested, but because of the wide variation in fecal egg count (FEC) among animals, results will be less accurate and there is a greater chance for an erroneous result. Consequently, if fewer than 10 animals are included per group, it is necessary to balance the groups based on FEC. This can be done one of two ways. Pretreatment FEC can be performed, or if *Haemonchus* is the primary parasite (most common situation), animals can be assigned to treatment based on their FAMACHA scores (see Selective Treatment and FAMACHA later). Using pretreatment FEC has the disadvantage of requiring a considerable amount of extra labor and expense because the animals need to be worked an additional time and an additional set of FEC must be performed. In contrast, when using FAMACHA, allocation to treatment is made on the spot at the time of treatment, so fecals only need to be collected and analyzed once. If using pretreatment FEC for allocation, animals are ranked from highest to lowest eggs per gram (EPG) of feces and then blocked into groups of two, three, four, or five depending on how many drugs are being tested. Then within each block, animals are randomly assigned to treatment or control groups. If using FAMACHA, the same approach is used but animals are blocked by their FAMACHA eye score. For example, if four drugs are being tested, of the first five animals to come through the chute with the same FAMACHA score, each of the five will be assigned randomly to one of the five treatment/control groups. Therefore for each FAMACHA score, a group of five animals will each be assigned to a different treatment group, and then the process repeats itself for the next five with the same eye score. If more than 10 animals are included in each group, it is likely that random allocation will produce groups that are sufficiently balanced to obtain useful data, but assigning treatment based on the FAMACHA score will increase this likelihood and is recommended as a routine practice no matter how many animals are tested (but only when *H. contortus* is the primary parasite of concern).

FECs only need to be performed once 10 to 14 days after treatment using the McMaster method,* and calculations are made using the following formula:

$$\left(\text{FECR\%} = 100 \left[1 - Xt/Xc \right] \right)$$

where *Xt* and *Xc* are the arithmetic mean eggs per gram (EPG) in the treated *(t)* and untreated control *(c)* groups, respectively.

*McMaster slides are available from the Chalex Corporation, 5004 228th Ave. S.E., Issaquah, WA 98029-9224. Phone (425) 391-1169, fax (425) 391-6669, e-mail: chalexcorp@att.net, website: www.vetslides.com.

Free software (RESO FECR4) that performs all calculations and provides accurate data interpretation according to WAAVP standards is available.* If the RESO calculator is used, the assignment of resistance status is based both on percent reduction and the 95% confidence intervals. If the RESO calculator is not used, the following guidelines can be applied: reductions of greater than 95% indicate sensitivity, reductions of 90% to 95% indicate low or suspected resistance, and reductions of less than 90% indicate resistance. Control group mean FEC should be at least 150 EPG for the FECRT to yield reliable results. This is rarely an issue with animals infected with *H. contortus*, but group mean FEC of less than 150 EPG is common in adult ewes infected primarily with *T. colubriformis* or *T. circumcincta*. Therefore when FECRT is performed on a sheep farm, it is preferable to use weaned lambs if available. With goats, low FEC are usually not a problem.

Selective Treatment and FAMACHA

The most important factor affecting the rate at which anthelmintic resistance develops is the proportion of the total worm population on the farm that is under drug selection. The unselected portion of the population, referred to as *refugia*, provides a pool of drug-sensitive genes, which dilute any resistant genes that are beginning to increase in frequency. In practical terms, at the time an anthelmintic treatment is given, refugia include all the eggs and larvae already on pasture and all the worms in host animals that are left untreated. Most parasitologists now agree that the principal factors leading to the rapid and widespread development of anthelmintic resistance are the common practices of treating all animals in the herd at one time and treating at times of the year when there are few infective larvae on pasture. These practices leave few worms in refugia. If all animals are treated at the same time, then all eggs deposited onto the pasture for several weeks following treatment are from those worms that survived treatment. Likewise, when treatments are given when few infective larvae are on pasture (e.g., early in grazing season or during drought), then eggs produced by resistant worms that survived the treatment are not greatly diluted. In both situations, and especially when done together, the chances that resistant larvae will successfully reinfect a host animal are greatly increased. When this dynamic is combined with frequent treatments, drug resistance is almost certain to develop fairly rapidly.

Sustainable parasite control strategies based on these new concepts must balance the need to maintain adequate levels of refugia with the goal of limiting economic losses resulting from parasitic infections. Fortunately, this goal is achievable because worm burdens are not evenly distributed in animal populations; 20% to 30% of the animals harbor about 80% of the worms. Consequently, using a selective approach in which only those animals harboring worm infections that

*Cameron A: RESO fecal egg count reduction analysis spreadsheet, AusVet Animal Health Services, University of Sydney, Sydney, Australia, 2000. (Based on calculations developed by Martin PJ, Wursthorn L, 1991. RESO fecal egg count reduction test calculator, CSIRO, Animal Health, Melbourne, Australia). Available on request by contacting the laboratory of Dr. Ray Kaplan, University of Georgia.

are severe enough to cause significant health effects and production loss are treated, a similar level of overall herd parasite control is achievable as compared with when the entire herd is treated. But by not treating animals with low-level infections, the total number of treatments given on a herd basis is greatly reduced; thus significant refugia are maintained, greatly reducing the selection for resistance, as well as generating savings on drug costs.

A new clinical on-farm system for classifying sheep/goats into categories based on level of anemia was developed recently in South Africa. This system, called *FAMACHA*,* is an effective tool for identifying those animals infected with levels of *H. contortus* that require treatment. To use FAMACHA, farmers observe the color of ocular mucus membranes and compare this color to a laminated card with illustrations of eyes from sheep at different levels of anemia. The card is calibrated into five categories: 1 = red, nonanemic; 2 = red-pink, nonanemic; 3 = pink, mildly anemic; 4 = pink-white, anemic; 5 = white, severely anemic. In South Africa and the United States, FAMACHA has proven to be an accurate means of identifying sheep and goats that require anthelmintic treatment; PCV, FAMACHA score, and *H. contortus* worm counts are all highly correlated. Information on FAMACHA and guidelines for its use are available (see www.scsrpc.org).

Other effective selective treatment strategies for *Teladorsagia* and *Trichostrongylus* have been developed. Epidemiologic studies have demonstrated that dairy goats in their first lactation and multiparous goats with the highest level of milk production are the most susceptible to parasite infection. Studies in France have shown that by targeting the most susceptible animals within a flock rather than treating all the animals, efficient control of gastrointestinal nematodes can be achieved. In Australia, recent studies have demonstrated that short-term weight gains in growing sheep can be used as a strong indicator for the need for anthelmintic treatment. This approach has great potential on large farms because the weighing of sheep and separation into groups based on predetermined weight gain categories can be accomplished using systems that are practically completely automated.

Keep Resistant Worms off the Farm

Anthelmintic-resistant worms come from only two sources: either they are produced on the farm or purchased. Unfortunately, resistant worms commonly infect new additions; this is a common means of spreading the resistance problem. Therefore veterinarians should recommend quarantine of all new additions to the herd or flock, with aggressive treatment on arrival. On arrival, all new additions should be placed in a dry lot (without any grass) or on concrete, held without feed for 24 hours, and then dewormed sequentially on the same day with moxidectin, levamisole, and albendazole. An FEC should be performed at the time of treatment and again after 14 days together with a fecal flotation, and the animal should be allowed to enter the herd only if the fecal flotation is negative. If a 14-day quarantine is not possible, animals should be confined to pens for a minimum

of 48 hours following treatment before being moved to pasture. However, this is a risky approach. After the animal is released from quarantine, it should be placed on the most contaminated pasture available (large refugia) and should never be placed on a clean pasture.

Administer the Proper Dose

Every dose of anthelmintic should be given with the goal of maximizing the killing of worms. Several studies have demonstrated that sheep/goat producers often underestimate the weight of their animals and therefore underdose their animals. Underdosing exposes worms to sublethal doses of drug, which increases the selection for resistance. Animals should be weighed individually or dosed according to the heaviest animals in the group (except for levamisole in goats, in which overdosing can be risky). Dosing equipment also should be frequently checked for accuracy.

Use Host Physiology to Maximize Drug Availability and Efficacy

For most anthelmintic drugs, efficacy is directly related to the duration of contact between drug and parasite. With all other factors being constant, by simply extending the contact time, drug efficacy is improved. Knowledge of host physiology can therefore be used to increase drug efficacy. When orally treating a ruminant, it is critical that the full dose lodges in the rumen. Once in the rumen, the duration of drug availability as it is absorbed from the rumen and flows to more distal sites of absorption is largely dependent on the flow rate of the digesta. Because rumen volume remains relatively constant, there is an inverse relationship between feed intake and digesta residence time. Simply restricting feed intake for 24 hours before treatment decreases digesta transit and increases drug availability and efficacy. Withholding of feed should be done when using a BZ drug or ivermectin. With moxidectin and levamisole it is not necessary to withhold feed.

Proper technique when drenching animals is also important. All anthelmintics administered orally should be delivered over the back of the tongue. Presenting a drench to the buccal cavity, rather than into the pharynx/esophagus, can stimulate closure of the esophageal groove with significant drench bypassing the rumen. Absorbed drug concentrations may be higher initially but are of such short duration that efficacy is reduced. Special dosing syringes and extenders that attach to regular syringes are sold by several sheep supply companies and should be routinely used. Without any additional cost or effort, these two recommendations have the potential to significantly improve drug efficacy, thereby prolonging the useful life of today's anthelmintics, and should be used as a matter of course.

Split and Repeat Dosing

Increasing the duration of contact between drug and parasite can also can be accomplished by administering two doses 12 hours apart. Repeat dosing can be used as an alternative to withholding feed or, even better, in addition to withholding feed. This approach is most likely to yield benefit when using a BZ drug. With levamisole it is recommended to wait a full 24 hours before redosing.

---

*FAMACHA cards are available for sale through the laboratory of Dr. Ray Kaplan. For more information contact famacha@vet.uga.edu.

Dosing with Two Different Drugs at Same Time

When drugs are still effective, treating with two drugs of different anthelmintic classes simultaneously can delay the development of resistance. Once resistance is present, treating with two drugs of different anthelmintic classes can still be of great benefit. Anthelmintics given together will produce a synergistic effect, significantly increasing the efficacy of treatment compared with the individual drugs. This synergistic effect is most pronounced when the level of resistance is low. Once high-level resistance to both drugs is present, the synergistic effect is unlikely to produce an acceptable efficacy.

Rotation of Anthelmintics

Rotation is an exaggerated concept that gives farmers and veterinarians a false sense that they are actually doing something worthwhile in terms of resistance prevention. No direct evidence indicates that annual rotation of anthelmintics has any beneficial effects in delaying resistance, and the common practice of rotating drugs with each treatment actually appears to increase the rate at which resistance develops. Consequently, in recent years many parasitologists have concluded that rotation should not be used. Instead, it is recommended that an anthelmintic be used until it is no longer effective and then drugs should be switched (this obviously requires testing the efficacy of drugs on a farm). The main rationale behind this approach is that it will become obvious when a drug no longer works, and the farmer will always be aware of the level of resistance to a particular drug in his or her situation. If a rotation is used, resistance develops slowly to all drugs simultaneously and the farmer is unaware of this until multiple-drug resistance is a serious problem. Rotation also becomes moot when only one drug is effective, a situation that is becoming increasingly common.

Strategies for When There Is Resistance to All Available Drugs

In the past few years it has become increasingly common to find farms that have resistance to all three classes of anthelmintics plus moxidectin. So what can be done to deal with this situation? First, because resistance exists in gradations, it is important to know what the actual level of resistance is. Some drugs that are declared resistant may still be achieving 90% to 95% reductions in FEC. If this is the situation, then using a two-drug combination with the two most effective drugs would be a wise choice. However, if the situation has deteriorated even further, a triple combination of albendazole, levamisole, and moxidectin may be necessary. In either case, it is critically important to absolutely minimize the frequency of treatment. Unless selective therapy and other strategies to maintain significant refugia are instituted, the worms will fairly rapidly develop higher-level resistance, rendering these combinations ineffective. In addition to using drug combinations, it is critical that the overall management of the farm be evaluated. Reduced stocking rates and improved level of nutrition will be critical to helping to reduce the need for treatment. Furthermore, novel nonchemical worm control strategies should be implemented wherever practical. Without making the necessary management changes and adjustments to worm control strategy, it is not realistic to expect that the use of drug combinations will be anything more than a quick and temporary fix.

Summary—Sheep/Goats

The days of being able to control gastrointestinal nematode parasites in small ruminants by treating with anthelmintics at frequent intervals are at an end. Therefore, if anthelmintics are to remain a viable component of gastrointestinal nematode control, a fresh smart drenching approach is necessary. Because of the complexities of instituting such a program, successful implementation will only be possible with the help and active involvement of small ruminant veterinarians and other animal health professionals. A selective approach using FAMACHA should be implemented everywhere that *H. contortus* is the primary parasite of concern. Efficacy of anthelmintics should be tested on each farm and drug choices made based on the results. Where treatment must be performed without prior testing, it is incumbent on the veterinarian to know the prevalence of resistance in that geographic region and make decisions based on this data and the drug usage history on the farm. Farms that are down to their last effective drug should reserve this drug for life-saving purposes only (4s and 5s or just 5s on FAMACHA) to preserve its efficacy. On farms with resistance to all drugs but one, the less effective drugs may be used in animals with only a marginal need for treatment (e.g., 3s on FAMACHA). To improve the efficacy of drugs with known resistance, these drugs can be used in combination. No matter what strategy is used, surveillance of drug efficacy using FEC monitoring and improved farm management is necessary.

CONSIDERATIONS FOR CATTLE

Most drug-resistance issues that have changed the way parasite control must be practiced in small ruminants are not considered as highly important in the control of parasites of cattle. However, this may change in the near future because in recent years drug resistance in cattle parasites has been reported with increasing frequency. Despite this, most parasite problems in cattle continue to be related to animals being treated too infrequently and at the wrong times, rather than too often, as is the problem in small ruminants. Therefore anthelmintic resistance prevention in cattle operations is really only important where cattle are intensively managed, such as in stocker and backgrounding operations. In these types of operations where animals are intensively grazed at high stocking densities, frequent anthelmintic treatment has proven itself to have excellent cost-benefit returns. However, it is noteworthy that areas of the world (New Zealand and South America) that have embraced these types of operations are also reporting high levels of drug resistance.

Selective Treatment of Cattle

Strategies for selective treatment, as have been developed for sheep and goats, have not been tested in cattle. Consequently, no strategy can be broadly recommended for cattle. However, of the various strategies available, short-term weight gain seems to have the most promise for those intensively managed operations where treatment is given most frequently. Though no new drug classes have been developed for quite a while, new formulations of old drugs are continually introduced to the market. Currently, most pharmaceutical companies are developing long-acting forms of the AM drugs. This is particularly troubling with regard to resistance. The use of a long-acting drug, when administered to all cattle on a pasture, produces a situation in which there are almost no refugia. Where resistance is not yet diagnosed, we can assume that several decades of drug treatment on worm populations have produced significant preselection for resistance. Therefore, use of these long-acting products is likely to rapidly select for the final (clinical) stages of resistance. Therefore when these drugs become available, it is suggested that the heaviest 5% to 10% of cattle within a given age group not be treated. By not treating the heaviest animals, significant refugia is maintained, and the fact that these animals are the heaviest suggests that parasites have had less of an impact on their growth than most others within the herd.

Other Strategies to Minimize Resistance in Cattle Operations

In integrated systems in which there are cattle of different age classes, growing weaned calves should not be grazed on the same pasture each year. Rather, it is best to rotate pastures among the cattle so that first-year calves are infected with larvae that were shed from older animals that would have been treated at a reduced frequency. Just as with small ruminants, it is advisable to avoid the introduction of resistant nematodes. This is best achieved by treating newly arrived animals with more than one anthelmintic type and then holding them on concrete for 48 hours. Levamisole has excellent efficacy against *Cooperia,* but is not effective against arrested *Ostertagia* and usually provides a lesser treatment response in terms of weight gain than the AM drugs do. Because the greatest problem of resistance is with AM-resistant *Cooperia,* levamisole should always be included in this combination, most likely in combination with one of the AM drugs. As with small ruminants, these newly acquired cattle should be placed on contaminated pastures.

Diagnosis of Resistance in Cattle Parasites

No in vitro tests have been optimized and validated for use in cattle. Thus in vivo testing using the FECRT is the only test available. Unfortunately, standardized methods for FECRT in cattle have not yet been developed. Though the methods used in sheep are not optimal, until standardized methods are published, they can be used in cattle with reasonably accurate results. Additional points that should be adhered to in developing protocols for FECRT in cattle include (1) using a more sensitive method for FEC than McMaster; the modified Wisconsin centrifugal flotation

method is usually recommended; and (2) using an injectable product; with pour-ons there is great variation in drug levels between animals because of differences in absorption and the fact that a substantial amount of the dose is ingested as a consequence of licking. If a pour-on product is used, the treated animals must be kept in a separate pen/paddock from the rest of the cattle.

Summary—Cattle

The crisis in parasite management facing small ruminant production systems has not yet materialized in cattle. However, available evidence suggests that the problem is worse than is generally recognized. A long list of reasons explains why this is the case, but of greatest importance is the fact that most cattle are treated with anthelmintic at a much lower frequency than are sheep/goats. Consequently, on many cattle operations, particularly those with low management input, the problem is not one of resistance but rather of treating too infrequently. Thus proven increases in productivity are sacrificed. In contrast, intensive cattle production systems that rely heavily on the frequent administration of anthelmintics must begin to rethink their approach. Though anthelmintics can produce important improvements in the productivity of cattle, total reliance on anthelmintics for parasite control is not recommended and will not be sustainable into the future as drug resistance becomes a more serious problem.

Recommended Readings

Coles GC: Cattle nematodes resistant to anthelmintics: why so few cases? *Vet Res* 33:481-489, 2002.

Jackson R, Rhodes AP, Pomroy WE et al: Anthelmintic resistance and management of nematode parasites on beef cattle-rearing farms in the North Island of New Zealand, *N Z Vet J* 54:289-296, 2006.

Kaplan RM: Drug resistance in nematodes of veterinary importance: a status report, *Trends Parasitol* 20:477-481, 2004.

Kaplan RM: Update on parasite control in small ruminants 2006: addressing the challenges posed by multiple-drug resistant worms, *AABP Proceed* 39:1-11, 2006.

Mejia ME, Igartua BMF, Schmidt EE et al: Multispecies and multiple anthelmintic resistance on cattle nematodes in a farm in Argentina: the beginning of high resistance? *Vet Res* 34:461-467, 2003.

Mortensen LL, Williamson LH, Terrill TH et al: Evaluation of prevalence and clinical implications of anthelmintic resistance in gastrointestinal nematodes of goats, *J Am Vet Med Assoc* 23:495-500, 2003.

Van Wyk JA: Refugia—overlooked as perhaps the most potent factor concerning the development of anthelmintic resistance, *Onderstepoort J Vet Res* 68:55-67, 2001.

Van Wyk JA, Bath GF: The FAMACHA system for managing haemonchosis in sheep and goats by clinically identifying individual animals for treatment, *Vet Res* 33:509-529, 2002.

Waghorn TS, Leathwick DM, Rhodes AP et al: Prevalence of anthelmintic resistance on 62 beef cattle farms in the North Island of New Zealand, *N Z Vet J* 54:278-282, 2006.

Waller PJ: The future of anthelmintics in sustainable parasite control programs for livestock, *Helminthologia* 40:97-102, 2003.

CHAPTER 98

Antimicrobial Resistance in Human Pathogens and the Use of Antimicrobials in Food Animals: Challenges in Food Animal Veterinary Practice

BO NORBY

The emergence of antimicrobial resistance in commensal and pathogenic bacteria is a growing concern in both human and veterinary medicine,[1-7] and it has been suggested that the use of antimicrobials in humans and animals is the primary reason for emergence and spread of antimicrobial resistance.[8] Some studies have suggested that resistant bacteria from food animals may be transmitted to humans,[9-11] but the issue of resistant bacteria of animal origin and their consequences to human health and calls for restrictions on use of antimicrobials in agriculture and veterinary medicine is exceedingly controversial and the source of much debate.[1,4,5,12-20] Nonetheless, the use of antimicrobial drugs in livestock production and associated resistance in bacteria *of animal origin* is likely a minor player in regard to antimicrobial-resistant bacteria infecting humans.[21] Regardless, several measures to reduce the total amount of antimicrobial drugs used in animal agriculture and perhaps reduce the levels of antimicrobial-resistant bacteria have been implemented by governments or adopted on a voluntary basis by producers.[22-27]

Concluding that if there are resistant bacteria in animals and animal-derived products, there is an increasing risk to humans getting infected with such resistant bacteria is tempting. This is not necessarily so: The fact that animals harbor resistant bacteria does not establish a risk or consequence to human health.[28] This must be established by following the risks from bacteria in animals to the human health risk. First, does the use of antimicrobial drugs in animal agriculture result in emergence of resistance and in a reservoir of resistant bacteria in food animals and food animal products intended for human consumption? Second, can these bacteria reach the human population by either direct transmission between animals and humans and/or indirectly through the food chain and how often does that happen? Third, if humans are exposed to these bacteria by ingestion, what consequences might that have to the person ingesting them? This not only includes the scenario of resistant pathogens infecting humans, but also the issue of resistant commensals and pathogens that may pass on their resistance genes to commensals and pathogens already present in the human intestinal tract. The subject is further complicated because resistant bacteria may spread through the environment and among animal populations through national and international trade of food and animals.[29] And last, if all the preceding steps are traced and a risk is determined, if certain antimicrobial drugs are banned or withdrawn from use in animal production, what are the potential consequences for livestock and veterinary medicine? The intent here is not to review the origin, development, and dissemination of antimicrobial resistance in animal populations and what the consequences may or may not be to human health, but rather review what is being done to monitor antimicrobial resistance in enteric bacteria from food animals and humans, consequences that this debate on antimicrobial resistance has had on the availability of antimicrobial drugs for use in food animals, and the effect that the removal of some antimicrobial agents from the agricultural and veterinary markets has had on livestock production risk (and risk to food safety).

LEVELS OF ANTIMICROBIAL RESISTANCE IN BACTERIA OF FOOD ANIMAL ORIGIN

The question of whether or not antimicrobial-resistant bacteria are present in the feces of food animals and food animal–derived products is easily answered: They are.[30,31] However, the levels and patterns of antimicrobial resistance vary with the species of bacteria, antimicrobial agents tested, as well as the species of animals. In Denmark, for example, the percentage of tetracycline-resistant *Escherichia coli* isolated from healthy animals between 1996 and 2005 fluctuated between approximately 2% to 14%, 6% to 19%, and 26% to 46% for cattle, broilers, and swine, respectively.[30]

Over the past decade an increasing volume of scientific literature reporting on the levels and patterns of antimicrobial resistance in different bacteria isolated from cattle,[25,26,32,33] pigs,[27,34-40] poultry,[41-43] and food products[44-49] destined for human consumption has emerged. This body of literature originates from both "stand-alone" scientific studies and national monitoring programs of antimicrobial resistance[30,50,51] (see later discussion). Isolates from food animals have shown that both pathogens and commensal bacteria carry genetic material (resistance genes) that renders them resistant to one or more antimicrobial agents.* Most studies and monitoring programs focus on pathogens of zoonotic potential (*Salmonella* and *Campylobacter*) and so-called indicator organisms (*E. coli* and *Enterococcus*), which are considered to be good indicators for the selective pressure of antibiotic usage.

In stand-alone studies, the animal species from which bacteria are sampled, the bacterial species, culture methods of pathogens and commensals, and the number of antimicrobial agents to which resistance in bacteria are tested can vary greatly. The prevalences of resistance to different antimicrobial agents vary among different geographic areas, season, herd size, and age of the animals.[25] Hence inference to the general population of animals throughout larger geographic areas is difficult. The sampling frames and methods also frequently vary among studies, which makes it difficult, if not impossible, to compare levels and patterns of resistance and potential risk factors for resistance development, emergence, and dissemination of antimicrobial resistance among bacterial and animal species. In addition, the use of antimicrobial agents close to the time of sampling may alter the pattern of shedding of potential pathogens.[32]

National Antimicrobial Resistance Monitoring Programs

Although stand-alone studies as described earlier may be helpful in determining the levels and patterns of resistance to antimicrobial agents in different bacterial species and their presence in animals, food and humans, as well as emergence of new resistance determinants and patterns, they are usually limited to a smaller geographic area and are of a cross-sectional nature that only allows for a "snapshot" in time.[52] Because national monitoring programs sample animal populations repeatedly over time, they are generally better suited for providing data for comparison of trends in antimicrobial resistance over time and inputs for models to assess the potential risk to human health associated with use of antimicrobial agents in food animals.[15,52] Some of these programs are highlighted here.

"The Danish Integrated Antimicrobial Resistance Monitoring and Research Programme" (DANMAP)[30] was established in 1995[53] with the objectives to (1) monitor the consumption of antimicrobial agents for food animals and humans; (2) monitor the occurrence of antimicrobial resistance in bacteria isolated from food animals (cattle, swine, poultry), foods of animal origin, and humans; (3) study associations between antimicrobial consumption and antimicrobial resistance; and (4) identify routes of transmission and areas for further research studies.[30,54-62] Reports of DANMAP findings are available from 1996 through 2005. Bacteria monitored in animals, humans, and some foods through DANMAP include *Campylobacter, Salmonella, E. coli, Enterococcus faecalis,* and *Enterococcus faecium.* In addition, monitoring of antimicrobial resistance is

performed on selected animal pathogens from diagnostic submissions (i.e., *Staphylococcus hyicus* ssp. *hyicus, Staphylococcus aureus, Actinobacillus pleuropneumonia, E. coli* F5, and *E. coli* O149). Besides the prevalence of resistance of different bacteria over time, DANMAP also records the use of antimicrobial agents in animals and humans. The yearly prevalence data on antimicrobial resistance in different bacterial species have specifically been used to monitor the trends on antimicrobial resistance after the ban of antimicrobial growth promoters (AGPs). As an example, the DANMAP results show that the resistance to vancomycin in *E. faecium* has decreased considerably since the ban of avoparcin in 1995 (see later discussion).[30] The DANMAP reports are available at http://www.danmap.org.

In the United States the National Antimicrobial Resistance Monitoring System for enteric bacteria (NARMS) was established in 1996 as a collaborative effort among three branches of the U.S. government: the United States Department of Agriculture (USDA) (Food Safety Inspection Service [FSIS] and the Agricultural Research Service [ARS]), the Centers for Disease Control and Prevention (CDC), and the Food and Drug Administration (FDA) (Center for Veterinary Medicine [CVM]).[51] The main focus of NARMS is monitoring of resistant enteric pathogens in humans (CDC), animals (USDA), and retail food (FDA). The objectives of NARMS are to (1) provide descriptive data on the extent and temporal trends of antimicrobial drug susceptibility in *Salmonella* and other enteric bacterial organisms from human and animal populations, as well as from retail meats; (2) assist the identification of antimicrobial drug resistance in humans, animals, and retail meats as it arises; and (3) provide timely information to veterinarians and physicians on antimicrobial drug resistance patterns.[51] An overview of the samples collected by different agencies is presented in Table 98-1.

In addition to the aforementioned monitoring programs in the United States, the USDA recently launched the Collaboration in Animal Health and Food Safety Epidemiology (CAHFSE), with the Animal Health and Plant Inspection Service (APHIS), ARS, and FSIS.[63] A particular emphasis of CAHFSE is to address issues related to antimicrobial resistance. The food safety–related objectives of CAHFSE are to (1) describe the on-farm and in-plant trends in the prevalence of *Salmonella, Campylobacter,* generic *E. coli,* and *Enterococcus* spp.; (2) characterize isolates with particular emphasis on their susceptibility to antibiotics and genetic relatedness; and (3) relate findings to on-farm management practices including patterns of antibiotic use in market swine. The program will collect and link prevalence and antimicrobial resistance data obtained on *Salmonella, Campylobacter, E. coli,* and *Enterococcus* from samples collected on-farm and at slaughter houses, and it will in the future likely contribute valuable information necessary to assess the risk of antimicrobial use in food animals to public health.

Other Resistance Monitoring Programs

Monitoring of antimicrobial resistance is likely to be conducted by the pharmaceutical industry after release of new antimicrobial agents; however, results do not appear to have been published.

---

*References 25, 30, 31, 33, 35, 50.

Table 98-1

U.S. Agencies Participating in Monitoring of Antimicrobial Resistance in Commensal and Pathogenic Bacteria in Human, Animal, and Food Samples in the United States

Agencies	Sample Types	No. Bacterial Isolates Tested in 2003
Centers for Disease Control and Prevention, NARMS*	Monitors antimicrobial susceptibility to 16 antimicrobial agents in every 20th non-*typhi Salmonella* and *Escherichia coli* O157 isolate received from health departments in 50 participating states. (In 1999 *S. typhi* and *Shigella* were added to the list.) 10 states participating in FoodNet† provide one *Campylobacter* isolate every week for susceptibility testing to 8 antimicrobial agents.	1865 Non-*typhi Salmonella* 157 *E. coli* 334 *S. typhi* 495 *Shigella* 328 *Campylobacter*
U.S. Department of Agriculture NARMS‡ CAHFSE††	Monitors antimicrobial susceptibility to 16 antimicrobial agents in: 1. *Salmonella, E. coli,* and *Campylobacter*§ collected in on-farm studies and at federally inspected slaughter houses. 2. Diagnostic samples submitted to NVSL,¶ state, and research laboratories. This program is still in its early stages and samples from swine in 5 states are included. *Salmonella, E. coli,* and *Campylobacter* isolates were tested for susceptibility to 16, 16, and 9 antimicrobial agents, respectively.	2312 *Salmonella* isolates from slaughter: cattle (*n* = 672), swine (*n* = 211), chicken (*n* = 1167), turkey (*n* = 262) 1703 *E. coli*‖: avian (*n* = 1703) 1144 *Salmonella* samples from NVSL: cattle (*n* = 306), swine (*n* = 252), chicken** (*n* = 95), turkey** (*n* = 90) 83 *E. coli*: cattle (*n* = 52), swine (*n* = 18), ovine/caprine (*n* = 8), avian (*n* = 5) Between July 1, 2004, and June 30, 2005, a total of 48 sites were sampled. 359 *Salmonella*, 1488 *E. coli*, and 424 *Campylobacter* isolates were tested for antimicrobial susceptibility.
Food and Drug Administration‡‡ NARMS	FDA received 40 samples of ground beef, chicken breast, ground turkey, and pork chops from each of 8 FoodNet sites. A total of 3533 samples.	469, 83, and 396 were positive for *Campylobacter, Salmonella,* and *E. coli,* respectively.

*http://www.cdc.gov/narms/.[108]
†The Foodborne Disease Active Surveillance Network.[109]
‡http://www.ars.usda.gov/saa/athens/rbrrc/bear.[31]
§The total number of *Campylobacter* that were tested for susceptibility to 8 antimicrobial agents is not readily available from the reports.
¶National Veterinary Services Laboratory.
‖Results from chicken samples obtained at slaughter in 2004 (results from 2003 not available). Results from cattle, swine, sheep, and caprines were based on diagnostic samples.
**Chicken and turkey samples were primarily monitoring samples.
††The Collaboration in Animal Health and Food Safety Epidemiology. Collaboration among APHIS, FSIS, and ARS. http://www.aphis.usda.gov/cahfse/swine/CAHFSE_Swine.htm.[63]
‡‡http://www.fda.gov/cvm/narms_pg.html.[51]

LIMITATIONS IN AVAILABILITY OF ANTIMICROBIAL AGENTS AND CONSEQUENCES TO ANIMAL AGRICULTURE AND VETERINARY MEDICINE

Experts have suggested that the main exposure of humans to resistant bacteria of food animal origin is through the food chain.[64,65] Despite differing opinions on the effect that antimicrobial use in food animal agriculture may have on development of resistant bacteria in food animals, as well as on the risk it may pose to human health, it is indisputable that many food animals harbor resistant bacteria in their intestinal tract regardless of how they are reared or managed. The concern over emergence of antimicrobial resistance in bacteria of food animal origin and the potential negative consequences to human health, as well as the subsequent repeated calls for reductions of antimicrobial usage and antimicrobial-resistant bacteria in animals intended for food consumption, has led

legislative agencies in many countries to consider what may be done to halt or slow down the emergence and dissemination of resistant bacteria in food animals. As a response to this debate, many veterinary associations and countries have instituted guidelines for judicious use of antimicrobial therapy in food and companion animals.[66,67] However, in some countries the response has been firmer and has resulted in restrictions or bans on the use of some or all antimicrobial for growth promotion purposes (see later).[22-24,53,68-72] Furthermore, the use of antimicrobial agents in food animal production has been suggested as an area where large reductions in usage may be possible.[3,73-76] However, the question still remains if subtherapeutic as compared with therapeutic use of antimicrobial agents increases the risk of development of resistance in bacteria remains (assuming that a definition of subtherapeutic can even be agreed on).

To a large extent the argument is speculative.[77] Furthermore, in the United States, an antimicrobial approved for therapeutic use in chickens was withdrawn from the market[78] because of concerns of the proposed negative impact on human health.[78,79] In addition, the FDA has now recommended the approval process for antimicrobial agents intended for use in food animals to include an assessment of the safety of antimicrobial new animal drugs to human health (FDA-CVM Guidance 152).[64] At the other end of the spectrum, some livestock producers have voluntarily decided to raise food animals in accordance with organic or antimicrobial-free guidelines, with little or no use of antimicrobial agents in their production of food animals.[25-27,33,38,80,81]

Ban of Antimicrobial Growth Promoters

As a response to cross-resistance between some growth promoters and their analogs used in human medicine, as well as their potential propagating effect on antimicrobial resistance, several countries have suspended or banned the use of antimicrobial agents for growth-promoting purposes.[22,23,70,71,82] This was, in part, done because of a reported association between the use of avoparcin and vancomycin-resistant *E. faecium* isolated from food animals[41,83-92] and cross-resistance between virginiamycin and quinopristin/dalfopristin.[93,94]

Sweden imposed a ban on AGP use in 1986 partly to maintain consumer confidence but also as a precautionary measure.[22,24,71] In 1995 Norway and Denmark followed suit by banning the use of avoparcin as an AGP.[22,23,72,86] In Denmark the use of virginiamycin was furthermore banned in 1998, and the same year the poultry industry voluntarily discontinued use of all growth promoters. In 1997 the European Union imposed a ban on use of avoparcin, and in 1999 a temporary ban was placed on spiramycin, tylosin, bacitracin, and virginiamycin.[23] Switzerland also imposed a ban on AGPs in 1999.[70]

As a result of the ban of growth promoters in some countries and a more rigorous approval process of antimicrobial new animal drugs, producers and producer organizations have voiced concerns about the potential consequences of such bans and the future availability of certain antimicrobial agents in food animal practice.[52] The possible effects of imposed bans on food animal production were summarized by McEwen and Fedorka-Cray (2002) and include (1) decreased incentive for development of new antimicrobial agents, (2) reduction in production efficiency, (3) increase in prophylactic or therapeutic use, (4) increase in incidence of infectious diseases in animals, and (5) limitations in drugs available to veterinarians and farmers for treatment and prevention of bacterial diseases.[95]

Effects on Animal Agriculture and Veterinary Medicine of Banned or Limited Antimicrobial Agents

Because antibiotics can exert a selective pressure to promote the development and propagation of resistance,[3,9] the presumption is that withdrawal of antimicrobial agents leads to a reduction in rates of antimicrobial resistance. A relevant question to be asked is, "How has the discontinuation of AGP use affected the levels of antimicrobial resistance in animal populations affected by the bans?" The first accounts of the large-scale removal of AGPs from poultry and pig production was published by Aarestrup in 2001. According to DANMAP data, the ban of avoparcin in 1996 resulted in a drastic decrease in percent of *Enterococcus faecium* resistant to vancomycin in poultry isolates from 72.7% in 1995 to 5.8% in 2000.[82] A similar decline was not seen in isolates from pigs until the use of tylosin as an AGP was banned in 1997, after which the percentage of resistant isolates also decreased in pigs.[82] This phenomenon was attributed to a linkage of genes coding for glycopeptides and macrolide resistance that were located on the same plasmid.[96] The resistance to glycopeptides has remained low through 2005 in isolates from broilers and pigs.[30] Overall, the Danish experience with ban of AGPs in food animal production has resulted in a substantial reduction in the levels of resistance to vancomycin, erythromycin, and virginiamycin.[82] *E. faecium* isolates from humans were included in the DANMAP monitoring in 2002, and resistance to vancomycin in these isolates has remained at zero through 2004 with a few isolates detected in 2005.[30]

The effect of reducing or eliminating the use of antimicrobial agents in food animal production has also been assessed in several cross-sectional studies comparing the levels of antimicrobial resistance in enteric bacteria among farms that use antimicrobial agents in their production when indicated (conventional farms) and farms that do not (organic or antimicrobial free farms).[25-27,33,41,80] In general, these studies have shown that the discontinuation of antimicrobial use significantly reduced the levels of resistance to some antimicrobial agents but not to others when comparing the two farm types. However, the levels of antimicrobial resistance still remained relatively high to some antimicrobial agents (e.g., tetracycline and sulfa drugs) in organic or antimicrobial-free production (Table 98-2).

Although a decrease in resistance to vancomycin in enterococci has been reported from a large national monitoring program,[30,82] several stand-alone studies on poultry farms have reported that vancomycin-resistant enterococci still could be detected in environmental samples from poultry houses and from poultry several years after avoparcin was banned.[87-92] These studies show that vancomycin-resistant enterococci can persist in the environment without the selective pressure from avoparcin even after thorough cleaning of the production units and repopulation of the units with chicks in which vancomycin-resistant enterococci were unlikely to be present.[89,91] In a comparison of vancomycin resistance in poultry flocks that were previously exposed to avoparcin use and flocks established after the ban, higher concentrations of vancomycin-resistant enterococci were found in previously exposed flocks.[87] However, they were still isolated from flocks established after the ban.[87] Discrepancies between results from the monitoring program in Denmark,[30,82] which showed a dramatic decline in vancomycin-resistant enterococci in monitoring samples after the ban, and studies showing that vancomycin-resistant enterococci are still cultivable on farms[89,90] may in part be explained by less sensitive isolation methods used in DANMAP. Regardless, the decline in DANMAP

Table 98-2

Levels of Antimicrobial Resistance in Bacteria Isolated from Animals Reared on Conventional and Antimicrobial-Free or Organic Farms

Animal Species	Bacterial Species	No. Antimicrobials Used for Susceptibility Testing	Sample Type	No. Herds ABF/Conv.	No. Samples ABF/Conv.	Antimicrobial	Percent of Isolates Resistant to Selected Antimicrobial Agents — Organic or Antibiotic Free	Conventional	Odds Ratio*	Reference
Dairy cattle	Escherichia coli	17	Feces	30/30	596/595	AMP	9.4	16.3	2.1	25†
						STR	12.3	18.4	1.8	
						KAN	9.4	18.8	2.6	
						GEN	1.3	3.9	3.2	
						CHL	0.9	3.9	4.4	
						TET	21.1	31.4	2.0	
						SLM	11.4	15.8	1.5	
Dairy cattle	Campylobacter	18	Feces, environmental, milk filters	128 total	450/1525 8/33 2/12	TET	49.3	58.3	$P < 0.01$§	26,107 †,‡
Dairy cattle	Salmonella	16 or 17	Feces, environmental, milk filters	26/69	1243	STR	30.4	7.7	7.5	33,107 †,‡
Pigs	Campylobacter	6	Feces, Carcass swabs at slaughter	10/11	660/450 166/183	TET	56.2	83.4	$P < 0.05$§	40‖
						ERY	34.5	77.0	$P < 0.05$§	
						TET	36.6	80.8	$P < 0.05$§	
						ERY	40.4	81.4	$P < 0.05$§	
Pigs	Salmonella	10	Feces, Carcass swabs at slaughter	10/10	503/200	AMP	12.4	35.3	3.9	36‖
						AMO	0.7	14.1	16.1	
						CHL	10.6	25.9	2.8	
						KAN	1.4	18.8	23.2	
						STR	36.2	10.9	10.9	
						TET	88.3	93.0	¶	
						SLM	30.1	64.7	4.3	
						AMP	3.2	23.5	9.7	
						AMO	1.8	3.5	¶	
						CHL	0.0	21.7	56.1	
						KAN	0.0	17.4	40.8	
						STR	30.3	54.8	2.9	
						TET	55.7	97.4	25.4	
						SLM	25.3	50.4		
Pigs	E. coli	17	Feces	35/60	498/883	AMP	13.1	24.1	3.0	27**
						SLM	21.9	31.6	2.0	
						TET	71.3	90.9	1.6	
						CHL	3.2	8.2	2.8	
						STR	20.9	28.9	2.7	

*Only antimicrobials for which there was a statistically significant difference in prevalence of resistance between ABF and Conv. farms were included in this table.
†Cattle within organic farms may have been treated with antimicrobial agents according to specific organic organizations' guidelines.
‡14 of 15 organic herds reporting using antimicrobial agents separated treated cattle from the rest of the herd.
§Odds ratio not reported.
‖Samples were collected from farms where antimicrobial agents were not used postweaning.
¶Not significantly different.
**Antimicrobial agents had not been used for 1 to 14 yr.

ABF, Antimicrobial-free or organic farms; AMO, (amoxicillin/clavulanic acid); AMP, ampicillin; CHL, chloramphenicol; Conv., conventional farms; ERY, erythromycin; GEN, gentamicin; KAN, kanamycin; SLM, sulfamethoxazole; STR, streptomycin; TET, tetracycline.

shows a quantitative reduction in the numbers of cultivable vancomycin-resistant enterococci[90] and hence may reduce the exposure of humans to these organisms. Nevertheless, experiences from Norway and Denmark show that extensive management and hygienic measures should be used along with a ban to prevent cross-contamination between flocks and to prevent the environment from serving as a reservoir for colonization of chickens as they enter production.

Incentive for the Pharmaceutical Industry to Develop Antimicrobial New Animal Drugs for Use in Food Animal Agriculture and Veterinary Medicine

It is difficult to predict how, if at all, the incentive for the development of new antimicrobial agents may be affected in the future, and it may be questionable whether the development of new antimicrobial agents can continue with the development of multi-resistant bacteria.[82]

Although several countries have banned the use of AGPs in an effort to prevent a rise in bacteria of animal origin resistant to antimicrobial agents that are of increasing importance for treatment of multi-resistant infections in humans, measures have so far not been quite as drastic in the United States. In the United States, the use of AGPs is still permitted. However, the FDA recently withdrew the approval of a fluoroquinolone for therapeutic use in chickens.[97] This decision was based partially on results from Spain that showed an increase in fluoroquinolone-resistant *Campylobacter* in human isolates following the approval of fluoroquinolones for use in poultry in the 1980s[98-100] and on a risk assessment conducted by the FDA that estimated the use of fluoroquinolones in chickens would have a negative impact on human health.[79,101,102] As a response to the potential negative effect of antimicrobial use in animals on human health, the FDA has published guidance documents that reflect this concern. The documents are "A Proposed Framework for Evaluating and Assuring the Human Safety of Antimicrobial New Animal Drugs Intended for Use in Food-Producing Animals" and "Guidance for Industry #152" (Evaluating the Safety of Antimicrobial New Animal Drugs with Regard to Their Microbiological Effects on Bacteria of Human Health Concern).[103-105] According to the Federal Food, Drug, and Cosmetic Act, the FDA must determine if new antimicrobial agents intended for use in food-producing animals are safe with respect to human health (21 CFR 514.1[b][8]). The agency recognizes that there is no certainty that adverse effects will not occur from use of antimicrobial agents in food animals, and the agency is therefore considering establishing thresholds for antimicrobial-resistant bacteria in food animals.[106] This predetermined threshold, if reached, would indicate that a certain antimicrobial is no longer safe for use in a particular food animal species. The framework document outlines the potential strategies needed for managing the risk to human health of the use of antimicrobial agents in food animals.[104] Guidance #152,[103] which is meant to guide the pharmaceutical industry through a qualitative risk assessment of the effect of the transmission of resistant food-borne bacteria consumed from

animal-derived food products on human health, is built on the concepts of the framework document. This guidance outlines the agency's general strategy for ensuring that new antimicrobial agents for use in food animals are safe with respect to human health.[105] Nonetheless, it is important to recognize that both Guidance #152 and the framework document are not legally binding documents, and unless specific regulatory or statutory requirements are mentioned, the guidance only describes the FDA's current thinking on the topic and should be considered the agency's recommendations.[105]

Effect of AGP Ban on Productivity and Occurrence of Diseases

The ban of AGP use in Sweden and other countries is fairly recent and relatively few studies have examined the consequences on production efficiency. Wierup (2001) reviewed the effects on production and antimicrobial use in Swedish agriculture following the ban of growth promoters in Sweden in 1986. The overall conclusion from the Swedish experience was that competitive production can be accomplished without the use of AGPs.[24] The ban did not come without problems, however. Necrotic enteritis in poultry initially resulted in treatment of 90% of broiler chickens with virginiamycin and later phenoxymethylpenicillin (penicillin V). However, since 1995, the amount of antibiotics needed to treat or prevent necrotic enteritis has been insignificant.[24] In pig production the ban initially resulted in a significant increase in postweaning mortality in pigs, but preweaning mortality did not change significant before and after the ban. In addition, postweaning mortality and days to reach 25 kg decreased. Importantly, the ban of AGPs was complemented by numerous management measures to optimize the rearing and production systems for both poultry and pigs. However, not all producers have optimal production facilities and some production parameters have not reached the preban levels.[24] A Finnish study of the effect of AGP ban in 1999 showed no changes in the number of weaned pigs per sow per year, age at weaning, and diarrhea incidence following the ban.[69] However, this study was limited to farms that had no prior problems with postweaning diarrhea, and farms with major problems in their husbandry and management practices were excluded.

Few cross-sectional studies comparing the levels of antimicrobial resistance among conventional and antimicrobial-free/organic farms have assessed the differences in production levels between the farm types. Zwald and colleagues (2004) showed that the rolling herd average and daily milk yield per cow were higher on conventional farms as compared with organic farms. However, this is likely due to differences in feeding practices (conventional farms were more likely to feed total mixed rations) between the two herd types.[107] In many instances ABF and organic farms are smaller than conventional farms and smaller farms may be less likely to have extensive record keeping for their herds, making comparison of production performance between the two herd types difficult.

The available literature examining the effects on production and disease occurrence as result of imposing AGP bans and conversion to organic production is relatively limited, and more studies are necessary to thoroughly investigate which "good management" practices can be instituted to reduce potential negative effects of restrictions in use of some or all antimicrobial agents. The Swedish and Finnish experience shows that the programs emphasizing good management practices may not experience increases in disease incidence and decreases in production.[24,69]

AGP Ban and Use of Therapeutic Antimicrobial Agents

Experts have suggested that the ban of AGPs will lead to an increase in use of antimicrobial agents for preventive and therapeutic uses. The effect was recently reviewed for Denmark, Norway, and Sweden.[22] In Denmark, from 1996 to 2003, the therapeutic use of antimicrobial agents doubled, but the overall tonnage of active substance decreased by 35%; however, in the same period the broiler and pig production also increased by 20%. The increase in therapeutic antimicrobial agents is largely attributed to an increased use in weaning pigs.[22,30] The therapeutic use appeared to have stabilized in 2004 and 2005.[30] In Norway the total and therapeutic uses of antimicrobial agents decreased by approximately 49% and 39%, respectively, from 1993-2003, while the production of slaughter pigs increased 10% and broiler production doubled in the same period.[22] In Sweden, from 1984-2003, the therapeutic uses decreased 49%, while broiler production roughly doubled and pig production declined slightly. These results from Scandinavia can be difficult to interpret because they are reported as tonnage of active substance compared with increases or declines in total production. A more appropriate measure is the prescribed daily dosage (PDD) per population at risk because it takes into account both the amount of antimicrobial use and the size of the population it is used on. In a study in one canton in Switzerland from 1996-2001 that investigated the impact of AGP ban in 1999 on the use of therapeutic antimicrobial agents,[70] the PPD per population was calculated for 17 antimicrobial agents. The Swiss results show that the PPD per population decreased 56% in 2001 as compared with 1996.[70] Although some results are difficult to interpret because of the reporting method, studies from Europe indicate that the ban of AGPs has led to an overall decrease in use of antimicrobial agents in food animal agriculture despite some problems controlling diseases, particularly in weaning pigs.

SUMMARY

Whether or not one believes that antimicrobial resistance in bacteria or food animal origin contributes to or increases the risk of resistant infections in humans, the argument has been used by several countries to ban the use of antimicrobial growth promoters. In addition, the first example of withdrawal of a therapeutic antimicrobial for use in a food animal species on the basis of the risk of resistance has occurred in the United States. Evidence indicates that removal of the selection pressure exerted by antimicrobial agents on bacteria to a certain extent will decrease the levels of antimicrobial resistance; however,

it is currently impossible to thoroughly assess the impact on public health. The effects seem to have occurred relatively quickly as a response to the AGP bans in Europe. However, antimicrobial-resistant bacteria are still found on farms that have not used antimicrobial agents for years and generalizations among bacteria-antimicrobial combinations should not be made. Although some experiences from Europe indicate that a ban of AGPs in chicken and swine production can be accomplished without substantial losses in production, the effect of such bans and/or withdrawals should be assessed in controlled studies or trials beforehand. In addition, trials that examine specific methods to reduce the levels and stop the dissemination of antimicrobial agents in and among food animal populations are desperately needed.

Currently, several national programs around the world are in place to monitor antimicrobial resistance in enteric bacteria of food animal origin. This information may be used in making decisions on whether or not to withdraw currently approved antimicrobial agents from the market. Although the impact of resistance to antimicrobial agents on public health from enteric bacteria from food animals is small compared with the overall pressure of antimicrobial agents used in human medicine, resistance in foodborne pathogens will likely receive even more attention in the future and judicious and appropriate use of antimicrobial agents in food animals is recommended to secure them as available therapeutics in food animal practice.

References

1. World Health Organization: *The medical impact of the use of antimicrobials in food animals*, Geneva, 2000, WHO.
2. World Health Organization: *Impact of antimicrobial growth promoter termination in Denmark. The WHO international review panel's evaluation of the termination of the use of antimicrobial growth promoters in Denmark*, Foulum, Denmark, November 6-9, 2002, WHO, Department of Communicable Diseases, Prevention and Eradication & Collaborating Centre for Antimicrobial Resistance in Foodborne Pathogens, 2003.
3. Witte W: Medical consequences of antibiotic use in agriculture, *Science* 279:996-997, 1998.
4. van den Bogaard AE, Stobberingh EE: Antimicrobial usage in animals: impact on bacterial resistance and public health, *Drugs* 58:589-607, 1999.
5. Levy SB: Antibiotic resistance: an ecological imbalance. In Chadwick DJ, Goode J, editors: *Antibiotic resistance: origins, evolution, selection, and spread*, New York, 1997, John Wiley & Sons, pp 1-14.
6. Angulo FJ, Nargund VV, Chiller TM et al: Evidence of an association between use of antimicrobial agents in food animals and antimicrobial resistance among isolates from humans and the human health consequences of such resistance, *J Vet Med B* 51:374-379, 2004.
7. Greenlees KJ: Animal drug human food safety toxicology and antimicrobial resistance—the square peg, *Int J Toxicol* 22:131-134, 2003.
8. World Health Organization: *WHO global principles for containment of antimicrobial resistance*, Geneva, 2001, WHO/CDS/CSR/DRS/2001.1.
9. Levy SB: Antibiotic use for growth promotion in animals: ecologic and public health consequences, *J Food Protect* 50:616-620, 1987.

10. Fey PD, Safranek TJ, Rupp ME et al: Ceftriaxone-resistant *Salmonella* infection acquired by a child from cattle, *N Engl J Med* 342:1242-1249, 2000.

11. Mølbak K, Baggesen DL, Aarestrup FM et al: An outbreak of multidrug-resistant, quinolone-resistant *Salmonella enterica* serotype typhimurium DT104, *N Engl J Med* 341:1420-1425, 1999.

12. Levy SB: Multidrug resistance, a sign of the times, *N Engl J Med* 338:1376-1378, 1998.

13. Anderson AD, Nelson JM, Rossiter S et al: Public health consequences of use of antimicrobial agents in food animals in the United States, *Microb Drug Resist* 4:373-379, 2003.

14. Phillips I, Casewell M, Cox T et al: Does the use of antibiotics in food animals pose a risk to human health? A critical review of published data, *J Antimicrob Chemother* 53:28-52, 2004.

15. World Health Organization: *Joint FAO/OIE/WHO expert workshop on non-human antimicrobial usage and antimicrobial resistance: scientific assessment*, Geneva, 2003, WHO.

16. Chiller TM, Barrett T, Angulo FJ: CDC studies incorrectly summarized in critical review, *J Antimicrob Chemother* 54:275-276, 2004.

17. Jensen VF, Neimann J, Hammerum AM et al: Does the use of antibiotics in food animals pose a risk to human health? An unbiased review? *J Antimicrob Chemother* 54:274-275, 2004.

18. Karp BE, Engberg J: Comment on: Does the use of antibiotics in food animals pose a risk to human health? A critical review of published data, *J Antimicrob Chemother* 54:273-274, 2004.

19. Tollefson L: Factual errors in review article, *J Antimicrob Chemother* 54:271, 2004.

20. Phillips I, Casewell M, Cox T et al: Does the use of antibiotics in food animals pose a risk to human health? A reply to critics, *J Antimicrob Chemother* 54:276-278, 2004.

21. Aarestrup FM: Veterinary drug usage and antimicrobial resistance in bacteria of animal origin, *Basic Clin Pharmacol Toxicol* 96:271-281, 2005.

22. Grave K, Frøkjær Jensen V, Odensvik K et al: Usage of veterinary therapeutic antimicrobials in Denmark, Norway and Sweden following termination of antimicrobial growth promoter use, *Prevent Vet Med* 75:123-132, 2006.

23. Emborg H-D, Andersen JS, Seyfarth AM et al: Relations between the consumption of antimicrobial growth promoters and the occurrence of resistance among *Enterococcus faecium* isolated from broilers, *Epidemiol Infect* 132:95-105, 2003.

24. Wierup M: The Swedish experience of the 1986 year ban of antimicrobial growth promoters, with special reference to animal health, disease prevention, productivity, and usage of antimicrobials, *Microb Drug Resist* 7:183-190, 2001.

25. Sato K, Bartlett PC, Saeed MA: Antimicrobial susceptibility of *Escherichia coli* isolates from dairy farms using organic versus conventional production methods, *J Am Med Assoc* 226:589-594, 2005.

26. Halbert LW: Evaluation of antimicrobial susceptibility patterns in *Campylobacter* spp. isolated from dairy cattle and farms managed organically and conventionally in the Midwestern and northeastern United States, *J Am Vet Assoc* 228:1074-1081, 2006.

27. Bunner CA, Norby B, Bartlett PC, et al: Prevalence and patterns of antimicrobial susceptibility in *Escherichia coli* isolated from pigs reared under antibiotic-free and conventional production methods in the Midwestern United States, *J Am Vet Med Assoc* 231:275-283.

28. Barza M: Potential mechanisms of increased disease in humans from antimicrobial resistance in food animals, *Clin Infect Dis* 34(suppl 3):S123-125, 2002.

29. Aarestrup FM: The origin, evolution, and local and global dissemination of antimicrobial resistance. In Aarestrup FM, editor: *Antimicrobial resistance in bacteria of animal origin*, Washington, DC, 2006, ASM Press.

30. DANMAP: *Use of antimicrobial agents and occurrence of antimicrobial resistance in bacteria from food animals, foods and humans in Denmark*, Copenhagen, Denmark, 2005, Danish Zoonosis Center.

31. United States Department of Agriculture: *National Antimicrobial Resistance Monitoring System (NARMS)*, Washington, DC, 2005, USDA.

32. Warnick LD, Kanistanon K, McDonough PL et al: Effect of previous antimicrobial treatment on fecal shedding of *Salmonella enterica* subsp. *enterica* serogroup B in New York dairy herds with recent clinical salmonellosis, *Prevent Vet Med* 56:285-297, 2003.

33. Ray K, Warnick LD, Mitchell R et al: Antimicrobial susceptibility of Salmonella from organic and conventional dairy farms, *J Dairy Sci* 89:2038-2050, 2006.

34. Dunlop RH, McEwen SA, Meek AH et al: Prevalences of resistance to seven antimicrobials among fecal *Escherichia coli* of swine on thirty-four farrow-to-finish farms in Ontario, Canada, *Prev Vet Med* 34:265-282, 1998.

35. Gebreyes WA, Davies PR, Morrow WEM et al: Antimicrobial resistance of *Salmonella* isolates from swine, *J Clin Microbiol* 38:4633-4636, 2000.

36. Gebreyes WA, Thakur S, Morrow WE: Comparison of prevalence, antimicrobial resistance, and occurrence of multidrug-resistant *Salmonella* in antimicrobial-free and conventional pig production, *J Food Protect* 69:743-748, 2006.

37. Mathew AG, Saxton AM, Upchurch WG et al: Multiple antibiotic resistance patterns of *Escherichia coli* isolates from swine farms, *Applied Environ Microbiol* 65:2770-2772, 1999.

38. Mathew AG, Beckmann M, Saxton A: A comparison of antimicrobial resistance in bacteria isolated from swine herds in which antimicrobials were used or excluded, *Swine Health Prod* 10:7-13, 2001.

39. Mathew AG: Effects of antibiotic regimens on resistance of *Escherichia coli* and *Salmonella* serovar Typhimurium in swine, *J Swine Health Prod* 10:7-13, 2002.

40. Thakur S, Gebreyes WA: Prevalence and antimicrobial resistance of Campylobacter in antimicrobial-free and conventional pig production systems, *J Food Protect* 68:2402-2410, 2005.

41. Aarestrup FM: Occurrence of glycopeptide resistance among *Enterococcus faecium* isolates from conventional and ecological poultry farms, *Microb Drug Resist* 1:255-257, 1995.

42. Arvanitidou M, Tsakris A, Sofianou D et al: Antimicrobial resistance and R-factor transfer of salmonellae isolated from chicken carcasses in Greek hospitals, *Int J Food Microbiol* 40:197-201, 1998.

43. Cormican M, Buckley V, Corbett-Feeney G et al: Antimicrobial resistance in *Escherichia coli* isolates from turkeys and hens in Ireland, *J Antimicrob Chemother* 48:587-588, 2001.

44. Pavia M, Nobile CGA, Salpietro L et al: Vancomycin resistance and antibiotic susceptibility of enterococci in raw meat, *J Food Protect* 63:912-915, 2000.

45. Oliveira SDd, Flores FS, Santos LRd et al: Antimicrobial resistance in *Salmonella enteritidis* strains isolated from broiler carcasses, food, human and poultry-related samples, *Int J Food Microbiol* 97:297-305, 2005.

46. Johnson JM, Rajic A, McMullen LM: Antimicrobial resistance of selected Salmonella isolates from food animals and food in Alberta, *Can Vet J* 46:141-146, 2005.

47. Johnson JR, Kuskowski MA, Smith K et al: Antimicrobial-resistant and extraintestinal pathogenic Escherichia coli in retail foods, *J Infect Dis* 191:1040-1049, 2005.

48. Hayes JR, English LL, Carter PJ et al: Prevalence and antimicrobial resistance of *Enterococcus* species isolated from retail meats, *Applied Environ Microbiol* 69:7153-7160, 2003.

49. Busani L, Grosso MD, Paladini C et al: Antimicrobial susceptibility of vancomycin-susceptible and -resistant enterococci isolated in Italy from raw meat products, farm animals, and human infections, *Int J Food Microbiol* 97:17-22, 2004.

50. Canadian Integrated Program for Antimicrobial Resistance Surveillance: Public Health Agency of Canada, 2006.

51. Food and Drug Administration: National Antimicrobial Resistance Monitoring System (NARMS), Washington DC, 2006, FDA.

52. McEwen SA, Aarestrup FM, Jordan D: Monitoring antimicrobial resistance in animals: principles and practices. In Aarestrup FM, editor: *Antimicrobial resistance in bacteria of animal origin*, Washington, DC, 2006, ASM Press.

53. Aarestrup FM, Bager F, Madsen M et al: Surveillance of antimicrobial resistance in bacteria isolated from food animals to antimicrobial growth promoters and related therapeutic agents in Denmark, *APMIS* 106:745-770, 1998.

54. DANMAP: *Consumption of antimicrobial agents and occurrence of antimicrobial resistance in bacteria from food animals, foods and humans in Denmark*, Copenhagen, Danish Zoonosis Center, 2000.

55. DANMAP: *Use of antimicrobial agents and occurrence of antimicrobial resistance in bacteria from food animals, foods and humans in Denmark*, Copenhagen, 1998, Danish Zoonosis Center.

56. DANMAP: *Use of antimicrobial agents and occurrence of antimicrobial resistance in bacteria from food animals, foods and humans in Denmark*, Copenhagen, 1999, Danish Zoonosis Center.

57. DANMAP: *Use of antimicrobial agents and occurrence of antimicrobial resistance in bacteria from food animals, foods and humans in Denmark*, Copenhagen, 2001, Danish Zoonosis Center.

58. DANMAP: *Use of antimicrobial agents and occurrence of antimicrobial resistance in bacteria from food animals, foods and humans in Denmark*, Copenhagen, 2002, Danish Zoonosis Center.

59. DANMAP: *Use of antimicrobial agents and occurrence of antimicrobial resistance in bacteria from food animals, foods and humans in Denmark*, Copenhagen, 2003, Danish Zoonosis Center.

60. DANMAP: *Use of antimicrobial agents and occurrence of antimicrobial resistance in bacteria from food animals, foods and humans in Denmark*, Copenhagen, 2004, Danish Zoonosis Center.

61. DANMAP: *Consumption of antimicrobial agents and occurrence of antimicrobial resistance in bacteria from food animals, foods and humans in Denmark*, Copenhagen, 1996, Danish Zoonosis Center.

62. DANMAP: *Consumption of antimicrobial agents and occurrence of antimicrobial resistance in bacteria from food animals, foods and humans in Denmark*, Copenhagen, 1997, Danish Zoonosis Center.

63. U.S. Department of Agriculture: *Collaboration in Animal Health and Food Safety Epidemiology (CAHFSE)*, Fort Collins, Colorado, 2004, USDA.

64. Food and Drug Administration: *Guidance 152*, Washington, DC, 2003, FDA.

65. Tollefson L, Flynn WT, Headrick ML: Regulatory activities of the U.S. Food and Drug Administration designed to control antimicrobial resistance in food borne pathogens. In Torrence M, Isackson RE, editors: *Microbial food safety in animal agriculture*, Ames, Iowa, 2003, Iowa State Press, pp 57-63.

66. American Veterinary Medical Association: Judicious therapeutic use of antimicrobials, Schaumburg, Ill, 1998 (revised 2004), The Association.

67. Morley PS, Apley MD, Besser TE et al: Antimicrobial drug use in veterinary medicine. ACVIM Consensus Statement, *J Intern Med* 19:617-629, 2005.

68. Tornøe N: *Consequences of the termination of antimicrobial growth promoter use for broiler health and usage of antimicrobials for therapy and prophylaxis*. Working papers for the WHO international review evaluation, from the invitational symposium "Beyond antimicrobial growth promoters in animal production," Foulum, Denmark, 2002, WHO Collaborating Centre for Antimicrobial Resistance in Foodborne Pathogens.

69. Laine T, Yliaho M, Myllys V et al: The effect of antimicrobial growth promoter withdrawal on the health of weaned pigs in Finland, *Prev Vet Med* 163-174, 2004.

70. Arnold S, Gassner B, Giger T et al: Banning antimicrobial growth promoters in feedstuffs does not result in increased therapeutic use of antibiotics in medicated feed in pig farming, *Pharmacoepidemiol Drug Safety* 13:323-331, 2004.

71. Swedish Government Official Reports series (SOU): *Antimicrobial feed additives. Report from the commission on antimicrobial feed additives*, Stockholm, 1997, SOU.

72. Grave K, Kaldhusdal M, Kruse H et al: What has happened in Norway after the ban of avoparcin? Consumption of antimicrobials for poultry, *Prev Vet Med* 62:59-72, 2004.

73. Bates J, Jordens JZ, Griffiths DT: Farm animals as a putative reservoir for vancomycin-resistant enterococcal infection in man [see comments], *J Antimicrob Chemother* 34:507-514, 1994.

74. Swartz MN: Human diseases caused by foodborne pathogens of animal origin, *Clin Infect Dis* 34:S111-S122, 2002.

75. van den Bogaard AE, London N, Stobberingh EE: Antimicrobial resistance in pig faecal samples from the Netherlands (five abattoirs) and Sweden, *J Antimicrob Chemother* 45: 663-671, 2000.

76. van den Bogaard AE, London N, Driessen C et al: Antimicrobial resistance of fecal Escherichia coli in poultry, poultry farmers, and poultry slaughterers, *J Antimicrob Chemother* 47:763-771, 2001.

77. National Academy of Science Committee on Drug Use in Food Animals: *The use of drugs in food animals, benefits and risks*, Washington, DC, 1999, NAC.

78. U.S. Department of Health and Human Services Food and Drug Administration: *Withdrawal of approval of the new animal drug application for enrofloxacin in poultry*, Washington, DC, 2005, FDA.

79. Bartholomew MJ, Hollinger K, Vose D: Characterizing the risk of antimicrobial use in food animals: fluoroquinolone-resistant *Campylobacter* from consumption of chicken. In Torrence M, Isackson RE, editors: *Microbial food safety in animal agriculture*, Ames, Iowa, 2003, Iowa State Press, pp 293-301.

80. Heuer OE, Pedersen K, Andersen JS et al: Prevalence and antimicrobial susceptibility of thermophilic *Campylobacter* in organic and conventional broiler flocks, *Lett Appl Microbiol* 33:269-274, 2001.

81. Sato K, Bartlett PC, Kaneene JB et al: Comparison of prevalence and antimicrobial susceptibilities of *Campylobacter* spp. isolates from organic and conventional dairy herds in Wisconsin, *Appl Environ Microbiol* 1442-1447, 2004.

82. Aarestrup FM, Seyfarth AM, Emborg H-D et al: Effect of abolishment of the use of antimicrobial agents for growth promotion on occurrence of antimicrobial resistance in fecal enterococci in food animals in Denmark, *Antimicrob Agents Chemother* 45:2054-2059, 2001.

83. Klare I, Heier H, Claus H et al: *Enterococcus faecium* strains with *vanA*-mediated high-level glycopeptide resistance isolated from animal foodstuffs and faecal samples of humans in the community, *Microb Drug Resist* 1:265-272, 1995.

84. Klare I, Heier H, Claus H et al: *vanA*-mediated high-level glycopeptide resistance in *Enterococcus faecium* from animal husbandry, *FEMS Microbiol Lett* 125:165-171, 1995.

85. Bager F, Madsen M, Christensen J et al: Avoparcin used as growth promoters is associated with the occurrence of vancomycin-resistant *Enterococcus faecium* on Danish poultry and pig farms, *Prevent Vet Med* 31:95-112, 1997.

86. Aarestrup FM, Ahrens P, Madsen M et al: Glycopeptide susceptibility among Danish *Enterococcus faecium* and *Enterococcus faecalis* isolates of animal and human origin and PCR identification of genes within the VanA cluster, *Antimicrob Agents Chemother* 40:1938-1940, 1996.

87. Sørum M, Holstad G, Lillehaug A et al: Prevalence of vancomycin resistant enterococci on poultry farms established after the ban of avoparcin, *Avian Dis* 48:823-828, 2004.

88. Manson JM, Smith JMB, Cook GM: Persistence of vancomycin-resistant enterococci in New Zealand broilers after discontinuation of avoparcin use, *Appl Environ Microbiol* 70:5764-5768, 2004.

89. Heuer OE, Pedersen R, Jensen LB et al: Persistence of vancomycin-resistant enterococci (VRE) in broiler houses after the avoparcin ban, *Microb Drug Resist* 8:355-361, 2002.

90. Heuer OE, Pedersen R, Andersen JS et al: Vancomycin-resistant enterococci (VRE) in Broiler flocks 5 years after the avoparcin ban, *Microb Drug Resist* 8:133-138, 2002.

91. Borgen K, Sørum M, Kruse H et al: Persistence of vancomycin-resistant enterococci (VRE) on Norwegian broiler farms, *FEMS Microbiol Lett* 191:255-258, 2000.

92. Borgen K, Simonsen GS, Sundafjord A et al: Continuing high prevalence of VanA-type vancomycin-resistant enterococci on Norwegian poultry farms three years after avoparcin was banned, *J Appl Microbiol* 89:478-485, 2000.

93. Hammerum AM, Jensen LB, Aarestrup FM: Detection of *satA* gene and transferability of virginiamycin resistance in *Enterococcus faecium* from food-animals, *FEMS Microbiol Lett* 168:145-151, 1998.

94. Wegener HC, Aarestrup FM, Gerner-Smidt P et al: Transfer of antibiotic resistant bacteria from animals to man, *Acta Vet Scand* 92:51-57, 1999.

95. McEwen SA, Fedorka-Cray PJ: Antimicrobial use and resistance in animals, *Clin Infect Dis* 34(suppl 3):S93-S106, 2002.

96. Aarestrup FM: Characterization of glycopeptide-resistant *Enterococcus faecium* (GRE), from broilers and pigs in Denmark: genetic evidence that persistence of GRE in pig herds is associated with coselection by resistance to macrolides, *J Clin Microbiol* 38:2774-2777, 2000.

97. 556 DoHaHSFaDACPa: *Animal drugs, feeds, and related products; enrofloxacin for poultry; withdrawal of approval of new animal drug application*, Washington, DC, 2005, Federal Register.

98. Endtz H, Ruijs G, van Klingeren B et al: Quinolone resistance in *Campylobacter* isolates from man and poultry following the introduction of fluoroquinolones in veterinary medicine, *J Antimicrob Chemother* 27:199-208, 1991.

99. Smith K, Besser J, Hedberg C et al: Quinolone-resistant *Campylobacter jejuni* infections in Minnesota, 1992-1998, *N Engl J Med* 340:1525-1532, 1999.

100. Valenquez J, Jimenez A, Chomon B et al: Incidence and transmission of antimicrobial resistance in *Campylobacter jejuni* and, *Campylobacter coli*, *J Antimicrob Chemother* 35:173-178, 1995.

101. Bartholomew MJ, vose DJ, Tollefson LR et al: A linear model for managing the risk of antimicrobial resistance in food animals, *Risk Anal* 25:99-108, 2005.

102. Vose D, Hollinger K, Bartholomew M et al: *The human health impact of fluoroquinolone resistant campylobacter attributed to the consumption of chickens*, Rockville, Md, 2001, Food and Drug Administration.

103. Food and Drug Administration: *Guidance for industry #78. Consideration of the human health impact of microbial effects of antimicrobial new animal drugs intended for use in food-producing animals*, Rockville, Md, 1999, FDA, Center for Veterinary Medicine.

104. Food and Drug Administration: *A proposed framework for evaluating and assuring the human safety of antimicrobial new animal drugs intended for use in food-producing animals*, Rockville, Md, 1999, FDA, Center for Veterinary Medicine.

105. Food and Drug Administration: *Guidance for industry #152. Evaluating the safety of antimicrobial new drugs with regard to their microbiological effects on bacteria of human health concerns*, Rockville, Md, 2003, FDA, Center for Veterinary Medicine.

106. Food and Drug Administration: *An approach for establishing thresholds in association with the use of antimicrobial drugs in food-producing animals. A discussion document*, Rockville, Md, 2000, FDA, Center for Veterinary Medicine.

107. Zwald AG, Ruegg PL, Kaneene JB et al: Management practices and reported antimicrobial usage on conventional and organic dairy farms, *J Dairy Sci* 87:191-201, 2004.

108. Centers for Disease Control and Prevention: *National Antimicrobial Resistance Monitoring System for Enteric Bacteria (NARMS): 2003 Human Isolates Final Report*, Atlanta, 2006, U.S. Department of Health and Human Services, CDC.

109. Centers for Disease Control and Prevention: *Foodborne active surveillance network (FoodNet), population survey atlas of exposures, 2002*, Atlanta, 2004, CDC.

CHAPTER 99

Evidence-Based Veterinary Medicine: Therapeutic Considerations

ROBERT L. LARSON and VIRGINIA R. FAJT

Evidence-based medicine (EBM) was introduced to the medical literature in a 1992 article by the Evidence-based Working Group at McMaster University Health Sciences Centre in Canada to label the clinical learning strategy they had been developing for more than a decade.[1] The basic concepts of EBM are being applied to the veterinary profession under the term *evidence-based veterinary medicine* (EBVM).[2-4] The underlying concepts of EBM and EBVM are rooted in clinical epidemiology and are not new, but the formal and explicit incorporation of research evidence into practice settings has not previously been integrated into the veterinary profession.[5]

Sackett and colleagues[6] initially defined EBM as the "conscientious, explicit and judicious use of current best evidence from clinical care research in making decisions about the care of individual patients." Because of a need to highlight the role of clinical skills and patient values, the definition of EBM was later refined to "evidence-based medicine is the integration of best research evidence with clinical expertise and patient values."[7] Using this definition as a foundation, the definition of EBVM could be "evidence-based veterinary medicine is the integration of best research evidence with clinical expertise and owner/manager values."

Today's veterinarians are taught to practice based primarily on textbooks, expert opinions, veterinary journals, or experience. These sources often lack scientific scrutiny and frequently do not constitute the best evidence available. Failure to learn methods to find and evaluate evidence will make veterinarians poorly suited to providing accurate, up-to-date information about therapeutic and other aspects of veterinary medicine.

In the context of making therapeutic decisions, "best research evidence" means clinically relevant research that tests the efficacy and safety of therapeutics.[7] When possible, veterinarians should use evidence derived from systematic, rigorous, controlled clinical studies in the target species to make diagnostic and treatment decisions. Unfortunately, the best available evidence for veterinary practitioners often entails extrapolations of pathophysiologic principles, studies in other species, and logic rather than established facts based on data derived from clinical trials in the same species (modified from Rosenberg and Sackett[8]).

LEVELS OF EVIDENCE

Although all or most veterinary clinical decisions are based on evidence of some type, some evidence is strong (rigorously tested in the target species under natural conditions in experiments designed to prove a theory to be false), some is weak (not tested), and some is intermediate.[9-11] The hierarchy of evidence is based on the strength of evidence of causation, the ability of the study to control bias, and the similarity between the study population and the population currently being considered in a clinical setting. Sources regarded as strong evidence for therapeutic questions include randomized controlled clinical trials in the target species under a similar husbandry environment or systematic reviews of more than one trial (meta-analysis) that meet these criteria. These are followed by progressively weaker epidemiologic studies—cohort studies, case-control studies, and case-series—and then controlled experimental challenge trials. The weakest evidence includes opinions based on in vitro research, pathophysiologic rationale, and uncontrolled observations. Uncontrolled observations are often used as the rationale for making therapeutic decisions (e.g., "I treat with Drug A and the animals get better") but ought to be considered the weakest evidence. (See Table 99-1 for descriptions of study types.)

The body of evidence relevant to answering clinical questions is the sum of multiple studies investigating the same area of interest. Each research study contributes to that body of evidence and each publication can be ranked on a scale from weak to strong evidence. Traditional sources of evidence include printed material such as textbooks, personal journal collections, conference proceedings, and clinical guidelines. Unfortunately, the number of studies and amount of available literature decreases as one moves from weak to strong evidence.

Although a simple ranking of experimental trial types is helpful to describe ascending levels of evidence, by its simplistic nature, it incorrectly depicts levels of evidence as a one-dimensional and straightforward hierarchy. For example, veterinarians are often confronted with determinations such as, "Which is better evidence, a randomized trial in a related species, or a case-control study in the target species?" In these situations the clinical expertise and judgment of the veterinarian must be

Table **99-1**

Study Types

Experimental studies	Laboratory study	Investigator assigns subjects to study groups and rigorously controls the study conditions in a laboratory setting.
	Randomized controlled clinical study	Investigator assigns subjects to study groups randomly (i.e., one group gets treatment, the other does not). This is the best experimental design to study therapeutic interventions.
	Randomized controlled field study	Investigator assigns subjects to study groups randomly, but contrasted to clinical studies, the intervention is prevention rather than treatment (i.e., used to evaluate the effectiveness of vaccines or other preventive measures).
Observational studies	Prospective cohort study	Investigator clearly defines the study cohorts without the outcome (disease) in question. The study groups are alike in many ways, but different in one exposure factor. The groups are followed forward in time and compared for the outcome of interest. This study type provides good estimations of risk for the groups studied, but they are long, costly studies that can only evaluate the exposure factors identified at the start of the trial when data collection began. These types of trials are best suited for common outcomes (diseases).
	Retrospective (nonconcurrent or historical) cohort study	Investigator uses a database to look at cohorts where both the exposure and outcome have occurred before the study begins. This type of study is fast and inexpensive compared with a prospective cohort study and is useful to study rare exposures. However, because the data collection is not controlled by the investigator, selection bias, misclassification, and confounding are significant risks.
	Case-control study	Investigator chooses a case group and a control group based on a known outcome (i.e., those having the disease and those without the disease), and then the groups are compared as to frequency of exposure to past risk. This type of study is fast and inexpensive and is useful to study the association of many risk factors to rare diseases. But selection bias and recall bias are significant risks.
	Cross-sectional study	Investigator determines the exposure and risk at the same point in time. This fast and inexpensive study type can determine prevalence but cannot determine incidence or prove causes.
Literature review	Meta-analysis	A meta-analysis is a mathematic synthesis of the results of two or more primary studies that addressed the same hypothesis in the same way. Meta-analysis attempts to overcome the problem of reduced statistical power in studies with small sample sizes.
	Systematic review	A systematic review is an overview of primary studies that contains an explicit statement of objectives, materials, and methods and has been conducted according to explicit and reproducible methodology. The search for relevant articles must be thorough and objective, and the criteria used to reject articles as "flawed" must be explicit and independent of the results of those trials.

used to aid the ranking by questioning whether the differences between species are likely to affect the issues being studied.

Veterinarians considering the strength of evidence must use several perspectives to determine the reliability of research for clinical use. The first consideration is the internal validity of the research, which is determined by the study method and appropriate use of controls for bias. Research reports with good internal validity provide assurance that the results represent an unbiased estimate of the true direction and magnitude of the treatment effect. Types of bias and methods of controlling for bias are described in Table 99-2. The second consideration is the population used in the research and its appropriateness as a model for the population that generated the clinical question. Generally, the target species in similar housing and husbandry environments provides stronger evidence than the target species in significantly different housing and husbandry environments, related species, unrelated species, or in vitro methods. Thirdly, the clinical relevance of the outcomes of the research should be considered with patient-/herd-oriented outcomes providing more direct evidence than disease-oriented outcome measurements. Using these considerations, the highest

rating in all three dimensions would provide the highest level of evidence.

These three considerations can be used to evaluate the strength and quality of evidence in a published study, by asking the following questions: *"First, are the results of this individual study valid?"* This can be addressed by determining if the assignment of patients to treatments was randomized and if the caregivers and clinicians were blind to those assignments. Also important is that all animals in a group or treatment were evaluated (even dropouts, e.g., look for "intent-to-treat" or "deads-in and deads-out" analyses), and that all groups were treated equally except for the experimental therapy. Of additional importance is that the trial last long enough to recognize both potential positive and negative outcomes. Randomization of study subjects to treatment groups is critical for study validity. Studies in which treatment is allocated by any method other than randomization tend to show larger and frequently false-positive treatment effects than do randomized trials.[12-14]

If it seems that the study results are valid, the second question one needs to ask is, *"Are the valid results of this individual study important?"* Or asked another way, *"How large was the treatment effect?"* This question may be

Table 99-2

Bias

Types of bias	Selection bias	Selection bias occurs when factors affect the selection of study subjects so that the study groups are not similar. Allocation of subjects to groups in a nonrandom manner and nonresponse or missing data can lead to selection bias.
	Information bias	Information bias occurs when inaccurate information on the exposure, outcome, and covariates of interest is used in a study. Incorrect classification of categorical variables such as the presence or absence of risk factors or the presence or absence of outcome variables is *misclassification bias*. Incorrect classification of continuous variables is *measurement error*. And *recall bias* can occur in retrospective observational studies when study subjects with or without the outcome of interest systematically recall risk factors with different sensitivity or specificity.
	Confounding bias	Confounding bias is due to the effects of factors other than the exposure of interest on the observed measure of association. Confounding can obscure a true effect, create the illusion of an effect where none exists, or estimate an effect (i.e., benefit/cost analysis) that is artificially high or low. Proper randomization is the best method to deal with known and unknown confounding factors. In addition, blocking and restriction are methods of experimental design and regression models and stratified analysis are methods of statistical interpretation to control known confounding factors.
Control for bias	Randomization	Simple randomization involves a formal method to allocate subjects to study groups in a manner such that each subject has an equal chance to be in each study group. Randomization is an important safeguard to prevent selection and confounding bias.
	Blinding (also called masking)	Investigators and animal handlers do not know during the study which subjects are allocated to which study group. This is an important safeguard to prevent information bias.
	Intent-to-treat analysis	Because patients or their owner/managers in a clinical trial may fail to comply with the treatment to which they were randomly assigned, differences (bias) may cause the treatment groups to differ in ways other than the treatment effect. To maintain the integrity of the randomization scheme, an intention-to-treat analysis includes all randomized patients in the groups to which they were randomly assigned, regardless of their adherence with the entry criteria, the treatment they actually received, and subsequent withdrawal from treatment or deviation from the protocol. Contrary to intention-to-treat analysis would be to only include individuals who actually completed their assigned treatment properly and eliminate consideration of all individuals who failed to follow their assigned protocol.
	Sufficient study length	Studies must last long enough to recognize both potential positive and negative outcomes to avoid misclassification bias.
	Multivariable regression model	Multivariable regression models provide an estimate of the effect of the factor of interest on the outcome of interest after controlling for the effects of all the other factors in the equation. The outcome is not biased (confounded) by any variable included in the regression equation.

Box 99-1

Measuring the Commoness (Risk) of Categorical Outcomes

Proportion	Proportion is a ratio in which the numerator is a subset of the denominator.
Odds	Odds is a ratio in which the numerator is not a subset of the denominator.
Rate	Rate is a ratio in which the denominator is the number of animal-time units at risk.
Prevalence	Prevalence is the proportion of sampled individuals with an outcome of interest at a given point in time. A prevalence estimate includes both new and old cases and can be determined in cross-sectional and case-control studies.
Incidence risk	Incidence risk is the proportion of individuals that develop a condition of interest over a defined period of time and only measures cases that have their onset during the time specified. Incidence is used in cohort studies to measure the effect of risk factors but cannot be calculated in cross-sectional and case-control studies.
Incidence rate	Incidence rate (incidence density) is the number of new cases (events) in a population per unit of animal-time during a given time period.

addressed by a report of the magnitude of treatment effect, such as relative risk reduction, absolute risk reduction, or number needed to treat (see Box 99-1 for descriptions of measures of commonness of outcomes and Box 99-2 for descriptions of measures of association). To determine if a particular magnitude of effect is important, the effect produced by the therapy in question should be compared with the magnitude of effect for other interventions and durations of therapy. The true magnitude of

effect of a therapy can never be known, but a valid trial provides a point estimate around which the true effect is expected to lie. The 95% confidence interval (CI) of the point estimate of the treatment effect is commonly reported to communicate the precision of the estimate of the treatment effect and indicates the range that includes the true treatment effect 95% of the time. CIs reflect the level of uncertainty in point estimates and indicate the expected range of values within which the true effect is

Box 99-2

Measures of Association

Measures of association are used to assess the magnitude of the relationship between a risk factor and an outcome. Strength of association is usually measured by ratio measures such as risk ratio or odds ratio but can be measured by risk or rate differences. Larger associations are related to less likelihood that unknown or residual confounding might have produced the observed effect.

Absolute risk reduction (ARR)	ARR indicates the percentage of animals that are spared the outcome of interest as a result of the intervention being tested by simply calculating the difference in the risk of the outcome in the population with the intervention or risk factor subtracted from the risk of the outcome of interest in the control population. ARR becomes smaller as risk in the control population decreases.
Relative risk reduction (RRR)	The RRR is the difference in risk between the intervention population and the control population divided by the risk in the control population. The RRR tends to stay the same across populations with varying risk of the outcome and can therefore be quite large even in populations at low risk of the outcome in question.
Number needed to treat (NNT)	NNT indicates the number of animals needed to treat in a defined period of time to avoid one negative outcome and is calculated as 1/ARR. NNT is helpful for making clinical decisions because it includes the efficacy of the intervention and the risk of the outcome without the intervention.
Number needed to harm (NNH)	NNH indicates the number of animals treated in a defined period of time for each adverse outcome or side effect of that intervention.
Risk ratio (relative risk) (RR)	Used in cohort studies but not case-control and cross-sectional studies. An RR near 1 implies no association between the outcome and risk factor. The greater the deviation from 1, the greater the magnitude of association. RR does not consider the amount of outcome occurring in a population in that the outcome frequency could be low, but the RR high.
Incidence rate (IR) ratio	The IR ratio can only be computed from studies where an incidence rate is calculated such as cohort studies. IR is the ratio of the disease frequency measured as an incidence rate in an exposed group to the incidence rate in a nonexposed group.
Odds ratio (OR)	The OR can be used in logistic regression analysis and is the only choice for measuring association between an exposure or intervention and an outcome of interest in case-control studies. The OR is the odds of having the exposure or intervention in question in populations with the outcome in question divided by the odds of having the exposure or intervention in question in populations without the outcome of interest.
Survival analysis	Survival analysis is equivalent to time-to-event analysis. Because survival analysis data are censored and abnormal, they cannot be analyzed by traditional parametric and nonparametric tests. The life table, survival distribution, and Kaplan-Meier survival function estimation are all descriptive methods for estimating the distribution of survival times from a sample.

likely to fall. Exact CIs are based on the exact probabilities of the distributions (known variance) underlying the parameter (binomial for proportions, Poisson for rates, and hypergeometric for odds ratios). If variance is not known, an estimate of the variance can be obtained and then an approximate CI calculated. The larger the sample size and the larger the number of outcome events, the greater is one's confidence that the true treatment effect is near the point estimate (narrow 95% CI). To determine the importance of a reported positive treatment effect, one should look at the lower boundary of the CI. If this lower boundary is important to you as a clinician, then you are confident that the treatment in question only has a 2.5% chance of failing to reach this lower boundary and the treatment can be deemed important. In contrast, if the treatment effect indicated by the lower boundary is not clinically important to you, the study cannot definitively indicate an important treatment effect even if the results are statistically significant. Similarly, to determine the risk of a reported neutral or negative treatment effect, one should look at the upper boundary of the CI. If the upper boundary is clinically important, you cannot exclude the possibility that an important treatment effect is possible even though the trial indicated either no

difference between treatment and controls or a negative treatment effect.

And finally, if a study appears to be valid and important, *"Are the valid, important results of this study applicable to my client's patient or herd?"*[15] If the study animals or treatment setting is sufficiently different from your patient/herd that initiated the question, or if the treatment is neither feasible nor consistent with the client's/manager's values and expectations, a valid and important therapy would not be applicable in your current situation. For a reported trial to influence treatment strategies, one should ask whether all clinically important outcomes were considered. And most importantly, were the outcomes of most importance to you, the clinician, and the owner/manager reported? Trials that report substitute end points such as blood cell counts, blood chemistry, or body temperature are not as valuable for evaluating treatment options as indications of reduced mortality rates or improved production (e.g., weight gain, conception rates). Even when a report indicates one or more positive outcomes associated with a treatment, one should consider whether other negative outcomes are also associated with that treatment. This is particularly important if the negative outcomes are more important to the owner/manager than are the positive outcomes.

USING EBVM IN CLINICAL PRACTICE

Until recently, efficiently finding the current best evidence to a therapeutic question was a difficult challenge. However, developments have permitted a new reality. The first of those developments is the creation of searchable databases (e.g., Medline, CAB) that are continually updated and available via the Internet. The other development is the increased education of practitioners and veterinary students in the areas of experimental design, statistics, and epidemiology to be able to appraise evidence for its validity and relevance. *Practitioners must take the initiative in improving their understanding of these concepts through continuing education and further reading if the profession is to continue to provide accurate and up-to-date therapeutic interventions with confidence.*

In human medicine the creation of systematic reviews and evidence-based journals of secondary publication and the development of information systems that bring these reviews and journals to a practitioner's desktop computer have almost instantaneously greatly enhanced the ability of medical students and practitioners to practice EBM. A systematic review is a structured review of the literature that includes a clear statement of the purpose of the review; a comprehensive search and retrieval of the relevant research; explicit selection criteria; critical appraisal of the primary studies; and reproducible decisions regarding relevance, selection, and methodological rigor of the primary research.[16,17] In a systematic review, emphasis is placed on results from studies of higher quality in preference to results from lower-quality studies; and for questions with an adequate number of studies, the review may exclude lower-quality experimental designs. This rigorous method is in contrast to a traditional review whereby the completeness of the literature search and evaluation rigor of the primary research is not obvious to the reader. Veterinarians need to demand this level of rigor in systematic reviews in the veterinary literature, as well as be willing to pay for these types of resources for use in their day-to-day practice.

OPPORTUNITIES AND CHALLENGES OF EBVM

Although EBM has gained interest and integration into medical teaching and practice, EBVM has lagged behind because of several challenges. Compared with human-patient-centered clinical and field trials, veterinary-patient-centered clinical and field trials are rare.[3] In addition to the slight investment that veterinary medicine has made in research that creates the higher levels of evidence, veterinary medicine must stretch those investments over a great many species. Therapeutic questions that are investigated in one species may or may not provide accurate evidence in other, even related species. Also, in human medicine, there are two practical factors that would appear to favor the adoption of EBM, at least in the United States. One is the pressure of

cost efficiency by medical insurance and health maintenance organizations that restrict payment to procedures that have met some standard. The other is the cost of malpractice insurance and lawsuits, which have negative consequences for those using procedures that have not been validated by sound and scientifically based (EBM) research. These discrepancies and challenges are not new to veterinary medicine and the advent and development of EBVM has great potential to bring the best available evidence into use in veterinary practices, thereby improving the effectiveness of veterinary services to patients and clients.

References

1. Evidence-Based Medicine Working Group: Evidence-based medicine: a new approach to teaching the practice of medicine, *J Am Med Assoc* 268:2420-2425, 1992.
2. Keene BW: Towards evidence-based veterinary medicine (editorial), *J Vet Intern Med* 14:118-119, 2000.
3. Doig GS: Evidence-based veterinary medicine: what it is, what it isn't and how to do it, *Aust Vet J* 81:412-415, 2003.
4. Roudebush P, Allen TA, Dodd CE et al: Evidence-based medicine: applications to veterinary clinical nutrition, *J Am Vet Med Assoc* 224:1766-1771, 2004.
5. Naldi L, Braun R, Saurat J-H: Evidence-based dermatology: a need to reset the agenda, *Dermatology* 204:1-3, 2000.
6. Sackett DL, Rosenberg WA, Gray JA et al: Evidence-based medicine: what it is and what it isn't, *Br Med J* 312:71-72, 1996.
7. Sackett DL, Straus SE, Richardson WS et al: Introduction. In Sackett DL, Straus SE, Richardson WS et al, editors: *Evidence-based medicine: how to practice and teach EBM*, ed 2, Philadelphia, 2000, Churchill-Livingstone.
8. Rosenberg WM, Sackett DL: On the need for evidence-based medicine, *Therapie* 51:212-217, 1996.
9. Sackett DL: Rules of evidence and clinical recommendations, *Can J Cardiol* 9:487-489, 1993.
10. Dans AL, Dans LF, Guyatt GH et al: Users' guide to the medical literature. XIV. How to decide on the applicability of clinical trial results to your patient, *J Am Med Assoc* 279:545-549, 1998.
11. Berg AO: Dimensions of evidence. In Geyman JP, Deyo RA, Ramsey SD, editors: *Evidence-based clinical practice: concepts and approaches*, Boston, 2000, Butterworth-Heinemann.
12. Sacks HS, Chalmers TC, Smith H Jr: Randomized versus historical assignment in controlled clinical trials, *Am J Med* 72:233-240, 1982.
13. Chalmers TC, Celano P, Sacks HS et al: Bias in treatment assignment in controlled clinical trials, *N Engl J Med* 309:1358-1361, 1983.
14. Colditz GA, Miller JN, Mosteller F: How study design affects outcomes in comparisons of therapy. I: Medical, *Stat Med* 8:441-454, 1989.
15. Sackett DL, Straus SE, Richardson WS, et al: Diagnosis and screening. In Sackett DL, Straus SE, Richardson WS et al, editors: *Evidence-based medicine: how to practice and teach EBM*, ed 2, Philadelphia, 2000, Churchill-Livingstone.
16. Cook D, Sackett D, Spitzer W: Methodological guidelines for systematic reviews of randomized control trials in health care from the Potsdam consultation and meta-analysis, *J Clin Epidemiol* 48:167-171, 1995.
17. Cook D, Meade M, Fink M: How to keep up with the critical care literature and avoid being buried alive, *Crit Care Med* 24:1757-1768, 1996.

CHAPTER 100

Therapeutic Options in Organic Livestock Medicine

HUBERT J. KARREMAN

Editor's note: The use of any of the therapeutic options discussed in this chapter falls under the same rules and regulations as the use of any drug, whether natural or synthetic. Therefore readers are reminded to review the legalities of therapies and abide by all laws regarding extralabel use of drugs and adherence to appropriate withdrawal times. Withdrawal time data may be obtained from FARAD (see Chapter 96 for more information), although data on plant and herbal medicines are limited.

BACKGROUND

U.S. Department of Agriculture (USDA)-certified organic farming is a production system that strives to produce food without the use of synthetic inputs. The organic sector is strongly driven by consumer demand for products that are produced without routine reliance on petroleum-derived fertilizers, herbicides, insecticides, fungicides, and synthetic pharmaceutical inputs. With passage of the Organic Food Production Act of 1990 (OFPA) and its full implementation beginning in October 2002, the official "USDA Organic" seal has become familiar to many consumers throughout the United States. The official seal sets the minimum regulations to be a USDA-certified organic producer and processor. All "natural" materials are allowed unless specifically prohibited by the Secretary of the USDA, and all synthetic materials are prohibited unless specifically allowed by the Secretary. The National Organic Standards Board (NOSB) was created by OFPA and has statutory authority on recommending the inclusion of materials on the National List of substances that can be used in certified organic production. In fact, OFPA expressly prohibits the Secretary from adding or removing materials to the National List without due process by the NOSB.

OFPA AS APPLIED TO LIVESTOCK

As is evident by reading OFPA, livestock consideration was minimal when crafting the law. Three key phrases regarding livestock production in OFPA have been the source of much consternation within the industry. First is that beef cattle must be raised organically from the last third of gestation. Second, milk that is to be organic must come from animals managed organically for the past 12 months. And third, the subtherapeutic use of hormone and antibiotics for growth promotion or production purposes is illegal.

The first and second points have been the center of much controversy because dairy replacements may be reared conventionally until they are 12 months away from organic production. The third item, which is germane to the veterinary profession, is that subtherapeutic use of hormones and antibiotics for growth promotion is illegal. That OFPA remains silent on the *therapeutic* use of hormones and antibiotics has given some certifiers leeway to allow the therapeutic use of these compounds in animals longer than 12 months from lactation (i.e., calves). Thus some farms will use antibiotics in diagnosed disease conditions in young stock (e.g., antibiotics for respiratory disease and coccidiostats for coccidia problems) without their removal from the herd. However, 7CFR205.238(c) (7) states that an animal receiving a prohibited material must be removed from production (Box 100-1). What exactly is meant by an "appropriate medication" and who will say if and when it is going to be used? Is "appropriate medication" to mean only what is currently being taught in veterinary schools? The other problem with this statement is that animals removed from organic production can *never* be returned to organic production. Thus there is actually a disincentive for farmers to reach for well-proven medicines because most of the medicines that veterinarians reach for are synthetic antibiotics and hormones, which are not specifically allowed on the National List. Additionally, there exists an official NOSB policy from 2002 to not allow antibiotics in organic livestock production at all, which the NOP has agreed to uphold. So, even though OFPA does not expressly prohibit therapeutic use of antibiotics and hormones, the NOSB has created a stricter standard and the NOP has upheld it. Yet this policy runs

---

Box 100-1

U.S. Department of Agriculture National Organic Program Animal Health Care Standard

"The producer of an organic livestock operation must not withhold medical treatment from a sick animal in an effort to preserve its organic status. All appropriate medications must be used to restore an animal to health when methods acceptable to organic production fail. Livestock treated with a prohibited substance must be clearly identified and shall not be sold, labeled, or represented as organically produced." 7CFR205.238(c)(7)

counter to a couple of materials that the NOSB has formally voted on to be allowed: ivermectin (in 1999) and moxidectin (in 2004). Both of these well-known macrocyclic lactone anthelmintics are, technically, antibiotics due to their chemical nature as compounds produced by one organism that inhibit the growth of another organism.

Because of the original law, later added policies, and the National List, confusion exists about how to actually treat an animal needing medical attention. This confusion can encompass many parties—farmers; inspectors; certifiers; and, perhaps most importantly, those entrusted by society to care for animals, veterinarians. Farm animal veterinarians are in a unique position in that they have taken an oath to use scientific knowledge and skills for the benefit of society through the protection of animal health, relief of animal suffering, conservation of animal resources, promotion of public health, and advancement of medical knowledge (portion of American Veterinary Medication Association Veterinarian's Oath, adopted November 1999).

THERAPEUTICS AND THE NATIONAL LIST

With the strict prohibitions on what can be used to treat organic livestock, the question for veterinarians becomes: If no antibiotics and hormones, then what is there to use? The first place to look is the National List (Box 100-2). Secondly, although antibiotics and hormones may be expressly forbidden in U.S.-certified organic livestock health care, other synthetic substances that relieve pain and suffering are likely to be permitted for use by the time of publication. Such compounds include activated charcoal, atropine, bismuth subsalicylate, butorphanol, epinephrine, flunixin, furosemide, kaolin pectin, magnesium oxide/hydroxide, mineral oil, propylene glycol, tolazoline, and xylazine. Some of these have New Animal Drug Approvals (NADAs) and some do not. If the U.S. Food and Drug Administration (FDA) has not granted NADA status to a material, the question arises as to how the USDA can write them into law. Ironically, some materials used daily in the conventional livestock sector (e.g., propylene glycol, mineral oil) do not have NADAs; however, the FDA has allowed these for decades by "regulatory discretion."

Additionally, some of the NADAs (xylazine and butorphanol) may not have approval for use in lactating cattle. Although the Animal Medicinal Drug Use Clarification Act of 1996 (AMDUCA) permits the extralabel use of these particular compounds by duly licensed veterinarians exercising a valid veterinary-client-patient relationship (VCPR) in specific cases, applications of these kinds of legal nuances ("AMDUCA," "VCPR") are difficult to shepherd through the federal bureaucracy. For instance, because activated charcoal can be made of all natural materials of vegetable origin, some certifiers have decided to allow this form of it as a natural material. In the case of magnesium oxide, considered by the American Association of Feed Control Officials (AAFCO) as an approved mineral livestock feed rations, it is now allowed by some certifiers because the USDA National Organic Program (NOP, the regulatory overseers of organic production) officially accepts the entire AAFCO-approved mineral and vitamin list for use in organic livestock. Special mention

also needs to be made of liquid calcium products for IV treatment of milk fever (hypocalcemia/parturient paresis). These materials, which are synthetic, have never been granted NADA status by the FDA and have always been allowed by "regulatory discretion." It was officially petitioned to the NOSB and the Board voted to recommend its inclusion on the National List, yet it has yet to be given final approval by the Secretary. However, this material is an electrolyte. Electrolytes (without antibiotics) are categorically allowed under 7CFR205.603.

Thus if a veterinarian can technically call a substance an "electrolyte," it should be allowed by a certifier. This would include lactated Ringer's solution, hypertonic saline, and sodium iodide or any other salt that is dissolved in solution (electrolyte). Therefore a veterinarian might declare a substance to be an electrolyte—or any other generic category specifically allowed on 7CFR205.603—without drawing intense scrutiny from the certifier and without having the animal removed from the herd. Some examples of these categories include products containing iodine, chlorhexidine, and biologics. Finally, it should be noted that all vaccines are allowed, regardless of how produced. Although some vaccines are produced via genetically modified organisms (a prohibited method of production in certified organic agriculture), the vaccine end product is still allowed. This is probably due to the need for rapid vaccine production of vaccine if an exotic disease were to surface.

CONDITIONS AND TREATMENTS

Livestock on organic farms can experience each and every illness that livestock on conventional farms experience. Thus common illnesses such as mastitis, metritis, metabolic disturbances, digestive disturbances, pneumonia, lameness, and pinkeye are all encountered. However, it is possible that the overall prevalence of such conditions is low (my private practice data). Reaching for antibiotics and hormones will not be the organic farmer's first choice nor does it necessarily have to be the attending veterinarian's first choice either. Depending on the clinical presentation, treatments can include materials on the National List such as aspirin, biologics, electrolytes (without antibiotics), chlorhexidine, glucose/dextrose, glycerin, hydrogen peroxide, iodine, magnesium sulphate, oxytocin, ivermectin, lidocaine, mineral oil, procaine, and trace minerals. It should be kept in mind that when writing up the bill and listing the materials used, using generic terms (e.g., "biologic" or "electrolytes") will help the process of review by USDA Accredited Certifying Agents (ACAs). However, the veterinarian should also be prepared to answer questions from an ACA regarding the nature of any administered or dispensed material. Although answering questions about therapy from a medically naive reviewer can be irritating, this should not be seen as meddling in a valid VCPR because the avoidance of prohibited materials is paramount to the integrity of organic production.

A growing and sincere interest in the organic livestock industry by veterinary practitioners is apparent. In an informal survey undertaken by myself, 750 self-identified dairy practitioners from within the American Association

Box 100-2

Synthetic Materials Allowed for U.S. Department of Agriculture–Certified Organic Livestock Production

§ 205.603 Synthetic substances allowed for use in organic livestock production.

In accordance with restrictions specified in this section the following synthetic substances may be used in organic livestock production:
(a) As disinfectants, sanitizer, and medical treatments as applicable.
  (1) Alcohols.
    (i) Ethanol—disinfectant and sanitizer only, prohibited as a feed additive.
    (ii) Isopropanol—disinfectant only.
  (2) Aspirin—approved for health care use to reduce inflammation.
  (3) Biologics—vaccines.
  (4) Chlorhexidine—allowed for surgical procedures conducted by a veterinarian. Allowed for use as a teat dip when alternative germicidal agents and/or physical barriers have lost their effectiveness.
  (5) Chlorine materials—disinfecting and sanitizing facilities and equipment. Residual chlorine levels in the water shall not exceed the maximum residual disinfectant limit under the Safe Drinking Water Act.
    (i) Calcium hypochlorite.
    (ii) Chlorine dioxide.
    (iii) Sodium hypochlorite.
  (6) Electrolytes—without antibiotics.
  (7) Glucose.
  (8) Glycerine—allowed as a livestock teat dip; must be produced through the hydrolysis of fats or oils.
  (9) Hydrogen peroxide.
  (10) Iodine.
  (11) Magnesium sulfate.
  (12) Oxytocin—use in postparturition therapeutic applications.
  (13) Parasiticides. Ivermectin—prohibited in slaughter stock, allowed in emergency treatment for dairy and breeder stock when organic system plan–approved preventive management does not prevent infestation. Milk or milk products from a treated animal cannot be labeled as provided for in subpart D of this part for 90 days following treatment. In breeder stock, treatment cannot occur during the last third of gestation if the progeny will be sold as organic and must not be used during the lactation period for breeding stock.
  (14) Phosphoric acid—allowed as an equipment cleaner, provided that no direct contact with organically managed livestock or land occurs.
(b) As topical treatment, external parasiticide or local anesthetic as applicable.
  (1) Copper sulfate.
  (2) Iodine.
  (3) Lidocaine—as a local anesthetic. Use requires a withdrawal period of 90 days after administering to livestock intended for slaughter and 7 days after administering to dairy animals.
  (4) Lime, hydrated—as an external pest control, not permitted to cauterize physical alterations or deodorize animal wastes.
  (5) Mineral oil—for topical use and as a lubricant.
  (6) Procaine—as a local anesthetic, use requires a withdrawal period of 90 days after administering to livestock intended for slaughter and 7 days after administering to dairy animals.
(c) As feed supplements—milk replacers without antibiotics, as emergency use only, no nonmilk products or products from BST-treated animals.
(d) As feed additives.
  (1) DL-Methionine, DL-Methionine—hydroxy analog, and DL-Methionine—hydroxy analog calcium for use only in organic poultry production until October 21, 2005.
  (2) Trace minerals, used for enrichment or fortification when FDA approved.
  (3) Vitamins, used for enrichment or fortification when FDA approved.
(e) As synthetic inert ingredients as classified by the Environmental Protection Agency (EPA), for use with nonsynthetic substances or synthetic substances listed in this section and used as an active pesticide ingredient in accordance with any limitations on the use of such substances.
  (1) EPA List 4—Inerts of Minimal Concern.
(f)-(z) [Reserved]
§ 205.604 Nonsynthetic substances prohibited for use in organic livestock production.
The following nonsynthetic substances may not be used in organic livestock production:
(a) Strychnine.

[65 FR 80657, Dec. 21, 2000, as amended at 68 FR 61992, Oct. 31, 2003]

of Bovine Practitioners were contacted in December 2005. A letter of introduction was sent out regarding organic livestock and Complementary and Alternative Veterinary Medicine (CAVM), along with a survey consisting of six questions with yes/no or multiple-choice responses on a self-addressed, stamped return card. The 180 responses represented a 24% return rate and indicated an interest in information about treating organic livestock (Box 100-3). Based on the results of the survey, the following conditions and their treatments for organic livestock are discussed: mastitis, reproductive disorders, pneumonia, digestion, and lameness.

NOTE: Where few published data exist, the following treatment recommendations are based on my clinical impression.

Mastitis

General treatment guidelines for organic control of mastitis need to include identification of the pathogenic organism. This is the same as for conventional dairies, except the need for antimicrobial susceptibility testing of pathogenic organisms is questionable because it is unlikely an organic farmer will use antibiotics for mastitis. This

Informal Survey of Dairy Practitioners Who Are Members of the American Association of Bovine Practitioners (AABP)

Informal Survey of AABP Dairy Practitioners (N = 180)

1. Would you or your clients be interested in the use of Complementary and Alternative Veterinary Medicine (CAVM) for livestock?

   Yes: 111   Maybe: 59   No: 6   No response: 4

2. Would you be interested in CAVM products if they are presented from a rational, pharmacologic basis?

   Yes: 142   Maybe: 31   No: 4   No response: 3

3. In which diseases would you be most interested? (circle one or more)

   Mastitis: 108; *Calf scours:* 67; *Metritis:* 62; *Infertility:* 50; *Lameness:* 45; *Pneumonia:* 43; *All:* 39

   Other: pinkeye: 1; adult scours: 1; parasites: 1; acupuncture for down cows: 1

4. Do you work with any certified organic or transitioning-to-organic dairy herds?

   Yes: 98   No: 81   No response: 1

   If so, how many herds?

   0-3: 64   *4-6:* 16   *7-10:* 8   *11-20:* 6

   How many milking on average?

   0-40: 31   *41-100:* 42   *101-300:* 16   *301-500:* 1
   500-1000: 0   *>1000:* 3

5. Do you feel that any of your conventional herds would be interested in CAVM?

   Yes: 113   Maybe: 30   No: 34   No response: 3

6. Would you be interested in receiving more information for a few specific products?

   Yes: 170   No: 7   No response: 3

---

is because common forms of mastitis are not usually life threatening, and it is in life-threatening situations that a prohibited material like an antibiotic will be used. Once the organism is identified as contagious or environmental, basic milking procedures need to be discussed with the client to minimize new infections. Treatments may include systemic immune augmentation or stimulation via biologics, topically applied ointments, orally administered tinctures, and intramammary botanical infusions. When using biologics, the goal is to either stimulate non-specific immunity (interferon-gamma and natural killer cells) and/or deliver passive IgG antibodies systemically. One commercial biologic, derived from mycobacterial cell wall fractionates (Immunoboost), has the ability to stimulate interferon gamma and may be useful in reducing somatic cell counts (SCCs) in cows with subclinical mastitis for up to 2 months with one injection (providing it is not *Staphylococcus aureus*). In my experience, this product seems to work in cows with subclinical cases of various *Streptococcus* spp. and coagulase-negative *Staphylococcus* spp. (CNS).

The need for dry cow antibiotic treatment is questionable, based on data suggesting SCCs of organic and conventional cows are equivalent at 0 to 41 days in milk.[1]

If there are some individual cows with high SCC near dry-off, one injection of Immunoboost may be useful for the 2-month dry time. The usual dose is 5 ml per adult cow IM, SQ, or IV. Other biologics include colostrum-whey–derived products (also called *ultra-filtered whey products*). Although manufacturers cannot claim that these products are a source of antibodies (because of USDA labeling requirements), most farmers consider them as such because they are derived from colostrum. Some firms manufacture "specifics," naming the pathogen and thereby suggesting which type of infection may be helped by the product. Colostrum-whey derivatives are generated from animals infused or vaccinated with a modified pathogen during the dry period, although details are trade secrets. Regardless of possible antibody content, a significant increase of the in vivo neutrophil iodination activity of periparturient cows, as well as an increase in the total erythrocytes in periparturient cows, was demonstrated with one such product. The same product demonstrated that neutrophils from dexamethasone-suppressed calves had cytochrome C reduction significantly enhanced in vitro and neutrophils from non–dexamethasone-suppressed calves had significantly increased neutrophil random migration; cytochrome C reduction; iodination activity; antibody-dependent cell-mediated cytotoxicity; and antibody-independent, cell-mediated cytotoxicity.[2] Farmers often remark that they will see a "shed down" when using colostrum-whey product. A "shed down" is an increased amount of clots in the milk for a day or two and then rapidly normalizing while the udder also milks out more fully. The usual dose is 30 ml injected subcutaneously once daily for 3 consecutive days. Interestingly, injecting milk back into a cow was done before the advent of antibiotics.[3] Subcutaneous injection of botanicals has also been shown to stimulate the immune system. Ginseng *(Panax ginseng)* was shown to decrease milk SCCs and the number of *S. aureus*–infected quarters, possibly because of the significantly increased phagocytosis and oxidative burst of neutrophils. In the same study, monocytes and lymphocytes were significantly higher than controls for a few weeks after treatment.[4] In a follow-up study, crude ginseng extracts and purified ginsenoside R_{b1} were used as adjuvants when immunizing cattle against *S. aureus*. Both the crude extract and the R_{b1} were shown to be safe, and the crude extract produced a significant increase in milk antibody titers while the R_{b1} produced the highest antibody production and lymphocyte proliferation.[5]

Commercially available and USDA-licensed sources of passive antibodies for treatment of coliform mastitis are another biologic to have ready for use on organic farms. These include such products as Bovi-Sera, PolySerum, Bo-Bac-2X, and Quattracon. These all are labeled as sources of passive antibodies to *Arcanobacterium pyogenes, Escherichia coli, Mannheimia hemolytica, Pasteurella multocida,* and *Salmonella typhimurium.* In cases of hot coliform mastitis, these products can be helpful as the active therapeutic agent against the infection, and electrolytes can be used to correct fluid and/or metabolic imbalances (e.g., lactated Ringer's solution, hypertonic saline, calcium-magnesium-phosphorus-potassium). Because there is hemolysis within the product, these passive sources of antibodies should only be given subcutaneously or intramuscularly.

If it is possible to obtain a pure product with no red cells present, via plasmapheresis, this can be given intravenously with reduced potential for anaphylaxis as compared with the commercially available products, which are only labeled for IM and SQ use. The usual dose for an adult cow is about 120 ml, which can be repeated in 12 to 24 hours as needed. No withholding times are associated with these products.

Many organic farmers readily use topical liniments to cool an inflamed, hot udder. The most common commercially available products contain essential oil of peppermint. If applied without the use of latex gloves, higher quality peppermint lotions will leave the applicant's hands feeling cool for up to 2 hours. The effect on the cow's udder is likely the same. Absorption of menthol, the active ingredient of peppermint, is probable and knowledge of possible residue in milk is wise. Although no pharmacokinetic studies have been performed in cattle, when 500 mg menthol was administered orally to healthy human volunteers, no unchanged menthol and only traces of the sulphate conjugate were detected in the urine.[6] Most essential oils have at least a biphasic elimination pharmacokinetic profile, suggesting that essential oils are absorbed from the blood (when given orally) and go into other tissues. With high clearance and short elimination half-lives, accumulation is improbable.[7]

Intramammary therapy is embraced by most conventional farmers and accepted by many organic farmers. Various botanically based products are in the marketplace. In general, these probably act more as local irrigation antiseptics than as antibiotics against specific pathogens as understood in conventional therapy. Some of these contain essential oils, whereas others contain aqueous or oil-based botanicals. Using an infusion that is slightly hypertonic or isotonic is probably safe and beneficial. Derivatives from oregano and thyme are commonly used, most likely due to the historical use of thymol as an effective antiseptic in medical practice before the advent of antibiotics.[8,9] My clinical impression is that using a combination of a systemic immune stimulant and a local intramammary infusion works better than either alone.

One intramammary botanical combination I have employed has thymol and a glycyrrhiza derivative as active ingredients (with a few other botanicals present). It is recommended for common mastitis types such as *Streptococcus* spp. and CNS. It is given at the rate of one intramammary infusion every 12 hours for four doses. This product is currently undergoing in vitro culture and sensitivity studies, as well as pharmacokinetic elimination studies. In one clinical study, glycyrrhizin was shown to decrease the SCC and down-regulate inflammation in CNS cows, possibly through modulation of histamine.[10] In a human pharmacokinetic study, volunteers were given an oral thymol-containing product (equivalent to 1.08 mg thymol) and no unchanged thymol was detected in plasma or urine; however, the metabolite thymol sulphate (but not thymol glucuronide) was detectable in plasma at peak concentrations of 93 ng/ml and was reached after 2 hours, with a mean terminal half-life of 10 hours.[11]

As can be seen, biologic and botanical approaches are rational choices for organic livestock with mastitis, especially when considering systemic stimulation or augmentation of the animal's immune system along with local irrigation of the mammary gland with botanicals known for their antiseptic qualities.

Reproductive Disorders

Treating uterine infections on organic farms requires extra manual labor compared with injections of therapeutic hormones on conventional farms. The management principle behind organic treatment of metritis is lavage and the use of antiseptics. However, the cow herself can help the situation (to some extent) by exercising and grazing because this aids lymphatic drainage of the uterine area. With manual cleansing of the uterus, it does not matter which material is used as long as repeated cleansing of the uterine environment is carried out to dilute offensive material present, as well as employing antiseptic materials. Additionally, manual removal of the retained fetal membranes should not be discouraged. However, removal should *never* occur before 4 to 5 days after parturition and only if the membranes are decomposed enough so that only slight, gentle traction is necessary to remove them. Under no circumstances should cotyledons be removed manually from caruncles. As is taught conventionally, there is generally no need for any treatment of the uterus within the first 1 to 3 days after parturition.

By day 4 (and every 24-48 hours thereafter) the use of iodine as an antiseptic can be beneficial.

(*Editor's note:* The use of nonapproved drugs in an extralabel manner is prohibited by AMDUCA.)

This can be applied as a bolus or an infusion at the rate of 1 g per treatment. Once the membranes are removed, iodine pills can continue to be placed until the cervix becomes too closed to insert pills into the uterus. Rarely, siphoning excessive fetid uterine fluid may be necessary if the fetal membranes are not reachable, but this should only be attempted if the cervix is open enough to still pass the operator's hand. (This is to prevent the end of the tube from coming into direct contact with the uterine wall, potentially perforating it.) As the uterine discharge improves and becomes more mucoid, infusions of various liquid solutions will be of value. Commonly used lavage materials include colostrum-whey products combined with tincture of marigold *(Calendula officinalis)* or infusions of aloe juice alone. Using 40 ml of hypertonic saline with 20 ml of 7% iodine tincture may be considered, as well as commercially available dilute chlorhexidine solutions (e.g., extralabel use of chlorhexidine infusion tubes normally intended for mares).

Amounts to be infused vary between 60 ml and 300 ml every 24 to 48 hours, depending on character of discharge. It should be noted that once the discharge improves to the point of being only slightly cloudy or clear with a few white mucopurulent streaks, infusions should cease because the risk of introducing foreign material at this point outweighs any benefit of infusing. The goal is to help improve the uterine environment so that by about 3 weeks' fresh, the cow is normal or only slightly infected. All cows should be checked for reproductive health at 30 to 40 days in milk if they had metritis. Although iodine may be thought of as a uterine chemical irritant, its antiseptic benefits outweigh its possible risks when used early after calving. Chronic pyometra is to be avoided at all costs and can be if "aggressive" cleansing of an infected uterus is done within the first 2 weeks after calving. Although infusions can be employed for chronic pyometra when a cow is greater than 50 days in milk, they are only rarely completely effective.

Cysts causing infertility should be gently ruptured if possible. If not, there are two homeopathic treatments that appear to give positive results. This includes using apis mellifica (derived from honeybee venom) twice daily for 5 days, followed by natrum mur (derived from sea salt) twice daily for 3 days. This can be given orally as medicated pellets or as liquid drops. Using a spray of the liquid can be administered intranasally or in the vulva. Contact with a mucous membrane appears to be important for homeopathic remedy administration.

Cows that have a normal corpus luteum and that are in good body condition, but have not shown any visible estrus, can be encouraged to show behavioral estrus by orally administering a botanical combination of traditional "female herbs." This combination includes *Turnera diffusa, Dioscorea villosa, Mitchella repens, Viburnum opulus, Angelica sinensis, Oenothera biennis,* and *Lanum usitatissimum.* When administering about 750 mg of this combination every other day for six doses when a corpus luteum is present, cows will generally show visible estrus during the treatment days or shortly thereafter. The cow should be bred as usual. Occasionally a cow will show an exceptionally strong estrus 3 weeks later again. Rebreed if need be. In general, cows conceive well when this regimen is used. This botanical combination has proved useful for cysts that have not responded to other therapies. However, for a cyst, the treatment time should be doubled.

In general the reproductive treatments outlined can yield normal reproductive parameters (via DHIA) and give statistically equivalent results to those obtained by using standard antibiotic and hormonal therapy for metritis.[1]

Pneumonia

Pneumonia should be avoided at all costs on organic farms. This can be accomplished by sound prevention strategies such as vaccines and individual hutches for young calves. Dry bedding and fresh air are critical for prevention. Occasionally a fresh heifer will experience pneumonia when brought into a milking barn (especially in tie-stall barns in the winter). Distinguishing between a primary viral pneumonia versus a secondary bacterial pneumonia greatly aids in prognosis, although the natural treatment used may not vary between the pneumonia types. Because of the severe morbidity and mortality potential of pneumonia, antibiotic use should be considered if a presumptive diagnosis of bacterial pneumonia is made, especially if there is suspicion of pending consolidation. If there is a concurrent infection elsewhere in the animal (e.g., metritis, mastitis), it is best to go immediately to the antibiotic treatment for the best welfare of the animal. However, the animal will then need to be permanently removed from organic production. If there is predominantly a viral pneumonia (where antibiotics are of no value) or if the clinician is not sure and the animal is bright, alert, and still eating fairly well, use of hyper-immune serum or

plasma is indicated. This method of therapy has a long tradition in veterinary medicine and was the active medical treatment (along with supportive measures) before the antibiotic era.[12] Experimental infection of lambs with *Mannheimia hemolytica* supports the previous historical use of treatment with immune serum.[13] Commercially available biologic sources of passive antibodies against *M. hemolytica* and *Pasteurella multocida* are available (see commercial products listed earlier in the Mastitis section). Additionally, stimulating the nonspecific immune system would be beneficial. This can be accomplished with a commercially available intranasal vaccine for IBR/PI$_3$ if early in the infection process to stimulate local IgA and γ-interferon along the respiratory mucosa. If the case is advanced, this probably should not be used; instead, use of a systemic immune stimulant such be employed.

Administration of antioxidants such as vitamin E and selenium (1 ml/200 lb IM or SQ) or vitamin C (5 ml/100 lb IV) may be of value. The immune serum and vitamin C can be repeated every 24 hours as needed. Garlic *(Allium sativum)* is a time-honored antimicrobial that now has achieved official National Formulary status, thus being available in standardized forms. Oral use for follow-up to systemic immune stimulants is recommended. Garlic is easily absorbed from the gastrointestinal tract with a high bioavailability in rats, mice, and dogs[14] and may be similar in the bovine. In my experience, it is useful to blend botanical tinctures into a carrier (e.g., dextrose) and administer intravenously. Use of Goldenseal *(Hydrastis canadensis)* and Barberry *(Berberis vulgaris)* in infections is also rational because their berberine constituents are antimicrobial. Ginseng should also be considered. Mixing garlic, goldenseal, barberry, and ginseng may be synergistic (Table 100-1).[15]

It should be noted that animals treated with nonantibiotic approaches in the early stage of pneumonia have a good prognosis but recover more slowly than those given antibiotics. As long as an animal shows daily improvement, natural treatment should not be abandoned. It usually takes about 5 to 7 days for most pneumonia cases treated in this way to return to normal. The animal still may exhibit a slight cough by day 7 after initiation of treatment, but as long as it is eating well and showing normal behavior, it will probably become a productive animal. However, if there is a relapse in the future, the prognosis is poor because permanent damage to lung tissue has probably occurred.

Table **100-1**

General Dosage Table for Botanic Formulations

Preparation	Goat	Cow	Horse
Decoction	4 oz	12 oz	8 oz
Extract powder	1 tsp	2 Tbsp	2 Tbsp
Extract tablet	3-5	10-15	10-15
Freeze-dried granules	1 tsp	2 Tbsp	2 Tbsp
Tincture	1 tsp	2 Tbsp	2-3 Tbsp

From Schoen A, Wynn S: *Complementary and alternative veterinary medicine: principles and practice,* Philadelphia, 1998, Mosby.

Digestion

In cows, normal digestion can be enhanced by using a combination of essential oils (thymol, eugenol, vanillin, and limonene) to inhibit the deamination of amino acids by altering some ammonia-producing bacteria and anaerobic fungi.[16] This may in effect protect certain amino acids from ruminal degradation and deliver them to the lower gut to be absorbed and used by the animal. For cows off feed with slow gut motility, *Strychnos nux vomica* was used historically in conjunction with ginger (*Zingiber officinale*), gentian (*Gentiana lutea*), and sodium bicarbonate.[9] The ingredients are all still obtainable for licensed veterinarians in the tincture form and may help prevent pending abomasal displacement. Other existing conditions such as hypocalcemia or ketosis need to be corrected as well. Use of IV electrolytes for correction of hypocalcemia and dextrose IV with oral glycerin as a putative gluconeogenic agent to correct ketosis is recommended.

Calves with diarrhea should be examined, and identification of etiologic agent or presumptive diagnosis should be made. IV administration of fluids to correct dehydration and metabolic acidosis is warranted, and tube feeding oral liquids (if needed) for hydration maintenance is critical. Psyllium products to help gel the fecal contents are advisable. Biologics that contain passive antibodies and ones that stimulate the immune system (mentioned previously) should be used as the active medicine in place of antibiotics. The first dose should be given intravenously in addition to a subcutaneous dose for slower absorption. Orally administered botanicals that are high in tannin content should be used to help constrict the gut and cause constipation so that no more loss of fluids occurs. Obtaining a product that has tannins, iron, and minerals is ideal. Certain marcasite clays found in the southern United States contain these elements. Use of vitamin E and selenium in a calf formulation is also beneficial to enhance the general immune system via antioxidant activity.

Parasites are found on organic farms as on conventional farms, and management should strive to prevent infestations from occurring. The entire life cycle of the parasite should be considered for treatment, not just when it is in the animal but when it is free-living in the pasture. Therefore internal medicines are only half the answer when thinking in the organic realm. Additional attention must be paid to good nutrition for immunocompetence, as well as pasture management to discourage the free-living stages of parasites. Clipping pastures to splatter manure pies can lead to desiccation of larvae and eggs. The hyphae of the fungus *Duddingtonia flagrans* can be beneficial because it appears to strangle free-living helminth larvae. Certain forages have been found to have beneficial effects for the digestive system of ruminants as forages, whereas others have been found to be effective treatments against parasites. In comparison with alfalfa, ryegrass, and white clover, forages that reduce adult helminths internally and/or fecal egg counts include birdsfoot trefoil (*Lotus corniculatus*), chicory (*Cichorium intybus*), sulla (*Hedysarum coronarium*), and sanfoin (*Onobrychis vicifolia*).[17-20] Therefore it may be of benefit to suggest these in the ration or grow them in the paddocks of animals grazing. In comparison studies with chemotherapeutic agents, effective in vivo botanical treatment for ruminant parasites has been shown with pyrethrum,[21] *Tinospora rumphii*,[22] *Balanites aegyptiaca*,[23] and *Fumaria parviflora*[24] among others. In clinical case studies, an oleoresin derived from *Commiphora molmol* was shown to cure sheep of fascioliasis[25] and sheep, goats, and humans of *Dicroceliasis dendriticum*.[26]

Coccidia can also be found in organic livestock, mainly when housed indoors in the first few months of life and just past weaning. Although it did not shorten the period of diarrhea associated with coccidia, a garlic-derived product was shown to delay onset of diarrhea in calves exposed to *Cryptosporidium parvum* oocysts.[27] Research in poultry using a botanical formula of Uncaria, Agrimony, Sanguisorba, Yetbadetajo, Rehmannia, Pulsatilla, and flavescent Sophorae compared with diclazuril showed that both treatments yielded birds that were experimentally infected with *Eimeria tenella* to have significantly higher body weight gain than experimentally infected birds without any medication.[28] Although botanicals can be effective, proper management of animals is critical to prevent major infestations.

Lameness

Organic farmers may be more apt to treat a lame cow because they know cows must be sound to be efficient when grazing in pasture. The total prohibition of antibiotic usage applies to those applied topically as well. Therefore interdigital dermatitis (hairy heel wart) and necrotic pododermatitis (foot rot) must be managed differently. In my experience, a simple and effective treatment for foot rot is to mix povidone iodine with white table sugar to make a thick paste and apply it to the interdigital area after cleansing with 3% hydrogen peroxide. This must be repeated in 3 to 4 days. For hairy heel wart, paring away the surface layer of the lesion will greatly improve the situation by itself, and the previously mentioned peroxide and sugar-iodine can then be applied. Abscesses simply need to be opened up correctly and, again, cleansed and wrapped like foot rot and hairy heel wart. Prevention of these conditions should be emphasized. Stones submerged in the soil (either soft muck or hard soil with no "give") can lead to puncture abscesses and foot rot. Hairy heel wart may not only be the result of cows standing in mucky slurries. It may also be a consequence of acidotic rations, allowing potential toxins to slip into circulation from a compromised rumen wall and settle at the hoof-hairline junction. This may weaken the area and allow easier colonization by bacteria.

CONCLUSION

Treating organic livestock can be both an opportunity and a challenge. It is an opportunity to learn about nonantibiotic and nonhormonal treatments for infectious disease, but it is a challenge because there are few published clinical studies. By using botanical substances that have known pharmacologic actions, a clinician can proceed from a rational perspective. However, bioavailability and pharmacokinetic studies for residues in milk and meat of commonly used botanical medicines are definitely warranted.

References

1. Karreman HJ: *Treating dairy cows naturally: thoughts and strategies*, Paradise, Pa, 2004, Paradise Publications.
2. Roth JA, Frank DE, Weighner P et al: Enhancement of neutrophil function by ultrafiltered bovine whey, *J Dairy Sci* 84:824-829.
3. Alexander AS: *Udder diseases of the cow*, Boston, 1929, Richard G. Badger.
4. Hu S, Concha C, Johannisson A et al: Effect of subcutaneous injection of ginseng on cows with subclinical *Staphylococcus aureus* mastitis, *J Vet Med Series B* 48:519-527, 2001.
5. Hu S, Concha C, Lin F et al: Adjuvant effect of ginseng extracts on the immune response to immunization against *Staphylococcus aureus* in dairy cattle, *Vet Immuno Immunopath* 91:29-37, 2003.
6. Bhattaram VA, Graefe U, Kohlert C et al: Pharmacokinetics and bioavailability of herbal medicinal products, *Phytomedicine* 9(suppl III):1-33, 2002.
7. Kohlert C, van Rensen I, Marz R: Bioavailability and pharmacokinetics of natural volatile terpenes in animals and humans, *Planta Med* 66:495-505, 2000.
8. Winslow K: *Veterinary materia medica and therapeutics*, ed 8, Chicago, 1919, American Veterinary Publishing.
9. Milks HJ: *Practical veterinary pharmacology, materia medica and therapeutics*, ed 4, London, 1930, Bailliere, Tindall and Cox.
10. Kai K, Komine K, Asai K et al: Anti-inflammatory effects of intramammary infusions of glycyrrhizin in lactating cows with mastitis caused by coagulase-negative staphylococci, *Am J Vet Res* 64:1213-1220, 2003.
11. Kohlert C, Schindler G, Marz R: Systemic availability and pharmacokinetics of thymol in humans, *J Clin Pharmacol* 42:731-737, 2002.
12. Eichorn A: Biological therapeutics. In Winslow K: *Veterinary materia medica and therapeutics*, ed 8, Chicago, 1919, American Veterinary Publishing.
13. Jones GE, Donachie W, Sutherland AD et al: Protection of lambs against experimental pneumonic pasteurellosis by transfer of immune serum, *Vet Microbiol* 20:59-71, 1989.
14. Nagae S, Ushijima M, Hatano S: Pharmacokinetics of the garlic compound S-allylcysteine, *Planta Med* 60:214-217, 1994.
15. Schoen A, Wynn S: *Complementary and alternative veterinary medicine: principles and practice*, Philadelphia, 1998, Mosby.
16. McIntosh FM, Williams P, Losa R et al: Effects of essential oils on ruminal microorganisms and their protein metabolism, *Appl Environ Microbiol* 69:5011-5014, 2003.
17. Marley FM, Cook R, Keatinge R et al: The effect of birdsfoot trefoil and chicory on parasite intensities and performance of lambs naturally infected with helminth parasites, *Vet Parasitol* 112:147-155, 2003.
18. Niezen JH, Charleston WA, Robertson HA et al: The effect of feeding sulla (*Hedysarum coronarium*) or Lucerne (*Medicago sativa*) on lamb parasite burdens and development of immunity to gastrointestinal nematodes, *Vet Parasitol* 105:229-245, 2002.
19. Paolini V: In vitro effects of three woody plant and sainfoin extracts on third stage larvae and adult worms of three gastrointestinal nematodes, *Parasitology* 129:69-77, 2004.
20. Molan AL, Hoskin SO, Barry TN et al: Effect of condensed tannins extracted from four forages on the viability of the larva of deer lungworms and gastrointestinal nematodes, *Vet Rec* 147:44-48, 2000.
21. Mbaria JM, Maitho TE, Mitema ES et al: Comparative efficacy of pyrethrum mare with albendazole against sheep gastrointestinal nematodes, *Trop Anim Health Prod* 30:17-22, 1998.
22. Fernandez TJ: *The potential of* Tinospora rumphii *as an anthelmintic against* H. contortus *in goats* (website): www.vetwork.org.uk/pune13.htm. Accessed November 22, 2004.
23. Koko WS, Abdalla HS, Galal M et al: Evaluation of oral therapy on Mansonial Schiostosomiasis using single dose of *Balanites aegyptiaca* fruits and praziquantel, *Fitoterapia* 76:30-34, 2005.
24. Hördegen P, Hertzberg H, Heilman J et al: The anthelmintic efficacy of five plant products against gastrointestinal trichostrongylids in artificially infected lambs, *Vet Parasitol* 117:51-60, 2003.
25. Haridy FM, Garhy El, Morsy TA et al: Efficacy of Mirazid (*Commiphora molmol*) against fascioliasis in Egyptian sheep, *J Egypt Soc Parasitol* 33:917-924, 2003.
26. Massaud A, Morsy TA, Haridy FM: Treatment of Egyptian dicrocoeliasis in man and animals with Mirazid, *J Egypt Soc Parasitol* 33:437-442, 2003.
27. Olson EJ, Epperson WB, Zeman DH: Effects of an allicin-based product on cryptosporidiosis in neonatal calves, *J Am Vet Med Assoc* 212:987-990, 1998.
28. Du A, Hu S: Effects of an herbal complex against eimeria tenella infection in chickens, *J Vet Med B* 51:194-197, 2004.

CHAPTER 101

Decision Making in Mastitis Therapy

SARAH A. WAGNER and RONALD J. ERSKINE

Mastitis is the most common reason for antibiotic use on dairy farms.[1] Even farms with excellent mastitis prevention programs in place will be faced with some cases of mastitis and decisions about whether and how to treat them. Objectives of treatment include maximizing therapeutic success, minimizing expense, and minimizing factors that promote the development of antimicrobial resistance or the risk of violative residues in marketed milk.

CLINICAL MASTITIS OF MILD TO MODERATE SEVERITY

Most clinical cases of mastitis are mild to moderate in severity. Mild clinical mastitis is indicated by abnormalities in the milk such as changes in viscosity or the presence of flakes or clumps of material (garget). Mastitis of moderate severity results in swelling of the mammary gland in addition to abnormal milk. Severe mastitis is typically defined as systemic signs of illness such as depression, dehydration, or fever, in addition to abnormal milk and mammary swelling. Treatment of severe mastitis is discussed later in this chapter.

Cow Factors

Before deciding how to treat a case of mastitis of mild to moderate severity, one must decide whether or not to treat the case at all. A number of traits of the affected cow should be considered:

1. Is this a new case or a relapse? An acute case of mastitis is more likely to respond to therapy than an infection that has established itself in the gland and flared up repeatedly for months or even from one lactation to the next. Repeated treatment of a longstanding infection is unlikely to provide economic benefit to the farm or lasting improvement in the condition of the cow.
2. How many quarters are affected? A cow with all four quarters infected is less likely to have a successful therapeutic outcome than a cow with only one or two affected quarters. Infection in three or four quarters may indicate that the cow has an immune system or anatomic deficiency or an infection with an especially hardy microbe.
3. Does the cow have other problems? The cow's overall health and reproductive status should be considered before instituting therapy of mastitis. A cow that is many days in milk and not pregnant may not provide good economic return on investment in mastitis treatment. Animals with other health problems may be less likely to respond favorably to mastitis treatment. Ketosis and milk fever are associated with increased incidence of mastitis.[2] It seems likely that these and other conditions may contribute to immunosuppression and depress mastitis cure rates. Concurrent diseases should be addressed therapeutically at the same time as mastitis if therapy is undertaken. In some cases, culling may make the most economic sense for a cow with numerous health problems.
4. How many days in milk is the cow? If a cow is fresh, treatment of a new case of mastitis is a priority, to make her lactation as healthy and productive as possible. For cows in later lactation, however, treatment may be unnecessary or undesirable. More therapeutic and economic benefit may be achieved by drying the cow off early or on the scheduled dry-off date and treating her with an appropriate dry cow therapy instead of implementing therapy at the end of a lactation that is nearly over.

Microbial Factors

In addition to the cow factors discussed earlier, the traits of the microbe causing the infection should be considered. Some pathogens respond well to antimicrobial therapy, some are unlikely to respond to therapy (either because they are difficult to cure or because they will resolve spontaneously without treatment), and some pathogens resolve more quickly when antibiotic drugs are not administered (Box 101-1).

Decisions about whether or not to treat a particular case of mild to moderate mastitis, and which antibiotic to use if treatment is warranted, should be based on the probable pathogen causing the infection and the spectrum of activity of antimicrobial drugs under consideration. To determine which pathogen is causing a particular case of mastitis, microbial milk culture must be performed. An informed conjecture about the likely causative pathogens may be drawn based on previous culture results from the same farm. Obtaining this information requires a procedure for obtaining milk samples, culturing them, and recording the results. Milk cultures may be performed on the farm, sent to a diagnostic laboratory, or some combination of the two.

Box 101-1

Mastitis Pathogens Unlikely to Respond to Antimicrobial Treatment

Arcanobacterium pyogenes
Bacillus
Mycobacterium
Mycoplasma bovis
Nocardia
Pasteurella
Proteus
Prototheca (algae)
Pseudomonas
Serratia
Yeast (antibiotic treatment will delay spontaneous cure)

Reprinted by permission from Erskine R, Wagner S: Antimicrobial therapy of mastitis. In Giguere S, editor: *Antimicrobial therapy in veterinary medicine*, ed 4, Ames, Iowa, 2006, Blackwell Publishing.

Some farms have committed to microbial culture of every new case of mastitis, but even less extensive culture information can be useful for observing and recording trends in pathogens causing mastitis on a particular farm. When faced with an outbreak of clinical mastitis or a steadily rising bulk tank somatic cell count (SCC), extensive culturing of new or chronic cases may be necessary; protocols for investigation of such problems are available. One especially good source for information about investigating mastitis outbreaks or rising SCC is the NMC, formerly known as the National Mastitis Council.

On farms with sporadic incidence of mastitis, intermittent sampling of new cases may be sufficient to provide an ongoing idea of which mastitis pathogens are most prevalent on the farm. In addition to directing efforts at mastitis prevention and control, this information can be used to guide therapeutic decision making for cases where treatment is initiated before or without diagnostic microbial culture.

Pathogens that may respond to antibiotic therapy include many *Staphylococcus* and *Streptococcus* species and some Enterobacteriaceae (*Escherichia coli* and *Klebsiella* sp.). Chronic *Staphylococcus aureus* infections have a low cure rate, even with extended therapy. Some farms do not treat mild to moderate mastitis caused by gram-negative pathogens at all. Such infections may resolve on their own, but cows with naturally occurring gram-negative mastitis treated with antibiotics are less likely to develop severe disease and have a decreased risk of a recurrent or subsequent case of mastitis compared with mastitic cows not treated with antibiotic drugs.[3,4]

After the decision has been made to treat and a probable pathogen has been identified, an antimicrobial drug should be selected based on the antimicrobial spectrum of available drugs. Intramammary antibiotic therapy is indicated; parenteral therapy is generally not undertaken except in severe cases. For nonsevere cases that are unresponsive to label regimens of intramammary therapy, extending the duration of treatment with the intramammary drug may be more efficacious than administering parenteral therapy.[5] Achieving and sustaining

adequate drug levels in the mammary gland following parenteral administration may be difficult.

Antimicrobial susceptibility testing may be performed; however, this requires additional expense and time, and the sample for such testing must be submitted to a properly equipped diagnostic laboratory with appropriately trained personnel. In addition, recent investigations suggest that the predictive value of susceptibility testing in mastitis is limited to a few combinations of drug and microbe.[6] Until further research refines recommendations for drawing conclusions based on susceptibility testing, a prudent and simple approach is to keep and review farm records of which treatments have been used for which pathogens and which treatment-microbe combinations have been most successful.

Selecting an antibiotic for intramammary therapy should take into account the properties of the pathogen and the spectrum of activity of the drug. Drugs available in the United States for intramammary use, their drug class, and label indications for each are described in Table 101-1.

Designing a Regimen

The label regimen for most intramammary preparations indicates that they are to be administered once or twice daily for a period of 2 to 3 days. All of the antimicrobial drugs in intramammary preparations available in the United States act in a time-dependent manner; the efficacy of the drug against susceptible pathogens is achieved by maintaining the drug concentration at the site of infection at or above the minimum inhibitory concentration (MIC) for 50% to 100% of the treatment period. This is in contrast to concentration-dependent drugs in which efficacy against susceptible pathogens depends on achieving concentrations of a certain magnitude above the MIC at least once per dosing interval.

For acute mild to moderate cases of mastitis, treatment following the labeled regimen may be adequate. If it is found that such cases of mastitis are not responding well to therapy according to the label regimen, extralabel therapy may be considered. Because the antimicrobials available for intramammary use are time dependent in their activity, extending the duration of therapy is likely to improve outcome more than increasing the dose at any time point.

In summary, most cases of mastitis are of mild to moderate severity. Before treatment of such cases is undertaken, it is best to consider the likelihood and value of successful treatment based on such factors as stage of lactation, chronicity, treatment, number of quarters affected, and the health and reproductive status of the cow. Therapy is usually limited to intramammary administration of antibiotics. Selection of an antibiotic regimen should be based on the known or suspected pathogen causing the mastitis and the spectrum of activity of available antimicrobial drugs. If a case is unresponsive to initial treatment, extralabel extension of the duration of treatment may be warranted. Under the provisions of the Animal Medicinal Drug Use Clarification Act in the United States, such extralabel administration must be prescribed by a veterinarian for animals with which she or he is familiar

Table **101-1**

Intramammary Preparations Available for Lactating Cows in the United States

Although every effort has been made to ensure that the information presented here is accurate and complete, we cannot bear responsibility for any errors or omissions. Readers are advised to contact drug manufacturers and/or read package inserts for complete information about the products listed herein.

Drug Name and Class	Product Name	Label Regimen and Indications	Other Label Claims
Amoxicillin Aminopenicillin	Amoxi-Mast (Schering-Plough Animal Health)	3 treatments at 12-hour intervals Subclinical *Staphylococcus aureus* mastitis Subclinical *Streptococcus agalactiae* mastitis	Susceptibility shown by *Escherichia coli* in vitro Most *Pseudomonas, Klebsiella,* and *Enterobacter* are resistant
Ceftiofur Third-generation cephalosporin	Spectramast (Pfizer Animal Health)	2-8 treatments at 24-hour intervals Clinical coagulase-negative *Staphylococcus* mastitis Clinical *Streptococcus dysgalactiae* mastitis Clinical *Escherichia coli* mastitis	
Cephapirin First-generation cephalosporin	Today, Cefa-lak (Fort Dodge Animal Health)	2 treatments at a 12-hour interval Mastitis in lactating cows	Shown to be efficacious against susceptible strains of *S. agalactiae* and *S. aureus*
Cloxacillin Penicillin (penicillinase-resistant)	Dariclox (Schering-Plough Animal Health)	3 treatments at 12-hour intervals Clinical *S. aureus* mastitis (non–penicillinase-producing strains) Clinical *S. agalactiae* mastitis	Laboratory evidence indicates that cloxacillin is resistant to destruction by penicillinase-producing organisms
Erythromycin Macrolide	[1]Gallimycin-36 (Agri-Labs) [2]Gallimycin-36 (Durvet)	3 treatments at 12-hour intervals Clinical *S. aureus* mastitis Clinical *S. agalactiae* mastitis Clinical *S. dysgalactiae* mastitis Clinical *Streptococcus uberis* mastitis	Works against both acute and chronic cases
Hetacillin Aminopenicillin	Hetacin-K Intramammary Infusion (Fort Dodge Animal Health)	3 treatments at 24-hour intervals Acute, chronic, or subclinical mastitis	Shown to be efficacious in treatment of mastitis in lactating cows caused by susceptible strains of *S. agalactiae, S. dysgalactiae, S. aureus,* and *E. coli*
Penicillin G Penicillin	Masti-Clear (G.C. Hanford)	Not more than 3 treatments at 12-hour intervals Clinical *S. agalactiae* mastitis Clinical *S. dysgalactiae* mastitis Clinical *S. uberis* mastitis	
Pirlimycin Lincosamide	Pirsue Aqueous Gel (Pfizer Animal Health)	2 treatments at a 24-hour interval Clinical and subclinical mastitis	Has been proven effective only against *Staphylococcus* species such as *Staphylococcus aureus* and *Streptococcus* species such as *Streptococcus dysgalactiae* and *Streptococcus uberis*

Reprinted by permission from Erskine R, Wagner S: Antimicrobial therapy of mastitis. In Giguere E, editor: *Antimicrobial therapy in veterinary medicine,* ed 4, Ames, Iowa, 2006, Blackwell Publishing.

and the milk and meat withholding times before marketing must be extended. Chronic cases of mastitis that have been unresponsive to therapy should have antimicrobial culture performed to determine the causative pathogen; in such cases cessation of milking the affected quarter(s) is often the best option.

TREATMENT OF SEVERE CLINICAL MASTITIS

The major components of therapy for severe clinical mastitis are outlined in Box 101-2. Cases of clinical mastitis with systemic involvement (pyrexia, anorexia, depression,

Box 101-2

Components of Therapy for Severe Clinical Mastitis

1. Intramammary antibiotic therapy
   a. Commercial intramammary preparation
   b. Gram-positive spectrum required
   c. Gram-negative spectrum desirable
2. Systemic antimicrobial therapy
   a. Gram-negative spectrum required
3. Fluid therapy to maintain plasma volume and correct dehydration
   a. High-volume isotonic fluids intravenously OR
   b. Low-volume hypertonic saline intravenously + high-volume hypotonic fluids orally
4. Correction or prevention of hypocalcemia
   a. Calcium solution intravenously (especially if cow is recumbent) OR
   b. Calcium solution orally if cow is ambulatory
5. Correction or prevention of hypokalemia
   a. Oral potassium supplementation

shock, ruminal stasis, etc.) are termed *severe*. Coliform organisms (lactose-fermenting, gram-negative rods of the family Enterobacteriaceae) are the most common cause of this form of mastitis and more frequently result in cases in which the cow is lost to death or agalactia.[7,8] Thus primary therapy for severe clinical mastitis should be directed against coliform organisms, although consideration must be given for other causative agents. Supportive care, in addition to antibacterial drugs, may be the most beneficial part of a therapeutic regimen for coliform mastitis. The preferred basis for antibacterial therapy is knowledge of the causative pathogen, but this information is not attainable for some hours after initial case recognition. Thus the practical problem is to design a therapeutic regimen based on clinical impression.

Experimental challenge models have clarified much of the pathophysiology of mastitis resulting from infection with gram-negative organisms. Following infection, bacterial numbers in milk increase rapidly. Depending on the size of the challenge, peak bacterial concentrations in milk often occur within a few hours. Typically, a subsequent rapid decline in bacterial concentration follows neutrophil migration into the gland. Though often severe, experimental coliform infections usually clear spontaneously and are rarely more than 10 days in duration. The resulting inflammation and leukocytosis in the affected quarter may persist for several weeks, or the quarter may become agalactic, even when the bacteria are no longer isolated on milk culture.[9,10]

Many of the inflammatory and systemic changes observed during acute coliform mastitis result from the release of lipopolysaccharide endotoxin (LPS) from the bacteria. Most of the LPS release occurs following bacterial phagocytosis and killing by neutrophils. This results in activation of the cyclo-oxygenase and lipoxygenase pathways, producing prostaglandins, leukotrienes, and thromboxanes, compounds that are potent mediators of local inflammatory and systemic circulatory events. Endotoxin also induces the release of macrophage-derived cytokines, initiating fever, leukocytosis, protein synthesis and release by hepatocytes, and serum iron sequestration, collectively termed the *acute phase response*. To reduce the severity of acute coliform mastitis, either bacterial growth must be inhibited to reduce exposure of the quarter and the cow to LPS, or the effects of the LPS release must be neutralized. From a practical standpoint, therapy of severe coliform infections cannot begin until clinical signs appear. Clinical recognition of coliform mastitis usually occurs after peak bacterial numbers have been attained and maximal release of LPS has likely occurred. Therefore the primary therapeutic concern is the treatment of endotoxin-induced shock with fluids and other supportive care.

The objectives of supportive therapy for severe mastitis are to counteract endotoxin effects such as fever and inflammation and to correct dehydration and electrolyte imbalances. The cornerstone of supportive therapy in severe clinical mastitis is fluid therapy. Intravenous administration of large volumes of isotonic fluids (40-60 L in the first 24 hours) is ideal.[11] Administration of large volumes of intravenous fluids over a period of hours is frequently impractical in a farm setting. An alternative approach to support plasma volume and tissue perfusion while correcting dehydration is to administer 1 to 2 L of hypertonic saline solution (7.5% NaCl) intravenously followed by up to 10 gallons of hypotonic fluids per os. If the cow does not drink adequate oral fluids following administration of hypertonic saline IV, the remainder should be administered by orogastric intubation.

Cows with severe clinical mastitis are commonly hypocalcemic. Anorexia and diarrhea associated with the illness also predispose such animals to hypokalemia. Calcium solutions should be administered orally or intravenously. Calcium propionate is more easily absorbed from the gastrointestinal tract than other calcium salts.[12] Potassium deficits may be addressed by administering potassium chloride (KCl) at the rate of ¼ lb (100 g) in a water drench two to three times daily.

Antiinflammatory drugs have received much attention as a treatment for endotoxic mastitis. Benefits of antiinflammatory drugs on the key variables of survival and milk production have not been conclusively established, and improvement in clinical signs such as fever, local inflammation, and appearance of well-being have been observed primarily in studies in which antiinflammatory drugs were administered before the development of clinical signs.[13] Still, there is no evidence that administration of such drugs causes harm to cows with severe mastitis, and mastitis is a painful condition. Humane considerations therefore dictate that some pain relief should be provided. Flunixin meglumine has been approved for use in dairy cows in the United States. Intravenous administration is recommended because of the potential for significant tissue reaction following intramuscular administration and the highly unpredictable drug disposition and withdrawal time estimation following administration by other routes. Hydration must be maintained while any nonsteroidal antiinflammatory drug (NSAID) is being administered to minimize the risk of renal toxicity. In addition, prolonged NSAID therapy should be undertaken with caution because of the risk of gastric ulceration.

Antibacterial therapy may be of secondary importance relative to immediate supportive treatment of endotoxic shock, but it remains an integral part of a therapeutic regimen for severe mastitis. Although useful for determining the pathogenesis of coliform intramammary infection (IMI), experimental challenge models cannot be considered universally applicable for all cases. Most challenge models of infection do not include recently calved cows, use strains of bacteria that may not be as virulent as some of the wild types of pathogens, and are generally not administered if other possible immune stressors such as metabolic imbalance or heat stress are present.

Research from Colorado suggests that bacteremia may occur in more than 40% of severe coliform mastitis cases.[14,15] In addition, numerous other pathogens including gram-positive cocci may cause severe clinical mastitis, which can be difficult to distinguish from cases caused by coliforms at initial presentation. Chronic IMI caused by pathogens such as S. aureus can become acutely gangrenous at times of neutropenic dysfunction such as parturition.[16] The therapeutic objective is to attain effective concentrations of antibacterial drugs in the plasma of the cow and the mammary gland.

Intramuscular gentamicin was not more efficacious in preventing agalactia or death resulting from severe coliform mastitis, or in improving other clinical outcomes, as compared with cows receiving intramuscular erythromycin or no systemic antibacterials.[17] Cows experimentally challenged with E. coli and dosed with 500 mg of intramammary gentamicin every 12 hours did not have lower peak bacterial concentrations in milk, duration of infection, convalescent SCCs or serum albumin concentrations in milk, or rectal temperatures as compared with untreated challenged cows.[10] Additionally, gentamicin readily diffused through the milk-to-blood barrier as indicated by detectable concentrations in serum throughout the treatment period and the first 12 hours after the last dose. Consequently, urine gentamicin concentrations were detectable 14 days after the last infusion and concentrations of 1 μg of gentamicin/g in renal tissue were detected in cows 6 months after the trial.[10]

Three doses of parenteral sulfadiazine-trimethoprim have also failed to achieve clinical improvement in experimental E. coli infections.[18] However, three intramuscular doses of cefquinome, a fourth-generation cephalosporin with good tissue distribution, was found to improve clinical outcome of experimentally infected cows as compared with use of cloxacillin or ampicillin.[19] This is one of the few studies that has demonstrated efficacy for parenteral use of antibacterials in cows with experimental coliform mastitis; it also demonstrates the importance of selecting antibacterials with beneficial pharmacokinetic properties for which targeted organisms have a low MIC. Further research at Illinois confirmed this concept, as intravenous oxytetracycline was determined to improve clinical outcomes in cows with clinical coliform mastitis (not necessarily severe) compared with cows that did not receive systemic antibacterials.[20]

Mammary tissue and milk concentrations of ceftiofur following systemic treatment remain below effective concentrations for most mammary pathogens including Streptococcus agalactiae.[21-23] Parenteral administration of ceftiofur did not affect the outcome of mild clinical mastitis.[24] However, in a study of naturally occurring cases of severe coliform mastitis in Michigan, cows with severe coliform mastitis that were treated with ceftiofur at a dose of 2.2 mg/kg once per day were one third as likely to be lost from the herd and had significantly higher marketed milk than cows not receiving systemic antibacterials.[8] This strongly supports targeting the cow rather than the mammary gland with parenteral antimicrobials when coliform-induced bacteremia is suspected.

Despite the focus on coliform organisms, intramammary infusion of commercial products, particularly those that are active against gram-positive organisms, should be administered to any cow with severe clinical mastitis.

In summary, therapeutic regimens for severe clinical mastitis should include supportive care, especially for those cows displaying shock, broad-spectrum systemic antibacterial therapy that maintains effective concentrations in plasma, and intramammary antibacterials to reduce the effects of a gram-positive intramammary infection.

TREATMENT OF SUBCLINICAL INTRAMAMMARY INFECTION

Like mild clinical mastitis, subclinical mastitis does not present an urgent potential loss of gland function or the cow. Consequently, no significant economic losses will occur as a result of delaying initiation of therapy until bacterial culture can be completed. Antibacterial susceptibility testing of isolated pathogens often will suggest potentially beneficial therapy of gram-positive cocci. However, many subclinical intramammary infections (IMIs) selected as potential therapy candidates are chronic, and prediction of therapeutic outcome by in vitro testing is poor, especially in chronically infected quarters.[25]

Therapy is administered on the premise that treatment costs will be outweighed by compensatory production gains following elimination of infection. In the case of contagious pathogens, elimination of an IMI may also result in a decrease of the reservoir of infection and the risk to uninfected cows. Most often, the predominant pathogens causing subclinical mastitis are streptococci and staphylococci. The contagious pathogens S. agalactiae and S. aureus offer a study in opposites with respect to therapeutic strategies.

Prevalence of S. agalactiae IMI can be rapidly reduced by "blitz" treatment. With this method an entire herd or, more economically, all the infected cows in a herd, are treated with antibacterial drugs.[26-28] The most efficacious and cost-effective regimen is to employ intramammary beta-lactam therapy. All four quarters of infected cows should be treated to ensure elimination of the pathogen from the cow and prevent possible within-cow cross-infection of an uninfected quarter by an infected quarter. Cure rates range from 70% to 90%.[22,27] Commercial intramammary products are as efficacious as procaine penicillin G or florfenicol infusions derived from multiple-dose vials.[20,30] Intramammary preparations are preferred because of higher quality control for sterility and better reliability for predicting withholding periods for milk and meat discard after treatment. It is necessary to monitor treated herds by SCC and bacteriology to further identify and treat cows that were not identified as being infected initially. Usually, 30-day monitoring intervals after each treatment will be successful. A small percentage of cows will not respond to therapy and should be segregated or culled. Additionally, failure to use postmilking teat dipping and total dry cow treatment to prevent new IMI while eliminating existing IMI using blitz treatment will ultimately result in reinfection of the herd, as well as considerable expense and frustration on the part of the producer. Parenteral therapy is not likely to offer any benefit over intramammary therapy; in one study, 90% cure rates were achieved with intramammary penicillin-novobiocin therapy as opposed to 9% with intramuscular ceftiofur, illustrating the importance of pharmacokinetics in parenteral drug selection.[27]

Other common streptococci causing IMI are *Streptococcus dysgalactiae, Streptococcus bovis,* and *Streptococcus uberis.* As with *S. agalactiae,* most of these streptococci are sensitive in vitro to antibiotics, especially penicillin. Despite this apparent sensitivity, these streptococcal infections are not as easily cured as those caused by *S. agalactiae.* Controlled clinical data on the therapy of subclinical streptococcal infections are not extensive. Cure rates have ranged from 46% to 90%.[29,30] Much of the variation in cure rates is probably due to variable duration of infection before treatment.

Therapy of *S. aureus* IMI is difficult; experimentally induced infections have cure rates of 25% to 55% of infected quarters when evaluated for 21 to 60 days after infection.[31-33] However, natural infections are usually of longer duration before detection and subsequent therapy and thus are less responsive to therapy. Intramammary cefoperazone for the treatment of naturally occurring clinical *S. aureus* mastitis resulted in bacteriologic cures for only 39% of the cases when evaluated 14 days after treatment, and intramammary florfenicol or cloxacillin administered for three doses at 12-hour intervals resulted in only 9% cures.[30,34] Novel combinations of drugs including parenteral treatment regimens may be necessary to eliminate a higher proportion of infections. In experimental infections in lactating cows, the combined use of intramuscular procaine penicillin G and intramammary amoxicillin achieved a better cure rate (18/35 infected quarters) than intramammary amoxicillin did alone (10/40 infected quarters).[33] Lactating cows with *S. aureus* IMI had improved cure rates when administered 5 mg/lb of oxytetracycline in addition to intramammary antibacterial drugs as compared with cows administered intramammary infusions only.[35] Additionally, intramuscular penicillin administered for longer periods than those typical for labeled intramammary regimens (4 days as opposed to 2 days) maintained MIC in the gland for more extensive time periods, resulting in better efficacy.[36]

The concept of extending the duration of therapy to attain better efficacy was further supported by a recent Tennessee study that determined overall subclinical mastitis cure rates for all pathogens to be 10%, 39%, 54%, and 66% for untreated, 2-, 5-, and 8-day therapeutic regimens with intramammary ceftiofur. Following the 8-day regimen, the cure rate was 36% for *S. aureus* IMI and between 67% and 86% for other gram-positive cocci.[37]

Therapy of chronic, subclinical IMI may have the best probability of success by including parenteral, in addition to intramammary, therapy, and/or extending the duration of therapy beyond the usual two to three doses. The dosing regimen should ensure drug levels above MIC for periods long enough to allow effective killing of the pathogen. However, it must be remembered that cure rates attained may not be much better than those attained from spontaneous cure. Additionally, definitions of cure must be made critically, and affected quarters should be monitored for at least 30 days after the end of treatment to encompass the refractory period when bacteria may not be isolated.

ANTIBACTERIAL THERAPY OF PREGNANT HEIFERS

By convention, heifers have been considered essentially free of IMI before calving, and except for the rare case, to need little therapeutic attention until after lactation when the risk of infection increases. Many IMIs in calving heifers are caused by staphylococcal species other than *S. aureus,* which have a high rate of spontaneous cure. However, in some herds, a substantial portion of heifers at calving are infected, and additionally some of the IMI are caused by more diverse groups of pathogens including *S. aureus.*[38] A geographic element of risk to this problem exists, and dermatitis of the teat end caused by *Haematobia irritans* (horn fly), may play a role in the pathogenesis.[39] Clinical investigations have indicated that intramammary infusions pirlimycin, cephapirin, or penicillin-novobiocin at 7 or 14 days before expected calving reduced the prevalence of IMI in early lactation.[40,41] Treated heifers produced 531 more kg of milk than untreated heifers during the first lactation.[42] In a large multistation research study of 9 herds and 561 animals, prepartum treatment of heifers with cephapirin resulted in reduced IMI as compared with controls but did not affect milk production or SCCs in the first 200 days of lactation.[43] A significant herd interaction for milk production occurred.

Risk of residues in milk, especially in heifers that calve before expected calving dates, may be reduced if heifers are treated earlier rather than later. Administration of cephapirin 14 days before expected calving markedly reduced the occurrence of residues in milk by 3 days after calving without reducing therapeutic efficacy.[40] As with cows, strict teat end antisepsis should be followed before infusion to prevent any contamination and the restraint needed to handle young animals for treatment may be extensive.

Experts have not established that intramammary treatment of heifers with antibiotics before calving is more effective than treatment in early lactation. Some cases of mastitis acquired before parturition will resolve spontaneously. In addition, infusing drugs into the mammary glands of pregnant heifers is likely to be expensive in terms of drug costs, labor costs, and stress to both humans and animals. There is also a risk of introducing bacteria into a previously uninfected gland. For farms with severe problems with heifers calving with mastitis, precalving treatment may be worthwhile. But for most farms the benefit is unlikely to outweigh the financial and other costs of implementing such a program.

References

1. Mitchell JM, Griffiths MW, McEwen SA et al: Antimicrobial drug residues in milk and meat: causes, concerns, prevalence, regulations, tests, and test performance, *J Food Prot* 61:742-756, 1998.
2. Curtis CR, Erb HN, Sniffen CJ et al: Association of parturient hypocalcemia with eight periparturient disorders in Holstein cows, *J Am Vet Med Assoc* 183:559-561, 1983.
3. Morin DE, Shanks RD, McCoy GC: Comparison of antibiotic administration in conjunction with supportive measures versus supportive measures alone for treatment of dairy cows with clinical mastitis, *J Am Vet Med Assoc* 213:676-684, 1998.
4. Van Eeenanaam AL, Gardner IA, Holmes J et al: Financial analysis of alternative treatments for clinical mastitis associated with environmental pathogens, *J Dairy Sci* 78:2086-2095, 1995.
5. Hillerton JE, Kliem KE: Effective treatment of *Streptococcus uberis* clinical mastitis to minimize the use of antibiotics, *J Dairy Sci* 85:1009-1014, 2002.
6. Constable PD, Morin DE: Treatment of clinical mastitis: using antimicrobial susceptibility profiles for treatment decisions, *Vet Clin North Am Food Anim Pract* 19:139-155, 2003.
7. Anderson KL, Smith AR, Gustaffson BK et al: Diagnosis and treatment of acute mastitis in a large dairy herd, *J Am Vet Med Assoc* 181:690-693, 1982.
8. Erskine RJ, Bartlett PC, Van Lente J et al: Efficacy of systemic ceftiofur as a therapy for severe clinical mastitis in dairy cattle, *J Dairy Sci* 85:2571-2575, 2002.
9. Erskine RJ, Eberhart RJ, Grasso PJ et al: Induction of *Escherichia coli* mastitis in cows fed selenium-deficient or selenium-supplemented diets, *Am J Vet Res* 50:2093-2100, 1989.
10. Erskine RJ, Wilson RC, Riddell MG et al: Intramammary gentamicin as a therapy for experimental *Escherichia coli* mastitis, *J Am Vet Med Assoc* 53:375-381, 1992.
11. Anderson KL: Therapy for acute coliform mastitis, *Comp Cont Ed Pract Vet* 11:1125-1133, 1989.
12. Goff JP, Horst RL: Oral administration of calcium salts for treatment of hypocalcemia in cattle, *J Dairy Sci* 76:101-108, 1993.
13. Anderson KL, Smith AR, Shanks RD et al: Efficacy of flunixin meglumine for the treatment of endotoxin-induced bovine mastitis, *Am J Vet Res* 47:1366-1372, 1986.
14. Cebra CK, Garry FB: RP Dinsmore: Naturally occurring acute coliform mastitis in Holstein cattle, *J Vet Intern Med* 10:252-257, 1996.
15. Wenz JR, Barrington GM, Garry FB et al: Bacteremia associated with naturally occurring acute coliform mastitis in dairy cows, *J Am Vet Med Assoc* 219:976–981.
16. Kerhli ME Jr., Nonnecke BJ, Roth JA: Alterations in bovine neutrophil function during the periparturient period, *Am J Vet Res* 50:207-214, 1989.
17. Jones GF, Ward GE: Evaluation of systemic administration of gentamicin for treatment of coliform mastitis in cows, *J Am Vet Med Assoc* 197:731-736, 1990.
18. Pyorala S, Kaartinen L, Käck H et al: Efficacy of two therapy regimens for treatment of experimentally induced *Escherichia coli* mastitis in cows, *J Dairy Sci* 77:453, 1994.
19. Shpigel NY, Levin D, Winkler M et al: Efficacy of cefquinome for treatment of cows with mastitis experimentally induced using, *Escherichia coli*, *J Dairy Sci* 80:323, 1997.
20. Morin D, Shanks RD, McCoy GC et al: Comparison of antibiotic administration in conjunction with supportive measures versus supportive measures alone for treatment of dairy cows with clinical mastitis, *J Am Vet Med Assoc* 213:676, 1988.
21. Erskine RJ, Wilson RC, Tyler JW et al: Ceftiofur distribution in serum and milk from clinically normal cows and cows with experimental *Escherichia coli*-induced mastitis, *Am J Vet Res* 56:481-486, 1995.
22. Erskine RJ, Bartlett PC, Johnson GL II et al: Intramuscular administration of ceftiofur sodium versus intramammary infusion of penicillin/novobiocin for treatment of *Streptococcus agalactiae* mastitis in dairy cows, *J Am Vet Med Assoc* 208:258, 1996.
23. Owens WE, Xiang ZY, Ray CH et al: Determination of milk and mammary tissue concentrations of ceftiofur after intramammary and intramuscular therapy, *J Dairy Sci* 73:3449-3456, 1990.
24. Wenz JR, Garry FB, Lombard JE et al: Short communication: Efficacy of parenteral ceftiofur for treatment of systemically mild clinical mastitis in dairy cattle, J Dairy Sci 88:3496-3499.
25. Hoe FG, Ruegg PL: Relationship between antimicrobial susceptibility of clinical mastitis pathogens and treatment outcome in cows, *J Am Vet Med Assoc* 227:1461-1468, 2005.
26. Erskine RJ, Eberhart RJ: Herd benefit-to-cost ratio and effects of a bovine mastitis control program that includes blitz treatment of, *Streptococcus agalactiae*, *J Am Vet Med Assoc* 196:1230-1235, 1990.
27. Yamagata M, Goodger WJ, Weaver L et al: The economic benefit of treating subclinical *Streptococcus agalactiae* mastitis in lactating cows, *J Am Vet Med Assoc* 191:1556-1561, 1987.
28. Edmondson PW: An economic justification of "blitz" therapy to eradicate *Streptococcus agalactiae* from a dairy herd, *Vet Rec* 125:591-593, 1989.
29. Weaver LD, Galland J, Martin PA, Versteeg J: Treatment of *Streptococcus agalactiae* mastitis in dairy cows: Comparative efficacies of two antibiotic preparations and factors associated with successful treatment, *J Am Vet Med Assoc* 189:666-669, 1986.
30. Wilson DJ, Sears PM, Gonzalez RN et al: Efficacy of florfenicol for treatment of clinical and subclinical bovine mastitis, *Am J Vet Res* 57:526-528, 1996.
31. Owens WE, Ray CH, Watts JL et al: Comparison of success of antibiotic therapy during lactation and results of antibacterial susceptibility tests for bovine mastitis, *J Dairy Sci* 80:313-317, 1997.
32. Newbould FH: Antibiotic treatment of experimental *Staphylococcus aureus* infections of the bovine mammary gland, *Can J Comp Med* 38:411-416, 1974.
33. Owens WE, Watts JL, Boddie RL et al: Antibiotic treatment of mastitis: comparison of intramammary and intramammary plus intramuscular therapies, *J Dairy Sci* 71:3143-3147, 1988.
34. Wilson CD, Agger N, Gilbert GA et al: Field trials with cefaperazone in the treatment of bovine clinical mastitis, *Vet Rec* 118:17-22, 1986.
35. Sol J, Harink J, van Uum A: *Factors affecting the result of dry cow treatment.* Proceedings International Symposium on Bovine Mastitis, 1990, pp 118-123.
36. Ziv G, Storper M: Intramuscular treatment of subclinical staphylococcal mastitis in lactating cows with penicillin G, methicillin and their esters, *J Vet Pharm Ther* 8:276-282, 1985.
37. Oliver SP, Gillespie BE, Headrick SJ et al: Efficacy of extended ceftiofur intramammary therapy for treatment of subclinical mastitis in lactating dairy cows, *J Dairy Sci* 87:2393-2400, 2004.
38. Shearer JK, Harmon RJ: Mastitis in heifers, *Vet Clin North Am Food Anim Pract* 9:583-595, 1993.
39. Owens WE, Oliver SP, Gillespie BE et al: Role of horn flies (Haematobia irritans) in *Staphylococcus aureus*–induced mastitis in dairy heifers, *Am J Vet Res* 59:1122-1124, 1998.
40. Oliver SP, Lewis MJ, Gillespie BE et al: Antibiotic residues and prevalence of mastitis pathogen isolation in heifers during early lactation following prepartum antibiotic therapy, *Zentralbl Veterinarmed* B 44:213-220, 1997.

41. Oliver SP, Gillespie BE, Ivey SJ et al: Influence of prepartum pirlimycin hydrochloride or penicillin-novobiocin therapy on mastitis in heifers during early lactation, *J Dairy Sci* 87:1727-1731, 2004.

42. Oliver SP, Lewis MJ, Gillespie BE et al: Prepartum antibiotic treatment of heifers: milk production, milk quality and economic benefit, *J Dairy Sci* 86:1187-1193, 2003.

43. Borm AA, Fox LK, Leslie KE et al: Effects of prepartum intramammary antibiotic therapy on udder health, milk production, and reproductive performance in dairy heifers, *J Dairy Sci* 89:2090-2098, 2006.

CHAPTER 102

Respiratory Disease Treatment Considerations in Feedyards

DEE GRIFFIN

This chapter discusses proper approaches of dealing with bovine respiratory disease (BRD) in terms of antibiotic selection including a section on the pharmacologic basis for proper selection and use. This chapter also discusses treatment protocol design and considerations for posttreatment intervals (PTIs) with the newer ultra-long-acting (>3 days) antibiotics, evaluating BRD cases and their treatment response, and antibiotic residue avoidance strategies.

Veterinarians and the Cattle Industry Have Never Had It So Good

Considering the available antibiotics for treating BRD, the veterinary profession and cattle industry have never had it so good. In the past three decades the trend has gone from BRD treatment regimens that required daily treatments to therapies that have a labeled duration of more than a week, and from rather ordinary antibiotics such as penicillin, oxytetracycline, tylosin, erythromycin, and sulfas to phenomenal single-treatment selection choices that include ceftiofur, enrofloxacin, florfenicol, tilmicosin, and tulathromycin. Antibiotic sensitivity testing of BRD bacterial isolates suggests the available antibiotics should be adequate; however, BRD fatality rates continue to be troubling. Many veterinarians and producers remember a time when antibiotics seemed more effective. Antibiotic sensitivity data from my laboratory evaluated since 1991 for the major BRD bacterial pathogens, while variable from year to year, have not significantly changed. Perhaps the impression that antibiotics once worked better is because the cattle feeding industry is starting younger and lighter-weight cattle than in past decades. Three decades ago the feedyard industry started cattle that were 18 to 24 months of age, and currently cattle are only 18 to 24 months of age at the end of the finishing phase. Cattle age should not change the interpretation of antibiotic sensitivity test results. If antibiotic resistance and treatment or dose management is not the problem, what is? An adage about determinants of BRD treatment success goes something like, "any antibiotic will work if you catch the disease early enough and nothing will work if the disease gets a head start." This is as true today as it was decades ago.

Why an Antibiotic May Seem to Work on Some Sets of Cattle and Not Others

The biggest factor that influences success of a BRD treatment protocol is *timing*. How much of a head start does the bacterial infection have? This factor plus the animal's ability to help fight back (immune preparation and maturity), combined with differences in bugs, have a tremendous influence on clinical outcomes. Another major factor that is seldom considered in the treatment response is correctness of the clinical diagnosis. Misdiagnosis as a cause of BRD treatment failure is a common necropsy finding and is discussed later.

DEALING WITH BRD BEFORE IT GETS A HEAD START MAY BE THE MOST IMPORTANT CONSIDERATION

The best way to deal with BRD is to prevent it. Preventing BRD requires more than a well-designed vaccination program. Calf immune preparation management is a life-cycle endeavor. Having calves born to healthy mothers and getting a proper dose of colostrum are the first most important steps in immune management. Minimizing massive exposure to pathogens before proper vaccination programs have been implemented and proper nutrition are important next steps in immune management. A properly designed vaccination program that is properly administered is the next step. Giving BRD vaccinations that include a modified live viral component for IBR, BVD, PI3, and BRSV on arrival at feedyards is a standard operating procedure (SOP) for many, if not most, veterinary consultants. The immediate cell-mediated immune response decreases the movement of BRD viral agents among newly received cattle. Available data indicate longer-term protective value for the newer technology leukotoxin bacterial vaccines for *Mannheimia hemolytica*. The data supporting the use of *Pasteurella multocida* and *Histophilus somni* are less convincing. The last critical step is proper stress management. Thoughtful management decisions that make minimizing stress a priority and careful handling and transportation by kind, caring, and trained people are key components.

Purchasing cattle that have been prepared to deal with BRD exposure is the best BRD defense. The data are clear. Preconditioning and backgrounding programs such as the Iowa Green Tag Program and the Texas VAC 45 Program reduce BRD losses that include costs for treatment, death, and gain performance. Antibiotic metaphylaxis is the next best procedure if cattle that have been properly preconditioned are not available.

Antibiotic metaphylaxis has a proven history of reducing BRD losses, especially in cattle that are considered at "high risk" of developing BRD. The high-risk designation is typically given to younger cattle that are recently weaned, have not received BRD vaccination, and have commingled with other cattle that similarly have poor BRD defense preparation. The younger the cattle, the more deficient the health management history (including lack of castration), and the more convoluted the commingling or shipping history, the higher the risk status of the cattle. Although antibiotic metaphylaxis may be administered in the feed, strict usage guidelines prohibiting extralabel drug use (ELDU) of feed additives and the concern for individual animal feed consumption make this delivery mechanism less effective than if an appropriate antibiotic is administered to individual animals at arrival processing. Metaphylaxis protocols using long-acting antibiotics (those with prolonged dosing intervals) make the procedure much simpler. The majority of the debate around metaphylaxis deals with economic analysis of product selection. The Animal Medicinal Drug Use Clarification Act (AMDUCA) does not allow medication cost to be a consideration for ELDU. Additionally, the national Beef Quality Assurance (BQA) guidelines prohibit the ELDU of aminoglycosides because of the potential violative residue if an extremely long withdrawal (WD) time is not assigned to animals that have received parenteral administration. In general, metaphylaxis will reduce BRD losses by approximately 20%, but the variability in the benefits can make the specifics of the decision difficult. Product selection analysis should consider labor costs and reduction in sickness events, sickness relapse, death, growth,

and feed efficiency. Long-acting oxytetracycline continues to provide good metaphylaxis value in most groups of newly received feeder cattle. Newly received feeder cattle that have an especially high BRD risk, as judged by cattle source and past history, may be candidates for antibiotics that have long dosing intervals (PTIs) as predicted by an antibiotic's half-life ($T_{1/2}$) and/or antibiotics that have a high volume of distribution (Vd). Examples of these are the long-acting formulation of ceftiofur (Excede, Pfizer Animal Health, New York); florfenicol (Nuflor, Schering-Plough Animal Health, Union, N.J.); tilmicosin (Micotil, Elanco Animal Health, Greenfield, Ind.); and tulathromycin (Draxxin, Pfizer Animal Health, N.Y.). It should be noted that although enrofloxacin (Baytril, Bayer Animal Health, Shawnee Mission, Kan.) would fit the pharmacokinetics ($T_{1/2}$ and Vd) needed, giving a fluoroquinolone to all cattle on arrival is an ELDU and a violation of AMDUCA. An argument might be made to use enrofloxacin on arrival if all the cattle fit the visual BRD criteria. This would include taking a rectal temperature at the time of consideration. Only those that have a temperature greater than the temperature criteria included in the veterinarian's BRD treatment protocol would be treated with the fluoroquinolone.

Finding Sick Cattle Early Is Next on the List of Important Considerations

Decades ago a video titled "Pull'em Deep" (Elanco Animal Health, Greenfield, Ind.) was a hit for helping cattle health checkers (pen riders) learn to find cattle in the early stages of BRD. The film stressed the mantra, "if in doubt, pull'em out," as an important key to addressing the needs of sick cattle during the early stages of BRD. More recently a training program titled "D.A.R.T" (Pfizer Animal Health, N.Y.) focused on evaluating an animal's depression, appetite, respiration rate, and rectal temperature, which could be attributed to BRD. These and other training programs developed by veterinary consultants focus not only on spotting symptoms attributed to BRD, but on cattle behavior and the interaction between cattle and their environment. Historically the focus has been on finding cattle that do not look "normal" and treating them with an antibiotic if they have an undifferentiated fever. This poor BRD case definition is undoubtedly responsible for treating ugly cattle suffering from heat stress or subclinical acidosis. To minimize this problem it is critical for cattle health checkers to have plenty of time to observe the cattle for which they are responsible. Because cattle are extremely susceptible to heat stress, checking cattle for illness should occur early in the day during times of the year when ambient temperatures will reach or exceed 82° F, which is cattle's upper critical temperature, especially in those with black hair coats. For the same reason it is important for cattle being treated for BRD to be evaluated early in the day during the hot times of the year. The increase in body temperature and respiration rate associated with heat stress make BRD evaluation and/or its treatment difficult. Similarly, cattle suffering from subclinical acidosis frequently have an increased body temperature and respiratory rate.

ANTIBIOTIC BASICS

Four mechanisms of action identified by which antibiotics inhibit microbes are (1) crippling production of the bacterial *cell wall* (CW) that protects the cell from the external environment; (2) interfering with *protein synthesis* (PS) by binding to the machinery that builds proteins, amino acid by amino acid; (3) wreaking havoc with *metabolic processes* (MPs), such as the synthesis of folic acid, that bacteria need to thrive; and (4) blocking *genetic replication* (GR) by interfering with synthesis of DNA and RNA. Understanding the mechanisms of action of an antibiotic may not be as important as understanding how an antibiotic disperses to the target organ(s) and penetrates the tissues within the target organ. Three pieces of pharmacokinetic (PK) information useful in predicting theoretical antibiotic dispersion and penetration are (1) Vd; (2) lipid solubility (LS); and (3) plasma protein binding (PB). The relative degree (low, intermediate, or high) rather than the specific value of each of these PK indicators is adequate for clinical considerations (Table 102-1). Additionally, it is important to understand how to use other PK and pharmacodynamic (PD) parameters in developing effective antibiotic treatment protocols (Table 102-2). The PK/PD approach to antibiotic use targets relationships such as time above a target minimum inhibitory concentration (T > MIC) and antibiotic absorption and excretion area under the curve (AUC) to MIC (AUC/MIC). The maximum duration of bacterial exposure to the antibiotic is predicted by T > MIC and is critical for successful use of beta-lactams such as ampicillin, ceftiofur, and penicillin. The AUC/MIC is predictive of the success of tetracyclines and tulathromycin. When the AUC/MIC and the peak concentration are considered together, they are predictive for the success of aminoglycosides such as gentamicin and neomycin and for fluoroquinolones such as danofloxacin and enrofloxacin.

Antibiotic-Resistant Mechanisms

The mechanisms by which microbes resist antibiotics are also basic to the discussion. Although the antibiotics of different classes of antibiotics have a main mechanism of action (see Table 102-2), microbes may possess multiple mechanisms by which they resist antibiotics. Bacteria may defend aminoglycosides by decreasing cell wall uptake or decreasing permeability. Bacterial defense for macrolides, fluoroquinolones, and tetracyclines may include efflux or pumping the compound out. Enzyme induction as a mechanism of resistance occurs for compounds such as aminoglycosides, florfenicol, and beta-lactams. Microbes may alter ribosome target binding sites as a defense mechanism for macrolides and lincosamides. Altering their cell wall protein structure may be used to defend against beta-lactams and glycopeptides. Genes encoding for resistance can be carried on plasmids (beta-lactams, tetracyclines, macrolides, lincosamides, fluoroquinolones, and sulfas); carried on transposons (beta-lactams and glycopeptides); or carried on chromosomes (beta-lactams and fluoroquinolones).

NATURAL HISTORY OF BOVINE RESPIRATORY DISEASE

Designing the structure and flow of the BRD treatment protocol should coincide with the sequences and timing in BRD development caused by the most probable bacterial pathogens. This timeline is a foundation for selecting the appropriate response and medications at any point along the disease progression. Although a bit remedial, it seems important to review this sequence.

A susceptible animal is exposed. The incubation period is the time from the first replication of the disease-causing biologic agent until sufficient compromise of the target organ(s) occurs, causing loss of function of the target organ(s). Primary viral BRD incubation averages 3 days.

Table **102-1**

Antimicrobial Groups Approved for Cattle

Antibiotic Class	Antibiotics Within Class	Mechanism of Action	Volume of Distribution	Lipid Solubility	Approximate Protein Binding %
Aminocyclitols	Spectinomycin	PS	Low	Low	Low
Aminoglycosides	Gentamicin, neomycin	PS	Low	Low	Low
Beta-lactams	Penicillin G (P), ampicillin (A), ceftiofur (C)	CW	Low	Low	P & A low, C high
Chloramphenicol derivatives	Florfenicol	PS	Intermediate	High	Intermediate
Fluoroquinolones	Enrofloxacin, danofloxacin	GR	High	High	Low
Macrolides	Erythromycin, tilmicosin, tylosin, tulathromycin	PS	High	High	Intermediate
Sulfonamides	Sulfamethazine, sulfadimethoxine	MP	Low	Low	High
Tetracyclines	Oxytetracycline (O), chlortetracycline (C)	PS	Intermediate	Intermediate	O low, C intermediate

CW, Cell wall; *GR*, genetic replication; *MP*, metabolic process; *PS*, protein synthesis.

Table 102-2

Pharmacokinetic and Pharmacodynamic for Bovine Antibiotics

Generic Name	ACT	LS	Vd	TM	C_{max}	AUC	$T_{1/2}$	Dose	MIC_{90} Mh	MIC_{90} Pm	MIC_{90} Hs	WD
Ampicillin	C	L	L	*	10	*	1.2	10	32	8	4	6
Amoxicillin	C	L	L	*	10	*	5	5	16	16	8	25
Ceftiofur sodium	C	L	L	1.2	14	115	10	1	0.03 (0.2)tt	0.03 (0.2)tt	0.03 (0.2)tt	4
Ceftiofur hydrochloride	C	L	L	2.5	11	160	12	1	0.03 (0.2)tt	0.03 (0.2)tt	0.03 (0.2)tt	3
Ceftiofur crystalline acid	C	L	L	19	6.4	376	50	3	0.03 (0.2)tt	0.03 (0.2)tt	0.03 (0.2)tt	13
Chlortetracycline (feed)	S	M	M	10.2	0.21	4.3	15.7	10	12	12	12	0
Danofloxacin†	C	M§	H	3.2	1.3	9	4.5	2.7	0.06	0.02	0.06	4
Enrofloxacin†	C	M	H	5.8	1.8	19	6.4	5.7	0.06	0.03	0.03	28
Florfenicol	S	H	M	5.3	5.4	71	18.3	18	1	1	0.5	38
Gentamicin†	C	H	L	*	<8	*	2	1	8	4	16	>730§
Neomycin†	C	L	L	*	10	*	2.5	2	64	64	64	36
Oxytetracycline (LA)‡	S	M	M	1.8	3.6	72	21	9	12	12	12	0
Oxytetracycline (feed)	S	M	M	2	0.16	4	9	10	12	12	12	0
Penicillin G, Benzathine	C	L	L	*	1.7	*	70	10k	16	8	16	>180§
Penicillin G, Procaine	C	L	L	*	3.4	*	5.2	10k	16	8	16	>60§
Spectinomycin	S	L	L	1	20	77	1.8	5.5	96	96	96	11
Sulfadimethoxine (IV)	S	L	L	*	8.9	*	13.1	25	350	350	350	5
Sulfadimethoxine (oral)	S	L	L	*	8.9	*	13.1	62.5	350	350	350	21
Sulfamethazine	S	L	L	*	16	*	12.9	200	350	350	350	12
Tilmicosin (lung C_{max})	S	H	H	1.4	1 (9)	8	≈24	4.5	16	32	8	28
Tulathromycin	*	H	H	.25	3.5	16	90	1.1	2	1	4	18
Tylosin	S	H	H	1.3	4.7	29	24	8	32	32	16	28

Iowa State University 2000-2003 for 90% of isolates; FDA NADA FOI; and Shryock, *J Vet Diag Invest* 8:337, 1996.

*No available data.

†Not approved for AMDUCA ELDU or BQA ELDU.

‡LA = Long-acting or depo formulations designed for >72-hr PTI.

§WD estimates for extralabel use. These WDs should be verified by FARAD or other source.

ACT, Action listed as either (C) cidal or (S) static; *AUC,* area under the curve (µg × hr/ml); C_{max}, peak ppm concentrations (ppm = µg/ml);

dose, refers to typical dose (mg/lb body weight) and is listed as the maximum label approval; *LS,* lipid soluble (L = low, M = moderate, H = high); *TM,* T_{max}—time at which C_{max} occurs; $T_{1/2}$ life, half-life in hours ($T_{1/2}$); *tt,* therapeutic threshold; *Vd,* volume of distribution (L = <0.5, M = 0.5-1, H = >1) see *LS; WD,* withdrawal days before marketing for food. The longest label WD is listed.

AMDUCA ELDU requires the adjustment so that no violative residues would be detected.

NOTE: Use the PHARMACOKINETICS, PHARMACODYNAMICS, & MIC information only as a starting guide.

Therapeutic regimen management requires response monitoring through accurate case definition, protocol adherence, record examination, and outcome follow-up.

Secondary bacterial BRD incubation averages 3 to 5 days after the initial viral infection. The inflammation of the affected organa (trachea and lung) occurs in stages. At the onset, the body diverts white blood cells and blood into the affected area, typically causing swelling of tissue, both cells and spaces between cells. As the inflammation continues, the affected tissue loses function. The late stage of inflammation involves the body trying to clean up, remove, or repair the damaged tissue. This is the beginning of recovery, which is 7 to 10 days after the initial disease tissue damage has subsided. This phase will last for weeks.

SELECTING ANTIMICROBIALS

Bovine Respiratory Disease Pathogens

No data support treatment of or vaccination for the viral component of BRD once the animal has developed symptoms. Antibiotic therapy is the only intervention that has proven to lower the case relapse rate (CRR), lower the case fatality rate (CRF), and mitigate the gain performance loss. Targeting the most probable bacterial pathogen(s) is a critical step in designing a treatment protocol. The most common bacterial BRD pathogens to be considered in a treatment protocol are (1) *M. hemolytica;* (2) *P. multocida;* (3) *H. somni;* and (4) *Mycoplasma bovis.* The MIC for the population of pathogens for the antibiotic approved for cattle can be estimated from diagnostic reports and/or Food and Drug Administration Center for Veterinary Medicine (FDA-CVM) freedom of information (FOI) documents. Considering the population MIC, whether for 50% (MIC_{50}) or 90% (MIC_{90}) of the population of isolates, along with the $T_{1/2}$ and the Vd, allows the design of protocols that supply an effective level of antibiotic at a target tissue (see Table 102-2).

Antibiotic Selection Focused on BRD Bacterial Pathogens and the Animal's Ability to Respond to Antibiotic Therapy

The bottom-line goal of therapy is to affect recovery. The medication portion of this strategy is to reach the targeted bacterial pathogen with a reasonably predicted effective antibiotic level and maintain that level during the dosing interval. Antibiotics with C_{max} similar to the targeted MIC would not likely maintain effective concentrations during the dosing interval. Similarly, antibiotics with short elimination half-lives ($T_{1/2}$) might not be reasonable if the dosing interval were longer than the compound's $T_{1/2}$, which prevented an effective concentration of antibiotic during the dosing interval. An example would be single-day dosing with ampicillin, which has a C_{max} similar to the MIC of BRD pathogens listed in Table 102-2 and which has a $T_{1/2}$ of only 1.2 hours. A different antibiotic should be selected unless the clinician has reason to believe that there will be a significant postantibiotic effect (PAE) on the targeted pathogen. Antibiotics that are known to have significant PAE include aminoglycosides, florfenicol, fluoroquinolones, macrolides, and tetracyclines. Beta-lactams and sulfa drugs have minimal or no PAE.

BRD bacterial pathogens that live in cells need antibiotics that cross cell walls. Using the data listed in Table 102-2, for example, ceftiofur hydrochloride dosed at 1 mg/lb would peak at 11 µg/ml and with a 12-hour half-life, the level of antibiotic would be above the MIC_{90} for all of the listed BRD bacterial pathogens for greater than 2 days (in the average animal). However, because *H. somni* is an obligate intracellular pathogen and ceftiofur, a beta-lactam, would have limited ability to penetrate cell walls (low Vd and low LS), the antibiotic would likely not be as effective for *H. somni* in the lung tissue but very effective during the septicemic phase of the infection. An antibiotic that had a higher Vd and LS such as enrofloxacin, danofloxacin, florfenicol, tilmicosin, tulathromycin, or tylosin would be a better choice for the tissue phase of the disease. When considering the MIC_{90} listed in Table 102-2 for these possible selections, only enrofloxacin appears to meet both the Vd and MIC_{90} criteria, although the value of Vd does not indicate the location of the drug (i.e., which tissues it might concentrate in).

Considering the information in Table 102-2, there are several antimicrobials such as procaine penicillin G (especially long-acting penicillin) and sulfas, the selection of which for BRD is indefensible.

Considerations must be given to the animal's immune system and its ability to fight bacterial infection. Many of the available antibiotics do not need to destroy all bacterial pathogens. Merely slowing the pathogen's growth as would be the case for the antibiotic listed as "static" in Table 102-2 or weakening the pathogen as with the PAE for any number of antibiotics is frequently enough for the animal's immune system to affect recovery.

Additionally, considerations must be given to the nature of damage the bacterial pathogen causes, where in the organs the targeted pathogen may reside, and unique features about the pathogen that affect suitability of the particular antibiotics mechanism of action. For example, Mb has no cell wall, so antibiotics in the beta-lactam class should not be expected to be effective.

Antibiotic Selection Considerations Focused on the Stage of BRD

Antibiotic penetration (Vd and LS) early in a BRD infection is not as much of a concern in designing a treatment protocol as it is late in the infection. Antibiotic therapy initiated late in a BRD infection or in cattle that have only poorly responded to previous BRD antibiotic therapy is of questionable value. Overwhelming infections or infections in cattle that have depressed metabolic or immune function may respond to the cidal antibiotics better than static antibiotics (see Table 102-2), although scarce data support this.

Select Generic Antibiotics with Extreme Caution

The PK and PD information listed in Table 102-2 is taken from FDA FOI documents and published articles that used FDA-approved pioneer compounds. The generic antibiotic's potency and purity, as well as the manufacturing quality control, should be investigated before considering a BRD treatment protocol.

EVALUATING TREATMENT RESPONSE: LOOK, LISTEN, AND SMELL

I would recommend trusting the cattle health checker's evaluation of the animal the first day it is pulled to the hospital for BRD evaluation and treatment. If I am told the animal looks sick, I accept the evaluation. The animal may not have BRD, but if the health checker sees something in the animal that seems abnormal, I feel obligated to investigate the observation.

Do not let a thermometer do your thinking. Combining all your senses along with daily weights and rectal temperatures will improve BRD treatment response evaluation.

Cattle are extremely sensitive to heat stress. A comfortable temperature for humans is about 70° F, whereas for cattle it is approximately 55° F. The upper critical ambient temperature of cattle is reached at 82° F. The rectal temperature in the afternoon for cattle pulled from their home pen will almost always be above 104° F regardless of their disease status. This is especially evident in animals that are not handled quietly, gently, kindly, and respectfully. Making sense of a rectal temperature can and should be challenging. Using a visual appraisal such as the depression score outlined in the D.A.R.T system is thought by most veterinary feedlot consultants to improve BRD evaluations. Using a stethoscope to evaluate lung sounds combined with a rectal temperature and visual appraisal may improve BRD evaluation even more.

I recommend treating BRD with an appropriate antibiotic for all cattle pulled for BRD evaluation that have a depression score 3 or higher (on a scale in which 0 is normal, and 5 is moribund); a harsh bronchial vascular or friction sound; and a rectal temperature 104° F or greater that have no evidence of other primary body system disease that could explain the depression, lung sounds, and rectal temperature.

BRD treated cases should be visually assessed daily. The evaluation of the first three elements in the D.A.R.T. system (the animal's depression or alertness evaluated outside their flight zone, their appetite as judged by the shape of the abdomen or rumen fill, and their respiratory rate and character) are sufficient. If the animal being considered visually appears worse than the day before, it should be returned to the hospital chute for additional evaluation that includes auscultation of the lung fields and a rectal temperature. It is extremely important to remember that a treatment response failure of an animal pulled for BRD may be due to an inaccurate original diagnosis. Therefore reexamination of BRD treatment failures should be more inclusive and specifically target other body systems than the original respiratory system evaluation performed by feedlot personnel at the beginning of the BRD treatment cycle.

FDA-CVM regulations for both prescription medications and AMDUCA ELDU require poor BRD treatment response to be addressed by the veterinarian prescribing the medication rather than feedlot personnel. Noncompliance with the veterinarian's prescription medication use orders cannot be tolerated. Most modern feedyards have medication use records that would detect personnel noncompliance with medication use orders. Good medical practices of the veterinarian prescribing the medications, as required by AMDUCA, include regular visits to the feedyard and availability for follow-up evaluation for all poorly responding animals. Most consulting veterinarians spend a significant amount of time during each feedyard visit evaluating the cattle that have not had an adequate treatment response.

Failure to initiate antibiotic therapy early in the BRD event is the most common cause of BRD treatment failure. Cattle, as prey animals, have over the millions of years on earth made not appearing sick one of their most important survival instincts, especially when a predator was in the vicinity. Prey animals that fail to expertly master not appearing sick increase the likelihood of their being selected by a predator for predation. The majority of BRD cases in feedlots occur during the first weeks following arrival of new cattle. During this time cattle that view cattle health checkers as predators may expertly hide their BRD symptoms. Lung evaluations in packing plants indicate that a remarkable number of cattle with lung lesions resulting from bacterial infection have no record of being treated for BRD. Considering these items, most consulting feedyard veterinarians target two items: (1) improving the bond between the newly arrived cattle and their cattle health checker and (2) designing BRD treatment protocols that allow for some delay in BRD detection. To improve the bonds between cattle and their caretakers, veterinarians work diligently to promote the gentleness and ease of cattle handling, especially during the first days that the animals stay at the feedyard. They encourage cattle health checkers to spend quiet time with newly arrived cattle to allow the animals to become more at ease being around the health checker. The cattle becoming more comfortable with the health checker in their environment and the health checker becoming more familiar with the animals make it easier for the health checker to identify BRD cases earlier. To deal with delay in BRD detection, consulting veterinarians also assume newly recognized BRD cases may have a two or more day head start before initiating antibiotic therapy and therefore design aggressive BRD treatment protocols that use the most potent antibiotic choices relative to predicted BRD MIC and Vd requirements.

The BRD treatment response and prevention bottom line is improved performance. Although decreased days of therapy, relapse rates, and death loss of treated cattle are important, growth and the efficiency of growth are perhaps the most objective sensitive measures of BRD treatment response.

MINIMIZING TIME SPENT TREATING BRD POTENTIALLY IMPROVES BRD TREATMENT RESPONSE

Long-acting penicillin, a mixture of procaine and benzathine penicillin G, and long-acting sulfadimethoxine were the first long-acting medications available for BRD therapy, but neither provided levels of medication that approached useful MIC levels for common BRD bacterial pathogens. Liquamycin LA-200 was the first effective long-acting BRD treatment approved by the FDA-CVM, and with its approval came a revolution in the acceptance of a single antibiotic dose therapy as effective for BRD treatment, as well as metaphylaxis. A single dose of long-acting oxytetracycline improved BRD metaphylaxis over prior practices involving individually treating cattle for consecutive days or attempting to feed antibiotics to lessen the BRD impact on performance. Acceptance as a single-dose therapy was not as great as acceptance for metaphylaxis. It seems reasonable to think this may have partly been due to the severe injection site reaction and the subsequent soreness, making BRD treatment response evaluation difficulty. As veterinarians learned that moving injections to the neck and giving products subcutaneously would minimize soreness and subsequent BRD treatment response evaluation, acceptance of the compound as a single-dose BRD treatment increased. Currently there are six subcutaneous injectable antibiotics, approved as a single dose for 3 or more days BRD therapy because they reach and maintain a level of compound greater than the MIC_{50} for *M. hemolytica*, *P. multocida*, and/or *H. somni*. These are ceftiofur crystalline, enrofloxacin, florfenicol, long-acting oxytetracycline, tilmicosin, and tulathromycin (see Table 102-2).

Although once unsure, veterinarians have become mentally comfortable with a single antibiotic dose providing an effective level of the compound for 3 or more days. Several benefits have been recognized. Obvious labor savings is generally first on everyone's list, but decreasing animal handling stress is significant and perhaps maintaining a higher level of antibiotic during the course of BRD therapy may decrease the number of resistance microbes that survive antibiotic exposure, therefore possibly decreasing the BRD relapse rate. Two antibiotics, ceftiofur crystalline and tulathromycin BRD, are labeled for treatment intervals greater than 7 days. Although BRD management techniques when working with antibiotics that have a prolonged posttreatment interval (PTI) are still being refined, outcome data in recent years suggest BRD treatment protocols using antibiotics that allow a prolonged PTI can be successful.

DESIGNING BRD TREATMENT PROTOCOLS

Preventing BRD from getting ahead of one's treatment protocol is extremely important. Severely damaged lung tissue becomes the nidus for chronic bacterial infection that cannot be reached with any antibiotic. Treating cattle chronically ill with BRD following failed primary BRD treatment is futile. The majority of lung cultures from cattle suffering chronically from BRD seldom recover bacteria considered primary pathogens, but instead recover only opportunistic bacteria such as *Arcanobacterium pyogenes*. As noted earlier, understanding this potential makes it important to treat cattle suffering from BRD as early as possible in the course of the disease and furthermore makes the first antibiotic one includes in the treatment protocol important. A BRD treatment protocol should attempt to effect a cure with the first antibiotic selected. It is folly to design a BRD treatment protocol that begins with an antibiotic that would predictably have marginal effectiveness and is followed by an antibiotic that would predictably be much more effective. Additionally, of the antibiotics listed in Table 102-2, no data support the value to BRD recovery of using more than one properly selected antibiotic. Likewise, no data support the value to BRD recovery from using an antibiotic IV as compared with SC.

Metaphylaxis is an important part of the BRD treatment protocol. Experts may debate whether an antibiotic used in this situation be considered prophylactic rather than metaphylactic. When BRD is experimentally induced using an upper respiratory tract inoculation with a respiratory virus, clinical BRD has seldom been observed in less than 7 days. Therefore if cattle develop BRD within the first week of feedlot arrival, it seems appropriate to assume the disease process had begun at or before their arrival. If this postulation is acceptable, metaphylaxis, not prophylaxis, would be the proper term.

When designing protocols, the first and foremost consideration is the source history and age of the cattle. Younger cattle that have not had previous marketing or commingling are especially susceptible to potential BRD pathogens. When commingled with other cattle in the marketing system, they are considered high BRD risk. The longer the delay from the time cattle first enter the marketing system and arrive at their final destination, the higher the risk of developing life-threatening BRD. Cattle that fit these criteria can be extremely difficult for cattle health checkers to evaluate. Additionally, cattle that fit these criteria are likely to have individuals develop BRD within the first few days following feedlot arrival. For these reasons it may be advisable to use an appropriate metaphylactic antibiotic. Antibiotics that have high Vd and LS such as tilmicosin have had excellent historical metaphylactic response that included decreased subsequent morbidity and mortality, as well as improved growth and growth efficiency. BRD being treated during the first week of arrival in the feedyard is likely to be in the early stages of the disease. Early BRD is more likely to have a septicemic component than late-stage BRD and is less likely to have the severity of lung tissue damage that develops in later stages, which may interfere with an antibiotic's ability to penetrate tissues. In this circumstance it may be acceptable to select an antibiotic such as ceftiofur crystalline, even though it has a lower Vd and LS. Ceftiofur crystalline has a prolonged $T_{1/2}$, and high C_{max} relative to the MIC_{90} (see Table 102-2) may make it an acceptable metaphylactic choice that provides a reasonable medication level for

at least 7 days. This should be ample time for the cattle to acclimate to the feedyard environment and the cattle health checker to become familiar with the cattle.

Treatment protocols for cattle identified by the daily cattle health checker's evaluation as having BRD can be divided into three categories: (1) high-BRD-risk cattle as noted earlier; (2) cattle that have had their immune system previously managed such as those preconditioned or backgrounded or yearlings that have been pastured following weaning (normal risk); and (3) cattle that develop BRD after having been in the feedyard for several months (late stage).

Treatment protocols for high-risk cattle should be aggressive, meaning the antibiotic selection should have an above-average Vd and LS (see Table 102-1) and a high C_{max} relative to the predicted MIC_{90} for the most probable bacterial pathogens (see Table 102-2). An additional consideration may include minimal side effects such as stressful animal handling requirements, injection site reaction and soreness, potential for hepatic damage, renal damage in dehydrated animals, and appetite depression. Of the antibiotics listed in Table 102-2, ceftiofur crystalline, danofloxacin, enrofloxacin, florfenicol, and tulathromycin meet the C_{max} to MIC criteria and have labeling indicating a single dose provides multiple-day therapeutic medication levels. Danofloxacin will be selected less often than enrofloxacin because it requires dosing every 48 hours. All beta-lactams, as represented by ceftiofur in this list of proposed antibiotic choices, have relative low Vd and LS, making them less attractive when significant lung damage could exist or if obligate intracellular pathogens such as *H. somni* or *Salmonella* spp. were significant concerns. Additionally, beta-lactams, because their mechanism of action is against the microbe's cell wall, would have no predicted activity against microbes that do not have cell walls such as *M. bovis*. Using this logic, enrofloxacin, florfenicol, and tulathromycin would be the three remaining antibiotic choices. Enrofloxacin and florfenicol have high C_{max} to MIC_{90}; therefore the opportunity for resistant BRD bacterial pathogens to survive and subsequently participate as the principle cause for BRD relapse would be predictably minimal. The long PTI as predicted by the $T_{1/2}$ (see Table 102-2) and the high Vd and LS makes tulathromycin an attractive choice, especially considering the long PTI would minimize animal handling stress, which could potentially aid in the animal's recovery. Considering the $T_{1/2}$, the tulathromycin C_{max} relative to the MIC_{90} would predict an effective concentration against *M. haemolytica* for approximately 5 days and against Pm for approximately 10 days, but the time above the estimated MIC_{90} against *H. somni* would be minimal. The C_{max}-to-MIC ratio for all three antibiotics being considered (enrofloxacin, florfenicol, and tulathromycin) for *M. bovis* has been reported as excellent, although enrofloxacin is not labeled for *Mycoplasma* in the United States.

Treatment protocols for normal-risk cattle can be less aggressive than outlined for high-BRD-risk cattle. This is not to suggest antibiotic selection is any less important, but cattle in this category are immunologically and metabolically healthier and, therefore, less dependent on medical intervention. Perhaps more importantly, the well-being of these animals at feedlot arrival is such that it is much easier for cattle health checker's to evaluate cattle in the normal risk category. Because cattle are less stressed, cattle health checkers are less likely to confuse depression associated with stress with BRD depression. Feedyards and their veterinarians report excellent BRD treatment results with ceftiofur hydrochloride, ceftiofur crystalline, danofloxacin, enrofloxacin, florfenicol, long-acting oxytetracycline, tilmicosin, and tulathromycin. All of these antibiotics provide a PTI of at least 48 hours, which many feedlot veterinarians report is sufficient to set the animal's complete BRD recovery in motion. In addition, this removes the antibiotic selection pressure as soon as practical, which meets one of the American Veterinary Medical Association's (AVMA) prudent use guidelines. Even though the C_{max} to MIC_{90} ratio is not as favorable for long-acting oxytetracycline and tilmicosin, these continue to be useful selections for many groups of cattle in the normal-risk category, especially yearling pastured cattle.

Treatment protocols for late-feeding-stage BRD frequently focus on minimizing the treatment WD time. The antibiotics listed in Table 102-2 that fit the shorter WD requirement and have acceptable predicted C_{max} to MIC_{90} ratios include ceftiofur sodium, ceftiofur hydrochloride, ceftiofur crystalline, danofloxacin, and tulathromycin. One of the ceftiofur choices may be acceptable if the late-stage BRD case is the animal's first BRD event. Danofloxacin or tulathromycin might be better selections if the animal has had a previous BRD event.

Feeding Antibiotics to Aid in the Prevention or Treatment of BRD

Low-level feeding of chlortetracycline (CTC) with or without sulfamethazine was once a common practice. A great deal of data supported its use to decrease morbidity and increase gain during the first 1 to 2 months following weaning. These levels of antibiotics were frequently added to rations fed to sick cattle. The practice of low-level antibiotic feeding to aid in BRD control has gone out of favor, not because it failed to improve cattle health, but because the benefits could not be economically justified long term. More recently, CTC has been approved to be fed to cattle at a much higher rate (10 mg/lb) short term (5 days) to aid in BRD treatment. The practice, although useful in some situations, has not gained wide acceptance.

When to Switch BRD Antibiotic Selection, Which Antibiotic to Select Next, and When to Stop Antibiotic Treatments

Antibiotics selected for BRD therapy that achieve an MIC_{90} should be given at least 48 hours at this level before declaring the antibiotic choice and dose ineffective. Additionally, the "stress" effect of the antibiotic is an important item to assess when contemplating switching antibiotic therapy. Look for gut fill, soreness, tissue temp, etc. Do not switch medications just because of their stress effects. Monitor the animal, *not* the animal's temperature. Do not let the thermometer do your thinking. Use the rectal temperature to confirm your visual assessment. Recheck the diagnosis and evaluate the treatment supportive care.

If the BRD infection is judged to still be in the early stages and the severity of the infection is worsening, if possible get tougher with the infection. Select the most potent antibiotic available relative to mechanism of action, ability to penetrate infected lung tissue (Vd and LS), and predicted C_{max} to MIC_{90} ratio. Also, consider the antibiotic's potential for causing stress and other side effects. For example, giving oxytetracycline, which has a carrier that ruptures red blood cells on contact, intravenously to reach a higher C_{max} may be outweighed by the renal damage caused from hemoglobin released when red blood cells were lysed by the medication (my unpublished observations).

If the BRD infection is judged in the later stages of the disease process and the severity of the infection continues to worsen, it is reasonable to assume significant lung tissue damage has occurred. For BRD events that occur to newly arrived feeder cattle, ask the following questions to help decide if the BRD treatment cycle should continue relative to identifying the late stages of BRD. First, ask, "How many days ago did the stress start?" The answer to this first question will be the estimated number of days in the marketing channel before arriving at the feedyard plus the number of days since arrival at the feedyard. Second, ask, "How many days has the animal been treated with an appropriately selected and dosed antibiotic?" BRD can be judged to be in the late stages if the answer to the first question is more than 21 days and the answer to the second question is more than 7 days. At this point in the disease it is futile to continue antibiotic therapy. These cases should be allowed to humanely run their course. Supportive therapy for these advanced BRD cases should include providing a comfortable environment and high-quality feed. Continuing to individually treat these animals with injectable vitamins or antiinflammatories causes more stress than the potential benefit offered. Euthanasia should be considered if cattle with advanced BRD continue to suffer and do not improve.

Giving up on a sick animal that has failed to recover is one of the toughest things a veterinarian asks the treatment crew to do. Medications given to sick cattle that repeatedly fail to respond are extremely expensive. Recognizing when it is time to stop therapy is tough, but guidelines similar to those outlined earlier or as simple as being based on total number of treatments or treatment expenditures must be developed and enforced. Management should evaluate continued therapy on all sick cattle that fail to respond within 7 days.

Dealing with BRD Relapse

The following discussion does not solve the debate and consternation that occurs in the veterinary profession over diagnosing a subsequent BRD event in an animal as either a new BRD event or as a BRD relapse. Current standards of practice generally include declaring a BRD case adequately recovered to cease antibiotic therapy if (1) the animal appears to be making acceptable progress toward recovery; (2) the animal's rectal temperature has returned to within the normal range; and (3) the animal's growth or weight gain is returning to that which would be expected of its contemporaries.

Cattle previously treated for BRD that have met the recovery criteria and which are identified by a cattle health checker as again suffering from BRD should be closely examined. The criteria for a BRD event would be confirmed if the animal's depression score is 3 or higher (0 being normal, and 5 being moribund); it has harsh bronchial vascular or friction lung sounds; its rectal temperature is 104° F or greater; and there is no evidence of other primary body system disease that could explain the depression, lung sounds, and rectal temperature. In addition to the visual observation and clinical signs, the difference between considering such a case a new BRD event or a BRD relapse event is the number of days and growth or gain between the last BRD event and the current BRD diagnosis. BRD cases separated from the previous BRD event by less than 21 to 28 days are generally considered by feedlot veterinarians to be BRD relapse events. Equally important is evaluating the animal's growth between BRD events and the number of days between BRD events. Weight gain should be an objective measure, but the high variability of cattle intestinal fill can make this difficult. The average daily gain (ADG) should be within two thirds of the contemporaries.

Declaring such a respiratory case a new BRD event or a relapse may be of little practical value. The prognosis for an acceptable recovery is much better for new BRD events than for BRD relapse events. Additionally, new BRD events may be more responsive to antibiotics that have lower Vd and LS such as ceftiofur. The antibiotic selection for cases that are judged to be a BRD relapse should emphasize significant Vd and LS.

Reasonable BRD Treatment Protocol Response Expectations

The BRD treatment response can be difficult to predict. Most of the focus is on BRD that occurs during the first 30 to 60 days following feedlot arrival. A good rule of thumb is to obtain a 90% to 95% first BRD event recovery for cases that occur during this time period. If the observed recovery rate for this time period is above 95%, many feedlot veterinarians feel the cattle health checkers and hospital crew are treating more cattle for BRD than should be required. If the observed recovery rate is below 90%, many feedlot veterinarians feel the cattle health checkers may be having difficulty identifying BRD cases during the early stages of the disease process or that they need to adjust their BRD treatment protocol. Too frequently, management is quick to lay blame on either the veterinarian or the cattle health checkers. However, preexisting BRD in cattle at the time of arrival at the feedyard is the most likely cause for not identifying sick cattle in the early stages. Certainly the veterinarian should continuously monitor BRD prevention and treatment protocols. Everyone involved with the cattle health program should regularly review the steps needed to find BRD cattle early. Emphasis must be placed on evaluating the process by which cattle are acquired. Evaluate source, source, and source. Did the source of the cattle provide proper immune management before entering the marketing channel? Did the source commingle immunologically ill-prepared cattle from different sources for more than

24 hours while traveling in the marketing channel? Did the source potentially mishandle or add unacceptable stress that could weaken them metabolically or immunologically? If the answer is "yes" to any one of these three source questions, it is not the cattle health checker's or hospital crew's fault, and it is not likely the BRD treatment protocol.

ENVIRONMENTAL AND FEED MANAGEMENT OF SICK CATTLE

Antibiotic therapy is only part of the puzzle for tending the needs of cattle suffering from BRD. Data about environmental and feed management of sick cattle are scarce to allow for a rational discussion. Most cattle husbandry experts believe these are important items to include in sick cattle management.

Managing the flow of cattle through feedyard hospital pens can be difficult. The prolonged PTI offered by antibiotics that provide 3 or more days between BRD treatments provide the opportunity to return BRD treated cattle to their home pen without spending time in a hospital pen. For some feedyards this practice has worked well for uncomplicated BRD cases. A number of feedyards have set up a rotation of hospital pens that allow BRD-treated cattle to remain undisturbed over the PTI. If they are making adequate progress toward BRD recovery at the end of the PTI, they are returned to their home pen.

Sick cattle management protocols that use hospital pens should do the following:

- NOT commingle BRD cattle with cattle suffering from diarrhea.
- Provide at least 75 square feet per animal.
- Provide a minimum of 12 liner inches of feeding space per animal.
- Provide a feed with adequate nutrient density to meet low-intake cattle requirements.
- Provide at least than 2 liner inches of watering space per animal.
- Maintain the pens so that cattle are dry.
- Maintain adequate air flow.
- Provide protection from extreme environmental conditions.

ANTIBIOTIC RESIDUE AVOIDANCE STRATEGY

1. Identify all animals treated.
2. Record all treatments: Date, ID, Dose given, Route of administration, Who administered the treatment, WD time.
3. Strictly follow label directions for product use.
4. Use newer technology antibiotics when possible.
   a. Reduce unwanted depot effect. Select low-volume products when available.
   b. Select generic medications and vaccines with *extreme caution.*
   c. Avoid inferior products. They may cause performance loss or damage quality.
5. Select an antibiotic with short WD when antibiotic choice is equivalent.

Table **102-3**

Cattle Antibiotic Residue Tolerance and FAST/PHAST Detection Estimates

Generic Name	Example NADA#	Tolerance in Cattle Tissues	*Bm* Detect	WD
Ampicillin	055-030	0.01 ppm edible	0.2[a]	6
Amoxicillin	055-089	0.01 ppm edible	0.2[a]	25
Ceftiofur sodium	140-338	0.4 ppm kidney, 1 ppm muscle	~0.1[b]	4
Ceftiofur hydrochloride	140-890	0.4 ppm kidney, 1 ppm muscle	~0.1[b]	3
Ceftiofur crystalline acid	141-209	0.4 ppm kidney, 1 ppm muscle	~0.1[b]	13
Danofloxacin*	141-207	0.2 ppm liver, 0.2 ppm muscle	>0.1[b]	4
Enrofloxacin*	141-068	0.1 ppm liver, 0.1 ppm muscle	>0.1[b]	28
Florfenicol	141-063	3.7 ppm liver, 0.3 ppm muscle	~5.0[b]	38
Gentamicin*	101-862	No residue tolerance	0.13[a]	>730?
Neomycin*	200-113	7.2 ppm kidney, 3.6 ppm liver, 1.2 ppm muscle	0.06[a]	>730?
Oxytetracycline (LA)[†]	Many	12 ppm kidney, 2 ppm muscle	0.8[a]	36
Procaine Penicillin G	065-505	0.05 ppm edible	<0.01[a]	>60?
Spectinomycin	141-077	4 ppm kidney, 0.25 ppm muscle	6.2[a]	11
Sulfadimethoxine (IV)	041-245	0.1 ppm edible	≈1[b]	5
Sulfadimethoxine (oral)	093-107	0.1 ppm edible	≈1[b]	21
Sulfamethazine	140-270	0.1 ppm edible	?	12
Tilmicosin (lung C_{max})	140-929	1.2 ppm liver, 0.1 ppm muscle	≈5.0[b]	28
Tulathromycin	141-244	5.5 ppm liver, 18 ppm kidney	>0.1[b]	18
Tylosin	012-965	0.2 ppm kidney, 0.2 ppm liver	≈5.0[b]	28

[a]Korsrud J: *Food Protect* 51:1 43-46, 1988.
[b]Griffin DD: Univ of Nebraska, Great Plains Veterinary Educational Center, PO Box 148, Clay Center, NE 68933. USDA-CSREES Grant: WBS # 25-6239-0098-011 (Develop Pre-Harvest Version of the USDA-FSIS Fast Antibiotic Screening Test and Education).
NOTE: Use the RESIDUE DETECTION information only as a starting guide.
Bm (*Bacillus megaterium*, ATCC 9885), Microbe used in the FAST and PHAST antibiotic screening tests; *FAST* (Fast Antibiotic Screening Test), a microbial inhibition test used by USDA-FSIS to screen for antibiotic residues; *PHAST* (Pre-Harvest Antibiotic Screening Test), uses the FAST test to screen cattle urine for antibiotic presence; *Tolerance*, U.S. Food and Drug Administration permissible tolerance for the antibiotic in ppm (mg/kg) for target marker tissue listed; *WD*, withdrawal—days listed are the maximum from labeled products within the product class; *?*, the FARAD published estimate.
*Not approved for AMDUCA ELDU or BQA ELDU.
[†]LA = Long-acting or depo formulations designed for >72-hr PTI.

6. Never give more than 10 ml per intramuscular (IM) injection site.
7. Avoid ELDU of antibiotics.
   a. Use label dose and route of administration.
8. Avoid using multiple antibiotics at the same time.
9. Do not mix antibiotics in the same syringe, especially if given intramuscularly or subcutaneously.
10. Check all medication/treatment records before marketing:
    a. Do not market cattle with less than 60-day WD time without examining the treatment history.
    b. Extend the WD time if the route or location of administration is altered.
       i. Example; the WD time for ceftiofur crystalline free acid will be more than 120 days if given SC in the neck.
    c. Extend the WD time for multiple medications given by summing their label-recommended WD time.
       i. Example: If first medication has a 10-day WD time and second medication has a 28-day WD, assign a 38-day WD time.
       ii. Example: If first medication has a 10-day WD time and is repeated in 3 days, assign a 20-day WD time.
    d. Do not inject gentamicin or neomycin. The estimated WD time is more than 24 months (urine test may not detect a test-positive kidney).
    e. Do not market cattle that have relapsed without examining the treatment history.
    f. Do not market cattle with suspected liver or kidney damage without examining the treatment history.
    g. Do not market cattle with antibiotic injection site knots without examining the treatment history.
    h. Screen the urine for antibiotics of all cattle identified in steps a to d. It is best to use broad-spectrum microbial inhibition tests such as the Pre-Harvest Antibiotic Screening Test (PHAST), a microbial growth inhibition test that uses *Bacillus megaterium* as the test organism. Test sensitivity relative to FDA-CVM violative residue tolerances is listed in Table 102-3.

BEEF QUALITY ASSURANCE CONSIDERATIONS

All injections should be given ahead of the slope of the shoulder and, if possible, one should avoid products that require IM injections. IM injections not only increase soreness compared with SQ injections, but many of the products given intramuscularly cause significant muscle damage, which subsequently causes a significant amount of expensive carcass trim. In 1991 a national survey indicated that injection lesions were found in the sirloin and eye of round in more than 20% of all carcasses from fed cattle. The injection damage lesions were examined extensively for potential residues but none were found. The injection-site lesions caused an average of 44 cubic inches of trim and decreased meat tenderness as much as 4 inches from the center of the injection lesion. Subsequent research demonstrated damage was caused by all injections including sterile saline. The National Cattlemen's Beef Association's National Beef Quality Assurance (BQA) program adopted a policy that *all* injections (antibiotics, vaccines, parasiticides, vitamins, prostaglandins, hormones, and all other injectables) be given in front of the slope of the shoulder; that products with SC labeling be selected in preference to products labeled for IM use only; and that IM injections, if required, be limited to not more than 10 ml per injection site. The BQA injection-site policy was developed to eliminate injection-site damage to the expensive meat cuts taken from the hindquarter. All state BQA programs have adopted these injection-site guidelines. Almost all of our pharmaceutic and biologic product suppliers and government agencies responsible for those product approvals have worked diligently to design and label products to meet the national BQA program injection guidelines. Every antibiotic developed and approved by the FDA-CVM for use in the past two decades has included use approval other than for IM use including the development of injectables that may be given in the SQ space of the ear.

One should change the injection needle between every 15 animals or if it becomes contaminated or damaged.

Never straighten a bent needle and use it again. Animals that have an injection needle broken off in them cannot be marketed.

SUMMARY

Proper antibiotic selection and use involves more than treatment response clinical impressions. Dr. Dan Upson, a pharmacologist who mentors livestock veterinarians, offers important yet simple advice: "Read the labels on all the medications you use and prescribe." The information contained in antibiotic labels is useful. Basic PK and PD information can be powerful in designing treatment regimens and frequently provides important clues in troubleshooting treatment regimen success or failure. Beyond humane care and treatment success, veterinarians have an obligation to the safety of the nation's food supply. They should help clients develop residue-avoidance strategies, keep appropriate treatment records, and always check those records before marketing cattle that have had previous treatments.

Recommended Readings

National Cattlemen's Beef Association, Denver Colorado: *Beef quality assurance* (website): http://www.bqa.org. Accessed February 8, 2008.

University of Nebraska, Lincoln—GPVEC: *Pre-harvest antibiotic residue test and antibiotic residue avoidance strategies* (website): http://gpvec.unl.edu/bqa/ncbqa.htm. Accessed January 17, 2008.

CHAPTER 103

Antibiotic Treatment of Diarrhea in Preweaned Calves

JOACHIM F. BERCHTOLD and PETER D. CONSTABLE

PRELIMINARY REMARKS

A consensus statement of the American College of Veterinary Internal Medicine recently provided recommendations for the prudent use of antimicrobials in veterinary medicine.[1] Briefly, the statement recommends that veterinarians should use and prescribe antimicrobial drugs conservatively to minimize the potential adverse effects on animal or human health. Furthermore, veterinarians should develop formal infection control plans, identify common case scenarios (e.g., diarrhea, respiratory disease) in which antimicrobial drugs are often employed, develop antimicrobial use protocols for their practice, and categorize all antibiotics in primary, secondary, and tertiary use categories, besides appropriate diagnostic and sensitivity measures. Monitoring and surveillance for trends in the prevalence of resistant bacteria within a practice, a farm, a region, or a nation permits continual evaluation of antimicrobial drug use on various levels.

CLINICAL IMPORTANCE

Antimicrobial agents have been used for treating calves with diarrhea for more than 50 years. Diarrhea in preweaned calves is by far the leading cause of mortality in dairy heifer calves with no change in mortality rates between 1995 and 2001 in the United States.[2] Despite the widespread availability of vaccines against enterotoxigenic *Escherichia coli*, rotavirus, and coronavirus, as well as continued emphasis on optimizing colostral transfer of passive immunity, the oral and parenteral administration of antimicrobial agents continues to play an important role in the treatment of calf diarrhea.[3-7] Evidence-based recommendations for the administration of antimicrobial agents in diarrheic calves were recently developed based on a systematic review of randomized controlled studies published in peer-reviewed journals.[8,9] This chapter is based on those recommendations and the results of recent studies on the use of antimicrobials in calves with diarrhea during the first few weeks in life (preweaning period). For a complete historic background and reference list of antimicrobial use in the treatment of calf diarrhea, the reader is referred to these reviews.[8,9]

ETIOLOGY OF CALF DIARRHEA

Neonatal calf diarrhea is usually due to infection by at least one enteropathogen (enterotoxigenic *E. coli*, rotavirus, coronavirus, cryptosporidia, *Salmonella* spp.). In many herds several agents are usually present and can be detected in neonatal calves with and without diarrhea. If calf diarrhea occurs in an outbreak situation with high morbidity, *Salmonella* bacteria may be involved. Regardless of the etiology, calves with diarrhea often have increased coliform bacterial numbers in the small intestine and this colonization is associated with altered small intestinal function, morphologic damage, and increased susceptibility to bacteremia.[9] The importance of bacterial overgrowth in calf diarrhea recently gained attention when the role of D-lactic acid in the development of acidemia in calves with diarrhea was identified. Production of D-lactic acid results from bacterial fermentation in the gastrointestinal tract and is a common finding in neonatal calves with and without diarrhea.[10-12] D-lactic acid is a major component of acidemia in diarrheic calves[13-15] and is accompanied by systemic signs of weakness and ataxia.[16]

BACTERMIA IN CALVES WITH DIARRHEA

Calves with diarrhea are more likely to have failure of transfer or partial failure of transfer of passive immunity, and these calves are more likely to have bacteremia. Bacteremia, predominantly with *E. coli,* is present in approximately 20% to 30% of calves with diarrhea or systemic illness.[17-19] The frequency of bacteremia is considered sufficiently high that treatment of calves with diarrhea that are severely ill (as manifest by reduced suckle reflex, >6% dehydration, weakness, inability to stand, or clinical depression) should include routine treatment against bacteremia, with emphasis on treating potential *E. coli* bacteremia. A clinical sepsis score to predict bacteremia is not recommended to guide antibiotic treatment decisions until further validation of the score in different calf-rearing scenarios.[20] Bacteremia should be suspected to be present in all calves with clinical signs of *Salmonella* diarrhea, although the prevalence of bacteremia in affected calves has not been determined.[21]

ANTIMICROBIAL SUSCEPTIBILITY TESTING

Bacterial enteropathogens (enterotoxigenic *E. coli* and *Salmonella* spp.) are most commonly isolated from fecal samples or from specimens obtained during necropsy of a dead calf. Submission of appropriate specimens for bacterial culture, identification of pathogens, and susceptibility

520

testing by standardized methods has been widely recommended to allow an evidence-based approach for drug selection and justify antibiotic use.[1] Laboratory methods and standardized breakpoints need to be established for several bacteria-drug combinations.[1]

Several fecal isolates—*E. coli*, *Clostridium perfringens* type A, and *Campylobacter* spp.—are normal intestinal flora. Therefore diagnostic laboratories should clearly indicate normal bacterial growth in fecal culture samples, if the cultured bacteria cannot be distinguished from normal flora by identification of species, specific virulence factors or correlated markers, or clear demonstration of overgrowth.[1] When enterotoxigenic *E. coli* or *Salmonella* is isolated, susceptibility testing may provide a useful guide for treatment decisions and antimicrobial drug selection.

The most important determinant of antimicrobial efficacy in calf diarrhea is obtaining an effective antimicrobial concentration against bacteria at the sites of infection (small intestine and blood).[9] The results of fecal antimicrobial susceptibility testing in calf diarrhea probably have clinical relevance only when applied to fecal isolates of enterotoxigenic strains of *E. coli* or pathogenic *Salmonella* spp., and possibly blood culture isolates from calves with bacteremia. Current susceptibility testing methods have not been validated for predicting treatment outcome in calves with diarrhea.[9]

The ability of fecal bacterial culture and antimicrobial susceptibility testing using the Kirby Bauer technique to guide treatment in calf diarrhea is questionable when applied to fecal *E. coli* isolates that have not been identified as enterotoxigenic pathogenic strains. No reports have demonstrated a correlation between in vitro antimicrobial susceptibility of fecal *E. coli* and *Salmonella* spp. isolates and clinical response to antimicrobial treatment. Susceptibility results obtained from dead calves should be interpreted carefully because isolates obtained from dead calves are likely to be obtained from treatment failures, and calves that died from diarrhea are likely to have bacterial overgrowth in the intestines and many organs not representing the in vivo situation. Another concern with fecal susceptibility testing is that the Kirby Bauer break points (minimum inhibitory concentration [MIC]) are not based on typical antimicrobial concentrations in the small intestine and blood of calves. The practitioner should therefore evaluate the antimicrobial efficacy based on clinical response to antibiotic treatment.[9]

The Kirby Bauer technique for antimicrobial susceptibility test has theoretically more clinical relevance for predicting the clinical response to antimicrobial treatment when applied to blood isolates than fecal isolates. This is because the Kirby Bauer break points (minimum inhibitory concentration [MIC]) are based on achievable antimicrobial concentrations in human plasma and MIC_{90} (MIC for 90% of the isolates) values for human *E. coli* isolates, which provide a reasonable approximation to achievable MIC values in calf plasma and MIC_{90} values for bovine *E. coli* isolates.[9]

SUCCESS OF ANTIMICROBIAL THERAPY

Important considerations for treating calf diarrhea are (1) administering an antibiotic as directed on the label whenever possible, (2) using an antimicrobial agent with an appropriate spectrum of activity, (3) selecting an antimicrobial agent that attains and maintains an effective therapeutic concentration at the site of infection, (4) treating for an appropriate duration, and (5) avoiding adverse local or systemic effects and violative residues.[9] Important critical measures of success of antimicrobial therapy in calf diarrhea are (in decreasing order of importance) (1) mortality rate, (2) growth rate in survivors, (3) severity of diarrhea in survivors, and (4) duration of diarrhea in survivors.

Success of antimicrobial therapy varies with the route of administration and whether the antimicrobial is dissolved in milk, oral electrolyte solutions, or water. Oral antimicrobials administered as a bolus, a tablet, or in a gelatin capsule may be swallowed into the rumen and exhibit a different serum concentration-time profile to antimicrobials dissolved in milk replacers that are suckled by the calf or administered as an oral drench at the back of the pharynx. Antimicrobials that bypass the rumen are not thought to alter rumen microflora, potentially permitting bacterial recolonization of the small intestine from the rumen. The normal intestinal flora is always exposed to varying amounts of antimicrobial drugs regardless of the type of administration.[1] Historic studies reported that some orally administered antibiotics (e.g., potassium and procaine penicillin, neomycin sulfate, ampicillin trihydrate, tetracycline hydrochloride) may increase the incidence of diarrhea, produce malabsorption, and reduce growth rate.[9]

EVIDENCED-BASED RECOMMENDATIONS FOR ANTIMICROBIAL ADMINISTRATION IN CALF DIARRHEA

Oxytetracycline and sulfachlorpyridazine administered parenterally and amoxicillin, chlortetracycline, neomycin, oxytetracycline, streptomycin, sulfachlorpyridazine, sulfamethazine, and tetracycline administered orally have been labeled by the U.S. Food and Drug Administration (FDA) for the **treatment and aid in the control** of bacterial enteritis (scours, colibacillosis) caused by *E. coli* bacteria susceptible to the antimicrobial.[9] Four of the eight antibiotics (oral administration of chlortetracycline, oxytetracycline, tetracycline, and neomycin) approved for treatment of calf diarrhea are labeled by the FDA for the **control or aid in the control** of bacterial enteritis (scours, colibacillosis) caused by *E. coli* and *Salmonella* spp. bacteria susceptible to the antimicrobial.[8]

Studies supporting the efficacy of parenteral oxytetracycline and sulfachlorpyridazine, and of oral amoxicillin, chlortetracycline, neomycin, oxytetracycline, streptomycin, sulfachlorpyridazine, sulfamethazine, and tetracycline in treating calves with naturally acquired diarrhea do not appear to have been published in peer-reviewed journals.[9] Oral amoxicillin was effective in the treatment of experimentally induced diarrhea[22,23] but was not efficacious in the treatment of naturally acquired diarrhea in beef calves.[24] In view of the apparent lack of published studies documenting clinical efficacy of antimicrobials with a label claim for the treatment of naturally occurring calf diarrhea, and because the health of the animal is threatened and suffering or death may result from failure to treat systemically ill calves, extra-label antimicrobial use (excluding prohibited antimicrobials) is justified for the treatment of calf diarrhea.[9]

Antimicrobials for the treatment of calf diarrhea should have local (small intestine) and systemic efficacy because the predominant sites of infection in calf diarrhea are the small intestine and blood.[9] The antimicrobial must reach therapeutic concentrations at the site of infection for a long enough period and, ideally, have only a narrow gram-negative spectrum of activity in order to minimize effects on normal intestinal flora.

The results of several studies indicate that oral and parenteral administration of broad-spectrum β-lactam and fluoroquinolone antimicrobials is efficacious in treating naturally acquired and experimentally induced diarrhea. It must be highlighted that administration of fluoroquinolone antimicrobials in a extralabel manner is illegal in the United States.* Parenteral administration of trimethoprim/sulfadiazine and ceftiofur (high extralabel dose) has proven efficacy in treating experimentally induced infections with *Salmonella enterica* serotype Dublin and serotype Typhimurium, respectively.[21,25] Orally administered apramycin has proven efficacy in treating naturally acquired diarrhea but is poorly absorbed after oral administration (oral bioavailability <15%) and has relatively high MIC values against *Salmonella* spp. and *E. coli* (MIC_{90} >3 µg/ml) in the calf.[26] Based on these issues, treatment recommendations focus on the use of broad-spectrum β-lactam antimicrobials such as amoxicillin, ampicillin, ceftiofur, and potentiated sulfonamides (trimethoprim/sulfadiazine).

Administration of Oral Antimicrobials to Treat *E. Coli* Overgrowth of the Small Intestine

In neonatal calves with diarrhea and mild systemic illness (defined as depressed suckling but normal rectal temperature, hydration status, and heart rate), the veterinarian should continue to monitor the calf's health or orally administer amoxicillin trihydrate (10 mg/kg, q12h) or amoxicillin trihydrate-clavulanate potassium (12.5 mg combined drug/kg, q12h) for at least 3 days; the latter constitutes extralabel drug use. Oral amoxicillin trihydrate (10 mg/kg, q12h for 4 days) was efficacious in decreasing mortality rate and duration of diarrhea in two studies where diarrhea was experimentally induced with enterotoxigenic *E. coli* bacteria.[22,23] The absorption rate of amoxicillin trihydrate from the calf small intestine is 30% when administered in milk.[27] High amoxicillin concentrations are present in the bile and intestinal contents, with lower antimicrobial concentrations in serum.[21] Feeding of amoxicillin with milk does not change the bioavailability of amoxicillin, although amoxicillin is absorbed faster when dissolved in an oral electrolyte solution

than in milk replacer.[28] Amoxicillin absorption is slowed during endotoxemia, presumably because of a decrease in abomasal emptying rate.[29] Amoxicillin trihydrate is preferred to ampicillin trihydrate for oral administration in calves because it is labeled for the treatment of calf diarrhea in the United States and is absorbed to a much greater extent.[27,28,30] However, a field study comparing equal amounts (400 mg, q12h) of oral amoxicillin and ampicillin for the treatment of diarrhea reported similar proportions of calves with a good to excellent clinical response.[31] The addition of clavulanate potassium to amoxicillin trihydrate is recommended because clavulanate potassium is a potent irreversible inhibitor of β-lactamase, increasing the antimicrobial spectrum of activity.

Oral administration of potentiated sulfonamides is not recommended for treating calf diarrhea because of the lack of efficacy studies. Oral administration of gentamicin is not recommended because antimicrobials administered to calves with diarrhea should have both local and systemic effects, and orally administered gentamicin is poorly absorbed. No other orally administered antimicrobial currently available in the United States is likely to be effective in treating neonatal calves with diarrhea.[9]

Fluoroquinolones clearly have proven efficacy in treating calf diarrhea, and a label indication exists in Europe for oral and parenteral enrofloxacin, oral marbofloxacin, and parenteral danofloxacin for the treatment of calf diarrhea. In those countries where their administration is permitted to treat calf diarrhea, oral fluoroquinolones are recommended because of their high oral bioavailability. However, it must be emphasized that extralabel use of the fluoroquinolone class of antimicrobials in food-producing animals in the United States is illegal and obviously not recommended.

Experts currently believe that salmonellosis is more of a systemic infection than local (intestinal) infection. Accordingly, parenteral administration is preferred when treating calves with salmonellosis.

It is possible that the widespread use of antibiotics in milk replacer in the United States may lead to a decreased incidence of D-lactic acidosis in calves with diarrhea, when compared with calves in Germany and Canada. Both Germany and Canada have a milk quota system that promotes feeding whole milk instead of milk replacer to calves. Because D-lactic acidosis in calves results from bacterial fermentation of milk in the gastrointestinal tract,[10] feeding milk-replacer that contains antibiotics could decrease the generation of D-lactic acid in calf intestine, assuming that the antibiotic promotes growth of non–D-lactate–producing bacteria.

Administration of Parenteral Antimicrobials to Treat *E. Coli* Bacteremia and Salmonellosis

In calves with diarrhea and moderate to severe systemic illness, the predictive accuracy of clinical and laboratory tests for detecting bacteremia are too low assuming reasonable estimates for the prevalence of bacteremia (20%-30%) in the field.[18-20] Bacteremia constitutes a significant cause of mortality and threat to the life of the calf. Therefore the authors recommend that clinicians routinely assume 20% to 30% of ill calves with diarrhea

---

*Extralabel administration of fluoroquinolones in food-producing animals in the United States is prohibited by law because of concerns regarding assisting the emergence of bacteria with multiple antimicrobial resistance, particularly pathogenic enteric bacteria in humans.

are bacteremic. Parenteral antimicrobial treatment is required for these calves.

Administration of ceftiofur (2.2 mg/kg [1 mg/lb], SC/IM, q12h) for at least 3 days is the most logical parenteral treatment for *E. coli* bacteremia.[9] Treatment of experimental salmonellosis with high extralabel dose of ceftiofur (5 mg/kg, IM, q24h) for 5 days was recommended to maintain antimicrobial concentrations above the MIC_{90} (1 µg/ml) for the *Salmonella enterica* serovar Typhimurium challenge strain.[21] Because other *Salmonella* serotypes present on a farm may have much higher MIC_{90} values, determination of MIC values is recommended before the start of treatment.[21] Ceftiofur constitutes an extralabel drug use for the treatment of *E. coli* bacteremia and salmonellosis, and ceftiofur should not be administered to calves to be processed as veal.

The second recommended treatment for *E. coli* bacteremia is parenteral amoxicillin trihydrate or ampicillin trihydrate (10 mg/kg, IM, q12h) for at least 3 days.[9] Both drugs are theoretically inferior to ceftiofur because parenterally administered ampicillin and amoxicillin reach lower plasma concentrations and require a higher MIC than ceftiofur, and they are not β-lactamase resistant. Even though the rate and extent of absorption is reduced with subcutaneous (SC) injection, relative to IM injection of amoxicillin and ampicillin,[32] SC administration is preferred in order to minimize potentially more painful IM injections, especially when repeated doses are administered. The most crucial issue in sick calves with diarrhea is maintaining or restoring a good suckle reflex for successful and adequate intake of milk and oral electrolyte solutions. Calves suffering from pain from whatever reason probably have a weak or absent suckle response as compared with calves without pain.

A third recommended treatment for the treatment of *E. coli* bacteremia is parenteral potentiated sulfonamides (20 mg/kg sulfadiazine with 5 mg/kg trimethoprim; IV or IM depending on the formulation characteristics, q24h for 5 days). Efficacy of potentiated sulfonamides has only been proven when treatment commenced before clinical signs of diarrhea were present.[25] Therefore it is unknown whether potentiated sulfonamides are efficacious when administered to calves with diarrhea and depression, although potentiated sulfonamides are likely efficacious in the treatment of salmonellosis.

Oral administration of potentiated sulfonamides is not recommended for the treatment of bacteremia because of poor oral bioavailability. Oxytetracycline and chlortetracycline may have some efficacy for treating *E. coli* bacterial overgrowth of the small intestine but are not recommended for the treatment of bacteremia.[9] Oral bioavailability of tetracycline antimicrobials is significantly decreased because they are bound to calcium. Oxytetracycline must be administered at 20 mg/kg, q12h, PO to achieve minimal serum concentrations to treat *E. coli* bacteremia (MIC_{50} = 4 µg/ml).[33]

Parenteral administration of gentamicin and other aminoglycosides (amikacin, kanamycin) cannot be currently recommended as part of the treatment for calf diarrhea in the United States because of prolonged slaughter withdrawal times (15-18 months); potential for nephrotoxicity in dehydrated animals; and availability of ceftiofur,

amoxicillin, and ampicillin. However, in two studies from Europe parenteral administration of gentamicin was equally effective as danofloxacin or fourth-generation cephalosporin cefquinome for the treatment of diarrhea or calves with clinical signs of septicemia.[19,34] Both studies were conducted in the field and did not include a negative control group.

In Europe a label indication exists for parenteral fluoroquinolones for the treatment of *E. coli* diarrhea and salmonellosis in calves. In those countries where administration is permitted to treat calves with *E. coli* diarrhea and salmonellosis, parenteral fluoroquinolones are only recommended when specific evidence from culture and susceptibility results suggest that these drugs are necessary and efficacious. For these reasons, it is preferable that parenteral fluoroquinolone administration be reserved for critically ill calves such as those also requiring intravenous fluid administration. However, it must be emphasized that extralabel use of the fluoroquinolone class of antimicrobials in food-producing animals is illegal in the United States.

In calves with diarrhea but no evidence of systemic illness (i.e., normal appetite for milk or milk replacer, no fever), we recommend that the clinician monitor the health of the calf and not administer parenteral antimicrobials. A recent study from Sweden concluded that most calves with uncomplicated diarrhea (i.e., the absence of concurrent infections such as pneumonia or omphalophlebitis) do not benefit from antibiotic treatment.[4]

Long-Term Administration of Oral Antibiotics for Prevention and Therapy of Calf Diarrhea

Antimicrobials in milk replacer are intended to prevent or treat bacterial scours and decrease the incidence of other common calf diseases during the neonatal period. Dairy heifer calves were fed with milk replacer containing antibiotics on 56% of herds in 2001 in the United States.[6] Local surveys reported between 45% (Michigan, Minnesota, New York, Wisconsin)[7] and 70% (Pennsylvania)[5] of dairy herds are using medicated milk replacer. Oxytetracycline in combination with neomycin followed by oxytetracycline alone are the most common medications.[6] Several studies reported inconsistent results of the effects of antibiotics containing milk replacer on the incidence of diarrhea (scours). The incidence of diarrhea was not influenced when antibiotics in milk replacer were compared with oligosaccharides or bovine plasma as nonantibiotic alternative treatments.[35-37] A more extensive recent study found that the onset and overall morbidity of important diseases in calves during their first weeks of life (diarrhea, respiratory disease, navel infection) were significantly lower in calves receiving antibiotics neomycin sulphate (22 mg/kg/day) and tetracycline HCl (22 mg/kg/day) in milk replacer than in control calves without in-feed antibiotics.[38] This study did not exclusively consider diarrhea as the primary outcome, but the findings are valuable because they reflect the pattern of diseases in newborn calves in a specialized calf-rearing facility with high disease incidence in a stressful environment.

It should be recognized that in one report the use of antibiotics in milk replacer was associated with a decreased risk of infection with *C. parvum* in preweaning dairy calves,[39] even though cryptosporidia are not directly susceptible to antibiotics. Another study reported that lack of routine feeding of medicated milk replacer (name of antibiotics not presented) increased the odds for isolation of *Salmonella* bacteria from calves.[40]

ANCILLARY TREATMENTS FOR CALF DIARRHEA

Oral and Intravenous Fluids

Administration of oral and parenteral fluids to calves with diarrhea is essential for adequate rehydration and restoration of circulating blood volume, correction of acidemia, electrolyte abnormalities, energy deficits, and mental depression to restore the suckle reflex and assist repair of the damaged intestinal surface. Oral administration of electrolyte-containing solutions may cover episodes of diarrhea with minimal or moderate dehydration and good suckle reflex. Calves that are unable to suckle, recumbent, severely depressed, or comatose need intravenous fluids for effective resuscitation. (See Chapter 104 for further discussion of fluid therapy.)

Nonsteroidal Antiinflammatory Drugs

Flunixin meglumine is probably the most widely antiinflammatory treatment of diarrheic calves. The administration of a single dose of flunixin meglumine (2.2 mg/kg [1 mg/lb] IM) as an adjunct treatment for naturally occurring diarrhea resulted in fewer morbid-days and antimicrobial treatments only when calves had fecal blood in their feces.[41] In calves with experimentally induced enterotoxigenic *E. coli* infection, flunixin meglumine (2.2 mg/kg [1 mg/lb] q8h IM) reduced fecal output perhaps by acting as an antisecretory agent.[42] Flunixin meglumine (2.2 mg/kg [1 mg/lb] q12h) is indicated in severely sick calves with presumed endotoxemia when hydration status is adequate to prevent nephrotoxicity. A rule of thumb is to administer flunixin meglumine once at a dose 2.2 mg/kg (1 mg/lb) and not to exceed three doses of flunixin meglumine for the treatment of diarrhea and respiratory disease to avoid potential damage of the intestinal mucosa of the abomasum, especially in intensive calf-rearing facilities with a history of case fatalities from perforated abomasal ulcers. An important effect of flunixin meglumine administration is the clinical impression that calves show a better suckle behavior after therapy. This impression is supported by a recent statement that "the use of flunixin meglumine is valuable in improving the well-being of the calves."[38]

Motility Modifiers and Intestinal Protectants

Administration of intestinal protectants (e.g., kaolin-pectin, activated attapulgite) or motility modifiers (e.g., hyoscine N-butylbromide, atropine) is not recommended despite their widespread use. No data on efficacy are available, and a recent study showed that nonantibiotic treatments including bismuth, kaolin-pectin, activated attapulgite, and activated charcoal for calf diarrhea resulted in prolonged duration of treatment and increased risk for morbidity and mortality compared with oral antibiotics in milk replacer (neomycin sulfate and tetracycline HCl) and parenteral administration of ceftiofur hydrochloride (2.2 mg/kg, 3-5 days).[38]

Probiotics

Administration of probiotics to diarrheic calves is done in some dairy herds. A recent study under field conditions showed that prophylactic administration of the probiotic bacteria *E. coli* strain Nissle 1917 for the first 10 or 12 days of life to calves with unknown status of passive transfer was associated with a significant decrease in the number of calves developing diarrhea.[43] In calves with spontaneous diarrhea, *Lactobacillus rhamnosus GG* administration for therapy of diarrhea was not associated with lower mortality or a decrease of scours in a clinical setting.[44] Another recent study in neonatal foals documented that administration of a different *Lactobacillus* strain for the prevention of diarrhea was associated with the development of diarrhea and further clinical abnormalities requiring veterinary intervention.[45] Based on these reports, administration of *E. coli* strain Nissle 1917 may be of value for the prevention of diarrhea in calves.

Oligosaccharides

Oligosaccharides in milk replacer are minimally absorbed in the small intestine and are thought to decrease binding of bacterial pathogens to enterocytes. Studies in calves reported that prophylactic addition of oligosaccharides to milk replacer resulted in fecal scores (scours) in calves that were similar to those observed when calves were fed milk replacer containing antibiotics.[35,36,46] It must be noted that in these studies data on morbidity and mortality were either low or remained undetermined.[46] Likely observed scours resulted primarily from nutritional origin rather than from infectious origins.[36]

Vitamins

Administration of B vitamins and fat-soluble vitamins may have beneficial effects in colostrum-deprived calves and in calves with chronic diarrhea. However, data supporting the beneficial effects of vitamins in calf diarrhea are lacking.

References

1. Morley PS, Apley MD, Besser TE et al: Antimicrobial drug use in veterinary medicine, *J Vet Intern Med* 19:617, 2005.
2. U.S. Department of Agriculture: 2002. Part II: Changes in the United States Dairy Industry, 1991-2002 USDA:APHIS: VS:CEAH, National Animal Health Monitoring System, Fort Collins, Colo #N388.0603.
3. Busani L, Graziani C, Franco A et al: Survey of the knowledge, attitudes and practice of Italian beef and dairy cattle veterinarians concerning the use of antibiotics, *Vet Rec* 155:733, 2004.

4. Ortman K, Svensson C: Use of antimicrobial drugs in Swedish dairy calves and replacement heifers, *Vet Rec* 154:136, 2004.

5. Sawant AA, Sordillo LM, Jayarao BM: A survey on antibiotic usage in dairy herds in Pennsylvania, *J Dairy Sci* 88:2991, 2005.

6. USDA: 2005. Part IV: Antimicrobial Use on U.S. Dairy Operations, 2002 USDA:APHIS:VS:CEAH, National Animal Health Monitoring System, Fort Collins, Colo #430.0905.

7. Zwald AG, Ruegg PL, Kaneene JB et al: Management practices and reported antimicrobial usage on conventional and organic dairy farms, *J Dairy Sci* 87:191, 2004.

8. Constable PD: Use of antibiotics to prevent calf diarrhea and septicaemia, *Bov Pract* 37:137, 2003.

9. Constable PD: Antimicrobial use in the treatment of calf diarrhea, *J Vet Intern Med* 18:8, 2004.

10. Ewaschuk JB, Naylor JM, Palmer R: D-lactate production and excretion in diarrheic calves, *J Vet Intern Med* 18:744, 2004.

11. Navetat H, Biron P, Contrepois M et al: Les gastroentérites paralysantes: maladie ou syndrome? *Bull Acad Vet France* 70:327, 1997.

12. Schlecher F, Marcillaud S, Braun JP et al: Metabolic acidosis without dehydration and no or minimal diarrhoea in suckler calves is caused by hyper D-lactatemia, *Proc World Buiatrics Congress* 89:371, 1998.

13. Constable PD, Staempfli HR, Navetat H et al: Use of a quantitative strong ion approach to determine the mechanism for acid-base abnormalities in sick calves with or without diarrhea, *J Vet Intern Med* 19:581, 2005.

14. Ewaschuk JB, Naylor JM, Zello GA: Anion gap correlates with serum D- and DL-Lactate concentration in diarrheic neonatal calves, *J Vet Intern Med* 17:940, 2003.

15. Lorenz I: Influence of D-lactate on metabolic acidosis and on prognosis in neonatal calves with diarrhoea, *J Vet Med A Physiol Pathol Clin Med* 51:425, 2004a.

16. Lorenz I: Investigations on the influence of serum D-lactate levels on clinical signs in calves with metabolic acidosis, *Vet J* 168:323, 2004b.

17. Fecteau G, Van Metre DC, Paré J et al: Bacteriological culture of blood from critically ill neonatal calves, *Can Vet J* 38:95, 1997a.

18. Lofstedt J, Dohoo IR, Duizer G: Model to predict septicaemia in diarrheic calves, *J Vet Intern Med* 13:81, 1999.

19. Thomas E, Roy O, Skowronski V et al: Comparative field efficacy study between cefquinome and gentamicin in neonatal calves with clinical signs of septicaemia, *Revue Méd Vét* 155:489, 2004.

20. Fecteau G, Paré J, Van Metre DC et al: Use of a clinical sepsis score for predicting bacteremia in neonatal dairy calves on a calf rearing farm, *Can Vet J* 38:101, 1997b.

21. Fecteau ME, House JK, Kotarski SF et al: Efficacy of ceftiofur for treatment of experimental salmonellosis in neonatal calves, *Am J Vet Res* 64:918, 2003.

22. Bywater J: Evaluation of an oral glucose-glycine-electrolyte formulation and amoxicillin for treatment of diarrhea in calves, *Am J Vet Res* 38:1983, 1977.

23. Palmer GH, Bywater RJ, Francis ME: Amoxycillin: distribution and clinical efficacy in calves, *Vet Rec* 100:487, 1977.

24. Radostits OM, Rhodes CS, Mitchell ME et al: A clinical evaluation of antimicrobial agents and temporary starvation in the treatment of acute undifferentiated diarrhea in newborn calves, *Can Vet J* 16:219, 1975.

25. White G, Piercy DWT, Gibbs HA: Use of a calf salmonellosis model to evaluate the therapeutic properties of trimethoprim and sulphadiazine and their mutual potentiation in vivo, *Res Vet Sci* 31:27, 1981.

26. Ziv G, Bor A, Soback S et al: Clinical pharmacology of apramycin in calves, *J Vet Pharmacol Ther* 8:95, 1985.

27. Ziv G, Nouws JFM, Groothuis DG et al: Oral absorption and bioavailability of ampicillin derivatives in calves, *Am J Vet Res* 38:1007, 1977.

28. Palmer GH, Bywater RJ, Stanton A: Absorption in calves of amoxycillin, ampicillin, and oxytetracycline in milk replacer, water, or an oral rehydration formulation, *Am J Vet Res* 44:68, 1983.

29. Groothuis DG, van Miert ASJPAM, Ziv G et al: Effects of experimental *Escherichia coli* endotoxemia on ampicillin: amoxycillin blood levels after oral and parenteral administration in calves, *J Vet Pharmacol Ther* 1:81, 1978.

30. Larkin PJ: The distribution of a 400 mg dose of ampicillin administered orally to calves, *Vet Rec* 90:476, 1972.

31. Keefe TJ: Clinical efficacy of amoxicillin in calves with colibacillosis, *Vet Med Small Anim Clin* 72(suppl):783, 1977.

32. Rutgers LJE, Van Miert ASJPAM, Nouws JFM et al: Effect of the injection site on the bioavailability of amoxycillin trihydrate in dairy cows, *J Vet Pharmacol Ther* 3:125, 1980.

33. Schifferli D, Galeazzi RL, Nicolet J et al: Pharmacokinetics of oxytetracycline and therapeutic implications in veal calves, *J Vet Pharmacol Ther* 5:247, 1982.

34. Sunderland SJ, Sarasola P, Rowan TG et al: Efficacy of danofloxacin 18% injectable solution in the treatment of *Escherichia coli* diarrhoea in young calves in Europe, *Res Vet Sci* 74:171, 2003.

35. Donovan DC, Franklin ST, Chase CCL et al: Growth and health of Holstein calves fed milk replacers supplemented with antibiotics or Enteroguard, *J Dairy Sci* 85:947, 2002.

36. Heinrichs AJ, Jones CM, Heinrichs BS: Effects of mannan oligosaccharide or antibiotics in neonatal diets on health and growth of dairy calves, *J Dairy Sci* 86:4064, 2003.

37. Quigley JD III, Drew MD: Effects of oral antibiotics of bovine plasma on survival, health and growth in dairy calves challenged with, *Escherichia coli, Food Agric Immunol* 12:311, 2000.

38. Berge ACB, Lindeque P, Moore DA et al: A clinical trial evaluating prophylactic and therapeutic antibiotic use on health and performance of preweaned calves, *J Dairy Sci* 88:2166, 2005.

39. Mohammed HO, Wade SE, Schaaf S: Risk factors associated with Cryptosporidium parvum infection in dairy cattle in southeastern New York State, *Vet Parasitol* 83:1, 1999.

40. Fossler CP, Wells SJ, Kaneene JB et al: Herd-level factors associated with isolation of Salmonella in a multi-state study of conventional and organic dairy farms II. Salmonella shedding in calves, *Prev Vet Med* 70:279, 2005.

41. Barnett SC, Sischo WM, Moore DA et al: Evaluation of flunixin meglumine as an adjunct treatment for diarrhea in dairy calves, *J Am Vet Med Assoc* 223:1329, 2003.

42. Roussel AJ, Sriranganathan N, Brown SA et al: Effect of flunixin meglumine on *Escherichia coli* heat-stable enterotoxin-induced diarrhea in calves, *Am J Vet Res* 49:1431, 1988.

43. Buenau R von, Jaekel L, Schubotz E et al: *Escherichia coli* strain Nissle 1917: Significant reduction of neonatal calf diarrhea, *J Dairy Sci* 88:317, 2005.

44. Ewaschuk JB, Zello GM, Naylor JM: Lactobacillus GG does not affect D-lactic acidosis in diarrheic calves, in a clinical setting, *J Vet Intern Med* 20:614, 2006.

45. Weese JS, Rousseau J: Evaluation of Lactobacillus pentosus WE7 for prevention of diarrhea in neonatal foals, *J Am Vet Med Assoc* 226:2031, 2005.

46. Quigley JD III, Drewry JJ, Murray LM et al: Body weight gain, feed efficiency, and fecal scores of dairy calves in response to galactosyl-lactose or antibiotics in milk replacers, *J Dairy Sci* 80:1751, 1997.

CHAPTER 104

Fluid Therapy, Transfusion, and Shock Therapy

ALLEN J, ROUSSEL, JR., and CHRISTINE B. NAVARRE

Water and salt, known for centuries to be elements essential for life, are as critical to survival today as ever. Because of the extreme importance of water and electrolytes to biologic processes, many organ systems are involved in their regulation and balance. The gastrointestinal tract, kidneys, skin, and several endocrine glands function to maintain body water and electrolyte concentration in delicate balance despite large changes in intake and loss. However, life-threatening imbalances can occur rapidly when these homeostatic mechanisms are overwhelmed.

WATER AND ELECTROLYTE BALANCE

Total body water comprises approximately 60% of the mass of the adult ruminant. Total body water is inversely related to body fat; therefore fattened livestock have relatively less body water. On the other hand, neonates have relatively more body water, as much as 86% of body mass. Total body water is divided into two major physiologic compartments that have imperfect anatomic corollaries. The largest compartment is the intracellular fluid compartment (ICF), which accounts for about two thirds of total body water. The extracellular fluid compartment (ECF) makes up the balance. Extracellular water can further be divided into the intravascular fluid compartment and the interstitial fluid compartment. Intravascular fluid or plasma volume makes up about 5% of total body mass. Water and certain molecules such as urea move freely from one compartment to the next, but the movement of certain ions and molecules is restricted or controlled by membrane channels and pumps. The osmolality of body fluids is relatively constant in healthy animals, about 300 mOsm/kg. Sodium, the most important extracellular cation, constitutes about 95% of the total cation pool. Major ECF anions include chloride and bicarbonate. The most important intracellular cation is potassium. The inverse relation of sodium and potassium inside and outside of the cells is maintained by the Na+- K+-ATPase pump found in almost all mammalian cell membranes. Phosphates, proteins, and other anions balance the charge of K+ and the other cations inside the cells.

When dehydration occurs, all fluid compartments are affected, but not uniformly. Rapid dehydration causes disproportionate reduction in the intravascular compartment, followed by contraction of the interstitial fluid compartment, and finally by contraction of the intracellular fluid compartment. In time equilibration occurs, and all compartments become dehydrated.

Depletion of body water and electrolytes usually occurs simultaneously, but the relative amount of water and electrolytes lost is not constant. If excess free water is lost owing to evaporative loss or water deprivation, electrolyte *content* of the ECF will not increase, but electrolyte *concentration* will increase. Plasma osmolality rises and this can most easily be estimated clinically by measuring plasma sodium concentration, which will rise above normal concentration. If body water and electrolytes are lost in the same relative proportions as they are found in the ECF, volume contraction or dehydration will be iso-osmolar. Measuring plasma electrolytes will reveal a normal sodium concentration. In some situations, sodium loss may exceed water loss, which results in hypo-osmolar or at least hyponatremic dehydration. This is seen in ruminants with ruptured bladders when sodium ion moves into the peritoneal cavity and in some calves with diarrhea when sodium is lost in the feces. Most clinically dehydrated ruminants and swine have iso-osmolar or nearly iso-osmolar fluid losses. Therefore it is essential to supply electrolytes, particularly sodium, in addition to water for rehydration and volume replacement. Failure to do so will result in relative water excess, which will be quickly corrected by the kidneys, subsequently returning the animal to a volume-depleted state again.

FLUID AND ELECTROLYTE REPLACEMENT THERAPY

Fluid therapy in food animals is both challenging and rewarding. Although it is often technically difficult, labor intensive, and inconvenient, this basic therapeutic modality produces clinical results that no sophisticated surgical technique or expensive miracle drug can duplicate.

The principles of therapy are relatively simple: The physical, logistical, and economic constraints can be (and are) overcome by creative, resourceful practitioners. Administration of effective and economical fluid and electrolyte replacement therapy is achievable by every large animal practitioner.

Many of the principles of fluid therapy are the same for all classes of livestock. However, there are enough differences between neonatal and mature ruminants in terms of the abnormalities frequently encountered and solutions subsequently required to correct them to warrant separate discussions. Most of the research and clinical experience has been derived from cattle, but the same principles apply to other ruminants as well.

Fluid Therapy for Calves

The most frequent indication for fluid therapy for calves is neonatal calf diarrhea. Regardless of the etiologic organism, the metabolic changes resulting from diarrhea in calves are similar. They include (1) dehydration, (2) acidosis, (3) electrolyte abnormalities, and (4) negative energy balance and/or hypoglycemia.

The major cause of dehydration of these calves is fecal fluid loss, which can be as much as 13% of body weight in 24 hours. Compounding this problem is decreased intake from either anorexia or withdrawal of milk by the owner.

Acidosis results from bicarbonate and strong cation loss in the stool, lactic acid accumulation in tissues, decreased renal excretion of acid, and increased production of organic acid in the colon in malabsorptive diarrheas. Along with water and bicarbonate, sodium, chloride, and potassium are lost in the feces, which results in a total body deficit of these ions.

Negative energy balance can occur in diarrheic calves owing to decreased milk intake, decreased digestion or absorption of nutrients, or replacement of milk with low-energy oral rehydration solutions. In some calves with malabsorptive disease, acute hypoglycemia may occur. Increased energy demand, such as that resulting from cold weather or fever, exacerbates these problems.

Patient Assessment

Dehydration. Acute dehydration can most accurately be quantified by monitoring body weight. This is seldom possible except during rehydration because accurate baseline weights are not usually available. Serial measurement of packed cell volume (PCV) and total plasma protein (TPP) provide assessment of the relative state of hydration, but without baseline data, these measurements can be misleading. The range for PCV in healthy neonatal calves is 22% to 43%, much too variable to provide reliable quantitative information of hydration status, at least with a single sampling. The TPP is even more variable, depending greatly on the degree of colostral immunoglobulin absorption that occurred, as well as hydration. The PCV aids in assessment of rehydration efforts and can be used to help prevent overhydration, but TPP may be less useful. Proteins are contained in other fluid compartments, which makes the volume of distribution of plasma proteins larger than the plasma volume. Therefore PCV is a more reliable indicator of changes in blood volume than is TPP.

Without a reliable quantitative measure for hydration status, we must rely on estimates based on clinical signs. Table 104-1 provides a guideline for estimating the degree of dehydration in cattle.

This table is based on research conducted by Constable and colleagues[1] and is the most critically validated estimate of dehydration in calves. However, even in the absence of a validated system of estimating degree of dehydration, rehydration has been clinically successful, suggesting that precise estimates are not necessary. Rather than becoming

Table 104-1

Guide to Estimation of Fluid Replacement Requirement

% Dehydration	0	2	4	6	8	10	12	14
Eyeball recession (mm)	0	1	2	3	4	6	7	8
Skin tent duration (sec)	2	3	4	5	6	7	8	9

From Constable PD, Walker PG, Morin DE et al: *J Am Vet Med Assoc* 212: 991-996, 1998.

overly concerned with pinpointing the exact degree of dehydration, veterinarians should be concerned whether intravenous therapy is necessary or whether voluntary or forced oral supplementation will suffice. Rather than defining an exact long-term fixed plan for rehydration, we should begin with a reasonable plan and adjust it as needed. In other words, *guess and reassess.*

Empirically, 8% dehydration is the severity beyond which it is considered that oral fluid therapy will not suffice. According to the Table 104-1, 8% dehydration is characterized by eyeball recession of 4 mm in the skin tent duration of 6 seconds. Other clinical signs associated with severe dehydration include dry mucous membranes and moderate to severe depression. Calves displaying these signs will benefit the most from intravenous therapy. In general, calves that readily suckle quantities of rehydration solution sufficient to meet their replacement, maintenance, and ongoing loss needs will respond to oral solutions. Many of the more severely dehydrated calves will respond to forced oral solutions as well, but intravenous replacement is preferred.

Acidosis. Acidemia can quickly and accurately be assessed when a blood gas analyzer is available. These units are becoming more affordable, but access to such a unit is still not common in private large animal practice. Measurement and assessment of total carbon dioxide (TCO_2) will provide essentially equivalent clinical data in assessment of nonrespiratory acidosis or alkalosis, which is the type of acid-base disturbance most frequently encountered in conscious animals. TCO_2 measurement is available with many units that measure electrolytes. Blood tubes should be filled to capacity if TCO_2 is to be measured to avoid falsely low values. In most cases in practice, the degree of acidosis will be estimated. Naylor has developed a scoring system for this purpose (see Chapter 21). Naylor also determined that dehydrated calves older than 1 week of age had more severe acidosis (mean base deficit of 19.5 mEq/L) than did those younger than 1 week of age (mean deficit of 14.4 mEq/L). As a rule of thumb, severely diarrheic calves younger than 1 week of age can be assumed to have a base deficit of 10 to 15 mEq/L whereas those greater than 1 week of age can be assumed to have a base deficit of 15 to 20 mEq/L.

Electrolyte imbalance. Laboratory analysis of serum or plasma electrolytes can be of benefit in evaluating the replacement needs of diarrheic calves but, if misinterpreted, could lead to inappropriate therapy. Plasma represents a small portion of total body water, and the concentration of electrolytes in a blood sample must be interpreted in light of that fact. If sodium and chloride are within normal limits and a calf has lost 20% of ECF volume, then the calf has a total body sodium and chloride deficit of nearly 20%. Because sodium and chloride concentrations are often within or below the reference range in diarrheic calves, it is extremely important to provide these electrolytes in replacement solutions. Failure to do so will result in dilution of the already deficient ions.

A potentially more misleading laboratory value than plasma sodium and chloride is plasma potassium. Many dehydrated, acidemic calves are hyperkalemic, yet they have a total body potassium deficit. This paradox is the result of a shift of potassium out of the ICF compartment into the ECF compartment during acidemia. The ECF, which normally contains only about 5% of the body's total exchangeable potassium, has a greater than normal concentration of potassium. Because of the fecal and urinary losses, however, ICF potassium concentration and total body potassium content are decreased.

Blood glucose. Blood glucose determination can be made by a serum analyzer or by a rapid method using a handheld meter. Hypoglycemia in calves results in weakness, lethargy, coma, convulsions, and opisthotonos. Negative energy balance is not easily quantified because it can result from inadequate intake, malabsorption-maldigestion, or increased metabolic demand caused by fever or low ambient temperature. If milk is withheld for more than 48 hours, especially in cold weather, a serious energy deficit can occur. Weak or recumbent calves that do not appear to be dehydrated, but are emaciated, are usually suffering from malabsorption or malnutrition. Sometimes these calves respond, at least temporarily, to intravenous dextrose infusion.

Estimating Fluid and Electrolyte Replacement Requirements

The first priority in treatment of a dehydrated calf should be restoration of ECF volume. When estimating the volume of fluid needed by a patient, the veterinarian should consider not only the deficit, but also maintenance requirements and compensation for continuing loss. Daily maintenance fluid requirement for the neonatal calf is 50 to 100 ml/kg, whereas ongoing fluid loss can range from minimal amounts to as much as 4 L in 24 hours. One must avoid overemphasizing the estimate of the degree of dehydration and the calculation of volume *replacement* needed, while neglecting to include maintenance and ongoing losses into the calculations. In many cases the actual deficit is less than half of the total 24-hour volume requirement.

Second in priority to correcting ECF volume depletion is correcting acidosis. It has been suggested that the restoration of ECF volume alone would allow the kidneys to eliminate acid in sufficient quantity to restore normal acid-base balance. When time and money are not limiting factors, slow correction of acidosis can be accomplished in most cases with nonalkalinizing fluids. In most cases with baby calves it is necessary to treat the calf rapidly and, in beef calves, return them to the care of their mothers as soon as possible. The ability of nonalkalinizing fluids to *rapidly* correct moderate to severe academia in calves has been disproved. Neither intravenously nor orally administered solutions without alkalinizing agents resolved acidosis expeditiously even through ECF volume was restored.

Acidosis can be corrected by the administration of bicarbonate ions or so-called bicarbonate precursors, salts of weak organic acids. Alternatives to bicarbonate include lactate, acetate, gluconate, propionate, and citrate. Studies in calves have demonstrated the superior rapid alkalinizing efficiency of bicarbonate, compared with L-lactate and acetate.

Sodium bicarbonate is the most economical and readily available alkalinizing agent; however, it cannot be heat sterilized. It also should not be used in solutions containing calcium because an insoluble compound will form.

Alternative alkalinizing agents offer both advantages and disadvantages. Lactate is a widely used alkalinizing agent in veterinary medicine, although it has several shortcomings. Hepatic perfusion and function are necessary for its metabolism, and endogenous lactate (lactic acid) that accumulates during hypovolemia and shock can reduce its metabolism. Also, commercial preparations of lactated Ringer's solution contain racemic mixtures of D- and L-lactate. Only the L-isomer is metabolized efficiently, whereas most of the D-isomer is excreted in the urine unchanged. Therefore the alkalinizing potential of the racemic mixture is only about half of the alkalinizing potential of an equimolar amount of the L-isomer. The quantity written on the label of a bottle of commercial lactating Ringer's includes both isomeric forms. Acetate has the advantage of being metabolized by peripheral tissues and of having no significant endogenous source and no unmetabolized isomer. Citrate can be used in oral rehydration solutions, but its calcium-chelating properties preclude its inclusion in solutions for intravenous administration. Gluconate, an alkalinizing agent used in combination with acetate in some commercially prepared solutions for intravenous administration to people, dogs, and horses, has been shown to be ineffective as an alkalinizing agent in calves when administered intravenously, but it is effective when administered orally.

Rate of administration of alkalinizing agents, especially sodium bicarbonate, is a controversial subject. Some concern is warranted because rapid intravenous administration of 8.3% sodium bicarbonate can cause serious side effects and should not be used undiluted. Rapid injection of this solution can cause hypernatremia and hyperosmolality, as well as rapid alkalinizing. Another complication reported to be associated with the use of sodium bicarbonate for alkalinization is cerebrospinal fluid (CSF) acidosis. This condition was reported in 1967 in two human patients who received sodium bicarbonate infusions; however, whereas numerous warnings about CSF acidosis can be found in veterinary literature, we are not aware of a documented clinical case of CSF acidosis in domestic animals and therefore do not hesitate to replace the total calculated deficit of bicarbonate in the initial deficit replacement solution.

When blood gas analysis is available, the value for the base deficit (BD) can be used to calculate total base requirement by use of the following formula:

$$0.6 \times BD \times \text{body weight} = \text{Base requirement in mEq}$$

The estimate of the bicarbonate space in young calves is typically 0.5 to 0.6 of body weight, whereas 0.3 is recommended for mature cattle. When the value for TCO_2 or bicarbonate is known, it can be subtracted from 25 (the approximate normal value for plasma bicarbonate) and the difference can be used in place of BD in the formula. When it is not possible to quantify acid-base status, an estimate of 10 to 20 mEq/L may be used to formulate fluids for intravenous use for diarrheic calves. Remember that calves older than 1 week of age tend to become more severely acidotic.

The addition of glucose to rehydration solutions has three benefits. First, in orally administered solutions, glucose enhances sodium absorption in the small intestine via a transmembrane cotransport system. Second, once absorbed or injected, glucose also stimulates the release of insulin, which in turn enhances the movement of potassium from the ECF to the ICF. Third, glucose provides readily available energy. Glucose concentrations of 1% to 2% in intravenously administered solutions have produced favorable clinical results and usually do not result in significant glucosuria or osmotic diuresis. Additional glucose may be provided in oral solutions. In selected cases, total or partial parenteral nutrition may be beneficial to calves with severe prolonged malabsorptive diarrhea. In one study, calves receiving parenteral nutrition gained more weight but did not have better survivability than those receiving traditional therapy.

The importance of replacing sodium and chloride should not be overlooked. Remember that total body sodium and chloride are deficient in dehydrated calves, even when plasma concentrations are normal.

The administration of potassium to a hyperkalemic patient seems absurd at first, but the objective is to replace the total body potassium deficit that exists despite hyperkalemia. Administration of potassium to hyperkalemic acidemic calves can be accomplished safely if bicarbonate and dextrose are administered concurrently. As previously mentioned, dextrose and bicarbonate enhance the movement of potassium from the ECF to the ICF. Ideally, the initial liter or so of intravenously administered rehydration solution should contain less potassium than subsequent volumes. However, practicality often dictates the use of a single solution for rehydration. There seems to be little danger in including up to 20 mEq of potassium per liter if bicarbonate and dextrose are included in the solution.

Formulating a Solution for Intravenous Administration

As many correct ways to formulate solutions for intravenous administration in calves as one can imagine are available. The following is a list of suggested criteria for intravenously administered solutions.

1. Osmolality between 300 and 450 mOsm/L.
2. Sodium and chloride concentrations near or slightly less than normal plasma concentrations.
3. Potassium concentration 10 to 20 mEq/L. (Because 1 g of potassium chloride contains 14 mEq potassium, inclusion of 1 g of potassium chloride per liter fulfills this criterion.)
4. Dextrose at 10 to 20 g/L of solution (1%-2%).

5. Sodium bicarbonate or a suitable metabolizable base calculated to meet the measured deficit (or an estimated base deficit of 10 to 20 mEq/L if laboratory values are not available).

Of course, commercial solutions such as lactated Ringer's can be used. In most cases, sodium bicarbonate is required in addition to correct acidosis. Dextrose and additional potassium should also be added. Remember that bicarbonate should not be mixed in the same container with calcium-containing solutions, such as lactated Ringer's. Therefore one strategy using commercial solutions is to administer sodium bicarbonate solution initially (2 L of 1.3% sodium bicarbonate or 0.5 L of 5% sodium bicarbonate solution) followed by lactated Ringer's solution with added potassium and dextrose. Although it may be ideal to rehydrate a patient over 24 to 48 hours, bovine practitioners must often use the maximal safe infusion rate rather than the ideal. Overhydration and hypertension can be detected when central venous pressure is monitored, but this luxury is seldom available to the practitioner. A maximum of 80 ml/kg/hr has been suggested as a safe flow rate. A more conservative rate of 50 ml/kg/hr is probably a reasonable, relatively safe maximal infusion rate. With use of this infusion rate, most calves can be rehydrated in 2 to 3 hours. During rapid intravenous administration of fluids, the veterinarian or attendant should periodically monitor heart rate, respiratory rate and character, and attitude, adjusting the flow rate if necessary. Extra caution should be exercised when administering intravenous fluids to hypothermic calves.

When possible, it is desirable to administer approximately 1 L of the solution rapidly to reverse hypovolemic shock and then administer the balance over a period of hours. Doing this maximizes the benefit of the therapy by minimizing the diuresis that is sometimes induced by rapid fluid administration. If it is impractical or impossible to administer the total 24-hour requirement, or even the total deficit by intravenous infusion, 1 or 2 L of fluid administered intravenously may be enough to improve the circulatory status of a calf so that the balance of the calf's requirement may be provided by the oral route. In other words, a relatively small volume of fluids administered intravenously may convert a calf from the *intravenous fluid required* to the *oral fluid satisfactory* category. Fluids for maintenance and continued loss may be administered orally or by slow intravenous infusion. Alternatively, intravenously administered hyperosmolar saline solution combined with intraruminally administered electrolyte solution may be administered.

Oral Rehydration Therapy for Calves

The popularity of oral rehydration solutions (ORSs) for calves is an accurate reflection of the success of this therapeutic modality. Veterinarians and livestock producers alike have witnessed the results of oral rehydration and promoted its use. Many products are commercially produced, each with its advantages and shortcomings. The following discussion should help veterinarians make informed decisions concerning the use of these products.

Advantages of Oral Rehydration Solutions

Oral fluid therapy has several obvious advantages over intravenous fluid therapy. Economy of materials, time, and equipment is the major advantage in treating food animals. The ORS can be carried and stored in dry form, mixed with tap water, administered by nursing bottle or stomach tube, and administered as infrequently as every 12 hours. Whereas suckling delivers the solution more directly to the abomasum by inducing reticular groove closure, intubation is also an accepted means of delivery in neonatal calves. A slight delay in absorption may occur after intubation, which could be beneficial if a depot effect is desired rather than an immediate effect. Finally, the gradual absorption of the ORS allows more flexibility in the formulation of these solutions than of those for intravenous use. Greater concentrations of potassium, glucose, and total osmoles can be supplied in ORS than in intravenous solutions.

Characteristics of Oral Rehydration Solutions

Several types and numerous individual formulations of ORS are available commercially. Although a significant difference in constituents exists, all of these solutions can be used successfully. Included in all ORS formulations are substantial amounts of sodium, chloride, potassium, and glucose. Most contain bicarbonate or another alkalinizing agent. Many contain glycine, acetate, or citrate to enhance sodium and water absorption. Calcium, magnesium, and phosphorus are present in some. Additives such as psyllium are now included as antidiarrheal agents.

The major differences between formulations occur in the following constituents: glucose, alkalinizing agents, and total osmolality. The variety of combinations of constituents in today's commercial ORS market allows the veterinarian to choose the type of solution that will perform best in a given situation. High-energy solutions approach the maintenance needs of the calf and reduce weight loss, compared with low-energy solutions. However, if a significant amount of glucose reaches the colon, it may exacerbate diarrhea. If milk intake is withdrawn or reduced for more than 24 hours, moderate- to high-energy solutions should probably be used.

Whenever acidosis is moderate to severe, ORS with alkalinizing agents must be used to restore normal acid-base status in a timely manner. According to Naylor's work, alkalinizing solutions are more likely to be needed for older calves.[2] Nonalkalinizing solutions are indicated for clients who monitor calves closely and institute fluid therapy early in the course of disease before dehydration or acidosis becomes severe. Alkalinizing potential and alkalinity of solutions do not necessarily parallel each other. Solutions containing sodium bicarbonate as an alkalinizing agent are alkaline, whereas some solutions containing a metabolizable base are actually acidic when consumed. Bicarbonate-containing solutions are therefore more likely to alkalinize the abomasum and allow the proliferation of bacteria and possibly the passage of pathogens to the intestines. The clinical significance of this is unproven, but experimentally it is easier to produce colibacillosis in calves if sodium bicarbonate is administered before bacterial challenge. The high-energy solutions mentioned must also be hyperosmolar because the energy

source is glucose. Reasonable arguments can be made for both iso-osmolar and hyperosmolar solutions. Intuitively, it seems reasonable that consumption of hyperosmolar solutions would result in movement of free water into the gastrointestinal lumen along the osmotic gradient. Such a shift in water would exacerbate the preexisting dehydration. Evidence indicates that a slight transient shift occurs, but no adverse effects have been shown. On the other hand, a villus countercurrent mechanism causes the interstitium of the villus tip to become hyperosmolar during absorption, which makes a hyperosmolar solution *isosmotic* relative to the interstitial fluid in closest proximity. However, the merit of creating a luminal osmolality equal to the interstitium is questionable because one of the theories explaining the purpose of the countercurrent mechanism and resulting villus hyperosmolality is that the gradient established between the lumen and interstitium enhances water absorption from the lumen. If this gradient is reduced or negated by hyperosmolar solutions, water absorption could theoretically be reduced.

One *ideal* ORS for all situations probably does not exist. In addition to the medical and physiologic considerations, other factors (e.g., cost, convenience, palatability) must be considered when an ORS is chosen.

Using Oral Rehydration Solutions for Optimal Results

To maximize the benefit of ORSs, there are certain practices to adopt and others to avoid. The controversy over whether an ORS should be used as a supplement to milk feeding or as a replacement is still unsettled, but a consensus is forming on a few points. Evidence in people has shown that removing all food from the diet results in rapid loss of digestive and absorptive capability of the intestines. In calves, weight loss is accelerated by withdrawing milk and replacing it with an ORS, especially the lower-energy solutions. Therefore it is desirable to maintain calves on milk if the intestinal damage is not so great that a severe malabsorptive osmotic diarrhea results. However, studies show that consumption of bicarbonate-containing solutions interspersed between milk feedings results in decreased weight gain, possibly due to poor digestibility of the milk. Also, when ORS was mixed 1:1 with milk and fed to healthy calves, diarrhea was noted. From these studies, it can be concluded that ORS should probably not be mixed with milk or milk replacer and that non–bicarbonate-containing solutions may be preferred if calves are not taken off milk during the time that fluids are being administered. If milk is completely withdrawn from the diet, it should probably be reintroduced after 24 hours or less to avoid excessive weight loss. Reduction of daily intake of milk is preferable to complete withdrawal.

Parenteral Nutrition

When the gastrointestinal tract is unable to digest and absorb nutrients adequately and the patient is severely debilitated, parenteral nutrition is indicated.

Total Parenteral Nutrition

Total parenteral nutrition (TPN) should be considered in sick neonates experiencing weight loss or failure to gain weight such as calves with chronic diarrhea or septicemia.

Small amounts of milk should still be fed to help preserve the digestive functions of the enterocytes. Dehydration and electrolyte abnormalities should be addressed before beginning TPN. The following formula has been recommended and used with success:

1000 ml 50% dextrose
1000 ml 8.5% amino acids
500 ml 10% lipids

Start at one-fourth the target rate of 2.1 ml/kg/hr for the first 6 hours, and then measure blood glucose. If the blood glucose is less than 200 mg/dl, increase the rate by one fourth every 6 hours until the target rate is reached, trying to maintain blood glucose under 200 mg/dl during the initiation period of TPN, then under 150 mg/dl during maintenance. In my (CBN) experience, the target rate is rarely reached and many calves show clinical improvement (weight gain, increased appetite, and improved clinical condition) from administration of TPN solution at a rate less than that of maintenance for as little as 24 hours. Once a sustainable maintenance rate is established and blood glucose is consistently under 150 mg/dl, urine glucose can be monitored daily with urine dipsticks. If urine glucose is positive, blood glucose should be checked for hyperglycemia. The animal should also be monitored closely for signs of hypoglycemia.

Once TPN is no longer necessary, calves should be slowly weaned from TPN to prevent hypoglycemia. The rate can be decreased by one fourth of the maintenance rate every 6 hours while trying to maintain blood glucose above 70 mg/dl. During either introduction to or weaning from TPN, drastic changes in rate should be avoided.

Although double- and triple-bore catheters are often recommended for administration of TPN solution in other species, these are expensive and not readily available in most practices. A single-bore catheter can be used provided that the catheter and connecting lines are completely flushed of other fluids and medications before TPN solution is administered. Attention to sterility is crucial during catheter placement and during administration of TPN solution. The catheter site should be checked daily for signs of venous thrombosis. Although the jugular vein is preferred, TPN solution can be administered in other peripheral veins such as the ear, cephalic, or saphenous vein. A fluid pump is recommended for consistent administration to avoid drastic changes in blood glucose.

Potential metabolic complications include persistent hyperglycemia, hyperlipemia, hypokalemia, dehydration, or overhydration/hypervolemia. Avoid hyperglycemia and hyperlipemia by starting fluids slowly and monitoring urine or blood for glucose and serum for lipemia. If these complications occur, reduce the infusion rate and allow time for adaptation to the fluids. Twenty mEq of potassium can be added per liter of TPN solution to help prevent hypokalemia.

Partial Parenteral Nutrition

Adult ruminants suffering from metabolic diseases such as chronic ketosis, fatty liver syndrome, and pregnancy toxemia may benefit from PPN. Because lipid mobilization is often associated with these diseases, the lipids in TPN solution may be contraindicated. The following formula can be used in adult ruminants for PPN (Chris Cebra, personal communication).

5 L balanced isotonic fluid
500 ml 50% dextrose
1 L 8.5% amino acids

The solution is administered at 5% body weight per day (maintenance fluid rate). Potassium and calcium can be added to these fluids as needed. These can be administered through a venous catheter with a regular fluid administration set. Blood and/or urine glucose should be monitored but are usually easier to maintain in normal ranges with PPN than with TPN.

Fluid Therapy in Mature Ruminants

Although some of the principles of fluid therapy of mature ruminants are similar to those of calves and other species, many important exceptions exist. When assessing hydration status, one must remember that body weight and rumen fill can be misleading. Cattle with carbohydrate engorgement may not lose weight and may actually look full, but much of the fill is intraruminal water, which is unavailable to the animal. Also, skin tent and enophthalmos must be evaluated in light of the body condition. Emaciated cows may have sunken eyes and skin that tents, regardless of their hydration status. When deciding on route of administration, one should consider not only hydration status but cardiovascular status as well. For example, cattle with strangulating-obstructing gastrointestinal disease, especially those soon to undergo standing surgery, will benefit from intravenous fluid therapy even if they are not severely dehydrated because they may be in or near shock and cardiovascular collapse.

The volume required for complete rehydration of a large cow or bull is substantial and may dissuade practitioners from using this mode of therapy. It should be remembered that 10 to 20 L of fluid administered rather rapidly may be lifesaving, even though it represents less than half of the total fluid deficit. By use of at least some intravenous fluid (iso-osmolar or hyperosmolar), intravascular volume can be restored, an underlying problem can be remedied by surgical or medical means, and oral fluids can be supplied to replace the rest of the deficit. To reduce the cost of administering intravenous fluids, practitioners may consider formulating their own solutions. Dry ingredients can be preweighed and packaged and mixed with sterile distilled water immediately before administration. Another advantage of preparing custom solutions is that prepackaged solutions are expensive, and relatively few commercially available solutions are therapeutically appropriate for most cattle.

Unlike neonates, adult ruminants do not usually require alkalinizing fluids when they are dehydrated. A few conditions (such as choke, carbohydrate engorgement, and diabetes mellitus) are consistently associated with acidosis. Renal failure, fatty liver-ketosis, severe diarrhea pneumonia, and pregnancy toxemia are often associated with acidosis. Abomasal volvulus, displacement and impaction, intussusception, and cecal torsion are causes of moderate to severe alkalosis. In a study of mature dehydrated cattle, only about 22% had metabolic acidosis. Therefore nonalkalinizing solutions are the fluid of choice for most dehydrated mature ruminants. Usually accompanying alkalosis is hypochloridemia. Sequestration of chloride in the proximal small intestine, abomasum, and rumen results in hypochloridemic alkalosis. Alkalosis and anorexia contribute to hypokalemia in many sick cattle. Lactating dairy cattle are often hypocalcemic as well. To address these metabolic problems, we have used the following formulation at our hospital:

140 g NaCl
30 g Kcl
10 g CaCl$_2$
q.s. to 20 L

This solution may be administered intraruminally via tube or intravenously. If it is administered intravenously, 1 bottle of commercially prepared calcium borogluconate solution may be substituted for the calcium chloride, and up to a liter of 50% dextrose may be added if ketosis is a concurrent problem.

When administering solutions intraruminally, we prefer to pass a medium-sized nasogastric tube through the nasal cavity instead of using a Frick mouth speculum. The procedure is less stressful to the patient and allows the veterinarian to administer fluids unassisted. Be aware that on a relative weight basis, the nasal cavity of the cow is smaller than that of the horse, so a relatively smaller tube must be used. If nutritional supplementation is necessary, pelleted feed (with no large pieces of grain) can be soaked in warm water, made into a slurry, and pumped by use of a marine bilge pump or a commercially available cattle pump system.

Intravenous administration of fluids may be accomplished through a jugular catheter. A 10- to 14-gauge catheter is sufficient to permit rapid fluid administration. Cyanoacrylate glue is effective for affixing the catheter to the skin. The author prefers to use a 30-inch extension set connected to the catheter and held in place by elastic tape wrapped around the cow's neck. The extension set may be taped so that the end is positioned at the dorsum of the cow's neck to allow easy access for attachment to the intravenous administration set or for injections. An alternative to the jugular is the auricular vein. It is easily accessible and is more convenient to use if cattle must be restrained in a head catch during fluid administration. A 14- to 18-gauge 1- or 2-inch catheter is placed in the vein, glued, and taped in place, with or without an extension set (Fig. 104-1). Because of the smaller size of the vein, speed of fluid administration is limited; however, the rate of administration is great enough to rehydrate even a severely dehydrated cow in a reasonable amount of time. An auricular vein catheter can also be used as an access for repeated intravenous infusions. One must be aware that an auricular artery courses down the dorsum of the pinna. It should be identified by palpation of a pulse and avoided. Use of a rubber band as a tourniquet at the base of the ear usually collapses the artery and distends the veins.

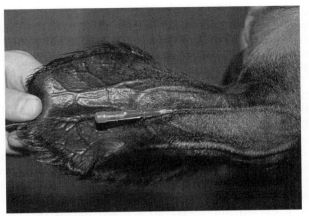

Fig 104-1 A 14-gauge auricular intravenous catheter in place.

Hypertonic Saline Solution

The sheer size of mature cattle and the great quantity of fluid required to resuscitate and rehydrate them has prevented many veterinarians from taking full advantage of intravenous fluid therapy. HSS (7.2% NaCl) offers the advantages of low cost and rapid administration, as well as efficacy, for treatment of shock and dehydration. HSS is commercially available, or it can be made by adding 72 g of NaCl to a liter of sterile distilled water. It should be administered at a dose of 4 ml/kg over 3 to 10 minutes. Rapid administration is essential because its effect is caused by transiently creating intravascular hyperosmolality. Intravascular volume increases by 3 to 4 ml per ml administered. The water is recruited from the interstitial and intracellular compartments. The effect of HSS is transient and must be supplemented by additional volume replacement. Colloids such as dextran and hetastarch enhance the efficacy of HSS by prolonging its effect. They add substantially to its cost, however. If HSS is administered to dehydrated cattle, it *must be accompanied by intraruminal water or followed by iso-osmolar crystalloid solutions.* The volume of intraruminal water that should accompany HSS administration to dehydrated cattle should be approximately eight times the volume of the HSS. Acidosis, hypokalemia, and hypocalcemia, if present, must be addressed separately by oral, intraruminal, or parenteral administration.

USE OF BLOOD AND PLASMA

Whole Blood

Whole blood is indicated when the red cell mass is below that necessary to carry an adequate amount of oxygen to the tissues. The point at which transfusion is necessary is determined in large part by the time course over which the red cells were lost or destroyed. The slower the process, the more tolerant the animal is to a low PCV. Cattle that become anemic can gradually tolerate a PCV as low as 8% if they are not stressed, and the author has seen parasitized goats with a PCV of 5% survive without transfusion. Transfusion has been recommended at a PCV of 12% to 15% if the anemia develops acutely. However, the most important indicator for determining if transfusion is indicated is the overall condition of the animal determined by respiratory rate and character, heart rate, and neurologic status. Another important fact to consider before deciding to transfuse is whether the stress of transfusion itself is likely to result in death.

Although plasma is more desirable, whole blood transfusion can be used to provide immunoglobulins to calves with failure of passive transfer. Achieving an adequate plasma immunoglobulin concentration in a calf with complete failure of passive transfer with the use of whole blood is difficult because the volume required may result in volume overload, polycythemia, and/or hemolytic icterus. Therefore whole blood is most useful in calves with partial failure of passive transfer. Up to 2 L of whole blood can be safely administered to a 45-kg calf.

Transfusion reactions are extremely rare in cattle that have not been transfused previously. A practical means of determining compatibility is to infuse a small quantity of blood, about 0.5 ml/kg body weight, and wait 10 minutes before proceeding with the transfusion. Blood should be administered slowly (10 ml/kg/hr or less) through a blood administration set with an appropriate filter. Usually, 10 to 15 ml/kg are administered. This dose can be expected to produce a rise of 3% to 4% in the recipient. Because the reticuloendothelial system is efficient at removing heterogenous red blood cells, only about 25% of the transfused cells remain after 4 days. Reported signs of transfusion reaction include hiccoughing, dyspnea, muscle tremor, salivation, lacrimation, and fever. Epinephrine hydrochloride 1:1000 should be administered (at 4-5 ml intramuscularly to an adult cow) if signs of anaphylaxis occur.

Although many diseases are transmissible by transfusion, bovine leukosis and anaplasmosis are two of the most important. If a known uninfected donor is unavailable, the donor should probably be a herdmate of the recipient. This will at least prevent inadvertent introduction of a new pathogen into the herd.

It is safe to remove 10 to 15 ml/kg of blood from a healthy donor. Remember, however, that if this same dose is given to a recipient, the rise in PCV will be small (3%-4%) and the duration short because exogenous red blood cells are rapidly destroyed by the recipient. Only 25% remain after the fourth day.

When blood is collected for immediate use, sodium citrate is an effective and inexpensive anticoagulant. It should be purchased or formulated to a 2.5% to 4% solution and added as one part solution to nine parts of blood. If blood is to be stored for more than a few hours, acid citrate dextrose solution should be used.

Plasma

Plasma is indicated in cases of hypoproteinemia and failure of passive transfer. Because ruminant red blood cells do not settle by gravity, centrifugation is required. The inconvenience of collection and harvesting along with the large volumes required to raise the recipient's plasma protein concentration significantly make plasma transfusion a relatively uncommon practice. If attempting to provide an acceptable immunoglobulin concentration to a calf with complete failure of passive transfer, 2 L of plasma should be administered. Commercially prepared plasma is currently available for purchase in certain locations.

SHOCK

Shock in its broadest sense is a condition in which there is decreased tissue perfusion, cellular hypoxia, and ultimately cell death.

Three major types of shock exist: hypovolemic, cardiogenic, and vasculogenic. The type of shock most commonly encountered in cattle is vasculogenic, specifically endotoxic or septic shock. Endotoxin is a constituent of the cell wall of gram-negative bacteria. It is released when bacterial cells die. Causes of endotoxic shock in cattle include colisepticemia, coliform mastitis, septic metritis, and pasteurellosis.

Endotoxic shock is characterized by dyspnea, depression, congested mucous membranes, recumbency, and death. Cardiovascular effects include decreased mean arterial blood pressure and cardiac output, as well as increased pulmonary arterial pressure. The most important treatment for shock in food animals is rapid intravenous infusion of crystalloid solutions. The rate of administration should be rapid, especially initially. In most cattle, 75 ml/kg/hr is probably safe for infusion of isosmotic solutions for at least 30 to 60 minutes. HSS has been used successfully to treat shock at the dose mentioned previously.

In endotoxic shock, corticosteroids and nonsteroidal antiinflammatory drugs have been shown to be effective in reducing the cardiopulmonary effects. The shock dose of corticosteroids used in research protocols for cattle has been 2 mg/kg for dexamethasone and 1.1 mg/kg for prednisolone sodium succinate, although many veterinarians use smaller doses. Flunixin meglumine and ketoprofen are approved for use in cattle in Europe at a daily dose of 2 mg/kg and 3 mg/kg, respectively. Flunixin meglumine is approved for use in cattle in the United States and Canada. More frequent dosing may be necessary in endotoxemia. These drugs must be used in an appropriate extralabel fashion.

Reference

1. Constable PD, Walker PG, Morin DE et al: Clinical and laboratory assessment of hydration status of neonatal calves with diarrhea, *J Am Vet Med Assoc* 212:991-996, 1998.

Recommended Reading

Roussel AJ, Constable PD: Fluid and electrolyte therapy, *Vet Clin North Am Food Anim Pract* 15:3, 1999.

CHAPTER 105

Pain Management in Cattle and Small Ruminants

ALEXANDER VALVERDE and THOMAS J. DOHERTY

Pain as defined by the International Association for the Study of Pain (IASP) is "an unpleasant sensory and emotional experience associated with actual or potential tissue damage, or described in terms of such damage."

Nociception is the perception of noxious stimuli and denotes activity of nerve pathways involved in the reception of such stimuli that could lead to the experience of local pain, referred pain, or visceral symptoms. Pain is in fact one potential manifestation of nociception; however, nociception does not imply pain. Deep noxious stimulation can reach lower central nervous system sites at the level of the hypothalamus and brainstem through second-order neurons in the anterolateral system, by means of the spinohypothalamic and spinoreticular tracts, and generate visceral symptoms associated with autonomic responses, independently of the relay of pain to conscious levels; thus there is nociception but not necessarily pain.[1] Assessing pain based on single responses alone, like changes in heart rate or behavior, could be misleading. Nevertheless, indicators of pain mentioned by practitioners in the United Kingdom included anorexia (45%), vocalization (45%), grinding teeth (38%), dullness and depression (32%), abnormal movements (30%), and abnormal posture (26%). Less frequently mentioned parameters included increased heart rate, respiratory changes, recumbency, reduced rumination, and reduced yield.[2]

Nociceptors are free nerve endings of neurons found in skin, periosteum, and joint surfaces. They are activated by mechanical, thermal, and chemical stimuli and project to the spinal cord through fast-conducting (A delta) and slow-conducting (C) fibers, where they release excitatory neurotransmitters such as glutamate and substance P to allow the relay of signals through specific pathways that connect to the thalamus, brainstem, and limbic system (Fig. 105-1). In the case of pain, nociception is relayed to the thalamus via neospinothalamic and paleospinothalamic tract cells or neurons. From the thalamus, certain thalamocortical fibers project to the limbic system, where the emotion of pain is generated and the individual becomes fully aware of the pain.

Pain recognition is difficult and considering the mechanisms involved in pain perception/nociception and the multiple autonomic responses that may be activated through nociception, but that may not cause pain, there is no correct way of assessing pain. A recent review describes the difficulties in assessing pain in cattle.[3]

However, changes in behavior, cardiorespiratory, and organ functions may indicate that nociceptive pathways are already activated and could potentially result in pain if untreated.

In a survey regarding the use of epidural analgesia and postoperative analgesia by bovine practitioners in the United Kingdom, analgesics were administered postoperatively to cesarean cases and other laparotomies in 68% and 57% of cases, respectively.[2] In Canada, more than 90% of veterinarians administered analgesics for cesarean

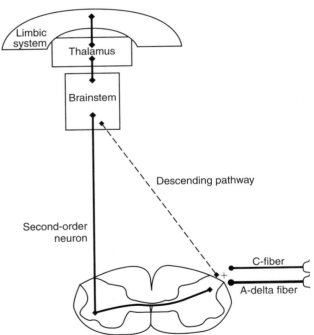

Fig 105-1 Stimulation of nociceptors results in release of excitatory (+) neurotransmitters (substance P, glutamate) from nonmyelinated C fibers and/or myelinated A delta fibers in the spinal cord and activates second-order neurons (spinohypothalamic, spinoreticular tracts) that reach the brainstem and thalamus for nociception. Further involvement of the limbic system results in pain perception. Descending inhibitory pathways are supraspinal in origin and use noradrenaline and serotonin as neurotransmitters to release endogenous opioids from spinal inhibitory interneurons. Inhibitory pathways are stimulated by activation of the brainstem and enhanced by centrally acting drugs (opioids).

sections, claw amputation, and omentopexies; however, the analgesics used were considered to be inadequate in some cases and the use of analgesics in younger animals was also less than optimal.[4] Similarly, in the United Kingdom even for those procedures considered more painful (cesarean cases and claw amputation) by practitioners, less than 68% of veterinarians used nonsteroidal antiinflammatory drugs (NSAIDs) to control postoperative pain, despite the availability of a wide variety of these drugs including flunixin meglumine, meloxicam, ketoprofen, and carprofen in their practices.[5]

The infrequent or inadequate use of analgesics in ruminants has multiple reasons, from difficulties in pain recognition to cost issues that preclude analgesic use. The lack of cost-effective analgesics, the limited duration of action of available drugs, the risk of side effects, and unknown withdrawal periods are reasons cited by veterinarians for limited use of analgesics.[4,5]

PAIN MANAGEMENT

Pain can be treated (1) locally at the site where the noxious stimulus occurs, (2) at any level of the pathways that transmit pain to the brain, or (3) at higher centers in the brain where pain recognition ultimately occurs. A particular analgesic drug may be effective at any or all of these three sites. In addition, different techniques can be employed to deliver the drug(s) to any of these sites to improve drug efficacy. Knowledge of the mechanism of action of analgesic drugs and the most appropriate route of administration is important to provide the best pain relief.

When considering pain management strategy, one should contemplate prevention (preemptive) and control of those pain pathways already activated in nociception. The different mechanisms of action of analgesic drugs may require more than one drug to effectively manage pain. Alternatively, a particular drug may be administered by different routes (e.g., intramuscular, epidural). Pain recognition and management should be intense to blunt hyperalgesic states and assist prompt and effective treatment.

The analgesic drugs most commonly used in ruminants include opioids, alpha-2 (α-2) adrenergic agonists, local anesthetics, and NSAIDs. These drugs may be administered alone or in combination.

Opioids

Opioid receptors are classified as mu, kappa, and delta (OP3, OP1, and OP2, respectively). These receptors may be present in the spinal cord, brain, and other tissues such as joints and cornea. The analgesic effects of opioids result from the interaction with receptors at the spinal level, where opioids modulate the release of excitatory neurotransmitters from nociceptive fibers. Peripherally, in tissues such as joints, opioids modulate the actions of C fibers already sensitized by inflammation. In the brain, opioids release adrenergic and serotonergic pathways from GABAergic inhibition, thereby increasing the activity of these descending inhibitory pathways and allowing the suppression of pain at the spinal level. Therefore opioids can act at all levels of the pain pathways and could potentially be administered close to the site of action such as intraarticularly for local actions in joints, epidurally for action on the spinal cord, and systemically for actions on the brain.

Despite the effectiveness of opioids for pain management in other species, their use in ruminants is infrequent. The schedule classification of opioids may preclude their regular use under farming conditions. In addition, the analgesic effects induced in other species appear to be less evident in ruminants and other pharmacologic groups including NSAIDs and α-2 agonists are often preferred and recommended in the literature. Opioids have proven to be useful analgesics in experimental settings using cutaneous thermal and mechanical stimulation models of pain. In sheep, most opioids including butorphanol, buprenorphine, fentanyl, and meperidine are effective analgesics against thermal stimulation when administered intravenously,[6-10] whereas fentanyl and, to a lesser extent meperidine, are effective against a pressure (mechanical) stimulus[8] (Table 105-1).

Table 105-1

Parenteral Analgesics Commonly Used in Ruminants

	Dose (mg/kg)	Route	Duration of Action (hr)	Species
Morphine	0.05-0.5	IM, IV	6	Cattle
	0.5	IM, IV	4-6	Goat
Meperidine	5	IM	0.25-0.5	Sheep, cattle
Butorphanol	0.05-0.2	IM, IV	1-3	Sheep, goat
Buprenorphine	0.0015-0.006	IM, IV	0.75-3.5	Sheep
Fentanyl	0.01	IV	1-2	Sheep
Xylazine	0.05-0.2	IM, IV	2-4	Sheep, goat, cattle
Detomidine	0.003-0.01	IM, IV	2-4	Sheep, goat, cattle
Medetomidine	0.005-0.01	IM, IV	2-4	Sheep, goat, cattle
Romifidine	0.003-0.02	IM, IV	2-4	Sheep, goat, cattle
Lidocaine	2.5	IV	1	Goat

Modified from Valverde A, Gunkel CI: *J Vet Emerg Crit Care* 15:295, 2005.

Morphine has been used less frequently in ruminants and a wide dose range has been suggested for cattle (0.05-0.5 mg/kg; intravenously [IV] or intramuscularly [IM]).[11,12] The authors use a dose of 0.25 to 0.5 mg/kg IM every 4 to 6 hours for cattle. In goats doses of up to 10 mg/kg have produced better analgesia than lower standard doses[12]; however, we recommend a dose of 0.5 mg/kg IM every 4 to 6 hours.

Morphine has been administered epidurally (0.1 mg/kg diluted in sterile saline) at the sacrococcygeal or first coccygeal space in cattle and at the lumbosacral space in goats to induce analgesia of 6 to 12 hours' duration[12-14] (Table 105-2). This dose is relatively low and despite systemic absorption from the epidural space will not result in marked cardiorespiratory effects or sedation. There appears to be no published report on the use of other opioids epidurally in these species. It is recognized that morphine, due to its low lipid solubility, has the longest duration of action; therefore other opioids may not provide a benefit over morphine.

Opioids, when administered epidurally, affect only sensory fibers (C fibers) and have no effect on other fiber types, thus avoiding the risk of ataxia caused by motor blockade and of hypotension caused by sympathetic blockade, as occurs with local anesthetics. However, morphine (0.1 mg/kg) administered by the intrathecal route at the lumbosacral space in sheep resulted in adverse effects including rear limb ataxia and licking and chewing of the flanks and hind limbs presumably because of pruritus or irritation.[15] These side effects are not expected using this dose by the epidural route. The dose used in these sheep was high for an intrathecal injection, and similar side effects have been reported in rats administered high intrathecal doses of morphine.[16] Thus intrathecal administration of the epidural dose of morphine is not recommended.

Table 105-2

Epidural or Intrathecal Analgesics Commonly Used in Ruminants

	Dose (mg/kg)	Route	Duration of Analgesia (hr)	Comments	Species
Morphine	0.1	Epidural	6-12	Diluted with 0.02-0.05 ml/kg of saline	Cattle
	0.1	Epidural	6-12	Diluted with 0.2 ml/kg of saline or combined with bupivacaine (1.5 mg/kg)	Goat
Medetomidine	0.015	Epidural	7	Diluted to 5 ml with saline	Cattle
	0.01-0.03	Epidural	>3	Diluted to 5 ml with saline	Goat
Xylazine	0.05	Epidural	2	Diluted to 5 ml with saline	Cattle
	0.07-0.4	Epidural	1-2	Diluted to 2.5 ml with saline	Sheep
	0.15	Epidural	3	Diluted to 5 ml with saline	Goat
	0.05	Epidural	0.5-1	Combined with ketamine (2.5 mg/kg) and diluted to 1.5 ml with saline	Goat
	0.05	Epidural	<1		
	0.05	Intrathecal	2	Diluted to 0.75 ml with saline	Goat
	0.1	Intrathecal	1.5	Diluted to 2 ml with saline	Sheep
	0.05	Intrathecal	3	Diluted to 4 ml with saline	Goat
				Combined with lidocaine (1.25 mg/kg) and diluted to 4 ml with saline	Goat
Detomidine	0.04	Epidural	3	Diluted to 5 ml with saline	Cattle
	0.01	Intrathecal	1	Diluted to 2 ml with saline	Sheep
Romifidine	0.05	Epidural	Up to 12	Combined with morphine (0.1 mg/kg) and diluted to 30 ml with saline	Cattle
	0.05	Intrathecal	1	Diluted to 4 ml with saline	Goat
	0.05	Intrathecal	2	Combined with ketamine (2.5 mg/kg) and diluted to 2 ml with saline	Goat
Ketamine	0.5-2	Epidural	1	Diluted to 5-20 ml with saline	Cattle
	1	Epidural	5	Diluted to 7-9 ml with saline	Sheep
	2.5	Epidural	0.25	Diluted to 0.75 ml with saline	Goat
	2.5	Epidural	0.5-1	Combined with xylazine (0.05 mg/kg) and diluted to 1.5 ml	Goat
	2.5	Intrathecal	2	Combined with romifidine (0.05 mg/kg) and diluted to 2 ml with saline	Goat
Lidocaine	0.2-0.4		1-2		Cattle
Bupivacaine	1.5-1.8		2-3		Goat
	0.05		2-3		Cattle

Modified from Valverde A, Gunkel CI: *J Vet Emerg Crit Care* 15:295, 2005.

The intraarticular use of morphine has not been described in ruminants, although its use has been proven effective and long acting in other species (rats, dogs, horses, humans) for inflammatory processes of the joint.[17-20] If opioid binding sites were determined to be present in inflamed joints in ruminants, this route of administration would be an effective and simple method of providing analgesia of relatively long duration (≥6 hours). The recommended dose in other species is 0.05 to 0.1 mg/kg diluted with sterile saline (5-15 ml according to the joint size).

Transdermal application of fentanyl has been studied in goats using patches of 50 μg/hr placed on the neck region. The bioavailability exceeds 100% because of the ruminosalivary cycle, and this predisposes to recycling of highly lipid-soluble drugs like fentanyl. Peak plasma concentrations are achieved in 8 to 18 hours and, because of the high bioavailability, animals should be monitored for adverse side effects associated with opioids (e.g., sedation, respiratory depression, mania).[21]

Alpha-2 Agonists

Commonly used α-2 agonists in ruminants include xylazine, detomidine, medetomidine, and romifidine. α-2 Adrenergic receptors are located supraspinally and spinally. In the spinal cord, α-2 receptors are found to be in the superficial laminae of the dorsal horn.[22] The central location mediates sedation, anxiolysis, and analgesia. More specifically, their location at the periaqueductal gray area of the midbrain, the site of origin of the descending inhibitory pathways of pain, results in the release of norepinephrine and modulation of pain at the spinal level.

Processing of nociception occurs via interaction of spinal receptors with the descending inhibitory pathways. The supraspinal and spinal distribution of adrenergic receptors results in the action of α-2 agonists at these two levels. Therefore systemic and epidural or intrathecal administration of α-2 agonists has been recommended in ruminants.

Systemic administration of α-2 agonists is commonly used to induce sedation and analgesia in ruminants (see Table 105-1). The α-2 agonists are associated with several cardiorespiratory effects including bradycardia, a transient initial arterial hypertension followed by hypotension, decreased cardiac output, hypoxemia, and hypercapnia.[23-26] These effects are more pronounced with intravenous administration and occur in cattle and small ruminants; however, respiratory changes such as increased respiratory resistance, decreased lung compliance, hypoxemia, and pulmonary edema are more evident in sheep.[27,28]

The α-2 agonists should be used with caution in the last trimester of pregnancy because xylazine has been shown to increase myometrial tone in the cow.[29,30] Detomidine appears to have less effect on uterine electrical activity in the cow.[31]

Pain models using cutaneous thermal, mechanical, and electrical stimulation have demonstrated the dose-dependent analgesic properties of α-2 agonists in ruminants after intravenous or intramuscular administration and the analgesia may last 60 to 90 minutes.[32,33] Epidural administration in the sacrococcygeal or first coccygeal space in cattle and sheep or the lumbosacral space in sheep and goats results in similar cardiorespiratory effects to systemic administration; however, analgesia tends to be of longer duration because of the interaction of larger amounts of the drug with α-2 adrenoceptors in the spinal cord because relatively similar doses are administered epidurally and systemically[34-42] (see Table 105-2). The analgesia after epidural administration is more profound in the hind limbs, perineum, and abdomen; however, systemic absorption may also result in generalized analgesia and sedation.[36,40,41] Sheep undergoing surgery appear to be less sedate than cattle and goats after epidural administration despite the use of higher doses in sheep.[37] Unlike epidural opioids that only provide analgesia, epidural α-2 agonists are capable of producing complete sensory blockade against surgical stimulation and have been used as the sole anesthetic to perform surgery including cesarean section in sheep.[37] In cattle, the combination of romifidine (0.05 mg/kg) and morphine (0.1 mg/kg) administered at the first coccygeal space provided analgesia for up to 12 hours against a noxious electrical stimulus applied to the flank[43] (see Table 105-2).

Paresis is common with epidural xylazine.[35-37] This latter effect is not documented for other α-2 agonists, although one goat that received epidural medetomidine exhibited hind limb paralysis for 3 days before being euthanized. Trauma to the spinal cord from the lumbosacral injection was suggested as the most likely cause of paralysis because other goats receiving two or three times the dose did not show complications.[41] In cattle the use of epidural xylazine has resulted in demyelination of lumbar spinal cord segments and irreversible paralysis in three cows.[12]

Epidural analgesia is commonly practiced in ruminants for replacement of uterine prolapses, calvings, cesareans, and perineal and tail surgery. In the United Kingdom, 99% of food animal practitioners use a variety of drugs by the epidural route including lidocaine (82% of the time); xylazine (50%); and, less frequently, detomidine, morphine, bupivacaine, meperidine, betamethasone, or mepivacaine.[2]

Intrathecal injection at the lumbosacral space is an alternative to epidural injection and is easy to perform in small ruminants. Intrathecal administration of xylazine has been reported in sheep and goats, and intrathecal administration of romifidine and detomidine has been reported in goats and sheep, respectively (see Table 105-2). Intrathecal xylazine (0.1 mg/kg) in goats provided analgesia caudal to the last rib and motor blockade for almost 90 minutes.[44] The duration of analgesia doubled when a lower dose of xylazine (0.05 mg/kg) was combined with 1.25 mg/kg of lidocaine; however, motor blockade also persisted for almost 120 minutes.[44] Intrathecal romifidine (0.05 mg/kg) provided moderate analgesia of the abdomen, perineum, and hind limbs for 60 minutes,[45,46] whereas the combination of romifidine (0.05 mg/kg) with ketamine (2.5 mg/kg) resulted in complete analgesia of the same anatomic areas and severe ataxia.[45] In sheep, detomidine (0.01 mg/kg) or xylazine (0.05 mg/kg) induced analgesia to electrical stimulation of the skin over the pastern of the hind limb; however, xylazine caused longer (2 hours vs. 1 hour) and superior analgesia and more ataxia than detomidine.[47]

Local Anesthetics

Local anesthetics (e.g., lidocaine, bupivacaine, ropivacaine, mepivacaine) block sodium channels and thereby prevent depolarization of nociceptors. Local anesthetics are used to provide anesthesia using regional blocks either by perineural injection, infiltration at nerve endings in the skin, or deposition near the spinal cord (epidural and intrathecal), all of which allow surgical procedures to be performed. More recently, the use of intravenous lidocaine has become common in several large and small animal species to provide systemic analgesia through its inhibitory actions on primary afferents A-delta and C fiber–evoked responses and spinal dorsal horn neurons, preferentially in painful conditions of visceral origin.[48,49] Therefore local anesthetics are similar to opioids in that they act at all levels of the pain pathways and can be administered locally, at the spinal cord, and systemically.

Perineural and skin infiltration are commonly used for local blocks of the structures of the head. Proparacaine drops may be instilled on the cornea for relief of pain during removal of foreign bodies and during diagnostics in the presence of corneal ulcers. Proparacaine should not be used repeatedly if an ulcer is present due to the interference with corneal epithelization. To assist enucleation of the eye, a retrobulbar block or Peterson's eye block can be performed using lidocaine and/or bupivacaine to cause blockade of the oculomotor, trochlear, abducens, and trigeminal branches (ophthalmic, mandibular, and maxillary nerves). Analgesia of the nasal structures can be achieved with an infraorbital block. Anesthesia for dehorning can be achieved by blockade of the cornual branch of the zygomaticotemporal nerve in cattle; however, for complete blockade in adult cattle it is necessary to block the infratrochlear nerve and the cervical nerves that supply the rostral area of the horn base.[50] In goats, it is necessary to block the cornual branch of the zygomaticotemporal nerve and the infratrochlear nerve. Anesthesia of the flank can be achieved by employing a line block; an "L" block; either a proximal or distal paravertebral block of T_{13}, L_1, L_2, and, occasionally, L_3; or epidural block. The duration of most of these blocks is 1 to 3 hours, with lidocaine and mepivacaine having the shorter duration and bupivacaine and ropivacaine having the longest duration due to the lower protein binding of lidocaine and mepivacaine. However, the onset of effect is faster for lidocaine and mepivacaine (5-10 minutes) than for bupivacaine and ropivacaine (10-30 minutes) because of a closer physiologic pH value of the constant of dissociation of lidocaine and mepivacaine. A complete description of these blocks is found elsewhere.[51]

Local anesthetics can cause complete blockade of sensory, motor, and sympathetic nerve fibers. However, bupivacaine and ropivacaine can provide sensory anesthesia with minimal impairment of motor function because of the diminished (dose-related) effect on motor A fibers. The epidural/intrathecal administration of local anesthetics could potentially lead to ataxia and paresis if the drug blocks sufficient motor fibers as it spreads rostrally in the spinal canal. Volume and concentration of the drug are factors that favor the spread within the spinal canal, and the possibility of excessive motor blockade increases as the volume and concentration are increased. Most ruminants tolerate recumbency because of motor blockade; however, to ensure that the patient will remain standing, lower doses can be titrated until the desired effect is achieved.

The epidural administration of low doses of local anesthetics, as is typically used, does not result in cardiorespiratory effects from the systemic effects of the drugs. Lidocaine doses for epidural administration in cattle and small ruminants are usually 0.2 to 0.4 mg/kg (see Table 105-2), whereas the intravenous dose is 2 to 3 mg/kg. In cattle the low-end epidural doses are useful for perineal analgesia in cattle because the injection is given at the coccygeal region, whereas high doses spread to more rostral dermatomes including the caudal abdomen. In small ruminants the spread of the block is also dose dependent; however, the lumbosacral injection favors coverage of more dermatomes than in cattle.

The combination of local anesthetics and opioids has been recommended in several species and the combination of bupivacaine (1.5 mg/kg) and morphine (0.1 mg/kg) has been recommended in goats[14] (see Table 105-2). Bupivacaine has also been used alone (1.8 mg/kg) in goats and resulted in longer-lasting analgesia of the flank for laparotomies than lidocaine, although the onset of analgesia was longer (up to 40 minutes) and goats were unable to stand for at least 11 hours.[52] The advantage of this combination is the relative rapid onset of bupivacaine's effect and the prolonged analgesic effects of morphine. In addition, combining two drugs with different mechanisms of action on pain pathways may result in more profound analgesia.

Local anesthetics have also been used intraarticularly in sheep undergoing stifle surgery. Lidocaine (40 mg) was administered before the start of surgery because of its fast onset of action and bupivacaine (10 mg) after joint closure because of its longer duration of action. The duration of analgesia was 3 to 7 hours.[53] In dogs and humans the intraarticular combination of local anesthetics and morphine has been recommended to provide better pain control than either drug alone.[19,54]

The intravenous use of lidocaine, although presently common in other species, has not been used routinely in ruminants. A recent study in goats demonstrated that as in other species, lidocaine at 2.5 mg/kg loading dose and 0.05 to 0.1 mg/kg/min decreased the inhalant anesthetic requirements (e.g., minimum alveolar concentration) necessary to prevent purposeful movement in response to a noxious stimulus.[55]

Nonsteroidal Antiinflammatory Drugs

This group of drugs was used more frequently than any other analgesics by veterinarians from the United Kingdom[2,5]; however, use by Canadian veterinarians was less frequent.[4]

NSAIDs are commonly used in ruminants for their analgesic effects. The analgesic actions of NSAIDs result mainly through the control of inflammation by inhibiting the production of prostaglandins, an effect that results from blocking the cyclo-oxygenase enzymes (COX). NSAIDs that specifically inhibit the COX-2 enzyme are

Table **105-3**

Nonsteroidal Antiinflammatory Drugs Commonly Used in Ruminants

	Dose (mg/kg)	Route	Duration of Action (day)	Comments
Phenylbutazone	2-6	PO, IV	1	Prohibited in dairy cattle older than 20 mo of age
Flunixin meglumine	1-2	PO, IV	0.5-1	
Ketoprofen	2-3	IV, PO	0.5-1	
Carprofen	0.7	IV	1-2	Sheep
Aspirin	100	PO	0.5	

Modified from Valverde A, Gunkel CI: *J Vet Emerg Crit Care* 15:295, 2005.

preferred over those that inhibit COX-1 because it is important to maintain homeostatic functions of COX-1; however, both enzymes are necessary for homeostasis. Furthermore, even supposedly COX-2 selective NSAIDs have sufficient anti-COX-1 enzyme activity to cause potent inhibition of homeostatic prostaglandins. Regardless, most NSAIDs used in ruminants are nonspecific for COX-2 inhibition. Therefore their potential benefit is lost and caution is advised to not overdose with this group of drugs.

The local antiinflammatory actions of NSAIDs reduce sensitization of nociceptors to noxious and nonnoxious stimuli peripherally. Also, a central antiprostaglandin effect may be present in the spinal cord that may be complementary to activation of descending inhibitory opioidergic and adrenergic mechanisms.[56] Despite their spinal actions and experimental use epidurally and intrathecally,[56] NSAIDs are only used systemically in ruminants, although peripheral and spinal actions should be expected from this route of administration.

The most commonly used NSAIDs in ruminants are phenylbutazone, flunixin, ketoprofen, and aspirin. Dosages and routes of administration of NSAIDs are outlined in Table 105-3. Carprofen and meloxicam have been used for bovine respiratory disease for their antiinflammatory properties, but there is no information on their analgesic effects. Similarly, in sheep the pharmacokinetics of carprofen has been determined but not the analgesic efficacy.[57] Conversely, the use of phenylbutazone is prohibited by the U.S. Food and Drug Administration in dairy cattle 20 months of age or older due to its prolonged half-life and the risk of toxicity from its metabolites in humans.[58]

Several studies have shown the benefits of preemptive use of NSAIDs in ruminants and the benefits of combining NSAIDs with local anesthetic blocks and sedatives. Combining ketoprofen administration with a cornual nerve block and/or xylazine sedation/analgesia alleviated the distress associated with pain in calves undergoing dehorning and disbudding and prevented or reduced the cortisol response.[59,60] In calves younger than 4 months old undergoing castration, ketoprofen and intratesticular lidocaine, but not lidocaine alone, blocked the cortisol response.[61] Therefore combining modalities of treatment may be more appropriate than relying on a single technique or drug.

Ketamine

Ketamine has analgesic properties at subanesthetic doses through its antagonism of the N-methyl-d-aspartate (NMDA) receptor. Such antagonism prevents presynaptic release of the excitatory neurotransmitter glutamate by A delta and C fibers, thereby preventing the relay of nociception from the periphery to the brain and the establishment of hyperalgesic states.[62] The epidural use of ketamine has been reported in cattle, sheep, goats, and buffaloes[36,63-65] (see Table 105-2). The intrathecal use of ketamine in combination with romifidine in goats provided complete analgesia of the tail, perineum, and hind limbs[45] (see Table 105-2).

Although systemic use of ketamine at subanesthetic doses should also be useful for pain management, there appears to be no published report on its use in these species.

A recent study in sheep undergoing orthopedic surgery indicated that epidural ketamine (1 mg/kg, diluted to a total volume of 7-9 ml) injected at the lumbosacral space resulted in less lameness and longer time to the first administration (at 5 hours postoperatively) of rescue analgesia than control sheep (at 3.3 hours).[64] In cattle, three different doses of epidural ketamine (0.5, 1 and 2 mg/kg, diluted to 5, 10, and 20 ml, respectively) injected into the first intercoccygeal space in standing animals caused dose-dependent analgesia for a maximum period of 1 hour. Sedation was not observed, although ataxia was present with the higher doses.[63]

Epidural ketamine (2.5 mg/kg), injected into the lumbosacral space, in goats induced complete abolition of response to perineal pin prick for 5 to 20 minutes, whereas combining ketamine with xylazine (0.05 mg/kg) extended the duration of analgesia for up to 1 hour.[36] Ataxia but no sedation was generally present by 5 minutes and reached maximum effects within 15 minutes for goats receiving ketamine alone, whereas both ataxia (for up to 60 minutes) and sedation (for up to 45 minutes) were observed with the ketamine/xylazine combination.[36]

WITHDRAWAL PERIOD

The withdrawal period is defined as the interval required after dosing for tissue concentrations of a drug or its metabolite to deplete to less than a specific concentration

Table 105-4

Suggested Withdrawal Periods for Analgesic Drugs Used in Ruminants

Drug	Withdrawal Period	Comment
Xylazine	3 days meat	Canada
	14 days meat	UK
	2 days meat	France
	3 days meat	Germany, Switzerland
	4 days meat	New Zealand, FARAD* recommendation for USA for cattle
	5 days meat	FARAD recommendation for USA for sheep and goats
	2 days milk	Canada, UK
	0 days milk	France
	3 days milk	Germany, Switzerland
	1 day milk	New Zealand, FARAD recommendation for USA for cattle
	3 days milk	FARAD recommendation for USA for sheep and goats
Detomidine	3 days meat	FARAD recommendation for USA
	3 days milk	FARAD recommendation for USA
Morphine	Cleared rapidly	No withdrawal time established
Meperidine	2-4 days	No withdrawal time established
Butorphanol	2 days	No withdrawal time established
Fentanyl	2-4 days	Sheep
Ketamine	3 days milk	Switzerland
	1 day meat	Switzerland
	2 days milk	FARAD recommendation for USA
	3 days meat	FARAD recommendation for USA
Lidocaine	1 day milk and meat	FARAD recommendation for USA
Bupivacaine	Cleared rapidly	No withdrawal time established
Phenylbutazone	Not recommended	Prolonged excretion
Flunixin meglumine	3 days milk	FARAD recommendation for USA
	4 days meat	FARAD recommendation for USA
Ketoprofen	1 day milk	FARAD recommendation for USA
	7 days meat	FARAD recommendation for USA
Aspirin	1 day milk	FARAD recommendation for USA
	1 day meat	FARAD recommendation for USA

From data in references 58, 67, 69, 70-72.
*Food Animal Residue Avoidance Databank.

that has been established to be safe for human consumption.[66] For drugs that exhibit a linear, first-order decay, multiplying the half-life of the drug (time required for 50% of the drug to be eliminated from the animal or tissue) by 10 will allow the assumption that 99.9% of the drug has been eliminated[66]; however, it must be ascertained that no metabolites exceed the half-life of the parent drug, that the determined half-life refers to the route of administration used, and that drug-clearance mechanisms are healthy.[67]

Current withdrawal times for analgesic drugs included in this review are shown in Table 105-4. Variability exists among countries; for example, in the United Kingdom lidocaine is prohibited from use in food animals due to the production of the intermediate metabolite 2,6 xylidine. This metabolite has been shown to be carcinogenic and possibly genotoxic in rats.[68] Interestingly, this metabolite also results from xylazine biotransformation. In North America, lidocaine is considered to undergo rapid clearance and achieves low drug concentrations in tissues after local infiltration; it is commonly used clinically.[67]

In conclusion, it is important that practitioners take a more proactive approach toward pain management in ruminants. This should include better methods of pain recognition and prompt instigation of analgesic techniques. Although many practitioners regard acquired experience and discussions with peers as the best source of knowledge about analgesic use, they also agree that lectures, wet laboratories, and review articles in journals are highly rated sources of continuing education on pain management.[4]

References

1. Feinstein B, Langton JN, Jameson RM, Schiller F: Experiments on pain referred from deep somatic tissues, *J Bone Joint Surg* 36-A:981, 1954.
2. Watts SA, Clarke KW: A survey of bovine practitioners attitudes to pain and analgesia in cattle, *Cattle Pract* 8:361, 2000.
3. Stafford KJ, Mellor DJ: *The assessment of pain in cattle: a review, perspectives in agriculture, veterinary science, nutrition and natural resources* (website): www.cababstractsplus.org 1, No. 013. Accessed June 2006.
4. Hewson CJ, Dohoo IR, Lempke KA et al: Canadian veterinarians' use of analgesics in cattle, pigs and horses in 2004 and 2005, *Can Vet J* 48:155-164, 2007.
5. Whay HR, Huxley JN: Pain relief in cattle: a practitioner's perspective, *Cattle Pract* 13:81, 2005.

6. Nolan A, Livingston A, Waterman AE: Investigation of the antinociceptive activity of buprenorphine in sheep, *Br J Anaesth* 92:527, 1987a.

7. Nolan A, Waterman AE, Livingston A: The correlation of the thermal and mechanical antinociceptive activity of pethidine hydrochloride with plasma concentrations of the drug in sheep, *J Vet Pharmacol Ther* 11:94, 1988.

8. Waterman AE, Livingston A, Amin A: Analgesia and respiratory effects of fentanyl in sheep, *J Assoc Vet Anaesth* 17:20, 1990.

9. Waterman AE, Livingston A, Amin A: Analgesic activity and respiratory effects of butorphanol in sheep, *Res Vet Sci* 51:19, 1991a.

10. Waterman AE, Livingston A, Amin A: Further studies on the antinociceptive activity and respiratory effects of buprenorphine in sheep, *J Vet Pharmacol Ther* 14:230, 1991b.

11. Pinheiro-Machado LC, Hurnik JF, Ewing KK: A thermal threshold assay to measure the nociceptive response to morphine sulphate in cattle, *Can J Vet Res* 62:218, 1998.

12. George LW: Pain control in food animals. In Steffey EP, editor: *Recent advances in anesthetic management of large domestic animals. International Veterinary Information Service* (website): www.ivis.org, A0615.1103. Accessed June 2006.

13. Pablo LS: Epidural morphine in goats after hindlimb orthopedic surgery, *Vet Surg* 22:307, 1993.

14. Hendrickson DA, Kruse-Elliot KT, Broadstone RV: A comparison of epidural saline, morphine, and bupivacaine for pain relief after abdominal surgery in goats, *Vet Surg* 25:83, 1996.

15. Wagner AE, Dunlop CI, Turner AS: Experiences with morphine injected into the subarachnoid space in sheep, *Vet Surg* 25:256, 1996.

16. Tang AH, Schoenfeld MJ: Comparison of subcutaneous and spinal subarachnoid injections of morphine and naloxone in analgesic tests in the rat, *Eur J Pharmacol* 52:215, 1978.

17. Nagasaka H, Awad H, Yaksh TL: Peripheral and spinal actions of opioids in the blockade of the autonomic response evoked by compression of the inflamed knee joint, *Anesthesiology* 85:808, 1996.

18. Day TK, Pepper WT, Tobias TA et al: Comparison of intraarticular and epidural morphine for analgesia following stifle arthrotomy in dogs, *Vet Surg* 24:522, 1995.

19. Reuben SS, Sklar J, El-Mansouri M: The preemptive analgesic effect of intraarticular bupivacaine and morphine after ambulatory arthroscopic knee surgery, *Anesth Analg* 92:923, 2001.

20. Sammarco JL, Conzemius MG, Perkowski SZ et al: Postoperative analgesia for stifle surgery: A comparison of intra-articular bupivacaine, morphine, or saline, *Vet Surg* 25:59, 1996.

21. Carroll GL, Hooper RN, Boothe DM et al: Pharmacokinetics of fentanyl after intravenous and transdermal administration in goats, *Am J Vet Res* 60:986, 1999.

22. Bouchenafa O, Livingston A: Autoradiographic localization of alpha-2 adrenoceptor binding sites in the spinal cord of sheep, *Res Vet Sci* 42:382, 1987.

23. Doherty TJ, Pascoe PJ, McDonell WN et al: Cardiopulmonary effects of xylazine and yohimbine in laterally recumbent sheep, *Can J Vet Res* 50:517, 1986.

24. Doherty TJ, Ballinger JA, McDonell WN et al: Antagonism of xylazine induced sedation by idazoxan in calves, *Can J Vet Res* 51:244, 1987.

25. Picavet MT, Gasthuys FM, Laevens HH, Watts SA: Cardiopulmonary effects of combined xylazine-guaiphenesin-ketamine infusion and extradural (inter-coccygeal) lidocaine anaesthesia in calves, *Vet Anaesth Analg* 31:11, 2004.

26. Kästner SB, Kutter AP, von Rechenberg B, Bettschart-Wolfensberger R: Comparison of two pre-anesthetic medetomidine doses in isoflurane anaesthetized sheep, *Vet Anaesth Analg* 33:8, 2006.

27. Celly CS, McDonell WN, Young SS et al: The comparative hypoxaemic effect of four α_2 adrenoceptor agonist (xylazine, romifidine, detomidine and medetomidine) in sheep, *J Vet Pharmacol Ther* 20:464, 1997.

28. Kästner SBR: A$_2$-agonists in sheep: a review, *Vet Anaesth Analg* 33:79, 2006.

29. Jansen CA, Lowe KC, Nathaielsz PW: The effect of xylazine on intrauterine activity, fetal and maternal oxygenation, cardiovascular function and fetal breathing, *Am J Obstet Gynecol* 148:386, 1984.

30. LeBlanc MM, Hubbell JA, Smith HC: The effects of xylazine hydrochloride on intrauterine pressure in the cow, *Theriogenology* 21:681, 1984.

31. Jedruch J, Gajewski Z: The effect of detomidine hydrochloride domosedan on the electrical activity of the uterus in cows, *Acta Vet Scand* 82(suppl):189, 1986.

32. Nolan A, Livingston A, Waterman AE: Antinociceptive actions of intravenous alpha 2-adrenoceptor agonists in sheep, *J Vet Pharmacol Ther* 10:202, 1987b.

33. Grant C, Upton RN: The anti-nociceptive efficacy of low dose intramuscular xylazine in lambs, *Res Vet Sci* 70:47, 2001.

34. St-Jean G, Skarda RT, Muir WW et al: Caudal epidural analgesia induced by xylazine administration in cows, *Am J Vet Res* 51:1232, 1990.

35. Aminkov BY, Hubenov HD: The effect of xylazine epidural anaesthesia on blood gas and acid-base parameters in rams, *Br Vet J* 151:579, 1995.

36. Aithal HP, Amarpal Pratap K et al: Clinical effects of epidurally administered ketamine and xylazine in goats, *Small Rumin Res* 24:55, 1996.

37. Scott PR, Gessert ME: Evaluation of extradural xylazine injection for cesarean operation in ovine dystocia cases, *Vet J* 154:63, 1997.

38. Lin HC, Trachte EA, DeGraves FJ et al: Evaluation of analgesia induced by epidural administration of medetomidine to cows, *Am J Vet Res* 59:162, 1998.

39. Prado ME, Streeter RN, Mandsager RE et al: Pharmacologic effects of epidural versus intramuscular administration of detomidine in cattle, *Am J Vet Res* 60:1242, 1999.

40. Mpanduji DG, Mgasa MN, Bittegeko SB et al: Comparison of xylazine and lidocaine effects for analgesia and cardiopulmonary functions following lumbosacral epidural injection in goats, *Zentralbl Veterinarmed* A46:605, 1999.

41. Mpanduji DG, Bittegeko SBP, Mgasa MN et al: Analgesic, behavioural and cardiopulmonary effects of epidurally injected medetomidine (Domitor) in goats, *J Vet Med A* 47:65, 2000.

42. Chevalier HM, Provost PJ, Karas AZ: Effect of caudal epidural xylazine on intraoperative distress and post-operative pain in Holstein heifers, *Vet Anaesth Analg* 31:1, 2004.

43. Fierheller EE, Caulkett NA, Bailey JV: A romifidine and morphine combination for epidural analgesia of the flank in cattle, *Can Vet J* 45:917, 2004.

44. DeRossi R, Junqueira AL, Beretta MP: Analgesic and systemic effects of xylazine, lidocaine and their combination after subarachnoid administration in goats, *J S Afr Vet Assoc* 76:79, 2005.

45. Aithal HP, Amarpal Kinjavdekar P et al: Analgesic and cardiopulmonary effects of intrathecally administered romifidine or romifidine and ketamine in goats *(Capra hircus)*, *J S Afr Vet Assoc* 72:84, 2001.

46. Amarpal Kinjavdekar P, Aithal HP et al: Analgesic, sedative and haemodynamic effects of spinally administered romifidine in female goats, *J Vet Med A* 49:3, 2002.

47. Haerdi-Landerer MC, Schlegel U, Neiger-Aeschbacher G: The analgesic effects of intrathecal xylazine and detomidine in sheep and their antagonism with systemic atipamezol, *Vet Anaesth Analg* 32:297, 2005.

48. Ness TJ: Intravenous lidocaine inhibits visceral nociceptive reflexes and spinal neurons in the rat, *Anesthesiology* 92:1685, 2000.
49. Ness TJ, Randich A: Which spinal cutaneous nociceptive neurons are inhibited by intravenous lidocaine in the rat? *Reg Anesth Pain Med* 31:248, 2006.
50. Butler WF: Innervation of the horn region in domestic ruminants, *Vet Rec* 80:490, 1967.
51. Skarda RT: Local and regional anesthetic and analgesic techniques. In Thurmon JC, Tranquilli WJ, Benson GJ, editors: *Lumb & Jones' Veterinary Anesthesia*, Baltimore, 1996, Williams & Wilkins.
52. Trim CM: Epidural analgesia with 0.75% bupivacaine for laparotomy in goats, *J Am Vet Med Assoc* 194:1292, 1989.
53. Shafford HL, Hellyer PW, Turner AS: Intra-articular lidocaine plus bupivacaine in sheep undergoing stifle arthrotomy, *Vet Anaesth Analg* 31:20, 2004.
54. Valverde A, Gunkel CI: Pain management in horses and farm animals, *J Vet Emerg Crit Care* 15:295, 2005.
55. Doherty T, Redua MA, Queiroz-Castro P et al: Effect of intravenous lidocaine and ketamine on the minimum alveolar concentration of isoflurane in goats, *Vet Anaesth Analg* 34:125-131, 2007.
56. Lizarraga I, Chambers JP: Involvement of opioidergic and α_2-adrenergic mechanisms in the central analgesic effects of non-steroidal anti-inflammatory drugs in sheep, *Res Vet Sci* 80:194, 2006.
57. Welsh EM, Baxter P, Nolan AM: Pharmacokinetics of carprofen administered intravenously to sheep, *Res Vet Sci* 53:264, 1992.
58. Haskell SRR, Gehring R, Payne MA et al: Update on FARAD food animal drug withholding recommendations, *J Am Vet Med Assoc* 223:1277, 2003.
59. Stafford KJ, Mellor DJ: Dehorning and disbudding distress and its alleviation in calves, *Vet J* 169:337, 2005.
60. Milligan BN, Duffield T, Lissemore K: The utility of ketoprofen for alleviating pain following dehorning in young dairy calves, *Can Vet J* 45:140, 2004.
61. Stafford KJ, Mellor DJ, Todd SE et al: Effects of local anaesthesia or local anaesthesia plus a non-steroidal anti-inflammatory drug on the acute cortisol response of calves to five different methods of castration, *Res Vet Sci* 73:61, 2002.
62. Himmelseher S, Durieux ME: Ketamine for perioperative pain management, *Anesthesiology* 102:211, 2005.
63. Lee I, Yoshiuchi T, Yamagishi N et al: Analgesic effect of caudal epidural ketamine in cattle, *J Vet Sci* 4:261, 2003.
64. Guedes AGP, Pluhar E, Daubs BM et al: Effects of preoperative epidural administration of racemic ketamine for analgesia in sheep undergoing surgery, *Am J Vet Res* 67:222, 2006.
65. Singh V, Amarpal Kinjavdekar P et al: Medetomidine with ketamine and bupivacaine for epidural analgesia in buffaloes, *Vet Res Commun* 29:1, 2005.
66. Riviere JE, Webb AI, Craigmill AL: Primer on estimating withdrawal times after extralabel drug use, *J Am Vet Med Assoc* 213:966, 1998.
67. Papich MG: Drug residue considerations for anesthetics and adjunctive drugs in food-producing animals, *Vet Clin Food Anim* 3:693, 1996.
68. U.S. National Toxicology Program: *Toxicology and carcinogenesis studies of 2,6-xylidine (2,6-dimethylaniline) (CAS No. 87-62-7) in Charles River CD Rats (Feed Studies)*. U.S. National Toxicology Program, Research Triangle Park, NC, NTP Technical Report No 278; NIH Publication No 90-2534, 1990.
69. FARAD: *Homepage* (website): www.farad.org. Accessed June 2006.
70. Craigmill AL, Rangel-Lugo M, Damian P et al: Extralabel use of tranquilizers and general anesthetics, *J Am Vet Med Assoc* 211:302, 1997.
71. Damian P, Craigmill AL, Riviere JE: Extralabel use of nonsteroidal anti-inflammatory drugs, *J Am Vet Med Assoc* 211:860, 1997.
72. Webb AI, Baynes RE, Craigmill AL et al: Drugs approved for small ruminants, *J Am Vet Med Assoc* 15:520, 2004.

SECTION XII

Chemical Restraint, Anesthesia, and Pain Management

Eric J. Abrahamsen

CHAPTER 106

Chemical Restraint in Ruminants

ERIC J. ABRAHAMSEN

Physical restraint is generally required when working with food animal patients. Adding a degree of chemical restraint can make many procedures more pleasant for both practitioner and patient. The enhanced level of patient cooperation improves efficiency, offsetting the modest additional cost of the drugs used.

Chemical restraint techniques used in ruminants range from mild sedation of standing patients to semianesthetized recumbency. When selecting a chemical restraint technique, one should first consider whether the patient must remain standing or recumbent for optimal completion of the procedure. Patient cooperation and systemic analgesia are generally greater with techniques that reliably produce recumbency. Instances in which either situation will facilitate successful completion of the procedure provide more latitude with regard to technique and doses.

Many of the drug combinations used to produce field anesthesia in ruminants are also used in chemical restraint. Drug doses are typically smaller when used in chemical restraint techniques, but the difference between these two applications is, at times, modest. The level of analgesia produced by chemical restraint varies with the technique and doses administered. Analgesia can approach surgical levels in some situations, but local anesthetic blockade should be used whenever feasible to reduce the risk of patient awareness and stress.

SITE SELECTION

Selecting a site that is quiet and free of distractions is important. The sedation produced by alpha$_2$-adrenergic agonists (α_2's) can be overridden by elevated "sympathetic tone" in anxious or unruly patients. This is especially true when a lower dose is administered, which is typically the case when using standing chemical restraint techniques in ruminants.

A flat, even surface that provides good footing should be selected. When chemical restraint is expected to result in recumbency, other factors must also be considered. A "soft" surface will reduce the chance of injury. The site selected should be free of hazards. Large ruminants are more difficult to physically control and require a somewhat larger "safety zone." Ruminants tend to be patient. They typically do not attempt to stand until they are awake and functional. Good footing is the primary requirement for achieving a good recovery. An open grassy area is generally ideal. A stall deeply bedded with shavings can be

used, but the confined space increases risk to personnel involved and may interfere with procedure. Proximity to water, electricity, and vehicle (containing emergency supplies) are also factors to consider when selecting a site.

PATIENT POSITIONING

Ruminants continue to produce a significant amount of saliva while sedated or anesthetized. The degree of protective laryngeal and eye reflexes retained will depend on the chemical restraint technique and drug doses selected. Milder levels of chemical restraint provide greater airway protection. When recumbency is produced, patients should be positioned so that saliva runs out of the mouth rather than pooling back near the larynx whenever possible. For patients in lateral recumbency this can be accomplished simply by placing a pad under the head-neck junction so that the opening of the mouth is below the level of the larynx.

Protecting the airway becomes much more challenging when the patient is placed in dorsal recumbency. Smaller ruminants placed in dorsal recumbency will typically be under the influence of a "potent" chemical restraint protocol. The body of these patients should be elevated using foam pads or some other method with the head resting on the floor or surgery table surface. Importantly, the head must be supported rather than hanging in space to prevent excessive tension on neck structures. The head and neck are rotated to place the opening of the mouth below the larynx to facilitate saliva egress. The short, thick neck of many cattle breeds can make proper orientation difficult to achieve. When the head cannot be positioned to facilitate saliva egress or the procedure is expected to produce a significant amount of blood or other material that could enter the airway, the patient should be intubated.

Positioning large ruminants in dorsal recumbency to facilitate saliva egress in a field setting is extremely difficult. The degree of sedation used determines how these patients are managed. Larger ruminant patients are often cast and physically restrained in dorsal recumbency. Chemical restraint will reduce the level of distress in these patients. Lightly sedated patients are typically able to protect their airway but should be monitored for signs of respiratory distress. Heavy sedation markedly depresses the cough and swallow reflexes, increasing the risk of aspiration. Unfortunately, patients must be fairly obtunded to tolerate intubation. If you suspect a large ruminant patient will require more than light sedation to tolerate restraint in dorsal recumbency, field anesthesia with intubation may be a better choice.

DRUGS USED IN CHEMICAL RESTRAINT

Alpha$_2$-Adrenergic Agonists (α_2's)

Xylazine is the most frequently used drug for sedation in large animals. Ruminants are 10 times more sensitive to xylazine than horses, whereas detomidine is dosed similarly in both species. Ruminants tend to lie down when dosed aggressively with α_2's, whereas horses exhibit increasing levels of ataxia.

The initial demeanor of the patient greatly influences the sedation produced by a given dose of an α_2. The sedative effect of α_2's can be overridden by elevated "sympathetic tone." This results in two characteristic features of α_2 sedation. The sedative effect produced by lower doses of α_2's is not as stable. Calm, quiet patients require smaller doses, whereas anxious or unruly patients require larger doses. This sounds easy, but selecting the incorrect dose may result in working on your knees or getting kicked in them. The ideal dose can be difficult to predict, especially when recumbency is not desired. Experience makes the necessary adjustments easier, but even seasoned practitioners get surprised at times.

Alpha$_2$-adrenergic agonists can be administered intravenously (IV), intramuscularly (IM), or subcutaneously (SQ) and produce a dose-dependent degree of sedation, muscle relaxation, and analgesia. Intravenous administration of α_2's provides a faster onset and more intense level of chemical restraint and analgesia. The fairly rapid onset time can be used to advantage, allowing multiple smaller intravenous doses of an α_2 to be administered in an attempt to titrate the effect to the desired level. Intramuscular administration results in a more gradual onset and provides a longer duration of less intense chemical restraint and analgesia. Intramuscular administration is often used when patient cooperation does not allow intravenous administration or when extended duration is desired. The intramuscular dose is traditionally twice the intravenous dose one would select for the patient based on the desired level of effect and the patient's initial demeanor. Subcutaneous administration results in the most gradual onset, longest duration, and mildest peak effect. Administering the intravenous dose IM or SQ is a method used to produce a degree of sedation with limited risk of recumbency.

Alpha$_2$-adrenergic agonist administration produces dose-dependent side effects. Decreases in gastrointestinal motility and cardiorespiratory function are the most serious. In compromised patients, α_2's should be avoided or used cautiously and should be reversed on completion of the procedure. Even in normal, healthy patients, when large doses of α_2's are administered (especially doses used to produce recumbency), reversal is advisable to minimize the risk of gastrointestinal complications. Xylazine has been reported to increase uterine tone in late gestation.

In tractable ruminants the response to xylazine is fairly predictable. Titrated administration (e.g., initial conservative dose that is supplemented if necessary) minimizes the incidence of unintended recumbency. Extremely anxious or unruly patients require larger doses of xylazine to achieve adequate control. In these patients the administration process often triggers even greater behavior problems, so they should be dosed fairly aggressively at the outset. Intramuscular administration is frequently the only option available in extremely anxious or unruly patients. A calm environment can also help to reduce the dose of xylazine required to calm the patient. Restraint or interaction should be minimized whenever possible until xylazine has produced a reasonable degree of patient control.

Additional information on the use of sedatives is provided in Chapters 107 and 108.

Alpha$_2$-Adrenergic Agonist Reversal

Yohimbine or tolazoline may be used to reverse the effects of α_2's at the end of a procedure to facilitate a quicker recovery and minimize the risks of gastrointestinal complications. Intramuscular administration of the reversal agent is preferred in all but emergency situations because it decreases the risk of central nervous system (CNS) excitement or cardiovascular complications. The shorter duration of action of reversal agents when administered IV can result in resedation in patients where the α_2 was administered IM, especially when larger doses were used. Reversal of α_2's should not be attempted until sufficient time has elapsed to allow any ketamine or Telazol used to resolve (15-30 minutes post-IV and 30-45 minutes post-IM, respectively) to reduce the chances of a rough recovery. The amount of reversal agent used depends on the dose of the α_2 and duration since administration. The recommended emergency intravenous doses for yohimbine (0.125 mg/kg) and tolazoline (2 mg/kg) are typically used as the maximum intramuscular dose and reduced to fit the circumstances. When dosed properly, the effects of reversal should start to become evident about 10 minutes following intramuscular administration. Splitting the reversal dose (using both intravenous and intramuscular routes) can produce a quicker recovery while minimizing the risk of resedation. Response to the small intravenous component will be fairly quick, so the primary intramuscular component should be administered first.

Anesthetic Agents

Ketamine and tiletamine are the injectable anesthetic agents used in large animal practice. Ketamine is by far the most common injectable anesthetic agent used in large animal practice. Tiletamine, a more potent and longer-lasting relative of ketamine, is available only in combination with the benzodiazepine zolazepam as Telazol. Subanesthetic doses of ketamine are also used in chemical restraint techniques. Because of the high cost of Telazol, it is primarily used in large animal practice for capturing intractable patients.

Both ketamine and tiletamine draw on sympathetic nervous system reserve to augment cardiac output and blood pressure. This effect helps counter their direct negative inotropic and vasodilatory effects, as well as the negative cardiovascular effects produced by xylazine. Cardiovascular function in normal healthy patients anesthetized with ketamine-based protocols is good to excellent.

Table **106-1**

Dose Range of Xylazine Expected to Produce Standing Sedation with a Low Incidence of Recumbency

Patient Type	IV*	IM
Quiet dairy breeds	0.0075-0.01 mg/kg	0.015-0.02 mg/kg
Tractable cattle	0.01-0.02 mg/kg	0.02-0.04 mg/kg
Anxious cattle	0.02-0.03 mg/kg	0.04-0.06 mg/kg
Extremely anxious or unruly cattle	0.025-0.05 mg/kg	0.05-0.1 mg/kg

*Administering the IV dose intramuscularly further reduces the possibility of recumbency.
IM, Intramuscular; *IV,* intravenous.

Table **106-2**

Dose Range of Detomidine Expected to Produce Standing Sedation with a Low Incidence of Recumbency*

Patient Type	IV†	IM
Tractable cattle	0.002-0.005 mg/kg	0.006-0.01 mg/kg
Anxious cattle	0.005-0.0075 mg/kg	0.01-0.015 mg/kg
Extremely anxious or unruly cattle	0.01-0.015 mg/kg	0.015-0.02 mg/kg

*Information regarding the use of detomidine in ruminants is limited. The dose ranges provided are estimates and should be adjusted on the basis of experience.
†Administering the IV dose intramuscularly further reduces the possibility of recumbency.
IM, Intramuscular; *IV,* intravenous.

I cannot emphasize enough the need for caution in dosing these seemingly safe drugs in compromised patients in which sympathetic reserve may be severely limited. An apneustic pattern of breathing is often observed in horses following induction with ketamine or Telazol, but is not common in ruminants.

CHEMICAL RESTRAINT TECHNIQUES

Xylazine

Xylazine sedation and its attendant analgesia are useful for facilitating short diagnostic or therapeutic procedures on less cooperative patients. Although patients will generally tolerate mildly uncomfortable stimuli, standing xylazine sedation should not be counted on to provide significant analgesia. Duration of xylazine sedation and analgesia is dose dependent, generally lasting about 30 to 40 minutes following IV administration in standing or laterally recumbent patients. In dorsally recumbent patients the duration of enhanced cooperation provided by IV xylazine may be as short as 20 minutes. Duration is typically doubled with IM administration, though intensity is commensurately reduced (Table 106-1). Clinicians who have tried the "ketamine stun" technique tend to prefer it to pure xylazine chemical restraint.

Xylazine (0.05 mg/kg IV or 0.1 mg/kg IM) will result in recumbency in 50% of tractable cattle. Xylazine (0.1 mg/kg IV or 0.2 mg/kg IM) will result in recumbency in most tractable cattle. Anxious or unruly patients are more resistant and somewhat higher doses of xylazine may be required to produce recumbency. Titrated administration (e.g., initial conservative dose that is supplemented if necessary) minimizes the amount of xylazine administered and, therefore, the degree of adverse side effects produced. Physical methods can also be used to produce recumbency once the patient is sufficiently sedated.

Detomidine

Detomidine is a more potent α_2. Because of increased sensitivity to xylazine, the dose relationship between xylazine and detomidine in ruminants does not reflect this difference (Table 106-2). Detomidine doses used in ruminants are similar to doses used in equine patients. Detomidine produces greater cardiorespiratory depression than xylazine and should not be used to produce recumbent sedation.

Alpha$_2$-Adrenergic Agonist and Opioid

An opioid (butorphanol, morphine) can be administered to augment the level of systemic analgesia in ruminants sedated with an α_2. Butorphanol (0.05-0.1 mg/kg IV or IM in smaller ruminants, 0.02-0.05 mg/kg IV or IM in larger ruminants) or morphine (0.05-0.1 mg/kg IV or IM) can be administered with the initial dose of α_2 or added in situations when patient cooperation needs improvement. The α_2 dose can typically be reduced somewhat when used in conjunction with an opioid.

Additional information on opioid use in ruminants is provided in Chapter 109, as well as chapters in the therapeutics section of this book.

"Ketamine Stun"

Ketamine is a dissociative anesthetic commonly used in veterinary medicine. Ketamine possesses potent analgesic effects when administered at subanesthetic doses. Adding a small dose of ketamine to more traditional chemical restraint combinations greatly enhances the level of patient cooperation. This technique is called the *ketamine stun* (or *stun*) because of the stunned effect it produces in patients when administered IV at doses that produce recumbency. These patients appear to be awake but seem oblivious to their surroundings and procedures being performed. The intravenous effect is quite brief (≈15 minutes) and patients typically stand and appear fairly normal at that time. I initially referred to this state as *semianesthetized,* but perhaps *chemical hypnosis* is more appropriate. The ketamine stun technique makes treating camelid patients, which are frequently uncooperative, much more pleasant.[1] Because of the success in camelid patients the stun technique was adjusted for use in ruminants (less xylazine) and proved to be just as useful. Dosing must be more conservative when using the ketamine stun technique in standing patients. This limits the degree of systemic analgesia relative to what we can achieve in recumbent patients but still provides improved patient cooperation when compared with more traditional methods of standing chemical restraint in both ruminants and horses.

The stun is basically the addition of a small dose of ketamine to any chemical restraint technique. In ruminants and camelid patients a combination of xylazine, butorphanol, and ketamine is typically used. In equine patients I generally use detomidine, morphine, and ketamine. I have used morphine (0.05-0.06 mg/kg) in ruminant stuns. Morphine is much cheaper than butorphanol. In standing adult cattle stuns a similar level of cooperation is achieved with either opioid, but patients appear less obtunded when morphine is used. Some practitioners may find the obtunded appearance useful, since it allows them to follow the decay over time in the level of chemical restraint. Deterioration in the level of patient cooperation can also be used to determine when supplemental drug administration may be required. Morphine is used to provide analgesic relief in food animal patients. More information on the use of morphine in ruminants can be found in Chapter 109.

Alpha$_2$-adrenergic agonists possess potent sedative and analgesic effects. Opioids are typically thought of as analgesic drugs, but they possess CNS effects that, when combined with a tranquilizer or sedative, produce a greater level of mental depression. Ketamine is an N-methyl-D-aspartate (NMDA) receptor antagonist that possesses potent analgesic effects at subanesthetic doses. Ketamine was initially included in the stun technique for its analgesic properties, but it likely contributes to the mental aspects of the enhanced cooperation exhibited by patients under the influence of the ketamine stun technique. By combining drugs, clinicians can use smaller doses of the individual components while still achieving the desired level of effect.

Ketamine stun techniques can be divided into two broad categories, standing and recumbent. The standing ketamine stun is used primarily in large ruminants and horses. The recumbent ketamine stun is used primarily in small ruminants, camelids, and foals. The level of effect achieved is determined by three variables (dose, route of administration, initial demeanor of the patient). The stun cocktail can be administered IV, IM, or SQ depending on the systemic analgesia, patient cooperation, and duration desired (Table 106-3).

Aggressive dosing increases the level of systemic analgesia and patient cooperation but also increases duration of recumbency or the risk of unintended recumbency. Xylazine is the most variable component of the stun combination. Initial patient demeanor plays a large role in the effect obtained from xylazine administration. Response to xylazine in tractable ruminants is fairly predictable. To minimize the incidence of unintended recumbency, a titrated approach (e.g., initial conservative dose that is supplemented if necessary) should be used. Extremely anxious or unruly patients require larger doses of xylazine to achieve adequate control. In these patients the administration process often triggers even greater behavior problems, so they should be dosed fairly aggressively at the outset.

Table 106-3

Route of Administration Determines the Relative Impact of the Ketamine Stun Technique

Parameter	Relative Ranking
Intensity (analgesia/cooperation)	IV >> IM > SQ
Onset	IV >> IM > SQ
Duration of effect	SQ > IM >> IV

IM, Intramuscular; *IV*, intravenous; *SQ*, subcutaneous.

Many permutations are possible when using the ketamine stun. Several years of experimentation in many different species have provided a great deal of insight into the potential of this technique but have not produced a definitive combination for all situations in each species. The following examples are provided as a guide and practitioners are encouraged to experiment with adjustments in doses. I thank Dr. David Anderson, who has used the ketamine stun technique extensively in food animal patients at Kansas State University, for his support during the development of the technique and his contributions to this section.

Clinical application of the ketamine stun in food animal patients can be divided into four basic categories.

Intravenous Recumbent Stun

The intravenous recumbent stun is used for short procedures or procedures requiring a high level of systemic analgesia and patient cooperation.

A combination of xylazine (0.025-0.05 mg/kg), butorphanol (0.05-0.1 mg/kg), and ketamine (0.3-0.5 mg/kg) is administered IV. Onset is approximately 1 minute. Patients gracefully become recumbent. Patients appear to be "awake" but seem oblivious to surroundings and procedure being performed. Mild random head or limb motion is not unusual, but purposeful movement and/or vocalization are signs of an inadequate stun level and additional drug should be administered. Half of the initial ketamine dose should be administered IV and is often effective. If, after allowing 60 to 90 seconds for onset, this additional half dose of ketamine fails to produce the desired level of analgesia, a second half dose of ketamine along with half of the initial dose of xylazine should be administered IV. The level of systemic analgesia produced varies depending on the doses administered but tends to be fairly intense. Surgical levels of analgesia have been achieved with this technique, but the use of local anesthetic blockade should be used whenever feasible to reduce the risk of patient awareness and stress. Duration of the stun effect is approximately 15 minutes and patients typically are able to stand and walk immediately or shortly after this point. The intravenous recumbent stun is designed for short procedures. The clinician should plan ahead and work quickly. Supplemental doses of ketamine and/or xylazine can be administered to extend duration, but this technique is not intended for procedures that are expected to last significantly beyond the 15- to 25-minute range. The degree of extension is relative to the amount of supplemental drug administered.

The recumbent intravenous stun has proved useful for facilitating a wide variety of short procedures in camelids and small ruminants.

Intramuscular or Subcutaneous Recumbent Stun

The intramuscular or subcutaneous recumbent stun is used for procedures requiring a longer duration of chemical restraint. The level of systemic analgesia is not as intense and local anesthetic blockade should be used to reduce the risk of patient awareness and stress. Umbilical hernia repair is an example of the procedures performed using this technique. This approach is also useful for improving cooperation in patients that have gone down before or during a surgical procedure.

A combination of butorphanol (0.025 mg/kg), xylazine (0.05 mg/kg), and ketamine (0.1 mg/kg) is administered IM or SQ. Subcutaneous administration is preferred because it provides a slightly longer duration of effect. Onset time is approximately 3 to 10 minutes. Patients are obtunded enough to require (and tolerate) intubation when placed in dorsal recumbency. Information on intubating and positioning patients to promote saliva egress is provided in Chapter 108. Duration of effect with SQ administration is approximately 45 minutes. Patients should be ambulatory within 30 minutes following this point.

The level of systemic analgesia produced by the intramuscular or subcutaneous recumbent stun is not as intense, but this approach does provide an enhanced level of patient cooperation that can make procedures much more pleasant for both patient and clinician.

Intravenous Standing Stun

The intravenous standing stun is typically used to provide a transient improvement in patient cooperation. Small intravenous boluses of ketamine have also been used to provide short periods of enhanced analgesia in equine colic patients.[2] Xylazine (0.02-0.0275 mg/kg), butorphanol (0.02-0.1 mg/kg; see later), and ketamine (0.05-0.1 mg/kg) can be administered individually or as a combination.

An example of the effectiveness of the intravenous standing stun technique is a 725- to 775-kg Charolais bull that was run into the chute for examination of a possible penile injury. He was extremely agitated and kept banging around inside the chute despite being left alone. Examination was impossible and patient injury was a valid concern. To calm him down, I administered 20 mg of IV xylazine (0.0275 mg/kg). This made him stand still when left alone, but he would not tolerate attempts to examine him. I then administered 40 mg of ketamine IV (0.055 mg/kg). The ketamine made him extremely cooperative, but the chute hampered full examination. A decision to place him on the tilt table was made. He was very compliant during the tabling process and subsequent examination. Intravenous xylazine boluses typically last approximately 15 minutes, though patients may remain more cooperative beyond this point when using the stun technique.

Small doses of intravenous ketamine can markedly improve the degree of patient cooperation in standing chemical restraint. Butorphanol (0.05-0.1 mg/kg IV or IM in smaller ruminants, 0.02-0.05 mg/kg IV or IM in larger ruminants) or morphine (0.05-0.1 mg/kg IV or IM) can be added to augment the level of analgesia and patient control.

Intramuscular or Subcutaneous Standing Stun

"5-10-20 Technique"
The intramuscular or subcutaneous standing stun is used for most standing procedures in ruminant patients. The level of systemic analgesia is limited and local anesthetic blockade should be used to reduce the risk of patient awareness and stress. Standing flank laparotomy is an example of the procedures performed using this technique.

A combination of butorphanol (0.01 mg/kg), xylazine (0.02 mg/kg), and ketamine (0.04 mg/kg) is administered IM or SQ. In a 500-kg cow this equates to butorphanol (5 mg), xylazine (10 mg), and ketamine (20 mg). For a 680-kg patient the doses are 7 mg butorphanol, 15 mg xylazine, and 25 mg ketamine.

The 5-10-20 combination has been used in student junior surgery laboratories at Kansas State to provide chemical restraint for standing cesarean sections in cattle. Patient weights varied from 340 to 660 kg, but no adjustments were made in the combination administered. The initial dose of 5-10-20 has not resulted in recumbency. Subcutaneous administration is preferred to minimize the risk of recumbency. In unruly cows intramuscular administration provides better patient control. Onset is 5 to 10 minutes with subcutaneous administration. Cows stood quietly during the cesarean sections (many were ill mannered before the ketamine stun). Duration of effect is approximately 60 to 90 minutes. Additional xylazine and ketamine can be administered SQ to extend the duration of chemical restraint. Recumbency has occasionally occurred with readministration of 50% of all three components. Current recommendation for supplemental drug administration is 25% to 50% of the initial xylazine and ketamine doses (0-2.5-5) and (0-5-10), respectively, depending on the degree of cooperation and time required to complete the procedure.

A similar approach (10-20-40 technique) has been used successfully in adult bulls. Preputial surgery (with a local anesthetic block) is an example of the procedures performed using this technique.

The intramuscular/subcutaneous standing stun is a simple method for improving the quality of standing procedures for both patient and clinician.

Intramuscular Xylazine—Ketamine

A combination of xylazine (0.05-0.1 mg/kg IM) and ketamine (2 mg/kg IM) is administered. This combination can be useful for subduing combative patients. It will generally produce recumbency, though extremely unruly patients may not go down in a timely fashion without some physical assistance. The degree of chemical restraint and systemic analgesia achieved with this technique varies markedly. Patients typically tolerate physical manipulation and mildly painful procedures but respond to more intense levels of stimulation. Additional intravenous ketamine, Double Drip, or Ruminant Triple Drip can be administered to enhance the level of patient cooperation and analgesia, if required. Reversal of xylazine should not be attempted until sufficient time has elapsed to allow the ketamine anesthesia to be resolved (30-40 minutes postintramuscular and 15-20 minutes postintravenous administration).

Intravenous Xylazine—Ketamine

Xylazine (0.025-0.03 mg/kg IV) is administered first. When marked sedation is evident or patient becomes recumbent ketamine (1 mg/kg IV) is administered. The addition of the ketamine markedly augments the level of analgesia, though it varies somewhat from patient to patient. This combination may provide a brief period (5-10 minutes) of surgical analgesia. A half dose of ketamine IV can be used to extend duration an additional 5 to 7 minutes.

Telazol-Ketamine-Xylazine

Telazol-ketamine-xylazine (TKX-Ru) is a modification of porcine TKX (TKX-P). TKX-Ru is used for capturing intractable ruminant patients and large exotic hoofstock. TKX-Ru is created by reconstituting a 500-mg vial of Telazol with 250 mg of ketamine (2.5 ml) and 100 mg of large animal xylazine (1 ml). As a result of the space occupied by the Telazol powder, the final volume is 4 ml. TKX-Ru is administered using a pole syringe or dart gun. The dosing protocol for TKX-Ru is still evolving. Current recommendations are 1.25 to 1.5 ml/110-115 kg for smaller ruminant patients and 1 ml/110-115 kg for larger ruminant patients. Patients should become recumbent and compliant approximately 5 (ideal) to 10 minutes following intramuscular administration. Onset significantly less than 5 minutes is indicative of an excessive dose or accidental intravenous administration. If onset has not occurred by 20 minutes, additional TKX-Ru (one quarter to half of the original dose, depending on the urgency of the situation and health of the patient) can be administered. The degree and duration of chemical restraint and analgesia varies markedly from patient to patient. Intravenous administration of Double Drip or Ruminant Triple Drip can be used to enhance and/or extend the systemic analgesia and patient cooperation produced by TKX-Ru.

Patients are typically awake and sternal by 40 to 60 minutes post-TKX-Ru administration. Due to the level of residual sedation, patients typically remain sternal for an additional 20 to 40 minutes (depending on demeanor and level of environmental stimulation) before attempting to stand. Recovery is generally smooth. Once the patient is awake and sternal xylazine can be reversed to speed the recovery process, though recovery quality may be reduced somewhat. Letting xylazine resolve on its own generally makes transporting unruly patients smoother.

TKX-Ru is fairly expensive. Leftover TKX-Ru can be frozen to preserve its function for up to 6 months.

Chemical Restraint Constant Rate Infusion

The level of patient cooperation and analgesia produced by bolus administration of intravenous drugs decays over time. For longer standing procedures in horses, I have been using a constant rate infusion (CRI) technique to deliver a steady state of chemical restraint and systemic analgesia.

This approach has proven extremely useful in equine patients. I believe a similar approach could work in ruminant patients, though I have not tried it yet. The drugs used in the equine chemical restraint CRI (typically detomidine, ketamine, and an opioid) are all used in various chemical restraint techniques in ruminants. Infusions containing ketamine and an opioid (butorphanol or morphine) have been used in managing severe pain in ruminant and camelid patients. The infusion rates of ketamine and the opioid in the ruminant pain CRI (Trifusion) are the same as those used in the equine standing chemical restraint CRI. Detomidine is the most commonly used sedative in the equine chemical restraint CRI technique. Ruminants are 10 times more sensitive to xylazine than horses, but detomidine is dosed similarly in both species. Because of ruminants' predilection for recumbency, the loading dose and infusion rate for detomidine (or xylazine) may need to be adjusted to adapt this technique to ruminant patients.

Practitioners interested in exploring this approach can find detailed information on the creation and delivery of standing CRI combinations in the following section written for equine presentations. Additional information on the creation and delivery of CRI combinations can be found in proceedings' notes on pain management and chemical restraint talks.[3-6] Greater detail on the ruminant pain CRI (Trifusion) can be found in the Chapter 109.

EQUINE STANDING CONSTANT RATE INFUSION TECHNIQUE

The standing chemical restraint CRI I have the most experience with is detomidine-morphine-ketamine. I have tried acepromazine-morphine-ketamine and detomidine-butorphanol-ketamine a couple of times each with good results. The presence of ketamine increases the level of analgesia provided and dissipates quickly once infusion is discontinued.

A CRI technique may seem complicated but is much easier than it appears. Using a stock solution with adjustments in delivery rate made to accommodate variations in patient size and/or alter the level of chemical restraint provided makes this technique much easier to apply. This simplified approach provides familiarity with the fundamentals behind the creation and delivery of drug mixtures by continuous infusion, allowing further exploration.

A stock solution is created for the prototypical 450-kg horse. The "450-kg base rate" of infusion is adjusted to patient size using ratios ("patient base rate" for a 337-kg horse is 75% or 0.75 of the "450-kg base rate"). The "patient base rate" determined in this manner can be further adjusted to alter the level of chemical restraint provided. An endless number of concentration and infusion rate combinations are possible. Selecting a rate of infusion first and then determining the appropriate concentrations for the drug(s) to be infused seems more intuitive, especially when multiple drugs are involved. An inverse relationship exists between infusion rate and drug concentration in the mixture. As the selected "450-kg base rate" of infusion decreases, the concentration of the stock solution must increase to maintain the same delivery of drug(s). How you intend to control the rate of infusion is one factor in solving the rate/concentration dilemma.

Stock solutions that are highly concentrated require precise control of infusion rate, necessitating the use of an infusion pump* or a flow control device such as a Dial-A-Flow.† Waste is more likely when using highly concentrated stock solutions unless small volumes are prepared (when mixed and stored in an aseptic fashion, chemical restraint CRI solutions can generally be safely stored for up to 2 weeks). Partially emptying a larger bag of fluids (NaCl is preferred, but lactated Ringer's seems to work) can be used to create smaller volumes of more concentrated stock solution.

Using an infusion pump or flow control device such as the Dial-A-Flow makes setting and adjusting the infusion rate much easier. The Heska Vet/IV 2.2 is a compact, rechargeable unit that is easy to use. Clients can be easily guided through changing the infusion rate using either of these devices, allowing the clinician to remain sterile. A solution administration set can be used to accurately control the infusion rate in certain ranges of concentration. The rapid drip rate required for very dilute solutions is difficult to count. The farther drip rate falls below one drop per second, the more time it takes to accurately set the infusion rate, making very concentrated solutions difficult to manage. A drip rate of one drop per second is the easiest to accurately set quickly using a solution administration set. This is the drip rate I prefer when creating infusion mixtures. Unfortunately, the drug concentrations required when using this drip rate in standing chemical restraint techniques will increase the likelihood of wastage if a large volume is mixed in practices not using this approach regularly. When using the CRI technique for standing chemical restraint at other equine hospitals, I frequently use two or three drops per second for the "450-kg base rate," which allows me to use the readily available liter bags of fluids without much waste. Drip rates above this level become increasingly difficult to count. Counting the number of drops per 10 seconds helps set the infusion rate more accurately when using solution administrations set to control delivery rate. The final determinant in selecting a "450-kg base rate" of infusion will be the expected duration of the procedure, plus a reserve to cover the unexpected. Selecting "1 hour" is probably the best choice when creating a stock 450-kg solution for standing chemical restraint. Volume mixed can easily be adjusted to fit the circumstances.

Sample protocol: "1 hour" infusion for a 450-kg patient using a 1-L bag of fluids
1000 ml/hr = 16.67 ml/min = 0.28 ml/sec. Drip sets come in 10, 15, and 60 drops/ml, with 10 being the most commonly used in equine practice.
(0.28 ml/sec)/10 drops/ml (invert and multiply) = 2.8 drops/sec

Rounding this value to 3 drops/sec makes adjustments in drip rate a little more intuitive. We must then determine the actual volume infused over time. Using a 10 drop/ml drip set, 3 drops/sec = 180 drops/min = 18 ml/min = 1080 ml/hr. The 1-L mixture will provide slightly less than 1 hour of coverage at the "450-kg base rate" of infusion.

The next step is to apply the drug delivery rates of the technique selected (in this example, detomidine-morphine-ketamine). The values provided in the recipe for this technique follow:

detomidine (0.022 mg/kg/hr) × 450 kg = 10 mg/hr
morphine (0.025-0.05 mg/kg/hr) × 450 kg = 11.25 mg/hr
ketamine (0.6 mg/kg/hr) × 450 kg = 270 mg/hr

We have now determined that 10 mg of detomidine, 11.25 mg of morphine, and 270 mg of ketamine must be added to 1080 ml to create the desired concentrations. Because only 1000 ml are in the bag of fluids, clinicians need to do some quick math to determine how much of each drug must be added. Yes, for those readers thinking hard, simply transferring 80 ml from another bag to create the 1080 ml volume (or solving the solution using the 2.8 drops/sec rate) would work, but the following conversion is quite simple:

10 mg/1080 ml = 0.009 mg/ml × 1000 ml = 9 mg of detomidine
11.25 mg/1080 ml = 0.01 mg/ml × 1000 ml = 10 mg of morphine
270 mg/1080 ml = 0.25 mg/ml × 1000 ml = 250 mg of ketamine

The drugs are injected into the liter bag of fluids (label appropriately) and a solution administration set is then inserted. Appropriate loading doses of detomidine and morphine should be administered before initiating the CRI.

This is just one of an endless number of solutions possible. Had a different "450-kg base rate" of infusion been selected, different values would have resulted. The advantage of this particular solution is that it satisfies many of the qualities desired when using the CRI technique. It uses the widely available liter bag of fluids, possesses a drip rate that allows reasonable control using a solution administration set, drug cost per bag is not excessive, and waste should be limited. The rate of infusion in this example far exceeds the 5- to 250-ml/hr range of the Dial-A-Flow.

The values obtained in this sample can be used to create other infusion combinations.

Doubling the drug amounts and still using a 1000-ml bag, the "450-kg base rate" of infusion decreases to 540 ml/hr and the mixture lasts nearly 2 hours. This rate of infusion still exceeds the capabilities of the Dial-A-Flow, but the drip rate (1.5 drops/sec, or 15 drops/10 sec) is easy to set with a solution administration set.

Doubling the drug amounts and switching to a 500-ml bag, the "450-kg base rate" of infusion rate decreases to 270 ml/hr and mixture lasts nearly 2 hours. This rate of infusion is just above the 250-ml/hr upper limit of the Dial-A-Flow and the drip rate (0.75 drops/sec, or 7.5 drops/10 sec) is close to the ideal rate of one drop per second.

Doubling the drug amounts and switching to a 250-ml bag, the "450-kg base rate" of infusion decreases to

---

*Heska Vet/IV 2.2, Heska Corporation, Loveland, Colo (made for the veterinary market, many other models of infusion pumps are available including used human units).
†Dial-A-Flow, Hospira Worldwide, Inc, Lake Forest, Ill (other manufacturers make similar products and prices vary).

135 ml/hr and the mixture lasts nearly 2 hours. This rate of infusion is well within the capability of the Dial-A-Flow, which is fortunate because the drip rate (0.375 drops/sec, or 3.75 drops/10 sec)* is too low for easy control with the solution administration set.

Additional information on the creation and delivery of CRI mixtures is provided in Chapter 109.

Detomidine-Morphine-Ketamine

The patient is sedated with detomidine (0.011-0.022 mg/kg IV, or 5-10 mg/450 kg) depending on its demeanor, with the higher dose generally providing a superior result. A loading dose of morphine (0.1-0.15 mg/kg IV, or 45-60 mg/450 kg) is then administered. Because of the higher loading dose of detomidine, I *do not* generally administer a loading dose of ketamine (0.22 mg/kg IV, or 100 mg/450 kg) when using the CRI technique. Starting the CRI early in the preparation phase allows adequate time for the ketamine levels to gradually build and begin exerting their analgesic effect. A CRI of detomidine (0.022 mg/kg/hr), morphine (0.025-0.05 mg/kg/hr), and ketamine (0.6 mg/kg/hr) is started and maintained throughout the procedure. The amount of morphine included in the CRI mixture depends on the level of noxious stimulation anticipated from the procedure. I have found that the lower dose of morphine (0.025 mg/kg/hr) infusion is sufficient for many procedures. A supplemental bolus can be administered and/or the bag can be spiked with additional morphine if the level of analgesic support is insufficient. In some instances where infusion time is prolonged, small doses of detomidine (0.0022-0.0044 mg/kg IV, or 1-2 mg/450 kg) and/or morphine (0.0167-0.034 mg/kg IV, or 7.5-15 mg/450 kg) have been required to fine-tune the level of patient analgesia or cooperation. Adjustments above (up to 1.3×) and below the "patient's base rate" of delivery can be made to alter the level of sedation and analgesia. Prolonged use of infusion rates above the "patient base rate" may produce weakness or ataxia in some patients. Response to reductions in infusion rate is fairly quick. Response to increases in infusion rate takes longer. A small top-up bolus of detomidine (sedation) or morphine (analgesia) can be used to shorten response time. Infusion rate should be reduced or temporarily discontinued if weakness or instability occurs during the procedure. The profound level of chemical restraint produced by the CRI resolves fairly quickly once the infusion is discontinued. Though somewhat ataxic, patients are typically walked back to their stall within minutes of completing the procedure. A residual level of sedation remains and gradually diminishes in 1 to 2 hours. I have used the CRI technique for a variety of standing procedures (e.g., laparoscopy, enucleations, sinus flaps) with good results.

Acepromazine-Morphine-Ketamine

Substituting acepromazine (0.055-0.088 mg/kg IV, or 25-40 mg/450 kg) tranquilization for the detomidine sedation in the previously mentioned combination can be used in patients when postural stability of the patient is more critical. A somewhat higher loading dose of morphine (0.1-0.2 mg/kg IV, or 45-90 mg/450 kg) can be used to replace the analgesia that would be provided by detomidine. I have found lower doses of morphine (0.1-0.15 mg/kg IV, or 45-60 mg/450 kg) are sufficient for many procedures. Delivery of morphine and ketamine in the CRI mixture remains as earlier. I have not included acepromazine in the infusion mix when using this combination because of its long duration of effect following intravenous bolus administration. Supplemental acepromazine has not been required in the small number of cases in which I have used this combination. If exceptionally long procedures are anticipated, acepromazine (1-2 mg/450 kg/hr IV) could be added to the infusion to help stabilize its effect.

Detomidine-Butorphanol-Ketamine

Butorphanol (0.011-0.016 mg/kg IV or 5-7 mg/450 kg) can be substituted in the standing chemical restraint CRI in situations when morphine is not available. Butorphanol (0.022 mg/Kg/hr) is substituted for the morphine in the previously mentioned mixture. Delivery of detomidine and ketamine in the CRI mixture remains as mentioned earlier. Supplements of butorphanol (0.005-0.007 mg/kg IV, or 2-3 mg/450 kg) and/or detomidine (0.0022-0.0044 mg/kg IV, or 1-2 mg/450 kg) may be required to fine-tune the level of patient analgesia or cooperation in some instances where infusion time is prolonged.

References

1. Abrahamsen EJ: *Sedation/chemical restraint/anesthesia.* Proceedings of the 2004, 2006, and 2008 International Camelid Health Conference for Veterinarians, Columbus, Ohio.
2. Abrahamsen EJ: *How to medicate a horse with colic before referral.* Proceedings of the 2005 British Equine Veterinary Association (BEVA) Congress, Harrogate, England, pp 45-46.
3. Abrahamsen EJ: *Constant rate infusion for standing surgery restraint and analgesia.* Proceedings of the 2007 BEVA Congress, Edinburgh, Scotland, pp 51-53.
4. Abrahamsen EJ: *Effective pain management in the acute stage of laminitis.* Proceedings of the 2007 BEVA Congress, Edinburgh, Scotland, pp 211-212.
5. Abrahamsen EJ: *Manage acute pain in laminitis.* Proceedings of the 2005 BEVA Congress, Harrogate, England, pp 195-196.
6. Abrahamsen EJ: Equine pain management. Proceedings of the 2005 BEVA Congress, Harrogate, England, pp 241-242.

*Drip rate: drops/sec = (ml/hr × 10 drops/ml)/3600 sec/hr (invert and multiply).

CHAPTER 107

Ruminant Field Anesthesia

ERIC J. ABRAHAMSEN

Ruminants can be safely anesthetized in a field setting. The higher level of analgesia provided by anesthesia eliminates the need for local anesthetic blockade. This can prove useful when a procedure is expected to produce a substantial level of pain and/or local anesthetic blockade is not feasible. Certain aspects of anesthesia place the patient at greater risk than chemical restraint techniques. Knowledge and vigilance reduce the additional risks associated with anesthesia.

PREANESTHETIC CONSIDERATIONS

Physical Examination

A brief physical examination should be performed. This should include an overall assessment of the patient's health status, auscultation of the cardiopulmonary systems, and evaluation of locomotor function. This helps determine whether the patient is a suitable candidate for field anesthesia and perhaps reduce liability should anesthetic complications occur.

Site Selection

A flat, even surface that provides good footing should be selected. The surface should be "soft," to help protect against injury during induction and recovery. The site selected should be free of hazards in all directions. Large ruminants are more difficult to physically control and require a somewhat larger "safety zone." Ruminants tend to be patient during recovery from anesthesia. They typically do not attempt to stand until they are awake and functional. Good footing is the primary requirement for achieving a good recovery. An open grassy area is generally ideal. A stall deeply bedded with shavings can be used, but the confined space increases risk to personnel involved and may interfere with procedure. Proximity to water, electricity, and vehicle (containing emergency supplies) are also factors to consider when selecting a site. A calm environment reduces patient anxiety and is always desirable.

Intravenous Catheters Are "Expensive" and Time Consuming—Are They Really Necessary?

A catheter should be placed before anesthesia in ruminant patients. The jugular vein is the most commonly used site for intravenous (IV) catheter placement. The thicker skin of ruminants makes catheter placement more difficult and accidental placement in the carotid artery has occurred. A 14-gauge, 5.5-inch catheter is used in most ruminant

patients. An 18-gauge, 2-inch catheter is sufficient for lambs and kids. The catheter should be secured to the neck with suture and/or bandage. The catheter should always be checked before anesthetic induction to ensure it is still functional. The veins on the external surface of the ear have been used as an alternative site for venous access in ruminant patients. An 18- or 20-gauge catheter should be used and secured with a combination of super glue and tape. These smaller catheters do not provide the flow rate of the 14-gauge catheter, but work well otherwise.

Endotracheal Intubation

Ruminants continue to produce a significant amount of saliva while anesthetized. The field anesthesia techniques covered in this chapter tend to leave a degree of laryngeal and eye reflexes in place, but they should not be counted on to protect the airway. Ruminants anesthetized in a field setting should be positioned so that saliva runs out of the mouth rather than pooling back near the larynx. For patients in lateral recumbency, this can be accomplished simply by placing a pad under the head-neck junction so that the opening of the mouth is below the level of the larynx.

Protecting the airway becomes much more challenging when the patient is placed in dorsal recumbency. Smaller ruminants placed in dorsal recumbency typically are under the influence of a "potent" chemical restraint protocol. The body of these patients should be elevated using foam pads or some other method with the head resting on the floor or surgery table surface. Importantly, the head must be supported rather than hanging in space to prevent excessive tension on neck structures. The head and neck are rotated to place the opening of the mouth below the larynx to facilitate saliva egress. The short, thick neck of many cattle breeds can make proper orientation difficult to achieve. When the head cannot be positioned to facilitate saliva egress or the procedure is expected to produce a significant amount of blood or other material that could enter the airway, the patient should be intubated. Larger ruminant patients are difficult to move, let alone lift while anesthetized and proper dorsal positioning is difficult to obtain in the field setting.

Many practitioners carry a selection of smaller endotracheal tubes and an Ambu bag for resuscitating newborn patients. The silicone endotracheal tubes used in larger ruminants are expensive (Bivona Air-Cuff Standard Silicone Endotracheal Tubes with Murphy Eye and Connector [Smiths Medical]).

Practitioners planning to anesthetize larger ruminant patients in dorsal recumbency should add a small selection of larger endotracheal tubes to the equipment in their vehicle. A compromise might be to add 12-, 16-, and 22-mm endotracheal tubes, which provides an adequate airway for a wide range of patient size. Patients weighing more than 680 kg experience increased work of breathing with a 22-mm endotracheal tube. Patients should be extubated with the cuff inflated in sternal recumbency to reduce risk of aspiration.

A brief period of apnea immediately following anesthetic induction with thiopental is fairly common. The central nervous system (CNS) depression produced by the thiopental bolus elevates the respiratory set point (the CO_2 level that initiates ventilation). The P_aCO_2 increases during the period of apnea, eventually reaching the new set point, and spontaneous ventilation resumes. Anesthetic induction with ketamine does not significantly alter the respiratory set point value and postinduction apnea is uncommon. Ketamine does affect the respiratory center. Irregular (apneustic) breathing is fairly common immediately following anesthetic induction with ketamine or Telazol in equine patients, though it is less common in ruminants. Apneustic breathing does not generally last long and is of little consequence in normal healthy patients unless uptake of inhalation anesthetics is involved. A 160 L/min demand valve (JDM-5041, JD Medical, Phoenix, Ariz.) and portable oxygen supply (tank and pressure regulator) are required to treat prolonged apnea. There is no substitute for this equipment on the rare occasions it might be required, but justification of the expense and space required varies from practice to practice. This equipment should be standard in all large animal clinics where anesthesia is regularly performed.

Oxygen Delivery, Muscle and Nerve Protection

Oxygen supplementation is not generally required during short-term field anesthesia in ruminants. Oxygen delivery, muscle and nerve protection are covered in greater detail in Chapter 108.

Fasting Before Anesthesia

Functioning ruminants should be fasted before anesthesia. Fasting reduces the volume of rumen contents, which reduces pressure on the diaphragm and the incidence of regurgitation. Ruminants properly fasted are less likely to bloat during recumbency and anesthesia. Withholding food and water for 24 hours before surgery has been traditionally recommended. Experience with nonfasted emergency cases has shown proper technique to be the most important factor in reducing the risk of regurgitation during induction and intubation. Attempting to intubate a patient with some degree of gag reflex present is more likely to result in regurgitation. Proper induction technique eliminates the gag reflex. Keeping the patient in sternal recumbency with the head elevated reduces the risk of passive regurgitation during intubation. Withholding food for 12 to 18 hours (access to water is permitted) has proved effective in minimizing problems during intubation and anesthesia while not producing the adverse effects on rumen motility and acid base status

associated with longer periods of fasting. Some abdominal procedures benefit from a greater reduction of rumen volume and a longer period of fasting is required in these cases.

Young animals have minimal energy stores. The risk of hypoglycemia in these patients increases with the duration of anesthesia. "Nursing" ruminants are typically anesthetized without fasting to reduce the risk of hypoglycemia. Ruminants younger than 2 months of age should be supplemented with dextrose during anesthesia. Adding 1.25% to 2.5% dextrose to the IV electrolyte solution (10 ml/kg/hr) is generally sufficient to ensure blood glucose levels are adequately maintained in these patients. Generally by 2 months of age most healthy ruminant patients no longer require dextrose supplementation during shorter anesthetic procedures. Adding 1.25% dextrose to the IV fluids is cheap insurance against hypoglycemia in ruminant patients 2 to 4 months of age when a long period of anesthesia is anticipated. Elevated body temperature increases metabolism and the risk of hypoglycemia in younger patients. Patients up to 4 months of age should be supplemented with dextrose when body temperature is significantly elevated.

Unless testing is performed during anesthesia, hypoglycemia is typically not recognized until the recovery period. Hypoglycemia produces a stuporous state and patients typically stall part way through the recovery process. Administration of dextrose has resulted in full recovery with no apparent adverse effects when this has occurred. As with most things medical, prevention is preferred to treatment. Protracted struggling during physical restraint of unruly young patients can produce substantial elevation of body temperature. Unruly patients should be sedated rather than battled.

Eye Protection

When ruminants are placed in lateral recumbency, care should be taken to ensure the lids of the down eye are closed. A towel or thin pad can be placed under the down eye to provide further protection. Ophthalmic ointment (bland or antibiotic) should be placed in the eyes to protect them during anesthesia. If the down eye ends up bathed in saliva or regurgitation, it should be rinsed out during recovery.

DRUGS USED IN RUMINANT FIELD ANESTHESIA

Alpha₂-Adrenergic Agonists

Xylazine is the most frequently used drug for sedation in large animals. Ruminants are 10 times more sensitive to xylazine than horses, whereas detomidine is dosed similarly in both species. Ruminants tend to lie down when dosed too aggressively with alpha₂-adrenergic agonists (α_2's), whereas horses exhibit increasing levels of ataxia.

The initial demeanor of the patient greatly influences the sedation produced by a given dose of an α_2. The sedative effect of α_2's can be overridden by elevated "sympathetic tone." This results in two characteristic features of α_2 sedation. The sedative effect produced by lower doses of α_2's is not as stable. Calm, quiet patients require smaller doses, whereas anxious or unruly patients require larger doses. This sounds easy, but selecting the incorrect dose may result in working on your knees or getting kicked in them. The ideal dose can be difficult to predict, especially when recumbency is not desired. Experience makes the necessary adjustments easier, but even seasoned practitioners get surprised at times.

Alpha$_2$-adrenergic agonists can be administered intravenously, intramuscularly, or subcutaneously and produce a dose-dependent degree of sedation, muscle relaxation, and analgesia. Intravenous administration of α_2's provides a faster onset and more intense level of chemical restraint and analgesia. The fairly rapid onset time can be used to advantage, allowing multiple smaller IV doses of an α_2 to be administered in an attempt to titrate the effect to the desired level. Intramuscular (IM) administration results in a more gradual onset and provides a longer duration of less intense chemical restraint and analgesia. Intramuscular administration is often used when patient cooperation does not allow IV administration or when extended duration is desired. The IM dose is traditionally twice the IV dose one would select for the patient based on the desired level of effect and the patient's initial demeanor. Subcutaneous administration results in the most gradual onset, longest duration, and mildest peak effect. Administering the IV dose intramuscularly or subcutaneously is a method used to produce a degree of sedation with limited risk of recumbency.

Alpha$_2$-adrenergic agonist administration produces dose-dependent side effects. Decreases in gastrointestinal motility and cardiorespiratory function are the most serious. In compromised patients, α's should be avoided or used cautiously and should be reversed on completion of the procedure. Even in normal, healthy patients, when large doses of α_2's are administered (especially doses used to produce recumbency), reversal is advisable to minimize the risk of gastrointestinal complications. Xylazine has been reported to increase uterine tone in late gestation.

Response to xylazine in tractable ruminants is fairly predictable. Titrated administration (e.g., initial conservative dose that is supplemented if necessary) minimizes the incidence of unintended recumbency. Extremely anxious or unruly patients require larger doses of xylazine to achieve adequate control. In these patients the administration process often triggers even greater behavior problems, so they should be dosed fairly aggressively at the outset. Intramuscular administration is frequently the only option available in extremely anxious or unruly patients. A calm environment can also help to reduce the dose of xylazine required to calm the patient. Restraint or interaction should be minimized whenever possible until xylazine has produced a reasonable degree of patient control.

Unless contraindicated, anxious or unruly patients should be sedated with xylazine 5 to 10 minutes before the anesthetic induction sequence. The dose of xylazine required will depend on the demeanor of the patient. It could easily be argued that all healthy ruminant patients might benefit from a small dose of xylazine (0.0075-0.01 mg/kg IV or 0.015-0.02 mg/kg IM) 5 to 10 minutes before anesthetic induction because even the calmest of patients experience some anxiety from the events surrounding anesthetic induction.

Additional information on the use of sedatives is provided in Chapters 106 and 108.

Alpha$_2$-Adrenergic Agonist Reversal

Yohimbine or tolazoline may be used to reverse the effects of α_2's at the end of a procedure to facilitate a quicker recovery and minimize the risks of gastrointestinal complications. Intramuscular administration of the reversal agent is preferred in all but emergency situations because it decreases the risk of CNS excitement or cardiovascular complications. The shorter duration of action of the reversal agents when given intravenously can result in resedation in patients in which the α_2 was administered intramuscularly, especially when larger doses were used. Reversal of α_2's should not be attempted until sufficient time has elapsed to allow any ketamine or Telazol used to resolve (15-30 minutes post-IV and 30-45 minutes post-IM, respectively) to reduce the chances of a rough recovery. The amount of reversal agent used depends on the dose of the α_2 and duration since administration. The recommended emergency IV doses for yohimbine (0.125 mg/kg) and tolazoline (2 mg/kg) are typically used as the maximum intramuscular dose and reduced to fit the circumstances. When dosed properly, the effects of reversal should start to become evident about 10 minutes following IM administration. Splitting the reversal dose (using both IV and IM routes) can produce a quicker recovery while minimizing the risk of resedation. Response to the small IV component is fairly quick, so the primary intramuscular component should be administered first.

Guaifenesin

Guaifenesin is a centrally acting muscle relaxant with mild to moderate sedative activity. At clinically used doses it produces minimal cardiorespiratory effects. Guaifenesin is used in combination with ketamine and in some cases xylazine to produce anesthetic induction in food animal patients. Guaifenesin-ketamine and guaifenesin-ketamine-xylazine combinations are also used in the IV maintenance of anesthesia in food animal patients.

Guaifenesin concentrations of 10% have been shown to cause hemolysis in ruminant patients. Practices mixing guaifenesin from powder stock should prepare solutions of 5%. Premixed guaifenesin solution (5%) is now commercially available in 1-L bottles.

Muscle relaxation and ataxia limit the amount of guaifenesin that can be administered before the induction bolus in large patients. In horses guaifenesin is typically preceded by xylazine, which also produces muscle relaxation and ataxia. The typically equine induction sequence delivers 40-50 mg/kg of guaifenesin. Anesthetic induction of small ruminants with Double Drip typically delivers 100 mg/kg. In larger cattle administration of Double Drip immediately preceding the induction bolus typically delivers 30 mg/kg.

Anesthetic Agents

Ketamine, tiletamine, and the ultra-short barbiturate thiopental are the injectable anesthetic agents used in large animal practice. Ketamine is by far the most common injectable anesthetic agent used in large animal practice. Thiopental is no longer generally used in large animal practice for induction or maintenance of anesthesia but remains the fastest option for restoring an anesthetized state when larger ruminant patients get too light during inhalation maintenance anesthesia. Thiopental (1.1 mg/kg IV) is also useful in dulling the protective swallowing reflex present during ketamine-based injectable anesthesia. Tiletamine, a more potent and longer-lasting relative of ketamine, is available only in combination with the benzodiazepine zolazepam as Telazol. Because of the high cost of Telazol, it is primarily used in large animal practice for capturing intractable patients.

Both ketamine and tiletamine draw on sympathetic nervous system reserve to augment cardiac output and blood pressure. This effect helps counter their direct negative inotropic and vasodilatory effects, as well as the negative cardiovascular effects produced by xylazine. Cardiovascular function in normal healthy patients anesthetized with ketamine-based protocols is good to excellent. I cannot emphasize enough the need for caution in dosing these seemingly safe drugs in compromised patients where sympathetic reserve may be severely limited. An apneustic pattern of breathing is often observed in horses following induction with ketamine or Telazol, but is not common in ruminants.

ANESTHETIC TECHNIQUES

"Ketamine Stun"

Ketamine is a dissociative anesthetic commonly used in veterinary medicine. Ketamine possesses potent analgesic effects when administered at subanesthetic doses. Adding a small dose of ketamine to more traditional chemical restraint combinations greatly enhances the level of patient cooperation. This technique is called the *ketamine stun* (or *stun*) because of the stunned effect it produces in patients when administered intravenously at doses that produce recumbency. These patients appear to be awake but seem oblivious to their surroundings and procedures being performed. The IV effect is quite brief ($\approx$15 minutes), and patients typically stand and appear fairly normal at that time. I initially referred to this state as *semianesthetized*, but perhaps *chemical hypnosis* is more appropriate. The ketamine stun technique makes treating camelid patients, which are frequently uncooperative, much more pleasant.[1] Because of the success in camelid patients, the stun technique was adjusted for use in ruminants (less xylazine) and proved to be just as useful. Dosing must be more conservative when using the ketamine stun technique in standing patients. This limits the degree of systemic analgesia relative to what we can achieve in recumbent patients but still provides improved patient cooperation when compared with more traditional methods of standing chemical restraint in both ruminants and horses.

The stun is basically the addition of a small dose of ketamine to any chemical restraint technique. In ruminants and camelid patients, a combination of xylazine, butorphanol, and ketamine is typically used. In equine patients, I generally use detomidine, morphine, and ketamine. I have used morphine (0.05-0.06 mg/kg) in

ruminant stuns. Morphine is much cheaper than butorphanol. In standing adult cattle stuns a similar level of cooperation is achieved with either opioid, but patients appear less obtunded when morphine is used. Some practitioners may find the obtunded appearance useful, since it allows them to follow the decay over time in the level of chemical restraint. Deterioration in the level of patient cooperation can also be used to determine when supplemental drug administration may be required. Morphine is used to provide analgesic relief in food animal patients. More information on the use of morphine in ruminants can be found in Chapter 109.

Alpha$_2$-adrenergic agonists possess potent sedative and analgesic effects. Opioids are typically thought of as analgesic drugs, but they possess CNS effects that, when combined with a tranquilizer or sedative, produce a greater level of mental depression. Ketamine is an N-methyl-D-aspartate (NMDA) receptor antagonist that possesses potent analgesic effects at subanesthetic doses. Ketamine was initially included in the stun technique for its analgesic properties, but it likely contributes to the mental aspects of the enhanced cooperation exhibited by patients under the influence of the ketamine stun technique. By combining drugs, clinicians can use smaller doses of the individual components while still achieving the desired level of effect.

Ketamine stun techniques can be divided into two broad categories, standing and recumbent. The standing ketamine stun is used primarily in large ruminants and horses. The recumbent ketamine stun is used primarily in small ruminants, camelids, and foals. The level of effect achieved is determined by three variables (dose, route of administration, initial demeanor of the patient). The stun cocktail can be administered intravenously, intramuscularly, or subcutaneously depending on the systemic analgesia, patient cooperation, and duration desired (Table 107-1).

Aggressive dosing increases the level of systemic analgesia and patient cooperation but also increases duration of recumbency or the risk of unintended recumbency. Xylazine is the most variable component of the stun combination. Initial patient demeanor plays a large role in the effect obtained from xylazine administration. Response to xylazine in tractable ruminants is fairly predictable. To minimize the incidence of unintended recumbency, a titrated approach (e.g., initial conservative dose that is supplemented if necessary) should be used. Extremely anxious or unruly patients require larger doses

---

Table 107-1

Effect of Route of Administration on Relative Impact of Ketamine Stun Technique

Parameter	Relative Ranking
Intensity (analgesia/cooperation)	IV >> IM > SQ
Onset	IV >> IM > SQ
Duration of effect	SQ > IM >> IV

IM, Intramuscular; *IV*, intravenous; *SQ*, Subcutaneous.

of xylazine to achieve adequate control. In these patients the administration process often triggers even greater behavior problems, so they should be dosed fairly aggressively at the outset.

Many permutations are possible when using the ketamine stun. Several years of experimentation in many different species have provided a great deal of insight into the potential of this technique but have not produced a definitive combination for all situations in each species. The following examples are provided guide and practitioners are encouraged to experiment with adjustments in doses. I thank Dr. David E. Anderson, who has used the ketamine stun technique extensively in food animal patients at Kansas State University, for his contributions to this section.

Clinical application of the ketamine stun in food animal patients can be divided into four basic categories.

Intravenous Recumbent Stun

The IV recumbent stun is used for short procedures or procedures requiring a high level of systemic analgesia and patient cooperation.

A combination of xylazine (0.025-0.05 mg/kg), butorphanol (0.05-0.1 mg/kg), and ketamine (0.3-0.5 mg/kg) is administered intravenously. Onset is approximately 1 minute. Patients gracefully become recumbent. Patients appear to be "awake" but seem oblivious to surroundings and procedure being performed. Mild random head or limb motion is not unusual, but purposeful movement and/or vocalization are signs of an inadequate stun level and additional drug should be administered. Half of the initial ketamine dose should be administered intravenously and is often effective. If, after allowing 60 to 90 seconds for onset, this additional half dose of ketamine fails to produce the desired level of analgesia, a second half dose of ketamine along with half of the initial dose of xylazine should be administered intravenously. The level of systemic analgesia produced varies depending on the doses administered but tends to be fairly intense. Surgical levels of analgesia have been achieved with this technique, but the use of local anesthetic blockade should be used whenever feasible to reduce the risk of patient awareness and stress. Duration of the stun effect is approximately 15 minutes, and patients typically are able to stand and walk immediately or shortly after this point. The IV recumbent stun is designed for short procedures. The clinician should plan ahead and work quickly. Supplemental doses of ketamine and/or xylazine can be administered to extend duration, but this technique is not intended for procedures that are expected to last significantly beyond the 15- to 25-minute range. The degree of extension is relative to the amount of supplemental drug administered.

The recumbent IV stun has proved useful for assisting short procedures in camelids and small ruminants.

Intramuscular or Subcutaneous Recumbent Stun

The IM or subcutaneous (SQ) recumbent stun is used for procedures requiring a longer duration of chemical restraint. The level of systemic analgesia is not as intense, and local anesthetic blockade should be used to reduce the risk of patient awareness and stress. Umbilical hernia repair is an example of the procedures performed using this technique. This approach is also useful for improving cooperation in patients that have gone down before or during a surgical procedure.

A combination of butorphanol (0.025 mg/kg), xylazine (0.05 mg/kg), and ketamine (0.1 mg/kg) is administered intramuscularly or subcutaneously. Subcutaneous administration is preferred because it provides a slightly longer duration of effect. Onset time is approximately 3 to 10 minutes. Patients are obtunded enough to require (and tolerate) intubation when placed in dorsal recumbency. Information on intubating and positioning patients to promote saliva egress is provided in Chapter 108. Duration of effect with SQ administration is approximately 45 minutes. Patients should be ambulatory within 30 minutes following this point.

The level of systemic analgesia produced by the IM or SQ recumbent stun is not as intense, but this approach does provide an enhanced level of patient cooperation that can make procedures much more pleasant for both patient and clinician.

Intravenous Standing Stun

An IV standing stun is typically used to provide a transient improvement in patient cooperation. Small IV boluses of ketamine have also been used to provide short periods of enhanced analgesia in equine colic patients.[2] Xylazine (0.02-0.0275 mg/kg), butorphanol (0.02-0.1 mg/kg; see later), and ketamine (0.05-0.1 mg/kg) can be administered individually or as a combination.

An example of the effectiveness of the IV stun technique is a 725- to 775-kg Charolais bull was run into the chute for examination of a possible penile injury. He was extremely agitated and kept banging around inside the chute despite being left alone. Examination was impossible, and patient injury was a valid concern. To calm him down, I administered 20 mg of IV xylazine (0.0275 mg/kg). This made him stand still when left alone, but he would not tolerate attempts to examine him. I then administered 40 mg of IV ketamine (0.055 mg/kg). The ketamine made him extremely cooperative, but the chute hampered full examination. A decision to place him on the tilt table was made. He was very compliant during the tabling process and subsequent examination. Intravenous xylazine boluses typically last approximately 15 minutes, though patients may remain more cooperative beyond this point when using the stun technique.

Small doses of IV ketamine can markedly improve the degree of patient cooperation in standing chemical restraint. Butorphanol (0.05-0.1 mg/kg IV or IM in smaller ruminants, 0.02-0.05 mg/kg IV or IM in larger ruminants) or morphine (0.05-0.1 mg/kg IV or IM) can be added to augment the level of analgesia and patient control.

Intramuscular or Subcutaneous Standing Stun

The IM or SQ standing stun is used for most standing procedures in ruminant patients. The level of systemic analgesia is limited, and local anesthetic blockade should be used to reduce the risk of patient awareness and stress. Standing flank laparotomy is an example of the procedures performed using this technique.

A combination of butorphanol (0.01 mg/kg), xylazine (0.02 mg/kg), and ketamine (0.04 mg/kg) is administered intramuscularly or subcutaneously. In a 500-kg cow this equates to butorphanol (5 mg), xylazine (10 mg), and ketamine (20 mg). For a 680-kg patient the doses are 7 mg butorphanol, 15 mg xylazine, and 25 mg ketamine.

"5-10-20 Technique"

An example of the effectiveness of the IV stun technique is the 5-10-20–mg combination has been used in student junior surgery laboratories at Kansas State to provide chemical restraint for standing cesarean sections in cattle. Patient weights varied from 340 to 660 kg, but no adjustments were made in the combination administered. The initial dose of 5-10-20 has not resulted in recumbency. Subcutaneous administration is preferred to minimize the risk of recumbency. In unruly cows IM administration provides better patient control. Onset is 5 to 10 minutes with SQ administration. Cows stood quietly during the cesarean sections (many were ill mannered before the ketamine stun). Duration of effect is approximately 60 to 90 minutes. Additional xylazine and ketamine can be administered subcutaneously to extend the duration of chemical restraint. Recumbency has occasionally occurred with readministration of 50% of all three components. Current recommendation for supplemental drug administration is 25% to 50% of the initial xylazine and ketamine doses (0-2.5-5) and (0-5-10), respectively, depending on the degree of cooperation and time required to complete the procedure.

A similar approach (10-20-40 technique) has been used successfully in adult bulls. Preputial surgery (with a local anesthetic block) is an example of the procedures performed using this technique.

The IM/SQ standing stun is a simple method for improving the quality of standing procedures for both patient and clinician.

Intravenous Xylazine-Ketamine

Intravenous xylazine and ketamine can be used to produce a short duration of injectable anesthesia in normal healthy ruminants. Because of the large dose of xylazine, this technique should not be used in compromised patients.

Xylazine (0.05 mg/kg IV) is administered first. When marked sedation is evident or the patient becomes recumbent, ketamine (2 mg/kg IV) is administered. This combination provides approximately 15 minutes of anesthesia. Administering one third to half of the original dose of each drug can be used to extend anesthesia, but recovery duration increases with the number of supplemental doses administered because of the slower clearance of xylazine. Gradually reducing the xylazine component in the supplemental doses reduces its adverse impact on cardiorespiratory function and recovery. Extending anesthesia with boluses of IV xylazine-ketamine should be limited to cases that require only a few supplemental doses or in emergency situations in which other options are not available. Double Drip or Ruminant Triple Drip is the preferred method for extending the duration of injectable anesthesia in ruminant patients.

Intramuscular Xylazine-Ketamine

Intramuscular administration of xylazine and ketamine can be used to produce an intermediate length of injectable anesthesia in normal healthy ruminants. Because of the large dose of xylazine, this technique should not be used in compromised patients.

A combination of xylazine (0.05-0.1 mg/kg IM) and ketamine (4 mg/kg IM) is administered. This combination generally produces 30 to 40 minutes of recumbency with a diminishing level of analgesia. A half dose of each drug can be administered intramuscularly to extend duration 15 to 20 minutes. A quarter dose of each drug can be administered intravenously to extend duration approximately 10 to 15 minutes.

Butorphanol-Ketamine-Xylazine

The butorphanol-ketamine-xylazine technique was developed by Dr. LaRue Johnson at Colorado State University. He prefers to call it *XKB*, but everyone else refers to it as *BKX*. A combination of xylazine, ketamine, and butorphanol is administered intramuscularly to produce an intermediate duration of injectable anesthesia in normal, healthy ruminants. Because of the large dose of xylazine, this technique should not be used in compromised patients.

A stock solution can be created to provide numerous doses. Add 100 mg of large animal xylazine (1 ml) and 10 mg of butorphanol (1 ml) to a bottle of ketamine (1000 mg). Administer mixture intramuscularly at a dose rate of 1 ml/20 kg. An alternative method is to draw up the individual components in a syringe as follows:

butorphanol (0.0375 mg/kg)
xylazine (0.375 mg/kg)
ketamine (3.75 mg/kg)

The patient should become recumbent within 3 to 5 minutes, with anesthesia lasting up to another 20 to 30 minutes. For procedures requiring considerable surgical preparation, the effective period of analgesia can be extended by administering half of the initial BKX dose IV before the start of surgery. Expect approximately 25 to 35 minutes of working time when the additional dose is used. Patients tend to remain laterally recumbent much longer following completion of the procedure when compared with the recumbent levels of the "ketamine stun."

Ruminant Triple Drip (GKX-Ru)

Ruminant Triple Drip is created by adding ketamine (1 mg/ml) and xylazine (0.1 mg/ml) to 5% guaifenesin.[3,4] Equine Triple Drip has a much higher concentration of xylazine (0.5 mg/ml). A constant rate infusion of Ruminant Triple Drip can be used to provide a stable plane of injectable anesthesia in normal, healthy ruminants. Compromised ruminant patients should be maintained with Double Drip to eliminate the cardiovascular depressant effects of xylazine.

In small ruminants, anesthetic induction is achieved by slowly infusing Ruminant Triple Drip to effect. A syringe should be used to administer Ruminant Triple Drip in very small patients to reduce the risk of overdosing because this combination has a somewhat slow onset. Muscle relaxation and sedation typically produce recumbency well before patient is anesthetized. Anesthetic induction generally requires administration of 1 to 1.5 ml/kg. Anesthesia can be maintained in normal, healthy ruminants by continued infusion of Ruminant Triple Drip at a rate of 2.5 ml/kg/hr without significant cardiorespiratory depression. Xylazine is cleared more slowly than ketamine. Because of this difference, postprocedure recumbency lengthens as the duration of Ruminant Triple Drip administration increases. Xylazine sedation can be reversed to speed the recovery process once the patient is awake. Additional information on the use of constant rate infusions can be found in Chapters 106 and 109.

In large ruminants, Double Drip is generally used to soften up the patient, but Triple Drip could also be used for this purpose. When early signs of sedation and muscle relaxation become evident, a combination of ketamine (1.5-2 mg/kg IV) and diazepam (0.06-0.1 mg/kg IV) is administered. This approach provides a more predictable and rapid drop, improving patient control and safety of personnel involved in the induction process. Cardiovascular function is good to excellent following induction with this combination in normal, healthy large ruminants.

Double Drip

Double Drip is created by adding ketamine (1 mg/ml) to 5% guaifenesin. Double Drip is the most commonly used method for inducing anesthesia to be maintained with inhalants in small ruminants. A constant rate infusion of Double Drip can be used to provide a stable plane of injectable anesthesia in ruminants. Because Double Drip does not contain xylazine, the level of analgesia provided is somewhat lower when compared with Ruminant Triple Drip. The absence of xylazine's cardiovascular depressant effects makes Double Drip a better choice for injectable maintenance in compromised ruminant patients. Butorphanol (0.05-0.1 mg/kg IV or IM in smaller ruminants, 0.02-0.05 mg/kg IV or IM in larger ruminants) or morphine (0.05-0.1 mg/kg IV or IM) can be administered to augment the level of analgesia when Double Drip is used to maintain anesthesia.

In small ruminants, anesthetic induction is achieved by slowly administering Double Drip to effect. A syringe should be used to administer Double Drip in very small patients to reduce the risk of overdosing because this combination has a somewhat slow onset. Muscle relaxation and sedation typically produce recumbency well before the patient is anesthetized. Anesthetic induction generally requires administration of 1.5 to 2 ml/kg. Anesthesia can be maintained by continued infusion of Double Drip at a rate of 2.5 ml/kg/hr without significant cardiorespiratory depression in normal healthy patients. In compromised patients sympathetic nervous system reserve may be limited. Though Double Drip is the most benign method of injectable anesthesia, care must be taken to minimize anesthetic depth in severely compromised

patients. Cardiorespiratory function should be monitored and supportive measures (IV fluids, dobutamine, oxygen, etc.) implemented as required. Additional information of the use of constant rate infusions can be found in Chapters 106 and 109.

Large ruminants should be managed as described in the section titled "Ruminant Triple Drip (GKX-Ru)."

Ketamine-Diazepam

Intravenous diazepam and ketamine can be used to produce a short duration of injectable anesthesia in normal, healthy ruminants. The absence of xylazine's cardiovascular depressant effects makes ketamine-diazepam (Ket-Val) a viable choice for injectable anesthesia of compromised patients. The same admonitions provided for Double Drip should be applied when using Ket-Val to anesthetize severely compromised patients. Titrated administration can be used to minimize the level of effect produced when administering boluses of Ket-Val. Double Drip provides a more stable plane of anesthesia than intermittent boluses of Ket-Val.

A mixture of equal volumes of ketamine (100 mg/ml) and diazepam (5 mg/ml) is administered intravenously at 1 ml/18-22 kg (which sounded better when it was 1 ml/40-50 lb). Anesthetic duration provided by a single bolus is approximately 15 to 20 minutes. Administering smaller boluses (one third to half of the original volume) can be used to extend anesthetic duration. The level of analgesia may not be as profound as injectable techniques that include xylazine. Butorphanol (0.05-0.1 mg/kg IV or IM in smaller ruminants, 0.02-0.05 mg/kg IV or IM in larger ruminants) or morphine (0.05-0.1 mg/kg IV or IM) can be administered to augment the level of analgesia.

Large ruminants should be managed as described in the section titled "Ruminant Triple Drip (GKX-Ru)."

References

1. Abrahamsen EJ: *Sedation/chemical restraint/anesthesia.* Proceedings of the 2004, 2006, and 2008 International Camelid Health Conference for Veterinarians. March 2004, 2006, 2008, Columbus, Ohio.
2. Abrahamsen EJ: *How to medicate a horse with colic before referral.* Proceedings of the 2005 British Equine Veterinary Association (BEVA) Congress, pp 45-46. September 2005, Harrogate, England.
3. Lin HC, Tyler JW, Welles EG et al: Effects of anesthesia induced and maintained by continuous intravenous administration of guaifenesin, ketamine, and xylazine in spontaneously breathing sheep, *Am J Vet Res* 54:1913-1916, 1993.
4. Thurmon JC, Benson GJ, Tranquilli WJ et al: Cardiovascular effects of intravenous infusion of guaifenesin, ketamine, and xylazine in Holstein calves, *Vet Surg* 15:463, 1986.

Suggested Reading
Veterinary anesthesia textbook(s) of your choice.

CHAPTER 108

Inhalation Anesthesia in Ruminants

ERIC J. ABRAHAMSEN

In large animal practice diagnostic and therapeutic procedures are generally accomplished with physical and/or chemical restraint techniques. When anesthesia is required, the choice of injectable or inhalation maintenance (commonly referred to as *general anesthesia*) must be made. Inhalation maintenance has been traditionally recommended for longer procedures, though the role of injectable maintenance is expanding in equine referral hospitals. Inhalation maintenance is cost effective if used frequently enough to offset the initial investment in equipment. With proper care, an anesthesia machine can outlast a veterinary career.

This chapter focuses on the principles and methods involved in applying inhalation maintenance techniques in ruminant patients. Information regarding patient preparation, induction, positioning, and recovery also apply to patients maintained with injectable techniques. Injectable maintenance techniques are covered in Chapter 107.

ANESTHESIA MACHINES

Most mixed animal practices have a small animal anesthesia machine that can also be used to provide inhalation maintenance in smaller ruminant patients. The machine should be thoroughly cleaned before returning it to small animal service. Large animal practices looking to add a small animal anesthesia machine or mixed practices wishing to obtain a separate unit dedicated to ruminant use have several options. Numerous companies sell anesthesia machines built for the veterinary market. Reasonably priced used human machines are available on the secondary market. For practices looking to spend even less money, a local hospital or medical clinic might have an outdated but serviceable anesthesia machine in storage that the staff would be willing to part with for little or no cost. Used machines obtained from hospitals or clinics should be carefully evaluated to ensure they are fully operational before placing them in service.

Modern large animal anesthesia machines are equipped with ventilators. These machines are fairly expensive when purchased new, though resourceful practitioners may find a secondhand unit available. Older large animal circle systems (not equipped with a ventilator) are generally much less expensive, though somewhat harder to find on the used equipment market. Constructing a To-and-Fro (Waters') canister is another option for providing inhalation maintenance in larger ruminant patients. Using a To-and-Fro canister for inhalation maintenance

in large ruminants provides practitioners with the ability to manually ventilate patients. Practices routinely using injectable maintenance techniques should invest in a selection of appropriately sized endotracheal tubes,* a 160 L/min demand valve,† and "portable" oxygen supply (tank and pressure regulator) to provide the ability to ventilate patients on the rare occasions it might be required.

The To-and-Fro canister was the first rebreathing method used to deliver inhalant anesthetic agents to patients. It is basically a container fitted with adapters to connect a rebreathing bag and endotracheal tube. Inhaled and exhaled gases travel through the carbon dioxide absorbent material contained in the canister. The original Waters' canister was horizontally oriented with the endotracheal tube, and rebreathing bag fittings were placed at opposite ends of the canister. The horizontal orientation of the canister creates the potential for a channel to open up at the upper surface as the absorbent load settles under the influence of gravity. The low resistance of this channel directs inhaled and exhaled gases around the absorbent material (channeling) rather than through it. Tightly packing the horizontal canister reduces the likelihood of channeling, but using a vertically oriented canister eliminates this potential problem. In a vertical To-and-Fro canister the endotracheal tube fitting is placed low on one side of the canister and the rebreathing bag fitting is placed high on the opposite side to maximize exposure to the carbon dioxide absorbent. The oxygen/inhalant gas mixture from the fresh gas outlet of a small animal anesthesia machine is delivered to a port on the endotracheal tube fitting. Alternatively, a dedicated system can be created to provide the oxygen/inhalant gas mixture. A pop-off valve must be included in the To-and-Fro system to vent excess gas volume. The pop-off valve can be located on either the endotracheal tube or rebreathing bag fittings or placed on the upper surface of the canister. The pop-off valve on the Waters' canister was placed on the endotracheal tube fitting, perhaps because this location tends to selectively vent end-expired gases. Unfortunately, this location also vents fresh gas flow at the same time. Placing the pop-off valve on the rebreathing bag fitting or the upper surface of the canister reduces loss of the fresh gas delivered from the anesthesia machine at

---

*Bivona Aire-Cuff Standard Silicone Endotracheal Tubes with Murphy Eye and Connector (Smiths Medical).
†JDM-5041 (JD Medical, Phoenix, Ariz.)

the end of expiration. The upper location also makes the pop-off valve easier to operate if manual ventilation of the patient is required.

A heavy-gauge, plastic, wide-mouth jug with screw-on cap is the type of container often used to create a To-and-Fro system. These jugs are available from laboratory and industrial suppliers. Plastic buckets with gasketed snap-on lids (commonly used to deliver feed supplements, etc.) have also been used to create To-and-Fro systems. A 12- to 15-L container provides the space required for the absorbent (generally 8-10 L for large ruminant patients) plus room for a plenum above and potentially below the absorbent material. Taller, narrower-diameter canisters use absorbent more efficiently but are more prone to tipping during use. A diameter of approximately 10 inches provides a reasonable compromise of efficiency and tip resistance. The fitting for the endotracheal tube is commonly placed near the bottom of the absorbent material. This location tends to produce a corridor of gas flow within the absorbent that prematurely reduces the chemical removal of carbon dioxide. Creating a plenum above and below the absorbent spreads the gas flow over a wider zone. The lower plenum also provides a space for exhaled moisture to collect. The lower plenum contributes to mechanical dead space, so its size must be kept small relative to patient tidal volume. Gluing small plastic blocks or dowels to the bottom of the canister to support the stiff screen required to contain the absorbent material could be used to create a lower plenum. The plastic blocks or dowels also reduce the volume of the lower plenum. The goal is to provide access to as much of the screen as possible while not introducing a significant volume of mechanical dead space. The absorbent material is the primary source of resistance in the To-and-Fro system. Creating a fairly tight maze of dowels to minimize volume of the lower plenum should not result in increased work of breathing. Placing the fitting for the rebreathing bag near the top of the container creates a plenum above the absorbent material. Though the pop-off valve introduces a subtle amount of positive end-expiratory pressure (PEEP) to help retain volume within the rebreathing bag, the fitting should be constructed to allow the bag to "hang" in a manner that reduces the likelihood of pinching. Incorporating a 45-degree elbow in the rebreathing bag fitting should provide the proper orientation. The inner surface of the rebreathing bag fitting should be screened to contain absorbent should the canister be tipped over. Size of the upper plenum will vary with the volume of absorbent used. The air-space within the absorbent (typically 50% of the volume) should ideally equal or exceed the patients' tidal volume. Eight to ten liters of absorbent should be sufficient for most adult cattle. Creating the fittings for the large animal endotracheal tube (with fresh gas inlet port) and large animal rebreathing bag (with pop-off valve) requires some creativity. Practitioners can contact a full-service veterinary anesthesia machine repair company* for assistance with developing these pieces or the entire apparatus.

The direct connection to the endotracheal tube places the To-and-Fro canister near the patient's mouth. This makes the To-and-Fro canister more cumbersome to use than a conventional circle system. Mechanical dead space increases in a To-and-Fro system as the carbon dioxide absorbent is consumed. Carbon dioxide retention (hypercapnia) increases over time when a To-and-Fro system is used. Ruminants tend to hypoventilate to a greater degree than other domestic species during anesthesia. Minimizing anesthetic duration reduces the degree of respiratory acidosis produced when using a To-and-Fro system. Inhaling caustic absorbent dust is frequently mentioned as a potential risk of the To-and-Fro canister. The addition of a lower plenum should reduce the risk of inhaling absorbent dust. Wetting the floor of the lower plenum before use should further reduce the risk of inhaling absorbent dust. Exhaled moisture quickly coats the interior surface of the lower plenum and lower regions of the absorbent material, eliminating the potential of inhaling absorbent dust.

In To-and-Fro canisters possessing a lower plenum, only the used (lower) portion of the absorbent material needs to be replaced. This must be done immediately following completion of the case because the color change typically exhibited by used absorbent is only evident for a short period of time following use. Used absorbent is also much harder than unused absorbent, making the transition zone easier to identify. Absorbent must be scooped out to preserve the layers present within the canister. In To-and-Fro canisters without a lower plenum the entire absorbent load should be changed following any significant use. Contents can be "stirred" following a short procedure, but absorbent capacity will be reduced and should be noted prominently on the canister. Fittings for the rebreathing bag and endotracheal tube should be capped when not in use to preserve the absorbent material contained in the canister.

For many mixed and large animal practices, the expense of adding a large animal machine may not be justifiable. Learning to fully use the capability of the small animal anesthesia machine will expand its role in large animal practice. Healthy patients exceeding the safe range of the small animal machine can be safely maintained with Ruminant Triple Drip (compromised patients should be maintained with Double Drip). Information on injectable maintenance techniques is provided in Chapter 107.

Several factors determine the upper limit of patient size that can be safely maintained using a small animal anesthesia machine. Resistance generated by gas flow along with the capacity of the reservoir bag and carbon dioxide absorbent canister must all be considered when deciding if a small animal anesthesia machine is suitable for a given patient. The anesthetic circuit and the endotracheal tube generate resistance. Small and large animal anesthesia machines use different adapters to connect the endotracheal tubes to the Y-piece. Endotracheal tubes up to 14 mm are equipped with small animal anesthesia machine adapters. Endotracheal tubes 16-30 mm* are equipped with large animal anesthesia machine adapters. In veterinary teaching hospitals where both small and

---

*Anaesthesia Equipment Service & Supply, Inc., Altamonte Springs, Fla, (800) 809-8499 or Anesthesia Service and Equipment, www.asevet.com.

*Bivona Aire-Cuff Standard Silicone Endotracheal Tubes with Murphy Eye and Connector (Smiths Medical).

large animal anesthesia machines are available, the endotracheal tube size appropriate for the patient determines which machine is used. The breakpoint, typically around 150 to 180 kg, places patients on the anesthesia machine best suited for their size.

Ruminants have a rapid, shallow pattern of breathing awake and under anesthesia. Deep sighs are unusual in anesthetized ruminants. In contrast, equine patients have a slower, deeper pattern of breathing awake and under anesthesia and often take deep breaths during anesthesia. The high gas flow velocity of ruminant ventilation generates significant resistance, but tidal volumes are relatively smaller and more easily accommodated by the small animal anesthesia machine. Tidal volume increases with patient size. The increased velocity of gas flow and resistance generated eventually results in an excessive level of respiratory effort. In ruminant patients this occurs at a level below the maximal tidal volume capacity of the small animal anesthesia machine. Ruminants up to 225 to 275 kg can generally be safely maintained using a small animal anesthesia machine. In contrast, the larger tidal volumes and sighs of equine patients exceed the capacity of the small animal anesthesia machine at a lower weight range.

The upper airway of ruminants is relatively large. Endotracheal tubes designed to fit a small animal anesthesia machine are often smaller than the patient's airway can accommodate. Using larger 16- or 18-mm endotracheal tubes* designed to fit large animal anesthesia machines can reduce resistance and the work of breathing. The 19-mm connector used to attach the scavenging hose to the pop-off valve outlet can also be used to adapt these larger tubes for use with a small animal anesthesia machine. The 19-mm connector fits snugly over the outside of the small animal Y-piece (small animal adapters go inside the Y-piece).

An appropriately sized reservoir bag (20-30 ml/kg for ruminants vs. 40-50 ml/kg for equine patients) ensures adequate reserve in the anesthetic circuit while not adding excessive volume that slows response to adjustments in vaporizer settings and/or oxygen flow rate. Reservoir bags for small animal machines come in 1-, 2-, 3-, and 5-L volumes.

The volume of the carbon dioxide absorbent canister varies between models of small animal anesthesia machines. The airspace within the absorbent volume should ideally be equal to or greater than the patient's tidal volume. When properly packed, the airspace is approximately 50% of the absorbent volume. Practitioners purchasing a small animal anesthesia machine for use in ruminant patients should look for models with a larger carbon dioxide absorbent canister volume. Practices using an existing small animal anesthesia machine with a marginally sized carbon dioxide absorbent canister volume should change absorbent before each ruminant case to achieve maximal possible functional volume (leaving the proper void above the absorbent to promote a wide zone of flow within the absorbent). Higher fresh gas (oxygen) flow rates reduce the rate of carbon dioxide absorbent consumption.

Mechanically ventilating a patient eliminates the work of breathing and can be used to extend the range of patient size that can be maintained using a small animal anesthesia machine. The tidal volume used to mechanically ventilate ruminant patients is typically 10 to 12 ml/kg. The size of the rebreathing bag becomes the "limiting" factor in mechanically ventilated ruminant patients. Patients with tidal volumes exceeding 4 L have been maintained using a small animal anesthesia machine with no apparent problems. Intermittent positive-pressure ventilation (IPPV) produces adverse mechanical (reduced venous return) and chemical (reduced $PaCO_2$) effects on cardiac output.[1,2] Global delivery of oxygen is generally reduced in mechanically ventilated patients. The adverse effect on cardiac output and tissue oxygen delivery should always be considered when contemplating the use of IPPV in anesthetized patients.

Management of the inhalation phase of anesthesia is similar whether using a small or large animal aesthetic machine.

PREANESTHETIC CONSIDERATIONS

Preanesthetic Examination

Assessment of the patient's overall health status should be done before anesthesia whenever possible. Economic considerations and the degree of patient cooperation determine the extent of the evaluation process. Because of the incidence of "subclinical" respiratory disease in ruminants, visual assessment of the patient can be misleading. Anesthetic risk is increased in patients with significant respiratory compromise, especially when its presence has not been detected.

Packed cell volume (PCV) and total protein (TP) values should be determined in all patients that can be reasonably sampled. In cooperative patients physical examination should include auscultation of the cardiopulmonary systems and patient temperature. Locomotor function should be evaluated to identify potential recovery problems. A complete blood count (CBC) and fibrinogen level determination can reveal the presence of "subclinical" infections. Additional laboratory work (e.g., serum chemistries) should be performed in all sick, debilitated, or depressed patients before anesthesia.

Unruly patients that cannot be evaluated before anesthetic induction should be considered to be at greater risk and treated accordingly. These patients can be examined and sampled once they are stabilized under anesthesia to identify potential problems.

Facility Requirements

An adequately sized area with resilient flooring (e.g., stall matting) is all that is required to safely anesthetize tractable ruminant patients. Ruminant patients induced with Double Drip, Ket-Val, or a combination of these two techniques tend to go down somewhat gracefully. Two or three individuals can induce and intubate smaller free-standing ruminants in the middle of the floor. The resilient flooring surface helps to reduce the risk of injury to larger ruminants, which are more difficult to physically

---

*Bivona Aire-Cuff Standard Silicone Endotracheal Tubes with Murphy Eye and Connector (Smiths Medical).

control as they go down. Ideally this space includes an unobstructed section of wall. Larger, freestanding ruminants can be positioned along the wall before anesthetic induction and pushed against the wall as they go down. This approach provides the best combination of patient control and personnel safety when dealing with larger freestanding ruminants, though it takes several strong individuals to hold 700 kg against the wall. Intubating ruminants in sternal recumbency reduces the risk of passive regurgitation and aspiration. Sliding larger ruminant patients down a wall improves the odds of maintaining sternal recumbency for the intubation process. Moving large, anesthetized ruminants is challenging, especially with limited personnel. A 1- or 2-ton overhead hoist can be used to move the patient into a better working position on the floor (preferably on a foam pad) or up onto a surgery table. If the ceiling will not support an overhead mounted hoist without extensive modification, a lateral pull using a wall-mounted winch system can be used to reposition larger patients. Multiple mounting points and a portable winch allow patients to be pulled to various areas of the operating theater. Using multiple lateral pulls to reposition a patient rather than a single pull that requires the patient to be rolled over reduces the risk of creating a displaced abomasum.

Two sets of hobbles connected by rings to the hook of the hoist or winch are used to move the patient. In horses hobbles are generally placed on the pastern. The ruminant pastern is shorter and the hoof to pastern diameter difference is modest, so hobbles are placed just above the fetlock. Due to the modest metacarpal/metatarsal to fetlock diameter difference in ruminants, care must be taken to ensure the hobbles provide a secure grip on the legs. Hobbles can be fashioned by splicing loops at each end of short segments of 1-inch cotton rope. Distance between the loops needs to be sufficient to make placing and removing the hobbles easy, but excessive length reduces the height patient can be lifted using an overhead hoist. Lifting large ruminants with cotton hobbles placed above the fetlock has not resulted in problems. Canvas strap hobbles (Shanks Veterinary Equipment, Inc., Milledgeville, Ill.) are available commercially. The wider, stiffer, canvas strap hobbles require somewhat more attention to attain a snug secure fit.

A tilt table can also be used to physically restrain tractable large ruminant patients before induction of anesthesia. This type of restraint induces a variable degree of patient distress, which is not desirable immediately before anesthetic induction. Sedative administration can be used to reduce the anxiety of patients restrained in this manner, but unless dosed fairly aggressively will generally not produce a significant centralization of cardiac output. Patients restrained in lateral recumbency are at somewhat greater risk of passive regurgitation. Large ruminants can be induced against a tilt table, but as they slump into the bellybands, abdominal pressure increases and passive regurgitation is more likely.

Unlike horses, ruminants generally stay recumbent during the recovery process until they are fully awake and functional. The most important requirement for achieving a smooth, uneventful recovery in ruminants is good footing. A calm recovery environment is always desirable, but only really necessary for anxious or unruly ruminant patients. Tractable ruminant patients can be recovered at the surgery site if the space is not required for other procedures. Ruminant patients that are not recovered in a confined space should be loosely tethered using the halter lead to prevent them from wandering after standing. If the surgery site is required for another procedure, a wall-mounted winch system can be used to pull the patient to an out-of-the-way spot in the surgery area for recovery.

Practices working primarily with beef cows will likely need a method of managing more unruly patients. One possible solution is to channel the patients into a chute to control them for intravenous (IV) catheter placement and examination. The patient is then released into an alleyway. The initial sections of the alleyway are swinging gates hinged to swing free of the front end of the chute providing full access to this area. A bar or section of pipe is inserted across the alleyway to confine the forward progress of the patient to the gated section. Anesthetic induction occurs in this segment of the alleyway. Large ruminants induced in the narrow alleyway generally remain in sternal recumbency. Following intubation the gates are swung open to allow the patient to roll into lateral recumbency. Midsized ruminants too difficult to manage freestanding may not always remain sternal with this method. These patients can be propped back up in sternal recumbency for intubation once the gates are swung open. A 1- or 2-ton overhead hoist is used to lift the patient and a transport device* or surgery table is moved under the patient. Clinicians can then move the patient to the surgery area. Placing a foam pad on top of the transport device allows it to be used as a surgery "table." Following the procedure, patients must be transported to an area where they can be safely managed once recovered. A confined space with good footing is all that is required for recovery. Bedded stalls are frequently used for ruminant recovery. The patient will need to be removed from the surgery table or transport device. A portable winch attached to the back wall of the stall can be used to pull the patient off the transport device or surgery table into the recovery area. A thick foam pad should be used to transition patients to the floor when pulling them off a lowered surgery table. A large opening makes moving the patient into the stall much easier. When loaded, the transport device or surgery table is heavy and bulky. Designing the recovery site(s) for easy access makes the chore more pleasant.

---

*A transport device can simply be a low gurney fashioned from reinforced aluminum plate with six to eight heavy-duty castors underneath and rope or chain pulls at each end. The large animal section of the Ohio State University College of Veterinary Medicine has designed a transport device that can also accommodate forks for lifting from all four sides. For more specifics on this device, contact Mr. Tom Burgett. Another option is the Custom Large Animal (padded or unpadded) Transfer Carts from Shanks Veterinary Equipment Inc. (Milledgeville, Ill.). An alternative method of moving large anesthetized ruminant patients is to create a movable platform that is lifted using forks mounted on a tractor's front-end loader. The platform is placed in the alleyway in front of the chute and the patient ends up anesthetized on top of it.

Fasting Before Anesthesia

Functioning ruminants should be fasted before anesthesia. Fasting reduces the volume of rumen contents, decreasing pressure on the diaphragm and the incidence of passive regurgitation. Properly fasted ruminants are less likely to bloat during recumbency and anesthesia. Withholding food and water for 24 hours before surgery has been traditionally recommended. Some authors have recommended even longer periods of fasting. Experience with nonfasted emergency cases has shown proper technique to be the most important factor in reducing the risk of regurgitation during induction and intubation. Attempting to intubate a patient with some degree of gag reflex present is more likely to result in regurgitation. Proper induction technique eliminates the gag reflex. Keeping the patient in sternal recumbency with the head elevated reduces the risk of passive regurgitation during intubation. Withholding food for 12 to 18 hours (access to water is permitted) has proven effective in minimizing problems during intubation and anesthesia while not producing the adverse effects on rumen motility and acid base status associated with longer periods of fasting. Some abdominal procedures benefit from a greater reduction of rumen volume and a longer period of fasting will be required in these cases.

Young animals have minimal energy stores. The risk of hypoglycemia in these patients increases with the duration of anesthesia. "Nursing" ruminants are typically anesthetized without fasting to reduce the risk of hypoglycemia. Ruminants younger than 2 months of age should be supplemented with dextrose during anesthesia. Adding 1.25% to 2.5% dextrose to the IV electrolyte solution (10 ml/kg/hr) is generally sufficient to ensure blood glucose levels are adequately maintained in these patients. Generally by 2 months of age most healthy ruminant patients no longer require dextrose supplementation during shorter anesthetic procedures. Adding 1.25% dextrose to the IV fluids is cheap insurance against hypoglycemia in ruminant patients 2 to 4 months of age when a long period of anesthesia is anticipated. Elevated body temperature increases metabolism and the risk of hypoglycemia in younger patients. Patients up to 4 months of age should be supplemented with dextrose when body temperature is significantly elevated.

Unless testing is performed during anesthesia, hypoglycemia is typically not recognized until the recovery period. Hypoglycemia produces a stuporous state and patients typically stall partway through the recovery process. Administration of dextrose has resulted in full recovery with no apparent adverse effects when this has occurred. As with most things medical, prevention is preferred to treatment. Protracted struggling during physical restraint of unruly young patients can produce substantial elevation of body temperature. Unruly patients should be sedated rather than battled.

Intravenous Catheters Are "Expensive" and Time Consuming—Are They Really Necessary?

A catheter should be placed before general anesthesia in ruminant patients. The jugular vein is the most commonly used site for IV catheter placement. The thicker skin of ruminants makes catheter placement more difficult and accidental placement in the carotid artery has occurred. A 14-gauge, 5.5-inch catheter is used in most ruminant patients. An 18-gauge, 2-inch catheter is sufficient for lambs and kids. The catheter should be secured to the neck with suture and/or bandage. The catheter should always be checked before anesthetic induction to ensure it is still functional. The veins on the external surface of the ear have been used as an alternative site for venous access in ruminant patients. An 18- or 20-gauge catheter should be used and secured with a combination of super glue and tape. These smaller catheters will not provide the flow rate of the 14-gauge catheter, but work well otherwise.

Eye Protection

When ruminants are placed in lateral recumbency, care should be taken to ensure the lids of the down eye are closed. A towel or thin pad can be placed under the down eye to further protect it when patients are anesthetized on the floor or ground. Ophthalmic ointment (bland or antibiotic) should be placed in the eyes to protect them during anesthesia. If the down eye ends up bathed in saliva or regurgitation, it should be rinsed out during recovery.

Oxygen Delivery and Muscle and Nerve Protection

Maintaining adequate delivery of oxygen to tissues during anesthesia is one of the most important goals of the anesthetist. Global oxygen delivery is determined by the combination of cardiac output and arterial oxygen content. Many sedative and anesthetic agents depress cardiac output. The partial pressure of oxygen in arterial blood (P_aO_2) is often decreased during anesthesia, especially in larger ruminants. The mass of the functioning ruminant stomach and/or bloating put pressure on the diaphragm, reducing tidal volume of the patient. Hypoventilation can also be caused by excessive anesthetic depth. Gravitational effects in larger patients redistribute pulmonary circulation to the more dependent regions of the lungs resulting in ventilation perfusion ($\dot{V}/\dot{Q}$) mismatch. Because of the influence of the oxygen-hemoglobin dissociation curve, arterial oxygen content is generally maintained at levels that are adequate when other aspects of oxygen delivery are properly managed. Anemic patients are the exception because they have a reduced oxygen carrying capacity.

Cardiac output (tissue flow) is the most important variable involved in tissue oxygenation. Tissues are able to cope with reductions in arterial oxygen content much better than they cope with reductions in blood flow. When arterial oxygen content is reduced, tissue oxygen tension falls and locally controlled vasodilation occurs. The resulting increase in tissue blood flow improves tissue oxygen delivery. When tissue blood flow is reduced, oxygen extraction from arterial blood is increased, but this mechanism is more limited in its ability to compensate.

Arterial blood pressure is monitored as a surrogate of cardiac output. Arterial blood pressure generally provides a reasonable estimation of cardiac output status, but large changes in cardiac output can occur without concomitant changes in arterial blood pressure. In anesthetized horses cardiac output has been shown to decrease 30% to 40% when IPPV is instituted.[1,2] Increased peripheral resistance maintains arterial blood pressure near preventilation levels, masking the serious decrease in cardiac output. Until clinically useful methods are developed to provide real-time cardiac output values, monitoring arterial blood pressure remains the best defense to poor tissue oxygen delivery during anesthesia.

Fortunately, global oxygen delivery is generally well maintained during anesthesia in normal, healthy ruminants. Conditions that compromise oxygen delivery status (e.g., hypovolemia, anemia, excessive anesthetic depth) require corrective measures. IV fluid administration can be used to reduce volume deficits. Patients should receive 10 ml/kg/hr of balanced electrolyte solution during routine general anesthesia. Higher delivery rates are used to restore blood volume in hypovolemic patients. PCV/TP should be periodically evaluated to guide fluid delivery in hypovolemic patients. Blood transfusions can be used to treat anemia. Properly monitoring anesthetic depth can reduce the negative cardiovascular effects of inhalant anesthetics. Inotropes such as dobutamine (1-3 μg/kg/min) can be infused in hypotensive patients to augment cardiac output and improve tissue oxygen delivery. In patients with persistent hypotension, deficits in arterial oxygen content become more important. Unfortunately, the ability to correct hypoxemia produced by pulmonary dysfunction in recumbent or anesthetized large animal patients is extremely limited. Methods such as IPPV or PEEP produce occasional improvement in P_aO_2 but also create adverse mechanical (decreased venous return) and chemical (decreased P_aCO_2) effects on cardiac output. Decreases in cardiac output typically exceed any improvements in arterial oxygen content and delivery of oxygen to tissues is reduced rather than improved. Anemic patients typically have elevated cardiac output due to peripheral vasodilation and reduced blood viscosity. When anemia cannot be corrected, maintaining a high level of cardiac output during anesthesia is vital to compensate for the reduced level of arterial oxygen content. Extreme cases of anemia require a complex blend of management techniques that are beyond the scope of this chapter.

Localized obstruction of blood flow is the typical cause of postanesthetic nerve or muscle complications in large animal anesthesia. Proper positioning of the patient is important to minimize compressive forces that can result in localized obstruction of blood flow. Placing ruminant patients on a thick foam pad during anesthesia distributes pressure of their weight more evenly, reducing the risk of localized obstruction of blood flow to dependent muscles. For patients in lateral recumbency, the down front leg should be pulled forward to reduce pressure on the radial nerve. The upper front leg should be propped up parallel to the floor or table surface to minimize the compressive force of its considerable mass. The upper rear leg should be supported in a similar manner. In situations where local tissue blood flow is partially obstructed, reduced arterial oxygen content may contribute to development of postanesthetic neuropathy or myopathy.

Airway Protection

Ruminants continue to produce a significant amount of saliva while anesthetized. Though patients are intubated during general anesthesia, it is still a good idea to position the head so that saliva runs out of the mouth rather than pooling back near the larynx whenever possible. For patients in lateral recumbency this can be accomplished simply by placing a pad under the head-neck junction so that the opening of the mouth is below the level of the larynx. This also reduces the risk of facial nerve injury.

Saliva egress during anesthesia becomes much more challenging when the patient is placed in dorsal recumbency. The body of smaller ruminant patients should be elevated using foam pads or some other method with the head resting on the floor or surgery table surface. Importantly, the head must be supported rather than hanging in space to prevent excessive tension on neck structures. The head and neck are rotated to place the opening of the mouth below the larynx to assist saliva egress. The short, thick neck of many cattle breeds can make proper orientation difficult to achieve. An overhead hoist system is required to achieve this positioning in larger anesthetized ruminant patients.

Keeping the opening of the mouth dependent to the larynx ("hanging the head") in patients hoisted into recovery helps to clear saliva or regurgitation from the oropharynx. Proper extubation technique further reduces the risk of aspiration.

PREMEDICATION

Why Is Premedication Necessary?

Veterinarians have been traditionally taught that ruminants do not generally require premedication before anesthesia. Actually, most ruminant anesthesia cases involve the use of premedication, but not in the traditional manner used in other veterinary species. Premedication is used to enhance patient control and modify the response to the induction bolus. Premedication can intensify or extend the effects of the induction bolus. Premedication can also minimize the adverse side effects of an induction drug.

Apprehension and activity alter the distribution of cardiac output, directing a greater portion of blood flow to skeletal muscles. Though many ruminant patients appear calm before anesthetic induction, some degree of apprehension likely exists. Extremely anxious or unruly ruminant patients experience a greater alteration in the distribution of cardiac output. Sedatives such as xylazine or guaifenesin produce a dose-dependent calming effect. Reducing the patient's anxiety and activity level directs a greater portion of the cardiac output to the vital organs (centralization of cardiac output). The degree of sedation determines the level of centralization achieved. Centralization of cardiac output does not occur instantaneously. It lags peak sedation by a few minutes in calmer patients and longer in extremely anxious or unruly patients. Centralization of cardiac output is desirable because it directs a greater portion of the intravenously administered anesthetic induction agent to the target sites in the central nervous system. When lipid-soluble drugs such as anesthetics induction agents are administered as an IV bolus, it is redistribution from the vital organs to skeletal muscle via continued circulation that ends the clinical effects of the drug. Any increase in the amount of drug sent directly to muscle will decrease the impact of the induction bolus (peak effect and duration).

Ruminants are typically induced using a combination of sedative and ketamine. In small ruminants Double Drip (5% guaifenesin with 1 mg/ml of ketamine added) is infused to effect. Small ruminants can also be induced with a combination of diazepam and ketamine (Ket-Val). In large ruminants Double Drip is slowly infused until the first signs of muscle weakness are apparent, and then a bolus of ketamine and diazepam (Ket-Val) is administered. Administering the sedative (guaifenesin or diazepam) along with the anesthetic induction agent (ketamine) does not provide the benefits achieved with the sedative first approach used in most other species. Double Drip administration produces obvious signs of sedation before actual anesthetic induction, but the short duration does not allow significant centralization to occur. When Ket-Val is used, the onset of diazepam's sedative effect is quick enough to prevent the neuroexcitatory effects produced by large doses of ketamine, but little centralization of cardiac output occurs. These techniques are generally effective in ruminants due in large part to the calm demeanor of these patients, but that does not mean they cannot be improved.

Unless contraindicated, anxious or unruly patients should be sedated with xylazine 5 to 10 minutes before the anesthetic induction sequence. The dose of xylazine required will depend on the demeanor of the patient. It could be argued that most healthy ruminant patients might benefit from a small dose of xylazine 5 to 10 minutes before anesthetic induction because even the calmest of patients will experience some anxiety from the events surrounding anesthetic induction.

Guaifenesin is a centrally acting muscle relaxant with mild sedative effects. Guaifenesin produces minimal cardiorespiratory effects at clinically used doses. Guaifenesin can be used to produce a degree of sedation in compromised patients that might not tolerate the adverse cardiovascular effects of xylazine. Guaifenesin is infused to effect. When a sedative effect is desired, a slow rate of infusion is used. As sedation builds, the rate of infusion should be decreased to avoid producing excessive muscle relaxation, which triggers corrective postural activity by the patient that negates some of the centralization produced by the sedation. Onset time for guaifenesin is approximately 1 minute. This delayed effect must be accounted for in determining the proper infusion rates and end points. This approach works better in calmer patients and should not be expected to provide significant centralization in extremely anxious or unruly patients. When using Double Drip, a slow initial rate of infusion extends the period of sedation somewhat, allowing a greater degree of centralization to occur before reaching the point of anesthetic induction.

Additional information on sedation of ruminants can be found in Chapter 106.

Adverse Side Effects of Premedications

The potential impact of adverse side effects produced by premedications must also be considered when developing an anesthetic plan.

Guaifenesin (also known as *GG*) is a milder sedative with strong muscle relaxant properties. Guaifenesin produces minimal cardiorespiratory or gastrointestinal effects at clinically used doses, making it a better sedative choice in compromised patients. Premixed guaifenesin is available as a 5% solution in 1-L bottles. Guaifenesin concentrations above 5% may cause hemolysis in ruminants. Guaifenesin is administered to effect by IV infusion. Excessive muscle relaxation generally limits the amount of guaifenesin administered.

Benzodiazepines (diazepam, midazolam) are moderate sedatives and centrally acting muscle relaxants. Benzodiazepines produce minimal cardiorespiratory or gastrointestinal effects at clinically used doses. The sedative effect of benzodiazepines does not produce a beneficial calming effect in most animal species, but ruminants do respond favorably. Midazolam is slightly more potent, but the two drugs are generally used interchangeably.

Alpha$_2$-adrenergic agonists (α_2's) possess potent sedative and analgesic properties. These desirable dose-dependent effects are accompanied by a myriad of dose-dependent side effects. The cardiovascular and gastrointestinal effects are the most important, though the dose-dependent muscle relaxation produced by α_2's likely contributes to the incidence of unwanted recumbency in ruminants. Cardiovascular side effects associated with IV xylazine include decreases in heart rate and cardiac output that can reach 25% when larger doses are administered. IV xylazine produces a biphasic change in blood pressure (initial increase in blood pressure produced by peripheral vasoconstriction, followed by a gradual decrease to below baseline values because of reductions in sympathetic nervous system tone). Xylazine administered intramuscularly does not produce vasoconstriction and arterial blood pressure gradually decreases as sedation occurs. Detomidine's cardiovascular effects are even more potent, producing larger decreases in heart rate and cardiac output. In contrast to xylazine, IV administration of detomidine results in prolonged elevation of blood pressure. Persistent peripheral vasoconstriction in the face of decreased cardiac output does not promote good tissue blood flow. Detomidine should not be routinely used as an anesthetic premedication for this reason. The cardiovascular changes produced by xylazine are generally well tolerated in the normal healthy ruminants but may be life threatening in patients suffering from hypovolemia. The sympatholytic effects of α_2's can exacerbate bradyarrhythmias, so they should be avoided in patients with hyperkalemia. Xylazine sedation decreases respiratory rate, whereas tidal volume seems to increase, resulting in only minor alterations in arterial blood gas values. Respiratory depression is greater with detomidine and extremely large doses have resulted in respiratory compromise in horses. The respiratory effects of α_2's are generally well tolerated in normal, healthy ruminants. In patients with respiratory compromise, α_2's should be used cautiously. They also produce a dose-dependent decrease in gastrointestinal motility. A large dose of an α_2 administered before anesthetic induction may depress rumen motility well beyond the anesthetic period. Rumen motility should always be evaluated following recovery in ruminant patients receiving larger doses of α_2's. Yohimbine or tolazoline can be used to reverse the effects of α_2's and restore rumen motility. Additional information on the use of α_2's can be found in Chapter 106.

Veterinarians should avoid using α_2's in compromised patients. In compromised ruminants a slow infusion of guaifenesin can be used in most cases to achieve the desired level of sedation and centralization before anesthetic induction. In situations where an α_2 must be used in a compromised patient, titrated administration minimizes the risk of overdosing the patient. Reversal of the α_2 should be done at the earliest point possible. Titrated reversal once the patient is anesthetized removes the adverse effects of the α_2 while minimizing the risk of the patient getting too light.

In the early days of ruminant anesthesia, atropine was recommended by several authors to counter the profuse salivation of these patients. Atropine administration does not eliminate salivation in ruminants during anesthesia. Atropine tends to reduce the aqueous component of saliva, making it more difficult to clear from the mouth and oropharynx. Atropine also reduces gastrointestinal motility. Routine administration of atropine before anesthesia in large animals is unnecessary and increases patient risk in my opinion. Atropine (0.01-0.02 mg/kg IV) can be used to treat bradycardia.

ANESTHETIC AGENTS

Ketamine, tiletamine, and the ultra-short barbiturate thiopental are the injectable anesthetic agents used in large animal practice. Ketamine is by far the most common injectable anesthetic agent used in large animal practice. Thiopental is no longer generally used in large animal practice for induction or maintenance of anesthesia but remains the fastest option for restoring an anesthetized state when larger ruminant patients get too light during inhalation maintenance anesthesia. Thiopental (1.1 mg/kg IV) is also useful in dulling the protective swallowing reflex present in ketamine anesthesia. Tiletamine, a more potent and longer lasting relative of ketamine, is available only in combination with the benzodiazepine zolazepam as Telazol. Because of its high cost, Telazol is primarily used for "capturing" intractable large animal patients.

Both ketamine and tiletamine draw on sympathetic nervous system reserve to augment cardiac output and blood pressure. This effect helps counter their direct negative inotropic and vasodilatory effects, as well as the negative cardiovascular effects produced by xylazine. Cardiovascular function in normal, healthy patients anesthetized with ketamine-based protocols is good to excellent. I cannot emphasize enough the need for caution in dosing these seemingly safe drugs in compromised patients in which sympathetic reserve may be severely limited. An apneustic pattern of breathing is often observed in horses following induction with ketamine or Telazol, but this is not common in ruminants.

Isoflurane is the most commonly used inhalant anesthetic in food animals. Halothane can be used, but recovery time may be somewhat longer due to its greater solubility. Both isoflurane and halothane depress myocardial function. Isoflurane produces a greater degree of vasodilation, a sparing effect on cardiac output, whereas halothane maintains better arterial (tissue perfusion) pressure at the expense of cardiac output. The extremely high cost of Sevoflurane makes its use in food animal patients difficult to justify. Sevoflurane also depresses respiratory function to a much greater degree than halothane or isoflurane, making spontaneous ventilation difficult to maintain.

ANESTHETIC INDUCTION TECHNIQUES

Double Drip

Double Drip is created by adding ketamine (1 mg/ml) to 5% guaifenesin. Ruminant Triple Drip is created by adding xylazine (0.1 mg/ml) to Double Drip. In normal, healthy ruminants either can be used for anesthetic induction, but Ruminant Triple Drip is generally only used for this purpose when it will also be used for IV anesthetic maintenance.

In small ruminants, anesthetic induction is achieved by slowly administering Double Drip to effect. A syringe should be used to administer Double Drip in very small patients to reduce the risk of overdosing because this combination has a somewhat slow onset. Muscle relaxation and sedation typically produce recumbency well before the patient is ready for intubation. Patients typically require 1.5 to 2 ml/kg of Double Drip for intubation. Double Drip is the most commonly used method for inducing anesthesia to be maintained with inhalants in small ruminants. Cardiovascular function is good to excellent in normal, healthy small ruminants following induction with Double Drip. Because of the absence of xylazine and titrated method of administration, Double Drip is considered the best choice for anesthetic induction in compromised small ruminants where sympathetic nervous system reserve may be limited. Although Double Drip is the most benign method of anesthetic induction available, care must be taken to minimize anesthetic depth in severely compromised patients. Cardiorespiratory function should be monitored and supportive measures (e.g., IV fluids, dobutamine, oxygen) implemented as required.

In large ruminants, Double Drip is generally used to soften up the patient. When early signs of sedation and muscle relaxation become evident, a combination of ketamine (1.5-2 mg/kg IV) and diazepam (0.06-0.1 mg/kg IV) is administered. This approach provides a more predictable and rapid drop, improving patient control and safety of personnel involved in the induction process. Cardiovascular function is good to excellent following induction with this combination in normal, healthy large ruminants. In compromised large ruminants the ketamine bolus dose should be reduced (0.75-1 mg/kg). Once recumbent, the patient's cardiorespiratory status should be evaluated (e.g., turgidity of the median auricular artery) and any supportive measures required (e.g., IV fluids, dobutamine, oxygen) should be initiated. Additional ketamine can be administered, if required, to facilitate intubation.

Ketamine and Diazepam

Intravenous diazepam and ketamine can be used for anesthetic induction of normal, healthy ruminants. The absence of xylazine's cardiovascular depressant effects makes ketamine-diazepam (Ket-Val) a viable choice for anesthetic induction of compromised patients. The same admonitions provided for Double Drip should be applied when using Ket-Val to anesthetize severely compromised patients. Titrated administration can be used to minimize the level of effect produced when administering Ket-Val.

In small ruminants a mixture of equal volumes of ketamine (100 mg/ml) and diazepam (5 mg/ml) is administered intravenously at 1 ml /18-22 kg (which sounded better when it was 1 ml/40-50 lb). Cardiovascular function is good to excellent following induction with Ket-Val in normal, healthy small ruminants. Additional Ket-Val may be required in some patients to assist intubation. If administered in a titrated fashion, Ket-Val can be safely used to induce anesthesia in compromised small ruminants.

In large ruminants, Double Drip is generally used to soften up the patient. When early signs of sedation and muscle relaxation become evident, a combination of ketamine (1.5-2 mg/kg IV) and diazepam (0.06-0.1 mg/kg IV) is administered. This approach provides a more predictable and rapid drop, improving patient control and safety of personnel involved in the induction process. Cardiovascular function is good to excellent following induction with this combination in normal, healthy large ruminants. In compromised large ruminants the ketamine bolus dose should be reduced (0.75-1 mg/kg). Once recumbent, the patient's cardiorespiratory status should be evaluated (e.g., turgidity of the median auricular artery) and any supportive measures required (e.g., IV fluids, dobutamine, oxygen) should be initiated. Additional ketamine can be administered, if required, to facilitate intubation.

Intravenous Xylazine and Ketamine

Xylazine (0.05 mg/kg IV) is administered first. When marked sedation is evident or the patient becomes recumbent, ketamine (2 mg/kg IV) is administered. Cardiovascular function is adequately maintained in normal, healthy patients. Because of the large dose of xylazine, this technique should not be used in compromised ruminant patients.

ENDOTRACHEAL INTUBATION

Smaller ruminants are intubated by direct visualization much like dogs or cats. Because of the small mouth opening and deep oral cavity, proper alignment is important to visualize the larynx. This is similar to looking through a long, narrow tube. A laryngoscope with an extra long blade aids visualization of the larynx by allowing greater control of the base of the tongue. An assistant straddling the patient's back holds the patient in sternal recumbency. The assistant extends the head and neck up toward the individual doing the intubation and holds the jaws apart. The assistant's knees can be used to help control the patient's head/neck. The head should not be elevated until the intubation process is imminent to minimize pooling of saliva back around the larynx. A reduced level of jaw tone and the absence of a chewing or lingual response to this manipulation can be used to determine when

intubation is appropriate. A stylet made from ⅛-inch aluminum rod is used to facilitate intubation of small ruminants. The thin rod does not obstruct the view of the larynx. The ends of the stylet should be smoothed or rounded to minimize the risk of damaging the mucosal surfaces of the airway. The stylet is guided into the larynx first and the endotracheal tube passed over it into the airway. The stylet must be long enough so that it can be grasped above the endotracheal tube as it is advanced down the rod and into the trachea. With practice, the endotracheal tube can be positioned on the stylet and held in place with the hand guiding the stylet into the airway, making the process less cumbersome. In somewhat larger ruminants, size of the oral cavity may be large enough to allow visualization of the larynx while the endotracheal tube is guided into the airway. The stylet is used to stiffen the endotracheal tube. Allowing the stylet to protrude slightly from the end of the endotracheal tube makes placement in the airway easier.

In large ruminants the depth of the oral cavity and the size of the endotracheal tube make direct visualization difficult. Large ruminants are intubated by manually guiding the tube in the airway. The anesthetist carries the endotracheal tube into the mouth with one hand and then uses his or her fingers to guide the tube between the arytenoids as the other hand advances the tube. A speculum is required for this technique. The arm/hand size of the individual performing the intubation is the limiting factor in determining the patient size in cases in which this approach becomes appropriate. The oral cavity must be large enough to accommodate one's arm and the endotracheal tube. The lower limit for this technique is generally around 300 to 350 kg, unless the operator has an exceptionally small arm and hand. A somewhat undersized endotracheal tube can provide additional room for the operator's arm in marginally sized patients. The operator should wash his or her arms off afterward because ruminant saliva tends to irritate the skin of most people.

A flexible endoscope can be used to guide the endotracheal tube into the larynx. The endoscope serves as both a stylet and visualization device. This technique has proven useful when traditional methods cannot be used. The endoscope must be small enough to fit inside the endotracheal tube.

Ruminants can be blindly intubated. With the head and neck extended, the endotracheal tube is gently advanced during inspiration. Repeated attempts will likely be required and care must be exercised to minimize the risk of producing laryngeal trauma. This technique is not always successful and should not be counted on for routine intubation of ruminants.

INHALATION MAINTENANCE

The principles are the same whether using a large or small animal machine. A high (5-10 L/min) oxygen flow is used initially to flush nitrogen from the circuit and patient. This high fresh gas flow rate also delivers large amounts of inhalant to the circuit to counter the rapid initial uptake by the patient. The high initial oxygen flow rate is generally reduced after 10 minutes. Maintenance oxygen flow rate can vary from 7 to 10 ml/kg (semiclosed circuit) down to 2 ml/kg (closed circuit). Initial vaporizer setting (generally 3%-5%) is reduced over time based on assessment of patient depth. The minimum alveolar concentration (MAC) values for halothane (0.9%) and isoflurane (1.4%) provide a comparison of their relative potencies. Because of dilution that occurs in the anesthetic circuit, vaporizer settings are generally much higher than these values during the maintenance phase of anesthesia, though the difference decreases as anesthetic duration lengthens. Greater dilution occurs when lower oxygen flow rates are used, and vaporizer settings must be subtly higher to maintain the proper anesthetic concentration in the circuit and patient.

Hypoventilation during anesthesia, as measured by the degree of carbon dioxide retention, varies by species. Small animal patients typically maintain normal physiologic $PaCO_2$ values during inhalation maintenance anesthesia. In horses $PaCO_2$ typically increases to around 60 mm Hg at a surgical plane of inhalation maintenance. In ruminants $PaCO_2$ typically increases to around 70 mm Hg at a surgical plane of inhalation maintenance. The mild metabolic alkalosis of normal, healthy ruminants allows them to tolerate this higher level of respiratory acidosis. Many anesthetists prefer to ventilate ruminants during inhalation maintenance anesthesia, feeling this level of respiratory acidosis is undesirable. Unfortunately, the use of IPPV produces adverse mechanical (decreased venous return) and chemical (decreased $PaCO_2$) effects on cardiac output.[1,2] Elevated levels of CO_2 produce a myriad of beneficial effects on tissue oxygen delivery. In my opinion, mechanical ventilation is not routinely necessary to correct this mild degree of hypoventilation in normal, healthy ruminants during inhalation maintenance.

The reduction in cardiac output (as much as 30%-40% in horse studies) typically exceeds any increase produced in arterial oxygen content and tissue oxygen delivery actually decreases. Changes produced by recumbency and anesthesia can result in hypoxemia, especially in larger ruminants. The degree of hypoxemia is typically well tolerated when all other aspects of tissue oxygenation are properly managed. Ensuring cardiac output is adequately maintained by minimizing inhalant levels and monitoring arterial blood pressure as a surrogate of cardiac output are the best methods for ensuring adequate tissue oxygenation during anesthesia. Severe hypoventilation produced by excessive abdominal pressure is one situation where the use of IPPV is warranted. A tidal volume of 10 to 12 ml/kg and respiratory rate of 6 to 10 breaths per minute are typically used when mechanically ventilating ruminant patients. Inspiratory pressure in nonbloated patients should be 25 to 30 cm of water, but higher levels may be required to deliver an adequate tidal volume when abdominal pressure is markedly elevated. Hypoventilation produced by excessive anesthetic depth should be corrected with the vaporizer rather than the ventilator. IPPV can also be used to reduce the degree of respiratory acidosis in ruminant patients with concurrent metabolic acidosis, though at the risk of reducing tissue oxygen delivery. Administration of sodium bicarbonate can be used to correct a metabolic acidosis, though it takes longer to affect a change in blood pH. Use of the ventilator to correct acidosis should be reserved for extreme cases where the combined effects of metabolic and respiratory acidosis threaten cellular integrity.

Smaller animals have a larger surface area for a given body mass. Very young animals have a reduced ability to regulate body temperature. A hot water blanket system should be placed under all young calves and small ruminant patients during anesthesia to reduce the risk of hypothermia. Minimizing wetting of the patient during the prep process whenever possible can also help reduce the risk of hypothermia in these patients.

MONITORING

Heart rate, respiratory rate, and tidal volume should be monitored at 5-minute intervals during routine periods of anesthesia and more frequently if problems occur. Recording data on an anesthesia record allows trends to be recognized more easily and may reduce liability should problems occur during anesthesia.

During anesthesia heart rate is typically 60 to 80 and respiratory rate is 20 to 30 in large ruminants. Rates are often slightly higher in small ruminants. Practices routinely anesthetizing ruminant patients should purchase a monitor capable of displaying an electrocardiogram (ECG) and blood pressure data. Direct measurement of arterial blood pressure is the more accurate method and is easily accomplished in ruminant patients. The median auricular artery running down the central ridge on the exterior surface of the ear can be easily cannulated with a 22- or 20-gauge over the needle catheter. A fluid-filled line from this catheter can be attached to a pressure transducer, mercury manometer, or modified aneroid gauge to monitor arterial blood pressure. In smaller ruminants blood pressure can also be monitored indirectly using a Doppler microphone and sphygmomanometer or oscillometric monitor. The inflatable cuff is typically placed on the forelimb just above the carpus. Digital evaluation of the turgidity of the median auricular artery can be used to provide an estimate of arterial blood pressure. Digital evaluation should not be considered an acceptable substitute for more traditional methods of monitoring arterial blood pressure in the hospital setting. Digital evaluation should be used when the auricular artery cannot be cannulated or a monitor fails. Digital evaluation can also be used to aid in evaluating the cardiovascular status in nonanesthetized patients. Developing good digital evaluation skills requires practice and known values for comparison.

Monitoring depth of anesthesia is best accomplished using a variety of parameters. Palpebral reflex, eye location, changes in ventilation, and arterial blood pressure are the most useful parameters. The palpebral reflex is typically brisk following anesthetic induction. During inhalation maintenance the palpebral reflex decreases as anesthetic depth increases. At the lighter end of the surgical plane the palpebral reflex is typically moderately brisk and at the deep end of the surgical plane the palpebral reflex is dull. Absence of a palpebral reflex generally indicates an excessively deep plane of anesthesia. The palpebral reflex remains strong during ketamine-based IV anesthesia maintenance techniques and changes with anesthetic depth are subtle. Eye position is the traditional method of evaluating anesthetic depth in ruminant patients. The eye is centralized following induction. The eye initially rotates ventrally as anesthetic depth increases and then returns toward its original centralized location. When the eye has progressed halfway back toward the central location from its most ventral position, surgical plane has been reached. As anesthetic depth increases, the eye returns to a central location and then repeats its ventral journey. An excessively deep plane of anesthesia can mimic the eye position of the desired surgical plane. Eye position must be evaluated periodically to follow the progression of movement. A single examination of eye position can be misleading.

Inhalant anesthetics produce a dose-dependent respiratory depression. Respiratory rate and/or tidal volume often increase as the plane of anesthesia is lightened. In most patients these changes are generally subtle until a light plane of anesthesia is reached. The rate of change in these parameters often increases at this point, warning the anesthetist to carefully evaluate anesthetic depth of the patient.

Inhalant anesthetics produce dose-dependent cardiovascular depression. Arterial blood pressure can provide useful information on anesthetic depth of the patient. Direct arterial pressure is more useful in this regard because the absolute value obtained is more reliable. Changes in arterial pressure can indicate a change in anesthetic plane, though decreasing blood pressure can also occur with conditions not related to anesthetic depth such as ongoing hemorrhage. Absolute arterial pressure can be a useful indicator of anesthetic depth in healthy ruminant patients. Unlike other species, ruminants generally have elevated blood pressure during anesthesia. Normal healthy ruminants generally have a mean arterial pressure of between 100 and 130 mm Hg at surgical plane (100 mm Hg is indicative of deep surgical plane, whereas 130 to 150 mm Hg indicates an extremely light plane of anesthesia). These absolute values will not work with all ruminant patients. Toxic patients or those with volume deficits may not be able to reach the values provided, though they should be kept in as light a plane of anesthesia as possible to minimize the adverse effects of the anesthetic agents. Extremely young ruminant patients often do not have the cardiovascular vigor to achieve to these high arterial pressure values. The rate of change in arterial blood pressure can also be used to evaluate anesthetic depth. Arterial blood pressure should increase as the plane of anesthesia is lightened. The rate of change will depend on the magnitude of the adjustment in anesthetic delivery. As the patient approaches a light plane of anesthesia, the rate of increase in arterial blood pressure will speed up, warning the anesthetist to carefully evaluate anesthetic depth of the patient.

RECOVERY

Ruminant patients should be placed in sternal recumbency for recovery whenever possible. Placing patients in sternal position assists venting of fermentation gas trapped in the rumen during recumbency and anesthesia. Sternal recumbency also allows saliva and any regurgitation to drain from the oral cavity. Patients may need to be propped up to maintain sternal recumbency early in the recovery period. Pulling the head around and tying the halter lead off to a hind leg temporarily can be used to keep larger cattle in sternal recumbency when left in the middle of a large space. Patients must be watched to make sure the rope is untied once they are awake enough to maintain the position on their own. It can be difficult to roll large ruminants into sternal recumbency with limited personnel. These patients should have a roll or pad placed under the head neck junction to assist drainage of the oral cavity until they are awake enough to roll up into sternal recumbency on their own.

Ruminant patients should be extubated in sternal recumbency with the endotracheal tube cuff inflated. This will squeegee any saliva or regurgitation trapped in the trachea above the cuff up into the oropharynx, where it can harmlessly drain from the mouth. Extubation should occur when the patient's chewing "threatens" the integrity of the endotracheal tube.

Ruminants generally stay recumbent during the recovery process until they are fully awake and functional. The most important requirement for achieving a smooth, uneventful recovery in ruminants is good footing. A calm recovery environment is always desirable, but only really necessary for extremely anxious or unruly ruminant patients. Ruminant patients that are not recovered in a confined space should be loosely tethered using the halter lead to prevent them from wandering after standing.

References

1. Steffey EP, Howland D: Cardiovascular effects of halothane in the horse, *J Am Vet Med Assoc* 39:611-615, 1978.
2. Hodgson DS, Steffey EP, Grandy JL et al: Effects of spontaneous, assisted and controlled ventilatory modes in halothane anesthetized geldings, *Am J of Vet Res* 47:992-996, 1986.

Recommended Readings

Lin HC, Tyler JW, Welles et al: Effects of anesthesia induced and maintained by continuous intravenous administration of guaifenesin, ketamine, and xylazine in spontaneously breathing sheep, *Am J Vet Res* 54:1913-1916, 1993.

Thurmon JC, Benson GJ, Tranquilli WJ et al: Cardiovascular effects of intravenous infusion of guaifenesin, ketamine, and xylazine in Holstein calves, *Vet Surg* 15:463, 1986.

CHAPTER 109

Managing Severe Pain in Ruminants

ERIC J. ABRAHAMSEN

The use of analgesic therapy in veterinary medicine has grown tremendously over the past two decades. The use of effective analgesic support is standard in the majority of small animal practices. Progress has been slower in the large animal sector of veterinary medicine. A combination of reasons is likely responsible for the reluctance to use effective analgesic therapy in large animal patients. The risk of adverse side effects associated with certain analgesic drugs such as morphine has been overstated for decades. Some clinicians are concerned that analgesic support will result in overuse of injured or recently repaired body components. Unfamiliarity with the use of newer or more potent analgesic agents in large animal patients amplifies these concerns.

Pain exhibited by ruminants can range from mild to debilitating. A wide array of options for providing analgesic support is available to the large animal practitioner. Local or regional techniques (local anesthetic blockade, epidurals, PainBuster) and systemic analgesic drug administration can be used alone or in combination to provide pain relief in large animal patients. Analgesic drugs available include nonsteroidal antiinflammatory drugs (NSAIDs), alpha$_2$-adrenergic agonists (xylazine, detomidine); opioids (morphine, butorphanol); N-methyl-D-aspartate (NMDA) receptor antagonists (ketamine); and local anesthetic agents. Drugs can be administered intermittently or, for a more consistent level of analgesia, delivered by constant rate infusion (CRI) or via a skin patch.

Providing an adequate level of analgesic support should be considered an essential part of patient care. Humane considerations are the primary reason for the explosive growth of analgesic therapy in veterinary medicine, but there are other benefits gained from the use of analgesic therapy. The general well-being of patients, as judged by appetite and demeanor, is improved with effective analgesic support. Reducing patient stress levels may aid the convalescence process. Effective analgesic support reduces the risk of overly stressing support limbs.

This chapter focuses on methods used to treat severe pain in ruminants. Additional information on pain management in food animal patients can be found in the therapeutic section of this book.

GENERAL CONCEPTS REGARDING ANALGESIC THERAPY

Preemptive treatment is more effective than treating pain once it becomes evident. Pain and inflammation produce activation of receptors in the central nervous system (CNS) that results in a phenomenon known as "wind up." The perception of pain is greater and more difficult to alleviate once "wind up" has taken place. When significant pain is anticipated from a diagnostic or therapeutic procedure, the administration of effective analgesic therapy before the perception of the pain will improve success in combating the discomfort and stress of the patient after the procedure. In my experience, the quality of recovery from general anesthesia in horses is improved when effective analgesic intervention is used.

COMBINATION THERAPY

Combining smaller doses of two or more analgesic drugs to provide relief in patients with mild to moderate pain reduces the level of side effects produced by each drug. Combining larger doses of two or more analgesic drugs may be required to provide adequate relief in patients with severe pain.

WHAT ABOUT THE RISK OF OVERUSE?

Long-term analgesic support is typically required in postoperative fracture patients to reduce stress levels in support limbs. Effective analgesic therapy also improves the general well-being of fracture patients. Heart and respiratory rates decrease while appetite and demeanor improve with effective analgesic therapy.

Intramuscular (IM) morphine (0.1 mg/kg IM q4h) does not totally eliminate pain during the early stages of convalescence in patients with more serious long bone fractures, and overuse has not been a problem. Morphine dose is reduced as the patient becomes more comfortable on the repaired limb to minimize the risk of overuse. Patients with less serious fractures still benefit from analgesic support, but the level must be titrated to the patient's condition to minimize the risk of overuse. Appropriate analgesic therapy should make the patient more comfortable while leaving enough pain to prevent overuse. The residual level of pain is also used to evaluate changes in patient status. It is important to compare equivalent points in the dosing interval to standardize the level of analgesia provided.

In equine patients we typically include a small dose of acepromazine (0.011-0.022 mg/kg IM, or 5-10 mg/450 kg) with each dose of morphine. Acepromazine was initially added to prevent any neuroexcitatory effects, though the presence of pain and smaller morphine dose make this unlikely. Ruminants do not seem to exhibit the same degree of sensitivity to this action of morphine. The small dose of acepromazine helps to minimize unnecessary activity in equine patients receiving analgesic support. Surgeons believe the calming influence of the acepromazine contributes to the successful recuperation of their orthopedic patients. The small dose of acepromazine does not typically produce overt tranquilization in equine patients and is reduced should this occur. I have not used acepromazine concurrently with morphine administration in ruminant patients. Ruminants tend to be less active than equine patients. Practitioners interested in limiting activity in a patient will have to experiment to determine if this dose of acepromazine is appropriate for ruminants.

OPIOIDS

The pain relief provided by NSAIDs is limited. Patients with moderate levels of pain require a greater degree of analgesic support. Systemic administration of an opioid can be used to increase the level of analgesic support for ruminant patients experiencing moderate levels of pain. Intravenous (IV) bolus administration provides a shorter, more intense analgesic effect. The higher peak blood levels achieved with IV bolus administration increase the risk of adverse side effects somewhat, though an initial IV bolus is often used to speed onset of relief in patients with more severe levels of pain. IM administration provides a longer duration of less intense analgesia. The lower peak blood levels produced by IM administration or CRI techniques reduce the risk of adverse side effects and are generally used to maintain analgesic support.

Butorphanol, an opioid agonist-antagonist, is the most widely used opioid in large animal practice. Butorphanol is a kappa and sigma opioid receptor agonist and a mu opioid receptor antagonist. Butorphanol (0.05-0.1 mg/kg IV or IM in smaller ruminants, 0.02-0.05 mg/kg IV or IM in larger ruminants) can provide total relief of milder levels of pain and a marked reduction in moderate levels of pain. Concomitant administration of an NSAID can be used to provide additional analgesic support in ruminant patients with moderate levels of pain.

Morphine, a mu opioid receptor agonist, is a more potent analgesic drug in most animal species, though it has traditionally been considered less effective in ruminant patients. Limited clinical experience indicates morphine (0.1 mg/kg IM) is capable of providing total relief of milder levels of pain and a marked reduction in moderate levels of pain in ruminant patients. Concomitant administration of an NSAID can be used to provide additional analgesic support in ruminant patients with moderate levels of pain.

Because of their competitive effects at the mu opioid receptor, butorphanol and morphine should not be used together. Butorphanol is quite expensive, whereas morphine is extremely cost effective. Given the economic nature of large animal practice, this price differential may be an important factor in determining which opioid is used, especially in larger ruminant patients.

The use of mu opioids is associated with several side effects, the most important being a negative impact on gastrointestinal (GI) motility. Morphine is also capable of producing CNS stimulation in many species. These adverse side effects are dose related. Much of the scientific literature regarding these complications involves doses much larger than we routinely employ for pain therapy in large animal patients. The presence of pain greatly reduces the incidence of CNS stimulation in patients receiving morphine. Unfortunately, veterinarians have been taught for decades that using morphine in large animal patients is likely to produce one or both of these adverse side effects. The incidence of GI complications (mild symptoms of colic and mild impactions) has been extremely low when smaller contemporary doses of morphine (0.1 mg/kg IV or IM) are used to provide analgesic support in equine patients. Persistent pain also decreases GI motility and likely contributes to the incidence of GI complications. I have maintained equine patients on morphine support for as long as 3 months without complications.

Large IV doses of morphine have been shown to reduce ruminoreticular contractions for up to 20 minutes. Administering an IV bolus of morphine (0.1 mg/kg) in nonanesthetized adult cattle has not resulted in rumen motility problems. Maintaining analgesic support with intramuscular administration or continuous IV infusion of morphine minimizes peak blood levels, reducing the potential for negative effects on rumen motility. Due to the more liquid nature of the colon contents in ruminants, impactions are less likely. I have not experienced a GI complication with morphine use in ruminants, but my experience is more limited in these patients.

The smaller contemporary doses reduce the clinical impact of morphine's GI effects but do not eliminate them. GI motility and fecal output (volume and moisture content) should be regularly monitored in patients receiving morphine. Morphine administration should be reduced or discontinued and medical treatment instituted if GI motility problems occur. A lidocaine-ketamine or lidocaine-ketamine-acepromazine infusion can be used to provide analgesic support in patients when morphine must be discontinued. The later section on Pentafusion provides information necessary to create these infusion mixtures.

Morphine (0.1 mg/kg IV or IM) can be administered to anesthetized ruminant patients expected to experience significant pain on recovery. Analgesic support can be maintained in ruminant patients with morphine (0.1 mg/kg IM q4h). Morphine doses in larger patients are often rounded to even milliliter increments to make the attendant paperwork easier. Morphine doses in smaller ruminant patients can often be rounded to 0.5-ml increments. Morphine onset is slow (10 minutes IV, 20 minutes IM). An initial IV bolus of morphine can be used to speed onset of relief in patients with more severe levels of pain with minimal risk of adverse side effects. If greater analgesic support is required, a higher dose of morphine (0.15 mg/kg IM) can be used transiently, but the combination of higher morphine and pain levels increases the risk of GI complications.

Morphine dose is reduced over time as patient comfort dictates. I have found morphine doses as small as 5 mg to make a difference in equine laminitis patients. Increasing the dosing interval reduces the mean analgesic effect, but peak effect remains unchanged and the risk of overuse increases. Analgesic support gradually declines over time following bolus administration of morphine, and extending the dosing interval drastically reduces the level of analgesia provided in the later stages of the interval.

TRIFUSION

In patients with severe pain, IM morphine in conjunction with NSAID administration does not provide sufficient relief. Increasing the dose of IM morphine can improve the level of relief provided, but the combination of higher morphine and pain levels increases the risk of GI complications. Using a CRI technique to deliver a steady state of analgesic support provided by a combination of drugs was the next logical step to try in these patients. The drug mixture used in the pain CRI was modified and refined over time. The five-drug mixture (Pentafusion) that resulted from this quest has been used in dozens of horses and proven to be effective in alleviating all but the most extreme pain in these patients. The Pentafusion mixture contains lidocaine, ketamine, morphine, detomidine, and acepromazine.

Food animal clinicians soon requested a similar approach but were concerned about the continuous delivery of the alpha$_2$-adrenergic agonist (detomidine) and acepromazine components of Pentafusion. Having no experience with continuous delivery of these drugs in ruminant patients to neutralize their concerns, I modified the technique, creating Trifusion.

Trifusion is a mixture of lidocaine, ketamine, and an opioid. I have used both butorphanol and morphine as the opioid component. I have used Trifusion in four adult cattle with severe to extreme pain. The first ruminant patient received a butorphanol-based combination, while the next three received a morphine-based combination. Trifusion provided obvious relief in these patients, though some pain remained. The small number of patients makes comparison of the opioid component difficult at this point. The initial pain level in these patients was quite high. Based on experience in horses, detomidine enhances the analgesic efficacy of the pain CRI and its inclusion may have provided greater analgesic support to these patients. Because detomidine is dosed similarly in cattle and horses, Pentafusion may eventually prove to be useful in ruminant patients as well. Trifusion was administered for several days in each of these patients with no adverse effects noted.

I have used a one-bag approach to deliver Trifusion to date. A two-bag approach would allow the opioid component to be delivered in a separate infusion. The two-bag approach typically used with Pentafusion allows greater flexibility in altering the levels of the drugs being delivered, which facilitates titration of the relief provided, adjustments to counter potential side effect produced by the drugs used, and eventual weaning when desired.

A CRI technique may seem complicated, but it is much easier than it first appears. One-bag administration of trifusion requires less equipment and simplifies application of this technique. Using a stock solution adjusted for patient weight further simplifies the use of Trifusion. Additional information on the creation and delivery of constant rate infusions is provided in Chapter 106.

Equipment Required for One-Bag Administration of Trifusion

1 Fluid pump*†
1 Solution administration set‡
2 Coiled extension sets§
1 L normal saline
1 Needle-lock device (if pain CRI is to be connected to IV fluid line)#

The following Pentafusion discussion provides the loading dose and infusion rate for morphine. Clinicians can use these doses when substituting butorphanol for morphine:

Loading dose of butorphanol (0.05-0.1 mg/kg IV or IM in smaller ruminants)
(0.02-0.05 IV or IM in larger ruminants)
Infusion rate for butorphanol (0.022 mg/kg/hr)

The loading dose for lidocaine is reduced in ruminant patients (1 mg/kg IV) and should be administered slowly to prevent adverse cardiovascular or CNS effects. Delivery of lidocaine and ketamine in the CRI mixture remains as described later.

TRIFUSION AND PENTAFUSION TECHNIQUE

The same basic approach is used to mix and deliver both Trifusion and Pentafusion. The following discussion on Pentafusion was written for equine presentations. It provides a background on the development, as well as a detailed explanation on how to create and deliver these analgesic mixtures.

PENTAFUSION

Lidocaine infusions (50 µg/kg/min) used to promote GI motility in postoperative colic patients do not seem to provide much systemic analgesia when used alone. Lidocaine becomes much more important when combined with other analgesic drugs. As an example, we had a horse with clostridial myositis that was extremely painful on presentation. IV and IM doses of detomidine and morphine had not produced much improvement when the primary clinicians on the case asked for a pain consult. I put the horse on a CRI of lidocaine (3 mg/kg/hr) and morphine (0.025 mg/kg/hr) (along with small doses of IM acepromazine). The horse remained uncomfortable, but there was a noticeable improvement with the infusion. Because higher blood levels of detomidine and morphine had not provided the same degree of relief, I surmised that the lidocaine contribution was much greater when it was combined with morphine. The lidocaine-morphine CRI did not provide the level of analgesia required to make this patient in extreme pain comfortable (it was eventually euthanatized), so I decided to add a small CRI of ketamine (0.6 mg/kg/hr) the next time I used the pain CRI technique. Ketamine is an NMDA receptor antagonist. Ketamine has been shown to possess potent analgesic effects when administered at subanesthetic doses. I was concerned about the potential for adverse behavioral effects (mania) resulting from morphine accumulation or excessive CNS stimulation from ketamine accumulation as infusion duration increased. I added a CRI of detomidine (0.0044 mg/kg/hr) to replace the small boluses of acepromazine I typically administer to equine patients receiving morphine. Detomidine possesses potent analgesic effects, and though the dose used was low, I hoped it would enhance the level of relief provided by the CRI technique while providing protection against drug-induced behavioral changes. This combination proved effective in treating severe laminitis pain (e.g., laterally recumbent with rapid heart and respiratory rates, "groaning" with each exhalation) in several patients.

Attempts to alter the rate of administration of some of the drugs contained in the pain CRI provided some insight as to the relative importance of those components in treating severe pain in the horse. In the next few laminitis patients I tried to substitute acepromazine (0.0022 mg/kg/hr) for the detomidine because it was being administered in IV boluses as part of the routine therapeutic approach in these patients, but I was not as satisfied with the relief provided. Detomidine was returned to the mix, but acepromazine was retained to help counter the vasoconstrictive effects of the detomidine and ketamine. A lower initial infusion rate of ketamine (0.3 mg/kg/hr) was tried in a couple of horses but yielded a less satisfactory level of relief. Patient pain also increased noticeably approximately 30 minutes following reduction or discontinuation of the ketamine component of the CRI, further indicating its importance and the potential for titrating the level of relief provided.

I use a two-bag approach when employing Pentafusion, though a one-bag approach could be used. The two-bag approach allows greater flexibility in altering the levels of the drugs being delivered, which facilitates titration of the relief provided, adjustments to counter potential side effect produced by the drugs used, and eventual weaning when desired. The ketamine and lidocaine are combined in one bag and the morphine, detomidine, and acepromazine combined in the second bag. Specific details regarding the creation and administration of Pentafusion are provided at the end of this section.

Pentafusion has been used successfully in dozens of horses to provide relief from severe pain at Ohio State. Many of these patients were facing imminent euthanasia when Pentafusion was instituted. The relief provided by Pentafusion allowed owners to be comfortable with continued treatment and several of these patients were eventually discharged from the hospital. A small number of the horses receiving Pentafusion have developed complications associated with decreased GI motility. Three horses developed mild impactions that were successfully resolved with the use of sodium sulfate and IV fluid therapy. One horse with extreme, uncontrollable pain developed severe abdominal bloating. Pain produces an adverse effect on GI motility and likely contributes to the GI complication rate in patients receiving opioid analgesic support. Careful monitoring of GI motility and fecal output (volume and moisture content) is vitally important when morphine or Pentafusion are used in the horse. Mineral oil should be administered via stomach tube if there is any question regarding GI motility or fecal

output to prevent an impaction from forming. Morphine and detomidine administration should be reduced or, if possible, eliminated when concerns regarding GI motility or fecal output arise. Lidocaine, ketamine, and acepromazine infusions can be maintained and seem to provide a reasonable amount of analgesia.

I have used Pentafusion for up to 17 days without complication, though the typical duration is shorter. I have encountered two horses to date with pain levels so severe that Pentafusion was not able to provide adequate relief. Clinical improvements such as return of appetite and the ability to get up for brief periods were evident in both of these patients with the use of Pentafusion, but even when a supersized rate (1.5×) of Pentafusion was used, adequate relief was not obtained. One of these patients experienced GI stasis and bloating during the enhanced rate of administration, though the problem persisted well beyond the discontinuation of the morphine and detomidine components of Pentafusion therapy and may have resulted, at least in part, from unrelenting pain. Both of these patients were eventually euthanatized.

When pain relief allows, we reduce the acepromazine-morphine-detomidine infusion rate (typically by half initially, and then perhaps by half again) before reducing the lidocaine-ketamine infusion rate. This allows us to alter the degree of analgesic support while at the same time reducing the administration rate drugs with the greatest concerns regarding GI motility.

PENTAFUSION: EQUIPMENT REQUIRED AND SAMPLE PROTOCOL

As mentioned earlier, Pentafusion is a mixture of ketamine, lidocaine, morphine, detomidine, and acepromazine. It is administered as a CRI for treating moderate to severe pain in equine patients.

Equipment Required for Two-Bag Administration

2 Fluid pumps*†
2 Solution administration sets‡
4 Coiled extension sets§
1-L normal saline
1 Needle-lock device (if pain CRI is to be connected to IV fluid line)#
1 High Flow Double T Extension Set¶
1 Sterile 1-L bag** (a liter bag of fluids can be emptied)

Equipment Required for One-Bag Administration

1 Fluid pump*†
1 Solution administration set‡
2 Coiled extension sets§
1 Sterile 1-L bag** (a liter bag of fluids can be emptied)
1-L normal saline
1 Needle-lock device (if pain CRI is to be connected to IV fluid line)#

I use a two-bag approach for the administration of Pentafusion. This approach allows greater flexibility and less waste when subsequent adjustments in drug administration are required to titrate the level of analgesia provided. A one-bag approach can be used, if required, by placing the morphine, ketamine, detomidine, and acepromazine in the bag containing the 2% lidocaine.

The drug volumes added to the bags are small enough to not alter the effective concentrations, and removal of a commensurate volume of carrier solution is not required when using this technique.

The infusion mixtures should be created in the bags before attaching and filling the lines. Otherwise, the extensive void volume of the lines will prevent delivery of medication for quite some time, limiting the usefulness of any loading boluses administered and delaying the onset of relief.

Sample Protocol (450-kg Patient)

The 450-kg mixture(s) can be used as a stock solution(s) with adjustments in delivery rate made to accommodate variations in patient size and/or alter the level of analgesic relief provided. The "450-kg base rate(s)" of infusion is adjusted to patient size using ratios (e.g., "patient base rate(s)" for a 337-kg horse is 75% or 0.75 of the "450-kg base rate(s)"). The "patient base rate(s)" determined in this manner can be further adjusted to alter the level of analgesia provided.

Bag #1

The empty sterile bag is filled with 1 L of 2% lidocaine. Lidocaine is administered at 50 µg/kg/min. For a 450-kg horse this is 22,500 µg/min, or 22.5 mg/min. Because 2% lidocaine is 20 mg/ml, one needs to administer 1.125 ml/min, or 67.5 ml/hr. This sets the flow rate for bag #1 at 67 ml/hr.

To bag #1 one adds the ketamine. Ketamine is administered at 10 µg/kg/min. For a 450-kg horse this is 4500 mcg/min, or 4.5 mg/min. The amount of ketamine required per hour is 270 mg, which must be contained in the 67 ml of lidocaine delivered per hour. The concentration of ketamine in the bag required to provide this level of administration is 4 mg/ml. I add 4 g of ketamine to the liter of 2% lidocaine.

Attach solution administration set and two coiled extension sets to bag #1 and fill the line. Set fluid pump for bag #1 at 67 ml/hr.

Bag #2

I typically set the infusion rate for bag #2 at the same level as calculated for bag #1. In this example it will be 67 ml/hr. Using the same infusion rate for bag #2 allows the drug amounts calculated for morphine, detomidine, and acepromazine to be added to the lidocaine solution for a one-bag technique. Morphine, detomidine, and acepromazine are added to a 1-L bag of normal saline in the following manner.

Morphine is dosed at 0.025 mg/kg/hr. One must administer 11.25 mg/hr, which must be contained in the 67 ml of saline delivered each hour. Concentration of morphine in the bag required to provide this level of administration is 0.17 mg/ml. Then 170 mg of morphine is added to the liter of normal saline.

Detomidine is dosed at 2 mg/450 kg/hr, or 2 mg/hr in this example. This amount must be contained in the 67 ml of saline delivered each hour. Concentration of detomidine in the bag required to provide this level of administration is 0.03 mg/ml. Then 30 mg of detomidine is added to the liter of normal saline.

Acepromazine is dosed at 1 mg/450 kg/hr, or 1 mg/hr. This amount must be contained in the 67 ml of saline delivered each hour. Concentration of acepromazine in the bag to provide this level of administration is 0.015 mg/ml. Then 15 mg of acepromazine is added to the liter of normal saline.

Attach solution administration set and two coiled extension sets to bag #2 and fill the line. Set the fluid pump for bag #2 at 67 ml/hr.

Constant Rate Infusion Technique

Create bags #1 and #2 based on patient body weight (or using the stock 450-kg approach). Fill lines and insert the administration sets in the fluid pumps and set volumes to be delivered. Attach the coiled extension sets leading from each of the treatment bags to the catheter or the IV fluid line using the High Flow Double T Extension Set. I use a needle-lock device to secure the High Flow Double T Extension Set to the Y-injection port of the primary fluid line if using that approach. Loading doses of several of the drugs can be given before starting the CRI to speed the onset of relief. I always administer a loading dose of lidocaine (1.3 mg/kg IV, administer slowly). If the patient has not recently received morphine as part of its prior therapeutic regimen, I generally give a loading dose of it as well (0.1 mg/kg IV) to speed onset of relief. I generally do not administer a loading dose of ketamine, detomidine, or acepromazine. Time to peak relief is typically several hours, so some patience is required.

When pain relief allows, I reduce the acepromazine-morphine-detomidine infusion rate (typically by half initially, and then perhaps by half again) before reducing the ketamine lidocaine infusion rate. This allows me to alter the degree of analgesic support while at the same time reducing the administration rate drugs with the greatest concerns regarding GI motility. Based on personal experience, the analgesic effects of the ketamine infusion are markedly diminished within 30 minutes of its discontinuation.

---

*Dial-A-Flow, Hospira Worldwide, Lake Forest, Ill. (flow control devices such as the Dial-A-Flow can be used to control infusion rates; other manufacturers make similar products).
†Heska Vet/IV 2.2, Heska Corp., Loveland, Colo. (compact rechargeable unit made for the veterinary market; many other models of infusion pumps are available including used human units).
‡Baxter Healthcare Corp., 10 drops/ml and approximately 68 inches long.
§CE8010, International Win, Ltd.
#2C7833, Baxter Healthcare Corp.
¶8575, Mila International, Inc.
**IntraVia Container, Baxter Healthcare Corp.

Cow-Calf Production Medicine

Brad J. White

CHAPTER 110

Marketing Beef Cow-Calf Production Medicine Programs in Private Practice

W. MARK HILTON

It is tremendous for a veterinarian to possess the skills necessary to help his or her clients achieve excellence in beef cow-calf production, but this knowledge is of no value if the client is unaware of this expertise. Veterinarians involved in production medicine need to be able to enunciate these skills and then market them to their producers so that both producer and veterinarian can be successful.

The first way the veterinarian can market these skills is through one-on-one communication. When a producer has a production-related problem, one must look at the problem and ascertain whether it could have been prevented. In most cases, the answer is affirmative. Depending on the urgency of the situation, now may be either a good time to discuss prevention or a poor time. If now is not the time, a callback or return trip in a few days would likely be appropriate. No matter, veterinarians must let the owner know that they are interested and available to provide consultative services. An example would be if a client were experiencing an outbreak of neonatal diarrhea in calves. Conditions that contribute to the disease need to be identified and corrected immediately to stop this disease from spreading. If, on the other hand, there is a 40% open rate in cows that just weaned their first calves, waiting a few days to discuss this problem may be best. The news of so many open cows may come as a shock and the owner may not be receptive to a discussion at this time.

As most veterinarians think about their own businesses or those of clients, they see owners and employees who are mostly overworked. Production medicine programs should not be overwhelming to the owner and, in fact, should help in doing the following:

1. Assist the owner in finding ways to decrease his cost of production per unit sold.
2. Assist the producer in adding value to the product he is selling.
3. Do both of the above with less time and labor.

One can devise the most complete beef cow-calf production medicine program in the world and have no one join the team if it is overwhelming in its scope. If it is not easy, it will likely not get done.

To make a program complete yet easy to implement, it should be broken down into a few parts. In my staff's program we identified the following as our seven areas of focus: herd health, records, fertility, nutrition, environment, genetics, and marketing.[1]

As we evaluate each herd we take notes and ask questions pertaining to these seven areas. In some herds we discuss only some of these areas and in others we touch them all. On an initial herd visit with a specific concern, we tend to discuss fewer areas of the program than if a herd has been a part of the program for many years. Because most problems are multifactorial, areas of concern frequently overlap.

In some herds, we develop a total beef herd health program in which all areas are covered at each consultation visit. Other herd owners may only want advice in a few areas of their operation. The program needs to be flexible for diverse producers. We find that achieving success in a limited program often leads to the addition of requests for advice in other areas.

MARKETING THE SEVEN AREAS OF BEEF COW-CALF PRODUCTION MEDICINE

Each herd health veterinarian has areas of strength and weakness in beef cow-calf production medicine. One should use areas of strength to build a program and either learn more about those areas in which expertise is lacking or build a team of experts for assistance. The best, of course, is to do both. Veterinarians should be comfortable using a team approach to help clients solve and prevent their problems. In fact, much of what we do as beef consultants is an evolution from the Integrated Resource Management Program initiated by the National Cattlemen's Association in the mid 1970s.[2]

HERD HEALTH

Herd health is the foundation of the veterinary business and training. Veterinarians need to be the experts and excellence is expected by clients. Questions to ask oneself include the following:

1. Does each herd have a custom-made herd vaccination and treatment program? This needs to be an easy-to-follow calendar that outlines all necessary health events.

2. Do herd owners understand herd biosecurity? Do they have a plan in place? A sign at the lane leading to the client's farm or ranch stating that one's clinic is in charge of herd biosecurity would be an excellent marketing tool.

3. Do your herds have specific disease control programs? Do producers understand diseases such as Johne's and bovine viral diarrhea? Veterinarians can hold meetings and write in newsletters about diseases that could affect herd health.

4. Are you the veterinarian who is called by the local or state cattlemen's association or extension service to speak at a beef meeting with health as the focus? If not, let them know you are available.

FERTILITY

Replacement Heifer Selection and Development

Proper management of replacement heifers provides a golden opportunity in many herds to make a positive impact on future production, and numerous veterinarians[1,3,4] have used this as a cornerstone to their production medicine programs. If herds experience poor rebreeding rates in nursing 2-year-old cows, many times this problem can be traced back to errors in selection and development of heifers younger than 2 years of age. A complete heifer program addresses all areas listed in Box 110-1.

Estrus Synchronization Programs

With about a dozen estrus synchronization programs available to clients, they are more than likely confused by all the choices.[6] Veterinarians can host meetings and write in newsletters about one or two of the programs that would best suit clients. Having an easy-to-follow handout with clinic information and a logo at the top is beneficial.

Extended Calving Season

For most herds, having a 65-day calving season for cows and a maximum 42-day calving season for heifers is ideal.[7] Herds calving for longer periods than these can be a source of financial loss and frustration for the owner. This is a prime example of how numerous areas of a production medicine program fit together to solve a larger problem. Explaining how health, nutrition, environment, records, and genetics affect fertility can be a real benefit to producers and would be a welcome educational topic at a beef field day.

NUTRITION

Dairy, swine, and feedlot clients may work closely with a livestock nutritionist. This is generally not the case in cow-calf operations. For the most part, nutrition companies supply salt, vitamins, and minerals to the cow-calf herd. Because these products amount to less than 5% of the yearly cost of keeping a cow, there is little financial incentive to spend much time with this segment of the industry.

Box 110-1

Components of Complete Replacement Heifer Program

- Selection
- Nutrition
- Prebreeding vaccinations
- Prebreeding reproductive tract scoring[5]
- Estrus synchronization recommendations[6]
- Determination of length of breeding season
- Selection of artificial insemination (AI) or natural service sires.

A great marketing tool for a veterinarian is to have a field day at a client's farm/ranch where he or she has developed a heifer program. Other clients will see that a dystocia rate of less than 15% and a rebreeding rate of 90% to 95% is not only possible, but expected.[7]

Although most veterinarians have limited training in cow-calf nutrition, the educational opportunities for them are almost endless. Using the expertise of extension or university-based faculty can be a real benefit to producers.

Cow Herd Nutrition

With yearly cow feed cost accounting for 56.7% of the variation in profitability of cow herds,[8] having a true nutrition program should be an absolute. Too many herds do not have an accurate inventory of feedstuffs available for winter feeding, nor do they have analysis for those feedstuffs. In a study in Nebraska, researchers showed that "forage testing and allocation of feeds for best use allowed producers to save an average of $25 per cow in feed supplements without jeopardizing performance or herd health."[9] With many computer ration-balancing programs available, formulating cost-effective yet simple rations can be an excellent practice builder. Veterinarians can take a laptop computer on all farm calls, and when a producer has a question about nutrition or one feels a more cost-effective ration can be formulated, a ration demonstration can be given to make a point. Charging an hourly fee to formulate rations that will save the owner thousands of dollars is cost effective for both the owner and the veterinarian.

Purchased Feed Consultation

Many herd owners purchase unnecessary supplemental feeds. The use of protein blocks and energy tubs are almost never cost effective. A veterinarian's advice here could be a real money saver for the producer. Time spent giving this advice can be charged as a part of the nutrition program.

Mineral Program

Standardized performance analysis (SPA) data show no correlation between dollars spent on cow minerals and total herd profit.[10] My experience is that those producers spending the most on minerals are wasting money. Instead of a haphazard nutrition program, one can offer a complete program that ties all elements together in one package.

GENETICS

As the concepts of value-based marketing and national animal identification continue to grow, producers need to improve quality if they expect to be paid a price above commodity beef. Producers are looking for an unbiased source of information when it comes to what genetics they should use. A veterinarian can be that source.

For a genetic program, the veterinarian can be compensated on a per-cow basis for helping to select artificial insemination (AI) sires or on a percentage basis of purchase price for natural service sires. If the genetic program is a part of the total beef herd health program, it is already calculated in that fee.

Heifer Program

Selecting AI sires to use on virgin heifers to reduce dystocia while maintaining adequate growth can be very beneficial to overall herd profit. If dystocia rates in heifers have exceeded farm/ranch goals of less than 15%, selecting bulls to reduce dystocia should be a short-term goal. Our recommendations based on heifer genetics are listed in Table 110-1. We want all AI sires used on heifers to be greater than .90 for birth weight (BW) expected progeny differences (EPD) accuracy for enhanced confidence. While giving recommendations, one should bear in mind that not all breeds have bulls that should be used on heifers.

Cow Program

Many herds have used breeds of bulls that have not necessarily improved their overall profitability. We have lost heterosis in the quest for the elusive carcass premium. Feed-out data from across the United States have shown that cattle of approximately 50% to 75% British and 25% to 50% Continental genetics are the most profitable.[11,12]

The largest benefit of heterosis, though, is realized via the cow herd. Research at Montana State University showed that crossbred cows netted $70 more profit per year than straight-bred cows.[13] With historic profit levels

Table **110-1**

Recommendations to Reduce Dystocia

Heifer Genetics	BW EPD Angus Bulls	BW EPD Red Angus Bulls
Primarily British heifers	<2	<−1
British × Continental or primarily Continental heifers	<0	<−3

BW EPD, Birth weight expected progeny difference.

of 2% return on assets, many cow-calf businesses have not shown enough profit to be sustainable.[14] So, with a concept such as improved heterosis showing such a huge financial impact, working with producers in this area seems beneficial.

ENVIRONMENT

Anything that involves the cattle's environment is included in this area. Concerns that fit here nicely are calving area, handling facilities, and management-intensive grazing.

Calving Environment

If neonatal disease exists, the first goal is to identify the environmental factors predisposing to disease. It takes time to formulate a plan to stop disease and then to prevent it. Writing up instructions for cow and calf flow during calving can be a significant benefit.

Handling Facilities

We kept numerous plans for cattle handling facilities in our office for clients to use. We never charged for this service, but I feel any improvement in facilities is a plus for the veterinarian.

Management-Intensive Grazing

Management-intensive grazing (MiG) can be viewed as a case of "where's the profit for the clinic?," but MiG fits nicely into our overall philosophy of making the beef herd a low-cost, low-maintenance business. If one has an interest in MiG, one will likely do work for clients who embrace this technology. I have found these producers to be excellent clients. Most are progressive and want to add more programs to their business.

This is an area in which it is likely that an extension specialist or Natural Resources Conservation System (NRCS) specialist will be the expert. This again builds a team for the owner and these specialists may be a source of marketing for one's program, because they generally deal with the most progressive owners.

RECORDS

Herd Production Records

The first program a veterinarian should offer clients is herd production records. As an industry, the beef cow-calf segment is woefully deficient in herd records.[15] If one begins a production medicine program without herd records, it will likely fail. Records indicate where things stand; records alone are not enough. Veterinarians need targets so that they know where to go, benchmarks to see how they compare, and analysis to see how they will get there. This is truly a key to any production medicine program. Most clinics charge for the records on a per-cow basis. By researching the commonly used computer programs (e.g., CowSense, CowCalf 5, CHAPS), one can see which is the best business fit. The most important factor is not which program a veterinarian purchases but the promptness of service the veterinarian provides. Records need to be entered soon after the clinic receives the information and then reports need to be generated and analyzed in a timely fashion. The veterinarian should write comments on the reports if it has been a full year since the last one; reminders of terms and concepts are appreciated. Appointments with key herd personnel should be made to go over all reports and answer questions. The time working on reports should be charged at the veterinarian's normal hourly rate. If the veterinarian simply sends the owner a stack of papers with many numbers, the program will fail.

Herd Financial Records

Although some clinics provide a financial records program that is done in-house for their clients, many use outside contractors for these services. Performing a full SPA for a herd can be a daunting task.[16] Many other programs are available and a cost-benefit analysis must be done before deciding to do this oneself or farm it out. One thing is certain—the owner has a high probability of learning much more about the herd from an economic standpoint. Ideally this should occur before the owner starts on a production medicine program so that the veterinarian can show financial progress as a result of his or her recommendations. If this service is performed, the normal hourly fee is appropriate to use. If an outside contractor provides the service, the owner pays the contractor directly. In either case, one's time spent on analysis is added to the production medicine fee.

MARKETING

Many beef herd owners tend to dislike the marketing aspect of their cattle business. They enjoy the production side, and marketing gets neglected. Does the herd health veterinarian have opportunities in this area?

Feeder Cattle Alliances

Much has been written lately about marketing alliances. Too much variation occurs in fed beef cattle, and programs to help reduce that variation are a real positive. A veterinarian who works with numerous herds could incorporate this concept into his or her total plan.

Organizing producers to sell cattle of similar health status, genetic base, and age in load lots could produce large financial benefits for clients. Networking with another veterinarian who has clients that custom feed cattle could be another opportunity. More and more cattle are being sold on a value-based market, and producers of high-health, high-quality cattle should benefit from this system. If producers do not know anything about their cattle

after they leave the farm or ranch, learning of their gain, health, and carcass data would greatly benefit herd owners. One client with 50 cows has little opportunity to capture these data, but 5 calves each from 35 herds make two potloads of calves for the custom feeder. In the Indiana Beef Evaluation and Economics Feeding (IBEEF) Program, producers pay $30/calf for this service.[12]

Replacement Female Alliances

As carcass premiums and discounts continue to widen, having a more uniform, profitable cow herd will become more important. Fewer herd owners should be trying to produce their own heifers and some herd owners may find this as a niche market. We have numerous clients who produce high-quality replacement heifers. Open heifers tend to sell for about $100 per head over market and bred heifers about $200 more than ones at the sale barn. We considered having our own bred female sale for our Total Beef Herd Health members but never did it mainly because of producers' success selling these females privately.

Replacement females could be advertised in one's clinic newsletter, or one could organize a replacement female sale once per year as another option. In both instances the client is paid adequately for his premium product and the veterinarian is compensated for the marketing component.

ADDITIONAL MARKETING IDEAS

Veterinarians who engage in production medicine see their clients' livestock enterprise as a business. To successfully market a production medicine program to clients, the clients must also see their enterprise as a business. As with any consultative service, the recommendations need to produce positive results.

These results must lead to additional profit or reduced expenses (or both) for the owner, and the fees charged by the veterinarian must equal value to the client. If all these things happen, the veterinarian has a successful program that he or she can demonstrate as a cost-effective option to his clientele.[1]

Some methods of marketing a cow-calf production medicine program have already been outlined: writing newsletters, having farm/ranch tours and field days, speaking at cattlemen's and extension meetings, having client education meetings, and having one-on-one discussions.

Additional ideas gained from personal experience or from talking to other veterinarians are listed in Box 110-2. Beef cow-calf producers are asking for additional services from their veterinarians. Developing a production medicine program is the first step in the process, but developing a marketing program is also essential.

Box 110-2

Additional Marketing Methods

- Only make two to three main recommendations at a time. Many times the owner can list a number of concerns for the herd in question, but prioritizing the list is difficult. We veterinarians can help by targeting the "weakest link in the chain" (i.e., the most economically important issue). If we overwhelm the owner, he or she will generally do the easiest thing first or do nothing.
- Develop a herd as your "pilot herd." Pick a client who asks questions, desires excellence, and accepts change. This herd owner must also allow you to have minor setbacks as you develop your program. Having a field day at this location can be a useful marketing tool for your program. Let the owner tell your clients what you have done for his herd.
- Write articles for your local newspaper that focus on production medicine topics.
- Take every opportunity to discuss production medicine. Always be aware of the correct timing.
- Have a client education meeting to specifically outline the costs and benefits of your program. Talk about financial gains and improving quality. Take few herds (≤10) the first year so that you do an outstanding job with each one.
- Use a questionnaire that will provide you with valuable information about the client's herd. Outline the questions in the seven areas mentioned earlier.
- Talk to other producers about your pilot herds and the changes you have recommended.
- Write about your production medicine program in your clinic newsletter. Do not hesitate to be a bit controversial on a subject—this is a great way to see if clients read the newsletter.
- Have your local newspaper do a story about your program, featuring your pilot herd.
- Target your good to excellent herd owners who are not on your program and ask them every year, "How can I assist you in the coming year to help make your beef business more successful?"

- Do not expect your bottom herds to join the program.
- Use experts in the field to assist you in building your program. There is no reason to reinvent the wheel and make every mistake yourself.
- Attend continuing education meetings that focus on herd health, production medicine, and integrated resource management.
- Have a yearly herd visit to answer questions, see updates in the operation, and review the yearly records. Write a follow-up report outlining successes and concerns in the seven areas.
- Before each yearly herd visit, ask the herd owner what the top three short-term (1-3 years) and top three long-term (5-10 years) goals are for the herd. Be sure to address how you will help the herd owner achieve those goals.
- Have a yearly meeting at your clinic for your production medicine clients. Poll your herd owners ahead of time to find out what subject(s) they would like addressed. Pick one and hire an expert in the field to be the morning speaker. After lunch have a roundtable discussion at which members of your production team (e.g., herd owners, forage specialists, nutritionists) share successes and failures of their own operations. This is a great opportunity for herd owners to learn from one another.
- Allow nonmembers to attend your production medicine meeting one time for free. If they want to attend the following year, you may want to assess a fee.
- Learn to say "no." You do not have to do everything for every herd. If it is not cost effective for you as the veterinarian, delegate it or do not do it.
- This is not a static program. As your clients demand more from you, you need to provide these services.

References

1. Hilton WM: *Delivery of a production medicine program in an Iowa veterinary practice.* Proceedings of the 110th Annual Meeting of the Iowa Veterinary Medical Association, Des Moines, January 1991.
2. Corah LR: The history of IRM and SPA, *Vet Clin North Am Food Anim Pract* 11:191-198, 1995.
3. Chenoweth PJ, Sanderson MW: Health and production management in beef cattle breeding herds. In Radostits OM, editor: *Herd health: food animal production medicine*, ed 3, Philadelphia, 2001, Saunders, p 509.
4. Larson RL: In Chenoweth PJ, Sanderson MW, editors: *Beef practice: cow-calf production medicine*, Ames, Iowa, 2005, Blackwell, p 127.
5. Anderson KJ, LeFever DG, Brinks JS et al: The use of reproductive tract scoring in beef heifers, *Agri-Practice* 12:19, 1991.
6. American Association of Bovine Practitioners North Central Region Reproductive Task Force publication.
7. Ringwall KA, Helmuth KJ: *1998 NCBA-IRM-SPA Cow-Calf Enterprise Summary of Reproduction and Production Performance Measures for CHAPS Cow-Calf Producers.*
8. Miller A, Knipe R: Characteristics of high profit cow herds, *Improving the Competitiveness of the Illinois Beef Industry*, March 2000.
9. Anderson B, Rice D, Kubik D et al: Forage analyses for dietary diagnosis and management, *Agri-Practice* 12:29-35, 1991.
10. Dunn B: *Factors affecting profitability of Northern Great Plains beef cow-calf enterprise.* SPA-EZ Seminar, American Association of Bovine Practitioners Meeting, Rapid City, SD, September 20, 2000.
11. Schiefelbein D: Data from the Gelbvieh Grid Feedlot Program. *Personal communication*, 2006.
12. *Indiana Beef Evaluation and Economics Feeding Program* (website): http://www.ansc.purdue.edu/ibeef. Accessed January 9, 2007.
13. Davis KC, Tess MW, Kress DD et al: Life cycle evaluation of five biological types of beef cattle in a cow-calf range production system: II. Biological and economic performance, *J Anim Sci* 72:2591-2598, 1994.
14. Dunn B: *Factors affecting profitability of the cow-calf enterprise.* Proceedings of the 35th Annual Convention of the American Association of Bovine Practitioners, Madison, Wis, September 2002.
15. Kniffen D: NCA-IRM desk record, *Vet Clin North Am Food Anim Pract* 11:215, 1995.
16. McGrann JM: Farm financial standards, *Vet Clin North Am Food Anim Pract* 11:279-291, 1995.

CHAPTER 111

Economic Analysis Techniques for the Cow-Calf Practitioner

THOMAS R. KASARI

Beef cattle producers are becoming increasingly more cost conscious about veterinary services. Veterinarians can provide a vital service to their clients if they are able to use economic analysis techniques to show them that it makes (or does not make) economic sense to implement a specific management procedure or accept a veterinary medical procedure. As a point of reference, a distinction is made between economic decision making and financial decision making. The former involves decisions concerning only the management (allocation) of scarce resources; in this case it is money, to achieve the farm's or ranch's desired goals,[1] whereas the latter involves decisions concerning the multiple facets of planning, acquiring, and using monetary funds in a way that achieves the farm's or ranch's desired goals.[2] This chapter focuses solely on economic decision-making analytic techniques.

Unfortunately, many, if not most, veterinarians have not received formal training in the various analytic techniques that are available to help answer specific questions that have short-term (≤1 year) operational or long-term (>1 year) strategic economic ramifications. This chapter is an attempt to describe some of these common techniques.

ECONOMIC TECHNIQUES TO USE FOR SHORT-TERM DECISION MAKING

Most farmers and ranchers do not have an endless supply of money with which to run their business each year. Operational decisions during the course of a year should be made based on expenditures that offer a monetary benefit that exceeds its cost of implementation. Analytic techniques that assist this short-term decision-making perspective include partial budgeting, decision trees, and standardized performance analysis (SPA).

PARTIAL BUDGETING

Partial budgeting is a tool that helps estimate the effect that the allocation of money to a management change for a current on-farm or on-ranch program will have on profitability to the operation. When developing a partial budget, only the revenue and costs affected by the specific change are considered. Consequently, this technique examines only a small part of business activities. If the proposed management change will affect the *entire* farm or ranch enterprise, a partial budget is inappropriate to use. Instead, a total enterprise budget is needed based on

a full cost analysis in which all variable and fixed costs are considered.

Typically, a partial budget assumes that the outcome of the analysis will occur exactly as calculated; thus variability in inputs and subsequently their effect on output of results is not considered. However, specialized computer software (e.g., @Risk, Palisade Corporation, Newfield, New York) is available that can evaluate the impact that variability in inputs has on partial budget results.

A partial budget is divided into two sections: *added returns* and *added costs*.[3] *Added returns* include (1) the increased revenue generated by the proposed management change and (2) decreased costs resulting from the proposed management change. *Added costs* include (1) the amount of revenue foregone because of the proposed management change and (2) the increased costs associated with the implementation of the proposed management change. The difference between *added returns* and *added costs* determines if the proposed management change is more profitable (>$0) or less profitable (<$0) than the status quo. Only profitable management changes should be considered for implementation.

The following scenario is presented to illustrate the construction and analysis of a partial budget:

A beef cow-calf producer comes to you as the veterinarian during the early summer to enlist your help in determining why over the past few years he has averaged 20 bred cows of various ages (out of 300 breeding cows) that are thinner than herdmates heading into the winter feeding period. In addition to their winter pasture, he can usually get some back in shape after segregating and feeding them 5 lb of 20% protein cubes per head daily for 100 days. The feed cost ($290/ton; $0.145/lb) and associated labor to feed and care for them ($12/hr; 0.50 hr) are estimated to be $1.025 per cow per day ([5 lb × $0.145/lb] + [($12/hr × 0.50 hr)/20 hd]). At the end of this feeding period, eight cows typically remain thin and are eventually culled because they do not breed back after calving. He buys young bred cows to replace these cull cows. He sold these cull cows last year at a loss of $550 ($1000 replacement cost and $450 salvage value per head) and expects these market prices to remain steady for the next 2 years.

After a visit to the ranch and a thorough investigation of all the factors that can be responsible for a "thin cow" problem, internal parasitism is determined to be the root cause. You recommend that this producer institute a deworming program for all his cows this winter and again sometime during the spring before turnout to grazing pastures. You believe this should essentially alleviate the reproductive failure observed in these problem "thin cows" and the necessity to cull them. Following anthelmintic treatment, body condition should improve enough to restore reproductive efficiency in these cows to that of the rest of the herd as well as follow their same culling pattern. His current weaned calf crop is 82% (500 lb average steer calf weaning weight; 480 lb average heifer weaning weight). He routinely keeps back around 30% (36 Hd) of the weaned heifers as replacements in order to keep his cow herd at a stable size (he shows you records that around 88% (264 Hd) of the cow herd calves each year). The owner is willing to spend the $5 per head (anthelmintic, labor, miscellaneous) to deworm the cow herd but inquires if other advantages will be gained by doing this. You tell him that a 20-lb increase in calf weaning weight is not unusual to see, presumably because the cows milk better after eliminating their internal parasite burden. The producer predicts that he will sell his steer calves next fall at $110/hunderweight (cwt) base price for a 500-lb calf along with an $8/cwt price slide. The heifer calves will likely sell at $102/cwt for a 480-lb calf along with the same price slide as steers.

Given the aforementioned information, the partial budget is constructed as follows:

Added Returns		$11801
Increased Revenue	$2751	
Increased steer weaning weight— 300 Hd × .82* × .5† × $13.68‡		
Increased heifer weaning weight— 300 Hd × .82 × .5 × .70§ × $12.40‖		
Decreased Costs	$9050	
Eliminate protein supplementation— 20 Hd × $1.025 × 100 Day		
Eliminate purchase of replacements for culled open thin cows— (8 Hd × .88¶ = ≅ 7) × $1000/Hd		
Added Costs		$6150
Increased Costs	$3000	
Management change of performing deworming procedure— 300 Hd × $5/Hd × 2		
Decreased Revenue	$3150	
Eliminate sales of culled open thin cows— (8 Hd × .88 = ≅ 7) × $450/Hd		
Added returns *less* added costs		$5651

Because the difference between added returns and added costs is a positive number (>$0), anthelmintic treatment is considered a profitable management change.

*Weaned calf crop percentage.
†Half of the calves are steers.
‡([500 lb + 20 lb]/100) × ($110/cwt − [($8/100) × 20 lb]) − ([500 lb/100] × $110/cwt).
§Only 70% of the heifers are sold; 30% are kept for replacements.
‖([480 lb + 20 lb]/100) × ($102/cwt − [($8/100) × 20 lb]) − ([480 lb/100] × $102/cwt).
¶Although this number represents calving percentage (pregnancy percentage + in utero losses), it is used as a proxy for pregnancy percentage in this example.

The partial budget analysis also shows the benefit to cost of the proposed short-term management change. In the previous example, the benefit to cost is approximately 1.92 ($11801/$6150), which means that nearly $1.92 is returned for every $1 allocated to the cost of this management practice. Partial budgeting is not the only method that provides information on the benefit to cost of a proposed management change. A Standardized Performance Analysis (SPA) of the producer's cow-calf operation can also be used for this purpose (see discussion below).

STANDARDIZED PERFORMANCE ANALYSIS

SPA was developed from an initiative of the National Cattleman's Beef Association in 1991.[6] As the name implies, SPA is an economic analysis tool and not an accounting or record keeping system. It focuses on financial/economic and production performance to determine the unit cost of production (UCP). The UCP is the cost incurred over time to produce each hundredweight (cwt) of calf up through weaning.

Because SPA is a standardized format, ranches can be more readily compared. The standard format also forces accurate input of data. Meaningful information cannot be expected to come out of incomplete or erroneous data. Therefore proper financial statement and production records are necessary to complete an accurate analysis. Once UCP is determined, the benefit to cost of management decisions can easily and confidently be answered (e.g., "Should steer calves receive a growth promotant implant?"; "Should calves be dewormed?"; Should a breeding soundness examination be done on a bull battery?").

An SPA analysis is based on historical data. This includes cattle and feed inventories, accounting data required for Internal Revenue Service (IRS) tax filings, a depreciation schedule, and accrual adjusted income statements. The SPA program is a computerized Windows-based system (Microsoft Corporation, Redmond, Wash.) that is divided into two parts: SPA production (breeding season to weaning) and SPA financial (for fiscal year calves are weaned). Numerous paper-based worksheets have been developed that can be used to help organize the data before entry into this computerized system.

STANDARDIZED PERFORMANCE ANALYSIS PRODUCTION

Every SPA analysis starts with the production section of the analysis.[6] The following production data are necessary to successfully complete this section:

- General ranch and herd descriptive data
- Cowherd management/production season
- Weaned calf production and value
- Cull or breeding cattle sales
- Owned and leased land use
- Raised and purchased feed use and inventory
- Purchased and raised breeding cattle inventories
- Number of breeding females "exposed" (i.e., the original number of females turned out with bulls at the start of the breeding season)

These production data are then organized into the following categories for analysis:

- Reproduction
- Production
- Marketing description
- Grazing and raised feed
- Amount of raised and purchased feed fed

The *reproduction* and *production* measures are determined using the same common denominator of "exposed" females.

Reproduction

The measures include pregnancy percentage, pregnancy loss percentage, calving percentage, calving distribution (day 1-21; 22-42; 43-63; >63 days); calf death loss percentage; calf crop percentage (weaning percentage); female replacement percentage (raised and purchased); cow death loss percentage; and calf death loss percentage based on the number of calves born.

Production

The measures include average calf weaned age (months), actual and average weaning weight for steers/bulls and heifers, and pounds of calf weaned per "exposed" female.

Cattle inventories are a critical element of this section of SPA. They are summarized by stage of production (beginning of the fiscal [accounting] year, beginning of breeding season, beginning of calving season). Other activities that are recorded include in and out movements of raised and purchased females; purchases, sales, and transfers of breeding females (and any calves at side); quantity of grazing land and raised land and their use; and quantity of feed fed.

Marketing Information

Marketing information that must be documented in SPA production includes method of marketing (e.g., private treaty, livestock auction, video auction, retained ownership); pricing method (e.g., cash, hedged); and dominant breed comprising the cowherd. Cattle prices ($/cwt) are segregated based on pay weight (not adjusted weaning weight) for bull calves, steer calves, and heifer calves (replacements and nonreplacements). In addition, a weighted average ($/cwt) price is used for cull mature breeding stock (cows and bulls) sold during the fiscal year.

Grazing and Raised Feed

The dominant grazing method for "exposed" females must be reported. Total grazed and raised feed acres are partitioned into grazing and raised feed acres per "exposed" female, grazing acres per "exposed" female, raised feed acres per "exposed" female, crop aftermath acres per "exposed" female, and pounds of calf weaned per acre used by the cow-calf enterprise.

Amount of Feed Fed

A beginning and ending (based on calendar year) raised and purchased feed inventory must be made. The quantity of raised and purchased feed must be determined based on the number of pounds of feed fed per breeding cow.

STANDARDIZED PERFORMANCE ANALYSIS FINANCIAL COMPONENT

The following data are necessary for the fiscal or tax year that calves are weaned in order to successfully complete the financial component of SPA[6]:

- IRS tax schedules for the fiscal year of analysis
  - Schedule F—Profit or loss from farming
  - Form 4562—Depreciation and amortization
  - Form 4797—Sales of business property
- Depreciation schedule for the producer's farm or ranch
- Loan payment schedules from each lender
- Beginning and ending balance sheet (BS) showing all business assets, liabilities, and owner's equity
- Income statement (IS)

A producer's accountant can be of great assistance in preparing the necessary financial data used in SPA financial.

Balance Sheet

The BS should show beginning and ending fiscal year amounts (note: the ending BS amount from the previous year serves as the beginning balance for the following year). An important aspect of the BS is that long-term asset values (e.g., buildings and equipment) reflect a historical cost basis adjusted downward each year for accumulated depreciation. Depreciation can be viewed as the amount ($) by which the asset is "used up" or "wears out" or "useful life disappears" each year. This new adjusted value is called the "book value" of the asset. Land is also recorded at its historical value but is not depreciated because land does not "wear out" or "disappear," per se.

A depreciation schedule should show separate categories for breeding livestock, buildings and improvements, and machinery and equipment. For IRS purposes, an accelerated depreciation schedule (e.g., MACRS) is probably used for depreciable assets, whereas for SPA purposes, a straight-line depreciation schedule is used. Any loan repayment schedules should include interest and principal payments, as well as inventory information (e.g., livestock, feed). For comparison to historical cost, the BS also reports items at fair market value.

Income Statement

The IS (also known as a profit and loss statement) is accrual based rather than cash based. The main difference between a cash-basis and accrual-basis approach is that with a cash-basis IS, income is recorded when cash, a check, or other monetary instrument is received for the product or service sold. An expense is recorded when the bill is actually paid by the producer. In contrast, accrual-basis income is recorded at the time the product is sold or service rendered, regardless of when cash is received from the buyer. An expense is recorded at the time that it occurs, regardless of when the bill is paid by the producer.

The IS prepared by most producers is almost entirely a cash basis because this is the form of submission the IRS prefers. Therefore a cash-basis IS must be reworked to yield an accrual-basis IS. Accrual adjustments are made for changes in inventory, accounts receivable, accounts payable, and prepaid expenses. Gains (revenue received is in excess of book value) and losses (revenue received is below book value) on sales of breeding livestock are also included in the IS.

Cow-calf financial cost elements in SPA include owners' labor and management (living cost), depreciation expense, raised replacement valuation, interest paid, and overhead. Opportunity costs (equivalent to the next best use of the asset) are also determined for capital, owned land (cost at cash lease rate), and raised feed (at market value) because these assets could be sold rather than used by the producer. The SPA financial component also inputs a cost for owner labor and management. The cost that is used is equivalent to what the salary would be to hire a non–family member to provide the equivalent service.

Standardized Performance Analysis Financial Reports

When completed, the most meaningful SPA results are reported on a per-cow basis. The actual SPA Financial and Economic Performance Summary (cost and fair market value) includes the following:

- Investment per breeding cow (average asset values)
  - Total investment per breeding cow
  - Debt per breeding cow (enterprise liabilities)
  - Equity-to-asset or percent equity
- Financial and economic performances
  - Total raised/purchased feed cost
  - Total grazing cost
  - Gross cow-calf enterprise accrual-basis revenue
  - Total financing cost and economic return
  - Total cost before noncalf revenue adjustment (i.e., revenue adjusted for cull cow and bull sales)
  - Net income
  - Return on assets (ROA) percentage
- Unit cost of weaned calf production (UCP)
  - Total noncalf revenue (i.e., revenue from cull cow and bull sales)
  - Total calf cost (adjusted for noncalf revenue)

Using UCP as the starting point for determining the benefit to cost of any short-term health management practices in the cow-calf operation is far superior to the aforementioned use of a partial budget.

Further information about SPA can be found on the Texas A&M University Extension Agricultural Economics website at http://agrisk.tamu.edu.

DECISION TREE ANALYSIS

A decision tree is a method of choice for making an informed decision about how to manage an animal health problem when several options are feasible, but each one has an uncertain outcome. Thus this decision-making technique is not focused on the prediction of an event but rather on weighing the outcome of the respective options in a relative sense.[3] The preferred action is chosen based on a predetermined decision criterion (e.g., highest expected monetary value or minimal losses).

A decision tree is constructed using lines (referred to as branches) that connect to squares (decision node), circles (chance node), and triangles (final outcome node).[4] As the name implies, a decision tree always begin with a decision node. Leading away from it in a rightward direction are two or more branches that comprise the various decisions to be made (e.g., medical treatment vs. surgical treatment vs. salvage). The decisions must be exhaustive (i.e., include all choices to be considered) and exclusive (i.e., only one choice is ultimately possible at a decision node).[4] Furthermore, each branch emanating away from a decision node can lead to one of three places: (1) to another decision node, which will then have two or more additional branches, representing decisions to be made, leading away from it; (2) to a chance node, which will then have two or more branches leading away from it representing potential outcomes (e.g., successful vs. unsuccessful; favorable vs. unfavorable); or (3) directly to a final outcome node.[5] Likewise, branches off a chance node can lead to one of three places: to another decision node, to another chance node, or directly to an outcome.[5] Associated with each branch emanating from a chance node is a probability that that specific outcome will occur. Mathematically, the probabilities are assigned to each branch in such a manner that they add up to 1.[4,5] These probabilities can be established based on personal experience, expert opinion, unpublished experimental or clinical data, and/or published literature.

Each branch of a decision tree will eventually end with a terminal node that signifies a final outcome. Each final outcome is expressed in monetary terms. Each monetary outcome (value) takes into account (1) the cost associated with implementing each intervention and any other associated losses and (2) either the animal (or herd) value associated with successful intervention or the animal (or herd) value associated with unsuccessful intervention.

A monetary outcome is not always automatically at its correct amount for subsequent comparison with the monetary outcomes determined for the other branches of the decision tree. A monetary value is at its correct amount if the branch of the decision tree to which it is assigned traces directly back from the terminal node to the original decision node without coursing through a chance node. In contrast, it is not at its correct amount if it was assigned to a branch of a decision tree that traced back from the terminal node through one or more chance nodes, with associated probabilities, to the original decision node. In the latter situation, to determine the correct amount, begin by multiplying the monetary value of the outcome

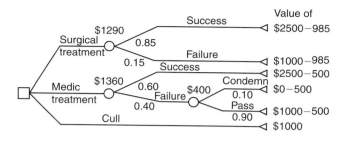

□ = Decision node   ○ = Chance node   ◁ = Outcome

Fig 111-1   Decision tree constructed to determine the best course of action (treat surgically, treat medically, cull) to follow for a bull that has sustained a preputial prolapse of traumatic origin.

at the terminal node by the probability associated with the branch leading from this node back to the first chance node that it connects to. Repeat this procedure for the remaining monetary values assigned to terminal nodes with branches leading back to this same chance node. These new "weighted" monetary values are then summed to provide a revised monetary value at the level of this chance node. Continue repeating this procedure for each of the other monetary outcomes with branches involving chance nodes, progressively working from right to left until all branches of the decision tree have been collapsed down to only the decisions that emanate from the original decision node and a single "weighted" monetary value is associated with each. These monetary outcomes are then compared against each other and only one is ultimately selected that satisfies the predetermined selection criteria of the decision maker.

Fig 111-1 shows a decision tree that has been constructed based on the information contained in the following scenario:

You, as the veterinarian, must help a producer make a decision whether to treat a bull with a preputial prolapse of traumatic origin or cull him. The bull is worth $2500. His slaughter value is $1000. Based on clinical experience, you estimate that 85% of your surgeries are successful, regardless of whether a reefing or circumcision operation is performed. The cost of surgery is $985. The bull will be worth the aforementioned $2500 if he recovers fully (i.e., can breed cows successfully again). If surgical treatment is unsuccessful, the bull can still be culled for $1000. You estimate that 60% of bulls treated medically with antibiotics, hydrotherapy, and a preputial sling recover fully (medical cost = $500). Similarly, if medical therapy fails, the bull can be culled for $1000, but only if antibiotic residues are *not* present in the meat (90% chance). Otherwise, the slaughter value is lost.

The decision tree tells you that, given the aforementioned economic values and probabilities, the expected value for this bull following surgical intervention is $1290, that is, (0.85 × [$2500 − 985]) + (0.15 × [$1000 − 985]), and $1360, that is, (0.60 × [$2500 − 500]) + (0.40 × [0.10 × ($0−500)]) + (0.40 × [0.90 × ($1000 − 500)]), following medical treatment. If no intervention is chosen, the value of the bull is its cull (slaughter) value of $1000. Because this

owner is interested in maximizing the value of the bull, the decision tree indicates that medical treatment should be the intervention of choice ($1360 > $1290 > $1000).

A decision tree can also be used to show what the expected value of the bull must be in order for a decision of pursuing medical or surgical intervention to be equivocal. This monetary point (breakeven point) equals the difference between surgical (C1) and medical (C2) treatment cost divided by the difference in the probability of a favorable outcome for surgical (P1) and medical (P2) treatment:

Breakeven (BE) = (C1−C2)/(P1−P2), where C1 = $985, C2 = $500, P1 = 0.85, P2 = 0.60
BE = ($985−$500)/(0.85−0.60) = $1940

LONG-TERM DECISION MAKING

A longer-term perspective (>1 year) is typically the focus when capital budgeting decisions are being made. Capital budgeting is the process of choosing an investment project based on a comparison of the initial investment cost of the asset with its expected future cash flows when put to use.[7] Central to a long-term decision is whether investing in the initial cost of the asset will outweigh the expected cash flow generated from its use. In other words, instead of investing in this asset, should the money be used for something else?

Numerous techniques have been employed to help answer this question including payback period, internal rate of return, book rate of return, and net present value (NPV).[8] The latter technique leads to better investment decisions than the other three methods because it takes into account the time value of money. Hence NPV is discussed next.

NET PRESENT VALUE

The NPV concept recognizes that a quantity of money received sometime in the future is worth less than the same amount of money received today. Alternatively, more money must be received in the future to equal the same amount of money today. But how much more? The answer is dependent on the discount (interest) rate chosen by the holder of this money.

The formula for NPV (Fig 111-2) takes into account (1) the initial outflow of cash (purchase price of asset and associated costs to put it into use), (2) yearly net cash inflows over the period of time under consideration, and (3) a discount rate. The discount rate should reflect a reasonable return on the monetary commitment. For production agriculture, a discount rate of 8% has been used historically for a long-term investment.[6]

$$NPV = (-\text{initial cash outflow}) + \sum \frac{\text{net cash inflow}}{(1 + R)^n}$$

where R equals the discount (interest) rate and n corresponds to the year number (1, 2, 3, etc.) associated with each net cash inflow.

Fig 111-2   Net present value formula.

The NPV value is determined by summing the discounted cash inflows obtained for each year and subtracting this dollar amount from the initial outflow of cash used to purchase and put the asset into service. Consistent with discounted cash flow, the further out in time that a series of net cash inflows goes, the lower the amount each contributes to total cash inflow.

The investment opportunity is deemed acceptable if NPV is greater than $0, whereas it should be rejected if NPV is less than $0. Indifference to the investment decision occurs if NPV equals $0. If several different scenarios are under consideration, the one with the highest NPV should be pursued.

The following example illustrates the use of NPV methodology:

A rancher is offered a parcel of grazing land for $200,000 (200 acres @ $1000/acre), which he can pay for with his own money. The only intended use of the land will be to lease it out for contract grazing over a 7-year period. The lessee's annual grazing fee will be $6000 ($30/acre/yr) to be paid at the end of each year. The tax obligation to the rancher (lessor) for the revenue received for each year of this lease is 28%. The lessee has responsibility for all maintenance of the property. At the end of the contract grazing period, the rancher can resell the property to another rancher for $1250/acre. Capital gains on the sale of the land are 15%. The discount rate is 8%. Inflation is not considered.

Is the investment in this parcel of land a good deal for its intended use? Without considering the time value of money, this investment appears to be a good deal because pretax net cash inflow is $92,000 (7 years @ $6000/yr lease income plus $50,000 appreciation in land value at time of resale) or $72,740 after-tax net cash inflow (7 years @ $4320*/year net income from leasing the land plus $42,500† net income from resale of the land). However, when the time value of money is considered, the net inflow of cash coming from this land investment is $36,013 less than the original amount of money used to purchase it:

$$
\begin{aligned}
NPV &= -\$200{,}000 + \$4320^*/1.08^1 + \$4320/1.08^2 + \\
&\quad \$4320/1.08^3 + \$4320/1.08^4 + \$4320/1.08^5 + \\
&\quad \$4320/1.08^6 + \$4320/1.08^7 + \$242{,}500^b/1.08^7 \\
&= -\$200{,}000 + (\$4000 + \$3704 + \$3429 + \$3175 + \\
&\quad \$2940 + \$2722 + \$2521 + \$141{,}496) \\
&= -\$200{,}000 + \$163{,}987 \\
&= -\$36{,}013
\end{aligned}
$$

---

*$6000 − ($6000 × .28) = $4320
†($1250/ac × 200ac) − {[($1250/ac × 200ac) − ($1000/ac × 200ac] × .15} = $242,500

Because NPV is negative, the land purchase price is not a good deal at $1000/acre under the current set of expected net cash inflows coming from its intended use.

SUMMARY

Admittedly, management decisions that are to be implemented must first be analyzed from a viewpoint of whether or not they make sense productivity-wise. However, a management change should not be pursued, no matter how good the improvement in productivity may look, if implementation costs exceed what will be realized monetarily.

Farmers and ranchers should be in business to make a profit. With this objective in mind, positive cash flow then becomes the lifeblood of their operations. With one's assistance as a veterinary adviser, the aforementioned analytic techniques should help them to make the best economic decisions possible, given his or her understanding of what cash outflows and cash inflows are expected to be.

References

1. McGuigan JR, Moyer RC, Harris FHdeB: Introduction and goals of the firm. In McGuigan JR, Moyer RC, Harris FHdeB, editors: *Managerial economics: applications, strategy, and tactics*, Cincinnati, 1999, South-Western College Publishing.
2. Baker HK: The finance function. In Baker HK, editor: *Financial management*, Mason, Ohio, 1987, Thomson South-Western.
3. Noordhuizen JPTM: Part IV. Analysis techniques commonly used in economics. In Noordhuizen JPTM, Frankena K, van der Hoofd CM et al, editors: *Application of quantitative methods in veterinary epidemiology*, Wageningen, The Netherlands, 1997, Wageningen Pers.
4. Weinstein MC, Fineberg HV, Elstein AS et al: The elements of clinical decision making. In Weinstein MC, Fineberg HV, Elstein AS et al, editors: *Clinical decision analysis*, Philadelphia, 1980, Saunders.
5. Radostits OM, Leslie KE, Fetrow J: Mathematical techniques for production medicine. In Radostits OM, Leslie KE, Fetrow J, editors: *Herd health food animal production medicine*, ed 2, Philadelphia, 1994, Saunders.
6. IRM-SPA Handbook: *Guide to Assembling Data for Cow-Calf Standardized Performance Analysis - SPA-38, 2000*, Texas Agricultural Extension Service, The Texas A&M University System.
7. Zimmerman JL: Opportunity cost of capital and capital budgeting. In Zimmerman JL, editor: *Accounting for decision making and control*, ed 3, Boston, 2000, Irwin McGraw-Hill.
8. Brealey RA, Myers SC: Why net present value leads to better investment decisions than other criteria. In Brealey RA, Myers SC, editors: *Principles of corporate finance*, ed 6, Boston, 2000, Irwin McGraw-Hill.

CHAPTER 112

Cow-Calf Operation Beef Quality Assurance

DEE GRIFFIN

The purpose of the beef quality assurance (BQA) program is to identify and avoid activities in beef production operations that can cause a quality or safety defect. The program encourages beef operations to seek all sources of information needed to accomplish the BQA goal and objectives. Although the BQA program started in the finish cattle feeding side of the industry, the BQA program today is a cooperative effort among beef producers in all segments, veterinarians, nutritionists, extension staff, suppliers, and other professionals. The program asks everyone involved with beef production to follow the government guidelines for product use and to use common sense, reasonable management skills, and accepted scientific knowledge to avoid product defects at the consumer level. The goals of the BQA program are to assure the consumer that all cattle shipped are healthy, wholesome, and safe and that their management has met all government and industry standards. Important points for a successful BQA program are included in Box 112-1.

The BQA objectives for the cow calf operation should be to do the following:

1. Set production standards that can be met or exceeded.
2. Establish systems for data retention and record keeping. Record keeping systems, which meet government and industry guidelines, allow validation of management activities and fulfill the program goal.
3. Provide hands-on training and education for participants to meet or exceed the guidelines of the BQA program and realize its benefits.
4. Provide technical assistance through cattlemen associations, veterinarians, and university staff. The veterinarian should serve as the facilitator of the BQA program and trainer of proper production management techniques that meet BQA standards.

QUALITY AND SAFETY CHALLENGES

The importance of beef quality assurance is obvious when analyzing the top eight quality challenges within the beef industry. These quality challenges include injection-site blemishes, rib brands, excessive fat, dark cutters, nonuniform cattle, and *Escherichia coli* O157:H7.

The U.S. Department of Agriculture–Food Safety Inspection Service (USDA-FSIS) reports beef to be below their chemical (residue) and physical (broken needles) defect targets. *E. coli* O157:H7 presents a difficult problem and at present effective on-farm control techniques have not

---

Box 112-1

Important Reminders for Beef Quality Assurance to Be Successful

1. The veterinarian, producer, and employees cannot foresee all potential problems. Identify one area at a time, then develop and implement a plan for assuring quality and safety in that area of production. The experience gained will make it easier to develop quality assurance in other areas of the operation.
2. Violative residues and product-related defects can be avoided if animal health products are administered according to government and industry standards and if BQA record keeping standards are maintained.
3. A number of safeguards are built into the beef feeding system to help avoid quality defects. These include handling of animals on an individual basis, the length of time required producing a finished product, and the quality and safety built into modern health-related technologies used in beef production.
4. Every producer and employee must be trained to know, understand, and identify areas where possible contamination with violative residues and/or where quality or hazardous physical defects may occur. Anyone who supplies services, commodities, or products to a producer must understand the producer's quality and safety assurance objectives.
5. The producer must be able to document all the steps of production. Good production records allow for documentation, analysis, and improved financial decisions.
6. Points in production must be monitored to ensure no residue violations or carcass defects occur. The critical points include, but are not limited to: cattle treated with any product; incoming products and commodities; cattle handling; and evaluation of outgoing cattle, particularly cull cows and bulls.
7. Some production areas have higher residue and carcass defect risks than others. High-risk production areas include, but are not limited to: nonperforming cattle cull cows and bulls; unusual single-source feed ingredients; and suppliers of nonstandard supplies.

---

been found. As soon as, even a partially effective control technique has been developed to control potential bacterial hazards, the technique will likely be incorporated into the BQA guidelines.

The BQA's challenge to improve beef quality are to eliminate side and multiple brands; remove horns; improve parasite control; improve red meat yield; improve handling/transport techniques; eliminate intramuscular injections; and measure traits that affect value and eliminate genetic and management systems that negatively affect tenderness, juiciness, and flavor.

BEEF QUALITY ASSURANCE HISTORY

Consumers have always wanted safe food. Because of concerns with additional government regulation and potential loss of modern production tools, in 1980 cattlemen began investigating ways to ensure that their production practices were safe and would satisfy consumer concerns.

In 1982 the USDA-FSIS began working with the beef industry in the United States to develop the Pre-harvest Beef Safety Production Program. Not wanting any additional governmental regulatory programs, the beef industry adopted the term *beef quality assurance*. BQA provided cattlemen an important key for avoiding additional government regulation. Currently there are 47 states and more than 90% of the U.S. beef production is involved with the voluntary program. Industry self-regulation has proven successful and will continue to allow industry the flexibility needed to produce safe and wholesome food in an economical manner. Success of the effort is clear; violative chemical residues have almost disappeared in fed beef cattle and injection site lesions have been reduced by almost 90%.

BEEF QUALITY ASSURANCE GOOD MANAGEMENT PRACTICES

Good management practices are an important part of a successful BQA program and Box 112-2 lists common BQA guidelines and agreements. Good management practices include having feed handling facilities designed to reduce the risk of feed contamination with chemicals, foreign materials, and disease-causing infectious agents. All chemicals (e.g., pesticides, lubricants, solvents, medications) should be stored away from feed supplies. Feed handling equipment should be routinely checked for fluid leaks. Avoid storing feedstuffs around electrical transformers. Dual-purpose equipment such as a loaders and shovels that handle feed and other materials (e.g., manure or dead animal removal), should be thoroughly cleaned before handling feed. No vehicles other than feed handling equipment should be allowed into feed storage areas such as silage pits. The most common source of infectious agent contamination comes from animal or human feces. Protecting feedstuffs, feed troughs, and water supplies from contamination with chemicals, foreign material, and feces is important. Control of rodents, birds, and other wildlife is important to avoid fecal contamination with many common infectious agents.

FEEDSTUFFS AND COMMODITY SOURCES GOOD MANUFACTURING PRACTICES

Monitoring Feedstuffs

Monitoring feed sources is essential. Producers purchasing outside feeds should maintain a sampling program to test for quality specifications of feedstuffs. This could include moisture, protein, and foreign material. Suppliers should be informed that sampling of delivered products will occur. A good business practice is to require all products to be accompanied by an invoice, which includes the date, amount, and signatures of both the person who delivered the product and the person who received the product. Most good suppliers have a quality control testing program of their own. Bonded suppliers often test for polychlorinated biphenyls, chlorinated hydrocarbons, organophosphates, pesticides and herbicides, heavy metals, and microbes (*Salmonella*). As part of the BQA program, the producer should ask for the test results.

A quality control program for feedstuffs aids in preventing chemical residues and ensures high-quality feeds. Visual inspection of feeds can be effective in avoiding some problems. Create a checklist, which includes such items as color (typical, bright, and uniform); odor (clean and characteristic); moisture (free flowing, no wet spots and moisture testing); temperature (no evidence of heating); and no evidence of foreign material or bird, rodent, or insect contamination.

Testing every load of grain or forage for contaminants is neither efficient nor economically feasible. However, a logical alternative is to obtain and store a representative sample of each batch of newly purchased feed. Commonly, a thorough investigation of suspected feed-related problems is not possible because no representative sample is available for testing. If feed sampling and storage is done on a routine basis and a suspected feed-related problem occurs, samples for appropriate laboratory testing will be available. A recommended sampling method for purchased grains, supplements, or complete feeds is to randomly sample each batch of feed in 5 to 10 locations and pool the individual samples into a larger sample of 2 to 5 lb. The pooled sample should be placed in a paper bag or small cardboard box, labeled, and frozen. Dry samples can be labeled and kept in a dry area. Higher moisture samples should be frozen. A feed tag should be attached to the sample for future reference if needed.

Forage samples should also be collected and stored. Representative samples should be obtained from several bales of purchased hay and mixed together before storage. Core samples are preferred over "grab" samples, particularly from large bales of hay. Most hay samples can be placed in a labeled paper bag and kept in a clean, dry area.

High-Risk Feeds

High-risk feeds are single loads or batches that will be fed to cattle over a prolonged period of time, thereby exposing large numbers of cattle. Examples of high-risk feeds include fats, rendered byproducts, plant byproducts, supplements, and additives. Typically, these feedstuffs are only a small percent of the total diet and are expensive to test. Suppliers should understand the producers' BQA concerns and provide quality specifications with the product. Doing business with a bonded supplier is best. One should find dependable suppliers and stay with them.

Ruminant Byproducts

Because of bovine spongiform encephalopathy (BSE) concerns, **certain ruminant-derived protein sources** such as meat and bone meal cannot be fed. Ruminant-derived

Box 112-2

Beef Quality Assurance Guidelines and Agreements

Feedstuffs

The producer should maintain records of any pesticide/herbicide use on pasture or crops that could potentially lead to violative residues in grazing cattle or feedlot cattle.

Adequate quality control program(s) are in place for incoming feedstuffs. Program(s) should be designed to eliminate contamination from molds, mycotoxins, or chemicals of incoming feed ingredients. Supplier assurance of feed ingredient quality is recommended.

Suspect feedstuffs should be analyzed before use.

Ruminant-derived protein sources cannot be fed per FDA regulations.

Feeding byproducts ingredients should be supported with sound science.

Feed Additives and Medications

Only FDA-approved medicated feed additives will be used in rations.

Medicated feed additives will be used in accordance with the FDA GMP regulation.

The veterinarian should follow judicious antibiotic use guidelines.

Extralabel use of feed additives is illegal and strictly prohibited.

To avoid violative residues, WDs must be strictly adhered to.

Complete records must be kept when formulating or feeding medicated feed rations.

Records are to be kept a minimum of 3 years.

The producer will ensure that all additives are withdrawn at the proper time to avoid violative residues.

Processing/Treatment and Records

Veterinarians and producers will follow all FDA/USDA/Environmental Protection Agency guidelines for product(s) used.

All products are to be used per label directions.

Extralabel drug use shall be kept to a minimum and used only when prescribed by a veterinarian working under a valid veterinary client patient relationship (VCPR).

Strict adherence to extended withdrawal periods (as determined by the veterinarian within the context of a valid VCPR) shall be employed.

Treatment records will be maintained with the following recorded:

1. Individual animal or group identification
2. Date treated
3. Product administrated and manufacture's lot/serial number
4. Dosage used

5. Route and location of administration
6. Earliest date animal will have cleared withdrawal period

When cattle are processed as a group, all cattle within the group shall be identified as such, and the following information recorded:

1. Group or lot identification
2. Date treated
3. Product administered and manufacturer's lot/serial number
4. Dosage used
5. Route and location of administration
6. Earliest date animal will have cleared withdrawal period

All cattle shipped will be checked by appropriate personnel to ensure that animals that have been treated meet or exceed label or prescription WDs for all animal health products administrated.

All processing and treatment records should be transferred with the cattle to the next production level. Prospective buyers must be informed of any cattle that have not met WDs.

Injectable Animal Health Products

Products labeled for subcutaneous (SC) administration should be administered subcutaneously in the neck region.

All products labeled for intramuscular (IM) use shall be given in the neck region only (no exceptions, regardless of age).

All products cause tissue damage when injected intramuscularly. Therefore all IM use should be avoided if possible.

Products cleared for SC, IV, or oral administration are recommended.

Products with low dosage rates are recommended and proper spacing should be followed.

No more than 10 ml of product is administered per IM injection site.

Care and Husbandry Practices

Follow a quality herd health plan that conforms to good veterinary and husbandry practices.

All cattle will be handled/transported in such a fashion to minimize stress, injury, and/or bruising.

Facilities (e.g., fences, corrals, load-outs) should be inspected regularly to ensure proper care and ease of handling.

The producer should strive to keep feed and water handling equipment clean, provide appropriate nutritional and feedstuffs management, and strive to maintain an environment appropriate to the production setting.

Biosecurity should be evaluated.

Records should be kept for a minimum of 3 years.

---

products such as tallow and blood byproducts are acceptable under the BQA program. Pure porcine and equine meat and bone meals can be fed to cattle.

Potential Feed Toxins

Importantly, producers and employees must have some knowledge about the relative toxicities of chemicals to livestock so that highly toxic chemicals such as soil insecticides can be handled and stored properly. All chemicals should be treated as potential hazards and stored away

from feed storage and mixing areas. If a feed-related poisoning is suspected, it is critical for the veterinarian to contact a diagnostic laboratory for assistance in confirming the suspicion. Some poisoning incidents may be reportable to the appropriate federal or state/provincial government agencies.

Naturally occurring mycotoxins also pose a threat to quality beef production. Mycotoxins can be found in grains and forages and, if present in sufficient concentrations, can cause reduced feed consumption, poor production, and adverse health effects. Mycotoxins can be produced in feedstuffs before harvesting or during storage. More commonly found mycotoxins include aflatoxin, vomitoxin, zearalenone, and fumonisins in grain, primarily corn and slaframine in red clover. Ergot alkaloids can be found in either grain or grass hays.

Fats

Steps should be taken to ensure that purchased fats and oils do not contain a residue. Discuss the quality of product with suppliers and request information concerning the sources, quality, stability, efficacy, and consistency of the product. Producers may be approached by brokers who offer a cheaper source of feed-grade fats; however, the potential for contamination increases with cheaper sources of fats.

A reputable dealer should be testing fats for such contaminants as polychlorinated biphenyls (PCBs), chlorinated hydrocarbons (CHCs), pesticides, heavy metals, *Salmonella* and tall oil (hydrocarbon). Verification of testing should accompany the product.

ANIMAL HEALTH MAINTENANCE AND TREATMENT GOOD MANUFACTURING PRACTICES

Quality Assurance Herd Health Plan

One should follow a "quality assurance herd health plan" that conforms to good veterinary and husbandry practices. Box 112-3 contains minimum guidelines for a quality assurance health plan.

The beef industry, largely through the efforts of feedlots, has done an excellent job of controlling violative drug residues. This been accomplished by placing emphasis on the identification of treated cattle and good record keeping. This includes identifying each animal treated, accurately recording the product (s) used, treatment date and treatment dosage, and following prescribed withdrawal times (WDs). The cow-calf industry is responsible for providing residue-free animals to the feeding industry. Of particular note are drugs with long WDs such as gentamicin. Gentamicin is also under a voluntary ban in use instituted by the Academy of Veterinary Consultants and American Association of Bovine Practitioners (AABP).

Treatment Protocol Book

The veterinarian should provide a treatment protocol book specific to the producer. This book should follow prudent antibiotic use guidelines and be reviewed regularly and updated at least every 6 months or more often if appropriate. One copy of the treatment protocol book should be kept at the operations headquarters and a second readily available at the working facilities. A written treatment protocol, along with current prescriptions, are important documents that the operation must have to outline drug usage procedures and residue avoidance plans. The treatment protocol book and prescription should meet Animal Medicinal Drug Use Clarification Act (AMDUCA) specifications. Box 112-4 lists National Cattlemen's Beef Association prudent

---

Box 112-3

Quality Assurance Herd Health Plan Minimum Guidelines

For All Cattle and Production Segments
- Provide appropriate nutritional feedstuffs.
- Handle cattle to minimize stress and bruising.
- Administer all injections administered in front of the shoulder.
- Individually identify any animals treated to ensure proper WD.
- Make records available to the next production sector.
- Always read and follow label directions.
- Keep records of all products administered including product used, serial number, amount administered, route of administration, and WD.

Heifers and Purchased Breeding Stock Entering the Cow Herd
- Vaccinate in front of the shoulder for viral and clostridial diseases.
  - Administer two vaccinations, 2 to 3 weeks apart.
- Control external and internal parasites.

Cow Herd
- Control external and internal parasites.
- Annually booster vaccinations in front of the shoulder.
- Consult with your veterinarian for additional health procedures appropriate to your area.

At Preweaning, Weaning, and/or Backgrounding
- If implanting, administer implants properly in a sanitary manner.
- Vaccinate in front of the shoulder for viral and clostridial diseases.
  - Administer two vaccinations, 2 to 3 weeks apart.
- Perform all surgeries such as dehorning and castration in a humane manner.
- Control external and internal parasites.
- Consult with your veterinarian for additional health procedures appropriate to your area.
- Keep records of all products administered including product used, serial number, amount administered, route of administration, and WD.
- Wean cattle (45 days recommended) to ensure cattle health and producer return on health management investment.

---

antibiotic use guidelines. Of greater significance, the treatment book provides written guidelines for animal health programs, thus minimizing chances of mistakes or misunderstandings.

Injections

A critical part of a BQA program is the proper administration of animal health products. Research has demonstrated injections given to calves at 50 days of age had injection-site lesions at 450 days of age that caused eatable tissue loss and loss of meat tenderness. Additionally, injection-site lesions in the hindquarter of culled cows historically decrease the value of the carcass by

Box 112-4

Prudent Antibiotic Use Guidelines from National Cattlemen's Beef Association BQA Program

1. **Prevent Problems:** Emphasize appropriate husbandry and hygiene, routine health examinations, and vaccinations.
2. **Select and Use Antibiotics Carefully:** Consult with your veterinarian on the selection and use of antibiotics. Have a valid reason to use an antibiotic. Therapeutic alternatives should be considered before using antimicrobial therapy.
3. **Avoid Using Antibiotics Important in Human Medicine as First-Line Therapy:** Avoid using as the first antibiotic those medications that are important to treating strategic human or animal infections.
4. **Use the Laboratory to Help You Select Antibiotics:** Cultures and susceptibility test results should be used to aid in the selection of antimicrobials, whenever possible.
5. **Combination Antibiotic Therapy Is Discouraged Unless There Is Clear Evidence the Specific Practice Is Beneficial:** Select and dose an antibiotic to effect a cure.
6. **Avoid Inappropriate Antibiotic Use:** Confine therapeutic antimicrobial use to proven clinical indications, avoiding inappropriate uses such as for viral infections without bacterial complication.
7. **Treatment Programs Should Reflect Best Use Principles:** Regimens for therapeutic antimicrobial use should be optimized using current pharmacologic information and principles.
8. **Treat the Fewest Number of Animals Possible:** Limit antibiotic use to sick or at-risk animals.
9. **Treat for the Recommended Time Period:** Minimize the potential for bacteria to become resistant to antimicrobials.
10. **Avoid Environmental Contamination with Antibiotics:** Steps should be taken to minimize antimicrobials reaching the environment through spillage, contaminated ground runoff, or aerosolization.
11. **Keep Records of Antibiotic Use:** Use accurate records of treatment and outcome to evaluate therapeutic regimens and always follow proper WDs.
12. **Follow Label Directions:** Follow label instructions and never use antibiotics other than as labeled without a valid veterinary prescription.
13. **Extralabel Antibiotic Use Must Follow FDA Regulations:** Prescriptions including extralabel use of medications must meet the AMDUCA amendments to the Food, Drug, and Cosmetic Act and its regulations. This includes having a valid VCPR.
14. **Subtherapeutic Antibiotic Use Is Discouraged:** Antibiotic use should be limited to prevent or control disease.

more than $25. To help avoid these production-induced quality defects, it is important, regardless of the animal's age, to give all injections in front of the shoulders and never in the rump or back leg. This includes approved subcutaneous ear routes of administration and subcutaneous dewlap injections. When possible, intramuscular (IM) injections should be avoided. However, some animal health products are labeled for IM use only. If IM medications must be used, administer them in the neck and never exceed 10 ml per IM injection site. As a rule, personnel should not inject more than 10 ml subcutaneously in each injection site; however, some products are labeled for use up to 20 ml per injection site and do not violate BQA guidelines. The subcutaneous space on either side of the tail head, although not approved as a BQA injection location, is a reasonable alternative that should not cause an injection-site lesion in eatable tissue in situations where giving an injection ahead of the shoulder would jeopardize safety. Safety of oneself, others working around the animal, the animal, and meat should always be foremost in your decisions.

Bent and Broken Needles

The veterinarian should train all producers and employees on the proper way to handle cattle, cattle restraint, and proper injection technique. Improper animal restraint is the cause of most bent needle problems. If a needle bends, it should never be straightened and reused. Although rare, a needle can break off in the muscle. A broken needle is an emergency and time will be of the essence. Broken needles migrate in tissue and if not immediately handled will be impossible to find, requiring the animal to be destroyed. Under no circumstances can animals with broken needles be sent to market. The veterinarian should outline procedures for handling such cases in the treatment protocol book. Purchasing high-quality needles, changing and discarding damaged needles, and providing proper restraint are all preventative measures.

Residue Avoidance

Avoiding violative residues depends on (1) using U.S. Food and Drug Administration (FDA)-approved medications; (2) following label directions when possible; (3) knowing that extralabel drug usage (ELDU) must have WDs appropriate for the dose, medication, and route of administration; (4) not exceeding dose per injection site recommendations; and (5) screening cattle that may not have cleared the antibiotics normally. A strategy for avoiding antibiotic residues is presented in Box 112-5.

Why Do We Need to Screen Selected Cattle Before Marketing?

First, nonperforming animals and cull cows and bulls that have been treated with an antibiotic should be considered "high risk for antibiotic residue violation" because of the potential for their poor performance associated with organ (liver or kidney) dysfunction. Liver and kidney function is vital to clearing antibiotics. Second, ELDU, by law, requires a veterinarian to adjust the WD from the label indications to a time more appropriate to the dose used. This includes using subcutaneous (SC) administration

Antibiotic Residue Avoidance Strategy

1. Identify all animals treated.
2. Record all treatments: date; animal ID; dose given; route of administration; the person who administered the treatment; WD.
3. Strictly follow label directions for product use.
4. Use newer technology antibiotics when possible.
   a. Reduce unwanted depot effect. Select low-volume products when available.
   b. Select generic medications and vaccines with *extreme caution.*
   c. Avoid inferior products. They may cause performance loss or damage quality.
5. Select with short WD when antibiotic choice is equivalent.
6. Never give more than 10 ml per IM injection site.
7. Avoid ELDU of antibiotics.
   a. Use label dose and route of administration.
8. Avoid using multiple antibiotics at the same time.
9. Do not mix antibiotics in the same syringe, especially if given intramuscularly or subcutaneously.
10. Check *all* medication/treatment records before marketing:
    a. Do not market cattle with less than 60 WD without examining the treatment history.
    b. Extend the WD time if the route or location of administration is altered.
       i. Example; the WD for ear route of administration of ceftiofur will be greater than 120 days if given subcutaneously in the neck.
       ii. Example; tissue irritation will cause the WD for Banamine to be Banamine 30 days if given intramuscularly or subcutaneously instead of IV.
    c. Extend the WD for multiple medications given by summing their label-recommended WD.
       i. Example; if the first medication has a 10-day WD and the second medication has a 28-day WD, assign a 38-day WD.
       ii. Example; if first medication has a 10-day WD and is repeated in 3 days, assign a 20-day WD.

d. Extend the WD for all penicillin given at doses that exceed the label dose.
   i. Example; the WD for Procaine Pen G given at 3 ml per CWT intramuscularly or subcutaneously is greater than 30 days.
   ii. Example; the WD for Procaine Pen G given at 4 ml per CWT intramuscularly or subcutaneously is greater than 30 days.
   iii. Example; the WD for long-acting Pen G given at 3 ml per CWT intramuscularly or subcutaneously is greater than 120 days.
   iv. Example; the WD for long-acting Pen G given at 4 ml per CWT intramuscularly or subcutaneously is greater than 180 days.
11. Testing urine test may not detect injection site residues and will test positive by the USDA-FSIS.
    a. Never inject gentamicin or neomycin. The estimated WD is greater than 24 months.
    b. Testing urine test may not detect a kidney that will test positive by the USDA-FSIS.
    c. Do not market cattle that have relapsed without examining the treatment history.
    d. Do not market cattle with suspected liver or kidney damage without examining the treatment history.
    e. Do not market cattle with antibiotic injection-site knots without examining the treatment history.
    f. Screen the urine for antibiotics of all cattle identified in steps a through d. It is best to use a broad-spectrum microbial inhibition test such as the Pre-Harvest Antibiotic Screening Test (PHAST), a microbial growth inhibition test that uses *Bacillus megaterium* as the test organism. Test sensitivity relative to FDA-CVM violative residue tolerances (Maximum Residue Limit or MRL).

when labels indicate IV or IM and increasing the dose above the label dose. Third, doses above 10 ml/site may depot and not be eliminated as rapidly as required to meet assigned WD. Perivascular injections are a frequent target for suspected residue violations.

SUMMARY

Remember the BQA basics:

- Recruit a BQA team: employees, family, affiliates, specialists, experts
- Take a look at what could go wrong
- Decide what will be done when something goes wrong
- How to avoid problems
- Validate the plan
- Train and educate, retrain, and reeducate

- Develop a timed checklist and then use it
- Document and double check (Box 112-6 and Box 112-7)

It is simple economics ... we sell performance. Animal performance can be optimized only if the people managing the animal respect the *animal, themselves,* and the *people they work with.* Following good manufacturing practices (GMPs) improves efficiency.

In addition, consumers buy what they trust. Confidence comes from trust ... a trust we have earned. A relatively small percentage of the population is involved in beef production, and consumers do not know us as they once did. Changes in demographics, government, media, etc. are making it even tougher and the standards required of us may seem impossible. But this is the life, the job God entrusted to us.

Box 112-6

BQA Cow-Calf Feed Checklist Example

Beef Operation _____ Date _____ Evaluator _____

Pasture Maintenance and Raised Feeds
- Protect water source and check yearly for contamination.
- Protect pastures from contamination.
- Undergo training for handling pesticides.
- Store pesticides in protected area away from feed or health products.
- Follow FDA/USDA/EPA guidelines for all product use.
- Check all pesticide handling equipment before each use for delivery accuracy and contamination.
- Establish cattle or harvest WD if needed before allowing cattle to graze.
- Properly dispose of used containers.

Purchased Feeds
- Develop and use evaluation, sampling, and sample storage protocol.
- Maintain receiving/inventory log/record: source (verified), date, description (name, invoice #).
- Undergo training for evaluating received/purchased feeds.
- Inspect feed storage for contamination before receiving new loads of ingredients.
- Use feed storage area only to store feed ingredients (e.g., no pesticides, solvents).
- Have procedures in place to protect feed-handling equipment contamination.
- Check all feed-handling equipment before each use for contamination.

Feed Additives
- Receiving log record: source (verified), date, description (including serial/lot #).
- Store feed additives separately from other feedstuffs.
- Maintain a use log record: date, dose per ton, ID of animals.
- Maintain a physical inventory log (can be column in use log).
- Undergo training for using feed additives.

Feed Formulas
- Record all feed formulas.
- Have medicated feed formulas checked by nutritionist or veterinarian for accurate dosing.
- Understand directions for use including WD.
- Undergo training for mixing and quality control sampling/ testing for feed mixing.

Batch/Load/Feed Delivery
- Batch/delivery log/load (delivery matches feeding plan if needed)
- Minimum/maximum and exception table or chart for ingredients and mixing
- Training (see earlier)

Cattle Release
- WD checked on all feed records.

Box 112-7

Beef Quality Assurance Cow-Calf Product Use Checklist Example

Beef Operation _____ Date _____ Evaluator _____

Cattle Handling Facilities
- Inspected for proper function for cattle and human safety before each use
- Handling facilities and equipment properly designed, maintained, and used

New Cattle Entering the Operation
- Receiving log record: source (verified), date, description
- Appropriate health/import/transfer/movement records
- Cattle handling training
- Basic quality control:
  1. Holding pens and handling alleys properly designed and maintained
  2. Clean feed and water as needed available to cattle on arrival
  3. Visual inspection of cattle on arrival

Health Management, Mass Medication, and Pesticide Products (Receiving, Storage, and Use)
- Receiving/inventory log/record: source (verified), date, description (name, serial/lot #)
- Stored in protected area: refrigerated as needed, sunlight controlled, locked if required
- Use (Health Management/Treatment) records for all cattle:
  - Date, animal(s) ID, diagnosis/reason, product, dose, withdrawal and release date
- Cattle product use maps used for health management (includes product and serial/lot #)
- Minimum/maximum and exception table or chart for product use
- Product handling and use training (including MSDS/Product Inserts)
- All injections given in the neck region, injectables given subcutaneously if possible
- Supplier agreements and veterinary drug order (as appropriate)
- Signed use protocols (health maintenance, treatment, premise pesticides)
- FDA/USDA/EPA guidelines followed for all product use
- Equipment for delivery properly designed, maintained, and used
  - Cattle: chutes, snakes, holding pens, syringes, needles
  - Feed and pesticides: scales, mixers, delivery system
- Proper disposal of used containers
- WD established and estimated date for release (injectables, see earlier)
- Residue screening of nonperformers (exceptions: reproduction and lameness if no prescription drugs taken)
- Training for processing, health management, mass medication, and pesticide products

Feed Management
- WD established, release date estimated
- Feed management, mixing, and delivery training
- FDA/USDA/EPA guidelines followed for all product use
- Training for feed management

Cattle Release
- WD checked on all products used (health management, and treatment records)
- All WDs met and PHAST test all nonperformers (except no prescription drugs for those with reproductive issues and lameness)
- Release/transfer form signed

Recommended Readings

Beef Quality Assurance: *National Cattlemen's Beef Association*, Denver, 2001 (website): http://www.bqa.org/. Accessed 2008.

Pre-Harvest Antibiotic Residue Test and Antibiotic Residue Avoidance Strategies: UNL-GPVEC, Clay Center, Neb, 2003 (website): http://gpvec.unl.edu/bqa/ncbqa.htm. Accessed 2008.

CHAPTER **113**

Biosecurity for Cow-Calf Enterprises

MIKE SANDERSON

The term *biosecurity* generally includes two components—preventing the introduction of new pathogens or toxins onto a farm and efforts to control spread of disease and/or intoxication within a herd. To be more exact, biosecurity is concerned with preventing the introduction of pathogens or toxins that have the potential to damage the health or productivity of a herd of cattle or the safety and quality of a food product. Biocontainment is a closely related concept and refers to efforts to control the spread of disease or intoxication within a herd. Biosecurity plans need to be based on the particular herd's current disease status, the particular disease to be controlled, cost of prevention, likelihood of an outbreak, impact of an outbreak, and risk aversion of the producer.

Multiple tools are available to decrease the risk of importing disease into a herd and include the following:

1. Only importing cattle from herds with known health status. That is, only import from disease-free herds or herds with an appropriate vaccination program and actual records of excellent health and performance.
2. Testing strategies for incoming cattle to identify those carrying infectious disease.
3. Quarantine strategies for incoming cattle to prevent contact with the resident herd until any incubating disease is manifest or acute disease is resolved.
4. Vaccination requirements for both incoming cattle before entry and the resident herd.
5. Management practices to control exposure of cattle to pathogens from other risk groups, neighboring herds, and wildlife reservoirs.

SOURCES OF EXPOSURE

Cattle are ruminant animals designed to consume forage and convert it to meat and milk. This is generally done in an extensive range environment, and in the course of doing so they are exposed to neighboring herds and a wide variety of wildlife that can expose the herd to disease. Biosecurity for cow-calf producers is challenging because of the extensive nature of cow-calf production and subsequent exposure to a complex and diverse environment (Box 113-1).

Most cow-calf herds allow entry of new animals. At a minimum, new bulls are imported and somewhat commonly other classes of cattle such as cows, heifers, and calves are imported as well. Semen and embryos are also potential sources of disease introduction if not handled correctly. Additionally, herds commonly have contact with other cattle over the fence between neighboring herds and through occasional breaches in the fence and intermingling of herds. Disease can also be introduced through wildlife contacts and contaminated feed or water sources. Finally, herd suppliers may introduce disease to the herd as well. Rendering trucks that pick up dead animals are a particular risk because they are carrying dead animals that are at high risk for carrying infectious disease. Visitors and perhaps especially veterinarians may introduce disease by coming onto the farm with dirty clothes and boots and by treating animals with inadequately cleaned and disinfected equipment.

The differences between herds lie in whether medical or production records from the source herd are known

---

Box 113-1

Sources of Exposure to the Cow-Calf Herd

1. New additions—bulls, replacement heifers, stockers, semen, embryos
2. Neighbors' herds—common grazing, fence-line contact, fence breaches, and commingling
3. Wildlife—deer, elk, rodents, birds, insects
4. Feed and water—imported feed, water drainage
5. Suppliers and visitors—rendering trucks, contaminated boots, contaminated equipment

and whether the imported animals are tested or quarantined for a period after arrival.

ASSESSING THE LEVEL OF RISK

Numerous risks for disease introduction exist, and the level of risk from particular sources varies in every herd because of their location and management practices. The risk from importing new cattle varies with the disease status of the source herd. Generally veterinarians do not have much, if any, documentation of the disease status of the source herd. If whole herd testing for particular pathogens is available from the source herd, it serves as the best evidence of disease freedom. A second source of information on disease status is documented herd health and performance records. If, for example, the herd has documented records of high reproductive performance, the likelihood of a reproductive pathogen in the herd is lessened. Similarly, if a herd has a documented biosecurity program, in addition to good performance and low morbidity and mortality levels, the risk of a significant pathogen is decreased. Source herds for semen and embryos are subject to the same concerns. Semen obtained from reputable sources that operate according to Certified Semen Services guidelines are a low risk for disease introduction, as are properly washed embryos for embryo transfer.

Imported feed is a risk for bovine spongiform encephalopathy and *Salmonella*, as well as potential toxic substances. Using reputable suppliers in compliance with federal guidelines for feed handling and ruminant protein and with on-site quality assurance programs will minimize risk. Risk of exposure by way of water depends on the amount of shared water source and the disease status of herds that share the water.

Risk level from suppliers and visitors depends on their practices and origin. Visitors or neighbors may introduce disease accidentally with dirty boots or clothes. Likewise, veterinarians can be a significant source of exposure because of their exposure to multiple herds and particularly herds with sick cattle. Veterinarians who arrive with dirty clothes, boots, and equipment increase the herd risk for disease introduction.

BIOSECURITY TOOLS

Several tools are available for the implementation of biosecurity programs. The implementation and importance of each depends on the individual farm and the importance of individual disease agents for that farm. They include the following:

- Quarantine
- Testing
- Vaccination
- Traffic control
- Environmental control

Quarantine

Quarantine is the separation of one group of cattle from another to prevent disease transmission. Complete quarantine of the resident herd from all outside herds is generally not practical for beef herds. We can, however, use short-term quarantine to control disease exposure.

Quarantine provides a period where incubating clinical disease, if present, may be expressed or detected before animals are introduced to the resident herd. As such, for acute diseases with short incubation times, and no inapparent carrier state, such as bovine respiratory syncytial virus (BRSV) and bovine viral diarrhea (BVD) in non–persistently infected animals, quarantine may be effective even when used alone. In contrast, for many diseases such as Johne's, brucellosis, leptospirosis, neosporosis, salmonellosis, BVD in persistently infected individuals, and leukosis, quarantine is not an effective biosecurity measure because of the inapparent carrier state. These animals can appear clinically normal but still carry and potentially shed the organism. In these cases the animals will need to be tested to detect the inapparent carrier state.

Proper quarantine involves preventing more than nose-to-nose contact between imports and the resident herd; drainage, distance, and duration need to be considered. For diseases that are shed in feces or urine such as *Salmonella*, *Leptospira*, and BVD, drainage from the quarantine site must not contact the resident herd. For diseases such as bovine leukemia virus or Anaplasma, which may have a significant insect vector, quarantine must be far enough away to prevent travel of vectors from quarantined cattle to the resident herd.

Duration of quarantine is again dictated by the disease of concern and its epidemiologic characteristics. For diseases where testing is undertaken, the quarantine period must last at least long enough for test results to return and establish the disease status of the cattle. If testing is not done, the quarantine period should at least exceed the incubation and shedding period of the diseases of concern. In general, the duration of the quarantine period should be 21 to 30 days.

Wildlife may be a source of exposure to *Leptospira*, *Salmonella*, and *Neospora*, but quarantine of cattle from wildlife is not likely possible or economically viable given the extensive nature of the cow-calf environment. Some practical steps, however, can be taken to minimize effective contact between the herd and local wildlife. Feedstuffs should be stored in a manner to prevent contamination by wildlife feces or urine. Control of standing water in corrals and pens and water sources will limit the environmental reservoir and decrease exposure to *Leptospira* spp. Population control of wild animals that are in contact with the herd may be prudent as well.

Testing

Testing of imported cattle can be useful in decreasing risk of introducing disease into the herd. Testing in addition to a quarantine period is required to prevent introduction of diseases with a clinically normal, inapparent carrier state such as Johne's, brucellosis, leptospirosis, neosporosis, salmonellosis, and leucosis. The quarantine period serves to prevent transmission to the resident herd while waiting for the test to establish disease status. Testing of imported animals is no panacea, however. Tests must be carefully evaluated for use to ensure they achieve the desired goal of decreasing risk of disease entry, and at an acceptable cost. Testing can be a valuable tool in a biosecurity program when appropriately applied. Test performance and utility will depend on the prevalence of the specific disease in the source herd and the sensitivity and specificity of the test.

Tests with high sensitivity will accurately identify a high proportion of positive animals. When applied to animals from a source herd with a low prevalence of disease, however, the positive predictive value will be poor, indicating a large proportion of the test-positive animals are false positives. This may be unacceptable if the cost of a false positive is high, resulting, for example, in the unnecessary exclusion of valuable genetics. Alternatively, if the cost of false negatives is high, then a significant level of false positives may be acceptable to exclude true positives. The negative predictive value is high when the test specificity is high and prevalence is low (i.e., negative test results are likely correct, but the test results provide little additional assurance that the animal is negative because the initial prevalence was low).

Tests with low sensitivity by definition fail to accurately identify a high proportion of true positive animals. When such tests are applied to individuals in populations with moderately low prevalence, the positive predictive value is low and the negative predictive value is approximately equal to 1-prevalence, so a negative test provides little information. The Johne's enzyme-linked immunosorbent assay (ELISA) test is just such a test. Prevalence of Johne's disease in beef cows is approximately 1%. The test is only about 25% sensitive in young preclinical cows, although sensitivity increases as the disease progresses. It is a specific test, correctly identifying about 97% to 99% of negative animals. When applied to a group of animals with a 1% prevalence of disease, the positive predictive value is 8% to 20%, so 80% to 92% of the positive test results are false positives. The negative predictive value is 99.2%, an excellent value until the veterinarian remembers that he or she was 99% sure any given animal was negative before the test was run (if 1% of cows were positive, then 99% were negative). Under these circumstances the test provides little useful information for the money that was spent and potentially provides false security that Johne's disease has been excluded from the herd. Further discussion of testing issues and test application are available (see Additional Resources on p. 599; Smith, Chapter 3, and Chenoweth, Chapter 3).

Vaccination

The use of vaccination for maintenance of immunity in the resident herd is another way to manage risk from imported cattle. It has probably been the most common way veterinarians and producers have attempted to mitigate biosecurity and biocontainment risks. Vaccination, however, should not be looked on as the only, or even primary, means of decreasing risk of disease. Clinical trial data on the effectiveness of most vaccines are limited. Even under optimal conditions, not all cattle will respond to vaccination, nor will all that respond to vaccination be protected from infection. In most cases vaccines do not prevent infection but work to decrease clinical disease and potentially shedding of pathogens. Vaccination

programs, however, can be useful adjuncts to other management practices. Producers may vaccinate the resident herd to increase immunity to pathogens that may be introduced by imported cattle or may require vaccination of imported cattle before entry into the herd to decrease introduction of disease agents.

Traffic Control

Traffic control has probably received little attention in the past but is important for both prevention of disease introduction to the herd (biosecurity) and control of disease transmission within the herd (biocontainment). Biosecurity traffic control involves controlling contact between visitors and the resident herd. Visitors and service providers can track manure and other biologic substances onto the farm, resulting in the introduction of disease. Agents such as *Salmonella* can survive for extended periods of time in dried manure, soil, etc. and in many cases have a relatively small infectious dose. Feed deliveries, vaccine deliveries, cattle deliveries, etc. should occur at the periphery of the farm and not contact cattle. Trucks delivering cattle may introduce disease because the truck was not cleaned between loads and the delivered cattle were exposed on the truck ride. Rendering truck pick-ups should especially be at the periphery of the farm.

Because of the nature of the profession in treating sick cows, veterinarians may also be a risk for disease introduction and should be especially careful to arrive with clean clothes, boots, and properly disinfected equipment. Equipment that is difficult to disinfect properly such as rope halters would best be provided by the producer rather than the veterinarian.

Environmental Control

Environmental control includes practices to decrease pathogen survival or accumulation in the environment and thus decrease disease exposure. For example, decreasing accumulation of standing water in corrals and pens will limit exposure of cows to *Leptospira* or other waterborne pathogens. Maintaining a well-drained and dry calving area will decrease pathogen survival and disease exposure in neonatal calves.

SPECIFIC BIOSECURITY APPLICATIONS

Sexually Transmitted Agents—*Campylobacter* and *Trichomonas*

Sexually transmitted diseases are perhaps the simplest to establish biosecurity for. Only one portal of entry is possible, so veterinarians can concentrate efforts on it. Artificial insemination using semen from reputable bull studs is an excellent way to decrease risk from sexually transmitted disease; however, each organism can contaminate semen collections and can survive freezing if proper precautions are not taken.

The primary reservoir for both *Trichomonas* and *Campylobacter* is the persistently infected bull. Importation of infected bulls or infected cows is the main source of introduction to the herd. Exposure to neighbor's bulls through communal grazing or fence breaks may also serve as a source of exposure. Ideally, only truly virgin bulls and females should be imported. If any breeding animal imports are not virgin, a quarantine and testing program should be established. Because both *Campylobacter* and *Trichomonas* are persistent infections that show no clinical signs in the infected bull or cow, quarantine alone is not effective in preventing introduction into a herd. Quarantine and testing of all nonvirgin bulls before contact with the herd can effectively prevent introduction of colonized bulls. Serial cultures should be taken for *Campylobacter* and *Trichomonas* at 1-week intervals for 3 weeks to increase the likelihood that infected bulls will be identified. The sensitivity of *Trichomonas* culture in commercial media has been estimated at 70% to 97%.

Vaccines for *Campylobacter* and *Trichomonas* are available either alone or in combination with *Leptospira*. Field trial data suggest that *Campylobacter* vaccination is effective in decreasing the effect of disease on the herd. *Campylobacter* vaccine efficacy has been estimated at 38% to 67% in cows. In bulls vaccination provides protection from persistent colonization. Trichomonas vaccine trials suggest the vaccine is effective in decreasing the duration of shedding and increasing pregnancy rates following exposure (vaccine efficacy 45%) in cows, but it does not appear to be effective in bulls.

Agents with Environmental Reservoirs— *Leptospira* and *Neospora*

Leptospira
Leptospirosis is an important cause of abortion and infertility in North American cattle. Cattle are the reservoir for the host adapted serovar *Leptospira borgpetersenii* serovar *hardjo*. All other serovars result in incidental infection in cattle and are adapted to and maintained in other species. Transmission of infections is through contact with a contaminated environment or by venereal transmission for the bovine host-adapted serovar. Survival of and exposure to leptospires in the environment is assisted in moderate temperatures and standing water.

Cattle infected with the serovar *hardjo* are typically normal clinically and continue to shed for months to years, so quarantine alone is not effective in preventing introduction of this form of leptospirosis. Quarantine could be effective in segregating imported animals until testing could determine their infection status. Additionally, runoff from the quarantine area must be controlled and not allowed to contact the resident herd. Utilization of polymerase chain reaction (PCR) to detect leptospires in urine and serology to identify the most likely serovar is the most practical testing strategy. Alternatively, one dose of long-acting oxytetracycline at 20 mg/kg eliminated renal shedding of *L. borgpetersenii* serovar *hardjo* in experimentally infected cattle. It may be helpful to treat all imported cattle with antibiotics to clear any infection during a quarantine period.

Vaccination of the resident herd and imported animals may be a useful way to provide some level of protection for the herd. Required frequency of vaccination varies with the level of exposure from one time per year in semiarid regions to two to three times per year in wetter environments with higher exposure.

Particularly in wetter climates, control of the environment may be important in reducing the exposure level of cows by decreasing the environmental survival of leptospires. Corrals should be graded to prevent the accumulation of standing water as a suitable environment for leptospires. A mild slope to the corral and a relatively impervious surface will aid water drainage. A program to limit contact between wildlife and cattle, pens, feed, and water may also be helpful.

Neospora
Neospora caninum has become a commonly recognized cause of bovine abortion in cattle. Evidence of *Neospora* infection is common in U.S. beef and dairy herds. Vertical transmission is common; transmission occurs between dam and fetus in approximately 90% of cases. Positive cattle are at increased risk for an abortion. Available evidence indicates horizontal transmission also occurs but less commonly. Dogs and coyotes are definitive hosts for *N. caninum* and deer appear to be able to serve as intermediate hosts. Dogs and wild canids should be prevented from consuming placenta and fetal tissues from abortions. Placentas and fetuses should be collected and disposed of as promptly as possible. Cattle feed sources should be protected from dogs and wild canids to prevent them from defecating in feed.

N. caninum causes no disease in the mature animal, so quarantine alone will not identify positive animals. An ELISA test kit is commercially available to identify infected animals for exclusion.

Recently, a vaccine for *N. caninum* received full approval for commercial availability in the United States (Neogaurd, Intervet Inc., Millsboro, Del.). Limited efficacy data from experimental studies or controlled clinical trials are available, so the efficacy of the vaccine is uncertain. A vaccination program could complicate differentiation of naturally infected animals from vaccinates and limit culling options.

Ubiquitous Agents—Bovine Viral Diarrhea and Infectious Bovine Rhinotracheitis

Bovine Viral Diarrhea
Seroprevalence studies indicate that BVD infection is widely distributed in cattle herds. The primary source of infection in an endemic herd is the persistently infected animal, which sheds high numbers of viral particles. Importation of a new animal, persistently or acutely infected, to the herd frequently precedes an outbreak of BVD. BVD can be introduced to the herd by any class of cattle. Exposure of pregnant cows or heifers to BVD virus (BVDV) from this imported animal from approximately 45 to 125 days of gestation may result in persistently infected calves that expose the rest of the herd well after the initial outbreak. Contact with neighboring cattle herds also provides some risk to the resident herd.

Preventing BVDV from entering a herd revolves around identification of acute and persistent infections in imported animals before introduction into the herd. Quarantine alone is not adequate to exclude BVDV from a herd because persistently infected animals may appear normal and not manifest disease during a quarantine period. Diagnostic testing is necessary in conjunction with quarantine during the time that tests are pending. Several good options exist for testing animals for BVD. If a persistently infected animal is identified during quarantine, it should be immediately culled. Acutely infected animals do not remain viremic, and when the acute infection has passed, the animal will be safe to add to the herd. Once a herd has a BVDV infection, biocontainment depends on identification and removal of PI animals. Specific testing strategies for identification and removal depend on the specific circumstances of the herd.

Vaccination can be a useful adjunct to proper management in the control of reproductive disease from BVDV. The vaccination must provide fetal protection to be useful in a control program focused toward reproductive disease. Available evidence suggests that vaccination may provide some level of fetal protection. Published reports of vaccine efficacy in preventing PI calves range from 57% to 82%. Clearly, vaccination alone will not prevent the birth of persistently infected calves if biosecurity methods allow introduction of infected cattle. It will, however, limit the effect of an inadvertent introduction of BVDV whether from imported cattle, contact with neighboring cattle, or an outside reservoir.

Infectious Bovine Rhinotracheitis

Seroprevalence studies suggest that bovine herpes virus (BHV)-1 infection is widely distributed in cattle herds. In susceptible herds 25% to 60% of cows may abort following exposure during pregnancy. BHV causes latent infection in cattle, and these latent infections may be reactivated by stressful conditions. Because of this latent reactivation, cattle previously exposed to BHV-1 can serve as a source of infection for susceptible animals. Persistence of infection in the herd is a result of both acute infections in susceptible animals and reactivation of shedding in latently infected animals.

A period of quarantine to allow possible acute or reactivated infections to manifest and resolve may be useful to avoid introducing active infection. It also allows time for vaccination and development of immunity in incoming cattle. Any seropositive animal may serve as a source of infection to a negative herd when reactivation of shedding occurs. Testing and exclusion of seropositive animals to establish a negative herd is not likely to be practical in a cow-calf herd.

Maintenance of immunity in individuals and the herd through vaccination is a crucial factor in an infectious bovine rhinotracheitis biosecurity program. Both modified live virus and killed products are available. Vaccine efficacy of a modified live virus vaccine in an experimental study was 90% 7 months after vaccination. Vaccination will not prevent establishment of latency, and modified live virus vaccination may induce latency.

Enteric Disease Biosecurity

In beef cattle operations the primary risk from enteric disease is in calves. Calf diarrhea is a multifactorial disease resulting from the interaction of host, agent, and environmental factors. Numerous agents are associated with diarrhea in calves including *Rotavirus, Coronavirus, Escherichia coli, Salmonella, Cryptosporidia, Coccidia,* and potentially BVDV. They share a common fecal-oral transmission route, so the methods of controlling disease introduction and spread are also substantially common between them. Most agents of calf enteric disease are ubiquitous organisms, present in the gastrointestinal tract of a large proportion of animals within a herd. In many cases the mature animals are the reservoir and calves are exposed as they enter the herd. The difference in disease rates between herds is due to differences in management practices and generally not the presence or absence of disease agents. In beef herds *Salmonella* and some specific strains of *E. coli* are not ubiquitous but may be introduced to herds from outside making biosecurity an important issue. Introduction of calves for grafting onto cows that have lost their calves is probably the greatest risk. This is particularly true for calves purchased through auction markets.

The two main enteric diseases of biosecurity and biocontainment interest in adult cattle are *Salmonella* and *Mycobacterium avium* ssp. *paratuberculosis* (MAP, or Johne's). Numerous *Salmonella* serotypes can infect cattle and may originate from multiple different reservoirs. Generally it is introduced to a herd by importation of a subclinical carrier animal. Calves or adult cows purchased through salebarn channels may be of particular risk due to the extensive exposure they have had to other cull cattle. Dairy source animals may present an increased risk as compared with beef animals. Wildlife exposure may also be a source of exposure for beef operations. Anecdotal evidence in the United States suggests turkeys and geese may carry strains that can subsequently infect cattle. *Salmonella* are hardy in the environment and may survive for years to produce infections. Salmonella are also a zoonotic concern and clients should be warned of the potential for infection, especially if immunocompromised persons are in the household.

Mycobacterium avium ssp. *paratuberculosis* has been considered more of a problem in dairy cattle but is receiving increasing attention in beef herds. Sero-prevalence estimates based on ELISA serology in beef cattle have ranged from 0.4% to 3% at the individual cow level and 8% to 44% at the herd level. Prevalence is higher in dairy herds. Adult cattle imported to the herd may introduce MAP and subsequently spread it to calves, resulting in establishment in the herd. Once MAP is in the herd, biocontainment practices to control contact of calves with adult manure is critical to minimize transmission. In a beef operation efforts should be focused on keeping a clean environment so that calves are not exposed to excess adult manure on udders, around feeding areas, or in feed or water. Use of dairy animals for nurse cows, embryo recipients, or as a source of colostrum may increase risk of importing MAP to the herd. Testing individual animals before entry into the herd is not a useful technique to prevent introduction of MAP as discussed earlier under testing. Alternately, importing cattle only from herds with a whole herd testing program in place for MAP provides some level of certainty that they are negative or low-prevalence herds and can substantially decrease risk.

SUMMARY

Rational biosecurity programs are a function of effectiveness and economics. Biosecurity is ideally implemented in a risk-analysis approach that assesses the risk of introducing disease, consequences of introduction (e.g., economic, reputation, labor), cost of a mitigation program, and effectiveness of the mitigation program (amount of risk is decreased). Adequate understanding of the epidemiology and ecology of the particular disease agent is necessary to strategically identify effective control points.

Additional Resources

Smith RD: Evaluation of diagnostic tests. In Smith RD, editor: *Veterinary clinical epidemiology,* ed 2, Boca Raton, Fla, 1995, CRC Press, pp 31-52.

Sanderson MW: Records and epidemiology for production medicine. In Chenoweth PJ, Sanderson MW, editors: *Beef practice: cow-calf production medicine,* Ames, Iowa, 2005, Blackwell Publishing, pp 29-64.

CHAPTER 114

Management of Neonatal Diarrhea in Cow-Calf Herds

DAVID R. SMITH

Diarrhea is one of the most likely reasons young beef calves become sick or die.[1] Besides its detriment to calf health and well-being, neonatal calf diarrhea is an economic burden to cattle producers due to poor calf performance, death, and the expense of medications and labor to treat sick calves.[2,3] In addition, catching and treating young calves puts herd owners and their employees at risk of physical harm, and many producers become disheartened after investing long hours to treat scouring calves during an already exhausting calving season.

INVESTIGATING OUTBREAKS OF NEONATAL CALF DIARRHEA

Cattle producers may not discuss neonatal calf diarrhea with a veterinarian until a serious outbreak occurs. Veterinarians investigating outbreaks of neonatal calf diarrhea must first make recommendations for therapy of affected calves, then take action to protect susceptible and unborn calves from ongoing exposure and illness. Finally, attention should focus on determining what future actions might prevent the disease in subsequent calving seasons. The outbreak investigation sometimes becomes sidetracked in the pursuit of an etiologic agent rather than identifying more useful explanations for the outbreak. Knowing the etiologic agent may provide an explanation for the proximal cause of a calf's illness or death (although that knowledge rarely explains the outbreak) or provide a solution for treatment, control, or prevention.

Neonatal calf diarrhea is a complex, multifactorial, and temporally dynamic disease.[4-6] Agent, host, and environmental factors collectively explain neonatal calf diarrhea,

and these factors interact dynamically over the course of time. Veterinarians must understand the relationships among these factors within the production system to control the disease or prevent its occurrence.[7]

AGENT FACTORS

Numerous infectious agents have been recovered from calves with neonatal diarrhea.[4,5,7,8-14] Common agents of neonatal calf diarrhea include bacteria such as *Escherichia coli* and *Salmonella,* viruses such as rotavirus and coronavirus, and protozoa such as cryptosporidia. Bovine rotavirus, bovine coronavirus, and cryptosporidia are ubiquitous to most cattle populations and can be recovered from calves in herds not experiencing calf diarrhea.[7] Further, multiple agents can be recovered from herds experiencing outbreaks of calf diarrhea; suggesting that even during outbreaks more than one agent may be involved. The adult cow herd commonly serves as the reservoir of pathogens from one year to the next.[15-20]

HOST FACTORS

Calves obtain passive immunity against common agents of calf diarrhea after absorbing antibodies from colostrum or colostrum supplements shortly after birth.[21-23] The quantity of antibodies absorbed is determined by the quality and quantity of colostrum the calf ingests, as well as how soon after birth it is ingested. In colostrum the presence of maternal antibodies against specific agents requires prior exposure of the dam to antigens of the agent. Vaccines are sometimes used to immunize the dam against specific agents, and some commercially available colostrum supplements contain polyclonal or monoclonal antibodies directed against specific agents. Unfortunately, the use of vaccines or colostrum supplements has not always prevented undifferentiated neonatal calf diarrhea.

Calves typically become ill or die from neonatal diarrhea within 1 to 2 weeks of age.[4,8,10,24] The narrow range of age within which neonatal calf diarrhea occurs is not explained solely by the incubation period of the agents. Diarrhea is observed in colostrum-deprived and gnotobiotic calves within a few days of pathogen challenge regardless of age.[25-27] Calves may have an age-specific susceptibility to neonatal diarrhea that occurs as lactogenic immunity is waning and before the calf is fully capable of developing an active immune response.[21]

Regardless of the reason for the age-specificity of neonatal calf diarrhea, this period defines the age of susceptibility, as well as the age calves are most likely to become infective and shed the agents in their feces.[28-32] Age specificity of susceptibility and infectivity has important implications for controlling transmission of the pathogens of neonatal diarrhea because in some calving systems the number of susceptible and infective calves can change dynamically with time. At times the number of potentially infective calves may greatly outnumber the number of susceptible calves, resulting in widespread opportunity for effective contacts.

The dam's age also explains a calf's risk for undifferentiated neonatal diarrhea. Calves born to heifers are at higher risk for neonatal diarrhea and have lower maternal antibody levels than calves born to older cows.[33] Calves born to heifers are probably more susceptible to disease because heifers produce a lower volume and quality of colostrum, may have poor mothering skills, and are more likely to experience dystocia.[34,35]

ENVIRONMENTAL FACTORS

The environment may influence both the level of pathogen exposure and the ability of the calf to resist disease. Exposure to pathogens may occur through direct contact with other cattle or via contact with contaminated environmental surfaces. Establishing environmental hygiene has long been recognized as important for controlling neonatal calf diarrhea,[36,37] but doing so is often a challenge. An effective contact is an exposure to pathogens of a dose-load or duration sufficient to cause disease. Crowded conditions increase opportunities for effective contacts with infected animals or contaminated surfaces. Ambient temperature (e.g., excessive heat or cold) and moisture (e.g., mud or snow) are important stressors that impair the ability of the calf to resist disease and may influence pathogen numbers, as well as opportunities for oral ingestion.

TEMPORAL FACTORS

Host susceptibility, pathogen exposure, and pathogen transmission occur dynamically over time within the calving season.[7] Although the adult cow-herd likely serves as the reservoir of neonatal diarrhea pathogens from year

to year,[15-20] the average dose-load of pathogen exposure to calves is likely to increase over time within a calving season because calves infected earlier serve as pathogen multipliers and become the primary source of exposure to younger susceptible calves. This multiplier effect can result in high calf infectivity and widespread environmental contamination with pathogens.[38] Each calf serves as growth media for pathogen production, amplifying the dose-load of pathogen it received.[27-29] Therefore calves born later in the calving season may receive larger dose-loads of pathogens and, in turn, may become relatively more infective by growing even greater numbers of agents. Eventually the dose-load of pathogens overwhelms the calf's ability to resist disease. These factors alone or in combination may explain observations that calves born later in the calving season are at greater risk for disease or death (Smith and colleagues, unpublished).[24]

BIOCONTAINMENT OF NEONATAL CALF DIARRHEA

Biosecurity is the sum of actions taken to prevent introducing a disease agent into a population (pen, herd, region), whereas biocontainment describes the actions taken to control a pathogen already present in the population.[39] In theory outbreaks of undifferentiated neonatal calf diarrhea could be prevented by eliminating the pathogens, decreasing calf susceptibility, or altering the production system to reduce opportunities for pathogen exposure and transmission. However, the endemic nature of the common pathogens of neonatal calf diarrhea makes it unlikely that cattle populations could be made biosecure from these agents. Maternal immunity is clearly important to calf susceptibility to enteric agents,[6,40] but lactogenic immunity wanes with time[21] and managers of extensive beef cattle systems have limited practical opportunities to improve rates of passive antibody transfer. In addition, vaccines are not available against all pathogens of calf diarrhea, they may not induce sufficient cross-protection,[32] and pathogens may evade the protection afforded by vaccination by evolving away from vaccine strains.[41] For these reasons, a biocontainment approach to control neonatal calf diarrhea seems prudent and logical.[39,42]

SANDHILLS CALVING SYSTEM FOR PREVENTING NEONATAL DIARRHEA

Effective contacts with pathogens can be prevented by physically separating animals, reducing the level of exposure (e.g., through the use of sanitation or dilution over space), or minimizing contact time. These principles have been successfully applied in calf hutch systems to control neonatal diseases in dairy calves.[43] Various biocontainment systems for beef herds have been developed to prevent neonatal calf diarrhea.[44-46] Each of these are strategies to manage cattle in a system that prevents calves from having effective contacts with pathogens by reducing opportunities for exposure and transmission. The management actions defined as the Sandhills Calving System prevent effective contacts among beef calves by (1) segregating calves by age to prevent direct and indirect transmission of pathogens from older to younger calves and (2) moving pregnant cows to clean calving pastures to minimize pathogen dose-load in the environment and contact time between calves and the larger portion of the cow herd. The objective of the system is to recreate the more ideal conditions that exist at the start of the calving season during each subsequent week of the season. These more ideal conditions are that cows are calving on ground that has been previously unoccupied by cattle (for at least some months), and older, infective calves are not present.

The Sandhills Calving System uses larger, contiguous pastures for calving, rather than high-animal-density calving lots. Cows are turned into the first calving pasture (Pasture 1) as soon as the first calves are born. Calving continues in Pasture 1 for 2 weeks. After 2 weeks the cows that have not yet calved are moved to Pasture 2. Existing cow-calf pairs remain in Pasture 1. After a week of calving in Pasture 2, cows that have not calved are moved to Pasture 3 and cow-calf pairs born in Pasture 2 remain in Pasture 2. Each subsequent week cows that have not yet calved are moved to a new pasture and pairs remain in their pasture of birth. The result is cow-calf pairs distributed over multiple pastures, each containing calves within 1 week of age of each other. Cow-calf pairs from different pastures may be commingled after the youngest calf is 4 weeks of age and all calves are considered low risk for neonatal diarrhea.

It can be difficult to manage many cattle groups in intensive grass management systems; therefore the Sandhills Calving System in these herds is modified to reduce the number of groups. Cattle are moved to different pastures throughout the calving season as appropriate for forage utilization; however, every 10 days, or whenever 100 calves are born, the herd is divided by sorting cows that had not calved from the cow-calf pairs of the preceding group. In this manner, fewer cattle groups are required, although the number of calves within any pasture group never exceeds 100, and all calves within a group are within 10 days of age of each other.

The Sandhills Calving System prevents effective contacts by using clean calving pastures, preventing direct contact between younger calves and older calves and preventing later-born calves from being exposed to an accumulation of pathogens in the environment. The specific actions to implement the system may differ between herds to meet the specific needs of each production system. Key components of the systems are age segregation of calves and the frequent movement of gravid cows to clean calving pastures. Age segregation prevents the serial passage of pathogens from older calves to younger calves. The routine movement (every 7-10 days) of gravid cows to new calving pastures prevents the buildup of pathogens in the calving environment over the course of the calving season and prevents exposure of the latest born calves to an overwhelming dose-load of pathogens.

Development of a ranch-specific plan for implementing the Sandhills Calving System must take place well in advance of the calving season, in some circumstances in consultation with a range specialist. Available pastures must be identified and their use coordinated with the calving schedule. Water, feed, shelter, and anticipated weather conditions must be considered. The size of the pastures should be matched to the number of calves expected to be born in a given week. Use of the pastures must not be damaging to later grazing.

The Sandhills Calving System may offer additional benefits to labor management. For example, there may be some efficiency because cattle movement could be scheduled once a week as labor is available. Moving cows without calves to a new pasture is often easier than sorting and moving individual cow-calf pairs. Also, the workload is partitioned between pasture groups such that cows at risk for dystocia are together in one pasture while calves at risk for diarrhea are in another. Information from pregnancy examination, when available, enables sorting cows into early and later calving groups. Cows expected to calve later in the season can be maintained elsewhere and added to the calving pasture as appropriate, thereby reducing the number of cattle moving through the initial series of pastures.

Ranchers using the Sandhills Calving System have observed meaningful and sustained reductions in morbidity and mortality caused by neonatal calf diarrhea and greatly reduced use of medications.[47] Although the system was tested and initially adopted in ranches typical of the Nebraska Sandhills, it has been useful elsewhere because the principles on which it is based are widely applicable.

CONCLUSIONS

Understanding the multifactorial, temporally dynamic nature of neonatal calf diarrhea in cattle populations is the basis for developing strategies for control and prevention. The common pathogens of neonatal calf diarrhea are endemic to most cattle herds, and it is unlikely that cattle populations could be made biosecure from these agents. Managers of extensive beef cattle systems have few opportunities to improve rates of passive transfer, and vaccines are not always protective. Lactogenic immunity wanes, making calves age susceptible and age infective. Each calf serves as growth media for pathogen production, amplifying the dose-load of pathogen it received and resulting in high calf infectivity and widespread environmental contamination over time in a calving season. For these reasons it is logical to apply biocontainment strategies to prevent effective transmission of the pathogens causing neonatal diarrhea. Cattle management systems based on an understanding of infectious disease dynamics have successfully reduced sickness and death caused by neonatal calf diarrhea.

References

1. USDA: *Part II: Reference of 1997 beef cow-calf health and management practices, 1997,* USDA: APHIS, VS, CEAH, National Animal Health Monitoring System.
2. Anderson DC, Kress DD, Bernardini MM et al: The effect of scours on calf weaning weight, *Prof Anim Sci* 19:399, 2003.
3. Swift BL, Nelms GE, Coles R: The effect of neonatal diarrhea on subsequent weight gains in beef calves, *Vet Med Small Anim Clin* 71:1269, 1272, 1976.
4. Acres SD, Laing CJ, Saunders JR et al: Acute undifferentiated neonatal diarrhea in beef calves. I. Occurrence and distribution of infectious agents, *Can J Comp Med* 39:116, 1975.

5. Acres SD, Saunders JR, Radostits OM: Acute undifferentiated neonatal diarrhea of beef calves: the prevalence of enterotoxigenic *E. coli*, reo-like (rota) virus and other enteropathogens in cow-calf herds, *Can Vet J* 18:274, 1977.

6. Saif LJ, Smith KL: Enteric viral infections of calves and passive immunity, *J Dairy Sci* 68:206, 1985.

7. Barrington GM, Gay JM, Evermann JF: Biosecurity for neonatal gastrointestinal diseases, *Vet Clin North Am Food Anim Pract* 18:7, 2002.

8. Bulgin MS, Anderson BC, Ward AC et al: Infectious agents associated with neonatal calf disease in southwestern Idaho and eastern Oregon, *J Am Vet Med Assoc* 180:1222, 1982.

9. Mebus CA, Stair EL, Rhodes MB et al: Neonatal calf diarrhea: propagation, attenuation, and characteristics of coronavirus-like agents, *Am J Vet Res* 34:145, 1973.

10. Trotz-Williams LA, Jarvie BD, Martin SW et al: Prevalence of *Cryptosporidium parvum* infection in southwestern Ontario and its association with diarrhea in neonatal dairy calves, *Can Vet J* 46:349, 2005.

11. Athanassious R, Marsollais G, Assaf R et al: Detection of bovine coronavirus and type A rotavirus in neonatal calf diarrhea and winter dysentery of cattle in Quebec: evaluation of three diagnostic methods, *Can Vet J* 35:163, 1994.

12. Naciri M, Lefay MP, Mancassola R et al: Role of *Cryptosporidium parvum* as a pathogen in neonatal diarrhoea complex in suckling and dairy calves in France, *Vet Parasitol* 85:245, 1999.

13. Morin M, Lariviere S, Lallier R: Pathological and microbiological observations made on spontaneous cases of acute neonatal calf diarrhea, *Can J Comp Med* 40:228, 1976.

14. Lucchelli A, Lance SA, Bartlett PB et al: Prevalence of bovine group A rotavirus shedding among dairy calves in Ohio, *Am J Vet Res* 53:169, 1992.

15. Crouch CF, Bielefeldt Ohman H, Watts TC et al: Chronic shedding of bovine enteric coronavirus antigen-antibody complexes by clinically normal cows, *J Gen Virol* 66:1489, 1985.

16. Collins JK, Riegel CA, Olson JD et al: Shedding of enteric coronavirus in adult cattle, *Am J Vet Res* 48:361, 1987.

17. Crouch CF, Acres SD: Prevalence of rotavirus and coronavirus antigens in the feces of normal cows, *Can J Comp Med* 48:340, 1984.

18. McAllister TA, Olson ME, Fletch A et al: Prevalence of *Giardia* and *Cryptosporidium* in beef cows in southern Ontario and in beef calves in southern British Columbia, *Can Vet J* 46:47, 2005.

19. Watanabe Y, Yang CH, Ooi HK: Cryptosporidium infection in livestock and first identification of *Cryptosporidium parvum* genotype in cattle feces in Taiwan, *Parasitol Res* 97:238, 2005.

20. Ralston BJ, McAllister TA, Olson ME: Prevalence and infection pattern of naturally acquired giardiasis and cryptosporidiosis in range beef calves and their dams, *Vet Parasitol* 114:113, 2003.

21. Barrington GM, Parish SM: Bovine neonatal immunology, *Vet Clin North Am Food Anim Pract* 17:463, 2001.

22. Besser TE, Gay CC: The importance of colostrum to the health of the neonatal calf, *Vet Clin North Am Food Anim Pract* 10:107, 1994.

23. Besser TE, Gay CC, McGuire TC et al: Passive immunity to bovine rotavirus infection associated with transfer of serum antibody into the intestinal lumen, *J Virol* 62:2238, 1988.

24. Clement JC, King ME, Salman MD et al: Use of epidemiologic principles to identify risk factors associated with the development of diarrhea in calves in five beef herds, *J Am Vet Med Assoc* 207:1334, 1995.

25. El-Kanawati ZR, Tsunemitsu H, Smith DR et al: Infection and cross-protection studies of winter dysentery and calf diarrhea bovine coronavirus strains in colostrum-deprived and gnotobiotic calves, *Am J Vet Res* 57:48, 1996.

26. Heckert RA, Saif LJ, Mengel JP et al: Mucosal and systemic antibody responses to bovine coronavirus structural proteins in experimentally challenge-exposed calves fed low or high amounts of colostral antibodies, *Am J Vet Res* 52:700, 1991.

27. Saif LJ, Redman DR, Moorhead PD et al: Experimentally induced coronavirus infections in calves: viral replication in the respiratory and intestinal tracts, *Am J Vet Res* 47:1426, 1986.

28. Kapil S, Trent AM, Goyal SM: Excretion and persistence of bovine coronavirus in neonatal calves, *Arch Virol* 115:127, 1990.

29. Uga S, Matsuo J, Kono E et al: Prevalence of *Cryptosporidium parvum* infection and pattern of oocyst shedding in calves in Japan, *Vet Parasitol* 94:27, 2000.

30. Nydam DV, Wade SE, Schaaf SL et al: Number of *Cryptosporidum parvum* oocysts of *Giardia* spp. cysts by dairy calves after natural infection, *Am J Vet Res* 62:1612, 2001.

31. O'Handley RM, Cockwill C, McAllister TA et al: Duration of naturally acquired giardiosis and cryptosporidiosis in dairy calves and their association with diarrhea, *J Am Vet Med Assoc* 214:391, 1999.

32. Murakami Y, Nishioka N, Watanabe T et al: Prolonged excretion and failure of cross-protection between distinct serotypes of bovine rotavirus, *Vet Microbiol* 12:7, 1986.

33. Schumann FJ, Townsend HG, Naylor JM: Risk factors for mortality from diarrhea in beef calves in Alberta, *Can J Vet Res* 54:366, 1990.

34. Odde KG: Reducing neonatal calf losses through selection, nutrition and management, *Agri-Practice* 17:12, 1996.

35. Odde KG: Survival of the neonatal calf, *Vet Clin North Am Food Anim Pract* 4:501, 1988.

36. Law J: *Special report on diseases of cattle*, Washington, DC, 1916, U.S. Department of Agriculture, Bureau of Animal Industry.

37. Van Es L: *The principles of animal hygiene and preventive veterinary medicine*, New York, 1932, John Wiley & Sons.

38. Atwill ER, Johnson EM, Pereira MG: Association of herd composition, stocking rate, and duration of calving season with fecal shedding of *Cryptosporidium parvum* oocysts in beef herds, *J Am Vet Med Assoc* 215:1833, 1999.

39. Dargatz DA, Garry FB, Traub-Dargatz JL: An introduction to biosecurity of cattle operations, *Vet Clin North Am Food Anim Pract* 18:1, 2002.

40. Nocek JE, Braund DG, Warner RG: Influence of neonatal colostrum administration, immunoglobulin, and continued feeding of colostrum on calf gain, health, and serum protein, *J Dairy Sci* 67:319, 1984.

41. Lu W, Duhamel GE, Benfield DA et al: Serological and genotypic characterization of group A rotavirus reassortants from diarrheic calves born to dams vaccinated against rotavirus, *Vet Microbiol* 42:159, 1994.

42. Larson RL, Tyler JW, Schultz LG et al: Management strategies to decrease calf death losses in beef herds, *J Am Vet Med Assoc* 224:42, 2004.

43. Sanders DE: Field management of neonatal diarrhea, *Vet Clin North Am Food Anim Pract* 1:621, 1985.

44. Radostits OM, Acres SD: The control of acute undifferentiated diarrhea of newborn beef calves, *Vet Clin North Am Large Anim Pract* 5:143, 1983.

45. Thomson JU: Implementing biosecurity in beef and dairy herds, *Proc Am Assoc Bov Pract* 30:8, 1997.

46. Pence M, Robbe S, Thomson J: Reducing the incidence of neonatal calf diarrhea through evidence-based management, *Compend Contin Educ Pract Vet* 23:S73-S75, 2001.

47. Smith DR, Grotelueschen DM, Knott T et al: Prevention of neonatal calf diarrhea with the Sandhills calving system, *Proc Am Assoc Bov Pract* 37:166, 2004.

CHAPTER 115

Calf Preweaning Immunity and Impact on Vaccine Schedules

JAMES A. ROTH

The goal in vaccinating young calves is to induce protective levels of active immunity before they lose maternal antibody protection and are exposed to infectious agents. Accomplishing this means facing many challenges: maternal antibody derived from colostrum may inhibit the immune response to a vaccine; calves have reduced immune responses as compared with older animals; calves are born immunologically naive and therefore have no immunologic memory to any pathogens and must mount a primary immune response against all pathogens for which they are at risk; multiple vaccines administered at the same time have the potential to interfere with each other; infestation with internal and/or external parasites may alter the immune response to a vaccine; multiple management factors may induce stress, which impairs the response to vaccination; and optimal nutrition is essential for an optimal immune response. All of these factors must be considered in order to design an effective vaccination program for preweaning calves.

IMMUNE COMPETENCE OF THE NEONATAL CALF

Native Defense Mechanisms

All of the components of native immunity begin to develop in utero and are functional at birth in calves. However, they do not function as efficiently as in the adult animal. They continue to mature and become more effective during the first weeks and months of life. Neutrophils, macrophages, complement, interferon production, and natural killer cells all have been shown to have reduced activity in young calves as compared with adults. In addition, stress or inadequate nutrition can further suppress native defense mechanisms, leading to increased susceptibility to infection. The subsequent viral, bacterial, or parasitic infections may further reduce native defense mechanisms, leading to even more severe disease. Calves that are sick are not as able to produce an optimal immune response to vaccines. It is extremely important to optimize management to avoid stress, provide adequate nutrition, and reduce exposure to infectious agents to keep the calf healthy so that it can respond to vaccination. Colostral antibody helps the calf to resist infection until it is older and its immune system is more mature and able to mount an effective resistance.

Bovine colostrum has been shown to contain high levels of several cytokines including interleukin 1 (IL-1), tumor necrosis factor alpha, and interferon gamma. These cytokines have been shown to enhance neutrophil, macrophage, and natural killer cell function. Colostrum management plans should be optimized to ensure that calves get an adequate supply of fresh colostrum so that they benefit from not only the antibodies in the colostrum, but the cytokines as well. Cytokines are more labile than antibody and may be destroyed by fermentation, pasteurization, improper storage, or overheating when thawing. Fresh colostrum should be frozen after collection from individual cows (not pooled) and slowly thawed immediately before use, to preserve the activity of the cytokines. Under some circumstances, it may be necessary to pasteurize colostrum to kill infectious agents. Higher levels of management should be used to compensate for any loss of immune stimulation from the cytokines in pasteurized colostrum.

Acquired Defense Mechanisms

Calves have at least three major disadvantages as compared with more mature animals when attempting to mount an immune response to a vaccine:

1. Antigen-presenting cells, cytokine production, B cells, and T cells do not function as efficiently in young calves as compared with adults. Newborn calves are capable of mounting an immune response to vaccines, but the response is often suboptimal, even in the absence of maternal antibody. The cytokines present in colostrum may help to enhance lymphocyte maturation and function. Proper colostrum management is essential for optimizing immune responsiveness in young calves.
2. Calves are born immunologically naive, so they do not have any memory B or T cells. They have to mount a primary immune response to all of the antigens that they are exposed to starting at birth including normal flora and environmental antigens. Minimizing exposure to pathogens for as long as possible is essential to give the immune system time to mature and respond to the myriad of novel antigens present after birth. The primary immune response is more susceptible to suppression by stress and other

factors than is the secondary immune response. Therefore the initial exposure to vaccine is more likely to be interfered with than booster doses of a vaccine. Every effort should be made to give the initial immunization at a time of minimum stress, even if maternal antibody is present and may partially interfere with the response to the vaccine. The initial dose may prime the immune system by stimulating production of memory B and T cells so that a more rapid and vigorous response can occur to a subsequent dose of vaccine.

3. Maternal antibody interferes with antibody responses to vaccines. The antibody in colostrum inhibits the calves' B cells from responding to specific antigen by producing antibody. In addition, the antibody may inhibit modified live vaccines from replicating to increase the mass of antigen that the calf is exposed to and may act to remove the antigen present in killed vaccines. This results in reduced antigen mass to stimulate immunity. Although colostral antibody inhibits the calf from producing its own antibody, it may not inhibit the development of memory B and T cells, which can be important for priming the immune system for subsequent vaccination or exposure to pathogens.

VACCINATION OF THE PREWEANING CALF

Acquired immunity is due to the actions of antibody and memory B, T helper, T cytotoxic, and gamma delta T cells. Recent advances in immunologic assays have made it possible to monitor the presence of antigen-specific memory T cell subsets. This is important in order to fully understand the immune response induced by a vaccine.

Even though maternal antibody passively transferred to a calf is known to inhibit antibody production in response to vaccines, there is evidence that exposure to antigen is capable of inducing T cell–mediated immunity and B cell memory, which may help to protect the calf from challenge with the infectious agent. Challenge of calves with high maternal antibody titers to bovine viral diarrhea virus (BVDV) during the first 2 to 5 weeks of life with virulent type 2 BVDV failed to induce an antibody response in the calves but did induce memory B cell, T helper cell, T cytotoxic cell, and gamma delta T cell responses to BVDV and protected the calves from challenge with BVDV type 2 after their maternal antibody titers had dropped to undetectable levels. Calves have also been observed to have B and T cell subset memory for bovine respiratory syncytial virus in the absence of detectable serum antibody. An anamnestic antibody response to bovine respiratory viral vaccine has been documented after a second immunization, despite the fact that no antibody response was measurable after the initial immunization. These observations prove that calves are capable of developing B cell memory and T cell–mediated immunity to pathogens even if colostral antibody prevents the calf from producing an antibody response to the pathogen.

The amount of specific antibody a calf receives through colostrum depends on the titer of antibody in the colostrum and the amount of colostrum that the calf receives during the first few hours of life. A calf that does not receive any maternal antibody to a specific pathogen is capable of mounting an immune response to that pathogen if vaccinated in the first few days of life. Importantly, the newborn calf is immune competent, but its immune system will continue to mature and become more efficient over the next few months. In addition, the newborn calf is immune suppressed due to high cortisol levels at the time of birth and for a few days afterward. The calf is capable of responding to antigen, but the response will not be optimal. Therefore if a calf is vaccinated as a newborn, it should receive a booster dose of vaccine a few weeks later.

Maternal antibody has a half-life of approximately 16 days in calves. Calves that have a high titer of colostral antibody may not be able to produce an antibody response to a vaccine for several months, but they may develop a memory B and T cell response. Calves that receive no colostral antibody, or only a small amount, will be susceptible to infection and ready to produce antibody in response to vaccine at a much earlier age. Because it is not possible to know how much colostral antibody a calf received without testing for titers in their serum, one should assume that some calves in a group may not have received adequate colostral antibody. If a production system has a history of disease outbreaks in young calves that is not controlled by a single administration of vaccine, it may be helpful to start vaccinating at a few weeks of age and to revaccinate at approximately 3-week intervals to booster the B and T cell memory. The first dose may prime B and T cell memory, even in calves with high titers of colostral antibody. The calves with low titers should respond to the first or second dose of vaccine by producing antibody. Every 3 weeks, additional calves will have reduced colostral antibody titers and will be capable of producing antibody in response to revaccination. The additional doses should boost the antibody response and the strength of the T cell–mediated immune response. Vaccination every 3 weeks from approximately 6 through 15 weeks of age has worked well to optimize the immune response of young puppies and kittens to vaccines. A similar vaccination schedule may occasionally be justified to help control refractory disease outbreaks in food animals.

The presence of internal or external parasites at the time of first exposure to antigen may be an especially important factor leading to interference with vaccine efficacy. In other species it has been shown that parasites stimulate a Th2-type immune response, which is important for resistance to parasitic diseases. However, a Th2-type immune response has also been shown to inhibit a Th1-type immune response, which is important for resistance to most viruses and bacteria. A calf that is parasitized at the time of vaccination may fail to mount an effective Th1 response to the vaccine. Therefore it is important to treat the animal for parasites and give the immune system 2 or 3 weeks to recover before vaccinating the calf, especially the first time that the calf is vaccinated, because the primary immune response is more susceptible to misdirection toward a Th2 response than is the secondary immune response. This misdirection of the immune response could also potentially occur when two different vaccines that induce different types of immune responses are used at the same time. Vaccines that are not manufactured to be given in a single dose have not been tested to see if they interfere with each other.

Vaccines are developed and tested to prove safety and efficacy in healthy calves, free of parasites, under minimal stress, with no concurrent infections or other vaccinations, and with optimal nutrition. This results in a U.S. Department of Agriculture license, which assures that the vaccine is safe and effective when used as directed in healthy animals. Vaccines used under suboptimal conditions in the field may not perform as well. Vaccines have the greatest safety and efficacy if they are used in animals under conditions similar to the animals they were tested in. Although it is often not possible to achieve those conditions in the field, it is important for animal producers to use the best management possible to get the greatest benefit from the vaccine. The best response to a vaccine should occur if the calves are free of parasites or are treated for parasites 2 or 3 weeks before vaccination; stress factors are minimized (no branding, weaning, or surgery within 2 weeks of vaccination); there is no concurrent infection at the time of vaccination; and only one vaccine is given at a time. It is unlikely that the ideal

can be achieved in most management situations. However, it is important to understand the ideal so that when management compromises must be made, these factors are considered.

Recommended Readings

Barrington GM, Parish SM: Bovine neonatal immunology, *Vet Clin North Am Food Anim Pract* 17:463-476, 2001.

Endsley JJ, Ridpath JF, Neill JD et al: Induction of T lymphocytes specific for BVD virus in calves with maternal antibody, *Viral Immunol* 17:13-23, 2004.

Menanteau-Horta AM, Ames TR, Johnson DW et al: Effect of maternal antibody upon vaccination with infectious bovine rhinotracheitis and bovine virus diarrhea vaccines, *Can J Comp Med* 49:10-14, 1985.

Ridpath JF, Neill JD, Endsley J et al: Effect of passive immunity on the development of a protective immune response against bovine viral diarrhea virus in calves, *Am J Vet Res* 64:65-69, 2003.

Sandbulte MR, Roth JA: T-cell populations responsive to bovine respiratory syncytial virus in seronegative calves, *Vet Immunol Immunopathol* 84:111-123, 2002.

Sandbulte MR, Roth JA: Methods for analysis of cell-mediated immunity in domestic animal species, *J Am Vet Med Assoc* 225:522-530, 2004.

CHAPTER 116

Beef Heifer Development

ROBERT L. LARSON

Veterinarians should take an active role in developing and administering replacement heifer management strategies for their beef-producing clients. Successful heifer development should result in a high percentage of heifers becoming pregnant early in the breeding season, a manageable risk of dystocia, and a high percentage of primiparous females rebreeding early in their second breeding season. Proper heifer development requires knowledge and experience in animal breeding and genetics, nutrition, reproductive endocrinology, and familiarity with parasite and infectious disease control.

Productivity for beef cattle herds has been shown to be increased when a high percentage of heifers become pregnant early in the first breeding season, and economic return is enhanced when more primiparous heifers conceive for a second pregnancy as 2-year-olds.[1,2] Heifer development should result in most heifers in the replacement pool reaching puberty before the start of breeding because the percentage conceiving to first service is lower on the puberal estrus compared with the third estrus.[3,4]

Putting additional pressure on heifers to reach puberty at a young age is the fact that many producers breed heifers 3 to 4 weeks earlier than the mature cow herd. The risk of calving difficulty is greater with heifers than older cows; thus breeding replacement heifers essentially one heat cycle earlier than the mature cows allows the producer to concentrate available labor on heifers at calving. In addition, the length of time from calving to the resumption of cycling is longer in heifers than in cows.[5] Therefore calving heifers earlier than mature cows gives the heifers the extra time they need to return to estrus and be cycling at the start of the subsequent breeding season.

To calve at approximately 24 months of age and to reach puberty the equivalent of three heat cycles before the start of the mature cow breeding season, heifers must become puberal by 11 to 13 months of age. Once puberty is attained, nutrition must be at a level that allows the heifer to continue cycling, ovulate a viable oocyte, and establish pregnancy. Deficiency of energy or protein for extended periods of time during any production phase during the first 2½ years of life negatively affects fetal development, calf viability, milk production, and/or rebreeding for the next pregnancy.

SELECTION OF REPLACEMENT HEIFERS

Conformation

Decisions about the suitability of individual heifers to enter the replacement pool should begin early in life. Heifer calves from early-maturing cows requiring minimal nutritional supplementation to conceive early in the calving season should be identified as possible replacements. These heifers should be from dams that have excellent udder, foot, and leg conformation. Structural correctness is critical in female selection because of the importance of longevity on cowherd efficiency and profitability.[6-8]

Breed/Type

Although great differences in fertility and growth occur within breeds, there are differences among breeds of beef cattle that should be considered when selecting replacement heifers. Mature cow size and milking ability are important considerations in matching breed and type to production environment. Producers should choose breeds and biologic types that will optimize milk production without sacrificing reproductive efficiency or increasing nutritional requirements above that provided by available grazed forages. In general, faster-gaining breeds that mature at a larger size (e.g., Charolais, Chianina) reach puberty at an older age than slower-gaining breeds with a smaller mature size (e.g., Hereford, Angus).[9] Researchers have also shown that breeds selected for milk production (e.g., Gelbvieh, Brown Swiss, Simmental, Braunvieh, Red Poll, Pinzgauer) reach puberty at younger ages than do breeds of similar size not selected for milk production (e.g., Charolais, Chianina, Limousine, Hereford).[9,10]

Researchers have also found that *Bos indicus* (Brahman-derivative) breeds and breed crosses are older at puberty than British-breed heifers.[9,11,12] British-breed heifers reach puberty at lighter weights than Brahman × British heifers.[11] However, once *Bos indicus* heifers reached puberty, percent conceiving is not different from *Bos taurus* heifers. Also, *Bos indicus* cows have been shown to have longevity that is greater compared with purebred *Bos taurus* cows.[12,13] Therefore the slow onset of puberty seen in *Bos indicus* heifers does not extend to decreased fertility as cows.

For commercial operators, crossbred heifers should be preferred because of their inherent hybrid vigor and greater fertility, longevity, and lifetime production.[14-17] In the U.S. Gulf Coast and in other less temperate environments, some influence from Brahman, Brahman-derivative (e.g., Beefmaster, Brangus), or other heat-tolerant (e.g., Senepol, Tuli) breeds may be necessary for heat tolerance and parasite resistance.

Expected Progeny Differences

Expected progeny differences (EPDs) predict the transmitting ability of a parent animal or how a bull's or cow's progeny will compare with other animal's progeny for various traits. They allow producers to make valid comparisons between purebred bulls and replacement heifers of the same breed raised in different herds, even under differing environmental and management conditions. The traits measured vary slightly between breeds but generally include birth weight, calving ease, weaning weight, yearling weight, and a prediction of daughter's milking ability. Some breeds have expanded their evaluation programs to include traits such as scrotal circumference, mature size, and carcass characteristics.

Producers should use EPDs to select sires that will add the optimum level of growth, milk production, and other economically important traits. Geneticists are finding that the heritability of reproductive traits is higher than previously assumed ($h^2 \approx 0.20$) and that using EPDs for selection for heifer fertility will allow herds to make genetic progress toward greater pregnancy proportions for heifers.[18,19] In response to this information, some breed associations are either currently or planning to report an EPD for heifer pregnancy percentage.

Selection Criteria at Weaning

A rigorous selection standard should be set at weaning time for prospective replacements based on available records and visual appraisal. Complete records of calf, dam, and sire performance are ideal; however, selection pressure can be applied to the herd simply by knowing a potential replacement's weaning weight, week of birth, and dam's identity. Heifers identified at birth as unsuitable replacements because of either sire or dam shortcomings should not be allowed in the selection pool.

Producers should select heifers born early in the calving season because older females are more likely to have reached puberty by the start of the breeding season and consequently to become pregnant early in the breeding season.[20] The rate of gain needed to reach the target weight that coincides with puberty by the start of the breeding season is less for older, heavier heifers compared with younger calves in the same herd. These older calves will then allow greater feeding and management flexibility than lighter, younger heifers.

Selection Criteria at Yearling Age

Meeting but not grossly exceeding a yearling target weight is important for heifer fertility and production. Developing heifers on a high plane of nutrition (both energy and protein) from weaning to breeding results in earlier puberty,[21,22] improved udder development,[23] and increased conception rates[24,25] compared with a low plane. The target-weight concept is based on reports that *Bos taurus* breed heifers such as Angus, Hereford, Charolais, and Limousine are expected to reach puberty at about 60% of mature weight.[26] Dual-purpose breed heifers such as Braunvieh, Gelbvieh, and Red Poll tend to reach puberty at about 55% of mature weight, and *Bos indicus* heifers, most commonly Brahma or Brahma-cross, are older and heavier at puberty than the other beef breeds; about 65% of mature weight.[27,28] However, in well-managed herds, opportunities may exist to lower heifer development costs by lowering traditional target breeding weights.

Funston and Deutscher[29] found that spring-born composite (MARC II: ¼ Gelbvieh, ¼ Simmental, ¼ Angus, ¼ Hereford) heifers reaching 53% or 58% of mature body weight at breeding had similar reproduction and first calf production traits.[29] Similarly, Clark and colleagues[30] showed that MARC II heifers that were targeted to achieve 50% to 55% of mature body weight at first breeding had equal reproductive performance and superior economic performance when compared with heifers targeted to achieve 65% of mature body weight.[30]

Heifer replacement pools can be evaluated with a reproductive tract scoring (RTS) system developed to subjectively classify puberal status using size of the uterus and ovaries estimated by palpation per rectum.[31] The system assigns a score to each heifer using a 5-point scale where a score of 1 is considered an immature tract and a score of 5 is considered a cycling tract.

An RTS of 1 is used to describe heifers with infantile reproductive tracts that are estimated to not be near the onset of puberty when palpated. These heifers have small, flaccid tracts and small ovaries with no significant structures. Heifers assigned an RTS of 1 are assumed to be either too young to fit into the breeding season being planned or too light to reach their target weight and are not able to express their genetic potential for reaching puberty. Heifers assigned an RTS of 2 have a slightly larger uterine diameter, but tone is still lacking and the ovaries have small follicles. Heifers described as having an RTS of 3 have some uterine tone and a larger uterine diameter than heifers with more immature scores. These heifers are assumed to be nearly puberal and many will begin cycling within 6 weeks. Heifers assigned either a score of 4 or 5 are considered cycling as indicated by good uterine tone and size and easily palpable ovarian structures. RTS 4 is assigned to heifers that, despite having large follicles present, do not have a palpable corpus luteum (CL) either because they are in their pubertal cycle or they are in a stage of the estrous cycle where a CL is absent. Heifers with an RTS of 5 are similar in uterine and ovarian size, tone, and structure when palpated per rectum as compared with RTS 4 heifers except that a CL is palpable.

Studies have reported sensitivity of ovarian palpation per rectum for the presence of a functional corpora lutea to be between 70% and 90%, and specificity has been reported to be between 50% and 84%.[32-35] False positives may have several explanations. A developing corpus luteum may be palpable between days 1 through 4 of the estrous cycle and mistaken for a mature corpus luteum, though it is not yet producing large quantities of progesterone.[36] Regressing corpus lutea may be palpable well into the next cycle, even though they cease to produce progesterone beyond day 17 of the estrous cycle.[37] Kelton suggested that the high false-negative percentage may be due to luteal tissue deeply embedded in ovarian stroma being difficult to palpate and/or small, progesterone-producing corpora lutea being mistaken as atretic.[38] Veterinarians should recognize that there is no correlation between size of corpus luteum and level of progesterone secretions.[34]

Rosenkrans and Hardin[35] report that the RTS system is repeatable within and between palpators. Substantial agreement (kappa = 0.6-0.8) was found within palpator (same palpator evaluating the same heifer twice a few hours apart), and moderate agreement (kappa = 0.4-0.6) was found between palpators in determining individual tract scores. The Rosenkrans study demonstrates that the RTS system can be used as a screening test for herds. But because the sensitivity of uterine palpation per rectum for the presence of progesterone-producing corpora lutea is 70% to 90% (i.e., 10%-30% false negative), many heifers classified as prepubertal will actually be pubertal, and therefore the RTS system is not sensitive enough for individual animal culling.

The scores assigned with the RTS system are retrospectively correlated with reproductive performance of yearling heifers, especially for pregnancy percentage to synchronized breeding and to pregnancy percentage at the end of the breeding season. Heifers with more mature reproductive tracts as yearlings had higher pregnancy percentage and calved earlier.[39]

Heifers should be evaluated for tract score about 6 to 8 weeks before the onset of breeding. If deficiencies are found, management changes instituted more than 6 weeks ahead of the breeding season can result in an increased number of heifers reaching puberty by the start of the breeding season. If the heifers are evaluated too far ahead of the breeding season (>8 weeks), the heifers are likely to be young and to have lower tract scores than what is a true reflection of their potential to reach puberty before the breeding season.

If a low percentage of heifers are cycling at the time of RTS evaluation and many of the heifers are scored as 2, management changes must be instituted immediately. These changes may include (1) increasing the plane of nutrition so that increased weight gain will allow the heifers to reach target weight by the start of the breeding season, (2) increasing the plane of nutrition and delaying the start of the breeding season by several weeks, (3) holding the heifers over to breed 6 months later to calve in the fall (for spring-calving herds), and (4) marketing the heifers for feeder cattle and finding another source of replacements.

Selection Criteria After the Breeding Season

The final culling of prospective replacement heifers is done once pregnancy status is determined soon after the end of the breeding season. By selecting only those heifers that conceive to a proven artificially inseminated (AI) sire or to natural service during a short breeding season, producers can be assured of selecting for females that reach puberty at a young age and conceive early in the breeding season. Lesmeister and colleagues[1] showed that heifers that conceive early in their first breeding season have greater lifetime productivity than do their counterparts that conceive later in their first breeding season.

PUBERTY

Puberty in the beef heifer is reached when she is able to express estrous behavior, ovulate a fertile oocyte, and obtain normal luteal function.[40] The maturing of the neuroendocrine system that induces maturation and ovulation of the first oocyte, as well as the hormonal changes that induce the first expression of behavioral estrus, are the result of a gradual increase in gonadotropic (luteinizing hormone [LH] and follicle stimulating hormone [FSH]) activity. This increased gonadotropic activity near the time of puberty is due to a decreased negative feedback of estradiol on the hypothalamic secretion of gonadotropin-releasing hormone (GnRH).[41-43] As puberty approaches, the gradually increased frequency of LH pulses results in increased secretion of LH, which enhances development of ovarian follicles that produce enough estradiol to induce behavioral estrus and a preovulatory surge of gonadotropins.[43] Wavelike patterns of follicular development can be detected as early as 2 weeks of age in heifer calves, and the duration of follicular waves increases and the maximum diameter of dominant follicles increases with age through puberty.[44-46]

The onset of puberty is primarily influenced by age and weight within breed.[21,22,47,48] Age of puberty in other species such as humans and rats is influenced by percent body fat or by body fat distribution[49-51]; however, in cattle, fatness is not the sole regulator of puberty because puberty does not occur at a constant percentage of body fat and age and breed appear to be important contributing factors.[52-56]

High-starch diets appear to influence the age and/or weight of puberty. Ciccioli and colleagues[57] reported that heifers with a higher starch intake had lower weight at puberty compared with an isonitrogenous-isocaloric diet with higher fiber even though the two diets resulted in the same body weight and fat reserves.[57] Similarly, Gasser and colleagues[58] found that heifers fed a higher-starch diet were younger and lighter at puberty than heifers fed a lower net energy (NE) control diet when the treatments were started at 99 days of age. In contrast, Marston and colleagues.[59] reported that heifers fed a high-concentrate diet reached puberty at the same weight but at a younger age than heifers raised on lower energy diets. And other studies have shown that although high-grain diets decrease the age at puberty, weight at puberty was increased.[24,56] Some investigators have hypothesized that increased propionate production is associated with the positive effects of starch supplementation on puberty; however, Lalman and colleagues[60] demonstrated that supplementing heifer diets with propionic acid did not hasten puberty.

Although it has been shown that undernutrition can delay puberty in heifers,[61] short-term fasting is generally less disruptive to the hypothalamic pulse generator and gonadotropin secretion in previously well-nourished ruminants compared with monogastrics, but this observation appears to be less consistent in heifers compared with mature cows.[62,63] In cycling heifers receiving an acutely decreased energy diet (0.4× maintenance), growth rate and maximum diameter of the first dominant follicle were less than in heifers fed above maintenance, but the LH pulse frequency and amplitude were not affected by diet.[64] In long-term studies with chronically nutrient-restricted heifers in which heifers lost 17% to 18% of their body weight, the heifers became anestrus.[65,66] The concentration of LH was lower, the maximum diameter of the dominant follicle was less, and FSH was higher during the cycle preceding anestrus compared with estrous cycles preceding dietary restriction.[65]

The latest edition of the National Research Council (NRC) Nutrient Requirements of Beef Cattle expresses protein requirements as absorbed protein, also known as *metabolizable protein* (MP).[67] Metabolizable protein replaces the earlier use of crude protein (CP) and is defined as the true protein absorbed by the intestine, supplied by microbial protein and undegraded intake protein (UIP).[67] The MP system separates and accounts for the two components of protein nutrition of importance to the animal—the needs of the rumen microorganisms and the needs of the beef animal. Lalman and colleagues[60] showed that feeding UIP in excess of NRC requirements may improve energy utilization of heifers fed mature forage but may delay the onset of puberty compared with heifers fed monensin. Kane and colleagues[68] found that in cycling beef heifers supplemented with high levels of UIP, anterior pituitary gland synthesis, storage, and secretion of gonadotropins was decreased, and they suggest that these changes may impair follicular growth and development.

Fat supplementation of heifer diets is generally restricted to less than 5% of the total dry matter intake (DMI) because of potential negative effects of higher inclusion on fiber digestibility and reduction in DMI.[69] In a review of fat supplementation and its effect on beef female reproduction, Funston[70] reported that nutritionally challenged replacement heifers may experience reproductive benefits from fat supplementation, but there is limited benefit of fat supplementation in well-developed heifers.

Some researchers have reported that supplemental fatty acids had positive effects on ovarian function and reproductive performance that was independent of energy source.[71,72] In contrast, Howlett and colleagues[74] reported that adding oilseeds or soybean hulls to corn silage–based diets did not affect reproductive performance of heifers. Lammoglia and colleagues[73] found that a high-fat diet fed for 162 days to beef heifers did not affect age at puberty, AI services per pregnancy, or final pregnancy percentage. Mattos and colleagues[75] concluded that a mechanism for dietary fatty acids to affect LH secretion that is independent from energy has not been established. A potentially negative consideration for feeding oilseed sources of fat is that phytoestrogens, which have been shown to negatively affect reproduction in cattle, can be present.[76]

The major minerals that need supplementation in heifer diets are sodium, calcium, and phosphorus. Magnesium and potassium require supplementation under certain circumstances. Because salt is deficient in most natural feeds, it should be supplemented by either including it with the concentrate or feeding it free-choice. The level of salt needed in the diet can vary depending on the diet, type of cattle, and environmental conditions, but a general rule is to supply 0.25% to 0.5% of the diet on an as-fed basis (1-2 oz) per day.

Calcium metabolism and phosphorus metabolism are interrelated and complex. Controlling factors include vitamin D, parathyroid hormone, thyrocalcitonin, and the dietary levels of calcium and phosphorus. The absorption of calcium is regulated to a large extent by calcium intake. The higher the intake of calcium, the less that is absorbed.[67] The extent of dietary phosphorus that is absorbed depends not only on the source of phosphorus, but also on vitamin D levels and the levels of other minerals such as aluminum, manganese, and potassium in the diet.

Cattle require 15 trace minerals. Of these, six may be deficient in forage-based diets. These are copper, cobalt, iodine, selenium, zinc, and manganese. Some researchers have seen a positive reproductive effect associated with trace mineral supplementation, whereas others have not. Saxena and colleagues[77] found a correlation between serum copper and zinc concentrations and age at puberty in heifers. DiCostanzo and colleagues[78] reported improved first-service conception percentage in heifers fed corn silage diets either with manganese or manganese, copper, and zinc compared with unsupplemented controls. In contrast, others have failed to observe a response to trace mineral supplementation on reproductive performance in cattle.[79-81]

PROGESTOGENS

Progesterone and synthetic progestogens induce puberty in heifers, and management systems that capitalize on this result have been used for more than 30 years. Short and colleagues[82] showed that more prepuberal heifers (8.5 months old and 249 kg) given a progesterone implant for 6 days plus an injection of estradiol-17β 24 hours after implant removal showed estrus and ovulated within 4 days than heifers treated with estradiol-17β alone.[82] Gonzalez-Padilla and colleagues[83] also used progesterone or norgestomet (a synthetic progestogen) in conjunction with estradiol valerate to induce estrus in prepuberal beef heifers in a series of experiments. Gonzales-Padilla and colleagues[83] were able to induce estrus in approximately 93% of heifers treated with either a 9-day, 6-mg norgestomet implant coupled with an injection of 3 mg norgestomet plus 5 mg estradiol valerate at the time of implant insertion or daily intramuscular (IM) injections of 20 mg progesterone for 4 days plus 2 mg estradiol-17β 2 days after the last progesterone injection. Pregnancy percentage ranged from 43% to 73%.

A progesterone-impregnated intravaginal device known as a CIDR (Pfizer Animal Health, Exton, Pa.) is available in the United States. The CIDR is a T-shaped device with a nylon spine covered by a progesterone impregnated silicone skin. On insertion, blood progesterone concentration rises rapidly. Maximal concentration is reached within an hour. Progesterone concentration is maintained at a relatively constant level during the 7 days the insert is in the vagina. On removal of the insert, if a CL is not present, progesterone concentration in the bloodstream drops quickly. This product is labeled for its ability to cause suckled beef cows to show estrus sooner after calving and will cause replacement heifers to express heat at a younger age and weight than nontreated animals. Research using CIDR in beef heifers and cows was conducted over several years at a number of universities and those trials indicate that use of CIDR did not decrease fertility compared with untreated females and was successful in inducing almost 50% of noncycling females to show signs of a fertile heat following removal of the CIDR in the herds tested.[84]

Another commercially available synthetic progestogen is melengestrol acetate (MGA, Upjohn Company,

Kalamazoo, Mich.). Work has also demonstrated the ability of MGA to induce puberty in heifers, especially heifers near the age and weight requirements for spontaneous induction of puberty. Percent pregnant at first service for heifers that attained puberty while being treated with MGA administered orally for 14 days followed by prostaglandin $F_{2\alpha}$ given as an IM injection 17 days after the final day of MGA feeding was not different from that of control heifers that attained puberty during the same period.[37]

IONOPHORES

Ionophores were originally cleared for use to improve the feed efficiency of feedlot cattle on high-concentrate diets and to improve pasture cattle gains.[85-87] Now ionophores are cleared for use in replacement heifers. Inclusion of ionophores in heifer diets has been shown to increase the number of heifers that had reached puberty by the start of the breeding season, decrease the age at puberty, decrease the weight at puberty, increase the corpora luteal weight, and increase the amount of progesterone produced.[88-92] The decrease in age at puberty was independent of improved average daily gain and increased body weight.

GROWTH IMPLANTS

Implanting suckling calves with anabolic growth promotants is a practice used by cow-calf operators to increase weaning weights of calves intended for slaughter. Research on the effect of implanting heifers who are later saved for replacements on percentage cycling and conceiving has been somewhat inconsistent, with results ranging from negative to positive.[93-97] When nutritional levels are adequate to sustain the anabolic effects on weight gain, implants have been reported to have no negative effects.[98,99] Negative results were most likely to occur when implants were placed at birth or when heifers were implanted with anabolic agents three times between birth and puberty.[93,94]

However, one paper revealed possible negative effects of a progesterone and estradiol implant that is approved for use in heifers intended to be retained as heifers.[98] Bartol and colleagues[98] implanted some heifers according to label directions at 45 days of age. Other heifers in the experiment were implanted at birth, at 21 days of age, or remained as unimplanted controls. All the implanted heifers had reduced uterine weight, decreased myometrial area, decreased endometrial area, and reduced endometrial gland density compared with the control heifers.[98] The effects were greatest in heifers implanted at birth.

Numerous studies have shown that heifers implanted with anabolic growth promotants at 2 to 3 months of age have a larger pelvic area as yearling than controls without implants. A few studies have followed the heifers to calving at 2 years of age to determine whether the larger pelvic areas were maintained. These studies showed that much of the advantage for implanted heifers seen as yearlings was lost by the time they were ready to calve; the advantage was only 3 to 9 cm² compared with controls with no implants.[93,97,99]

Some implants are approved for use in suckling heifers that are to be retained as replacements, but I do not recommend implanting calves that can be identified at a young age as likely replacements. There are no benefits to implanting replacement heifers because producers do not benefit economically from maximum growth. Instead, economic benefits from replacement heifers occur because of early onset of puberty, high fertility, and a long productive life in the cowherd.

ANTHELMINTIC TREATMENT

Internal parasites can have a negative impact on virtually all production characteristics of beef cattle including gains from weaning through the first pregnancy.[100-103] Presence of internal parasites affects nutrient utilization and possibly alters metabolism in infected animals. Minimizing the negative impact of internal parasites with the use of broad-spectrum anthelmintics that are able to kill inhibited stages of *Ostertagia ostertagi* improves the efficiency of gain for replacement heifers. Improved gain increases body weight and hence the number of heifers cycling at the beginning of the breeding season.[89,100] But it is interesting to note that improvements in reproductive response in replacement heifers treated with anthelmintics may not be solely due to reaching target weights faster than nontreated heifers. Of note, Larson and colleagues[100] found the correlations between weight gain or prebreeding heifer weight and puberty in ivermectin-treated heifers approached zero, indicating that the gain response does not fully explain the earlier onset of puberty. Purvis and Whittier[89] also showed that decreased age and weight at puberty in ivermectin-treated heifers compared with controls was not due to improved average daily gains. Therefore other pathways affecting onset of puberty, besides weight gain, are being stimulated due to treatment with ivermectin and possibly other anthelmintics.

HEIFER HEALTH PROGRAM

Biosecurity is the attempt to keep infectious agents (e.g., bacteria, virus, fungi, parasites) away from a herd. One aspect of biosecurity is a vaccination program that improves the immunity of cattle against the infectious agents that they may contact. Not all diseases of cattle have commercial vaccines available, and no vaccine is completely effective at preventing disease in all situations. Therefore other aspects of disease prevention and biosecurity are at least as important as a vaccination program. A vaccination program should be tailored for specific risk factors and should be designed and then rigorously applied to the herd. For most beef herds in the United States, the potential list of pregnancy-wasting diseases to be considered in a vaccination program would include brucellosis, vibriosis (campylobacteriosis), leptospirosis, infectious bovine rhinotracheitis (IBR), and bovine viral diarrhea (BVD). Other diseases for which vaccines are available include *Histophilus somnus* and trichomoniasis.

SUMMARY

Veterinarians should be actively involved in planning and implementing management systems on their clients' farms to evaluate and plan intervention as needed for heifer development. A good heifer development system will ensure that a high percentage of heifers in the replacement pool become pregnant early in their first breeding season, continue to grow adequately during gestation, have a healthy calf unassisted at 24 months of age, and rebreed for a second pregnancy early in the second breeding season. Proper selection of replacement candidates; adequate nutritional development to reach target weights; and utilization of commercially available ionophores, anthelmintics, and progestogen-containing estrous synchronization systems will ensure that a high percentage of heifers are puberal and available for breeding at the start of the breeding season. In addition, a herd biosecurity program that includes stringent vaccination and quarantine protocols for replacements will minimize the risk of pregnancy-wasting diseases.

References

1. Lesmeister JL, Burfening PJ, Blackwell RL: Date of first calving in beef cows and subsequent calf production, *J Anim Sci* 36:1, 1973.
2. Patterson HH, Adams DC, Klopfenstein TJ et al: Supplementation to meet metabolizable protein requirements of primiparous beef heifers: II. Pregnancy and economics, *J Anim Sci* 81:563, 2003.
3. Byerley DJ, Staigmiller RB, Berardinelli JG et al: Pregnancy rates of beef heifers bred either on puberal or third estrus, *J Anim Sci* 65:645, 1987.
4. Perry RC, Corah LR, Cochran RC et al: Effects of hay quality, breed and ovarian development on onset of puberty and reproductive performance of beef heifers, *J Prod Agric* 4:13, 1991.
5. Short RE, Bellows RA, Staigmiller RB et al: Physiological mechanisms controlling anestrus and infertility in postpartum beef cattle, *J Anim Sci* 68:799, 1990.
6. Arthur PF, Makarechian M, Berg RT et al: Longevity and lifetime productivity of cows in a purebred Hereford and two multibreed synthetic groups under range conditions, *J Anim Sci* 71:1142, 1993.
7. Tanida H, Hohenboken WD, DeNise SK: Genetic aspects of longevity in Angus and Hereford cows, *J Anim Sci* 66:64, 1988.
8. Rogers LF: Economics of replacement rates in commercial beef herds, *J Anim Sci* 34:921, 1972.
9. Martin LC, Brinks JS, Bourdon RM et al: Genetic effects on beef heifer puberty and subsequent reproduction, *J Anim Sci* 70:4006, 1992.
10. Gregory KE, Lunstra DD, Cundiff LV et al: Breed effects and heterosis in advanced generations of composite populations for puberty and scrotal traits in beef cattle, *J Anim Sci* 69:2795, 1991.
11. Gregory KE, Laster DB, Cundiff LV et al: Characterization of biological types of cattle-cycle III: II. Growth rate and puberty in females, *J Anim Sci* 49:461, 1979.
12. Stewart TS, Long CR, Cartwright TC: Characterization of cattle of a five breed diallel. III. Puberty in bulls and heifers, *J Anim Sci* 50:808, 1980.
13. Rohrer GA, Baker JF, Long CR et al: Productive longevity of first-cross cows produced in a five breed diallel: II. Heterosis and general combining ability, *J Anim Sci* 66:2836, 1988.
14. Bailey CM: Lifespan of beef-type *Bos taurus* and *Bos indicus × Bos taurus* females in a dry, temperate climate, *J Anim Sci* 69:2379, 1991.

15. Steffan CA, Kress DD, Doornbos DE et al: Performance of crosses among Hereford, Angus, and Simmental cattle with different levels of Simmental breeding. III. Heifer postweaning growth and early reproductive traits, *J Anim Sci* 61:1111, 1985.

16. Núñez-Dominguez R, Cundiff LV, Dickerson GE et al: Heterosis for survival and dentition in Hereford, Angus, Shorthorn, and crossbred cows, *J Anim Sci* 69:1885, 1991.

17. Cundiff LV, Núñez-Dominguez R, Dickerson GE et al: Heterosis for lifetime production in Hereford, Angus, Shorthorn, and crossbred cows, *J Anim Sci* 70:2397-2410, 1992.

18. Evans JL, Golden BL, Bourdon RM et al: Additive genetic relationships between heifer pregnancy and scrotal circumference in Hereford cattle, *J Anim Sci* 77:2621, 1999.

19. Doyle SP, Golden BL, Green RD et al: Additive genetic parameter estimates for heifer pregnancy and subsequent reproduction in Angus females, *J Anim Sci* 78:2091, 2000.

20. Bergman JAG, Hohenboken WD: Prediction of fertility from calfhood traits of Angus and Simmental heifers, *J Anim Sci* 70:2611, 1992.

21. Oeydipe EO, Osori DIK, Aderejola O et al: Effect of level of nutrition on onset of puberty and conception rates of Zebu heifers, *Theriogenology* 18:525, 1982.

22. Wiltbank JN, Kasson CW, Ingalls JE: Puberty in crossbred and straightbred beef heifers on two levels of feed, *J Anim Sci* 29:602, 1969.

23. Bond J, Wiltbank JN: Effect of energy and protein on estrus, conception rate, growth and milk production of beef females, *J Anim Sci* 30:438, 1970.

24. Short RE, Bellows RA: Relationships among weight gains, age at puberty and reproductive performance in heifers, *J Anim Sci* 32:127, 1971.

25. Patterson DJ, Corah LR, Kiracofe GH et al: Conception rate in *Bos taurus* and *Bos indicus* crossbred heifers after postweaning energy manipulation and synchronization of estrus with melengestrol acetate and fenprostalene, *J Anim Sci* 67:1138, 1986.

26. Wiltbank JN, Roberts S, Nix J et al: Reproductive performance and profitability of heifers fed to weigh 272 or 318 kg at the start of the first breeding season, *J Anim Sci* 60:25, 1985.

27. Stewart TS, Long CR, Cartwright TC: Characterization of cattle of a five-breed diallel. III. Puberty in bulls and heifers, *J Anim Sci* 50:808, 1980.

28. Sacco RE, Baker JF, Cartwright TC: Production characteristics of primiparous females of a five-breed diallel, *J Anim Sci* 64:1612, 1987.

29. Funston RN, Deutscher GH: Comparison of target breeding weight and breeding date for replacement beef heifers and effects on subsequent reproduction and calf performance, *J Anim Sci* 82:3094, 2004.

30. Clark RT, Creighton KW, Patterson HH et al: Symposium paper: economic and tax implications for managing beef replacement heifers, *Prof Anim Sci* 21:164, 2005.

31. Anderson KJ, Leferver DG, Brinks JS et al: The use of reproductive tract scoring in beef heifers, *Agri-Practice* 12:19, 1991.

32. Ott RS, Bretzlaff KN, Hixon JE: Comparison of palpable corpora lutea with serum progesterone concentrations in cows, *JAVMA* 188:1417, 1986.

33. Watson ED, Munro CD: A reassessment of the technique of rectal palpation of corpora lutea in cows, *Br Vet J* 136:555, 1980.

34. Boyd H, Munro CD: Progesterone assays and rectal palpation in pre-service management of a dairy herd, *Vet Rec* 104:341, 1979.

35. Rosenkrans KS, Hardin DK: Repeatability and accuracy of reproductive tract scoring to determine pubertal status in beef heifers, *Theriogenology* 59:1087, 2003.

36. Hansel W, Concannon PW, Lukaszewka JH: Corpora lutea of the large domestic animal, *Biol Reprod* 8:222, 1973.

37. Jaeger JR, Whittier JC, Corah LR et al: Reproductive response of yearling beef heifers to a melengestrol acetate-prostaglandin $F_2\alpha$ estrus synchronization system, *J Anim Sci* 70:2622, 1992.

38. Kelton DF, Leslie KE, Etherington WG et al: Accuracy of rectal palpation and of a rapid milk progesterone enzyme immunoassay for determining the presence of a functional corpus luteum in subestrous dairy cows, *Can Vet J* 32:286, 1991.

39. Patterson DJ, Bullock KD: *Using prebreeding weight, reproductive tract score and pelvic area to evaluate prebreeding development of replacement beef heifers,* Proc Beef Improvement Federation Annual Meeting, Sheridan, Wyo, 1995, pp 174-177.

40. Moran C, Quirke JF, Roche JF: Puberty in heifers: a review, *Anim Reprod Sci* 18:167, 1989.

41. Niswender GD, Farin CE, Braden TD: Reproductive physiology of domestic ruminants, *Proc Soc Theriogenol* 116-136, 1984.

42. Foster DL, Yellon SM, Olster DH: Internal and external determinants of the timing of puberty in the female, *J Reprod Fert* 75:327, 1985.

43. Kinder JE, Bergfeld EBM, Wehrman ME et al: Endocrine basis for puberty in heifers and ewes, *J Reprod Fertil* (suppl) 49:393, 1995.

44. Gasser CL, Burke CR, Mussard ML et al: Induction of precocious puberty in heifers II: advanced ovarian follicular development, *J Anim Sci* 84:2042, 2006.

45. Evans ACO, Adams GP, Rawlings NC: Follicular and hormonal development in prepubertal heifers from 2 to 36 weeks of age, *J Reprod Fertile* 102:463, 1994.

46. Bergfeld EGM, Kojima FN, Cupp AS et al: Ovarian follicular development in prepubertal heifers is influenced by level of dietary energy intake, *Biol Reprod* 51:1051, 1994.

47. Nelsen TC, Short RE, Phelps DA et al: Nonpuberal estrus and mature cow influences on growth and puberty in heifers, *J Anim Sci* 61:470, 1985.

48. Nelsen TC, Long CR, Cartwright TC: Postinflection growth in straightbred and crossbred cattle. II. Relationships among weight, height and puberal characters, *J Anim Sci* 55:293, 1982.

49. Kennedy GC: Interaction between feeding behavior and hormones during growth, *Ann N Y Acad Sci* 157:1049, 1969.

50. Frisch RE, McArthur: Menstrual cycles: fatness as a determinant of minimum weight necessary for their maintenance or onset, *Science* 185:949, 1974.

51. de Ridder CM, Bruning PF, Zonderland ML et al: Body fat mass, body fat distribution, and plasma hormones in early puberty in females, *J Clin Endocrinol Metab* 70:888, 1990.

52. Brooks AL, Morrow RE, Youngquist RS: Body composition of beef heifers at puberty, *Theriogenology* 24:235, 1985.

53. Baker JF, Long CR, Posada GA et al: Comparison of cattle of a five-breed diallel: Size, growth, condition and pubertal characters of second-generation heifers, *J Anim Sci* 67:1218, 1989.

54. Hopper HW, Williams SE, Byerley DJ et al: Effect of prepubertal body weight gain and breed on carcass composition at puberty in beef heifers, *J Anim Sci* 71:1104, 1993.

55. Yelich JV, Wettemann RP, Dolezal HG et al: Effects of growth rate on carcass composition and lipid partitioning at puberty and growth hormone, insulin-like growth factor I, insulin, and metabolites before puberty in beef heifers, *J Anim Sci* 73:2390, 1995.

56. Hall JB, Staigmiller RB, Bellows RA et al: Body composition and metabolic profiles associated with puberty in beef heifers, *J Anim Sci* 73:3409, 1995.

57. Ciccioli NH, Wettemann RP, Spicer LJ et al: Influence of body condition at calving and postpartum nutrition on endocrine function and reproductive performance of primiparous beef cows, *J Anim Sci* 81:3107, 2003.

58. Gasser CL, Grum DE, Mussard ML et al: Induction of precocious puberty in heifers I: enhanced secretion of luteinizing hormone, *J Anim Sci* 84:2035, 2006.

59. Marston TT, Lusby KS, Wettemann RP: Effects of postweaning diet on age and weight at puberty and milk production of heifers, *J Anim Sci* 73:63, 1995.

60. Lalman DL, Petersen MK, Ansotegui RP et al: The effects of ruminally undegradable protein, propionic acid, and monensin on puberty and pregnancy in beef heifers, *J Anim Sci* 71:2843, 1993.

61. Day ML, Imakawa E, Zalesky DD et al: Effects of restriction of dietary energy intake during the prepubertal period on secretion of luteinizing hormone and responsiveness of the pituitary to luteinizing hormone-releasing hormone in heifers, *J Anim Sci* 62:1641, 1986.

62. Amstalden M, Garcia MR, Stanko RL et al: Central infusion of recombinant ovine leptin normalizes plasma insulin and stimulates a novel hypersecretion of luteinizing hormone after short-term fasting in mature beef cows, *Biol Reprod* 66:1555, 2002.

63. Boland MP, Loneragan P, O'Callaghan D: Effect of nutrition on endocrine parameters, ovarian physiology, and oocytes and embryo development, *Theriogenology* 55:1323, 2001.

64. Mackey DR, Wylie ARG, Sreenan JM et al: The effect of acute nutritional change on follicular wave turnover, gonadotropin, and steroid concentration in beef heifers, *J Anim Sci* 78:429, 2000.

65. Rhodes FM, Fitzpatrick LA, Entwistle KW et al: Sequential changes in ovarian follicular dynamics in *Bos indicus* heifers before and after nutritional anestrus, *J Reprod Fert* 104:41, 1995.

66. Bossis I, Wettemann RP, Welty SD et al: Nutritionally induced anovulation in beef heifers: ovarian and endocrine function preceding cessation of ovulation, *J Anim Sci* 77:1536, 1999.

67. National Research Council: *Nutrient requirements of beef cattle*, ed 7, Washington, DC, 1996, National Academy of Sciences.

68. Kane KK, Hawkins DE, Pulsipher GD et al: Effect of increasing levels of undegradable intake protein on metabolic and endocrine factors in estrous cycling beef heifers, *J Anim Sci* 82:283, 2004.

69. Coppock CE, Wilks DL: Supplemental fat in high-energy rations for lactating cows: effects on intake, digestion, milk yield, and composition, *J Anim Sci* 69:3826, 1991.

70. Funston RN: Fat supplementation and reproduction in beef females, *J Anim Sci* (suppl):E154, 2004.

71. Thomas MG, Bao B, Williams GL: Dietary fats varying in their fatty acid composition differentially influence follicular growth in cows fed isonitrogenous diets, *J Anim Sci* 75:2512, 1997.

72. Bellows RA, Grings EE, Simms DD et al: Effects of feeding supplemental fat during gestation to first-calf beef heifers, *Prof Anim Sci* 17:81, 2001.

73. Lammoglia MA, Bellows RA, Grings EE et al: Effects of dietary fat and sire breed on puberty, weight, and reproductive traits of F1 beef heifers, *J Anim Sci* 78:2244, 2000.

74. Howlett CM, Vanzant ES, Anderson LH et al: Effect of supplemental nutrient source on heifer growth and reproductive performance, and on utilization of corn silage-based diets by beef steers, *J Anim Sci* 81:2367, 2003.

75. Mattos R, Staples CR, Thatcher WW: Effects of dietary fatty acids on reproduction in ruminants, *Rev Reprod* 5:38, 2000.

76. Adams NR: Detection of the effects of phytoestrogens on sheep and cattle, *J Anim Sci* 73:1509, 1995.

77. Saxena MS, Gupta SK, Maurya SN: Plasma levels of macro and micro-elements in relation to occurrence of pubertal estrum in crossbred heifers, *Indian J Anim Nutr* 8:265, 1991.

78. DiCostanzo A, Meiske JC, Plegge SD et al: Influence of manganese, copper and zinc on reproductive performance of beef cows, *Nutr Rep Int* 34:287, 1986.

79. Vaughan L, Poole DBR, Smith FH et al: Effect of low copper status and molybdenum supplementation on pregnancy in beef heifers, *Ir J Agric Food Res* 33:121, 1994.

80. Small JA, Charmley E, Rodd AV et al: Serum mineral concentrations in relation to estrus and conception in beef heifers and cows fed conserved forage, *Can J Anim Sci* 77:55, 1997.

81. Grings EE, Hall JB, Bellows RA et al: Effect of nutritional management, trace mineral supplementation, and norgestomet implant on attainment of puberty in beef heifers, *J Anim Sci* 76:2177, 1998.

82. Short RE, Bellows RA, Carr JB et al: Induced or synchronized puberty in heifers, *J Anim Sci* 43:1254-1258, 1976.

83. Gonzalez-Padilla E, Ruiz R, LeFever D et al: Puberty in beef heifers. III. Induction of fertile estrus, *J Anim Sci* 40:1110, 1975.

84. Lucy MC, Billings HJ, Butler WR et al: Efficacy of an intravaginal progesterone insert and an injection of PGF2a for synchronization of estrus and shortening the interval to pregnancy in postpartum beef cows, peripubertal beef heifers, and diary heifers, *J Anim Sci* 79:982, 2001.

85. Raun AP, Cooley CO, Potter EL et al: Effect of monensin on feed efficiency of feedlot cattle, *J Anim Sci* 43:665, 1976.

86. Oliver WM: Effect of monensin on gains of steers grazed on Coastal bermudagrass, *J Anim Sci* 41:999, 1975.

87. Potter EL, Cooley CO, Richardson LF et al: Effect of monensin on performance of cattle fed forage, *J Anim Sci* 43:665, 1976.

88. Moseley WM, McCartor MM, Randel RD: Effects of monensin on growth and reproductive performance of beef heifers, *J Anim Sci* 45:961, 1977.

89. Purvis HT, Whittier JC: Effects of ionophore feeding and anthelmintic administration on age and weight at puberty in spring-born beef heifers, *J Anim Sci* 74:736, 1996.

90. Sprott LR, Goehring TB, Beverly JR et al: Effects of ionophores on cow herd production: a review, *J Anim Sci* 66:1340, 1988.

91. Moseley WM, Dunn TG, Kaltenbach CC et al: Relationship of growth and puberty in beef heifers fed monensin, *J Anim Sci* 55:357, 1982.

92. Bushmich SL, Randel RD, McCartor MM et al: Effect of dietary monensin on ovarian response following gonadotropin treatment in prepuberal heifers, *J Anim Sci* 51:692, 1980.

93. Rusk CP, Speer NC, Schafer DW et al: Effect of Synovex-C implants on growth, pelvic measurements and reproduction in Angus heifers, *J Anim Sci* (suppl 1)70:126, 1992 (abstract).

94. King BD, Bo GA, Lulai C et al: Effect of zeranol implants on age at onset of puberty, fertility and embryo fetal mortality in beef heifers, *Can J Anim Sci* 75:225, 1995.

95. Whittier JC, Massey JW, Varner GR et al: Effect of a single calfhood growth-promoting implant on reproductive performance of replacement beef heifers, *J Anim Sci* (suppl 1) 69:464, 1991 (abstract).

96. Deutscher GH: Growth promoting implants on replacement heifers—a review, *Proc Range Beef Cow Sym* XII:169, 1991.

97. Larson RL, Corah LR: Effects of being dewormed with oxfendazole and implanted with Synovex-C as young beef calves on subsequent reproductive performance of heifers, *Prof Anim Sci* 11:106, 1995.

98. Bartol FF, Johnson LL, Floyd JG et al: Neonatal exposure to progesterone and estradiol alters uterine morphology and luminal protein content in adult beef heifers, *Theriogenology* 43:835, 1995.

99. Hancock R, Deutscher G, Nielson M et al: Synovex-C affects growth, reproduction, and calving performance of replacement heifers, *J Anim Sci* 72:292, 1994.

100. Larson RL, Corah LR, Spire MF et al: Effect of treatment with ivermectin on reproductive performance of yearling beef heifers, *Theriogenology* 44:189, 1995.

101. Williams JC, Knox JW, Marbury KS et al: Effects of ivermectin on control of gastrointestinal nematodes and weight gain in weaner-yearling beef cattle, *Am J Vet Res* 50:2108, 1989.

102. Wohlgemuth K, Melanconn JJ, Hughes H et al: Treatment of North Dakota beef cows and calves with ivermectin: some economic considerations, *Bov Pract* 24:61, 64, 1989.

103. Lacau-Mengido IM, Mejia ME, Diaz-Torga GS et al: Endocrine studies in ivermectin-treated heifers from birth to puberty, *J Anim Sci* 78:817, 2000.

CHAPTER 117

Investigation of Abortions and Fetal Loss in the Beef Herd

WILLIAM DEE WHITTIER

SCOPE OF THE PROBLEM

Many authors have documented that reproductive losses are the most economically significant of all losses that accrue to beef cattle operations in North America.[1,2] This being so, the portion of losses associated with pregnancy wastage may be the greatest. Late-term abortions typically occur after beef females have been either totally developed, in the case of replacement heifers, or after cows have been maintained through the dry period. In many cases these losses occur after the cows have been through the winter, so the expense of winter feeding has been incurred. Although cows that fail to conceive can be rebred to fit into another calving season, cows that have aborted typically face either being culled or maintained an entire year without production.

Fetal loss has been divided into the categories of early gestation, midgestation, and late-term abortion.[3] Another view of losses classifies them as either apparent or inapparent. Apparent abortions involve the discovery of a fetus, placental membranes, or vaginal discharge of a nature that suggests fetal loss. Inapparent fetal loss results when cows that are either assumed to be pregnant or have been diagnosed pregnant fail to deliver a calf or are observed to return to estrus. Early-term fetal loss is, of course, associated with an inapparent presentation more frequently because pregnancy tissues are either small or may be absorbed rather than expelled. The extensive conditions under which many beef cows are kept lead to more classification of fetal loss as inapparent because many aborted tissues are never observed by management.

The extent to which fetal loss occurs throughout the North American beef industry remains largely unknown. Surprisingly little published information about abortion rates in U.S. beef cow herds is available. Several authors suggest that a 1.5% to 2% rate is expected and that there is little to be gained by investigating pregnancy losses that are in this range.[1,4] North Dakota State University at the Dickinson Research Extension Center processed 220 beef cow herds with the Specific Performance Analysis (SPA) computer software and reported only a 0.7% pregnancy loss with a standard deviation of 1.4%.[5] In these same herds there was an open rate of 6.8% with a standard deviation of 4.5%.

The extent to which fetal loss contributes to failures in season-long pregnancy percentages is also an unknown, but the use of ultrasound pregnancy diagnosis provides some interesting data. The University of Minnesota Beef Team reports a 4.2% incidence of embryonic loss in beef heifers initially ultrasounded at day 30 of gestation and subsequently palpated rectally at between days 60 and 90 after insemination.[6] The same group reports that in mature beef cows embryonic loss has ranged from 3% to 8% from 30 to 75 days of gestation. In another study, pregnancy was diagnosed by transrectal ultrasonography between 30 and 35 days after insemination to determine the presence of a viable fetus, thereby assessing artificial insemination (AI) pregnancy rates.[7] A second pregnancy diagnosis was performed in 835 cows between 80 and 100 days after AI to determine overall pregnancy rates. Embryonic survival among theses cows between the first and second diagnosis of pregnancy was 96.7%. In our records of 451 cows that were diagnosed pregnant at 30 days (of 821 inseminated) by ultrasound, 7 (1.55%) did not calve to the AI date and 5 of these were diagnosed open, having lost their pregnancies. The other two calved at the end of the breeding season, having gotten reimpregnated by clean-up bulls. The five open cows represented about 5% of the total open cows (12.5%) for the breeding season. Had the overall season-long pregnancy rate been higher, the percentage of early pregnancy loss would have contributed more to the overall open rate. This demonstrates that early fetal loss can be a significant contributor to open rates and erroneously assumed to be due to decreased fertility (failure to conceive) rather than to pregnancy wastage.

CHALLENGE OF DIAGNOSING CAUSES OF FETAL LOSS

Diagnosis of the causes of fetal loss in beef cattle is an inherently challenging proposition. As has already been mentioned, much of the diagnostic material goes undetected in most operations. Even when the abortive fetus is discovered, it is often grossly contaminated and may have been passed some time before discovery occurs. Despite the fact that most pathologists suggest that examination of placental membranes often offers more diagnostic hope than examination of the fetus, it is difficult to get producers to collect the placental tissues and submit them for diagnostic examination.

Another major challenge to the successful diagnosis of the cause of abortion is the fact that fetal death and resultant tissue deterioration typically precede significantly the expulsion of the fetus. During the days between fetal death and expulsion the tissues typically deteriorate to a considerable degree, thus making their examination less fruitful.

Still a third impediment to diagnosis of abortion is the subtlety of lesions that are present in the aborted fetus. This is true for at least three reasons: (1) the fetus has often not developed its immune system to the extent that it is capable of mounting an immune response that can be observed as part of the pathologic examination; (2) fetal death occurs quite readily before the development of significant observable lesion; and (3) fetal lesions develop in an environment that is different enough that they may not be recognized as being associated with the causative disease agent.

A PRACTICAL APPROACH TO ABORTION DIAGNOSIS

From a practical perspective it is useful to divide fetal loss into four epidemiologic presentations, each of which lends itself to a different diagnostic approach. The four epidemiologic presentations of abortion are as follows:

- A baseline level of fetal loss
- An endemic level of fetal loss in which losses that are judged to exceed baseline occur chronically in a herd
- An epidemic level of fetal loss in which the incident in the herd is explosive

- Losses in which fetal loss may be confused with either conception failure or neonatal losses

Defining an individual fetal loss situation as probably fitting into one of these categories is useful because it allows exclusion of certain etiologies and aids in focusing diagnostic efforts on those causative agents that are most likely to be the ones involved in a given herd.

Baseline Level of Fetal Loss

A general consensus of the baseline level of fetal loss that should be anticipated in a typical herd exists.[3,4] Fetal losses between 1% and 3% are assumed by most authors to be relatively unavoidable. These are probably due to congenital lethals, fetal injuries, and sporadic dam illnesses.

Two different approaches to dealing with the baseline level of fetal losses are common. Some authors suggest that monitoring these losses is important.[1] They suggest that any aborted fetus discovered should be submitted for diagnostic examination. This effort is justified in the idea that either (1) the loss might be part of an endemic loss and its examination might lead to an intervention that will reduce future losses or (2) the individual loss might be the beginning of an epidemic so that its diagnosis allows intervention earlier in the course of the outbreak and thus limits the losses that will occur.

The counterargument to examination of each aborted fetus is that it is relatively unrewarding and carries a cost. Worldwide, diagnostic laboratories only make a specific diagnosis in about one third of submissions (range of 23%-46% in five studies).[4] Alternatively, a diagnosis of a single abortion suggests an etiology that is not representative of a true herd problem and resources are expended in preventive actions that are not economically justified.

If the decision is made not to diagnostically pursue losses that seem to be baseline in nature, it should be done with the caveat that a monitoring system in place quantifies ongoing losses. In the absence of such monitoring, at least two risks are taken. One risk is that an opportunity is missed to define an endemic problem, the correction of which might allow increased productivity in a herd. Second, the abortion might be the beginning of an epidemic and failure to pursue diagnosis early postpones intervention that could limit losses from the epidemic.

Endemic Fetal Loss

Chronic, low-level but excessive losses of pregnancy are seen on some herds and have significant ongoing influences in herd productivity. The recognition of such losses is, of course, a prerequisite to taking steps to limit these losses.

Careful record keeping and analysis is frequently necessary to illuminate the fact that these losses are occurring. Such monitoring is difficult without accurate pregnancy diagnosis. Such monitoring may be justification enough to prompt that pregnancy diagnosis be routinely performed. At the end of every calving season an analysis of cows that either had frank abortions or failed to calve should be performed.

Box 117-1

Disease-Causing Agents Associated with Endemic Fetal Loss

Hemophilus somnus
Listeria monocytogenes
Corynebacterium pyogenes
Bluetongue virus
Bovine viral diarrhea virus
Leptospira species
Cache Valley virus
Ureaplasma diversum
Neospora caninum
Foothill abortion (epizootic bovine abortion)
Mycotic agents
Inbreeding
Sires transmitting lethal traits
Robertsonian defect
Feed estrogens (silage/poultry litter)
Progesterone aberrations (high pasture protein reported to affect synthesis or clearance)
Protein deficiency
Vitamin A deficiency
Iodine deficiency
Selenium deficiency
Protein/urea excess
Copper excess
Iodine excess
Endotoxins associated with bacterial infections in dams
Endotoxin in gram-negative bacterial vaccines, especially in first 2 months and last 2 months of gestation
Pine needle toxicity
Broomweed toxicity
Locoweed toxicity
Narrow leaf sumpweed toxicity
High plant estrogens
Aflatoxin
Ergotamine
Fusarium toxin (zearalenone)
Nitrate fertilizer
Organophosphate toxicity

As in any clinical setting, an organized diagnostic approach should be pursued. This includes collecting a careful history, doing a thorough physical examination of both individual animals and the herd as a whole, and performing appropriate laboratory testing.

Box 117-1 contains a list of disease-causing agents that have been suggested to be associated with endemic fetal loss. Obviously, testing for all of these agents is not practical. Timing of fetal loss, results of pathology performed on aborted fetuses and placentas, and examination of the herd and its management will guide further testing.

Because of their current interest in bovine viral diarrhea (BVD) virus, neosporosis and leptospirosis are discussed in more detail in terms of their potential to cause endemic fetal loss.

Significant progress in the understanding of BVD disease has occurred in recent years.[8] With the elucidation of the existence and mechanisms creating the persistently infected (PI) animal, a leap in understanding the epidemiology of the disease has occurred. These animals are created when the fetus is infected in utero, a stage of development when it accepts the virus as part of itself and thus lives the balance of its life infected with and shedding the virus. It is now easy to understand how a herd that has not been exposed to other cattle can have PI calves born each year that shed virus during the breeding and gestation period so that fetal loss is precipitated. It has still not been totally explained why some herds with PI calves seem to have optimal reproduction outcomes. Recently, vaccines that claim protection for the fetus against infection with BVD virus have been approved. A near universal consensus is that testing calves as opposed to their dams is the more effective approach to diagnosing the disease on a herd basis. Most authors also recommend that culling PI calves before the breeding season is a necessary adjunct to vaccination to achieve complete control of the disease.

Neosporosis, caused by a protozoan parasite, is a particularly challenging disease as related to bovine abortion.[9] *Neospora caninum* infection has emerged as an important reproductive disease in cattle throughout the world, often shown in surveys to be the major diagnosed cause of abortion in cattle. Abortion, occurring during the middle of gestation, is the primary clinical sign of the infection in cattle. Widespread presence of titers in beef cattle in North America is apparent.[10] Both endemic and epidemic patterns of abortion may occur in herds associated with the demonstration of *Neospora* organisms in fetal tissues. Two methods for transmission of the infection in cattle exist. Horizontal transmission uses a two-host life cycle whereby the cow is infected from ingestion of coccidial oocyst stages shed by the definitive host (dogs and probably other carnivores). Vertical transplacental transmission of the infection is an important route of infection in many herds. Vertical transmission occurs because fetal infection frequently does not result in abortion, but rather the fetus survives to be a PI animal. A heifer calf that is born congenitally infected is capable of transmitting the infection to the next generation when she becomes pregnant, thus maintaining the infection in the herd. The clinical outcome of transplacental fetal infection with *N. caninum* is likely determined by maternal and fetal immune responses that involve humoral and, most important, cell-mediated immune factors. The diagnosis of the infection is assisted through histopathology and immunohistochemical examination of aborted fetuses and serologic testing of cattle for evidence of infection. It should be noted that *Neospora* organisms can be demonstrated in normal neonates, so there exists the possibility that some *Neospora* diagnoses in aborted fetuses are false positives.[10,11] Suggested control methods for the prevention or treatment of neosporosis include reducing the number of congenitally infected animals retained in the herd and minimizing the opportunity for postnatal transmission from the environment, perhaps including vaccination.

Leptospirosis in cattle has long been considered a principle cause of fetal loss in cattle. This has precipitated widespread use of a five-antigen multivalent vaccine in U.S. beef herds. A recent reclassification of leptospira types has focused attention on *Leptospira borgpetersenii* serovar *hardjo*, commonly referred to as *Lepto hardjo-bovis*.[12] This is reputed to be the host-adapted strain of leptospira for cattle, residing in the carrier state in the kidneys and invading the uterus to cause fetal loss. Its presence in beef herds throughout the United States has been documented. Because the organism is host adapted, there is little humoral response to its presence, so serologic testing as a means of documenting infection is reported to be unrewarding. Instead, a technique for diagnosis involving urine collection and centrifugation and the demonstration of leptospires in the urine is recommended.[13] This is coupled with serologic testing to rule out the presence of other leptospires because the urine testing is relatively nonspecific. Several vaccines that are documented to prevent the shedding of *Lepto hardjo-bovis* are now available in the United States. These do not, however, cure animals already infected, so treatment with oxytetracycline is also recommended in a herd control program. The extent to which fetal loss occurs in beef herds infected with the organism has not been elucidated, nor has the benefit to vaccination and oxytetracycline treatment in reducing fetal loss.

In summary, endemic fetal loss can be one of the greatest diagnostic challenges in a beef herd. It must first be recognized that excessive losses are occurring and that these losses are due to fetal loss and not to infertility. Because there are many possible etiologic agents, the history and examination of fetal material and the herd environment must be carefully examined to guide diagnostic sampling. Especially difficult diseases such as BVD virus, neosporosis, and leptospirosis offer special diagnostic challenges.

Epidemic Fetal Loss

Epidemic fetal loss can result from most of the same agents listed as causes of endemic abortion earlier. Whether the abortions occur with an endemic pattern or as an epidemic depends on herd immunity to the abortive agent, the level of exposure to the agent, the virulence of the agent, and the stage of pregnancy of the females in the herd.[14] A herd with a tight pregnancy pattern is more susceptible to an abortion epidemic than one that has cows in all stages of pregnancy.

Investigation of an abortion epidemic is assisted by the time pattern of the event. Investigation of the agents on the list of potential causes of the abortion can be prioritized by the time and spatial pattern of the abortions. The explosive nature of an abortion storm often stimulates an earnestness in the investigation that is difficult to engender with endemic abortion, even when the losses may be similar in amount.

Although tittering dams that have aborted is common practice, it is not a highly rewarding approach to investigating an abortion epidemic.[15] Interpreting results of serologic examination of maternal serum is difficult in cases of abortion. So many animals have had an inapparent infection with or have been vaccinated for many of the common abortifacient infection such as infectious bovine rhinotracheitis, BVD, and leptospirosis. Therefore the mere presence of antibodies to these infections is not proof of their involvement in the abortion. The lack of antibody to a specific infection may be helpful in excluding a specific infection as the cause of an abortion. However, in the case

of BVD, low titers or the lack of antibody may indicate immunotolerance and persistent infection. Most systemic maternal infections that result in abortion occur at least 10 days before the abortion. Therefore the antibody level in the dam's serum has reached its maximum or near its maximum by the time the abortion occurs. Because of this, one should not expect titer rises in serum taken 10 to 21 days after abortion. The possible exception to this is abortions caused by chlamydial infection.

Sample submission to a diagnostic laboratory in an appropriate manner is crucial.[16] Following are recommendations for a generic set of samples that should generally be submitted or at least collected and preserved so that an analysis can be done at a later date if preliminary investigation suggests such.

The veterinarian should submit entire aborted calves and their fetal membranes to the laboratory. Fetal tissues usually are not difficult to preserve. Fetal carcasses are usually not contaminated with large numbers of bacteria from the intestine, as are postnatal animals. Therefore refrigerating the tissues or fetus is sufficient to maintain their condition. Freezing is objectionable because (1) it often ruins tissues for histologic examination; (2) some infectious agents are killed by freezing; and (3) when fetuses arrive at the laboratory frozen, necropsy cannot be done until they thaw. This may delay results a day or more. Frequently, fetuses are retained in the uterus a few days or more after they die. Obviously the autolysis that results cannot be avoided, but it should not deter submitting the specimen.

If calves in the late stages of gestation are too large to ship conveniently, an on-farm necropsy can be performed and specimens submitted. Box 117-2 describes a generic set of samples submitted to or processed in a laboratory that will allow a thorough examination for the most common causes of abortion in beef cattle.[16]

Defining the temporal, animal, and spatial patterns of abortions increases the success in obtaining a diagnosis.[14,15] Case-control analyses wherein aborting females are sampled and the results of their analyses are compared with the same analyses from nonaborting females can be useful.[17] This technique is capable of identifying the degree of association of a variety of risk factors with abortions.

An important question to be answered when investigating an abortion storm is whether dams of the aborted fetuses are apparently clinically normal. Not included in the earlier list are a number of systemic diseases of dams that result in either death of the fetus or such severe stress that premature parturition is induced. Any endotoxemia from conditions such as salmonellosis, mastitis, peritonitis, or any number of other conditions can result in abortions.

Are Excessive Numbers of Open Cows a Result of Infertility or Fetal Wastage?

Early embryonic death is a diagnosis that has historically been made only in theory, especially in the beef herd. Because the conceptus is generally absorbed rather than expelled in the first 60 days of pregnancy, there is little outside evidence that fetal death occurred as opposed to

---

Box 117-2

Generic Listing of Samples, Their Preservation and Preparation, for Pathologic and Clinical Pathologic Diagnosis of Abortion in a Beef Herd

Refrigerated or frozen:

1. Stomach content (1-3 ml collected with a sterile syringe and needle)

   Contents are used for bacteriologic culture. It is the amniotic fluid that has been ingested by the fetus and usually contains those organisms that have infected the placenta, which is the most common entrance to the fetus.

2. Kidney, spleen, lung, and liver (⅛ to ¼ of the organ)

   Fluorescent antibody examinations for IBR, BVD, and leptospirosis are done on the kidney, and FA for BVD is done on the spleen. These organs are also cultured for viruses. The kidney must be fresh in order to do FA examinations for IBR and leptospirosis. Lung and liver are cultured for viruses. Large enough portions of each of these organs are necessary so that they can be divided into several parts.

3. Placenta—three or more cotyledons, especially any with lesions

   Most infectious bovine abortions result from blood infections transmitted through the placenta to the calf. Therefore the placenta is usually the first and most consistently affected organ. The effects on the bovine placenta usually are general and the entire organ often has lesions.

Formalin fixed:

1. Lung, liver, kidney, and any other organ (especially with lesions) that the situation suggests should be examined histologically. Sections about ¼-inch thick should be immersed in 10% formalin (10× the volume of tissue) in a warm area overnight; pour off 90% of the formalin, and ship the tissues in the remainder.
2. Placenta. One or more cotyledons in 10% formalin as described earlier. As indicated earlier, selecting an area of placenta to be examined histologically is not terribly important.

Blood:

1. Dam's serum (3-5 ml) ships with less risk than whole blood. The lack of antibody to a specific infection may be helpful in excluding a specific infection as the cause of an abortion.
2. Fetal serum should be 3-5 ml of body cavity fluid or fetal heart blood.

---

the chance that the female never conceived. With the advent of routine ultrasonography, fetal death loss that occurs following 26 to 28 days of gestation can, in theory, be diagnosed. Thus pregnancy diagnosis by ultrasonography in early gestation followed by a second examination at a later date or comparison with calving records allows one to rule out fetal loss from 26 to 28 days to the stage at which expelled fetuses would be observed (60-plus days but perhaps much later if careful observations are not being made).

Employing ultrasonography followed by a second pregnancy diagnosis would probably only be justified after other causes of failure to conceive have been explored.

Herd pregnancy rates are a function of female cyclicity at the beginning of the breeding season, female fertility (the likelihood of conceiving at each estrus) and male fertility. Female cyclicity is a function of time postpartum, body condition (body fat reserves) at calving, age of the female, exposure to a bull, whether the female is suckling, and the influence of any exogenous hormone usage (e.g., use of progestins). Female fertility is a function of time postpartum and energy balance near the time of breeding. Male fertility is strongly influenced by bulls' scrotal circumference, semen normalcy, libido, and physical normalcy as it influences mating ability. The presence of venereal diseases should be considered when herd pregnancy rates are unexpectedly low. Heat stress, especially coupled with tall fescue endophyte toxicity, results in embryo death early enough that the length of the estrous cycle is not disturbed. In general, exploring these common contributors to decreased herd pregnancy rates will be more productive than trying to rule early fetal loss in or out.

Fetal Loss or Perinatal Loss

The U.S. Department of Agriculture's National Health Monitoring System (NAHMS) asked producers in a computer-assisted telephone interview how much death loss occurred at calving time.[18] Producers reported 2.9% of calves are born dead, with 6.4% of replacement heifers and 2.3% of mature cows losing calves at birth. The 220-herd North Dakota herd analysis showed a 4.3% (standard deviation 3.8%) level of perinatal death loss.[5] Almost certainly some of this loss occurs because diseased fetuses have either died near term and are then expelled or die during the birthing process because they are diseased.

Late-term abortion should be considered as one of the causes of death loss at calving time. A careful examination of losses will help elucidate causes for death loss. If artificial insemination was performed, gestation length will help elucidate whether calving losses have an abortion component. The early initiation of the calving season with associated calf death loss would also signal late-term fetal disease.

SUMMARY

In summary, fetal loss can be a financially devastating occurrence in a beef cow herd. Baseline levels of loss occur in all herds and their occurrence should be monitored, if not routinely investigated. Because of the extensive conditions under which beef cattle are kept, aborted materials often go undetected.

Two major patterns for abortion occur in beef cattle herds: endemic and epidemic. An endemic pattern, even if the loss accumulation is eventually quite large, often receives less diagnostic attention than when abortions are manifest in an epidemic. Investigation of fetal loss should include an epidemiologic approach, as well as a laboratory approach.

Two often unrecognized patterns for fetal loss include early losses near the time of conception and late-term losses near calving. Fetal deaths that occur during the early postconception period are often mistaken as conception failure. Ultrasonography is a tool that can now be used to investigate early-term abortions that occur after 26 to 28 days. The possibility that late-term abortions are part of a calving death loss problem should be considered.

References

1. Radostits OM, Fetrow J, Leslie KE: Profitability in beef cattle production. In *Herd health food animal production medicine,* ed 2, Philadelphia, 1994, Saunders.
2. Ramsey R, Dove D, Ward C et al: Factors affecting beef cow-herd costs, production, and profits, *J Agri Appl Econ* Apr 2005, pp 91-99.
3. Miller RB: Diagnosis of abortion, *Vet Clin North Am Food Anim Pract* 10:3, 1994.
4. Wikse SE: Practitioner's approach to investigation of abortions in beef cattle, *Proc Soc Theriogenol* 214-221, 2004.
5. Ringwall KA, Helmuth KJ: *1998 NCBA-IRM-SPA Cow-calf enterprise summary of reproduction and performance measures for CHAPS cow-calf producers* (website): http://www.ag.ndsu.nodak.edu/dickinso/research/1998/beef98a.htm. Accessed January 29, 2008.
6. Lamb GC: *Pregnancy diagnosis for the beef herd. University of Minnesota Beef Team Newsletter* (website): http://www.extension.umn.edu/beef/components/releases/09-13-05-Lamb.htm. Accessed September 13, 2005.
7. Larson JE, Lamb GC, Stevenson JS et al: Synchronization of estrus in suckled beef cows for detected estrus and artificial insemination and timed artificial insemination using gonadotropin-releasing hormone, prostaglandin F2*a*, and progesterone, *J Anim Sci* 84:332-342, 2006.
8. Wittuma TE, Grotelueschen DM, Brock KV: Persistent bovine viral diarrhoea virus infection in US beef herds, *Prev Vet Med* 49:83-94, 2001.
9. Anderson ML, Andrianarivo AG, Conrad PA: Neosporosis in cattle, *Anim Reprod Sci* 60:417-443, 2000.
10. Waldner CL, Janzen ED, Ribble CS: Determination of the association between *Neospora caninum* infection and reproductive performance in beef herds, *J Am Vet Med Assoc* 213:685-690, 1998.
11. Thurmond MC, Hietala SK: Effect of congenitally acquired *Neospora caninum* abortion and subsequent abortions in dairy cattle, *Am J Vet Res* 58:1381-1385, 1997.
12. Bolin CA, Alt DP: Use of monovalent leptospiral vaccine to prevent renal colonization and urinary shedding in cattle exposed to *Leptospiral borgpetersenii* serovar *hardjo, AJVR* 62:995-1000, 2001.
13. Nervig RM, Garrett LA: Use of furosemide to obtain bovine urine samples for leptospiral isolation, *AJVR* 40:1197-1200, 1979.
14. Kinsel ML: *An epidemiologic approach to investigating abortion problems in dairy herds.* Proceedings of the 32nd Annual Convention of the American Association of Bovine Practitioners, 152-160, 1999.
15. Miller RB: Diagnosis of abortion, *Vet Clin North Am Food Anim Pract* 10:3, 1994.
16. Zeman DH: *South Dakota animal disease research & diagnostic laboratory user guide,* Brookings, SD, Department of Veterinary Science, Animal Disease Research and Diagnostic Laboratory, South Dakota State University.
17. Hurd HS: *Bovine abortion: the case-control study as a different approach to diagnosis.* Proceedings of the 23rd Annual Convention of the American Association of Bovine Practitioners, 31-33, 1991.
18. USDA Animal and Plant Health Inspection Service: Calving management in beef cow herds, Washington, DC, 1998, USDA, Info Sheet Veterinary Services.

CHAPTER 118

Addressing High Dystocia Incidence in Cow-Calf Herds

MEREDYTH L. JONES and ROBERT L. LARSON

Significant economic losses are associated with dystocia in beef cow-calf herds. These include direct calf loss, failure of passive transfer of immunoglobulins from weakened calves and poor mothering, poor production in surviving calves, and reduction in dam fertility. Target dystocia percentage has been discussed and is typically set around 10% for first calf heifers and 2% for mature cows. Although it would seem logical to aim for 0% dystocia, this is likely an unattainable goal because of the multifactorial nature of the condition. A selection strategy to attain a 0% dystocia rate, such as selecting replacements likely to support low birth weight, negatively affects other production parameters, including calf growth rate and weaning weight. Target dystocia percentage for individual herds varies greatly depending on the tolerance level of the producer and the consulting veterinarian. For this reason, this chapter does not focus on determining whether a problem exists, but rather on the many factors to investigate and address when a problem is perceived.

Most dystocias are due to maternal-fetal misproportion, 99% in one study,[1] with the remaining due to malpresentation of the fetus. Clinical and research observations indicate that maternal-fetal misproportion is primarily due to fetal oversize rather than maternal undersize.[1-3]

SIRE-RELATED FACTORS

The high frequency of dystocia caused by large fetal size requires that an investigation of an unacceptable frequency of dystocia on a farm or ranch focus on sire selection initially. This may be the single most important step in evaluation of a herd experiencing a high dystocia rate. In reviewing records, look for patterns of large calves resulting from the same sire. Many times, producers will look at the sire's birth weight or his mature body size as a determinant of the size of calves he will produce. These are both ineffective. The birth weight of the sire may have some ability to determine the size of his calves but, if used alone, is an inadequate measure of his calving ease potential.

A more accurate means of evaluating sires relative to dystocia prevention is expected progeny difference (EPD).[4,5] EPD values predict the performance of progeny of selected individuals relative to other individuals of the same breed. Three EPD measures are specifically related to calving: birth weight EPD, calving ease EPD (direct), and maternal calving ease EPD.[6] Birth weight EPD defines the difference in birth weight, in pounds, of a particular sire's calves relative to those of other sires within the same breed. Calving ease EPD reflects the ease of which a sire's calves are born. This EPD may be divided by some breeds into values for first-calf heifers and mature cows, indicating the ease with which the sire's calves are born to each female group. Maternal calving ease EPD indicates the relative ease of calving experienced by the daughters of that sire as heifers or cows. Both calving ease EPD and maternal calving ease EPD are reported as differences in percentages of unassisted births, with higher values being associated with higher calving ease. When interpreting EPDs, it is important to remember that each breed publishes its own summary and that bulls can only be directly compared within each breed, although there are tools that have been used to evaluate bulls across breeds. Also, the accuracy measure of the EPD should be evaluated. This ranges from 0 to 1 and indicates the reliability of the EPD, with higher accuracy increasing the predictability of that bull. The accuracy increases as a higher volume of information is available on that bull and his relatives, so young bulls will have inherently lower accuracy scores. Selection of bulls with high calving ease scores and low birth weight scores may result in long-term dystocia relief.

DAM-RELATED FACTORS

Second, an evaluation of dam-related factors should be undertaken, first determining whether the problem lies primarily with first-calf heifers, mature cows, or both.

Heifers

For first-calf heifers, many factors contribute to their inherent higher risk of dystocia, the greatest of which is body weight and size. Body size is a reflection of the nutritional development of a heifer. It is advised that replacement heifers weigh 65% to 70% of their anticipated mature weight at the time of breeding and 85% to 90% of their mature weight at first calving. Using these targets, periodic weight determination of a subset of heifers during the growth phase would be advisable to monitor that heifers are at an appropriate weight for their day of age in relation to their target breeding dates and mature weight. At 7 through 12 months of age, heifers should be fed to gain 0.1% of their anticipated mature weight per day.[7] At 18 months of age, they should gain 0.06% of their mature weight daily and at 24 months, gain 0.04% of mature weight daily.[7] Gain at higher rates than these may result in deposition of fat into the pelvis, leading to calving difficulty. When evaluating rates of gain in growing heifers, particular attention should be paid to parasite control programs, as well as to macromineral and micromineral balance, for their particular influence on skeletal growth.

To increase body weight, some may consider the use of growth-promoting implants and creep feeding. Implanting may increase weaned and yearling body size and pelvic area over nonimplanted heifers, but this difference has been shown to be minimized by the time of calving. Implants have mixed results in the ability to reduce calving difficulty and have been shown to inhibit reproductive tract function and impair fertility.[8-10] It is recommended that implanting replacement heifers be avoided, and if implants are used in replacement heifers, increased numbers of replacements should be retained as compensation for reduced pregnancy percentage. Similarly, creep feeding of replacement heifers increases weaning weight, but this difference is absent by 1 year of age. Creep feeding of heifers significantly reduces reproductive productivity and should not be practiced if additional energy results in fat deposition in the udder.[11]

Pelvic area is a specific, calving-oriented assessment of skeletal size. Pelvimetry involves measurement of the internal height and width of the bony pelvis in yearling heifers, with subsequent calculation of the pelvic area. Pelvimetry is often used as a means of predicting whether an individual heifer will experience dystocia. Under this concept, a threshold pelvic measurement, usually 140 to 170 cm^2, is preset, and any heifer smaller than that area is culled. Pelvimetry suffers from poor sensitivity and specificity,[5,12] likely as a result of its use to try to predict dystocia on an individual animal basis. Its utility may be improved when it is used to describe the status of the population rather than the individual.

When selecting heifers for the replacement pool of animals, both management and genetic decisions are being made and it should be remembered that phenotype is not a perfect predictor of genotype. Veterinarians are often confined to selecting animals based on phenotype for many traits because it is their only readily accessible estimation of genetic potential. In using pelvimetry, veterinarians are selecting genotypic contribution to herd dystocia risk based on phenotypic expression. When making genetic decisions for the herd, the genetic diversity of the evaluated population should be considered when evaluating phenotypic characteristics such as pelvic area, reproductive tract score, and body weight. Because pelvimetry is known to better evaluate the group rather than the individual, the population diversity influences the interpretation of the data obtained. If an unacceptably large percentage of genetically similar heifers falls below the predetermined pelvic area cutoff, one has evidence

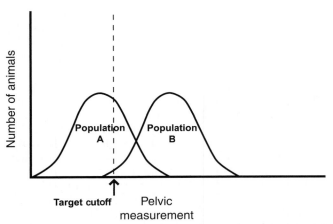

Fig 118-1 Two groups of heifers. Evidence of genetic potential for a small pelvic area exists in Population A. Evidence of genetic potential for a larger pelvic area is present in Population B.

that the genetics of that group does not support adequate pelvic area and the entire group should be culled (assuming the population is relatively homogeneous). Another way to look at it is that even though there will be individual heifers that exceed the cutoff (phenotypic acceptability), they share the genetic potential to have offspring with unacceptable pelvic area (genotypic unacceptability). In Fig. 118-1, populations A and B represent two groups of heifers; heifers within each population are genetically similar. Population A shows genetic potential for small pelvic area, even though some heifers are above the acceptable threshold. If those above-threshold heifers are retained, there is a high risk that their offspring will express small pelvic areas because that is their genetic potential. Population B, however, shows evidence of a genetic potential that trends for larger pelvic area, even though a few heifers fall below the threshold.

Pelvic measuring used to predict individual risk of dystocia is ineffective and is an inferior predictor of dystocia when compared with prebreeding body size. Because pelvic area is of moderate high heritability,[13-16] selection based on this can allow for a herd genetic change over time. This genetic change over time should result in a phenotypic change in dams but not necessarily a reduction in dystocia incidence. As with most parameters, the decision to select for larger skeletal size of replacement heifers should not occur in a vacuum. Selection for greater pelvic area, and therefore skeletal size, will also select for calves with larger skeletons, requiring a balance between dam skeletal size and fetal skeletal size.

A more appropriate evaluation of heifers is the maternal calving ease EPD of their sire. This EPD encompasses a number of criteria that contribute to dystocia, including calf shape and size, sire selection, heifer skeletal size, metabolism, and uterine environment. There exists significantly more literature on this trait in dairy cattle, but its use in beef cattle could be equally valuable.

The age of dam is a well-recognized factor in dystocia rate.[1,17] Skeletal growth, evidenced by growth in pelvic area, increases through 4 years of age.[14] Dystocia risk decreases as the age and parity of the dam increases, but this applies to heifers as well. Age at time of first calving influences odds of an unassisted birth, increasing

1.24 times each month from the ages of 22 to 29 months.[18] Because heavier calves may be tolerated by older heifers,[18] replacement heifers should be selected from those born early in the calving season.

Mature Cows

For mature cows, fetal-maternal mismatch may occur as in heifers, but typically only with extremely large calves. Pelvic trauma and malformation, previous dystocia, and fetal malpresentation predispose to dystocia in the individual mature cow but will not result in an increased incidence on a herd basis. Dam nutrition may be the most significant contributor to a high dystocia incidence in mature cows on a herd basis. Specifically, energy, protein, calcium, and trace mineral status should be considered.

NUTRITION DURING PREGNANCY

In assessing nutrition of pregnant heifers and cows during pregnancy, it should be noted that restriction of nutrition in late pregnancy does not reduce dystocia risk.[19] Within reasonable limits, energy intake does not alter fetal weight, but dam weight loss of 0.5 kg/day in the last trimester in beef heifers is associated with weakened labor and dystocia.[19-21] So, even if fetal weight could be restricted nutritionally, the restriction would have to be so extreme that dystocia would still likely occur from a weakened dam. In heifers, high planes of energy increase pelvic size but do not decrease dystocia rate because of increased fetal weight and pelvic fat deposition.[22] It is much easier to make a larger calf with increased planes of nutrition than it is to make a smaller calf by restricting nutritional intake. Thus it has been recommended that nutrition during late pregnancy target only a moderate weight gain of 0.5 kg/day.[6]

Significantly inadequate protein nutrition in late pregnancy, in conjunction with cold stress, can induce "weak calf syndrome."[23] Otherwise, protein level does not seem to significantly alter calf birth weight or dystocia rate. Geographic area and ambient conditions should always be considered when evaluating a herd's nutritional needs as weather and shelter availability significantly alter requirements.

Overall, the highest incidence of dystocia caused by maternal factors appears to be in dams that are small and weak or those that are overfat. Extreme nutritional manipulation during pregnancy can be expected to have significant effects on the dam, with little effect on fetal size or dystocia.

The herd should be regularly evaluated during gestation for body condition score (BCS). Cows should be at a target BCS of 6 on a 9-point scale at the time of calving. If, during gestation, a number of cows are at a BCS of less than 4/9 or greater than 8/9, then nutrition should be adjusted accordingly, perhaps to involve the feeding of those animals separately. For heifers, it is prudent not to allow them to fall below a BCS of 5/9.

If uterine inertia is determined to contribute to a number of dystocias on a farm, several factors should be considered. Uterine inertia on a herd basis may result from hypocalcemia, trace mineral deficiencies, and myometrial exhaustion. Calcium is important at the time of parturition in that it is required for functioning of oxytocin receptors of the uterus. Although hypocalcemia is not as widely encountered in beef as in dairy production, subclinical hypocalcemia may occur in mature, heavily lactating beef cows or in cows grazing forages high in potassium in late pregnancy. Deficiencies of the trace minerals zinc and iodine have been directly correlated with uterine inertia and prolonged calving.[24,25] Deficiencies of selenium, copper, cobalt, and vitamins A, D, and E have been associated with delayed uterine involution and therefore are considered important for proper uterine function.[25] Secondary uterine inertia results from myometrial exhaustion as a result of prolonged dystocia.[26] When this is suspected, the focus should be placed on producer interventional strategies during calving, discussed later in this chapter.

Additional dam factors include inadequate cervical dilation, inadequate vulvar relaxation because of immaturity or heredity, uterine torsion, and hormonal imbalances, specifically low estrogen levels. These are frequently uncontrollable and occur as a single-animal problem.

CALF-RELATED FACTORS

Calf-related factors have been partially addressed because birth weight is the main contributor to dystocia, particularly in heifer dams. It should be noted that a calf's genotype is contributed to equally by the dam and sire, and additionally, the environment provided by the dam contributes to expression of the genetic basis. Frequently, this is forgotten and sire selection is the only factor addressed in herds with dystocia problems. Dam and sire selection may be altered for future calving seasons but does not provide immediate relief from large fetuses.

Sex also plays a role in the birth weight of the calf, with bull calves weighing 4 kg (8.8 lb) heavier than heifer calves in one study.[1] The odds of an unassisted birth are 1.45 times higher for heifer calves than bull calves.[18] The technology to determine calf sex is not widespread, but some producers use fetal sexing by ultrasound during early development (55-85 days), and sorting of dams by fetal sex allows for closer monitoring of dams carrying bull calves as a dystocia management tool.

Fetal malpresentation, as noted earlier in the chapter, does not usually cause a significant rise in herd dystocia rate. Fetal presentation is a factor for which there is no known management control, except possibly for some that may be due to oversized calves that may become malpresented as a result of uterine contraction against a relatively undersized pelvis.

Some evidence suggests that cold weather during late gestation increases calf birth weight and dystocia rate, whereas warmer temperatures decrease calf body weight[4] because of differential blood flow from the dam to fetus. For winter- and spring-calving herds, as winter temperature increases, calf birth weight and calving difficulty decrease. Although controlling the weather is not an option, this may help to explain minor year-to-year fluctuations.

One final point about fetal factors involves the production of calves by artificial means such as embryo transfer and cloning. These calves tend to be much larger than their natural counterparts and with the use of these technologies come an increased risk of dystocia. When these technologies are required as part of individual producer production goals, selection of the recipient dam must be carefully performed to accommodate such fetuses.

PRODUCER INTERVENTION

Finally, direct human factors should be considered when there is an increase in particularly complicated dystocias or in stillborn calves.[17] Evaluation of the interventional strategies of the producer should include the timing of heifers calving relative to the mature cow herd, the length of the heifer calving season, and the duration of stage II labor allowed before intervention. It is recommended that heifer calving be initiated before the mature cow calving season. And, ideally, the heifer calving season should be limited to less than 45 days, which can be achieved with cycling heifers when an estrous synchronization program is used. Both of these strategies have many positive effects, including the ability to concentrate labor efforts toward closer monitoring of first-calf heifers. Producers should be encouraged to provide assistance 1 hour after the appearance of membranes in heifers and 30 minutes in mature cows.[27,28] Although this seems shorter than traditionally thought, when time of decision to time of actual intervention and frequency of observation are considered, particularly in the situation in which a herd is experiencing significant problems, these times may be appropriate. Additionally, the practice of maintaining specialized calving areas for heifers also allows for close monitoring and timely intervention.

References

1. Nix JM, Spitzer JC, Grimes LW et al: A retrospective analysis of factors contributing to calf mortality and dystocia in beef cattle, *Theriogenology* 49:1515, 1998.
2. Bennett GL, Gregory KE: Genetic (co)variances for calving difficulty score in composite and parental populations in beef cattle: I. Calving difficulty score, birth weight, weaning weight, and postweaning gain, *J Anim Sci* 79:45, 2001.
3. Rice LE, Wiltbank JN: Factors affecting dystocia in beef heifers, *J Am Vet Med Assoc* 161:1348, 1972.
4. Colburn DJ, Deutscher GH, Nielsen MK et al: Effects of sire, dam traits, calf traits, and environment on dystocia and subsequent reproduction of two-year-old heifers, *J Anim Sci* 75:1452, 1997.
5. Cook BR, Tess MW, Kress DD: Effects of selection strategies using heifer pelvic area and sire birth weight expected progeny difference on dystocia in first-calf heifers, *J Anim Sci* 71:602, 1993.
6. Chenoweth PJ, Sanderson MW: Health and production management in beef cattle breeding herds. In Radostits OM, editor: *Herd health: food animal production medicine*, ed 3, Philadelphia, 2001, Saunders.
7. Fox DG, Sniffen CJ, O'Connor JD: Adjusting nutrient requirements of beef cattle for animal and environmental variations, *J Anim Sci* 66:1475, 1988.
8. Anthony RV, Kittok RJ, Ellington EF et al: Effects of zeranol on growth and ease of calf delivery in beef heifers, *J Anim Sci* 58:1325, 1981.

9. Hancock RF, Deutscher GH, Nielson MK et al: Effects of Synovex C on growth rate, pelvic area, reproduction, and calving performance of replacement heifers, *J Anim Sci* 72:292, 1994.

10. Staigmiller RB, Bellows PA, Short RE: Growth and reproductive traits in beef heifers implanted with zeranol, *J Anim Sci* 57:527, 1983.

11. Martin TG, Lemenager RP, Srinivasan G et al: Creep feed as a factor influencing performance of cows and calves, *J Anim Sci* 53:33, 1981.

12. Van Donkersgoed J, Ribble CS, Booker CW et al: The predictive value of pelvimetry in beef cattle, *Can J Vet Res* 57:170, 1993.

13. Benyshek LL, Little DE: Estimates of genetic and phenotypic parameters associated with pelvic area in Simmental cattle, *J Anim Sci* 54:258, 1982.

14. Green RD, Brinks JS, Denham et al: Estimation of heritabilities of pelvic measures in beef cattle, *J Anim Sci* 59(suppl 1):174, 1984.

15. Morrison DG, Williamson WD, Humes PE: Heritabilities and correlations of traits associated with pelvic area in beef cattle, *J Anim Sci* 59(suppl 1):160, 1984.

16. Naazie A, Makerechian M, Berg RT: Genetic, phenotypic, and environmental parameter estimates of calving difficulty, weight, and measures of pelvic size in beef heifers, *J Anim Sci* 69:4793, 1991.

17. Dargatz DA, Dewell GA, Mortimer RG: Calving and calving management of beef cows and heifers on cow-calf operations in the United States, *Theriogenology* 61:997, 2004.

18. Berger PJ, Cubas AC, Koehler KJ et al: Factors affecting dystocia and early calf mortality in Angus cows and heifers, *J Anim Sci* 70:1775, 1992.

19. Kroker GA, Cummins LJ: The effect of nutritional restriction on Hereford heifers in late pregnancy, *Aust Vet J* 55:467, 1979.

20. Bellows RA, Short RE: Effects of precalving feed level on birthweight, calving difficulty and subsequent fertility, *J Anim Sci* 46:1522, 1978.

21. Corah LR, Dunn TG, Kaltenback CC: Influence of prepartum nutrition on the reproductive performance of beef females and the performance of their progeny, *J Anim Sci* 41:819, 1975.

22. Arnett DW, Totusek R: Some effects of obesity in beef females, *J Anim Sci* 33:1129, 1971.

23. Olson DP, Bull RC, Kelley KW et al: Effects of maternal nutritional restriction and cold stress on young calves: clinical condition, behavioral reactions, and lesions, *Am J Vet Res* 42:758, 1981.

24. Corah LR, Ives S: The effects of essential trace minerals on reproduction in beef cattle, *Vet Clin North Am Food Anim Pract* 7:41, 1991.

25. Graham TW: Trace element deficiencies in cattle, *Vet Clin North Am Food Anim Pract* 7:153, 1991.

26. Youngquist RS: Parturition and Dystocia. In Youngquist RS, editor: *Current therapy in large animal theriogenology*, ed 1, Philadelphia, 1997, Saunders.

27. Doornbos DE, Bellows RA, Burfening PJ et al: Effects of damage, prepartum nutrition and duration of labor on productivity and postpartum reproduction in beef females, *J Anim Sci* 59:1, 1984.

28. Rice LE: Dystocia-related risk factors, *Vet Clin North Am Food Anim Pract* 10:53, 1994.

Recommended Readings

Larson RL: Heifer development: reproduction and nutrition, *Vet Clin North Am Food Anim Pract* (in press).

Sanderson MW, Dargatz DA: Risk factors for high herd level calf morbidity risk from birth to weaning in beef herds in the USA, *Prev Vet Med* 44:97, 2000.

Larson RL, Tyler JW: Reducing calf losses in beef herds, *Vet Clin North Am Food Anim Pract* 21:569, 2005.

Patterson DJ, Perry RC, Kiracofe GH et al: Management considerations in heifer development and puberty, *J Anim Sci* 70:4018, 1992.

Van Donkersgoed J: Pelvimetry. In Youngquist RS, editor: *Current therapy in large animal theriogenology*, Philadelphia, 1997, Saunders.

CHAPTER 119

Carcass Ultrasound Uses in Beef Cattle Production Settings

SHELIE LAFLIN

Utilization of real-time ultrasound (RTU) technology to obtain noninvasive, antemortem carcass data has been available since the 1950s, when it was first used in the swine industry. Significant progress has been made in the software and equipment used for this purpose since its initiation. Regulation of data collection and interpretation has led to high accuracy in data and the ability to provide reliable information on which to evaluate individual animals.

Accuracy and predictability of carcass data obtained via ultrasonic examination has proven to be highly precise and allows for rapid evaluation of an individual's carcass merits. Several separate images are collected on an individual to be analyzed and provide the necessary information to evaluate percent intramuscular fat (PIMF), rump fat thickness (RF), rib fat thickness (BF), and rib eye area (REA). These measurements are then used to determine other market potential and are often expressed in estimated progeny differences (EPDs). Information obtained from EPDs and RTU carcass information can aid in genetic and marketing decisions.

Carcass EPDs have been developed for several breeds and now play an important part in replacement stock selection. Determining how to evaluate and implement carcass EPDs versus actual carcass data is becoming an important focus point for producers and veterinarians assisting their clients.

DATA COLLECTION AND ANALYSIS

Image Collection

According to the Beef Improvement Federation (BIF), four traits can be accurately measured via ultrasonography and therefore used in antemortem analysis of carcass disposition. These traits include twelfth to thirteenth rib fat thickness (RF), rump fat thickness (UF), REA, and PIMF.[1]

Fig. 119-1 illustrates proper orientation of an ultrasound probe to collect required images. The RF measurement is obtained from a transverse image of the longissimus dorsi (LD) between the twelfth and the thirteenth ribs. REA is a measurement taken from the same image as the RF in which the actual outline of the LD is traced by the laboratory technician. PIMF is obtained from a sagittal image of the LD over the twelfth and thirteenth ribs. UF is obtained from an image taken between the tuber coxae and the tuber ischium.

For optimal image collection, the animal to be scanned should be well restrained in a squeeze chute. The hair needs to be shaved to be no longer than ½ inch in the following three areas: (1) over the hip between the tuber coxae and the tuber ischium, (2) along the spine over the LD between the twelfth and thirteenth ribs and parallel to the spine over the LD. All debris needs to be removed from the areas to be scanned via a curry comb or a blower.

A couplant is then applied for maximum contact. Any oil such as vegetable oil or sunflower oil works well as an economical couplant. Mineral oil is typically not advised because it can erode the covering on the ultrasound probe over extended use. Equipment needs to maintained at 45° F or greater. The couplant needs to be kept at 55° F or greater. The warmer the couplant, the quicker the penetration and possibly the better the image one will achieve.

The optimal age to ultrasound and the age limit instituted by breed associations differ among breeds. However,

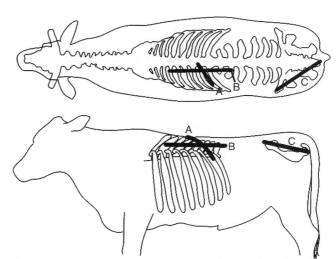

Fig 119-1 Probe placement to obtain the percent intramuscular fat and rib fat thickness measurements is over the twelfth and fourteenth ribs covering the longissimus dorsi (LD) muscle *(A)*. Probe placement to obtain the rib eye area and rib fat is between the twelfth and thirteenth ribs parallel to the ribs and over the LD muscle *(B)*. Probe placement to obtain the rump fat and muscle depth is over the medial gluteal and bicep femoris muscles in a line between the tuber coxae and tuber ischium *(C)*.

most breeds analyze individuals around 360 days of age for bulls and around 400 days of age for heifers.

Equipment

Several different ultrasound machines can be used in collection of carcass data. However, the software being used to interpret the data may limit which ultrasound machine is used. Currently, most images are captured using an Aloka 500 with a 3.5-MHz, 17-cm linear array probe or a Classic Scanner 200 with a 3.5-MHz, 18-cm linear array probe.[2] However, several other equipment combinations are allowed by the Ultrasound Guidelines Council (UGC).[3]

Transducer/probe size is important in data collection. First-generation ultrasound equipment could only accept a 12.5-cm transducer. This was not long enough to obtain the entire image of the LD in one image. Capture of two images, also known as *split screen imaging,* that were overlain was required to obtain one complete image traced to attain the area of the muscle.[4] This provided opportunity for error in reading the image and required extreme skill in image collection. Second-generation equipment uses a transducer that is typically 17 to 18 cm in length and is capable of capturing the entire LD outline in one image. This probe provides a single image and removes many of the obstacles in image interpretation previously encountered with the shorter probes.

Image Analysis

Most breed associations are requiring that field technicians be UGC certified and that data be submitted to one of four centralized processing laboratories recognized by the UGC. Centralized laboratories provide the added benefit of image analysis performed by trained technicians specializing in image interpretation. Breed associations not requiring adherence to UGC standards may allow images to be collected and interpreted by technicians who are not UGC certified and data analysis companies that are not UGC approved.

The UGC regulates consistency and quality in technician certification and is responsible for maintaining testing and certification standards for ultrasound technicians. Technicians who are UGC certified have passed strict testing criteria and are required to maintain high levels of accuracy on submitted data or have their certification revoked.

To maintain UGC certification, technicians are required to ultrasound approximately 20 head of cattle every 2 years. Technician accuracy is evaluated by comparison to reference images (obtained at the same time) and individual animal carcass information. Image quality, accuracy, and a written examination are required for certification. Technicians are required to obtain a minimum of 80% acceptable images per trait evaluated (REA, PIMF, RF, UF).[3,5]

Specific ultrasound equipment systems are required for the certification process. A total of either 40 or 80 images (depending on the type of certification sought) for each trait will be evaluated during the certification procedure.[3] The laboratory technician is required to obtain 95% accuracy on image interpretation.[3] Images interpreted are judged against actual carcass comparisons.

FUNCTIONALITY OF CARCASS ULTRASOUND DATA

The initiation of value-based marketing has led the cattle industry to focus less simply on external evaluation of an animal and emphasize carcass value. The dilemma faced with this shift in paradigm involved the time and expense required to evaluate potential breeding animals. Historically, progeny testing required 3 to 5 years for the individual to reach breeding age and produce a significant number of offspring, with subsequent maturation and slaughter of those progeny. This accumulated a cost of approximately $5000 per sire.[6] By using ultrasound evaluation, progeny testing can be achieved in as little as 2 years with a significant reduction in cost and the accuracy of the actual data collected has proven reliable.[6]

Correlation and Heritability

Ultrasound carcass traits have moderate to high correlation, depending on the trait, and are moderately heritable.[6,7] Research has demonstrated high correlation between ultrasound and actual RF and moderate heritabilities of 0.57 and 0.38, respectively.[8] Ultrasound REA and actual REA are moderately correlated (0.59) and the ultrasound area of the longissimus muscle is moderately heritable (0.28).[8] Research results have a wide range on the correlation of ultrasound PIMF and actual PIMF. Although the range is extensive, all values have demonstrated moderate to high correlation between the two. Ultrasound PIMF is also moderately heritable (0.23).[9]

Revealing the correlation between ultrasound and actual carcass information within one animal is significant and extremely helpful to the industry. However, for this information to be useful in affecting genetic improvement within the industry, the correlation between sire or dam EPDs and carcass characteristics in progeny needs to be understood. Crews[10] performed a study evaluating 15 Charolais sires and the resulting 273 progeny of those animals to determine the correlation between sire EPDs and progeny phenotype. In this research, fat thickness related as a 1-mm increase in EPD resulted in a 1.27-mm increase in progeny carcass fat thickness. REA showed an increase of 1.23 cm^2 in progeny carcass for each 1 cm^2 EPD increase in the parent. Crews also showed positive correlations between other sire ultrasound and progeny carcass traits including hot carcass weight, percent lean yield, and marbling.

A study done by Sapp and colleagues[11] involving 20 Angus bulls and 188 steer progeny focused on ultrasound PIMF and carcass marbling in progeny. This study grouped cattle into high and low marbling groups. It was noted that the progeny of high marbling bulls typically demonstrated lower REA (74.89 cm^2) than those progeny of low marbling sires (77.86 cm^2).[11] This relationship has been previously reported with correlations ranging from −0.12 to −0.01.[12]

Understanding the degrees of correlation associated with ultrasound data to progeny carcass traits has unveiled a whole new science for producers to use in making genetic decisions in their herd. However, for this information to become practical to the beef industry, a uniform method of comparing individuals within a breed needs to be developed.

Expected Progeny Differences

EPDs are used to compare traits between two individuals and predict the performance differences in their offspring. EPDs exist for many traits that can be passed on to offspring. Many EPDs have been in use for decades, whereas newer EPDs such as for carcass traits have only recently been added to an individual's reports. Box 119-1 contains brief descriptions of EPDs currently used by several breed associations.[13] Although the definitions remain constant among breeds, it is important to not compare EPDs among breeds unless it is noted that the EPDs are across-breed or an across-breed EPD adjustment table is used.

Carcass EPDs versus Ultrasound EPDs

Carcass EPDs for an individual are derived from actual carcass information obtained from that individual sire, maternal grand sire, maternal great grand sire, and slaughtered progeny. Carcass EPDs are adjusted for a slaughter endpoint of 480 days.[14] Ultrasound EPDs are obtained from ultrasound data from that individual; that individual's parents, if available; and any scanned yearling progeny. Although the two different EPDs are both useful and important, it is imperative to remember that the two may vary greatly. The reason for this is that although there is a genetic correlation between the two, ultrasound EPDs are only a partial reflection of carcass EPDs. This is due to the external impacts (e.g., feed, environment, disease) that can potentially have impacts on carcass attributes.

EPD Accuracy and Interim EPDs

Accuracy indicates to what extent one can have confidence that the EPD numbers are truly indicating the animal's genetic potential. Accuracy increases with the number of individuals (progeny and ancestors) evaluated. Importantly, carcass EPDs typically have higher accuracy ratings than ultrasound EPDs because the industry has significantly more individual carcass data than individual ultrasound data. This is particularly true for young animals that may not have many progeny that have been ultrasounded. Accuracy rises as an individual has more offspring that are subsequently ultrasounded.

An interim value is indicated by an uppercase "I" preceding the EPD value. This is true for any EPD and indicates only that individual's information is being included in the formulation of the EPD value. Interim values should be used accordingly, recognizing that only that individual's information is being used. The accuracy of an interim is low and may not accurately reflect genetic potential.

Using EPDs for Sire Selection

The sheer volume of information available for cattle breeders to use in making breeding decisions can be quite overwhelming. As with any genetic change, it is important to focus on the entire picture, not just one part of it.

Box 119-1

Relevant Estimated Progeny Difference Definitions

$Value Indexes:
These are estimates expressed in dollar value of how progeny will perform in comparison with progeny of other sires. Calculation includes many different traits and their individual impact on the performance of that individual in the given circumstance.

$W (Weaned Calf Value): Indicates average dollars per head that an individual is expected to demonstrate for preweaning value. It takes into consideration birth weight, weaning direct growth, maternal milk, and mature cow size.
$F (Feedlot Value): Indicates average dollars per head that an individual is expected to demonstrate for postweaning merit.
$G (Grid Value): Indicates average dollars per head that an individual is expected to demonstrate for carcass grid value. This is further broken down into quality grade ($QG) and yield grade ($YG).

Carcass:
CW (Carcass Weight): Used to predict the number of pounds difference in carcass weight.
Marb (Marbling): Indicates the expected difference of U.S. Department of Agriculture (USDA) marbling score. It is expressed as a fraction of a USDA marbling score.
Rib Eye Area (RE): Indicates the expected difference of rib eye area in square inches.
Fat Thickness (Fat): Indicates the expected difference of external rib fat thickness in inches.

Ultrasound:
Intramuscular Fat (%IMF): Indicates the expected difference of intramuscular fat in the longissimus dorsi.
Ribeye Area (RE): Indicates the expected difference of ultrasound REA in square inches.
Fat Thickness (FT): Indicates the expected difference in ultrasound rib fat thickness. This is a weighted average of 60% rib fat and 40% rump fat and is expressed in inches.

As mentioned earlier, if a decision is made to use only high-marbling bulls, over time the REA of offspring will be significantly reduced. Many correlations are yet to be uncovered. Therefore focusing on a single trait may rapidly lead to a reduction in other desirable traits that a producer has spent years trying to develop within the herd.

Contemporary groups should be considered when evaluating EPDs. The number of contemporary groups and the total number of individuals evaluated in these groups are expressed for both carcass and ultrasound EPD information. A contemporary group is a group of peer animals of the same breed, age, and sex that have been managed similarly. Accuracy of EPDs increases with the number of animals evaluated in a contemporary group and the number of sires evaluated within the group.

Definition of goals for progeny is an important first step. A breeder who is intending to retain ownership in his calves and market them on a grid may desire to increase PIMF and decrease RF in his calves. A seedstock producer who will be marketing bulls may seek to improve all or select carcass traits based on what the individual's carcass values currently are. The environment, management, and marketing future of animals determines specific EPDs that should be evaluated.

SUMMARY

Carcass ultrasound is a useful tool to obtain antemortem carcass data for cow-calf producers. When properly collected and evaluated, this information can be an important part of the genetic planning process for the beef herd. Veterinarians can assist their clients by assisting in collection and interpretation of information gained through this process.

References

1. Beef Improvement Federation: *Guidelines for uniform beef improvement programs,* ed 8, Athens, Ga, 2002, University of Georgia, pp 41-44.
2. Wilson DE: Beef improvement federation certification criteria, Ames, Iowa, 1993, Iowa State University.
3. Ultrasound Guidelines Council: *The beef cattle ultrasound technician annual proficiency and certification program: certification procedures and policy* (website): http://www.aptcbeef. org/Portals/aptcbeef/Documents/UGC%20Certifcation%20 Guidelines.pdf. Accessed October 1, 2006.
4. Perkins TL, Paschal JC, Tipton NC et al: Ultrasonic prediction of quality grade and percent retail cuts in beef cattle, *J Anim Sci* 75(suppl 1):178, 1997 (abstract).
5. Perkins T, Meadows A, Hays B: *Study guide for the ultrasonic evaluation of beef cattle for carcass merit. Ultrasound Guidelines Council Study Guide Sub-Committee* (website): http:// www.aptcbeef.org/Portals/aptcbeef/Documents/UGC%20 STUDY%20GUIDE.pdf. Accessed October 1, 2006.
6. Williams AR: Ultrasound application in beef cattle carcass research and management, *J Anim Sci* 80(suppl 2):E183-E188, 2002.
7. Greiner SP, Rouse GH, Wilson DE et al: The relationship between ultrasound measurements and carcass fat thickness and longissimus muscle area in beef cattle, *J Anim Sci* 81: 676-682, 2003.
8. Moser DW, Bertrand JK, Mitsztal I et al: Genetic parameter estimates for carcass and yearling ultrasound measurements in Brangus cattle, *J Anim Sci* 75(suppl 1):149, 1997 (abstract).
9. Devitt CJB, Wilton JW: Genetic correlation estimates between ultrasound measurements on yearling bulls and carcass measurements on finished steers, *J Anim Sci* 79:2790-2797, 2001.
10. Crews DH Jr: The relationship between beef sire carcass EPD and progeny phenotype, *Can J Anim Sci* 82:503-506, 2002.
11. Sapp RL, Bertrand JK, Pringle TD et al: Effects of selection for ultrasound intramuscular fat percentage in Angus bulls on carcass traits of progeny, *J Anim Sci* 80:2017-2022, 2002.
12. Bertrand JK, Green RD, Herring WO et al: Genetic evaluation for beef carcass traits, *J Anim Sci* 79(suppl):E190-E200, 2001.
13. American Angus Association: *How to read the report: EPDs* (website): http://www.angus.org/sireeval/howto.html. Accessed September 29, 2006.
14. Greiner SP: *Understanding expected progeny differences (EPDs), Virginia Polytechnic Institute and State University Virginia Cooperative Extension Publication 400-804,* Blacksburg, Va, 2002, Virginia Polytechnic Institute and State University.

Recommended Readings

CUP training material (website): www.cuplab.com. Accessed October 1, 2006.

Gwartney BL, Calkins CR, Rasby RJ et al: Use of expected progeny differences for marbling in beef: II. Carcass and palatability traits, *J Anim Sci* 74:1014-1022, 1996.

Hassen A, Wilson DE, Rouse GH: Evaluation of carcass, live and real-time ultrasound measures in feedlot cattle: I. Assessment of sex and breed effects, *J Anim Sci* 76:273-282, 1998.

Hassen A, Wilson DE, Rouse GH et al: *Accuracy evaluation of real-time ultrasound measurement for fat thickness and ribeye area on feedlot cattle. Beef Research Report. Iowa State University Extension Publication AS-630,* Ames, Iowa, 1995, Iowa State University.

Herring WO, Miller D, Bertrand J et al: Evaluation of machine, technician, and interpreter effects on ultrasonic measures of backfat and longissimus muscle area in beef cattle, *J Anim Sci* 72:2216-2226, 1994.

Izquierdo MM, Zhang H, Wilson DE et al: Development and validation of a model to predict percentage of intramuscular fat in live animals by using ultrasound techniques. In *Beef research report. Iowa State University Extension Publication AS-624,* Ames, Iowa, 1994, Iowa State University.

Smith MT, Oltjen JW, Dolezal HG et al: Live animal measurement of carcass traits by ultrasound: assessment and accuracy of sonographers, *J Anim Sci* 70:1667-1676, 1992.

Wilson DE: Application of ultrasound for genetic improvement, *J Anim Sci* 70:973-983, 1992.

SECTION XIV

Feedlot Production Medicine

Daniel U. Thomson

CHAPTER 120

Preconditioned Calves in the Feedyard

BRAD J. WHITE and ROBERT L. LARSON

Preconditioning is intended to prepare calves for the postweaning phase of cattle production by using management practices to reduce the negative impacts of disease and to assist adjustment to new management and nutritional situations. Programs designed to decrease morbidity in feeder calves are not a new concept; variations on the theme have been around since the 1960s. Vaccine technology has improved, but the idea remains relatively simple: prepare unweaned beef calves to thrive in the next phases of their lives even when faced with health and nutritional challenges.

New technologies typically have uptake curves related to the usefulness of the methodology. Industry-wide utilization of preconditioning programs has been slow. Adoption of preconditioning programs is based not only on the potential value added through these procedures but also on the economic signals between market segments. Therefore the challenge becomes not only how to add value by preventing health problems but also how to capture value and provide appropriate incentives to achieve goals.

Cattle often change ownership between production phases. The cow-calf owner is in possession of the cattle at the most opportune time to precondition, yet feedyards often own animals when benefits of preconditioning are reaped. The decision to precondition or purchase calves that have been managed in a specific manner is based on the expected return on investment, or rather, the ability to capture value from the health program. Full benefits can only be gained when preventive health measures are effective and the animals are marketed in a manner that rewards the seller for improved health status.

Accurate conveyance of the potential value between seller and buyer is a critical step in capturing the increased worth of preconditioned animals. Current marketing structures make communication between production segments difficult in many cases. Expending large efforts for direct communication is difficult to justify if disclosing the immunization program is the only goal. Beef production is shifting toward a consumer focus and new areas are achieving more attention including individual animal identification; value-based marketing; food safety; and source, process, and age verification. These recent developments in the beef industry are compatible with concepts of preconditioning and should serve to generate further interest by the feedlot sector in these management techniques.

Feedyards purchase preconditioned calves based on yard-specific profit influencing factors. The value of preconditioned cattle to the feedyard is determined by two major factors: 1) the cattle growth and health performance impact resulting from a specific preconditioning program and 2) the methodology used to incorporate preconditioned cattle into the current management system. Procedures included in preconditioning programs differ and an accurate definition is critical to generate valid expectations. Specific components (i.e., length of weaning, type of feeding and use of vaccinations) likely impact the outcomes of animal health and performance. Differing management of preconditioned cattle modifies expectations for cattle in the program and the potential value that could be captured from these animals.

PRECONDITIONING PROGRAMS

Alliances and vertical integration have been greatly discussed in recent years as methods to increase communication through the production chain and foster consumer-driven economic signals. Although the industry is evolving, the majority of cattle still have multiple owners throughout their productive lifetime with poor transfer of information between owners. Segmentation results in different production end points (and thus economically driven performance targets) for owners in each section of the chain. Cow-calf producers precondition to add value to their animals and the feedyard must determine how much they can pay for the additional procedures the animals received. This calculation is based on the expected improvement in health and performance relative to animals that were not preconditioned.

A comprehensive preconditioning program increases resistance to disease through preventative measures and reduces stressors associated with transition between production phases. Ideally, many of the preconditioning events occur before the traditional sale point between the cow-calf and feedyard phases (at or near maternal separation). One challenge in evaluating impact from preconditioning programs is the widely varied definitions of what preconditioning entails. Programs have been designed by universities, pharmaceutic and biologic companies, marketing groups, and integrated production chain alliances. The overall target of maintaining animal wellness is shared by all programs, yet specific requirements are influenced by internal program factors. For example, preconditioning programs for cattle entering an all-natural program may differ slightly from cattle in a traditional management scheme. Other examples include the utilization or prohibition of specific biologic and pharmaceutic products.

Preconditioning guidelines range from requiring castration and one viral immunization before sale to more complex management regulations. The most comprehensive programs include initial and booster immunizations, acclimation of calves to eating specific ration types from a bunk, and weaning for 45 days on farm of origin before sale. The cost of preconditioning calves is based largely on the complexity of the requirements and dictates the breakeven value for the calves.

If the term "preconditioned" is applied generically to all calves that had some procedure performed before sale, the brand, or perceived value, is diluted. Logically, the likelihood of reducing disease incidence varies in each set of calves based on specific procedures performed. King and Seeger[1] analyzed 10 years of data from Superior Livestock Auction sales and found that the percentage of nonviral vaccinated calves has decreased significantly relative to the percent of sale lots with some value-added procedures. In this work, 55% of sale lots had at least one vaccination in 1995 and 95% of all sale lots met this same criteria in 2005. However, expected health and performance for a set of unweaned calves with one vaccination are different than for a set of weaned animals with two vaccinations and adjusted to feeding conditions. Specific preconditioning program descriptions should adequately differentiate on the basis of the level of management, yet in many cases buyers view preconditioning as a binary (yes/no) descriptor. This binary view of the preconditioning state results in unrealistic expectations for some sets of calves that received relatively few preconditioning procedures.

Preconditioning programs are often categorized into levels based on specific procedures required. Further analysis of the data from King and Seeger[1] reveals that the largest increase in value-added participation was generated from increases in the percent of lots that were vaccinated, but not weaned (12.7% in 1995 to 49% in 2004) (Fig. 120-1). Sale lots of cattle that were weaned and immunized twice also increased during the period from 3.2% of lots in 1995 to 25.2% of lots in 2004. The majority of cattle sold in 2004 had at least one vaccination but were unweaned and presumably not acclimated to a feeding program consistent with a commercial feedyard. If unweaned calves are sold as preconditioned and perform poorly, they diminish the reputation of all preconditioned calves.

Variations in the specific protocols affect health and performance outcomes, yet when the animals are marketed in a similar manner, the predictability of the cattle described as preconditioned is decreased. Buyers discriminate between specific programs based on level of payment, yet independent worth of each procedure in the protocol is impossible to determine. If value capture from a preconditioned calf is based on product differentiation, each additional management procedure should provide an incremental decrease in disease risk for that group. Each feedyard should evaluate specific components of preconditioning programs and determine which techniques are most important to their management system.

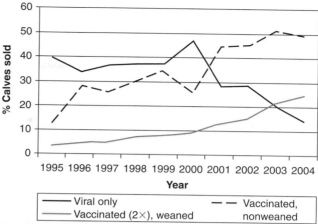

Fig 120-1　Superior Livestock Auction 10-year trend within value-added calves sold. (From King ME, Seeger JT: Ten-year trends at Superior Livestock Auction: calves in value-added health programs consistently receive higher prices, *Pfizer Anim Health Tech Bull,* 2005.)

COMPONENTS OF PRECONDITIONING PROGRAMS

Preconditioning programs have been promoted to improve feedlot performance, decrease morbidity and mortality, and improve profits. Well-controlled, large-scale, randomized trials evaluating the effects of preconditioning in the feedyard are scarce, and the ability of preconditioning programs to consistently provide an advantage has been questioned.[2,3] More research needs to be performed to evaluate preconditioning health and performance impact and to more specifically define relative importance of specific preconditioning management procedures. In lieu of definitive numbers, managers must still make decisions based on available information. One method is to evaluate individual components of the preconditioning program and compare relative worth.

Castration of male calves before shipment is one of the oldest and most straightforward methods of preconditioning. Bull calves castrated on feedyard arrival have higher morbidity and decreased performance relative to comparable steer mates. Pinchak and colleagues[4] recently described that castration at arrival resulted in a 13.5% reduction in daily gain and a significantly ($P < 0.05$) greater morbidity in bulls castrated after arrival (60%) than purchased steers (28%) during a backgrounding period. Gonadal status of male animals is easy to visually confirm and castrated males typically garner higher prices than comparable intact males.

Prevention of disease through proper immunizations is a mainstay of preconditioning protocols. Bovine respiratory disease complex (BRD) is the most common and economically important disease affecting cattle after weaning.[5] The total economic influence of this disease complex is even greater than the sum of treatment cost and death loss because of the impact on animal performance and carcass characteristics. The literature illustrates that when compared with nondiseased animals, BRD-affected calves have a lower rate of weight gain,[4,6,7] smaller carcass weights, and a decreased likelihood to grade U.S.D.A. Choice.[8,9]

In addition to calves identified and treated for illness, subclinical disease plays a role in economic loss associated with sickness. Wittum and colleagues[6] studied steers from birth to harvest and found that although only 35% of the animals were treated for respiratory disease, 72% of the population had pulmonary lesions at slaughter. The authors concluded that treatment of clinical disease may not prevent significant economic losses associated with the bovine respiratory disease complex. Therefore efforts should be concentrated on prevention of disease to minimize economic losses during the feeding phase.

Cattle may take 7 to 14 days postvaccination to stimulate immunity to infectious etiologic agents. Nonspecific immune responses may occur sooner, but in general the vaccination schedule should be completed at least 1 week before shipment or exposure to disease challenge. Killed vaccines require a booster and the booster immunization should be completed at least 7 to 14 days before disease challenge. Preconditioning programs assist immunization programs in a timely manner to generate immunity before disease exposure.

Fulton and colleagues[10] evaluated animal health status in 417 calves from 24 herds from feedyard arrival through harvest relative to individual farm vaccination schedules before arrival. The three herds with highest morbidity received killed viral vaccines without a booster or with a second dose given immediately before shipment. The herds with lowest morbidity used modified live viral vaccine and gave the second dose 3 weeks before arrival. Effective immunization must be performed in time for the animal to mount an appropriate response before challenge to confer health benefits to the animal.

Weaning on the cow-calf farm of origin for 30 to 45 days is a component of some preconditioning programs. Cattle in these systems face relatively low levels of disease challenge during the stressful period of maternal separation and tend to have comparatively low rates of illness. The feeder still faces disease risk after this phase, but it is decreased because of the removal of the weaning stress factor. In addition to health parameters, postweaning grazing or backgrounding periods influence subsequent animal performance. Sending calves directly from the cow-calf farm to the feedyard may be the most biologically efficient method of beef production.[11] Yet feedlot managers must consider the potential benefits to on-farm weaning and growing related to animal health and performance in the postweaning phase.

Preconditioning programs may also include a postweaning dietary acclimation period for the calves to allow adjustment to both ration and feeding behavioral changes. Most health problems occur soon after arrival to the feedyard, and adequate nutrition in the first weeks is critical to allow the animal to overcome stress and disease challenges. Low intakes in the arrival period are somewhat influenced by the fermentative and digestive capacity of the calves, but behavioral characteristics may be the most important factors that influence appetite.[12] Inclusion of a period allowing cattle to understand the procedure for eating from a bunk in a low-stress environment is a valuable component of a complete preconditioning program.

Feeder calf nutritional status is difficult to evaluate visually, but body condition is often used as a gauge of previous management. Preconditioning programs that incorporate weaning and feeding for a period of time may result in cattle with good flesh scores at the time of sale. Fleshy cattle may be viewed as healthier yet still garner a price discount because buyers will be unable to capture compensatory gains. The goal is to find a balance between healthy calves with adequate nutritional status and the potential for rapid, efficient weight gains.

Preconditioning programs based on a combination of castration, vaccination, weaning, and nutritional management can provide benefits to feedyards. In a study of heifers from a single ranch comparing preconditioned (modified-live vaccines and boosters, 45-day wean) and calves weaned at time of shipment, preconditioned animals had improved performance and feed efficiency.[13] Mortality in this research was dramatically different in preconditioned (1.3%) and nonpreconditioned (4.4%) calves. The medicine costs were also different with almost $30 per head higher costs for the nonpreconditioned calves. The preconditioned calves in this trial had an overall improvement in net return of $60 per head, illustrating a benefit to preconditioning. However, the trial design did not test which component was most important.

Preconditioning feeder calf programs represent the most comprehensive tool to prevent morbidity because they increase resistance to appropriate pathogens and reduce stress surrounding transport.[14] More research is necessary to evaluate the true worth of individual components of the preconditioning program and how response varies based on cattle type, seasonality, geographic region, and management style. Based on limited data, preconditioning using castration, weaning, and vaccinations appears to reduce animal health problems in the feeding phase. This reduction should translate into improved animal performance; the question for the manager is the economic return versus the input costs to procure preconditioned calves.

PURCHASING PRECONDITIONED CALVES

The potential value of purchasing preconditioned calves is improved performance, decreased health problems, and increased predictability. Capturing the value of these traits is based on placing the preconditioned calf in the appropriate management scheme. Specific benefits related to preconditioning cattle vary by feedyard based on the unique profit drivers, goals, facilities, and labor restraints of the operation.

Calves are an input into the feeding phase and the purchase price is influenced by expected expenses and animal performance. Purchasing preconditioned calves for the feedyard is a risk management tool to increase predictability of animal health and performance. The literature has defined relatively few traits that explain a large percentage of the variability in calf feedlot profitability. Schroeder and colleagues[15] evaluated data to find that variability in fed and feeder prices explained 70% to 80% of profit variability. Thus accurately estimating performance and generating a realistic breakeven purchase price is critical to help decrease uncertainty regarding economic outcomes. Purchase of preconditioned calves with expected lower health costs and more accurate breakeven values limits the feedyard's investment risk.

Buyers often expect to pay moderate premiums for preconditioned feeder calves, and the purchase decision shifts to comparing the expected performance increases versus the higher input costs associated with these calves. Based on limited data, the value of preconditioned calves in the feedyard appears to be between $40 and $75 per head greater than calves where vaccination, weaning, and other preconditioning procedures occur at feedyard arrival.[16,17]

In the literature regarding market valuation of preconditioned calves, it appears that buyers pay the minimum necessary amount to purchase preconditioned calves and this premium is less than the expected value of these calves.[18] The difference in payment price and expected value is logical based on the inherent risk associated with owning calves through the finishing phase. The risk is related to information regarding the expected versus actual performance of the calves and variability in animal health performance.

INCORPORATION OF PRECONDITIONED CALVES IN THE FEEDYARD

Purchasing calves with proper preweaning health programs can increase net returns in some feeding situations through better calf performance and decreased disease expenses. Preconditioning is a herd concept and cannot be applied effectively to individuals or sale lots within pens. Animals in feedlots are managed on a pen, or large group, basis. Uniformity of the management unit affects both health and nutritional recommendations. A subpopulation of animals within the pen that has been weaned and acclimated to feed may adjust to a feedlot ration more quickly, yet feeding decisions are made on a pen level. Therefore a subset of preconditioned calves within a pen does not capture the full benefit of preparation for the feeding program.

The goal of preconditioning is not to prevent illness in an individual animal but rather to minimize disease in the group. Collective resistance of the population must be greater than the expected disease challenge to prevent disease spread. In feedyards, herd immunity is gauged by the number of animals with effective immunity within a pen. Depending on the level of biosecurity, infectious diseases may spread between pens and contiguous pens could be viewed as a single herd. Vaccination of only 50% of cattle on arrival would not be efficient at eliminating disease outbreaks, and purchasing partial pens of preconditioned calves also reduces the value and predictability from prior management procedures.

All preconditioning programs are not equal and level of value added by specific practices is not adequately quantified in the literature. The ability to measure performance of preconditioned calves in a specific management system allows the feedyard to generate a breakeven purchase price for preconditioned calves.

The value of a preconditioning program may even change depending on season as the yard population changes. For example, consider a yard where decreased labor cost (because of expected lower illness rates) is the major benefit of preconditioned calves. The rewards may be greater during a busy season (such as the fall receiving period when labor is limited) than during a slow period when labor is more abundant.

SUMMARY

Calves entering the feeding phase are adjusting to nutritional and environmental changes, placing them at risk for diseases that negatively affect performance. The owner immediately before this transition is in a unique position to reduce these disease risk factors. Utilization of preventative immunization and health management programs can reduce the risk of disease, yet the producer may not receive adequate incentive in the current calf marketing system.

References

1. King ME, Seeger JT: Ten-year trends at Superior Livestock Auction: calves in value-added health programs consistently receive higher prices, *Pfizer Anim Health Tech Bull* 2005.
2. Pritchard RH, Mendez JK: Effects of preconditioning on pre- and post-shipment performance of feeder calves, *J Anim Sci* 68:28-34, 1990.
3. Cole NA: Preconditioning calves for the feedlot, *Vet Clin North Am Food Anim Pract* 1:401, 1985.
4. Pinchak WE, Tolleson DR, McCLoy M et al: Morbidity effects on productivity and profitability of stocker cattle grazing in the Southern Plains, *J Anim Sci* 82:2773-2779, 2004.
5. Smith RA: Impact of disease on feedlot performance: a review, *J Anim Sci* 76:272-274, 1998.
6. Wittum TE, Woollen NE, Perino LJ et al: Relationships among treatment for respiratory tract disease, pulmonary lesions evident at slaughter, and rate of weight gain in feedlot cattle, *J Am Vet Med Assoc* 209:814-818, 1996.
7. Thompson PN, Stone A, Schultheiss WA: Use of treatment records and lung lesion scoring to estimate the effect of respiratory disease on growth during early and late finishing periods in South African feedlot cattle, *J Anim Sci* 84:488-498, 2006.
8. Gardner BA, Dolezal HG, Bryant LK et al: Health of finishing steers: effects on performance, carcass traits, and meat tenderness, *J Anim Sci* 77:3168-3175, 1999.
9. Busby WD, Strohbehn DR: Effect of postweaning health on feedlot performance and quality grade, *Iowa State University Animal Industry Report 2004*, Ames.
10. Fulton RW, Cook BJ, Step DL et al: Evaluation of health status of calves and the impact on feedlot performance: assessment of a retained ownership program for postweaning calves, *Can J Vet Res* 66:173-180, 2002.
11. Williams CB, Bennett GL, Keele JW: Simulated influence of postweaning production system on performance of different biological types of cattle: III. Biological efficiency, *J Anim Sci* 73:686-698, 1995.
12. Loerch SC, Fluharty FL: Physiological changes and digestive capabilities of newly received feedlot cattle, *J Anim Sci* 77:1113-1119, 1999.
13. Cravey MD: Preconditioning effect on feedlot performance, *Proc Southwest Nutr Manage Conf 1996*.
14. Speer NC, Young C, Roeber DL: The importance of preventing bovine respiratory disease: a beef industry review, *Bov Pract* 35:189-196, 2001.

15. Schroeder TC, Albright ML, Langemeier MR et al: Factors affecting cattle feeding profitability, *J Am Soc Farm Man Rural Appras* 57:54-58, 1993.
16. Lalman DL, Ward CE: *Effects of preconditioning on health, performance and prices of weaned calves,* Salt Lake City, Utah, 2005, American Association of Bovine Practitioners.
17. Dhuyvetter KC: Preconditioning beef calves: are expected premiums sufficient to justify the practice? Honolulu, 2004, Western Agricultural Economics Association Annual Meeting.
18. Avent RK, Ward CE, Lalman DL: Market valuation of preconditioning feeder calves, *J Agr Appl Econ* 36:173-183, 2004.

CHAPTER 121

Low-Stress Livestock Handling

TOM NOFFSINGER and LYNN LOCATELLI

People can improve the level of animal welfare in cattle operations by learning, applying, and teaching low-stress handling methods. Currently, measures of morbidity and mortality are used to describe production successes of cattle class when in fact they should be assessed as an index of failure of cattle care. The speed at which a caretaker completes a task has overshadowed the emphasis of providing proper care to production animals. Expectations focus on "which animals are sick" and "which antibiotic regimen should be used." It is time to shift efforts from damage control to creating good health and performance. Shifting caregiver priorities from disease detection to performance enhancement results in new levels of cattle welfare and the appropriate realignment of animal husbandry.

Webster defines welfare as "health, happiness, and general well-being." We have a responsibility to provide cattle with physical comfort, disease protection, nutritional needs, and emotional stability. Little is truly understood about affecting the emotional stability of animals, and even less effort is placed on creating emotional stability. The human impact on the health and well-being of production animals is far more influential than most people realize. This concept is quite difficult to measure, so there is variable skepticism and belief in its truth. The cornerstone of low-stress cattle handling focuses on creating an emotionally strong animal that can thrive in the rigors of confinement and the modern production system. Veterinarians understand that physical and psychologic stress play important roles in cattle disease resistance and performance levels. Psychologic stress can become overwhelmingly negative, resulting in the inability of some animals to integrate into certain production systems. Psychologic stress can be dissipated by caregivers or amplified. Caregivers can be trained to realize that ALL human contact with cattle affects animal well-being and subsequent behavior. Because human impact shapes the subsequent behavior of the animals, caregivers can make future production events either more difficult or less difficult. Mutual trust, respect, and communication are necessary for a successful animal production. Cattle that are simply "petlike" are desensitized and not emotionally fit. Emotionally fit animals will work for their handlers, making production events a pleasure, not a challenge. With understanding of low-stress handling techniques, human contact can create a positive impact on health, performance, and cattle and human safety.

Veterinarians must improve their abilities to train caregivers to encourage cattle to communicate their true state of health. Cattle exhibit strong prey animal instincts. Prey animals have survived in nature, aware that predators select the lame, depressed, and weak to harvest. The natural behavior of many people trends toward predator tendencies. Proper low-stress handling allows veterinarians to override predator tendencies and convince cattle that caregivers can be looked to for guidance, trust, and understanding. If caregivers behave like predators, cattle will hide signs of depression and disease from these people as long as possible. Cattle are so proficient at hiding weakness that in many cases the pathology is too advanced for any treatment regimen to be effective. Understanding more about the inherent differences between cattle and people including visual, auditory, and sensory differences encourages handlers to override their predator tendencies. Understanding how to create successful interaction between cattle and people and developing mutual respect and communication enables a successful partnership, which also enables the early detection of disease.

Cattle are not a verbally based species. Therefore effective handlers are proficient at communicating with body language. Everyone has observed really good stockmen communicate effectively with cattle—without words, with subtle body movements, and without additional labor. These handlers exhibit a calm, confident demeanor and possess the ability to translate their body language into clear messages to the cattle. Body language is a melding of body position, angle, distance, timing, and pressure. Pressure is used as a motivator. The release of pressure is used as the trainer. Handlers that reward cattle motion with release of pressure can quickly train cattle, and in doing so create mutual respect and develop trust between themselves and the cattle.

Whenever cattle undergo a change of address, it is imperative that the new caregivers implement the process of acclimation. Animals whose surroundings and social fabric change are in a vulnerable state and are therefore quite impressionable. Cattle inherently learn quickly, so the process of acclimation can be accomplished with minimal time investment. This process dissipates stress, dissipates threat, develops trust, and establishes the basis of communication between the handlers and the animals. Caregivers effectively "read" the cattle and use proper body language to establish this foundation.

Understanding that cattle like to see what is pressuring them and like to see where they can go is fundamental to low-stress handling. Cattle that trust handlers volunteer to move away from handlers and will walk straight away and move as directed, in response to proper body language. Understanding low-stress handling techniques and being able to successfully communicate with cattle allows handlers to become comfortable in positions that may be counterintuitive and previously overlooked. This attitude of willingness has a positive effect on herd social interaction. Sensitive cattle are more content and timid cattle are more willing to compete for feed and water. The integration of exercise into confinement operations has shown tremendous benefit on the health, behavior, and performance of the confined animals. Handling opportunities become positive to cattle health and performance instead of a stress.

Focus on low-stress cattle handling encourages caregivers to engage their brains and further develop their observation skills, lessen tolerance for mild depression, and build diagnostic skills that refine therapy. Sources of depression include psychologic causes such as confinement anxiety, social disruption, feed and environmental unfamiliarity, as well as pathologic causes (i.e., infectious diseases of the respiratory, locomotive, and digestive systems). Understanding animal behavior in greater depth encourages us to look beyond pathologic reasons as the sole cause of depression or poor performance.

Caregivers can have a positive impact on cattle health and performance. Cattle are easily trained to respond to the release of pressure and become more willing to communicate their true state of health when they realize that handlers are not predators. Caregivers who concentrate on low-stress handling skills increase their powers of observation, recognize abnormal behavior and attitude, and develop the confidence and skill to manipulate behavior to improve levels of animal welfare.

CHAPTER 122

Biosecurity for Feedlot Enterprises

MIKE SANDERSON

The term *biosecurity* generally includes two components—preventing the introduction of new pathogens or toxins onto a feedyard and efforts to control spread of disease and/or intoxication within the yard. Specifically, biosecurity is concerned with preventing the introduction of pathogens or toxins that have the potential to damage the health or productivity of the cattle or the safety and quality of a food product. Biocontainment is a closely related concept and refers to efforts to control the spread of disease or intoxication within the yard. Biosecurity/Biocontainment programs in the broad sense may be efficiently integrated in a hazard analysis critical control point (HACCP)-like program to control food quality and safety and minimize antimicrobial use. Essentially the hazards for introduction or transmission are identified, and the critical control points to prevent or minimize that risk are implemented. In many cases implemented control points may not technically be "critical control points" because data proving their effectiveness in preventing disease introduction may be lacking. Practical controls may still need to be implemented, but recognition of this fact highlights specific research needs. Historically, production medicine programs have not emphasized biosecurity or preventing the introduction of disease into the herd except for encouraging vaccination programs. Biosecurity has become an increasingly important component of an integrated production management program, however.

Responsibility for biosecurity depends on the disease. For exotic diseases such as foot-and-mouth disease (FMD), contagious bovine pleuropneumonia, or rinderpest, government agencies have responsibility for establishing import procedures and guarding the national borders to prevent the introduction of disease. The individual producer is only responsible for obeying the import control regulations. Veterinarians in the field are the first line of defense in quickly recognizing a foreign animal disease and involving appropriate governmental agencies to investigate.

For endemic diseases with established eradication programs, veterinarians have responsibility for administration of the program and producers are responsible for adhering to the program rules. These may include testing and quarantine procedures to prevent transmission of the agent from one herd to another, as well as identification and removal of positive individuals or herds. For the feedyard enterprise, the most relevant example of an endemic agent with an eradication program is tuberculosis. For all other endemic diseases, responsibility for biosecurity lies largely with individual producers and is driven by the cost of disease and the cost and effectiveness of prevention plans. Producers must decide what procedures to implement to prevent disease introduction to their herd. The veterinarian is a critical resource for producers desiring to implement biologically and economically appropriate programs.

Biosecurity is a challenge for feedlot enterprises. Once at the feedyard, resident cattle generally do not have direct contact with neighboring cattle; however, wildlife and people with curious or nefarious motives may have access to the cattle. The large number of cattle confined in a relatively small space may also be attractive for individuals desiring to make a statement against production agriculture. Feedlot operations in the United States are generally carried out in a relatively unsecured premises where these risks may be difficult to control. Further, because of the large number of cattle imported onto the feedyard each year, exclusion of endemic diseases is, in general, not practical. Recognition of likely risks, practical controls, and good training of feedlot employees can result in a valuable biosecurity program. In each instance discussed, employee training and recognition of the importance of biosecurity procedures is critical to a successful biosecurity program.

BIOSECURITY—CONTROL OF DISEASE INTRODUCTION

Biosecurity and biocontainment programs for feedyards must account for accidental or natural, as well as intentional, introductions of both biologic and toxicologic agents. Accidental or natural introductions (hereafter referred to as *accidental*) include those that occur in the course of operation, either as the result of importing cattle to the lot or because of wildlife exposure or visitor exposure. A key determinant of accidental introduction is that there is no intent to introduce the agent or toxin to a specific feedyard. Intentional introductions include those where there is specific intent to introduce disease

or toxin to the specific feedyard. The security practices to control risk from each of these are different and are considered separately.

Intentional Introduction

Intentional introductions are the result of a harmful agent being purposefully introduced to a particular feedyard. This could be the work of a disgruntled neighbor, employee, or domestic or international terror group. The current encroachment of suburbia into areas near production agriculture has the potential to expose feedyards to substantial populations of people with little knowledge of, or support for, production agriculture. Terrorists include international groups but perhaps more significant domestic groups such as the People for the Ethical Treatment of Animals (PETA), the Animal Liberation Front (ALF), and the Earth Liberation Front (ELF). Intentional introductions could potentially include a foreign animal disease agent such as FMD or a ubiquitous endemic agent such as *Salmonella*. It seems more likely that a savvy terrorist, domestic or international, would introduce FMD into the beef cattle distribution system via salebarns rather than an individual feedyard. Alternately, a terrorist group could introduce the bovine spongiform encephalopathy agent into feed, followed by a public announcement that the feed had been contaminated. The claim could be real or spurious and still result in substantial effects related to public confidence and the potential need to destroy the supposedly exposed cattle. A potentially more likely intentional scenario is introduction of a toxicologic agent into feed or water. Though not a biosecurity matter per se, a general "rescue" or "liberation" of cattle within the yard could also occur. Which methods might be chosen could depend on the philosophy and goals of the organization (e.g., animal rights vs. saving the environment). Protection against intentional acts requires methods and procedures designed to prevent access by deception. Individuals and groups intending to harm will not announce their presence, so preventive techniques must be focused on preventing undisclosed access such as at night, through unsecured or unmonitored access points. As such, deterrents that prevent unauthorized human access such as a secure perimeter fence, entry gates that are locked when not in use and lighted at night, and a night watchman may be useful. Secure and lockable feed storage areas and water sources may also decrease risk. Any security that increases the barriers to an intentional introduction may make a feedyard a less attractive target and cause a potential terrorist to move on to another target. "Undercover" domestic terrorists could potentially gain access to the feedyard through employment and thus have increased access and opportunity for harm. Thorough checking of backgrounds, references, and experience should decrease the likelihood of this occurrence.

Accidental Introduction

Accidental introductions are the result of everyday activities of the feedyard including the import of cattle and feed and the arrival of employees, consultants, and visitors. Accidental introductions are not purposeful but are the inadvertent result of business practice. As such, their control depends on the recognition and control of everyday events that pose risk. Incoming cattle may bring disease to the feedyard. Because of the large number of cattle imported to the yard every year, this is a near certainty for ubiquitous endemic agents such as bovine viral diarrhea (BVD) and *Salmonella*. Testing may be a useful biosecurity intervention for identifying and excluding cattle persistently infected with BVD (PI-BVD). Test procedures for detection of PI-BVD cattle are sensitive, specific, and relatively inexpensive. Exclusion of PI-BVD cattle may improve overall pen morbidity rates.[1] In contrast, testing of incoming cattle for identification and exclusion of *Salmonella* carriers is likely not practical or effective. Similarly, although disease from *Mannheimia, Pasteurella,* infectious bovine rhinotracheitis, bovine respiratory synctial virus, and parainfluenza virus type 3 are important causes of morbidity and mortality, biosecurity efforts to exclude them are also not likely practical or effective. Visitors including consultants may introduce disease by coming on the yard with dirty boots or cloths. Visitors who are unaware of proper biosecurity procedures may be a particular risk for introduction if they step in feedbunks or walk in feed storage areas. There is potential for introduction of both *Salmonella* and FMD by this route.

Enteric agents such as *Salmonella* may be accidentally introduced to the yard by imported feedstuffs. Toxins could also be introduced to a feedyard accidentally in purchased feeds. Accidental toxin contamination at the feed mill or intentional contamination by a terrorist organization would allow for increased distribution and impact. This possibility highlights the need for feed suppliers to have an HACCP plan in place to prevent accidental or intentional contamination of feeds. Feedyards should preferentially work with feed suppliers that have an HACCP plan in place and should keep a frozen sample of purchased feedstuffs for later evaluation if needed.

For both ease of introduction and level of impact, FMD is the foreign animal disease most likely to be intentionally introduced to the United States. To maximize impact, it seems most likely that terrorists would introduce FMD into the livestock marketing system. Subsequent introduction of FMD to the feedyard would be an accidental introduction in the normal course of procuring and importing cattle. Livestock auction markets are congregation points for livestock including cattle, sheep, and hogs, which are subsequently sold and dispersed widely across the country. Introduction of FMD into the livestock marketing system could result in multiple simultaneous outbreaks across the country, maximizing impact. If this is true, then purchase of cattle from live auction markets may pose more risk of FMD introduction. This scenario is difficult for the individual feedyard to control because cattle might arrive at the feedyard healthy and develop FMD in 1 to 3 days. Purchase of auction market cattle from markets with good security systems to make introduction of a pathogen or toxin difficult may be prudent. Auction security systems may need to include a secure perimeter fence and night watchman to decrease the probability that livestock could be covertly exposed.

A valid health certificate should be required on all incoming cattle and they should be unloaded at the periphery of the feedyard and kept isolated at least until a health inspection can be performed. Ideally incoming cattle would remain isolated from the resident feedyard population for 1 week to assess health status. Individual cattle that arrive sick should be kept separate from the feedyard cattle population or sent back to the origin.

Traffic coming onto the yard poses a significant risk of introducing a pathogen. Traffic includes both foot traffic and vehicle traffic. All visitors, vendors, and consultants should check in at the feedyard office and sign into a log book. Ideally all service personnel and consultants would use feedyard vehicles for transportation around the feedyard. In general, visitors should not have contact with cattle or feed and should be supervised while on the feedyard to prevent driving or tracking into feed or cattle areas. Feed delivery trucks must contact feed storage areas and may be a risk for contamination that should be controlled. They visit other livestock operations and may arrive with contaminated tires, which may need to be washed before driving to the feed area. If a rendering company picks up "deads" at the yard, they should do so at the periphery of the yard to avoid driving through and contaminating cattle or traffic areas shared with other vehicles. Of particular importance would be avoiding common traffic patterns between renderers and feed delivery trucks.

BIOCONTAINMENT—CONTROL OF TRANSMISSION WITHIN THE YARD

Biocontainment programs for feedyards must also account for accidental and intentional introductions of both biologic and toxicologic agents, although once on the premises the methods are largely the same. Biocontainment on the feedyard is achieved by isolation and segregation, cleaning and disinfecting equipment and facilities, and controlling vehicle and foot traffic on the yard.

Isolation and Segregation

Segregation is the long-term physical separation of groups of cattle within herds and generally not practiced in feedyards. Isolation is the physical separation of individuals or groups to prevent disease transmission. It may be carried out by isolating incoming cattle from the resident population until an initial assessment of their health status can be made. This may be effective in controlling the exposure of resident cattle to incoming pathogens. Ideally incoming cattle would be unloaded in separate working facilities from the processing and hospital facilities for the yard and remain there for approximately 1 week to assess their health status. Isolation could also involve separation of sick cattle from the yard population in hospital pens away from healthy cattle. This pulling of sick cattle from healthy cattle may help decrease the number of infective cattle in a pen and blunt a disease outbreak, but it may also allow pathogen transmission within the hospital pens and subsequent dispersal around the feedyard. If hospital facilities are to be managed to assist biocontainment, care must be taken to ensure they are not a focus of disease transmission and dispersal. Managing contact between sick animals by sorting according to the region or alley of origin or maintaining multiple hospitals serving regions of the feedyard may be helpful in limiting the dispersal of infectious agents from the hospital system. Disinfection of treatment equipment is also an important method of maintaining isolation within the hospital as discussed later.

Cleaning and Disinfection

Cleaning and disinfection of facilities and equipment can break the cycle of transmission within livestock premises. Ideally, arrival and processing facilities should be cleaned and disinfected between common source groups of cattle. At times this may be difficult to achieve, but at least daily cleaning is prudent. Hospital facilities should be cleaned daily and oral treatment equipment should be cleaned and disinfected between each animal. This can be effectively accomplished by rinsing the equipment clean and then placing it in a bucket of disinfectant to soak between uses. The disinfectant should be changed regularly (at least daily) and anytime it is visibly contaminated with organic matter. Equipment should not be stored overnight in disinfectant solutions. Depending on the disinfectant, used equipment should be rinsed before reuse on cattle. Ideally, trucks and loaders that are used for moving manure or mortalities would never be used to handle feed. If they must be, they should be thoroughly washed and disinfected, focusing particularly on buckets, beds, and tires before reuse for feed.

Commercially available disinfectants are generally effective against a broad range of viruses and bacteria. They have variable effectiveness against bacterial spores and fungi. In general disinfectants do not work well in the presence of organic matter such as dirt, feces, and blood. For full effect they should be applied to clean surfaces and allowed 10 to 30 minutes of contact time. Product label directions should be checked for specific use recommendations. Information about disinfectants is available on the product label and from the U.S. Department of Agriculture, *Compendium of Veterinary Products*,[2] and extension bulletins.[3]

Traffic Control Within the Yard

Traffic within the yard is also a significant risk for disease transmission and should be controlled to minimize contamination of feed and cattle. Direct travel from high-risk areas (e.g., dead pile, hospital, or incoming cattle areas) to feed areas or healthy cattle areas should be prevented without cleaning and disinfection. Equipment used for handling deads or manure should not be used for feed handling or entering healthy cattle pens without thorough washing and disinfection. Traffic into silage pits or other feed storage areas should be strictly limited. Feed trucks should park outside the silage pit and be filled by a designated (or cleaned and disinfected) loader. No other vehicles should be allowed into the pit. Foot traffic should not track through feed storage areas or step in feedbunks. Animals including dogs, cats, birds, rats, mice, and flies are another source of potential transmission within the feedyard. They may be biologic carriers of disease agents or mechanically transmit it on their feet as they travel around the yard. Having a bird, rodent, and fly control program, as well as limiting access of cats and dogs to the feedyard, is prudent.

SUMMARY

The tools of biosecurity and biocontainment are not new. They require a clear understanding of the transmission of infectious agents in feedlot production systems but also of the risks and likely methods for intentional acts against the feedlot. The implementation of specific management practices to control this risk is different for each feedlot based on its particular situation. No one is more suited than the practicing veterinarian to identify the hazards and their likelihood and potential impact on the feedlot and then implement this into a cost-effective security program. In some cases some level of risk analysis or decision analysis may be helpful to assist in identifying optimal security practices. Veterinarians can seek this training for themselves or seek out assistance when necessary.

References

1. Loneragan GH, Thomson DU, Montgomery DL et al: Prevalence, outcome and health consequences associated with persistent infection with bovine viral diarrhea virus in feedlot cattle, *J Am Vet Med Assoc* 226:595-601, 2005.
2. Anonymous: 2004 *Compendium of veterinary products*, Bayer Animal Health.
3. Kennedy J, Bek J, Griffin D: Selection and use of disinfectants, *NebGuide University of Nebraska Extension Bulletin G1410*, 2000.

CHAPTER 123

Use of Statistical Process Control in Feedlot Practice

ROBERT L. LARSON and BRAD J. WHITE

Statistical process control (SPC) was developed by Dr. Walter A. Shewhart while working in the Bell Telephone Laboratories starting in 1918.[1] Shewhart developed SPC methods for the purpose of improving quality and reducing costs in manufacturing settings by accounting for the variation that exists within any process. Shewhart looked at variability as being either within the limits set by chance or outside those limits. If it was outside the limits set by chance, he believed that the source of the variability could be identified and potentially managed. Shewhart taught that data contains both signals and noise.[2-4] Noise variation is due to usual day-to-day fluctuations in process output, whereas signals are due to special causes such as changes in the material, people, equipment, or method in which the process was performed.[5] To be able to extract information, one must be able to separate a signal from the noise within the data.[2-4] Process control charts are one of the main tools of statistical process control. A control chart is a graphical representation of the process output over time and displays the amount of noise inherent in the system (which does not need to be investigated) and can display a signal if present (which does need to be investigated). During the 1990s, Shewhart's work was repackaged and promoted as the "Six Sigma" approach to business and manufacturing management.

The goal of using process control charts is to make real-time decisions about an ongoing production process. Other statistical tools are more appropriate when looking at data retrospectively. For feedlot managers and veterinarians to use process control charts properly, the information gleaned from the feedyard data should be used to make immediate decisions to change the production process for the population that generated the data. Feedyard health and production data are different than most data used in manufacturing environments that use process control charts. In manufacturing, data measured is directly related to a change that can be made in the process. For example, if a process control chart indicates that the length of a manufactured rod is too long and outside the length variation inherent in the system, the action to correct rod length is most likely directly related to measuring and cutting. In contrast, most feedyard production and health data does not indicate a direct action. For example, if feed efficiency is found to be poorer than can be explained by the variation inherent in the feedyard system, there is no direct action a decision maker can make to immediately correct the signal.

In addition to the lack of direct correlation between measured feedyard production and health data and desired outcomes, current feedyard data reflect a great deal of complexity (lack of standardization) and variation that is translated as wide control limits, making it difficult to detect a signal. Despite these limitations, the key concept of statistical process control that both signals and noise cause variation in data is applicable to feedlot production and data evaluation. Understanding these two causes of variation in cattle feeding should influence the type of strategies used by veterinarians and managers to reduce variation or improve performance of feedyard production systems.

DATA DISTRIBUTION

One of the foundational tenets of feedlot management is to realize that all processes (e.g., feed manufacturing, animal growth, animal health, economic return, human behavior) result in a distribution rather than a single level of output[6] (Fig. 123-1). Even if every aspect of production is managed so that inputs are precisely defined, employees are fully trained, the environment is constant, and all equipment is perfectly designed and maintained, the output will not all be identical. Many feedlot outputs have a normal (bell-shaped curve) distribution, meaning that the output is symmetrical around the mean (half of the output is above the mean and half of the output is below the mean). The mean is also called the *average* and is calculated by adding all the observations and dividing by the number of observations. Other outputs may be skewed (greater than half of the output is either above or below the mean).

Standard deviation is a mathematical depiction of the amount of variation in the output of interest.[7] If the standard deviation is small, each individual output measurement is similar to the mean of all the output measurements. If the standard deviation is large, any individual measurement may be different (higher or lower) than the mean of all the measurements. Regardless of the amount of variation in the output, in a normal distribution, roughly 68% of all the output falls within one standard deviation of the mean, 95% fall within two standard deviations of the mean, and 99.7% fall within three standard deviations of the mean. With skewed output, the percentage of data that falls within a given standard deviation to the mean is not grossly dissimilar from a normal distribution.

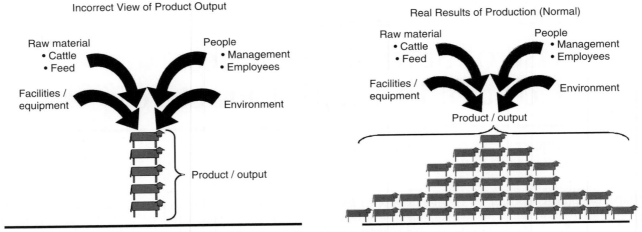

Fig 123-1   Incorrect and actual depictions of product output.

When managing any process, one must understand the expected distribution in output and be able to identify when the current output is within or outside the expected outcome. In controlled experimental situations, the goal is determining whether or not a sample or group of samples fall outside the expected distribution (the control), and this evaluation takes place with a statistical test after all the data have been collected; in contrast, in feedlot production settings, the job of a manager or consultant is to determine whether or not the data one sees today is within the expected distribution and to make an accurate and timely decision whether or not to take action.

PROCESS CONTROL CHARTS

A process control chart is a line graph used to study a process by plotting data in time order, with time on the x-axis. A control chart always has three lines that are determined by historical data: a central line (usually mean or median), an upper line for the upper control limit, and a lower line for the lower control limit. The control limits are always set at a distance of three sigma units on either side of the central line, and sigma can be determined using an estimate of the dispersion parameter of a homogenous set of data (i.e., standard deviation).[8] It is common to wait until several data points are available before calculating control limits, but when limited amounts of data are available, one may calculate control limits with whatever data are available.[9] The plotted points are usually averages of subgroups (when plotted on a chart depicting the center of the output) or ranges of variation between subgroups (when plotted on a chart depicting the distribution of the output) but can be individual measurements. Different types of control charts are used for different types of data. The two broadest groups are for variable data and attribute data.[10] Variable data such as weight, time, or temperature are measured on a continuous scale. Control charts for variable data are used in pairs with one chart monitoring the average, or centering of the distribution, and the other chart monitoring the range, or width of the distribution. Some common variable charts include averages and range charts (X and R charts) and cumulative sum charts (CUSUM charts). Attribute data are counts such as

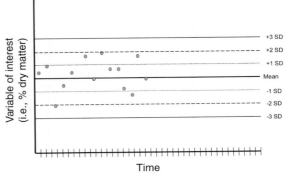

Fig 123-2   Process control chart.

when determining the presence or absence of something (i.e., treatment success or failure, dead or alive). Control charts for attribute data depict the center of the output and include proportion charts (p charts), count charts (c charts), and np charts.

By the 68%, 95%, 99.7% rule, it is clear that almost all of the output values should fall within three standard deviations of the mean if a process is stable. Lines representing the third sigma unit are the "control limits" (Fig. 123-2). Data that fall within the control limits will vary around the mean, but the variation is expected even if the process has not changed and is considered noise. A process that operates with only noise is described as "in control." In contrast, any output outside the control limits is an immediate signal that the production process has changed and if the change is negative, the signal should be investigated. A process that displays a signal is described as "out of control."

The three sigma upper and lower control limits are used to determine if a single measurement indicates that a signal is occurring. Three other indicators, which use multiple measurements, are also used to determine the presence of a signal; the first is if two of three consecutive points fall between two and three standard deviations on the same side of the mean. In other words, the chances that two out of three consecutive measurements would fall that far into the tail of a bell-shaped curve by chance is small. More likely, the mean or distribution of

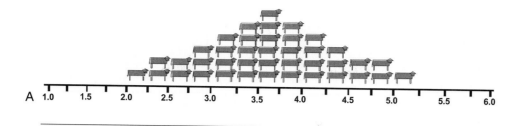

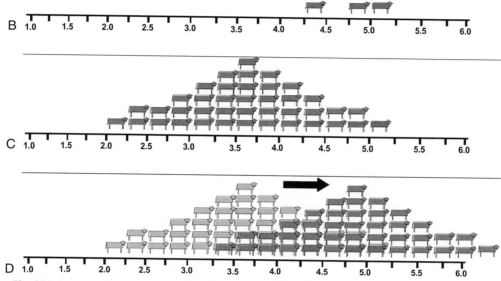

Fig 123-3 If the historical output (mean and distribution) of a variable is known **(A)** and then two out of three consecutive measurements fall more than two standard deviations from the mean of that historical output **(B)**, it would be unlikely that an interpretation that the output had stayed the same **(C)** is true. More likely, the output had changed **(D)** (i.e., a signal).

the bell-shaped curve changed (i.e., a signal that the system changed) (Fig. 123-3). The other signals are four of five consecutive points falling between one and two standard deviations on the same side of the mean, and eight consecutive points falling on the same side of the mean[10] (Fig. 123-4). Using these rules for detecting a signal, process control charts will, over time, assess any process's variation.[2,10]

TWO CAUSES OF VARIATION—NOISE AND SIGNALS

Noise stays the same from day to day and produces output over a long period that falls inside the control limits of the process.[10,11] If all the output falls within the control limits over a long period of time, one can assume that all the variation found is just noise. Examples of noise include variation among cattle; normal weather variation; employee turnover; quality of employee training; facilities (e.g., amount of shade, dust); accuracy of ration measuring and mixing; and level of biosecurity. Many of the causes of noise are completely under the responsibility and control of management, but some noise variability is

inherent to biology. To noticeably reduce the amount of noise, management must control causes of variation that occur day to day and affect most or all groups, rather than specific causes of variation that only affect a few groups. Reducing noise usually involves increasing standardization of the animals, environment, and/or processes of the feeding system.

A signal indicates that something unusual has occurred. Previous performance is not able to predict the current or future performance of a process if a signal is present. The first time a signal is present may not cause enough variation to be detected with a process control chart, particularly if the control limits are wide (large standard deviation), indicating a great deal of noise. However, if a signal is present over time, the process control chart will eventually indicate a change has occurred in the process. Causes of a negative signal could include a malicious employee; a toxicologic event; a natural disaster (e.g., lightning, flood); a ration error; or a particularly virulent or novel infectious agent. A signal is one not typically found in the process and needs to be investigated. Signals can be divided into two different groups, transient signals and persistent signals. Transient signals are those signals that

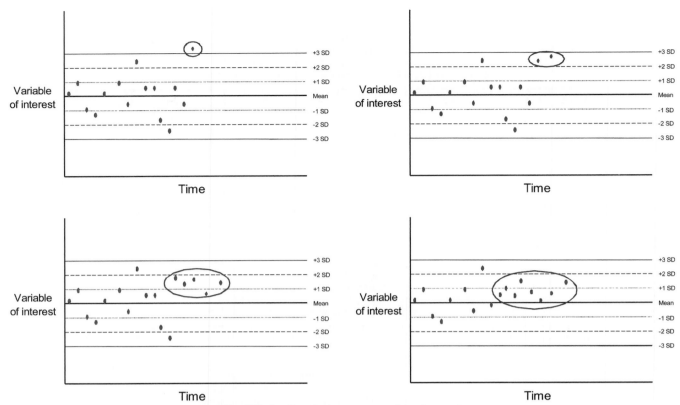

Fig 123-4   Signals that a process has changed.

affect a process for a short time, disappear, and then may reappear at a later time. Persistent signals are those signals that stay in the process until they are detected and removed. If a signal can be addressed with a management intervention, a cost-benefit analysis should be done.

When called to a feedlot to investigate any problem that is perceived by the client to warrant a veterinarian's attention, one's thought process should first be focused on determining if the output in question is noise or a signal (outside the control limits if you constructed a control chart). If the veterinarian determines that in fact the current problem is a signal, he or she should focus on the cause of this particular problem and not be concerned with the mean and dispersion of the feedlot's output over time. In contrast, if the veterinarian determines that the current problem is within the noise of the feedlot (albeit perceived as unusually negative by the client) but does point out that the variation on this feedlot is too great or the mean performance needs improvement, he or she should further investigate the root cause of the unacceptability of the current situation. Is it due to an unacceptable mean, an unacceptable distribution around the mean, or both? In these cases, the specific output that caused the client to call a veterinarian is not more important than the mean and distribution of many instances of the output over time and should not be investigated as a single-point-in-time problem.

The same cause of variation may be classified as noise on one feedlot with a great deal of variability but a signal on another feedlot with more standardization to reduce complexity and variation. An example could be percent morbidity on a pen basis. On a feedlot that feeds only low-risk yearlings and manages for high health, procurement and arrival management is developed to support low morbidity and ensure high correlation between the expected and actual morbidity. In this case, pen morbidity would only affect the feedlot in exceptional situations such as severe weather or a highly pathogenic infectious agent. On a feedlot that feeds high-risk calves, the fluctuation in percent morbidity by pen is wide and some pens with high morbidity are part of the normal process.

In this example, percent morbidity is a signal on the low-risk yearling feedlot that has little day-to-day fluctuation, but it is noise on the feedlot feeding high-risk calves. Because the classification of percent morbidity as a source of variation is different between the two feedlots, the veterinary response to the two feedlots should be different. Additional management of day-to-day health on the yearling feedyard may not be warranted or economically rewarded, but addressing a morbidity signal and then returning to the previous management is likely to be beneficial. In contrast, failing to address the entire management strategy on the feedlot feeding high-risk calves will fail to significantly change the amount of variation in percent morbidity. If the veterinarian investigates the noise of percent morbidity on the second feedyard as if it were a signal, he or she will focus on a single output and will not succeed in reducing variation or changing the mean.

Two mistakes are possible when investigating causes of variation. The first mistake is to react to an outcome as if it came from a signal, when it actually came from

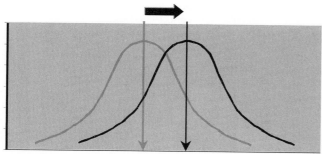

Fig 123-5   Improving a process by management changes that affect all groups equally results in a more optimum mean, but the distribution is unchanged.

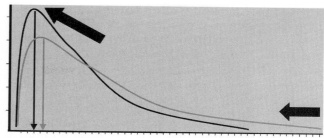

Fig 123-6   Improving a process by management changes that only affect poor-performing groups results in a more optimum mean and a narrower distribution.

noise. This often results in tampering with the system without making improvements in the output. The other possible mistake is to treat an outcome as if it came from noise, when actually it came from a signal. Either mistake causes loss. By taking one or the other extreme responses to data variation, one could consistently avoid either mistake, but not both (it is impossible to reduce both mistakes to zero). The best that we can do is to make each type of mistake occasionally, following rules that over the long run minimize the net economic loss from both mistakes.

IMPROVING THE SYSTEM

If signals are occurring in a feedlot, those causes of variation must be investigated and, if likely to reoccur, be resolved. Once a feedlot is stable (no indication over time of the existence of signals), management must decide if the current mean or level of noise of an output has an acceptable effect on the profitability or other goal of the feedlot. If it is, the process is stable and should be monitored to keep it that way. In contrast, if improvement is possible and desirable, changes in management must be initiated to reduce variation or move the mean.

Some management interventions will affect all groups equally. If this is the situation, the mean is changed but range is unchanged (Fig. 123-5). Examples are improved nutrition, more accurate micro-ingredient inclusion, and improved animal husbandry because of better employee training and performance.

In contrast, if a management intervention only affects some groups of cattle (i.e., poor performers), the variation is reduced because the tail of the distribution is removed. The mean is improved because fewer poor performers are present to pull the mean away from optimum (Fig. 123-6). Examples of management changes that only affect some individuals or groups are improved facilities and improved vaccination and other disease prevention strategies. Improved facilities only affect some groups because environmental affecters such as heat stress, windchill, or mud are not present at all times nor do they affect all groups equally; therefore improved facilities that would minimize these negative environmental situations would only benefit some groups of cattle. Similarly, because many groups of cattle under current management have low morbidity and mortality, management changes to improve disease

prevention only have the opportunity to affect those groups with morbidity and mortality present.

USE OF PROCESS CONTROL CHARTS IN FEEDLOTS

Statistical process control charts are used extensively in both manufacturing and service industries, and they are being adapted for use in dairy and swine production to monitor health, reproduction, and serologic indices.[5,12-15] Once established, control charts are easy to use by laborers, managers, and consultants. Software to create process control charts is readily available. In U.S. feedlots, process control charts are being used in areas such as feed mills, where standardized inputs and direct correlation between measurements and actions make process control charts easily applicable, but challenges limit their use for health and performance monitoring.

Process control charts are most commonly used when the data measured are directly related to a change that can be made in the production process. For example, if a feed mill is supposed to produce a feed with a certain dry matter or particle size and a process control chart signals that the percent moisture or particle size is changing, one of only a few direct actions can be applied to the system to restore a stable production system. In contrast, if feedlot data such as morbidity percent, mortality percent, average daily gain, or feed efficiency indicate a potential signal, a specific action is not obvious. The complexity of factors affecting morbidity, mortality, average daily gain, and feed efficiency does not allow one to directly translate a signal into an action that will lower morbidity or mortality or improve average daily gain or feed efficiency. Veterinary, nutritional, and management expertise are required to make sense of the complexity of feedlot production when statistical process control methods fail.

A conceptual foundation of control charts is homogenous subgroups where the variation within subgroups is a logical and proper yardstick for setting limits on the variation between groups.[8] Because of the lack of homogeneity within and between pens of cattle based on age, days on feed, genetics, and prior management, this foundation is currently lacking in U.S. feedlots. Current feedlot information systems for health, gain, and efficiency measures that could generate data for process control charts do not adequately capture the complexity of feedlot production, resulting in difficult or inconsistent interpretation of the system using that data. Swine and dairy producers have decreased the complexity of their systems so that available information systems can capture more of the remaining complexity; therefore process control charts have gained quicker adoption in these animal industries.

Despite these challenges, feedlot consultants and managers should look for opportunities to develop and test process control charts as a method to monitor certain production processes within feedlot production. In addition, the key statistical process control concepts of understanding the difference between signals and noise as causes of variation in feedlot data, as well as the differing response to an unusual event versus a response to a stable process with an unacceptable variation or average outcome, are applicable and valuable as feedlot veterinarians intervene to improve health and productivity.

SUMMARY

Improving the success of any feedlot involves having a method to accurately evaluate the production process and a mechanism to continually remove barriers to efficiency and quality. Statistical process control is a set of tools used by many industries to harness the power of statistical evaluation of processes to improve quality and reduce total cost. Statistical process control has led many companies to concurrently improve quality, efficiency, and performance. These tools and principles can be used by feedlots to improve the quality and efficiency of beef production.

References

1. *Walter A. Shewhart*, Wikipedia online encyclopedia (website): http://en.wikipedia.org/wiki/Walter_A._Shewhart. Accessed July 31, 2006.
2. Shewhart WA: *Economic control of quality of manufactured product*, New York, 1931, D Van Nostrand.
3. Shewhart WA: *Statistical method from the viewpoint of quality control*, Mineola, New York, 1939, Dover Publications.
4. Wheeler DJ: *Understanding variation: the key to managing chaos*, ed 2, Knoxville, Tenn, 2000, SPC Press.
5. Lukas JM, Hawkins DM, Kinsel ML et al: Bulk tank somatic cell counts analyzed by statistical process control tools to identify and monitor subclinical mastitis incidence, *J Dairy Sci* 88:3944-3952, 2005.
6. Scherkenbach WW: *Deming's road to continual improvement*, Knoxville, Tenn, 1991, SPC Press.
7. Petrie A, Watson P: *Statistics for veterinary and animal science*, Oxford, England, 1999, Blackwell Science.
8. Wheeler DJ: *Advanced topics in statistical process control. The power of Shewhart's charts*, Knoxville, Tenn, 1995, SPC Press.
9. Wheeler DJ, Chambers DS: Understanding statistical process control, ed 2, Knoxville, Tenn, 1992, SPC Press.
10. Tague NR: The quality toolbox, ed 2, Milwaukee, Wis, 2005, ASQ Quality Press.
11. Deming WE: *Out of the crisis*, Cambridge, Mass, 1986, MIT Press.
12. de Vries A, Conlin BJ: Design and performance of statistical process control charts applied to estrous detection efficiency, *J Dairy Sci* 86:1970-1984, 2003.
13. Niza-Ribeiro J, Noordhuizen JPTM, Menezes JC: Capability index: a statistical process control tool to aid in udder health control in dairy herds, *J Dairy Sci* 87:2459-2467, 2004.
14. Rademacher C: Use of statistical process control in finishing records, *J Swine Health Prod* 12:158-159, 2004.
15. Baum DH, Ward S, Baum CL et al: Statistical process control methods used to evaluate the serologic responses of pigs infected with three *Salmonella* serovars, *J Swine Health Prod* 13:304-313, 2005.

CHAPTER **124**

Growth Promotants for Beef Production: Anabolic Steroids: Performance Responses and Mode of Action

BRADLEY J. JOHNSON and CHRISTOPHER D. REINHARDT

Although discussed in the third and fourth editions of this book, the dynamic nature of growth promoting technology deems this topic worthy of continued study. Changes in the economic and political environment of animal production require that professionals within the industry stay attuned to subtle changes in how products may be used to benefit producers, and how those products may be perceived by those outside the industry.

HISTORY OF ANABOLIC STEROID USE AND PRODUCT SAFETY

The age of anabolic growth promotant use in the cattle industry dawned with the published observations by Dinusson and coworkers,[1] who, in 1948, presented their findings of increased rate and efficiency of gain of heifers implanted with diethylstilbestrol (DES) versus their nontreated counterparts. Burroughs and others[2,3] later reported that feeding DES to steers also improved rate and efficiency of gain. U.S. Food and Drug Administration (FDA) approval of DES was obtained in 1954. Following DES approval and 18 years of successful implementation by the cattle feeding industry, both as an implant and a feed additive, the FDA was forced to reevaluate the approval of DES. The Delaney Amendment of 1958 precluded the use of known carcinogens in the production of food animals. In 1971 a link was formed between adenocarcinoma in female offspring of women who took exceptionally high doses of DES[4] during pregnancy, and Cole and colleagues[5] reported that DES caused carcinoma in rats that were genetically predisposed to cancer. Thus after years of deliberation, DES was finally withdrawn in 1979.[6] Other anabolic growth promotants were subsequently approved by the FDA for use in feedlot and pasture cattle (Table 124-1). All of the listed growth promotants other than DES remain approved for use as of this writing. Because of the great furor surrounding withdrawal of DES approval, subsequent product approvals have been subject to much greater scrutiny to prevent similar controversy.

Although much discussion still surrounds the human health implications of anabolic steroid use in cattle, hard scientific data on the subject is nearly unequivocal. The estrogen content of beef implanted using currently available technology, although fractionally higher than nonimplanted beef, is actually two to three orders of magnitude lower in estrogenic activity than nonmeat items such as dairy foods, peas, or cabbage.[7] Biologic systems, both animal and vegetable, require, produce, and contain biologically active compounds. Their consumption is unavoidable.

MODE OF ACTION OF ANABOLIC STEROIDS[8-13]

Classification of Compounds

Steroid hormones commonly used in beef production can be categorized as estrogenic, androgenic, or progestinic in nature. Typically, used compounds may also be

Table **124-1**

Chronologic Sequence of Growth Promotant Approval by U.S. Food and Drug Administration (FDA)

Growth Promotant	Year of FDA Approval
Oral diethylstilbestrol (DES)	1954
DES implant	1955
Estradiol benzoate/progesterone (steers)	1956
Estradiol benzoate/testosterone propionate (heifers)	1958
Oral melengestrol acetate (heifers)	1968
Zeranol (36 mg) implants (cattle)	1969
Silastic estradiol implant (cattle)	1982
Estradiol benzoate/progesterone (calves)	1984
Trenbolone acetate (TBA) implants (cattle)	1987
Estradiol (17-β)/TBA implants (steers)	1991
Bovine somatotropin (lactating dairy cows)	1993
Estradiol (17-β)/TBA implants (heifers)	1994
Zeranol (72 mg) implants (cattle)	1995
Estradiol (17-β)/TBA implants (stocker cattle)	1996
Ractopamine (cattle)	2004
Zilpaterol (cattle)	2006

From Raun AP, Preston RL: *J Anim Sci* 2002 (website): http://www.asas.org/Bios/Raunhist.pdf. Accessed November 28, 2006.

Table 124-2

Naturally Occurring and Synthetic Forms of Steroid Hormones

	Naturally Occurring	Synthetic
Estrogens	Estradiol	Zeranol
Androgens	Testosterone	Trenbolone
Progestins	Progesterone	Melengestrol acetate

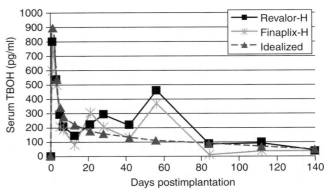

Fig 124-1   Serum trenbolone (TBOH) concentration following implantation. (Modified from Henricks DM, Edwards RL, Champe KA et al: *J Anim Sci* 55:1048-1056.)

classified as synthetic or naturally occurring (Table 124-2). Estradiol is administered either as E_2 or, alternatively, as estradiol benzoate (71% estradiol). Trenbolone (TBOH) is originally manufactured as trenbolone acetate (TBA; 80% trenbolone). Testosterone is primarily produced as testosterone propionate.

Within steroid classes, there are differences in the biologic activity of individual compounds. For example, estradiol is more potent than zeranol, which simply means that a greater dose of zeranol is required to produce a similar anabolic response when compared with estradiol. For this reason, zeranol-containing implants have a greater dosage of active compound than do estradiol-containing implants. Secondarily, zeranol is also less estrogenic than estradiol. Testosterone is much less potent than trenbolone but only slightly less androgenic. Various implants used in heifers contain testosterone; however, TBA is more economical and is used in a greater variety of products. Another major factor that may affect potency for growth promotion is that trenbolone is not converted to estradiol as is testosterone.

Delivery to Target Cell Types

It can be expected that circulating levels of implanted hormones will decrease over time as the implant is depleted.[14] With this reduction in circulating hormones over time comes a concomitant reduction in feedlot performance as days on feed advances. This suggests that a certain level of circulating anabolic steroid is required to maintain optimal performance and that the potential to observe biologic responses caused by anabolic steroids should be predicted from postimplantation levels of circulating E_2 or TBOH.[15] Circulating E_2 levels indicate a burst effect for about 30 days followed by decreasing E_2 levels.[16] Implantation of E_2 alone results in this burst effect for 30 days and a decrease to baseline levels by 60 days.[10] Heitzman and colleagues[17] suggested that if TBA is implanted in combination with E_2, the circulating E_2 levels can be maintained for approximately 100 days. However, implantation with E_2 alone resulted in baseline E_2 levels after 60 days postimplantation. Hayden and colleagues[15] observed similar patterns with E_2 delivery; E_2 implants elevated circulating E_2 for the first 31 days, but between the period of 31 days and 72 days the E_2 levels began to decline. The authors also noted that TBOH was not beneficial in maintaining E_2 levels as seen previously by Heitzman and colleagues.[17]

Hancock and colleagues[18] reported that infused E_2 has a short half-life of 7.7 minutes in the fast pool and a longer half-life of 41.5 minutes in the slow pool. Therefore once E_2 enters the circulation, it is cleared rapidly. The increased circulating E_2 level observed following implantation is most likely a result of release rate from the implant rather than slow clearance rate from plasma.[18] However, the animal must have a mechanism for compensating for increased E_2 concentrations. Moran and colleagues[19] reported no significant differences in circulating E_2 (13.1 pg/ml vs. 16.8 pg/ml) in heifers implanted with either one or two E_2 implants. Circulating TBOH levels follow similar patterns after implantation compared with E_2. Henricks and colleagues[20] reported that on the day following implantation, plasma TBOH rose to greater than 900 pg/ml in heifers implanted with 300 mg TBA. The circulating levels gradually decreased to 400 pg/ml on day 90 postimplantation (Fig. 124-1). MacVinish and Gaibraith[21] found that TBOH levels peaked between weeks 1 and 3 in lambs implanted with 35 mg TBA and 5 mg of E_2. In bulls, Istasse and colleagues[22] reported that TBOH increased to about 1000 pg/ml and was sustained at that level until week 8 and then began to decline until week 11 when the bulls were reimplanted and the circulating TBOH levels were again elevated.

Administration of E_2 simultaneously with TBA has been shown to affect circulating TBOH levels compared with animals implanted with TBA alone. Hunt and colleagues[23] observed that serum TBOH was greater than 1000 pg/ml in steers implanted with TBA alone. However, in steers implanted with TBA/E_2 the serum TBOH was approximately 550 pg/ml, or almost half the concentration of steers receiving TBA alone. In contrast, Istasse and colleagues[22] found that plasma concentrations of TBOH tended to be higher with higher doses of E_2. Bulls implanted with 200 mg TBA + 60 mg E_2 had 964 pg/ml compared with 844 pg/ml in bulls implanted with 200 mg TBA + 40 mg E_2. Similarly, Hayden and colleagues[15] reported that TBOH levels in TBA/E_2 implanted steers were twice as high as those in steers implanted with TBA alone (1672 pg/ml vs. 652 pg/ml). The authors suggested that this may be because of E_2 competition with hepatic TBOH metabolism. In addition, the half-life of one steroid is often influenced by simultaneous administration of another steroid.[24]

Previous studies have shown that the combined administration of TBA/E$_2$ can have interactive effects on payout from the implant, which in turn can result in different circulating levels of the steroid postimplantation. In addition, these changes in circulating steroid concentrations then in turn could affect clearance rate of the individual steroid and major metabolites of these steroids. Previous plasma kinetic studies have revealed that hydrolysis of a single IV injection of radiolabeled TBA to the alcohol derivative, TBOH, was extremely rapid.[14] Trenbolone was estimated to have a half-life of 1.5 hours following a single IV injection.[14] These authors followed up their initial study, which used only a single dose of TBA with an experiment describing plasma kinetics following administration of an ear implant containing radiolabeled TBA. The half-life of radiolabeled TBA in the implant was estimated between 68 and 84 days.[14] The authors reported that the majority of steroid was excreted in the bile and urine with only traces excreted in milk from a lactating cow. Total radioactivity recovered at slaughter indicated approximately two thirds of activity was in the bile fraction and one third in the urine component. In agreement with these findings, another study reported that in beef calves implanted with TBA and tritiated E$_2$ (^{3}H) for 100 days, nearly 100% of the steroid could be accounted for in accumulated excretion from feces and urine.[25] Furthermore, approximately two thirds of accumulated excretion over the 100-day period was in the feces (bile) and one third in urine.[25]

Circulating hormone concentrations are not valid for assessment of duration of implant product payout and such values are often misinterpreted. The circulating level is a function of the difference between two rates: the rate at which compound enters the animal's bloodstream and the rate at which it is cleared, by the liver or kidneys, rather than simply payout from the implant. The minimum effective concentration is not known for all animal types and production situations, so assessing the concentration in the blood does not provide sufficient information to assess the function of the implant. Performance and circulating steroid concentration are not highly correlated. The correlation between weight gain and serum TBOH concentration has been reported to be no greater than 0.29. Other studies have reported little to no relationship between circulating steroid hormone levels and rate and efficiency of gain in animals treated with steroid hormones. In growing bulls, circulating steroid concentration had little correlation to growth rate.

Receptor-Mediated Genomic Steroid Actions

Receptors for estrogens, androgens, and progestogens are located in most cell types but in vastly different proportions. The concentration and binding affinity of these receptors affects the ability of the steroid to elicit a response in that cell type.

Steroid hormone receptor proteins act as transcription factors. These receptors recognize specific cis-acting DNA sequences referred to as *hormone response elements* (HRE) on target genes. The HREs are located on the 5' promoter region of hormone-responsive genes. A general schematic of classical genomic steroid action follows.

- Steroid hormones, which are lipophilic, gain entry into a target cell by simple diffusion.
- Receptors are often associated with other cytosolic proteins such as chaperone and heat-shock proteins that help stabilize the receptor.
- Once the steroid binds to the receptor, these heat-shock proteins dissociate.
- The above transformation results in increased affinity of the receptor for the HRE.
- Some receptors are found in the cytosol and translocate to the nucleus after ligand binding (glucocorticoid and mineralocorticoid receptors), whereas others (estrogen, androgen, and progesterone receptors) are located in the nuclear region.
- Following ligand binding, the ligand-receptor complex binds to palindromic DNA sequences in the promoter regions of hormone-responsive genes.
- Binding of the ligand-activated receptor to HRE on hormone-responsive genes either initiates and upregulates transcription or can cause a down-regulation of transcription.

Receptor-Mediated Nongenomic Steroid Actions

The previously mentioned sequence is often referred to as *genomic steroid action* because gene transcription must be up- or down-regulated as a result of hormone action. This process can take many hours after initial exposure to the steroid.

Recently, nongenomic mechanisms of steroid hormones have been investigated. A nongenomic steroid action is a rapid intracellular response caused by steroids but inconsistent with the classic genomic model. These changes can occur within seconds to minutes following steroid administration and are insensitive to transcription and translation inhibitors, suggesting this signaling pathway may involve a classical second messenger cascade such as phospholipase C, cAMP/cGMP changes, protein kinase C, etc. Nongenomic effects may be mediated by a receptor type other than the classic steroid hormone receptor because antisteroid molecules like the potent antiglucocorticoid, antiprogesterone, RU 486, do not block these nongenomic effects. For many peripheral tissues such as skeletal muscle, these nongenomic steroid actions appear to be important signaling mechanisms compared with classic genomic effects.

Effects of Steroids on Skeletal Muscle

Muscle tissue contains both androgen and estrogen receptors, but the concentrations of these receptors in muscle are often 1000 times less than in reproductive tissues. However, the relative binding affinity for the androgen receptor in skeletal muscle and prostate is identical. Androgen receptors in muscle tissue have been characterized in several species including rat, porcine, bovine, ovine, and human. Similarly, estrogen receptors in muscle tissue have also been characterized in rat and bovine.

The level of circulating steroid has been reported to be an important determinant in the amount of unoccupied steroid receptors. In sheep, implantation with TBA appeared to reduce the number of detectable androgen receptors as compared with those in nonimplanted lambs. TBA implantation decreased the binding affinity of cytosolic androgen receptors. Implantation of calves with TBA/E_2 reduced the number of free estrogen receptors approximately sixfold as compared with nonimplanted calves. Up- or down-regulation of steroid receptors may occur via gene transcription. Androgen withdrawal via castration resulted in 1.5- to 3-fold increase in androgen receptor mRNA in the rat prostate. Testosterone propionate injections in castrated rats 24 hours before tissue removal reduced androgen receptor mRNA to the level of intact males.

Steroids have both direct and indirect effects on muscle growth. In the case of estrogens, the direct effects are thought to be secondary to indirect effects, mediated by changes in other hormone profiles. The primary effect of estrogens is through an altered somatotrophic axis. Estrogens increase pituitary size and increase the proportion of somatotrophs in the pituitary. The pituitary is also more responsive to somatotropin releasing factor (SRF). Insulin-like growth factor-I (IGF-I) production is increased and both somatotropin (ST) and IGF-I binding characteristics are altered. These changes work together to produce higher circulating ST, a more efficacious release pattern, and a more responsive muscle, resulting in stimulus of muscle growth.

Increased ST does not explain all of the effects of estradiol. Exogenous ST has been shown to increase growth of estradiol-implanted cattle and estradiol and SRF are additive in affecting circulating metabolites and growth factors. Effects of estradiol and ST are nearly additive when calorie consumption is restricted to the level of cattle without estradiol implants. Other hormones such as insulin and thyroid hormones are also altered, supporting the increased muscle growth.

The direct effects of androgens are significant. Trenbolone works directly on the muscle cell to stimulate muscle protein synthesis and deposition. The specific gene products that respond to trenbolone have not been fully characterized.

Androgens have significant indirect effects as well, primarily through altered glucocorticoids. Circulating cortisol is reduced in TBA-implanted steers and both cortisol binding and response to ACTH are diminished as well. Androgens also produce an altered ST profile (higher, more frequent peaks and lower troughs). These changes make the circulating hormone profile of TBA-implanted steers more like that of bulls and result in increased muscle deposition.

The effects listed earlier can be observed within days after implant administration. Early muscle growth stimulus is primarily hypertrophic in nature, which has been shown by depressed DNA/protein ratios. Prolonged (weeks) exposure to combined estrogenic/androgenic implants produces hyperplasia (increase in satellite cell nuclei) as well. In this case, quantity of muscle protein is increased but normal DNA/protein ratios are observed, indicating that proliferation of satellite cells resulted in increased quantity of DNA in the muscle. Cell culture studies have shown that the mitogenic activity of sera from implanted steers is increased, providing support for the line of thinking that implants initially increase hypertrophy and ultimately increase hyperplasia to support increased muscle mass.

Combined TBA/E_2 implants increase carcass protein by approximately 10% when compared with nonimplanted steers. Much of this increase occurs the first 40 days following implantation. Increases in circulating and locally produced IGF-I have been reported during this time period of rapid muscle growth in TBA/E_2 implanted steers. Because IGF-I is known to be a potent stimulator of both proliferation and differentiation of satellite cells, locally produced IGF-I could act through autocrine and/or paracrine mechanisms to promote the proliferation and differentiation of muscle satellite cells, thus enhancing skeletal muscle hypertrophy. In fact, satellite cells isolated from the semimembranosus muscle of TBA/E_2-implanted steers after 35 days of steroid exposure exhibited a shorter lag phase and began proliferating sooner when placed in culture than cells from nonimplanted steers. TBA/E_2 either directly or indirectly activates quiescent satellite cells in vivo or maintains them in a proliferative state, supporting muscle hypertrophy.

Effects of Steroids on Adipose Tissue

Steroid hormones are not thought to have significant direct effects on adipose tissue. Estrogen receptors are present in low concentrations and presence of androgen receptors in adipose tissue has not been demonstrated. Indirect effects are likely due to altered ST, which would impede fat deposition, and increased caloric consumption, which would enhance fat deposition. The net effect is that fat deposition rate in food-producing animals is not largely altered by exogenous steroids. Carcasses may be leaner at harvest, but this is due to increased quantity (and concentration) of muscle, not decreased quantity of fat.

There may be some fat depot specificity because many studies have shown reduced intramuscular fat (marbling) in implanted cattle, especially males. This could be a true effect of the steroids but it could also be an artifact. Most studies have harvested implanted and nonimplanted cattle at similar time end points. In these studies chemical composition usually differs between treatments, so marbling would be expected to differ as well. Investigators who chose end points other than time have typically observed less marbling reduction.

Effects of Steroids on Bone Growth

Sex steroids are vitally involved in control of skeletal growth. Adult levels of sex steroids are required for a pubertal growth spurt (velocity) to occur in both males and females. Prolonged exposure to these adult steroid levels results in closure of the epiphyseal growth plate (cessation). Thus steroids can be positive (velocity) or negative (cessation) in bone growth. As a practical matter in animal agriculture, effects of implants on bone growth are modest. Limited work has shown that long bone growth

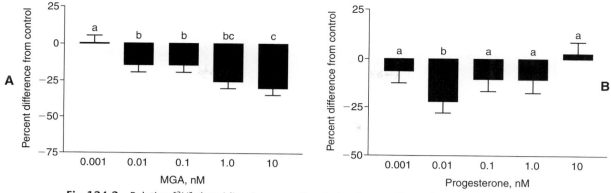

Fig 124-2   Relative [^{3}H]-thymidine incorporation in bovine satellite cells treated with various doses of melengestrol acetate (MGA) **(A)** or progesterone (P4) **(B)**. Bars represented as percent difference from control. Bars with different superscripts differ (P < 0.05). (Modified from Sissom EK, Reinhardt CD, Johnson BJ: *J Anim Sci* 84:2950-2958, 2006.)

of females can be increased by exogenous estradiol, either preweaning or postweaning. Theoretically, excess steroid levels could limit bone growth by hastening growth plate closure but there is no research to prove that this has occurred and steroid levels required are likely greater than used in production agriculture. Exogenous steroids appear to have little effect on bone growth of steers.

Melengestrol Acetate

Melengestrol acetate (MGA) suppresses estrus in cycling females, and the resulting behavioral change is favorable for animal performance. In addition, MGA induces a hyperestrogenic state in the static ovary,[26] which in some ways mimics use of an estrogenic implant. Numerous studies have demonstrated that feeding MGA in the absence of an estrogenic implant enhances feedlot performance, and the performance response from MGA is additive to the response from TBA.[27-30] However, when implanted with E$_2$, performance response to MGA is nominal.[31] This may simply be redundancy in the growth promotion mechanisms of MGA and exogenous E$_2$. However, when MGA is fed carcass, fatness increases and ribeye area decreases.[31] Suggesting a putative mechanism for this increase in adiposity of MGA-fed cattle, Sissom and coworkers[32] reported that inclusion of either MGA or progesterone to bovine satellite cell and myoblast cultures resulted in a reduction in DNA synthesis as measured by incorporation of [^{3}H]-thymidine (Fig. 124-2). This suggests that progestins may act directly on muscle cells, causing a reduction in muscle cell proliferation, ultimately reducing muscle growth and advancing the onset of physiologic maturity.

PERFORMANCE RESPONSE TO STEROIDAL GROWTH PROMOTANT IMPLANTS

In the period since publication of the aforementioned pioneering studies with DES, results of hundreds of implant trials have been published from around the world. For the purpose of this chapter, we attempt to focus on current trends in growth promotant use.

Currently 32 growth promotant implants are approved for use and marketed in the United States (Table 124-3).[33] These products vary in active ingredients, dosage, and carrier. Theoretically, dosage of active hormone is the primary determinant of performance response. However, if nutrients (primarily protein and/or energy) are limiting, response to a greater dosage of hormone will not be observed. Another determinant of the absolute response to implants is the inherent genetic potential for growth of each animal. As the growth rate of the nonimplanted animals increases, so does the added benefit from the implant (Fig. 124-3).[34] However, the percentage response to the implant may not change dramatically (Fig. 124-4).[34] Therefore regardless of cattle genetics or pasture conditions, expected average daily gain response to implants will be in the range of 10% to 15%.

With respect to feedlot performance, Duckett and coworkers[35] reviewed 33 independent implant studies, which compared performance of nonimplanted cattle to those given a combination androgenic/estrogenic implant. Implanting increased average daily gain 21% and improved feed efficiency 11%, with a 7% increase in carcass weight. The majority of feedlot implant studies have been conducted using a time-constant termination point for all treatments. Given this restriction, the aforementioned review also reported a 5% increase in ribeye size, 7% reduction in fat cover, a 5% reduction in marbling score, and a 17% reduction in percent of carcasses grading Choice or above. This indicates that, although implanted cattle gain faster than nonimplanted cattle, they do not accumulate fat at a rate proportional to their increased growth. If cattle are harvested at different fat-content end points, lower marbling content is normally expected.

A small number of studies have been conducted where cattle, having been treated with different dosages of implant, are harvested at multiple times and, hence, fat-content end points. Hutcheson and colleagues[36] reported that when the dosage of TBA/E$_2$ implant was increased by 50% (120/24 vs. 80/16 mg TBA/mg E$_2$), an additional 22 days on feed resulted in similar ADG, F:G, and similar percent of carcasses grading Choice and Prime for

Table 124-3
Currently Approved Implants

| APPROVED USES | | | | | | Implant Companies | | | | | | |
| Suckling Calves <400 lb | | Stockers >400 lb | | Feedlot Confinement | | | | | | | | |
Steer	Heifer	Steer	Heifer	Steer	Heifer	Fort Dodge*	Intervet†	Schering-Plough‡	Merial§	VetLife‖	Ingredients	Dose (mg)
x	x					Synovex-C				Component E-C	Estradiol benzoate	10
											Progesterone	100
x	x	x	x	x	x			Ralgro			Zeranol	36
		x		x		Synovex-S				Component E-S	Estradiol benzoate	20
											Progesterone	200
			x		x	Synovex-H				Component E-H	Estradiol benzoate	20
											Testosterone propionate	200
					x				Duralease		Estradiol benzoate	20
x	x			x					Duralease		Estradiol benzoate	10
		x	x		x	Synovex T40	Revalor-G			Component TE-G	Estradiol	8
											Trenbolone acetate	40
		x		x	x					Encore	Estradiol	43.9
		x		x	x					Compudose	Estradiol	25.7
					x		Finaplix-H			Component T-H	Trenbolone acetate	200
					x		Revalor-H			Component TE-H	Estradiol	14
											Trenbolone acetate	140
					x		Revalor-IH			Component TE-IH	Estradiol	8
											Trenbolone acetate	80
				x	x		Revalor-200			Component TE-200	Estradiol	20
											Trenbolone acetate	200
				x	x	Synovex Plus					Estradiol benzoate	28
											Trenbolone acetate	200
				x	x	Synovex Choice					Estradiol benzoate	24
											Trenbolone acetate	100
				x		Synovex T120	Revalor-S			Component TE-S	Estradiol	16
											Trenbolone acetate	120
				x		Synovex T80	Revalor-IS			Component TE-IS	Estradiol	16
											Trenbolone acetate	80
				x	x					Component T-S	Trenbolone acetate	140
				x	x			Ralgro Magnum			Zeranol	72

Modified from Selk GE, Reuter RR, Kuhl GL: *Vet Clin North Am Food Anim Pract* 22:435-449, 2006.
*Fort Dodge Animal Health (Subsidiary of Wyeth), Madison, NJ.
†Intervet, Inc., Millsboro, Del.
‡Schering-Plough Animal Health Corp., Union, NJ.
§Merial Ltd., Duluth, Ga.
‖All component products available with Tylan pellet; VetLife, West Des Moines, Iowa.

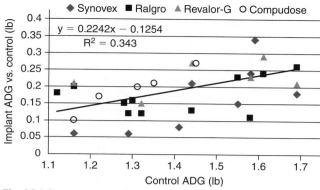

Fig 124-3 Average daily gain response to pasture implants over a range of control average daily gain. (Modified from Kuhl GL: *P-957, May,* Stillwater, 1997, Oklahoma Agric Exp Sta, Oklahoma State University.)

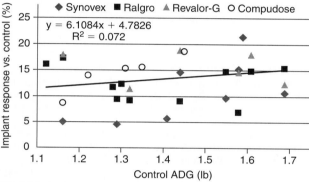

Fig 124-4 Percentage response to pasture implants over a range of control average daily gain. (Modified from Kuhl GL: *P-957, May,* Stillwater, 1997, Oklahoma Agric Exp Sta, Oklahoma State University.)

Table 124-4

Effect of Implant Dosage and Additional Days on Feed on Performance and Carcass Traits

Days on feed	123	123	145	145
Implant dosage*	80/16	120/24	80/16	120/24
ADG, lb	3.81	3.96	3.74	3.85
F:G	5.57	5.46	5.73	5.54
HCW, lb	847	858	895	902
Pr+Ch, %	53	48	57	56

Modified from Hutcheson JP, Nichols WT, Reinhardt CD et al: *J Anim Sci* 82(suppl 1):350, 2004 (abstract).
*Implant dosage=mg trenbolone acetate/mg estradiol.

implant on tenderness.[40] As described previously in this chapter, implants exert their influence on animal growth through numerous complex mechanisms involving various tissues and organs. Understanding that these mechanisms are the same systems by which growth is mediated in all animals, regardless of implant status, is important. The presence of an anabolic implant simply increases the amounts of hormones that stimulate the existing metabolic pathways for growth. Montana State University[41] researchers compared animals given a combination TBA/E_2 implant to negative controls, as well as large-frame to moderate-frame cattle, in a factorial experiment. They reported that breed-type effects on growth performance and beef tenderness were similar to the effects of implant. These results suggest that implants influence both growth and beef tenderness in a similar pattern and to similar magnitude to that realized by using higher-growth genetics. But also, they suggest that any presumed effects of implants on beef tenderness may simply be a function of increased muscle protein deposition, rather than a specific, direct effect of exogenous hormone administration.

Behavior

Buller steer syndrome has been linked to multiple factors and conditions at the feedyard. In cattle that all received a common terminal feedlot implant, Canadian researchers have documented greater incidences of bullers from August through October and in yearling steers versus steer calves.[42] Incidence of bullers in Colorado feedyards increases 70% in summer and fall versus winter and spring,[43] and incidence in Kansas feedyards roughly doubles from July through August compared with the average of the rest of the year.[44]

Total implant dosage used, especially for yearling steers, may contribute to the buller syndrome. Research from a commercial feedyard in Texas suggests that buller incidence in yearling steers may be related to the dose of estrogenic implant given, whether given as the initial implant or reimplant,[45] and a review of commercial feedyard data suggests that yearling steers implanted on arrival and reimplanted with estrogenic implants will have twice the cumulative buller rate as those only implanted on arrival.[46]

Although 70% of bullers occur within 30 days of initial processing and implantation, reimplantation of steer

the higher dosage compared with the lower dosage at the earlier time end point. However, at the higher dosage and the later time point, hot carcass weight was also increased by 55 lb (Table 124-4). Preston and colleagues[37] reported that, based on a review of 24 studies, steers and heifers implanted with combination TBA/E_2 implants required an additional 12 and 15 days on feed, respectively, to attain a similar degree of marbling compared with nonimplanted animals. Cornell University researchers[38] calculated that live empty body weight of steers implanted twice in the feedyard with combination TBA/E_2 implants would be 97 lb heavier at comparable body fatness compared with steers that receive no feedyard implant, and steers would have similar-quality grade. Anderson reported that the difference between implanted and nonimplanted feedyard cattle would be 128 lb.[39]

Another common issue surrounding the use of implants in beef cattle is the potential impact on meat tenderness. Of 32 published comparisons that have evaluated tenderness using either Warner-Bratzler Shear Force or trained sensory taste panel, 6 have shown a decrease in tenderness as a result of implanting, 3 have shown an improvement in tenderness because of implanting, and the remaining 23 comparisons have shown no effect of

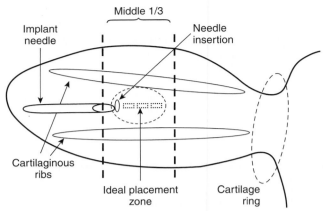

Fig 124-5   Preferred placement of implant.

calves 90 days postarrival fails to initiate a similar occurrence, exonerating the implant as the sole causative agent and raising questions as to further contributing factors surrounding the transition from pasture to feedlot.

Buller steers have been shown to have greater concentrations of plasma estrogen[24] and serum testosterone[44] and depressed serum progesterone.[47] Although the urine of buller steers is higher in estrogen,[44] endogenous production of estradiol and testosterone is actually lower in buller steers.[48]

Kansas State research has shown that bullers have elevated monoamine oxidase-A activity in the frontal cortex of their brain.[47] These data suggest that bullers are inherently different from their penmates and not simply responding to a greater estrogen supply.

Application

The implant should be placed in the back of the ear, subcutaneously in the middle one third of the ear, between the two longitudinal cartilaginous ribs (Fig. 124-5). Care should be taken that the implant is placed distal on the ear from the cartilage ring at the base of the ear, and to avoid placement immediately adjacent to old implant sites or ear tag scars; 1 inch separation from such areas should suffice. Sanitation is important in any surgical procedure. Do not implant into an area with visible fecal contamination. It has been demonstrated that implanting into a freshly contaminated area will lead to infection and abscess formation within the implant site.[49] Clean the area with a brush and dilute aqueous chlorhexidine solution. Remove as much excess solution as possible after cleaning. If the ear is dry and free from obvious contamination, there is no need to clean the ear as excess moisture on a relatively clean ear may assist wicking of infectious organisms through the incision.

To alleviate concerns about infection within the implant site, inclusion of an antibiotic pellet with the implant has been advocated; however, efficacy of an integral antibiotic pellet in reducing the incidence of implant abscesses has been equivocal.[50] Although there has been great interest surrounding implant placement and the potential impact that implant site abnormalities may have on animal performance, Berry and coworkers[51] reported that abnormal implant sites (abscesses, bunched pellets,

separated pellets, partial retention, and poor placement) had no correlation to reduced performance.

SUMMARY

Steroid hormones increase production and improve efficiency of food-producing animals. This results in economic benefit to livestock producers and influences relative price competitiveness of protein sources for consumers, favorably influencing market share for those species in which they are used. Consumers benefit from reduced costs and, in some cases, improved nutrient content of the meat. Most consumers accept products from animals produced with prudent use of metabolic modifiers. The variety of compound and dosage choices available to producers allows for specific "targeted outcome" programs to fit the production and marketing objectives of individual operations. The next decade of research will likely focus on production aspects of concurrent use of steroids with β-adrenergic agonists and the influence of these products on consumer acceptance of meat.

References

1. Dinusson WE, Andrews FN, Beeson WM: The effects of stilbestrol, testosterone, and thyroid alterations on growth and fattening of beef heifers, *J Anim Sci* 7:523-524, 1948 (abstract).
2. Burroughs W, Culbertson CC, Kastelic J et al: The effects of trace amounts of diethylstilbestrol in rations of fattening steers, *Science* (Washington, DC) 120:66-67, 1954a.
3. Burroughs W, Culbertson CC, Kastelic J et al: *Hormone feeding (diethylstilbestrol) to fattening cattle II. A.H. Leaflet 189,* Ames, 1954b, Anim Husb Dept, Agric Expt Sta, Iowa State College.
4. Herbst AL, Ulfelder H, Poskanzer DC: Adenocarcinoma of the vagina, *N Engl J Med* 284:878-881, 1971.
5. Cole HH, Gass GH, Gerrits RJ et al: On the safety of estrogenic residues in edible animal products, *Bioscience* 25:19-25, 1975.
6. Raun AP, Preston RL: History of diethylstilbestrol use in cattle, *J Anim Sci* 2002 (website): http://www.asas.org/Bios/Raunhist.pdf. Accessed November 28, 2006.
7. Preston RL: *Impact of implants on performance and carcass value of beef cattle. P-957,* Stillwater, 1997, Oklahoma Agric Exp Sta, Oklahoma State University.
8. Anderson PT: Trenbolone acetate as a growth promotant, *Compend Cont Educ Pract Vet* 13:1179, 1991.
9. Anderson PT: Mechanisms by which metabolic modifiers alter growth rate and carcass composition of meat animals, *Proceedings of the 53rd Annual Reciprocal Meat Conference,* 2000.
10. Hancock DL, Wagner JF, Anderson DB: Effects of estrogens and androgens on animal growth. In Pearson AM, Dutson TR, editors: *Growth regulation in farm animals* 7:255-297, 1991.
11. Johnson BJ, Halstead N, White ME et al: Activation state of muscle satellite cells isolated from steers implanted with a combined trenbolone acetate and estradiol implant, *J Anim Sci* 76:2779, 1998.
12. Preston RL: Hormone containing growth promoting implants in farmed livestock, *Adv Drug Del Rev* 38:123-138, 1999.
13. Tucker HA, Merkel RA: Applications of hormones in the metabolic regulation of growth and lactation in ruminants, *Fed Proc* 46:300, 1987.

14. Pottier J, Busigny M, Grandadam JA: Plasma kinetics, excretion in milk and tissue levels in the cow following implantation of trenbolone acetate, *J Anim Sci* 41:962-968, 1975.

15. Hayden JM, Bergen WG, Merkel RA: Skeletal muscle protein metabolism and serum growth hormone, insulin, and cortisol concentrations in growing steers implanted with estradiol-17 beta, trenbolone acetate, or estradiol-17 beta plus trenbolone acetate, *J Anim Sci* 70:2109-2119, 1992.

16. Lee CY, Henricks DM, Skelley GC et al: Growth and hormonal response of intact and castrate male cattle to trenbolone acetate and estradiol, *J Anim Sci* 68:2682-2689, 1990.

17. Heitzman RJ: The absorption, distribution and excretion of anabolic agents, *J Anim Sci* 57:233-238, 1983.

18. Hancock DL, Preston RL, Bartle SJ: Estradiol clearance rate in feedlot steers, *Texas Tech Anim Sci Res Rep* No:T-5-233:22-23, 1987.

19. Moran C, Quirke JF, Prendiville DJ et al: The effect of estradiol, trenbolone acetate, or zeranol on growth rate, mammary development, carcass traits, and plasma estradiol concentrations of beef heifers, *J Anim Sci* 69:4258, 1991.

20. Henricks DM, Edwards RL, Champe KA et al: Trenbolone, estradiol-17 beta and estrone levels in plasma and tissues and live weight gains of heifers implanted with trenbolone acetate, *J Anim Sci* 55:1048-1056, 1982.

21. MacVinish LJ, Gaibraith H: The effect of implantation of trenbolone acetate and oestradiol-1713 in wether lambs at two initial live weights on concentrations of steroidal residues and blood glucose, urea and thyroid hormones, *Anim Prod* 47:75, 1988.

22. Istasse L, Evrard P, Van Eenaeme C et al: Trenbolone acetate in combination with estradiol: influence of implant supports and dose levels on animal performance and plasma metabolites, *J Anim Sci* 66:1212, 1988.

23. Hunt DW, Henricks DM, Skelley GC et al: Use of Irenbolone acetate and estradiol in intact and castrate male cattle: effects on growth, serum hormones, and carcass characteristics, *J Anim Sci* 69:2452, 1991.

24. Harrison LP, Heitzman RJ, Sansom BF: The absorption of anabolic agents from pellets implanted at the base of the ear in sheep, *J Vet Pharmacol Ther* 6:293-303, 1983.

25. Riis PM, Suresh TP: The effect of a synthetic steroid (trienbolone) on the rate of release and excretion of subcutaneously administered estradiol in calves, *Steroids* 27:5-15, 1976.

26. Zimbelman RG, Smith LW: Control of ovulation in cattle with melengestrol acetate: II. Effects on follicular size and activity, *J Reprod Fert* 11:193-201, 1966.

27. Macken CN, Milton CT, Klopfenstein TJ et al: Effects of final implant type and supplementation of melengestrol acetate on finishing feedlot heifer performance, carcass characteristics, and feeding economics, *Prof Anim Sci* 19:159-170, 2003.

28. Trenkle A: *Evaluation of feeding MGA and implanting Finaplix-H, and Synovex-H in feedlot heifers*, 1992 Beef & Sheep Research Report—Iowa State University. A.S. Leaflet R910, 1992, pp 73-75.

29. Stanton TL, Birkelo CP, Hamilton R: Effects of Finaplix-H and Synovex-H with MGA on finishing heifer performance. 1989 Beef Program Report. Fort Collins, Colo, 1989, Colorado State University, pp 71-77.

30. Clay BR, Koers WC, Turgeon OA et al: Comparison of MGA premix and Rumensin in beef heifers implanted with Synovex-H or Finaplix-H. Upjohn Technical Report No. 76, 1991.

31. Hutcheson DP, Rains JR, Paul JW: The effects of different implant and feed additive strategies on performance and carcass characteristics in finishing heifers: a review, *Prof Anim Sci* 9:132-137.

32. Sissom EK, Reinhardt CD, Johnson BJ: Melengestrol acetate alters carcass composition in feedlot heifers through changes in muscle cell proliferation, *J Anim Sci* 84:2950-2958, 2006.

33. Selk GE, Reuter RR, Kuhl GL: Using growth-promoting implants in stocker cattle, *Vet Clin Food Anim* 22:435-449, 2006.

34. Kuhl GL: *Stocker cattle responses to implants. P-957, May*, Stillwater, 1997, Oklahoma Agric Exp Sta, Oklahoma State University.

35. Duckett SK, Owens FN: *Effects of implants on performance and carcass traits in feedlot steers and heifers. P-957, May*, Stillwater, 1997, Oklahoma Agric. Exp. Sta., Oklahoma State University.

36. Hutcheson JP, Nichols WT, Reinhardt CD et al: Evaluation of implant strategy and days on feed on performance and carcass merit of finishing yearling steers, *J Anim Sci* 82 (suppl 1):350, 2004 (abstract).

37. Preston RL, Bartle SJ, Brake AC et al: No differences found in feeding time among implants, *Feedstuffs* August 20, 1990, p 17.

38. Guiroy PJ, Tedeschi LO, Fox DG et al: The effects of implant strategy on finished body weight of beef cattle, *J Anim Sci* 80:1791-1800, 2002.

39. Anderson PT: Effects of combined use of trenbolone acetate and estradiol on crossbred steers slaughtered at three weight endpoints, 1991 Minnesota Beef Cattle Research Report. B-372, 1991.

40. Nichols WT, Galyean ML, Thomson DU et al: Review: effects of steroid implants on the tenderness of beef, *Prof Anim Sci* 18:202-210, 2002.

41. Boles JA, Neary KI, Boss DL et al: Growth implants' effect on tenderness and protein degradation, *J Anim Sci* 82 (suppl 2):121, 2004 (abstract).

42. Taylor LF, Booker CW, Jim GK et al: Epidemiological investigation of the buller steer syndrome (riding behaviour) in a western Canadian feedlot, *Aust Vet J* 75:45-51, 1997.

43. Pierson RE, Jensen R, Braddy PM et al: Bulling among yearling feedlot steers, *J Am Vet Med Assoc* 169:521-523, 1976.

44. Brower GR, Kiracofe GH: Factors associated with the buller-steer syndrome, *J Anim Sci* 46:26-31, 1978.

45. Voyles BL, Brown MS, Swingle RS et al: Case study: effects of implant programs on buller incidence, feedlot performance, and carcass characteristics of yearling steers, *Prof Anim Sci* 20:344-352, 2004.

46. Turgeon A, Koers W: *Effects of pen size on the implant response of feedlot cattle. P-957, May*, Stillwater, 1997, Oklahoma Agric Exp Sta, Oklahoma State University.

47. Epp MP, Blasi DA, Johnson BJ et al: Steroid hormone profiles and brain monoamine oxidase type A (MAO-A) activity of buller steers. 2004 Cattlemen's Day Report, *Kansas Agricultural Experiment Station Report of Progress #923*.

48. Irwin MR, Melendy DR, Amoss MS et al: Roles of predisposing factors and gonadal hormones in the buller syndrome of feedlot steers, *J Am Vet Med Assoc* 174:367-370, 1979.

49. Zollers Jr WG, Cook DL, Janes TH et al: Effects of a tylosin tartrate pellet added to cattle growth implants on the incidence of implant site abscesses, *Prof Anim Sci* 18:258-261, 2002.

50. Anderson PT, Botts RL: Evaluation of the ability of implants containing a pellet of tylosin tartrate (Component with Tylan) to prevent implant site abscesses under field conditions, *Prof Anim Sci* 18:262-267, 2002.

51. Berry BA, Perino LJ, Galyean ML et al: Association of implanting abnormalities with growth performance of feedlot steers, *Prof Anim Sci* 16:129-133.

CHAPTER 125

Feedlot Vaccination Protocols

JANEY L. GORDON and DANIEL U. THOMSON

In the fall of 1999 the U.S. Department of Agriculture (USDA)'s National Animal Health Monitoring System (NAHMS) conducted a study of vaccination usage on feedlots for the prevention of respiratory disease. Their results are indicated in Table 125-1 and Fig. 125-1.[1] The majority, 95.7% of small and 100% of large feedlots, vaccinated cattle with an injectable vaccine for IBR. Overall, between 86% and 94% of feedlots vaccinated cattle against diseases caused by bovine viral diarrhea (BDV), parainfluenza virus type 3 (PI3), and bovine respiratory syncytial virus (BRSV). Nearly two thirds (62.1%) of the feedlots used *Haemophilus somnus* bacterins and more than half (53.3%) of feedlots used *Pasteurella* spp. bacterins.

Vaccination protocols for feeder cattle are a primary discussion point between practitioners and producers (Table 125-2). Producers and practitioners vaccinate cattle with many different antigens based on cattle history and the risk of elevated morbidity and mortality. This chapter reviews the published evidence for use of vaccines to protect cattle from viral and bacterial pathogens.

BOVINE VIRAL DIARRHEA VIRUS

BVD virus (BVDV) is an economically important disease to all aspects of cattle production including the feedlot segment of our industry. BVD persistently infected (PI) cattle are a major reservoir of virus among newly arrived feedlot cattle and pose a significant threat for viral exposure and causing transient infections in naive cattle.[2] Transient infections can lead to immunosuppression of infected cattle. This may predispose cattle to a variety of secondary respiratory and enteric infections. Field investigations have indicated that BVDV is causally related to the occurrence of undifferentiated bovine respiratory disease, particularly chronic, unresponsive pneumonia.[3] Furthermore, Brodersen and colleagues[4] demonstrated cattle experimentally infected with BVD and BRSV resulted in a more severe respiratory disease than did infection with either virus alone. Therefore a strategic vaccination program should be in place at every feedlot to minimize the effects of BVDV.

Antigenic diversity of BVD can play a role in deciding a BVD vaccination protocol. BVDV isolates are divided into two biotypes (groups of viruses with the same genetic constitution), which include cytopathic and noncytopathic. Cytopathic strains cause vacuolization and lysis in host cells. In contrast, noncytopathic isolates do not cause destruction on host cells and are the most prevalent form in nature. Additionally, noncytopathic strains are responsible for persistent infections. BVD isolates are

further divided into two genotypes, type I and type II. Type I is further divided into type Ia and type Ib. Type I is commonly used as a laboratory reference and vaccine strain.[2] It has been demonstrated that type Ib is responsible for chronic unresponsive pneumonia associated with BVD.[5] Type II isolates are associated with high mortality acute and peracute infections.[2]

Like most RNA viruses, the BVDV has a high mutation rate, resulting in an almost unlimited antigenic diversity among isolates.[6] Apparently no one vaccine strain of BVDV (or even a combination of vaccine strains) is capable of providing cross-protective serum neutralizing antibody titers against all potential virulent BVD virus isolates. The question is what vaccine, or what combination of vaccines, should be used in a feedlot setting.

BVDV vaccines should protect against systemic infection with a range of antigenic variant strains of BVDV isolates. Important variables to consider when selecting a vaccine for use in a feedlot protocol include immune response, cross-reactivity, duration of immunity, immunosuppression, and reversion to virulence.[2] There has been some skepticism in the past regarding using

Table 125-1

Percent of Feedlots That Gave Any Cattle the Following Injectable Vaccines by Feedlot Capacity and Region

	CATEGORIZATION				
	Feedlot Capacity (No. Head)		**Region**		
Pathogen	1000-7999	8000 Or More	Central	Other	All Feedlots
BVDV	93.5	96.8	94.5	94.2	94.4
IBR	95.7	100	97.4	95.7	96.9
PI3	86.2	86.6	82.6	94.3	86.3
BRSV	87.3	87.6	87	88.3	87.4
Haemophilus somnus	65.1	54.1	56.9	72.9	62.1
Pasteurella spp.	52.9	54.3	51	58.3	53.3

From USDA: *Part II: baseline reference for feedlot health and health management, 1999. USDA:APHIS:VS, CEAH, National Animal Health Monitoring System,* Fort Collins, Colo, 2000, USDA #N335.1000.
BRSV, Bovine respiratory syncytial virus; *BVDV,* bovine viral diarrhea virus; *IBR,* infectious bovine rhinotracheitis; *PI3,* parainfluenza virus type 3.

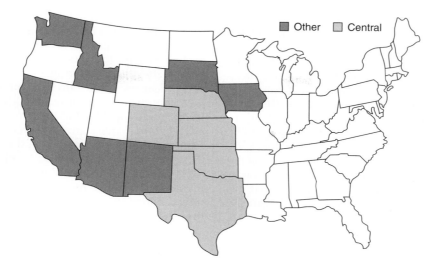

Shaded states = participating states

Fig 125-1   Feedlot 1999 study regions. (From USDA: *Part II: Baseline Reference for Feedlot Health and Health Management, 1999. USDA:APHIS:VS, CEAH, National Animal Health Monitoring System,* Fort Collins, Colo, #N335.1000, 2000, USDA.)

Table 125-2

Recommendations for Feeder Cattle Vaccinations

	Comments
IBR	All cattle on arrival, MLV
BVD	Types I and II, all cattle on arrival, MLV
BRSV	All cattle
PI3	Default because it is included in most multivalent vaccines
Mannheimia haemolytica	Neutral for high-risk cattle on arrival; not recommended in low-risk cattle
Pasteurella multocida	Neutral for high risk cattle on arrival; not recommended for low-risk cattle
Histophilus somnus	Not recommended at this time
Mycoplasma bovis	Not recommended at this time
Clostridial species	All cattle that have not received a dose before entry or history is unknown
Tetanus toxoid	Recommended if calves are castrated by banding
Moraxella bovis	Not recommended at this time for all cattle
Fusobacterium necrophorum	Recommended for cattle not receiving Tylosin in the finish ration

BRSV, Bovine respiratory syncytial virus; *BVDV,* bovine viral diarrhea virus; *IBR,* infectious bovine rhinotracheitis; *MLV,* modified-live virus; *PI3,* parainfluenza virus type 3.

modified-live vaccines (MLVs) in stressed feedlot cattle. However, the cell-mediated immune response stimulated by MLV vaccines is advantageous for calves entering the feedlot. Because of current marketing strategies of feeder cattle, immune protection is required quickly.[7] On the other hand, killed vaccines are fairly safe in that they are not typically immunosuppressive[2] but they generally induce a weaker neutralizing antibody response and a shorter duration of protection. The shorter duration of protection leads to increased frequency of administration

with killed BVD vaccines, which is generally not practical in the modern feeding facility.

Grooms and colleagues[8] examined the effects of exposure to PI calves during transport and subsequent arrival vaccination on calf morbidity rates. Two groups of 92 cattle were purchased in Alabama. Each group was placed on a truck for shipment to a feeding facility in Michigan. One truck contained two PI animals (types I and II) and the other truck contained no PI cattle. On arrival, half in each truck were vaccinated with MLV BVD vaccine. An exposure to PI by vaccine interaction occurred. Cattle exposed to PI cattle during transport had higher morbidity rates for the first 28 days postarrival compared with cattle not exposed to PI cattle. Cattle exposed to PI calves during transport and vaccinated with an MLV BVD vaccine on arrival had lower morbidity rates than the cattle exposed to PI calves and not vaccinated for BVD on arrival. Vaccine had no effect in cattle that were not exposed to BVDV.

The second variable to consider when designing a BVDV vaccination program is the cross-reactivity of the vaccine. Inactivated BVDV vaccines induced antibodies with equivalent cross-reactivity to modified-live BVDV vaccines, which neutralized representative strains of type II BVDV isolates in vitro.[9] Another study assessing the cell-mediated immune response in cattle vaccinated with either a BVDV type I MLV or a BVDV type I and II MLV demonstrated increased type II cell-mediated immune memory response in the animals vaccinated with both strains.[10] However, in a number of challenge studies the best protection rates were achieved with homologous strains of BVDV.[11] Along these lines it has been demonstrated that most cattle respond with higher SN titers to the genotype of BVDV with which they are vaccinated or inoculated, and with lower cross-reactive titers to other genotypes.[12]

Duration of immunity is the third thing to consider in a vaccination program. MLV vaccines generally have advantages with respect to duration of immunity because they tend to induce a stronger neutralizing antibody response and require fewer administrations of vaccine compared with inactivated vaccines. One study showed a decline in antibody titers at 4.7 months following vaccination with MLV.[9] To optimize duration of immunity, booster vaccinations should be administered at the frequency recommended by the manufacturer.[2]

Immunosuppression and reversion to virulence should be taken into consideration. A commercial MLV BVDV vaccine has been shown to induce prolonged suppression of host defense mechanisms in stressed and nonstressed cattle.[2] However, the stronger immune response that is received with an MLV vaccine must be weighed against this immunosuppression. The potential risk for shedding of vaccine virus from animals vaccinated with modified-live BVDV vaccines, followed by transmission to susceptible contact animals and reversion to virulence, has been examined experimentally.[13] Calves vaccinated with modified-live BVDV vaccines did develop transient viremia; however, the BVDV vaccine virus was not transmitted from calves receiving the modified-live BVDV vaccine to susceptible cohort calves.

Perino and colleagues[14] concluded that there were no reliable peer-reviewed reports of field trials examining clinical effects of BVDV virus vaccines in North American beef cattle based on research that uses scientifically valid methods with clinically relevant outcomes. Veterinarians still must make a vaccine choice to prevent the economic impacts of clinical disease. Although not documented, the use of different strains or serotypes of MLV BVD vaccines for each injection has been proposed so as to expand the range of cross-protection. In addition, to develop high levels of protection in the field, choosing a modified-live BVD vaccine that includes both type I and type II isolates may also widen the elicited protection. Currently there are more than 180 USDA-licensed BVDV vaccines available commercially, and because there is no current consensus on their use, the BVD virus will continue to be one of the most controversial topics in the feedlot industry.

BOVINE HERPES VIRUS-1: INFECTIOUS BOVINE RHINOTRACHEITIS

Bovine herpes virus-1 (BHV-1) is considered the most important respiratory virus in feedlot cattle. The typical presentation of infectious bovine rhinotracheitis (IBR) in feedlot cattle is often referred to as "red nose."[15] Clinical syndromes in the feedlot are often associated with respiratory infections and eye lesions. BHV-1 is harbored in a latent state in animals that have recovered from an initial infection. Any type of stress that increases endogenous cortisol levels including administration of exogenous corticosteroids can lead to recrudescence of the virus.[6] Once the virus is reactivated, the infected animal sheds IBR virus through eye, nose, and reproductive secretions.

Large numbers of cattle in close contact provide an ideal situation for rapid spread of the shedding IBR virus. Unfortunately, a serum-neutralizing antibody can prevent infection but it cannot prevent recrudescence and shedding of the latent BHV-1. In fact, an MLV vaccine

strain can be reactivated and shed under the influence of glucocorticoids.[16] Therefore it is beneficial for feedlots to prevent this disease before it occurs and becomes latent.

A vaccine for the prevention of BHV-1 should be based on the effectiveness during a certain scenario. Fairbanks and colleagues[17] concluded that administration of a commercially available multivalent MLV vaccine (IBR-BVD [types I and II], PI3, BRSV) to nonvaccinated calves at arrival will provide significant weight gain benefits while reducing clinical signs and viral shedding if given as early as 72 hours before exposure. Another field trial used an MLV IBR vaccine at arrival and demonstrated a reduced incidence of upper respiratory disease (17.2% in 3371 unvaccinated calves to 1% in 3345 vaccinates).[18] Therefore the consensus is to include the IBR virus in arrival vaccine regimens.

IBR vaccines are available in both MLV and killed forms. Killed vaccines have a higher cost and shorter duration of immunity, and they require two doses in a 14- to 28-day period, which makes them less practical for use in a feedlot. MLV BHV-1 vaccines can be administered either through parenteral or intranasal (IN) routes. Intramuscular (IM) MLV vaccines are thought to quickly induce immunity following proper administration of a single dose[6]; however, IN vaccinations have an advantage over parenteral vaccination in the provision of a shorter period from vaccination to stimulation of active immunity.[17] In a recent comparison of intranasal and intramuscular vaccinations of MLV IBR-PI3, there were no differences in average daily gain, dry matter intake, or morbidity in cattle vaccinated with either route of administration.[19] Today, there is not enough evidence to promote the usage of IBR intranasal vaccines with concurrent use of intramuscular vaccinations of IBR or PI3 in newly received cattle.

IBR infections in calves and feedlot cattle can lead to BRD and secondary bacterial infections that can cause significant economic losses. Although current vaccine protocols recommend vaccination of calves before weaning or commingling to provide maximum protection against IBR,[17] many feedlots are using IBR vaccine on arrival with success. This can be attributed to less antigenic diversity between BHV-1 isolates. Therefore one vaccine strain of BHV-1 appears to provide cross-protection against all field isolates.

BOVINE RESPIRATORY SYNCYTIAL VIRUS

BRSV is typically considered a primary pathogen in newly weaned cattle. Serologic studies suggest that BRSV is also common in incoming feedlot cattle.[20] Typically, affected cattle show signs within the first 7 days after arrival; however, reports of BRSV "breaks" in cattle over 30 days on feed have been reported.[15] Recovery from natural infection with respiratory syncytial virus does not induce protective immunity in most species, so it is unlikely that vaccination can prevent subsequent infections.[6] However, it may be possible for vaccination to attenuate clinical signs of subsequent infections and reduce recovery time.

Literature on the use of BRSV vaccination in feedlot cattle has produced differing results. Vaccinating calves for BRSV was shown to be beneficial in auction market–derived calves. Calves vaccinated with BRSV were two times less likely to be treated for BRD than the nonvaccinated controls.[21] However, a statistically significant benefit of BRSV vaccination was not shown in two classes of calves with low morbidity rates, which included preconditioned calves, and freshly weaned calves that were not transported.[21] This was reconfirmed in another study that observed no benefit for BRSV vaccination on arrival of yearling cattle.[22]

MacGregor and colleagues[23] used 19,099 cattle in a field setting to examine the effects of a four-way MLV virus vaccine (IBR-BVD-PI3-BRSV) versus a three-way viral with no BRSV virus included. Four-way vaccination revealed several benefits when compared with the three-way vaccination group including a decrease in respiratory morbidity, respiratory mortality, and overall mortality. This study leads to the conclusion that the inclusion of BRSV in a vaccination program can lead to economic benefits in the feedlot.

The choice must still be made whether to use an MLV or killed BRSV vaccine. Just like the short-duration killed vaccines, many MLV BRSV vaccines currently marketed require both an initial BRSV dose and revaccination with BRSV vaccine for adequate protective immunity.[23] Because duration of protection is similar between MLV and killed BRSV vaccines, the actual strength of the immune response must be considered. Kerkhofs and colleagues[24] tested the relevant antibody responses, lymphoproliferation, and gamma interferon responses to BRSV after administration of either an inactivated combination vaccine containing BRSV, PI3, and *Mannheimia haemolytica* or a modified-live vaccine combining BRSV and BVDV. Two single doses, 4 weeks apart, of one of the two vaccines were administered. The inactivated vaccine tested gave as good of a response as the MLV vaccine.

Cattle entering the feedlot are at significant risk of becoming exposed to BRSV and although there is evidence to support BRSV vaccine usage in naive or mismanaged calves, inclusion in vaccine regimens is not universal.[6] However, the previously cited studies indicate that a significant decrease in respiratory morbidity and mortality is seen when BRSV is included in the vaccination program.

PARAINFLUENZA VIRUS TYPE 3

PI3 is generally considered to be a severe respiratory pathogen in young cattle. Usually the disease is self-limiting and uncomplicated, but as with all of the bovine respiratory viruses, PI3 can be associated with severe secondary bacterial infections.[25] As was the case with BVD, a 1997 literature review on the efficacy of PI3 vaccines revealed there were no reliable peer-reviewed reports of field trials examining clinical effects of PI3 virus vaccines in North American beef cattle based on research that used scientifically valid methods with clinically relevant outcomes.[14] Furthermore, because many older cattle arriving at feedlots are likely to be immune, the value of PI3 virus vaccination in yearling cattle is questionable.[6] On a practical note, it is difficult to select a multivirus BRD vaccine that does not include the PI3 virus, making its inclusion in a vaccination program less of an issue.

PASTEURELLOSIS

Pasteurellosis is caused by *Mannheimia (Pasteurella) haemolytica* and *Pasteurella multocida*. These bacteria can be isolated in low numbers from the upper respiratory tract but are typically considered secondary invaders of the lower respiratory tract following a primary respiratory viral infection and stressors that cripple the innate respiratory immune mechanisms. *P. multocida* may be a more important cause of respiratory disease in younger feedlot cattle and is thought to cause less fulminating respiratory disease than *M. haemolytica*. Additionally, *P. multocida* requires more organisms to initiate a primary infection.[26]

M. haemolytica serotype 1 (S1) is by far the most important and commonly isolated bacterial pathogen in development of the often fatal fibrinous pleuropneumonia in beef cattle known as *shipping fever*.[27] Reports indicate that antibodies to *M. haemolytica*, as well as immune complexes that result from the interaction between the bacteria and the antibodies in the lung, may be a component of the pathogenesis of BRDC.[28]

Antibody against *M. haemolytica* leukotoxin (LKT) and surface capsular antigens is important in the prevention of pneumonic pasteurellosis and should be kept in mind when choosing a vaccine. The vaccines available today vary greatly in composition and can include the following components: bacterins, bacterins with LKT, bacterial extracts, culture supernatants containing LKT, or live streptomycin-dependant mutant.[29] Currently available *M. haemolytica* vaccines contain serotype 1 exclusively and may or may not provide efficacious immunity against other serotypes; however, vaccines containing antileukotoxin antibodies should provide some cross-protection.[30]

With all the available choices on the market today it is important to look at the efficacy of the vaccines. Field studies of a streptomycin-dependent live *Pasteurella* spp. vaccine[31] and an intradermally administered live *P. haemolytica* vaccine demonstrated efficacy.[32] Studies of a *P. haemolytica* capsular antigen vaccine failed to show significant health effects,[33] as did a study using a tissue-cultured *P. haemolytica* bacterin.[34] A review of literature indicated that three studies showed statistically significant reduction in morbidity and/or mortality in calves administered a *P. haemolytica* toxoid on arrival, whereas two trials showed no significant effects when the same vaccine was given at arrival or 3 weeks before shipment and on arrival.[14] A more recent study used a commercial bacterin-toxoid whole cell product and revealed there was a statistically significant reduction in crude mortality in the vaccinated group as compared with the unvaccinated cattle.[35]

When Perino and Hunsaker[14] reviewed published field studies on commercial *M. haemolytica* vaccines and found that efficacy could be established in only 50% of the trials, it was obvious that there is a continued need for additional well-controlled field studies to compare the efficacy of available vaccines. However, the previously cited references support the use of an *M. haemolytica* toxoid on arrival. To optimize immunity, special attention should be paid to the label requirements on the vaccine because some are required to be boostered, which may not be practical for the feedlot setting.

HAEMOPHILUS SOMNUS

H. somnus is hard to distinguish from other causes of BRD, but it has been implicated in its cause. It tends to be more of a problem in Canadian feedlots rather than U.S. feedlots and infected calves typically become ill and die later in the feeding period.[15,36] The septicemic form of the disease can be devastating, leading to such conditions as thromboembolic meningoencephalitis (TEME), myocarditis, pericarditis, pleuritis, polyarthritis, and diphtheria.[37] Little is known about the protective immunity to *H. somnus,* which makes understanding vaccine efficacy difficult. A study showed there were negative effects with a single dose of an *H. somnus* bacterin. Specifically, a higher number of single-dose vaccinated calves were treated for respiratory disease as compared with groups of unvaccinated control calves or groups of calves vaccinated twice at a 21-day interval.[38] Currently there is no clear consensus on the usage of *H. somnus* in a feedlot vaccination program. In addition, modern technology vaccines for this disease have not been sufficiently evaluated and the common bacterins available have not at this time proven to be effective, which leads us to believe that there is not a need for them in a receiving cattle program.[15]

MYCOPLASMA BOVIS

M. bovis is an emergent or at least better-recognized respiratory pathogen in feedlot cattle with mycoplasma-like lesions frequently observed in finished cattle.[15] A postnecropsy study using 500 lungs from feedlot pneumonia deaths were cultured for mycoplasmas, and 86% percent of the lungs were positive for mycoplasma, with *M. bovis* being the predominant isolate.[39] A more recent study of chronic, antibiotic resistant pneumonia in feedlot cattle demonstrated that 44/48 cases submitted for postmortem analysis were positive for *M. bovis.*[40] Normal cattle harbor *M. bovis* in the upper respiratory tract with no apparent detrimental effect. However, once a lower respiratory tract infection occurs, *M. bovis* can be spread hematogenously to the joints of affected cattle, which can cause severe arthritis and tenosynovitis.[41] *M. bovis* has a detrimental effect on the feedlot industry, which costs the United States an estimated 32 million dollars a year in mortality and setback losses.[42]

M. bovis, like all mycoplasmas, is naturally resistant to antibiotics because of its lack of cell wall.[43] Management of *M. bovis* should focus on augmentation of immune system function to reduce infections. Few reliable field trials have evaluated the efficacy of mycoplasma vaccines in cattle.[14] On the other hand, studies completed and published in the United Kingdom in the 1980s documented the efficacy of combination vaccines containing *M. bovis* in reducing respiratory disease that was associated with *M. bovis* infection alone or together with BRSV.[44] A more recent study suggested that even a single dose of vaccine prepared from saponised *M. bovis* cells may provide effective control against mycoplasma-induced calf pneumonia.[43] Some feedlots have used autogenous vaccines for the prevention of *M. bovis,* but there is a severe need for more field trials to determine the efficacy of these vaccines. Currently there is no direct consensus on whether using mycoplasma vaccines in the feedlot setting is beneficial.

FUSOBACTERIUM NECROPHORUM AND THE CONTROL OF LIVER ABSCESSES

Liver abscesses are a major economic liability, because of liver condemnation, reduced feed intake, reduced weight gain, decreased feed efficiency, and decreased carcass yield, with the incidence averaging from 12% to 32% in most feedlots.[45] Liver abscesses are formed secondarily to acidosis and rumenitis when *F. necrophorum* and/or *Arcanobacterium pyogenes* disperse from focal abscesses in the rumen wall and enter the portal circulation, subsequently seeding themselves in the liver and forming abscesses. Although *F. necrophorum* is the primary etiologic agent in this disease, *A. pyogenes* is thought to work synergistically to form abscesses. In the past, feeding of antimicrobials such as tylosin has decreased the incidence of liver abscesses by 40% to 70%. Importantly, these antimicrobial compounds reduce the incidence of liver abscesses but do not eliminate the problem.[46] Therefore an effective vaccine would be highly desirable in the feedlot industry.

Although the pathogenicity and virulence factors of *F. necrophorum* have been studied widely for years, attempts to develop an effective vaccine against liver abscesses have not been successful commercially. Jones and colleagues[47] reviewed the efficacy of an *A. pyogenes–F. necrophorum* bacterin-toxoid in the prevention of liver abscesses in a feedlot setting. They concluded that a single dose of the bacterin-toxoid given to cattle entering a feedlot reduced the prevalence and severity of liver abscesses in an antigen dose-dependent manner. Additionally, high antigen dose vaccinates had a more favorable USDA yield grade than placebo vaccinates. Interestingly, the liver abscess scores of the steers in the high antigen dose vaccine group did not differ from those of steers fed tylosin-medicated feed. Also, the number of steers with the most severe and the most economically important liver lesions (A+ or A++) was greatest in the nonvaccinates and least in the tylosin-medicated group. This study suggests that the high antigen dose bacterin-toxoid demonstrated efficacy in reducing the incidence and severity of liver abscesses. However, accurate estimation of the potential economic benefits of the bacterin-toxoids has not yet been determined. A vaccine approach may alleviate public health concerns associated with the use of subtherapeutic levels of antibiotics in the feed rations.

MORAXELLA BOVIS AND THE PREVENTION OF INFECTIOUS BOVINE KERATOCONJUNCTIVITIS

Hemolytic strains of piliated *Moraxella bovis* cause conjunctivitis and ulcerative keratitis in cattle. Environmental factors such as ultraviolet radiation, dust, blowing feed, and the face fly *(Musca autumnalis)* are also a crucial part of pathogenesis for this disease. Even though *M. bovis* does not cause systemic disease, the economic impact of infectious bovine keratoconjunctivitis (IBK) on feedlot cattle is considerable due to the ultimate reduction in weight gains.[15] Elimination of this disease would be economically beneficial.

M. bovis bacterins currently marketed in the United States contain high concentrations of bacterial pilus attachment antigens and are designed to produce concentrations of antibodies in the tears that will prevent attachment of *M. bovis* to the cornea and conjunctival epithelium, thereby preventing damage to the eye.[48] Some experimental cytolysin and autogenous vaccine trials have resulted in partial protection or no protection from IBK, respectively.[3,49] Vaccine failure in these instances may have resulted from usage of a vaccine strain of *M. bovis,* which did not provide protection against challenge from an antigenically different strain of *M. bovis.*

Prevention of IBK is difficult because of the high attack rate and the sporadic lack of efficacy of commercially produced vaccines. However, IBK is generally not a problem in feedlot cattle after the first few weeks on feed. Therefore present vaccines have limited utility in a feedlot setting.[15] On the other hand, IBK is available in combination with clostridial bacterins and could be used in this fashion.

CLOSTRIDIAL DISEASES

Clostridial disease in feedlots may be rare because of the extensive use of clostridial vaccines in cattle before entering the feedlot. However, clostridial diseases that can found in the feedlot include malignant edema *(Clostridium septicum),* blackleg *(Clostridium chauvoei),* black disease *(Clostridium novyi type B),* redwater disease *(C. novyi type D),* enterotoxemia *(C. perfringens type D),* bacillary hemoglobinuria *(Clostridium hemolyticum),* and tetanus *(Clostridium tetani).*[50,51] Some clostridial vaccinations have been associated with injection-site lesions, so concerns have developed for prudent use of these vaccines. Despite the potential for injection-site lesions, the 1994 National Animal Health Monitoring System report indicated that 34.4% of feedlots with fewer than 1000 head used clostridial vaccines, whereas 91% of larger feedlots vaccinated against one or more clostridial agents. To respond to the topic on injection-site lesions with clostridial vaccines, the National Cattlemen's Beef Association's Beef Quality Assurance task force released recommendations, which include the use of subcutaneous injections whenever possible. Furthermore, after the primary immunization with clostridial bacterins, repeat or multiple injections should be discontinued, especially late in the feeding period.

A common consensus among feedlot veterinarians is to administer a clostridial vaccine to calves on arrival. However, it is probably not advantageous to administer more than one clostridial vaccine after arrival to the feedlot. Several studies have shown detrimental effects on feedlot performance after a booster of clostridial vaccine. One such study reported a 20% decrease in feed consumption in response to a second vaccination with a multivalent vaccine.[52] Additionally, another study indicated there was no effect on the incidence of sudden death syndrome after a second vaccination.[19]

SUMMARY

The increasing concerns over the use of antibiotics in livestock and the perceptions of possible negative implications of animal agriculture-related antimicrobial resistance for human medicine indicate that the manipulation of the bovine immune system may become increasingly important in disease management in the future. Preventing disease in the feedlot is of huge economic benefit when compared with treatment cost and production loss in cattle. An effective vaccination program relies on identifying which pathogens the cattle are likely to be exposed to and then choosing a vaccine that will provide the most effective immunity. Veterinarians should remember that just because cattle are vaccinated does not mean they are immunized. The two key components required for successful immunization are an efficacious vaccine and an immunocompetent animal. Unfortunately in a feedlot setting it is usually not possible to know which vaccines have been given before arrival. Therefore communication with previous owners would be ideal.

References

1. USDA: *Part II: baseline reference for feed lot health and health management, 1999. USDA:APHIS:VS, CEAH, National Animal Health Monitoring System,* Fort Collins, Colo, #N335.1000, 2000, USDA.
2. Kelling CL: Evolution of bovine viral diarrhea virus vaccines, *Vet Clin North Am Food Anim Pract* 20:115-129, 2004.
3. Haines D, Martin K, Clark E et al: The immunohistochemical detection of *Mycoplasma bovis* and bovine viral diarrhea virus in tissues of feedlot cattle with chronic, unresponsive respiratory disease and/or arthritis, *Can Vet J* 42:857-860, 2001.
4. Brodersen B, Kelling C: Effect of experimentally induced concurrent bovine respiratory syncytial virus and bovine viral diarrhea virus infections on respiratory and enteric diseases in calves, *Am J Vet Res* 59:1423-1430, 1998.
5. Fulton R, Ridpath J, Saliki J et al: Bovine viral diarrhea virus (BVDV) 1b: predominant BVDV subtype in calves with respiratory disease, *Can J Vet Res* 66:181-190, 2002.
6. Roth JA, Perino LJ: Immunology and prevention of infection in cattle, *Vet Clin North Am Food Anim Pract* 14:233-256, 1998.
7. Bolin SR: Control of bovine viral diarrhea infection by use of vaccination, *Vet Clin North Am Food Anim Pract* 11:615-621, 1995.
8. Grooms DL, Brock KV, Norby B: *Performance of feedlot cattle exposed to animals persistently infected with bovine viral diarrhea virus,* St Louis, November 11, 2002, Abstract #186. Proceedings of the 83rd Annual Meeting of the Conference of Research Workers in Animal Diseases.
9. Fulton R, Burge L: Bovine viral diarrhea virus type 1 and 2 antibody response in calves receiving modified live virus or inactivated vaccines, *Vaccine* 19:264-274, 2000.
10. Endsley JJ, Quade MJ, Terhaar B et al: Bovine viral diarrhea virus type 1- and type 2-specific bovine T lymphocyte-subset responses following modified-live virus vaccination, *Vet Ther* 3:364-372, 2002.
11. Chase CL, Elmowalid G, Ausama AA: The immune response to bovine viral diarrhea virus: a constantly changing picture, *Vet Clin North Am Food Anim Pract* 20:95-114, 2004.
12. Jones L, Campen HV, Xu Z et al: Comparison of neutralizing antibodies to type 1a, 1b and 2 bovine viral diarrhea virus from experimentally infected and vaccinated cattle, *Bov Pract* 35:137-140, 2001.

13. Fulton R, Saliki J, Burge L et al: Humoral immune response and assessment of vaccine virus shedding in calves receiving a modified live virus vaccines containing bovine herpesvirus-1 and bovine viral diarrhea virus 1a, *J Vet Med B* 50:31-37, 2003.

14. Perino LJ, Hunsaker BD: A review of bovine respiratory disease vaccine field efficacy, *Bov Pract* 31:59-63, 1997.

15. Griffin DD: Feedlot diseases, *Vet Clin North Am Food Anim Pract* 14:199-231, 1998.

16. Pastoret PP, Babiuk LA, Misra V et al: Reactivation of temperature sensitive and non-temperature sensitive infectious bovine rhinotracheitis vaccine virus with dexamethasone, *Infect Immune* 29:483, 1980.

17. Fairbanks KF, Campbell J, Chase CL: Rapid onset of protection against infectious bovine rhinotracheitis with a modified-live virus multivalent vaccine, *Vet Ther* 5:17-25, 2004.

18. York CJ, Schwarz AJF, Zirbel L et al: Infectious bovine rhinotracheitis vaccine, *Vet Med* Oct:522-524, 1958.

19. De Groot BD, Dewey CE, Griffin DD et al: Effect of booster vaccination with a multivalent clostridial bacterin-toxoid on sudden death syndrome mortality rate among feedlot cattle, *JAVMA* 211:749-753, 1997.

20. Yates WDG, Kingscote BF, Bradley JA et al: The relationship of serology and nasal microbiology to pulmonary lesions in feedlot cattle, *Can J Comp Med* 47:375-378, 1983.

21. Hansen DE, Syvrud R, Armstrong D: Effectiveness of a bovine respiratory syncytial virus vaccine in reducing the risk of respiratory disease, *Agri-Practice* 13:19-22, 1992.

22. Van Donkersgoed J, Janzen ED, Townsend HG et al: Five field trials on the efficacy of a bovine respiratory syncytial virus vaccine, *Can Vet J* 31:93-100, 1990.

23. MacGregor S, Wray MI: The effect of bovine respiratory syncytial virus vaccination on health, feedlot performance and carcass characteristics of feeder cattle, *Bov Pract* 38:162-170, 2004.

24. Kerkhofs P, Tignon M, Petry H et al: Immune responses to bovine respiratory syncytial virus (BRSV) following use of an inactivated BRSV-PI3-*Mannheimia haemolytica* vaccine and a modified live BRSV-BVDV vaccine, *Vet J* 167:208-210, 2004.

25. Griffin DD: *Bovine respiratory disease: source book for the veterinary practitioner*, Trenton, NJ, 1996, Veterinary Learning Systems, pp 6-11.

26. Mosier DA: Bacterial pneumonia, *Vet Clin North Am Food Anim Pract* 13:483-493, 1997.

27. Purdy CW, Raleigh RH, Collins JK et al: Serotyping and enzyme characterization of *Pasteurella haemolytica* and *Pasteurella multocida* isolates recovered from pneumonic lungs of stressed feeder calves, *Curr Microbiol* 34:244-249, 1997.

28. McBride JW, Wozniak EJ, Brewer AW et al: Evidence of *Pasteurella haemolytica* linked immune complex disease in natural and experimental models, *Microb Pathog* 26:183-193, 1999.

29. Loan RW, Rung H, Payne JB: Comparative efficacy and duration of immunity of commercial *Pasteurella haemolytica* vaccines, *Bov Pract* 32:18-21, 1998.

30. Confer AW, Ayalew S, Panciera RJ et al: Immunogenicity of recombinant *Mannheimia haemolytica* serotype I outer membrane protein PipE and augmentation of a commercial vaccine, *Vaccine* 21:2821-2829, 2003.

31. Kadel WL, Chengappa MM, Herron CE: Field-trial evaluation of a *Pasteurella* vaccine in preconditioned and nonpreconditioned light-weight calves, *Am J Vet Res* 46:1944-1948, 1985.

32. Smith RA, Gill DR, Hicks RB: Improving the performance of stocker and feedlot calves with a live *Pasteurella* haemolytica vaccine, *Vet Med* 81:978-981, 1986.

33. Hill WJ, Kirkpatrick J, Gill DR, et al: The effects of Septimmune on health and performance of stressed stocker cattle, *Ok State Univ An Sci Res Rep* P-933:301-303, 1993.

34. Frank GH, Briggs RE, Loan RW et al: Respiratory tract disease and mucosal colonization by *Pasteurella haemolytica* in transported calves, *Am J Vet Res* 57:1317-1320, 1996.

35. MacGregor S, Smith D, Perino LJ et al: An evaluation of the effectiveness of a commercial *Mannheimia (Pasteurella) haemolytica* vaccine in a commercial feedlot, *Bov Pract* 37:78-82, 2003.

36. Guichon PT, Jim GK, Booker CW et al: *Haemophilus somnus*: important feedlot pathogen. In *Bovine respiratory disease: sourcebook for the veterinary professional*, Yardley, Pa, 1996, Veterinary Learning Systems, 1996, pp 12-17.

37. Lechtenberg KF, Smith RA, Stokka GL: Feedlot health and management, *Vet Clin North Am Food Am Pract* 14:177-197, 1998.

38. Morter RI, Amstutz HE: Evaluating the efficacy of a *Haemophilus somnus* bacterin in a controlled field trial, *Bov Pract* 18:82-83, 1983.

39. Hjerpe CA: The role of mycoplasma in bovine respiratory disease, *Vet Med* 75:297-298, 1980.

40. Shahriar FM, Clark EG, Janzen E et al: Coinfection with bovine viral diarrhea virus and *Mycoplasma bovis* in feedlot cattle with chronic pneumonia, *Can Vet J* 43:863-868, 2002.

41. Stokka GL, Lechtenberg K, Edwards T et al: Lameness in feedlot cattle, *Vet Clin North Am Food Anim Pract* 17:189-201, 2001.

42. Rosengarten R, Citti C: The role of ruminant mycoplasmas in system infection. In *Mycoplasmas of ruminants: pathogenicity, diagnostics, epidemiology and molecular genetics*, vol 3, Brussels, 1999, European Commission, pp 14-17.

43. Nicholas RAJ, Ayling RD, Stipkovits LP: An experimental vaccine for calf pneumonia caused by *Mycoplasma bovis*: clinical, cultural, serological and pathological findings, *Vaccine* 20:3569-3575, 2002.

44. Howard CJ, Stott EJ, Thomas LH et al: Protection against respiratory disease in calves induced by vaccines containing respiratory syncytial virus, parainfluenza type 3 virus, *Mycoplasma bovis* and *M. dispar*, *Vet Rec* 121:372-376, 1987.

45. Brink DR, Lowry SR, Stock RA et al: Severity of liver abscesses and efficiency of feed utilization of feedlot cattle, *J Anim Sci* 68:1201-1207, 1990.

46. Nagaraja TG, Chengappa MM: Liver abscesses in feedlot cattle: a review, *J Anim Sci* 76:287-298, 1998.

47. Jones G, Jayappa H, Hunsaker B et al: Efficacy of an *Arcanobacterium pyogenes–Fusobacterium necrophorum* bacterin-toxoid as an aid in the prevention of liver abscesses in feedlot cattle, *Bov Pract* 38:36-44, 2004.

48. Pugh GW, Hughes DE, Booth GD: Experimentally induced infectious bovine keratoconjunctivitis: effectiveness of a pilus vaccine against exposure to homologous strains of *Moraxella bovis*, *Am J Vet Res* 38:1519-1522, 1977.

49. Callan RJ, Garry FB: Biosecurity and bovine respiratory disease, *Vet Clin North Am Food Anim Pract* 18:57-77, 2002.

50. Thompson GB, O'Mary CC: *The feedlot*, ed 3, Philadelphia, 1983, Lea & Febiger, pp 183-195.

51. In Howard JL, editor: *Current veterinary therapy: food animal practice*, ed 3, Philadelphia, 1993, Saunders.

52. Stokka GL, Edwards J, Spire MF et al: Inflammatory response to clostridial vaccines in feedlot cattle, *J Am Vet Med Assoc* 204:415-419, 1994.

An Economic Risk Assessment Model for Management of Pregnant Feeder Heifers

MARILYN J. CORBIN and LAURA L. HUNGERFORD

UNDERSTANDING RISK ASSESSMENT MODELING

In 1897 Ronald Ross made the discovery that mosquitoes were the vector for malaria. This discovery led Ronald Ross to begin publishing epidemic models concerning the prevention of the disease of malaria. Ross communicated, "All epidemiology, concerned as it is with the variation of disease from time to time or from place to place, must be considered mathematically, however many variables are implicated, if it is to be considered scientifically at all. To say that a disease depends upon certain factors is not to say much, until we can also form an estimate as to how largely each factor influences the whole result. And the mathematical method of treatment is really nothing but the application of careful reasoning to the problem at issue."

Susser[1] describes the concept of modeling well. He states that the purpose of a model is to take a complex biologic system and reduce it to a model of related variables within the system. This helps to develop and clarify variables and statements concerning causal relationships. Susser[1] believes models serve one of two functions: They are either predictive or representative. The predictive function model uses present and past trends to exemplify the relationship between variables in the model. From this model the trends are extrapolated to predict future results with a certain degree of uncertainty or a margin of error around these results. The representative function model represents existing or hypothesized relationships in a simpler form.[1] According to Susser[1] the representative function model serves at least three additional functions of organizing, mediating, and analyzing.

Horst and colleagues[2] extensively discuss an outline for a modeling approach for contagious animal diseases. Three decisions, concerning the fundamental properties of the model, must be made. The modeler must decide to represent the model as static or dynamic, stochastic or deterministic, and optimization or simulation. A static model does not contain time as a variable. A dynamic model contains time as a variable needed to help define the problem.[2] Stochastic models such as those built with Monte Carlo simulation reveal the expected resulting value along with an expected variation of this resulting value.[2] Models of the deterministic nature reveal an outcome based on an assumed certainty about the input variables and their relationships.[2] Optimization models determine the optimal solution given the independent variables' restrictions.[2] Simulation modeling will determine the resulting effects of predefined strategies and scenarios resulting from manipulation of the input variables.

The usefulness of a biologic model is directly related to how well the model reflects reality in the population. Many focus on the process of building the model. Typically, a great deal of time is devoted to identifying the input variables, defining the input variables, constructing feedback loops associated with the input variables, and obtaining mathematical values for the input variables. A thorough modeler also allows for verification and validation of the model. Verification consists of understanding, interpretation, and clarification of the computer system, code, and analysis. Validation is an attempt to demonstrate that the biologic model behaves as the real biologic system.

Modeling, in particular, dynamic stochastic modeling, allows for the epidemiologist to take a complex biologic system and reduce it to a model of related variables within the system. This helps to develop and clarify variables and statements concerning causal relationships. Modeling has a number of advantages when compared with traditional statistical methods.

The first advantage of modeling is the ability to model uncertainty and variability. Vose[3] defines uncertainty as the researcher's lack of knowledge about the parameters characterizing the biologic system being modeled. Uncertainty may be reducible by further experimentation, literature reviewing, or consultation with experts of the system. Variability is the effect of chance or inherent randomness of the biologic system.[3] It is not able to be reduced by further experimentation, literature reviewing, or consultation with experts of the system. Dynamic stochastic modeling allows each independent variable to have a corresponding probability distribution associated with it. This probability distribution allows for variability in the data or for uncertainty in the biologic system to be modeled via many iterations of the model.

Dynamic, stochastic, simulation modeling has the advantage of eliminating much of the guesswork of traditional statistical analysis involving one answer.

Traditional statistical analysis provides one answer, an answer that may be the most likely, minimum, or maximum, depending on the external validity of the collected data. Simulation modeling relies on the use of many iterations (runnings) of the model, until a static outcome is achieved. In many cases this is 1000 or more iterations. In essence the computer has randomly selected a number from the probability distribution for each independent variable and input the number into the model 1000 times. This allows us to determine the most likely outcome based on multiple iterations of the model.

On completion of the dynamic, stochastic, simulation model the researcher has the ability to detect which independent (exposure or study) variables have the most effect on the dependent outcome (morbidity or mortality). Numerous charts, graphs, and tables can be constructed to demonstrate which independent variables are "driving" the model. For example, tornado charts provide a pictorial of the sensitivity analysis.[3] They illustrate the degree of correlation between the independent variable and the dependent variable. Spider plots offer an illustration of the degree of uncertainty in the model.[3] Variability of each independent variable is demonstrated on the x axis with the dependent value on the y axis.[3] An independent variable with a large amount of variability will have a greater effect on the dependent variable, represented by a larger vertical line distance.[3]

Dynamic modeling allows for interactions within independent variables. Models may include complex feedback loops involving multiple variables, which may have multiple effects on the biologic system at multiple locations or levels. Using modeling allows the feedback mechanism to demonstrate the effect of changing one independent variable.

A fifth advantage of dynamic, stochastic, simulation modeling is the ability to simulate with predetermined criteria. Most simulation modeling is run with many iterations, allowing each iteration to randomly sample a number from each probability distribution. Running simulations requesting minimum, maximum, or most likely values to be selected from each probability distribution is possible, however. This feature of modeling allows the researcher to predict best, worst, and most likely scenarios.

Dynamic, stochastic, simulation modeling is not without limitations. Perhaps the most severe limitation is human error. Each independent variable may have a probability distribution determined via data, literature, or expert opinion. It is plausible for some error to exist as a result of the use of inappropriate usage of probability distributions. Recognition of which independent variables are driving the model is a benefit of modeling; however, there is a limitation to how useful this is. Unfortunately, identification of "driving" independent variables may not lead to our ability to understand the biologic reasons of why certain independent variables are "driving" the model.

The purpose of modeling is to take a complex biologic system and reduce it to a model of related variables within the system.[1] This helps to develop and clarify variables and statements concerning causal relationships.[1] Modeling is of paramount importance in understanding, demonstrating, and communicating biologic systems. The following article is an example of how to apply economic risk assessment modeling to a biologic system.

ABSTRACT

Pregnant heifers in the feedyard present a challenge that can significantly affect an individual feeder's sustainability. We applied simulation modeling to a partial budget model to compare alternative strategies for managing pregnant heifers in feedyards. The model was developed with input costs (cattle, processing, health, and performance); input benefits (sales of chronics, baby calves, normal heifers, recently calved heifers, and pregnant heifers); and net returns as the output. Mean net returns for feeding either open heifers or aborted heifers averaged more than $100 (live basis sales) to $200 (rail basis sales) higher than for pregnant heifers. There was substantial variability in net returns for all three types of heifers, indicating the importance of other economic factors for profitability. Net returns, when heifers were sold on live or rail basis, were compared among three decision choices: (1) palpate all heifers on arrival and inject with abortifacient only those pregnant, (2) inject all heifers with abortifacient on arrival without determining pregnancy status, and (3) do not palpate or administer abortifacient to any of the heifers on arrival. At high pregnancy levels (≥49%), it was more cost effective, 95% of the time, to nondifferentially administer abortifacient to all heifers on arrival. For heifer lots with pregnancy rates less than or equal to 36%, palpating all heifers and aborting those found pregnant yielded highest net returns, 95% of the time. Doing nothing was economically beneficial, 95% of the time, only if pregnancy rates were less than 1.5% (live basis) or less than 0.5% (rail basis). In this study, sensitivity analyses and graphic representations of results were useful in developing recommendations. The true power of modeling may be that it yields both clearer understanding of implications of alternative management strategies and a tool for context-specific decision making.

Pregnant heifers present a management dilemma for feedyards. Pregnancy rates have been reported to range from approximately 3% to 20% on arrival at the feedyard.[4] Differences in income have been estimated to be $66.35 for pregnant heifers relative to open heifers and $26.41 for pregnant compared with aborted heifers.[5] Pregnant heifers in the feedyard may have increased health costs (e.g., dystocias, cesarean sections, death loss, palpation, abortifacient, abortifacient related morbidity), as well as losses resulting from decreased harvest prices for pregnant and recently calved heifers. Healthy pregnant heifers may have decreased dressing percentages.[6] Problems associated with pregnant heifers can also have a negative effect on morale among feedyard employees.

Feedyards have several options to manage pregnant heifers. For example, some only feed ovariectomized or otherwise guaranteed nonpregnant heifers or do not feed heifers at all. Other strategies include observing and shipping heifers before calving, palpating all new heifers for pregnancy and aborting pregnant heifers, giving abortifacients to all incoming heifers, and palpating a percentage of the lot and basing the decision on pregnancy status of those heifers palpated.[7,8]

New tools and approaches have been developed to model production systems and compare the feasibility and economics of different management options. Partial budget analyses provide a framework to compare returns for sets of interventions under fixed input conditions.[9] Dynamic models expand on this base to incorporate uncertainty, variability, interactions, and feedback loops.[3] We used these techniques to compare net returns for multiple health management decisions concerning pregnancy in the cattle feeding industry. Our secondary objective was to identify input variables strongly influencing per head profitability of various alternative strategies.

MATERIALS AND METHODS

Model Construction

The model was developed using a template[10] of a partial budget spreadsheet (Box 126-1) (Excel 5.0, Microsoft Corporation, Redmond, Wash.), on an individual lot basis, with inputs of costs (cattle, processing, health, and performance); inputs of benefits (sales of chronics, baby calves, normal heifers, recently calved heifers, and pregnant heifers); and the output of net return. Three decision choices were evaluated for each lot of heifers: (1) palpate all heifers on arrival and inject with abortifacient only those pregnant (PALABT), (2) inject all heifers with abortifacient on arrival without determining pregnancy status (ABTALL), and (3) do not palpate or administer abortifacient to any of the heifers on arrival (NOTHING). Simulation software (@Risk, Palisade Corporation, Newfield, N.Y.) was used to incorporate distributions around model inputs and to generate ranges of expected net returns under each scenario. Data entry fields were provided for input variables that feeders could control or that might be yard specific. Values derived from the industry, literature, existing data sets, or expert opinions were provided as defaults when no custom input was entered. Distributions were defined to include variability and uncertainty around these inputs when generating values in the simulations.

Base Heifer Population

Users were able to specify lot size and efficacy of abortifacient used (Fig. 126-1). Lot size default was set to 200 head to provide model robustness. Abortifacient efficacy was 95% based on a single prostaglandin injection.[11,12] The percentage of heifers pregnant on entry into the feedyard could be specified either directly as an estimated percentage or based on the month of entry into the feedyard. Each month was linked to a corresponding estimated pregnancy rate of heifers.[4] Estimated pregnancy rate was the producer's informed parameter estimate of pregnancy rate for a lot. A binomial distribution was used to describe uncertainty in the actual rate that might be observed in lots of heifers. When actual pregnancy rates, rather than producer estimates, were of interest, this stochastic component could be disengaged. The percentage of pregnant heifers that would calve in the feedyard was also user specified with a default value of 50%. This accounted for

the differing stages of gestation that would be represented at entry with recently bred heifers not at risk to calve in the feedyard and some heifers spontaneously aborting in the feedyard environment.[5,13] Variability around the specified rate was based on a binomial distribution.

Costs

Cattle costs were specified by the user or drawn from default values. The baseline simulation was conducted for heifers with a mean of 318 kg at entry. A large national

Please Fill in the Variables in Column B	User Inputs
Pen Size	200
Fill in % pregnant (if unknown enter "0" and then fill in month)	
% Pregnant	10.00%
Month in (Jan = 1…Dec = 12)	0
% Pregnant	0.00%
Abortifacient efficacy	95.00%
Percent pregnant threshold	10.00%
Based on threshold and pen size—<u>PALPATE</u> (% hd)	27
Please answer "1" = yes or "0" = no	
Were any of the palpated heifers pregnant?	
Pregnant heifers that calve in feedlot (% of pregnant heifers)	50.00%
<u>CATTLE COSTS</u>	
Purchase weight (lb)	700
Total delivery cost ($/hd)	$537.88
Yardage ($/hd)	$0.05
<u>PROCESSING COSTS</u>	
Nonpregnancy related ($/hd)	$17.75
Pregnancy—mass medication	$0.00
Palpation charge	$2.00
Abortifacients	$3.50
<u>HEALTH COSTS</u>	
Nonabortifacient-related BRDC morbidity (% of all heifers)	15.00%
Treatment cost ($/sickhd)	$13.00
Non-abortifacient BRDC morbidity relapse rate (% of BRDC pulls)	30.00%
Relapse treatment cost ($/sickhd)	$16.00
Chronic rate (% of all heifers)	2.00%
Abortion-related BRDC morbidity, above normal morbidity (% of those aborting)	5.00%
Treatment cost ($/sickhd)	$13.00
Abortion-related BRDC morbidity relapse rate (% those aborting and pulled for BRDC)	20.00%
Relapse treatment cost ($/sickhd)	$16.00
Direct abortion-related morbidity (% of those aborting)	2.00%
Treatment cost ($/sickhd)	$3.00
Pregnancy-related dystocia (% of pregnant heifers)	15.00%
Treatment cost ($/sickhd)	$13.00
Pregnancy-related C-sections (% of pregnant heifers)	3.00%
Treatment cost ($/sickhd)	$85.00
Respiratory death loss (% of total BRDC pulls)	5.00%
Pen (BSA) death loss (% of all heifers)	0.02%
Pregnancy-related death loss (% of pregnant heifers)	6.00%
Other death loss (% of all heifers)	0.00%
<u>PERFORMANCE GAIN COSTS</u>	
Feed cost/DM ton	$114.57
Days on feed (normal)	160
Total DM consumed 1-14 DOF (lbs/DM/hd)	15
Total DM consumed 14-28 DOF (lbs/DM/hd)	18
Total DM consumed 28—finished (lbs/DM/hd)	25
<u>INCOME FROM CHRONICS</u>	
Income from chronics ($/cwt)	$42.00
<u>SALE OF BABY CALVES</u>	
Heifers that produce a live saleable calf (% of heifers that calve)	50.00%
Price received for live baby calf ($/hd)	$100.00

Fig 126-1   Pregnant feeder heifer model.

survey established that the median arrival weight for heifers was 318.18 kg.[14] Total delivery costs[15] and yardage fee on a per-head basis were also included.

Processing costs included the general processing program used with all heifers on entry. The default value for this was $17.75 per head. General processing charges are highly variable; however, this value was based on summation of estimated charges for viral, clostridial, and bacterial vaccines; parasite control; labor; identification; and mass medications. Additional costs that could be incurred with specific interventions included a palpation and abortifacient charge of $2 and $3.50 per head, respectively. The model allowed mass medication charges to be allocated to the general processing program (default) or to pregnancy.

Health costs could be accrued because of respiratory disease, induction of abortion, dystocias, cesarean

Please Fill in the Variables in Column B	User Inputs
SALE OF NORMAL HEIFERS	
Estimated finish weight to the packer (lb/hd)	1200
Estimated dressing percentage (%)	63.50%
Live bid (normal) (%/cwt)	
Rail bid (normal) (%/cwt)	
SALE OF PREGNANT HEIFERS	
Estimated finish weight to the packer (lb/hd)	1200
Estimated dressing percentage (%)	59.80%
Live bid (pregnant) ($/cwt)	
Rail bid (pregnant) ($/cwt)	
SALE OF RECENTLY CALVED HEIFERS	
Estimated finish weight to the packer (lb/hd)	1000
Estimated dressing percentage (%)	63.50%
Live bid (calved) ($/cwt)	
Rail bid (calved) ($/cwt)	

Fig 126-1—cont'd   Pregnant feeder heifer model.

sections, pen deaths, and other death losses. Users could enter rates and costs to customize analyses. Binomial distributions, based on the specified pregnancy rate and lot size, were used to generate actual numbers of affected heifers in each step of the simulation. The base rate of bovine respiratory disease complex (BRDC) morbidity was 15%, with relapses occurring in 30% of cases and 2% becoming chronic. The case mortality rate was 5%. Bovine respiratory disease complex morbidity has been estimated, in a large national survey, to be 14.4% of all cattle on feed.[16] Feedyard veterinary consultants provided expert opinion to formulate ranges for default values of relapse rate, chronic rate, and case mortality rate. Bovine respiratory disease complex treatment costs were $13 for initial treatments[16] and $16 for treatment of relapses. The rate of BRDC, among heifers that aborted, was specified to be 5% higher, because of stress-related immune depression.[17] Aborted heifers had a slightly lower relapse rate to account for the more intense observation of these heifers, increasing the probability of earlier detection of BRDC. Treatment costs for BRDC remained the same as for nonaborting heifers. For pregnant heifers, those that remained pregnant had a 15% risk for dystocia with a 3% risk for cesarean sections, at a cost of $13 and $85, respectively, and a 6% additional risk of mortality.[18] A 2% rate of morbidity was directly related to the abortifacient, for aborted heifers. Pen death and other death loss had default values of 0.02% and 0%. Heifers were only eligible for pregnancy mortality if they had survived bovine respiratory disease complex, pen deaths, and other mortalities.

Cost of gain was determined from average feed cost per dry matter kilogram and average days on feed (DOF). Users were able to directly supply values for each component. Feed costs are highly variable; however, this cost was based on summation of estimated ration components and allocated $0.13/dry matter kilogram. Variability in days on feed was introduced through a Gaussian distribution around the average value. Default values for kilograms of feed consumed per head per day were compiled from feedyard records and feedyard veterinarians (6.82 kg DM/hd/day for 1-14 DOF, 8.18 kg DM/hd/day for 14-28 DOF, and 11.36 kg DM/hd/day for balance of feeding period).

Returns

Income was from sale of normal, pregnant, recently calved, and chronically ill heifers. Income could also be derived from the sale of baby calves if heifers calved in the feedyard. Heifer prices were based on bid price per kilogram, estimated harvest weight, and dressing percentage. Returns were calculated on a live and rail bid basis for each decision choice. Normal and pregnant heifers were finished to the same industry standard weight of 545 kg but differed in dressing percentage.[5] Live bid prices were drawn from a beta distribution, which was built using historical data,[15] and were the same for all heifers. Rail prices were drawn from a triangular distribution, which also used historical data.[15] Rail prices were $10 lower for pregnant heifers; however, all other heifer prices were the same. Default values for the sale of chronically ill heifers and baby calves were $0.92/kg and $100/hd, respectively.

Simulation

Net return per head for each decision choice and pairwise differences in per head net returns between choices were computed through computer simulation. Latin Hypercube sampling was used to derive input values from distributions. Simulation continued until changes in percents, means, and standard deviations of each outcome converged at 1.5% or less or until 15,000 iterations and two of the three parameters converged at 1.5% or less. Estimated pregnancy rates of 0% and 100% were used to generate overall net returns for pregnant, open, and aborted heifers. The default value of 10% pregnancy with binomial variability was thereafter used for baseline simulations.

Default values (see Fig. 126-1) were used to generate distributions of pairwise differences in net returns between all possible combinations of the three decision choices on live and rail bases. For each decision comparison, mean, median, and 5 to 95 percentile range in per head net return differences were determined by repeated iteration. Distributions were graphed. The 5 to 95 percentile

Table 126-1			
Input Parameters for Sensitivity Analyses			
Input Variable	5 Percentile	50 Percentile	95 Percentile
% Pregnant	6.5%	10%	13.5%
Pregnant heifers that calve in feedlot (%)	44%	50%	55.5%
Non–abortifacient-related BRDC morbidity (%)	11%	15%	19%
Abortifacient-related BRDC morbidity, above normal	2.5%	5%	7.5%
Direct abortifacient-related morbidity (%)	0.5%	2%	4%
Pregnancy-related dystocia (%)	11%	15%	19.5%
Pregnancy-related cesarean sections (%)	1%	3%	5%
Respiratory death loss (% of BRDC pulls)	2.5%	5%	7.5%
Pregnancy-related death loss (% of pregnant heifers)	3.5%	6%	9%
Days on feed	148.4	160	171.4
Pregnant heifers that produce a live saleable calf (%)	44%	50%	56%
Live bid (normal) ($/cwt)	$60.34	$69.38	$79.30
Rail bid (normal) ($/cwt)	$96.95	$110.03	$127.76

BRDC, Bovine respiratory disease complex; *cwt,* hundredweight.

range was used to summarize spread, capturing 90% of the total values for differences in mean net return per head. Tornado graphs of regression correlations between outcome (net return per head) and input distribution values were assessed to identify influential inputs. Sensitivity and threshold analyses were performed and graphed for each decision choice, independently fixing one input and sampling all others from their default distributions (Table 126-1). Curves comparing net returns per head for different decision choices, over the range of possible pregnancy rates, were generated to illustrate thresholds for reversal of decision choices and slopes of relationships between pregnancy rates and net returns. Pregnancy rates that yielded equal mean net returns for two decision options were determined through repeated substitution and simulation. Threshold pregnancy rates, in which each decision generated higher net returns than the others at least 95% of the time, were also identified.

RESULTS

Base Simulation

The baseline simulation for the pregnant feeder heifer model had less than a 1.5% change in percent, mean, and standard deviation of each outcome, thereby meeting convergence criteria. Open heifers had a higher mean net return per head than pregnant heifers on both a live ($113.18 increase) and rail basis ($235.68 increase). The 5 to 95 percentile ranges for mean net returns were –$58.14 to $170.57 per head for open heifers on a live basis and –$45.01 to $192.50 per head on the rail. Equivalent ranges for pregnant heifers were –$162.36 to $43.57 per head (live) and –$267.57 to –$66.60 per head (rail). Aborted heifers also had a mean per head advantage of $100.18 and $215.89 over pregnant heifers, on a live and rail basis, respectively. The 5 to 95 percentile ranges for returns were –$69.75 to $152.02 per head for aborted heifers on a live basis and –$63.70 to $171.16 per head on the rail. Differences were smaller between open and aborted

Table 126-2				
Comparisons of Baseline Mean, Median, 5 Percentile Level, and 95 Percentile Level Differences in Mean Net Returns (Dollars Per Head) for Each Pairwise Comparison of Decision Choices				
Decision Choice	Levels	ABTALL[†] (live)	(rail)	NOTHING[‡] (live)	(rail)
PALABT*	Mean	$1.15	$1.15	$7.96	$19.59
	Median	$1.15	$1.15	$7.68	$19.36
	5 percentile level	$1.03	$1.03	$3.61	$11.48
	95 percentile level	$1.27	$1.27	$13.22	$28.21
ABTALL[†]	Mean	—		$6.81	$18.44
	Median			$6.55	$18.20
	5 percentile level			$2.37	$10.23
	95 percentile level			$12.14	$27.17

*Palpate all heifers on arrival and inject with abortifacient only those pregnant.
†Palpate none, but inject all heifers with abortifacient on arrival.
‡Palpate none and inject none of the heifers on arrival.

heifers, although open heifers still had an advantage for both live ($13 more per head) and rail ($19.79 more per head) comparisons. In all three cases, bid price for finished cattle (regression coefficient = 0.93-0.99) and days on feed (regression coefficient = –0.18 to –0.14) had the largest effects on per head net return. Pregnancy-related death loss (regression coefficient = –0.29 to –0.30) was also important for pregnant heifers, with a stronger effect than days on feed.

Mean differences in net return, for the baseline simulation, varied among the three pregnancy management choices, ranging from $1.15 to $19.59 on a per-head basis (Table 126-2). Means, 5 and 95 percentile ranges for differences in net return per head, were generally larger for comparisons involving rail prices than live prices. Based on mean net return differences, the decision choices could be ranked from most to least profitable as: PALABT, ABTALL, NOTHING. In the baseline simulation, with a pregnancy rate of 10% and a palpation charge of $2, decision choice PALABT always gave a higher net return per head than ABTALL, for both the live and rail bids. For all other decision contrasts, input combinations existed that could reverse the direction of net benefit between the two options.

Decision Choice PALABT versus ABTALL

The distributions of net returns per head were virtually identical for PALABT (live basis, mean = $48.66, 90% range = −$60.84-$167.60; rail basis, mean = $57.82, 90% range = −$47.82-$186.54) and ABTALL (live basis, mean = $47.50, 90% range = −$61.96-$166.44; rail basis, mean = $56.67, 90% range = −$48.95-$185.41), although offset by a constant amount. Decision choice PALABT yielded at least a $1.03 greater net return per head, 95% of the time, on both a live and rail basis. Sensitivity analysis revealed that no input variables, except estimated pregnancy rate, were correlated with differences in net return. An almost perfect negative correlation (regression coefficient = −1 [live basis] and −0.9 [rail basis]) occurred between these two variables.

When estimated pregnancy rates were 36% or less, PALABT was more profitable 95% of the time. At 36% pregnancy, median net returns were $45.79 (PALABT) and $45.55 (ABTALL), on a live basis, and $51.76 (PALABT) and $51.52 (ABTALL), on a rail basis. When input pregnancy rates were above 49%, ABTALL was more profitable 95% of the time. At 49% pregnancy, median net returns were $44.17 (PALABT) and $44.38 (ABTALL), live basis, and $49.34 (PALABT) and $49.55 (ABTALL), rail basis. A pregnancy rate of 43% gave equal mean net returns for these two decisions at $44.92 (live basis) and $50.46 (rail).

The impact of palpation charge per head was assessed by increasing the $2 palpation fee to $3. Decision PALABT still yielded positive net returns per head versus ABTALL on a live and rail basis 95% of the time with the default pregnancy rate of 10% or less. When heifer pregnancy rate was 19% or higher, net return per head was higher at least 95% of the time for ABTALL rather than PALABT on a live and rail basis. The per head net returns were equal when the estimated pregnancy rate was 14%.

Decision Choice PALABT versus NOTHING

Net returns per head for PALABT (live basis, mean = $48.66, 90% range = −$60.84-$167.60; rail basis, mean = $57.82, 90% range = −$47.82-$186.54) and NOTHING (live basis, mean = $40.65, 90% range = −$67.71-$157.76; rail basis, mean = $38.21, 90% range = −$65.38-$166.52) had overlapping distributions. In our baseline simulation with the estimated pregnancy rate set to 10%, the 5 to 95 percentile range of stochastically generated values of pregnancy rate was 6.5% to 13.5%. Over this range, PALABT was always more profitable than NOTHING. The most influential input variables for decision choice PALABT versus NOTHING were pregnancy rate, pregnancy-related

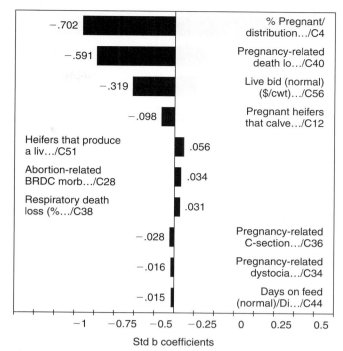

Fig 126-2   Regression correlation coefficients for decision choice NOTHING versus PALABT, on a live basis.

death loss, and bid price (Figs. 126-2 and 126-3). When pregnancy rates were varied, PALABT yielded a positive net return per head relative to NOTHING, 95% of the time, when estimated pregnancy rate was 5% or greater on a live basis, and 2.5% or greater on the rail. Median net returns were $49.67 for PALABT and $46.65 for NOTHING, on a live basis, at 5% estimated pregnancy and $58.01 for PALABT and $54.60 for NOTHING on a rail basis, at 2.5% estimated pregnancy. PALABT and NOTHING yielded equal net returns when estimated pregnancy rate was 2% for live sales (median net returns of $50.05) and approximately 0.9% for sales on a rail basis (median net returns of $58.36 [PALABT] and $58.30 [NOTHING]). Decision choice NOTHING attained a positive net return per head, relative to PALABT, 95% of the time only when input pregnancy rates were decreased to below 1.5% (live bid, median net returns of $50.11 for PALABT and $50.61 for NOTHING) and below 0.5% (rail, median net returns of $58.38 for PALABT and $59.30 for NOTHING).

When pregnancy-related death loss was decreased to 0%, instead of the default value of 6%, differences in mean net returns per head were $2.02 and $13.58 (live and rail basis, respectively) rather than $7.96 and $19.59. Although pregnancy-related death loss percentage was decreased by 6%, the actual number of heifer deaths decreased by only 1.19 head for decision choice NOTHING and 0.06 head for decision choice PALABT.

DISCUSSION

Dynamic modeling provides a conceptual means to reduce a complex system to a set of related variables,[1] from which qualitative and quantitative assessments of economic benefits can be made.[3] These methods allow

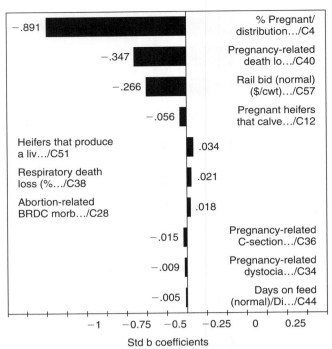

Fig 126-3 Regression correlation coefficients for decision choice NOTHING versus PALABT, on a rail basis.

for interactions and feedback among inputs to account for variables that may have different effects at multiple locations or levels. Estimates of uncertainty and inherent variability in the data can be incorporated to illustrate the range of likely outcomes rather than a single result. Simulation modeling also allows detection of those input variables with the greatest effect on the outcome. Charts, graphs, and tables can be constructed to identify independent variables that are "driving" the model. Finally, dynamic modeling allows prediction of best, worst, and most likely scenarios and determination of input conditions that define them.

These attributes of simulation modeling were exploited to evaluate programs to manage financial risk associated with pregnant heifers in the feedyard. Although recommendations abound in the lay press, there has been little application of tools to quantitatively compare management options. A partial budget-based simulation provides a means to gain understanding of the problem, as well as derive and explore management options. Such a model can allow customization to individual situations and incorporation of yard-specific and current production costs and returns. Expanding this tool further, by using risk assessment, produces a model that can incorporate uncertainty in producer estimates, biologic variation in health parameters, and fluctuations in economic inputs. The resulting distributions of net returns give a better summary of likely outcomes that will result from choosing each management option.

Base Simulation

Mean net returns were substantially higher for feeding open heifers and aborted heifers than for pregnant heifers. The large detrimental effects for pregnant heifers

were traced to costs of pregnancy-related deaths, dystocia, cesarean sections, and lower rail prices for pregnant heifers. Losses were accentuated for pregnant heifers sold on a rail basis because fetal weight decreased dressing percentages. Inputs that contributed to increased costs of production for aborted heifers included abortifacient cost, abortion-related BRDC morbidity, and direct abortion-related morbidity.

Output distributions for pregnant, aborted, and open heifers showed predicted net returns extending well into both positive and negative regions. Although this range could be summarized by the maximums and minimums of the distributions, these descriptors are unstable and fluctuated between simulations. The rare event of sampling an extreme value from the tail of an input distribution would unduly influence these values. The 5 and 95 percentile limits of net returns capture the degree of variability in expected performance of these three types of heifers as other inputs vary without this weakness. However, these values are less intuitive and must be clarified when presenting summaries and recommendations to feedyard managers.

The substantial overlap in net returns for all three types of heifers represents the large influence of other economic factors on net returns when feeding heifers. These effects would not have been apparent with a static, partial budget calculation, which would only compare means. Calculation of means alone does not allow integration of uncertainty, variability, and evaluation of best and worst case scenarios. Communication of the range of predicted net returns is important when recommending procedural changes to a feedyard. Normal temporal variability in other inputs, if not accounted for, could mask positive effects of a change in pregnant heifer management.

Even within a dynamic model, wide variability in inputs may hide differences in outcomes. In this model, variables were held constant for calculation of individual comparisons between decisions but were varied between iterations, allowing variability to be incorporated without allowing extraneous variables to control the model or obscure comparisons of interest. Examining effects of input variability on output net returns can provide insight into the relative importance of different health and productivity issues within the feedyard.[3]

Other authors, using limited partial budgets, have also found use of abortifacients to be more profitable than feeding pregnant heifers.[13,18] Ranking and direction of our results were similar to those reported in a previous Canadian study,[5] although the approaches and price scales differed. Jim and colleagues[5] assumed that health, treatment, and processing costs would be equal for pregnant and aborted heifers. We explicitly allowed variability in morbidity, mortality, and treatment rates among open, pregnant, and aborted heifers. The Canadian study specified different growth and efficiency values for these classes of heifers. Although rate of gain was modeled to be equal regardless of pregnancy status in our model, cost of gain was indirectly varied in each iteration by random selection of values from feed cost and days on feed distributions. This was reflected in the wide ranges between the 5 and 95 percentile net returns even under our constraints.

Both studies estimate complementary components of losses associated with feeding aborted and pregnant heifers. Simulation modeling further allowed for assessment of likely ranges of net returns as other inputs such as feed and bid prices changed rather than a single static net return value.

Decision Choice PALABT versus ABTALL

These two strategies differed only in costs for additional abortifacients given to nonpregnant heifers (ABTALL) and palpation to ascertain pregnancy status (PALABT). All pregnant heifers received abortifacients for both decision choices, which equalized costs and benefits associated with managing pregnant animals for both options. This led to extremely high negative correlation between percent pregnant heifers and net returns and a narrow distribution of differences in net return between decisions (see Table 126-2), although there was large variability in individual net returns for each decision.

All distributions in the model were bounded and most were symmetrical. The convergence criteria required that means and standard deviations stabilized. If the same decision choices were compared in a partial budget, values that set differences in net returns to zero in the partial budget were the same points for which 50% of the differences in net returns between the two decision choices were positive and 50% were negative in the simulation model. At this pregnancy rate, both decision options would be equally likely to yield higher net returns. The simulation provided additional information on expected variability in outcomes and identified values for which a particular decision choice was predicted to be profitable 95% of the time. Both of these aspects would be helpful when considering implementation of new management programs. In the range between 36% and 49% pregnancy rates, temporal variation in other inputs would have a larger effect on actual profitability of one decision over the other. Also, within this range, net returns differed by only $0.03 to $0.24 per head between decisions. For pregnancy rates above or below this range, expected benefits from a particular decision choice would be clearer and more consistent.

Other authors have suggested these two strategies for potential management of feedyard pregnancies.[7,8] However, this model provided a method to identify the economic thresholds between these plans. At higher pregnancy levels, it was more costly to palpate the entire lot of heifers than to nondifferentially administer abortifacient to all on arrival. When per-head palpation cost was $2, PALABT was a valuable strategy 95% of the time, until pregnancy rates exceeded 36%, which is above the range expected for usual heifer lots.[4] Costs for palpation and abortifacient would affect this decision choice, as illustrated by the decrease in the threshold from 36% to 10% when per head palpation fee was increased to $3. Feedlot managers can use knowledge of these thresholds to better plan interventions. Direct input of yard-specific values into the model would allow producers to balance palpation costs with estimated pregnancy rates on arrival and determine when PALABT would be advantageous in their yards.

Decision Choice PALABT versus NOTHING

If no heifers were pregnant, decision choice NOTHING would obviously be preferable. Determining the threshold at which pregnancy is high enough to justify intervention is an important management point. Our model found that decision choice PALABT would be advantageous 95% of the time when pregnancy rates were equal or above 5% on a live basis or equal or above 2.5% on a rail basis and 50% of the time when pregnancy rates were above 2% on a live basis or above 1% on a rail basis. Decision threshold values differed between live and rail analyses because pregnant, open, and aborted heifers had the same final live weight and bid price, whereas pregnant heifers received a discount and had a lower dressing percentage when sold on the rail. Several authors have stated that ignoring feedyard pregnancies is not the best management strategy.[4,19] A previously published partial budget[20] also found that largest losses occurring when no treatment was applied to pregnant heifers.

Although there was a moderately high correlation between pregnancy-related death loss and differences in net returns for PALABT and NOTHING, numbers of heifers that died because of pregnancy-related complications were low (1.19). This was because the baseline model simulated a population of 200 head with only a 10% pregnancy rate. Even when deaths caused by pregnancy-related complications were decreased to 0%, which would not be a biologically reasonable value nor an input producers could readily control, PALABT remained preferable on the live basis, with a mean difference of $2.02 per head favoring PALABT. Higher values for population size and pregnancy-related mortality could be evaluated through further simulation, but death loss would still not be directly controllable by feedyard managers. Influential variables must be examined in a biologic context to separate those that are strongly correlated but have limited practical effects from those that are modifiable with value for producers.

Bid price exemplified a different type of influential input, but also not directly controllable by producers. Cattle sales were the main source of income in the model, so changes in bid prices multiplied differences between decision choices. Normal heifer bid values were drawn from a distribution of annual mean prices in a 20-year historical database.[15] Variability would be reduced, while still using these real data, by using separate monthly mean price distributions linked to an input of month of harvest. Decreasing the range of possible bid prices could lead to a more robust model; however, variability at the current level may be more appropriate because it represents true fluctuations in prices faced by producers. For variables such as this one that are correlated with decision value, yet not available for producer intervention, the range of possible outcomes should be communicated to producers in outlining expected returns from management change.

Use of Dynamic, Stochastic, Simulation Modeling in Decision Making

Based on composite comparisons among the three strategies, under the defined input ranges, ignoring heifer pregnancy would not be economically advantageous unless

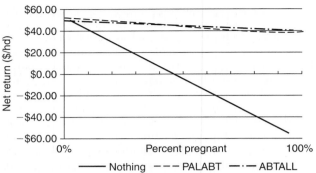

Fig 126-4   Net return (live basis) for PALABT, ABTALL, and NOTHING over a range of percent pregnant values.

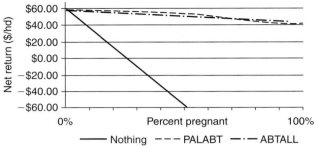

Fig 126-5   Net return (rail basis) for PALABT, ABTALL, and NOTHING over a range of percent pregnant values.

purchased groups were essentially guaranteed not to contain bred animals. Strategy NOTHING yielded higher returns 95% of the time only when pregnancy rates were below 1.5% (live) or 0.5% (rail), where pregnancy costs were balanced by palpation and abortifacient costs incurred under PALABT. Above these levels net returns dropped rapidly if pregnant animals were retained in the lot (Figs. 126-4 and 126-5). Although break-even pregnancy rates between PALABT and NOTHING were 2% (live) and 1% (rail), economic risk associated with underestimating pregnancy rate was much greater than overestimating pregnancy rate.

For the two other strategies, information on relationships between pregnancy rates and net returns and on thresholds between decision choices provided guidelines for managing risk. Feedyards purchasing groups of heifers likely to have high pregnancy rates (≥49%) would be best served by implementing ABTALL. At these pregnancy levels, the information cost incurred through palpation did not improve decision making. For heifer lots, pregnancy rates at or below 36% for PALABT would be most consistently profitable, even with wide variability in other inputs. This threshold should be useful for producers because most lots of heifers have pregnancy rates lower than 20%.[4] Although net returns increased for ABTALL and decreased for PALABT as pregnancy rates rose above 43%, differences between these strategies in the 36% to 49% pregnancy range were small, making choice of strategy less critical.

These general rules provide helpful guidelines and could also be easily modified to give more specific guidance to individual producers by running the model with custom inputs.

Lack of clear advantage to any one of the three strategies over the entire range of possible pregnancy rates suggests exploration of possible two-stage approaches to management of pregnant heifers. Palpation of a statistically based subsample of the lot could estimate pregnancy rate as either above 49% or below 37%. If no pregnancies were detected among palpated heifers, ABTALL would be ruled out as the decision of choice, with PALABT expected to yield higher net returns. This would provide an alternative plan for feedyards acquiring heifers with unknown and highly variable pregnancy rates.

Although this type of dynamic, stochastic, simulation modeling has promise, there are also limitations.

Complexity and clarity must be balanced to create a useful tool. Decision rules extracted from simulation analyses are predicated on those baseline inputs and specific scenarios examined. Selection of different defaults could change resulting recommendations. Inputs may be enhanced by incorporating real aspects of uncertainty and variability through probability distributions determined from data, literature, or expert opinion. But artifact can be introduced through inappropriate probability distributions. Recognition of variables that influence model predictions is an important step but may not lead to greater ability to understand biologic processes or make reasonable interventions. It is crucial that patterns observed in simulations be filtered through knowledge of biologic and production systems, if models are to be integrated into industry decision making.

Innumerable other feedyard management scenarios could be evaluated. These range from defining specific sets of inputs applicable to a single yard, time frame, and decision choice, to examining more generalized issues. Producer risk tolerance could be incorporated by varying confidence intervals generated around differences in net returns. Options external to the feedyard for managing risk such as negotiating discounted purchase prices for heifer lots of unknown pregnancy status could be explored. For all these applications, modeling explicitly defined variables in a spreadsheet format assists both customized and generalized decision making and risk analysis. This provides a tool for enhancing profitability in feedlots by helping managers explore alternative programs to optimize animal health, well-being, and productivity.

CONCLUSION

Modeling of management strategies for pregnant feeder heifers allowed for evaluation of modeling and risk assessment as compared with traditional methods.[3] Inclusion of inputs as distributions allowed integration of uncertainty, variability, and evaluation of thresholds and best and worse case scenarios. Sensitivity analyses provided a means to identify points for intervention, as well as to recognize sources of uncontrollable variability. Decision thresholds were identified as starting points to help producers better manage pregnant heifers in the feedyard. However, the model itself provides the most flexible means of decision making and enhanced risk management.

References

1. Susser M, editor: *Causal thinking in the health sciences*, New York, 1973, Oxford University Press.
2. Horst HS, Dijkhuizen AA, Huirne RBM: Outline for an integrated modeling approach concerning risks and economic consequences of contagious animal diseases, *Netherlands J Agri Sci* 44:89-102, 1996.
3. Vose D, editor: *Risk analysis: a quantitative guide*, Chicheester, NY, 2000, Wiley & Sons Ltd.
4. Edwards AJ, Laudert SB: Economic evaluation of the use of feedlot abortifacients, *Bov Pract* 19:148-150, 1984.
5. Jim GK, Ribble CS, Guichon T et al: The relative economics of feeding open, aborted, and pregnant feedlot heifers, *Can Vet J* 32:613-617, 1991.
6. Clayton P, Lloyd B: *Cost to the packer*, Dallas, 1984, Proceedings of the Academy of Veterinary Consultants, pp 28-43.
7. MacGregor S, Falkner TR, Stokka GL: Managing pregnant heifers in the feedlot, *Compend Cont Educ Pract Vet* 19:1389-1407, 1997.
8. Stanton TL, Birkelo CP, Flack DE et al: Effect of abortifacient on open, individually fed finishing heifer performance, *Agri-Practice* November/December: 27-30, 1987.
9. Martin SW, Meek AH, Willeberg P, editors: *Veterinary epidemiology principles and methods*, Ames, 1987, Iowa State University Press.
10. Griffin DD: In *Veterinary Clinics of North America Food Animal Practice*, Philadelphia, 1997, Saunders.
11. Arrioja-Dechert A: In Bayley AJ, editor: *Compendium of veterinary products*, ed 4, Port Hurson, 1997, North America Compendiums.
12. Barth AD, Adams WM, Manns JG et al: Induction of abortion in feedlot heifers with a combination of cloprostenol and dexamethasone, *Can Vet J* 22:62-64, 1981.
13. Stanton TL, Birkelo CP, Bennett BW et al: Effect of abortion on individually fed finishing heifer performance, *Agri-Practice* January/February:15-17, 1988.
14. USDA: *Part I: baseline reference of feedlot management practices, 1999. USDA:APHIS:VS, CEAH, National Animal Health Monitoring System*, Fort Collins, Colo, 2000a, USDA N327.0500.
15. Feuz DM, Burgener PA, Holmon T: *Historical cattle and beef prices, seasonal patterns, and futures basis for Nebraska, 1960-2000*, University of Nebraska Cooperative Extension Institute of Agricultural and Natural Resources Panhandle Research and Extension Center, PHREC 01-21, 2001.
16. USDA: *Part III: health management and biosecurity in U.S. feedlots, 1999. USDA:APHIS:VS, CEAH, National Animal Health Monitoring System*, Fort Collins, Colo, 2000b, N336.1200.
17. Borcher GM, Woollen N, Clemens E: An evaluation of dystocia and the endocrine response to stress in the primiparous heifer and calf, *Nebraska Beef Rep* 1994, pp 17-20.
18. Bennet B: *The liability of the pregnant heifer*, Dallas, 1984, Proceedings of the Academy of Veterinary Consultants, pp 14–27.
19. Woolen TS: Using prostaglandins in feedyard heifers, *Anim Nutr Health* May:22-25, 1985.
20. Bennet B: Economic liability: the pregnant feedlot heifer, *Anim Nutr Health* May:5-8, 1985.

CHAPTER 127

Investigating Lameness Outbreaks in Feedlot Cattle

JASON OSTERSTOCK

Lameness remains a substantial cause of morbidity in the cattle feeding industry and is associated with substantial economic losses resulting from treatment cost, decreased productivity, premature marketing, carcass defects, and labor costs associated with addressing lameness problems. The Feedlot 1999 survey performed by the National Animal Health Monitoring Service (NAHMS) found that 1.9% of all feedlot cattle suffered from at least one lameness event during the feeding period.[1] Additionally, the incidence of bullers, which may also be associated with lameness, was 2.2% of all fed cattle. Estimates suggest that lameness accounts for 15% to 45% of all morbidity and 1% to 5% of all mortality in feedlots with larger feedlots generally associated with a higher incidence of lameness and yearling placements having a lower incidence of lameness than lighter calves. Average treatment cost associated with lameness was $7.68 (USD) per head treated among U.S. feedlots surveyed. Of equal importance to the industry are the welfare concerns associated with lameness in cattle. Many causes of lameness in cattle are associated with pain that alters the normal behavior of animals.[2] Therefore every effort should be made to intervene and provide relief early in the disease process.

Although there are a multitude of causes of lameness in cattle, there are a more limited number of common etiologies in feedlot cattle. The most common cause of lameness in feedlots is interdigital necrobacillosis (foot rot) caused by the bacteria *Fusobacterium necrophorum, Bacteroides melaninogenicus,* and *Dichelobacter nodosus.*[3] This disease generally manifests with inflammation and swelling of the interdigital space with varying extension of swelling from the interdigital space and coronary band up the distal limb. Often, a fetid exudate can be appreciated in the interdigital space. Potential sequelae to this infection include tenosynovitis in the flexor tendon sheaths and deep digital sepsis. This is probably the most familiar of all the causes of lameness in feedlot cattle and probably is overdiagnosed because of familiarity with the condition and the term used to describe it. Another infectious disease commonly found in fed cattle is septic arthritis. Although this can be caused by direct trauma to joints in cattle or extension from foot rot, the most common route of infection is hematogenous, particularly associated with concurrent or prior respiratory disease, liver abscesses, or vegetative valvular endocarditis. The principal pathogen associated with septic arthritis in feedlot cattle is *Mycoplasma bovis.*[4] The diagnosis of this organism has increased with increased awareness of its role as a pathogen and advanced capabilities for identifying the organism in culture and with molecular techniques. In Clark's[4] report among specimens submitted to a diagnostic laboratory from feedlots in Western Canada, 10% of all cases where *M. bovis* was isolated from pneumonic lung had concurrent arthritis and 70% of all arthritis cases were associated with pneumonia. Anecdotal information supports a potential association between bovine viral diarrhea virus (BVDV) infection and mycoplasma pneumonia and polyarthritis.[4] The immunosuppressive role of BVDV presumably contributes to the development of opportunistic mycoplasmal infections. A potentially emerging lameness etiology in feedlot cattle is papillomatous digital dermatitis, commonly referred to as *hairy heel warts,* associated with superficial infection of the interdigital space and heel with *Treponema* spp.[5] The disease is common in confined dairy cattle and may have been introduced into feedlot environments by fed dairy steers.

Perhaps the most common potential cause of lameness in feedlot cattle is laminitis; however, the disease is often subclinical and rarely presents as the primary cause of lameness. It has been implicated as a contributing factor in the development of subsolar abscesses and sole ulcers and has been shown to compromise the integrity and strength of the bovine hoof, particularly along the white line and the junction with the sensitive lamina. Intensively reared cattle are predisposed to laminitis largely due to the relatively high concentration of rapidly fermentable starches and low amounts of effective fiber in conventional diets.[3] This represents a physiologic trade-off between performance and ruminal physiology. Rapid fermentation of carbohydrates in the rumen induces a decrease in ruminal pH and compromise of the rumen wall, a natural barrier to bacteria and toxins. Although the exact pathophysiologic link between ruminal acidosis and laminitis remains unclear, it has been suggested that lysis of gram-negative bacteria in the rumen provides

a source of endotoxin that, when absorbed into the systemic circulation, induces vascular changes in the lamina of the feet because of vasoconstriction and venous thrombosis.[6,7] The compromise of circulation in the lamina leads to hypoxic necrosis and subsequent laminitis.

Traumatic injuries remain common in feedlots, likely because of the social interactions of confined cattle and the frequency of processing used in conventional feedlot systems. Bullers remain one of the most significant causes of injuries, some of which are severe enough to warrant euthanasia. Unlike the infectious causes of lameness discussed here, injuries more commonly affect the proximal limb with hip and stifle injuries accounting for up to 50% of reported injuries in some populations.[3] Traumatic causes of lameness provide an additional challenge in that advanced methods of treatment necessary for some injuries (e.g., fractures) are cost prohibitive in most operations. Salvage or humane euthanasia is often the only feasible option for these patients given their poor prognosis and welfare concerns.

Outbreaks of lameness in populations of feedlot cattle may be difficult to identify early in the process because lameness is a routine occurrence in feedlot cattle. Many of the common causes of lameness including foot rot, laminitis, and septic arthritis are endemic in these populations. The incidence of many of the most common causes will vary during the feeding period based on environmental conditions, time of year, and days on feed. The end result is a complex, but regular, pattern of lameness in feedlot cattle that occurs at a relatively stable rate during the feeding period. Epidemic curves can help to graphically display the historical occurrence of lameness events and serve as a baseline for what might be expected under similar circumstances. However, several curves must be considered simultaneously including number of cases by days on feed, numbers of cases by month of the year, and stratification of these curves by host factors including age or weight at arrival and sex.

Investigation of lameness outbreaks in feedlots should be systematic and needs to contain several steps common to all outbreak investigations. If an outbreak is suspected, the diagnosis must be confirmed followed by careful consideration of the case definition. The magnitude and extent of the outbreak must be compared with historical levels to determine if the incidence of disease exceeds endemic levels. Assuming the outbreak has been well defined by these steps, investigation of risk factors can be used to modify the diagnosis and identify opportunities for intervention.

Diagnosis of the cause of lameness observed in a perceived outbreak is one of the most challenging aspects of the investigation. Two diagnostic steps need to occur. The first is the diagnosis made by the pen rider or hospital crew member identifying an animal demonstrating lameness and assigning a diagnosis to the condition. As stated previously, there is a tendency for overdiagnosis of diseases that are common or associated with common terminology. Consulting veterinarians and feedlot managers must make every effort to develop training programs and protocols to assist in this initial diagnosis. Visual inspection to examine for superficial lesions, determine the distribution of swelling, and identify exudates in combination with palpation of the affected limb can allow an accurate tentative diagnosis to be made in most cases of lameness. Employees participating in the diagnosis of lameness should be encouraged to take sufficient time to make the correct diagnosis. For example, deep digital sepsis and interdigital necrobacillosis can both be characterized by acute onset of lameness, swelling of the distal limb, and exudate. However, careful inspection of the distribution of swelling and degree of lameness should allow these two conditions to be correctly differentiated. To assist accurate diagnosis, facilities should be available for safe and effective restraint of the animal and the ability to wash off and palpate the affected limb. Feedlot personnel may also be responsible for diagnosis of lameness on the basis of postmortem examinations. A thorough necropsy and familiarity with common lesions associated with lameness are extremely important in helping make the correct diagnosis.

The second diagnostic step that must be made is the confirmation of the etiology by the consulting veterinarian. This may include examination of acutely affected animals and postmortem examination of representative animals. Submission of diagnostic specimens for lesions identified on postmortem examination for culture or histopathology becomes particularly important when investigating an outbreak because of the necessity for a definitive diagnosis. If postmortem examinations are not performed or if the examinations performed are incomplete, substantial amounts of potentially valuable diagnostic information are lost. If infectious diseases are suspected, fresh and fixed samples should be submitted for organism detection and histopathology. Tissues routinely selected for submission should include sterile samples of synovial fluid from affected joints; biopsy sections from synovial capsules and tendon sheaths; biopsies from acute, characteristic skin lesions; and culture samples from exudates.[8] Some causes of lameness in cattle including *M. bovis* polyarthritis and papillomatous digital dermatitis will not be identified using routine organism detection methods and must be communicated as suspected etiologies to diagnostic laboratory personnel to allow appropriate test selection. It may also be necessary to submit samples for infectious agents indirectly associated with the lameness (e.g., BVDV) to assist identification of underlying diseases that may have contributed to the development of the lameness.[4]

In addition to inspection of acutely affected animals and postmortem examination, additional sources of information can be used to help make an accurate diagnosis. Evaluation of response to therapy may be useful in making a diagnosis. Assuming animals were diagnosed with the correct cause of lameness, failure to respond to recommended therapy may indicate the presence of organisms that often respond poorly to therapy such as *M. bovis*, the emergence of new infectious agents, or the development of resistance to antimicrobial therapy among the population of bacteria associated with particular causes of lameness including resistant strains of *Fusobacterium necrophorum* identified in cases on foot rot in dairy cattle.[3,9] Anatomic location of lameness will also assist in making the correct diagnosis. As stated previously, most infectious causes of lameness are associated with

the distal limb, whereas most traumatic injuries are associated with the proximal limb. Additionally, if the same limb appears to be affected in all of the animals identified in a suspected outbreak, recent processing may be contributing to the lameness. Trauma caused by an undetected defect in the processing facilities or poor animal handling may show this pattern of localization. Shoulder injuries have been reported to be common among animals moving through hydraulic chutes at a high rate of speed.[10] Inappropriate vaccine administration may also contribute to the development of lameness. This has been reported following vaccine administration in the hip and I have observed this with vaccine administration in the axilla.[11] The latter case presented as a herd outbreak of left forelimb lameness.

Once a tentative diagnosis has been made, a clear case definition must be formulated. This will allow for data collection to further characterize the outbreak including information from those animals that appear to be associated with this outbreak while excluding those calves that are experiencing unrelated lameness. The case definition should be restricted to clinical features of the case presentation and should not include information regarding exposure history, environment, or host risk factors. This information will be reserved for analysis of risk factors associated with the outbreak.

The underlying goals of an outbreak investigation are to identify opportunities to mitigate the current outbreak and design protocols to prevent future outbreaks. A key component to being able to achieve these goals is characterization of the risk factors associated with the outbreak. At this point in the investigation, we have made a diagnosis and defined the clinical features of those animals involved in the outbreak. To identify risk factors for the outbreak, one needs to compile information regarding the host, environmental, spatial, and temporal characteristics of these individuals and the onset of lameness. This information can be used to define some basic epidemiologic measures of risk for involvement in the outbreak. A simple measure often used in preliminary outbreak investigations is the affected proportion (AP). The AP is the proportion of individuals with a given exposure that have the outcome of interest. An example is a simple feedlot consisting of two pens with 100 animals in each pen (Table 127-1). A lameness outbreak is suspected and the case is defined. Pen 1 has 30 animals with lameness

Table **127-1**

Selected Epidemiologic Measures for Evaluation of Pen of Origin as a Risk Factor for a Lameness Outbreak in a Feedyard*

	Affected	Unaffected	Affected Proportion	Attributable Risk	Relative Risk
Pen 1	30	70	0.3	0.2	3.0
Pen 2	10	90	0.1		
Total	40	160			

*Affected Proportion (AP) = Number Affected/Total In Pen; Attributable Risk = $AP_1 - AP_2$; Relative Risk = AP_1/AP_2.

Table **127-2**						
Selected Epidemiologic Measures for Evaluation of a Hypothetic Lameness Outbreak in an 800-Head Feedlot*						
		Affected	**Unaffected**	**Affected Proportion**	**Attributable Risk**	**Relative Risk**
Pen	1	16	184	0.08		
	2	18	182	0.09	0.01	1.13
	3	45	155	0.23	0.15	2.81
	4	21	179	0.11	0.03	1.31
Pneumonia	Yes	72	61	0.54	0.5	12.9
	No	28	639	0.04		
Proximal limb	Yes	36	4	0.9	0.82	10.69
	No	64	696	0.08		
Mycoplasma	Positive	12	2	0.86	0.75	7.66
	Negative	88	698	0.11		
BVDV	Positive	8	7	0.53	0.42	4.55
	Negative	92	693	0.12		

*The incidence of lameness in this outbreak is 12.5%. Note that some animals are listed as "unaffected" even though they suffered lameness events, presumably because they did not fit the hypothetic case definition. Based on this analysis, one would identify higher risk associated with concurrent respiratory disease, proximal limb lameness (vs. foot), and isolation of either Mycoplasma or bovine viral diarrhea virus (BVDV) from diagnostic specimens. A much smaller effect is observed by pen. This information would support the role of *Mycoplasma* spp. Associated pneumonia and polyarthritis in the lameness outbreak may implicate concurrent BVDV infection as a contributing factor.

and pen 2 has 10 animals with lameness. The AP for pens 1 (AP$_1$) and 2 (AP$_2$) would be 0.30 and 0.10, respectively. From these proportions, one can calculate the attributable risk (AR) by subtracting AP$_2$ from AP$_1$ (AP$_1$ − AP$_2$ = 0.30 − 0.10 = 0.20 = AR). The AR represents the increase in disease risk associated with the exposure, in this case the pen of origin. One can also calculate a relative risk (RR) associated with this exposure given by dividing AP$_1$ by AP$_2$ (AP$_1$/AP$_2$ = 0.3/0.1 = 3 = RR). This RR indicates that the risk of this disease is three times greater for animals from pen 1. In a more realistic and complex scenario, these calculations could be completed for a multitude of host and environmental risk factors to identify those that are most likely significant for the outbreak at hand (Table 127-2). An additional factor to consider when interpreting risk measures is the prevalence of the outcome among the different strata of exposure. A potential risk factor could conceivably have a large RR despite small AP. In other words, it would be of limited use to design an intervention strategy for an exposure not associated with a significant proportion of the outcome of interest.

One of the challenges to efficient data analysis is data capture. Outbreak investigations, by definition, are rapid responses to newly recognized problems. Therefore it would be too late in most instances to try to collect all of the necessary data after the investigation has been initiated. This underscores the importance of recording individual animal health events, response to therapy, and outcomes for use later in data analysis. NAHMS data reported in 1999 indicated that 57.6% of feedlots always recorded a diagnosis and 18.4% never recorded a diagnosis.[12] Outcome of treatment was recorded with similar frequencies. NAHMS data also suggests that electronic records were predominantly used for economic analysis and performance data, whereas only 58.8% of feedlots considered records important for comparison with historical data.[1] Although there have undoubtedly been

advances in the use of computerized records systems with the application of electronic identification and portable computer systems, the implementation of these technologies for monitoring health data needs to continue to be developed and used in decision making. Further, there are numerous software programs available that will assist in epidemiologic calculations for measures of risk and these programs are becoming increasingly user-friendly.

Although the different aspects of an outbreak investigation have been discussed as separate entities here for clarity, it is important to recognize how many of them overlap. For instance, analysis of trends in disease over time and during particular seasons of the year would be important in both recognizing that an outbreak existed, as well as to determine the effect of these exposures to risk in the current outbreak. The outcome of an outbreak investigation might be able to identify that additional exposure risks were present. Alternatively, the outbreak investigation might indicate that the typical risk factors remained the most significant in the current outbreak. Regardless of the specific risk factors identified, the completed investigation should allow appropriate intervention strategies to be employed and modifications of existing preventive medicine programs to reduce the risk of future outbreaks.

References

1. *Feedlot '99 part III: health management and biosecurity in U.S. feedlots* (website): http://www.nahms.aphis.usda.gov/feedlot/feedlot99/FD99pt3.pdf.
2. Vermunt JJ: The multifactorial nature of cattle lameness: a few more pieces of the jigsaw, *Vet J* 169:317-318, 2005.
3. Stokka GL, Lechtenberg K, Edwards T et al: Lameness in feedlot cattle, *Vet Clin North Am Food Anim Pract* 17:189-207, 2001, viii.
4. Clark T: *Relationship of polyarthritis and respiratory tract pathogens in the feedlot*, 4-9, 2001.

5. Lubbers BV, Apley M: *A case of papillomatous digital dermatitis in feedyard cattle*, St Paul, Minn, 116-118, 2006, Proceedings American Association of Bovine Practitioners 39th Annual Convention.
6. Brent BE: Relationship of acidosis to other feedlot ailments, *J Anim Sci* 43:930-935, 1976.
7. Bergsten C: Causes, risk factors, and prevention of laminitis and related claw lesions, *Acta Vet Scand Suppl* 98:157-166, 2003.
8. Adegboye DS, Halbur PG, Nutsch RG et al: *Mycoplasma bovis*–associated pneumonia and arthritis complicated with pyogranulomatous tenosynovitis in calves, *J Am Vet Med Assoc* 209:647-649, 1996.
9. Guard C: Super foot rot. In Howard JL, Smith RA, editors: *Current veterinary therapy IV: food animal practice*, Philadelphia, 1999, Saunders, pp 693-694.
10. Grandin T: Handling methods and facilities to reduce stress on cattle, *Vet Clin North Am Food Anim Pract* 14:325-341, 1998.
11. O'Toole D, Steadman L, Raisbeck M et al: Myositis, lameness, and recumbency after use of water-in-oil adjuvanted vaccines in near-term beef cattle, *J Vet Diagn Invest* 17:23-31, 2005.
12. *Feedlot '99 part I: baseline reference of feedlot management practices* (website): http://www.nahms.aphis.usda.gov/feedlot/feedlot99/FD99Pt1.pdf.

CHAPTER 128

Investigating Feedlot Respiratory Disease Outbreaks

LARRY C. HOLLIS

Respiratory disease in feedlot cattle is a common occurrence. In the most recent National Animal Health Monitoring Service (NAHMS) report, more than 14% of all cattle entering the feedlot were reportedly treated for respiratory disease.[1] The majority of bovine respiratory disease (BRD) problems are anticipated to occur within the first 30 days after arrival at the feedlot, usually as a sequela to the combination of events that occurred in the life of the animal shortly before and/or after arrival at the feedlot. The stresses of weaning; transitioning to and through the marketing channels; commingling; transportation to the feedlot; changing environment (not just from pasture to drylot conditions, but often including changes in range of daily temperature, humidity, solar radiation, wind exposure, dust, freezing rain or snow, elevation, etc.); being processed with a variety of vaccines, a parasiticide, an implant, and ear tag; possibly being castrated, dehorned, and branded; adapting to different feed types and water sources; establishing a new social order with unknown penmates; and dealing with a variety of strange vehicles and strange people on even stranger creatures called horses contribute to the development of physiologic changes within cattle. This stress allows previously innocuous bacterial inhabitants of the upper nasal cavity to proliferate, migrate to the lower respiratory tract, and cause disease in individual animals. This series of events is familiar to experienced feedlot operations, and the resultant BRD is normally anticipated once all risk factors are taken into consideration.

The problem arises when BRD occurs at an unexpectedly high rate or an unexpected time during the feeding period, or when treatment failures occur. When any of these situations arise, they can lead to great consternation and present a management crisis that sometimes leads to accusations and finger pointing. Where cooler heads prevail, they are the cause for critical investigation to determine (1) what is happening, (2) why is it happening, (3) what steps can be undertaken to correct the current situation, and (4) what can be done to prevent a similar recurrence in future groups of feeder cattle.

Investigating a feedlot respiratory disease outbreak is a process of looking through a series of potentially contributing or controlling factors. If one moves through the investigation in a stepwise fashion, it may help prevent overlooking some important piece(s) of information.

BE PREPARED

Preparation for investigating a respiratory disease outbreak actually occurs well before the initial crisis arises. The veterinarian should have an established working relationship with a veterinary diagnostic laboratory and be familiar with personnel, testing capabilities, sampling requirements, and normal turnaround time for samples submitted to the laboratory. The laboratory can serve as a vital resource, not only to perform the tests, but also as a source of well-educated colleagues to help brainstorm the situation. Having an established line of communication with appropriate laboratory personnel and incorporating them as diagnostic consultants can sometimes help in making sure appropriate tests and specialized handling requirements are considered, and it may even speed up the priority or rate of sample processing once samples reach the laboratory.

The next step is to have the equipment and supplies on hand that might be necessary in any disease investigation. Items such as necropsy equipment, sample collection supplies such as Whirl-Paks, 10% neutral buffered formalin, vacutainer tubes, blood collection equipment, tracheal or deep nasal swabs, tracheal wash supplies, special culture or transport media (viral and bacterial [anaerobic and aerobic]), pH strips, urine ketone and glucose strips, cooler and ice packs, and shipping containers are often vital to the success of any field disease investigation. Both digital still and video cameras may prove useful to document situations, lesions, or clinical signs, especially if they are unique.

GATHER THE PERTINENT HISTORY

The initial contact by feedlot personnel will describe the reason for their concern. As information about the cattle and situation is put together, a mental picture will begin to develop. Questions should move from general to specific. The normal starting point is a series of general questions, usually starting with asking about the region of the country where the cattle originated. The experienced feedlot veterinarian knows that a semiload of cattle purchased through an order buyer in a particular state may be made up of cattle originating from up to 40 different farms located in 10 different states. The "origin" just happens to be the home base for the order buyer who assembled the load. Gathering this type of history helps the veterinarian determine that the cattle may have come from an area where cattle are commonly mismanaged or undermanaged, a mineral-deficient area, an area where tall fescue frequently creates a toxicity problem, or where internal or external parasitism may be a major contributing factor.

Specific history of the cattle should be obtained. What is the age, sex, quality, and origin of the cattle? How were the cattle purchased or supplied to the feedlot—ranch/farm of origin, video auction, local auction barn, stocker or backgrounding operation, order buyer? If cattle were from multiple origins, how long did it take to put the load together? From which states were cattle assembled? Were cattle fresh at the time of purchase? Were cattle preconditioned? What products, procedures, and timing were included in any preconditioning program? Was anything requested to be done to cattle at an order buyer facility (e.g., castrated, dehorned, vaccinated, mass medicated, individuals treated for illness)? Were any things done that were not requested or anticipated before shipment? Were the trucks clean before the cattle were loaded? When did the trucks load up and leave for the feedlot? What was the distance between the origin and the feedlot? How long were the trucks en route? Did the trucks encounter any delays? Answers to these questions help develop the mental picture further and provide additional insight into the overall situation.

Arrival history at the feedlot should then be obtained. What time of day/night did the trucks arrive? Did a qualified person watch the cattle unload from the trucks? Did the cattle match the description of the order from a health status and freshness appearance, as well as number, sex, quality, etc.? Were there dead cattle on the truck or cattle that were obviously sick as they unloaded from the truck? What did the cattle do when they were placed in the receiving pen—explore the pen, search for feed and water, or lay down and rest? Did the cattle appear dehydrated? Were the cattle bawling? How much did the cattle shrink from payweight at the point of origin to the inweight at the feedlot? Were answers based on memory, or were these items routinely recorded for each set of cattle received at the feedlot? Again, answers to these questions provide additional insight.

Processing history should be obtained next. How long were the cattle rested between arrival at the feedlot and processing? Were backtags removed to see if the amount of hair retained on the backtag matched the amount of hair missing from the spot where the backtag was removed? Which vaccines were administered and what procedures were conducted during processing? How were the vaccines handled from the time of purchase until the actual time of administration to the animals? Were observations made for sick cattle before and during processing? Were temperatures taken as animals were being processed? Were any delays encountered during processing? Were cattle mass medicated and, if so, with what product and dose? Has the processing crew experienced problems in the past? Were new personnel working on the processing crew the day the problem cattle were processed? Were serial numbers recorded for products administered, as well as the name of the individual administering each product? Were answers based on memory, or were these items routinely recorded for each set of cattle processed at the feedlot? All of these answers lead to more insight.

Transitioning to feed history should be obtained. What is the general history of this feedlot's ability to mix rations properly and deliver the correct ration to the correct pen of cattle on a timely basis? Were there any problems getting the cattle started on feed? How does this feedlot transition cattle from starting ration to finishing ration? Which ration step were the cattle on when the respiratory outbreak started? If the problem occurred later in the feeding period, were there any problems getting the cattle to step up through the intermediate rations to the top ration? Were there any feed-related problems at any time before the time the respiratory outbreak occurred?

Time and location history should be obtained. Is there only a single pen or several groups of cattle affected? Is it a generalized problem or localized to a specific area within the feedlot? Is there a pattern in the age, sex, or arrival time of affected cattle? Is the affected section of the feedlot served by a specific treatment facility? Did the problem arise following a weekend, holiday, or major social event when feedlot employees might have been preoccupied? Are there new pen riders or new members of the treatment crew? How well do they know their jobs? Has the veterinarian observed them doing their jobs?

STOP, LOOK, AND LISTEN

An onsite visit is always desirable and often required to determine what is happening. Unless a veterinarian has trained the people he or she is talking to and knows their capabilities and limitations, he or she should resist the temptation to try to diagnose the situation by long distance. Most well-trained feedlot personnel are honest with themselves and know when they are seeing something out of the ordinary. However, they sometimes panic if they are surprised by an unexpected outbreak. The veterinarian should listen to what they have to say, then go look for himself or herself. What one hears over the phone and what one encounters in person are sometimes different.

The veterinarian should observe the cattle in question. He or she should look at the remaining cattle in the problem pen(s), first from a distance, then walk through the pen to look at individual animals and pen conditions, listen for abnormal respiratory sounds, and check for abnormal odors. If the veterinarian has trouble seeing the problem, he or she can have the pen rider show which animals fit the problem encountered or explain what was observed. Next, the veterinarian should look at problem cattle in the sick pen or hospital area, looking and listening to cattle that are currently being treated. He or she should check the treatment records, looking especially at recorded temperatures and to determine if the recommended treatment regimen is being followed. The lungs of typically affected animals should be auscultated.

The veterinarian should talk to the people: the processing crew, pen riders, treatment crew, feed truck drivers, and others who work directly with the cattle. This should not be done in the presence of management personnel. Ask them what they noticed. One may be surprised what can be learned from the lowest-paid employee on the feedlot.

SAMPLING

The veterinarian should sample live animals. The preferable animals for sample collection are acutely affected, recently selected live animals exhibiting typical symptoms of the respiratory disease problem in question. Samples should be collected before any antibacterial or symptomatic therapy. When collecting samples for culture purposes, laryngeal swabs or tracheal washes often provide samples with fewer contaminants than deep nasal swabs, which in turn have fewer contaminants that shallow nasal swabs. Blood for virus isolation and serology and other body fluids should be collected at this time. Unneeded samples can always be thrown away later.

The veterinarian should necropsy dead animals. The ideal animal to collect necropsy samples from would be an untreated animal that died shortly before the necropsy; however, any dead animal from the problem group will have a story to tell. Perform a *complete* necropsy, looking for any lesions or indicators of problems in other body systems that may have contributed to

the respiratory problem observed (e.g., systemic salmonellosis, *Histophilus somni* lesions in heart or brain). Observe the entire respiratory tract including nasal passages, trachea, and lungs. Observe the pattern of changes in the lungs including the color, weight, texture, and lobes affected. Check for the presence of verminous pneumonia. Collect a complete set of fresh tissue samples for bacterial and viral culture and formalin-fixed tissues for histopathology. Collect and retain samples of any abnormal fluids. Samples should be submitted to the diagnostic laboratory in a timely fashion, which often means being hand-carried to the laboratory on the day of collection. If in doubt, and fresh dead cattle are available, the veterinarian may want to send one or several intact animals to the laboratory for necropsy.

WHEN THINGS DO NOT ADD UP

When things a veterinarian is seeing do not add up mentally, he or she should dig deeper. Several consulting veterinarians have encountered situations where processing or treatment records were being falsely completed by feedlot personnel to cover up the theft of biologic or pharmaceutic products from the feedlot. When these products were diverted from use in the cattle, disease outbreaks or "treatment" failures occurred. Keeping products under lock and key, recording the serial numbers, checking these products out to the processing and treatment crews, and requiring them to check the empty bottles or containers back into the office where the serial numbers were rechecked, caused theft to go down and respiratory (and other) disease problems to improve.

In a somewhat similar situation, treatment records were being falsified to cover up the fact that the person in charge of treating sick cattle did not like the consultant's treatment regimen and chose instead to use his own favorite program. Because the individual "dry labbed" treatment records to indicate he was following the consultant's recommendations, his paperwork always looked correct. Reconciling product inventories against reported use and hiring an undercover agent to work with the treatment crew and document the falsified records were tools used to determine the reason behind the treatment failures experienced in this case.[2]

In another situation, a feedlot had been experiencing an unusually high frequency of injection-site abscesses. Feedlot management told the processing crew to clean up the problem, but gave no specific directions for how it was to be accomplished. Shortly thereafter, the feedlot started experiencing problems that were thought to be a vaccine failure caused by a series of laboratory-diagnosed infectious bovine rhinotracheitis (IBR) problems. When feedlot records were evaluated, the problem was not consistent across all pens processed with the same vaccine. When the sequence of processing was evaluated, it became obvious that pens of cattle processed early in the day were not having any IBR problems. Pens of cattle processed later in the day experiencing an increasing percentage of IBR problems directly correlated to the lateness of the hour when they were processed. When the entire processing procedure was observed, the cause became apparent. The crew had realized that their sanitation problems became steadily worse as the day progressed. As one potential solution, they decided to mix all modified live vaccines at the start of the day when everything was clean to prevent possible contamination during mixing later in the day. The vaccine obviously became more inactivated as the day grew longer. Changing their reconstitution procedures solved the IBR problem.[3]

In a different type of situation, a pen rider was making additional money by training horses for other people and riding them in the feedlot as he did his daily job. Management started noticing spikes in respiratory death losses in pens he was checking. Closer consideration suggested that these spikes correlated to the time when he started working with each new horse. Closer observation of this individual's work routine revealed that he initially spent more time in the pen teaching each new horse to rein than he did looking for sick cattle. His horseback activities would actually stir up the cattle in the pen, interfering with his ability to identify sick cattle when he finally started looking for them. Discontinuing the practice of allowing non–employee-owned horses in the feedlot stopped these spikes in death loss.

CONCLUSION

Investigating respiratory disease outbreaks in the feedlot takes preparation, planning, training, an inquisitive mind, a systematic approach, and perseverance. It takes an understanding of both the science and management factors associated with respiratory disease. And, sometimes, it takes a little luck.

References
1. National Animal Health Monitoring System: Health management and biosecurity in U.S. feedlots, *Feedlot '99* Part III:22, 2000.
2. Miles DG: Personal communication, circa 1989.
3. Hill WJ: Personal communication, circa 1985.

CHAPTER **129**

Feedlot Therapeutic Protocols

MICHAEL D. APLEY

Written protocols are essential to achieve consistent and accurate application of therapy for diseases commonly encountered in feedlots. This section addresses the structure of feedlot therapeutic protocols.

Protocol sophistication varies depending on the autonomy of the individuals treating cattle. Regardless of how extensive a protocol is, it is important that all of the people who will be using it have ownership in developing the contents, monitoring results, and updating the protocol. In addition to benefits to the production facility, detailed protocols and records of education and agreement related to the protocols are important to the veterinarian in the case of a violative drug residue or regulatory inspection.

A complete protocol should include the following diseases.

- Respiratory disease
  - Low risk (expected morbidity = 10%, case fatality 1%-2%)
  - High risk (expected morbidity > 10%, case fatality > 2% up to 10%)
  - Heavy cattle within 30 days of harvest (withdrawal times are now a primary consideration)
  - Acute interstitial pneumonia (AIP)
  - Tracheal edema (Honkers)
  - Diphtheria (relatively rare in the feedlot)
- Gastrointestinal disease
  - Acidosis
  - Bloat
  - Coccidiosis
- Musculoskeletal disease
  - Footrot
  - Sole abscesses
  - Undifferentiated lameness (e.g., sprains)
  - Hairy heel wart (Strawberry footrot)
- Central nervous system disease
  - Polioencephalomalacia
  - Thrombolic meningoencephalitis
  - Listeriosis
- Miscellaneous
  - Rectal, vaginal, and uterine prolapses
  - Calvers and abortions
  - Anaphylactic shock

- Bullers
- Pinkeye
- Abscesses

Each disease section should include the following comments.

- Case definition
- Population to which this regimen applies (e.g., low or high risk for respiratory disease, heavy cattle within 30 days of harvest)
- Regimen
  - Dose
  - Route
- Volume per injection site
- Needle gauge and length
  - Frequency of treatment application
  - Duration of treatment application
  - Slaughter withdrawal time
  - User precautions
- Posttreatment interval—the period from the last (or only) application of the treatment to when the determination of success or failure is made. This is also the time when the animal is eligible for further therapy.
- Success/failure definition that is applied at the end of the posttreatment interval
- Disposition of treatment successes and failures
- Regimen for continued therapy of treatment failures (may include multiple additional success/failure definitions, regimens, and dispositions)

After developing the protocols, the next challenge is to establish communication that will ensure both consistent application of the protocols and a means for modification in the case of new ideas or inadequate response. Without consistent protocol application, subsequent attempts to evaluate treatment outcomes are misleading at best and may result in continuation of ineffective therapeutic programs. Protocols that are accurate and up to date serve to train new employees, as a template for receiving feedback from the personnel evaluating cattle for disease and administering treatments and as a documented record of prescribed procedures for examination by regulatory authorities. A 6-month review cycle for protocols is a sound practice. These reviews should involve all of the personnel who apply the protocols. Individual conversations with these personnel in addition to a group meeting may solicit input that would not be offered to the entire group. Distributing a written protocol in the absence of initial and ongoing communication will lead to failure. A cardinal rule for working with production crews is that if they decide to make the veterinarian look like an idiot, they will get it done.

After the protocols have been developed and implemented, it is time to start a program of routine evaluation of the outcomes. A good practice for evaluating protocol adherence is to routinely evaluate the treatment histories of mortalities. Additional information may come from periodic reviews of treatment histories of groups of cattle with high morbidity rates. Evaluation of protocols hinges on several key parameters.

- **Morbidity:** The break for low- and high-risk cattle is commonly accepted to be at 10% morbidity.
- **Case fatality rate:** Rates of 1% to 2% for low-risk cattle and 3% to 5% (up to 10% in severe challenges) for high-risk cattle are typical.
- **Time from initial treatment to death:** Animals that die within 48 to 72 hours of initial therapy for infectious bovine respiratory disease are typically considered to be a result of the therapy being administered too late in the disease process.
- **Treatment success rate:** This characterizes the percent of cattle treated for a disease that do not die or require further treatment during the feeding period. Success rates of 65% to 85% are commonly encountered. Rates of 50% or less indicate definite problems in treatment response, whereas rates approaching 100% raise questions as to the rigor of the selection process for therapy.
- **Relapses or retreats:** These are cattle that were initially characterized as a treatment success but required further therapy for the same disease during the feeding period. These are typically considered to be cattle requiring additional therapy within 21 days of the initial therapy.
- **New episodes:** By convention, cattle requiring additional therapy for the same disease more than 21 days after the first therapy are considered to be a new episode of the disease as opposed to a relapse of the initial episode. This time frame is by convention and I am not aware of any data to support this cutoff.

Through routine evaluation of records resulting from consistently applied protocols, the veterinarian can establish typical performance parameters for a production site and the different sources of cattle encountered at that site. This then serves as a basis for comparison with other sites and past performance.

Other protocols related to therapy include preventive protocols (e.g., vaccination, mass medication criteria); necropsy protocols; and mechanisms for checking withdrawal times before shipment. Some computer record systems have mechanisms for checking withdrawal times on cattle lots before shipment. Other systems require manual record examination to make sure all cattle are clear of withdrawal time requirements before shipping. Whatever the method, this check should be performed before cattle go on the trailer. In my experience, one of many causes for a really bad day includes finding an animal with a withdrawal time still in effect as the truck heads to the processing facility.

Controlling therapy in a feedlot requires consistently addressing the correct diseases with the right regimens and then following up with evaluation of the outcome. For this approach to work, the people observing and treating the cattle must have ownership in all of the steps. The system will break down quickly without recurring communication. After all, protocols are just a method for managing the application of sound therapeutic principles through people.

CHAPTER 130

Feedlot Hospital Management

DANIEL U. THOMSON

The management of the hospital system is the center of all animal health programs for cattle on feed. Cattle suffering from respiratory disease, lameness, digestive upsets, and other conditions commonly wind up in the feedlot hospital setting. Little to nothing has been published on management of hospital systems in a cattle feeding operation. The employees working in the hospital setting are important to the overall health program. This chapter focuses on theories associated with managing sick or injured cattle in a feedlot hospital along with concepts for training feedlot employees.

HANDLING OF SICK CATTLE

Cattle handling and management is probably one of the most overlooked areas of animal health programs. Getting the sick cattle from the home pen to the hospital with low stress is crucial for treatment success. Sick cattle should walk, not run, to the hospital facility. In some instances, feedlot managers have found that hauling cattle from the alley to the hospital may be warranted to decrease stress of cattle suffering from bovine respiratory disease complex.

In larger feedyards, sick cattle may arrive at the hospital before the animal caregivers are available to diagnose and treat them. If cattle have to wait, it is recommended that a comfortable holding pen be available. The holding pen should have a source of water, shade, and a wind break to give comfort to the sick cattle. These holding pens have continuous cattle, horse, and people traffic daily. This causes erosion of the pen floor and the low spots become wet during precipitation events. Keeping these areas as dry as possible is important so that sick cattle have a place to lie down or rest while they are waiting for attention at the hospital.

Pull tickets serve an important piece of communication between hospital and pen riding crews. The pull tickets inform the hospital employees of the individual animal's lot number, pen number, animal number, reason for pulling, and the severity of the clinical signs in the home pen. Pull tickets aid the hospital employees by describing how the animal looked before removal from the home pen and placed in a commingled hospital holding pen. This process also enhances proper diagnosis and treatment of cattle suffering diseases or injuries (e.g., lameness, bulling) that are hard to visualize once the cattle are in the chute.

Moving cattle from the holding pen to the squeeze chute has to be delicate. Good facilities and cattle handling promote less stress when treating sick cattle. Cattle should not be left in the crowding tub or box. Only bring as many cattle to the tub or box as will fit in the snake at that given time. Another problem with moving cattle to the squeeze chute is filling the tub too full. When the tub is too full, the weak cattle will go down and can be trampled by the larger animals. Also, overcrowded tubs can decrease the ventilation to cattle that already have decreased respiratory capacity because of bronchopneumonia.

Downed animals are not easy or pleasant to deal with in the hospital setting. Downed cattle can be scared and therefore aggressive. Animal caregivers should approach these cattle with caution. All downed cattle should have access to feed, water, and shelter without exceptions. If a calf does not show improvement, it should be humanely euthanized. Also, not only is it unethical to drag a downed animal, it is against the law.

SANITATION IN THE HOSPITAL SETTING

Sanitation is probably important in feedlot hospital systems. Improper sanitation of facilities, convalescent pens, water tanks, and equipment can result in nosocomial infections in cattle and zoonotic illnesses in feedlot employees. Bacterial and viral infections can be caused by improper sanitation.

Bacterial infections not associated with direct cattle-to-cattle transmission are thought to be due to environmental contaminants such as *Escherichia coli* and *Salmonella* in a hospital system. Hancock[1] found that improper sanitation of equipment such as balling and drench guns increased the sickness and death loss in feeder cattle. This study found that cattle exposed to the hospital system had a high prevalence of *Salmonella* infection, whereas cohort calves not taken to the hospital had zero prevalence. The authors also found that *Salmonella* prevalence increased the longer cattle stayed in the hospital system.

Many viruses can cause illness in feeder cattle (e.g., IBR, BVD, BRSV). Most viruses do not survive if exposed in the environment. The effects of BVD virus have been researched extensively in feedlot operations.[2-4] Niskanen and Lindberg[5] ran a series of experiments to better understand the possibilities of environmental contamination caused by BVD virus. The first experiment looked at taking the nasal secretions from a calf persistently infected (PI) with BVD virus. They smeared the nasal secretions on the rubber surface of a vaccine bottle (Trichophyton vaccine) where a needle would be injected to draw a dose. They allowed the bottle to dry until the nasal secretions were undetectable. They then placed the bottle at room temperature for 80 minutes. A noncontaminated bottle of the same vaccine was used as a control.

The researchers then drew the vaccine through the contaminated area on the bottle and subsequently vaccinated two calves that were sero-negative for BVD virus. One calf housed in a separate room was vaccinated with the control vaccine. Both calves vaccinated with the contaminated bottle of fungal vaccine were sero-positive for BVD virus 21 days postvaccination. One of the two calves vaccinated from the contaminated bottle was viremic for BVD 7 days postvaccination. The calf vaccinated from the control bottle was neither viremic nor sero-positive for BVD during the study.

Next, Niskanen and Lindberg[5] looked at the ability of BVD virus to infect cattle in the environment. They conducted two experiments where PI BVD calves were placed in a pen for 1 week. Calves sero-negative for BVD were introduced 2 hours (Experiment 1) and 4 days (Experiment 2) after the PI BVD calves were removed from the pen. Two of the three BVD-negative calves sero-converted to BVD virus and were also viremic within 10 days after being introduced to the pen 2 hours after removal of the PI BVD calves. None of BVD-negative calves sero-converted or became viremic with BVD virus when introduced to the pen 4 days after the PI BVD calves were removed.

These experiments are relative to our understanding of biosecurity issues surrounding viral pathogens and feeder cattle. Hospital pens are rarely empty for 4 days. Cattle are constantly added and removed from these pens with little regard to home pen origination. Also, before arrival at the feeding facility, cattle are commingled in sale barns and order buyer stations. Many times these calves have naive immune systems and the calves are not vaccinated before entering the marketing channels. The control of viral pathogens and protection of our calf crop must start at the herd of origin.

EQUIPMENT

Equipment used to treat cattle needs to be sanitary. At the end of each day, crews need to take the time to clean the equipment before storage and the next day's usage. Needles, syringes, drench guns, balling guns, and other equipment need to be properly cleaned to decrease the chance of iatrogenic infections in the hospital system.

Needles penetrate the skin of cattle to deliver pharmaceuticals and biologicals. Needles need to be changed every 10 to 15 head of cattle when administering treatments. In between usage, needles need to be cold sterilized with chlorhexidine and a sponge. Also, one should be careful to never inject a used needle into a bottle of antibiotics. A new needle can be placed in the rubber stopper of the bottle or the plastic tip of the syringe can be placed through a hole in the rubber stopper after initially punctured by a new needle. Needles should be disposed in a designated container and never discharged in the general trash.

Syringes are used daily to make injections in the hospital system. Some feedyards use disposable syringes and change the syringes as often as they do needles. Disposable syringes should definitely be disposed at the end of the day. Some feedyard hospital crews use syringes that are not disposable. The daily care of these syringes is important in preventing localized and systemic infections in cattle. Griffin[6] has outlined the proper method for cleaning syringes at the end of the working day. First, the outside of the syringe should be scrubbed with a brush, soap, and water. At a minimum, syringes should be flushed with clean tap water numerous times. The inside of syringes can be heat sanitized by pulling water (without soap or disinfectants) into the syringe and heated for 5 minutes in the microwave through the syringe for a minimum of three cycles. Malfunctioning syringes should not be used; one should fix them or dispose of them.

HOSPITAL PEN MANAGEMENT

Cattle Comfort

The main reason why hospital pens systems fail is because the pens and overflow of sick cattle are not thought out when the facilities are being built. These pens are often built too small and subsequently become overcrowded. Also, many of the feedyard hospital systems were built with the yearling cattle (not calves) in mind. Therefore they never anticipated the number of pulls that can be seen daily when calves hit the operations in the fall. Hospital pens need to offer at least 150 to 200 sq ft per head. Feeding pens adjacent to hospital pens need to be made available for hospital overflow during times of high cattle turnover.

Cattle also need protection from the environment. Heat, humidity, cold, and wind can have negative effects on cattle that are trying to recover from respiratory disease. Cattle cool their bodies through respiratory evaporation. When their lung capacity is decreased as a result of respiratory disease, their ability to cool their bodies is decreased as well. In times of extreme heat it may be beneficial to supply shade (20 sq ft/head).[7] Also, during the winter, windbreaks for hospital cattle improve their comfort.

The pen floor maintenance is crucial. Manure needs to be hauled out of these pens on a regular basis. Also, care should be taken to remove low spots in the hospital floors because they will cause large water holes during the winter. Mapping hospital pens in the summer after a rain allows identification of low spots. This allows the crews to fill holes and build mounds to decrease moisture pooling in the fall and winter in the hospital pens. Bedding the hospital cattle is also important, but one should be sure to remove/change the bedding in a timely fashion or it could lead to a *Salmonella* outbreak.

Water Tanks

Water tanks in the hospital pen are a challenge to keep clean in a timely fashion. Cattle are constantly being added and removed from the hospital pen, which adds pressure to management to keep the water tanks scrubbed. Birds use the cattle water tanks as a drinking source and bathing area, which can contaminate the water tanks with bacterial pathogens. Also, the cattle in the hospital pen are there because they are sick or injured. No pen on the feedlot needs to have cleaner, fresher water than the hospital pen.

Hospital tanks should be washed every other day. Most feedyards set up a schedule in which half of the hospital water tanks are washed one day and the rest are washed the next. The use of bleach to clean water tanks does not improve the bacterial contamination for longer than 24 hours compared with just rinsing and scrubbing the water tanks.

Cattle Flow

Many methods are available to manage cattle flow through the hospital pens. Understanding cattle flow and when to return a calf to its home pen is important to the success of any animal health program. Three hospital management systems are discussed: (1) up and back, (2) two-day system, and (3) biocontainment system.[8] The first two of these systems are used on a regular basis in feedyards. The biocontainment system is used more in smaller operations and operations where all the cattle are owned by one entity.

Cattle are pulled, treated, and returned to their home pen without staying in the hospital system overnight in the up and back hospital program. This system eliminates hospital pens from the feedyard. A recovery pen is recommended for chronically ill animals. Another advantage of this system is that cattle do not miss ration changes and head counts are consistent for feed delivery. However, there are some negatives with this system. First of all, sick cattle do not always have the strength or will to compete with their penmates for food, water, or dry places to lay down. As mentioned before, some cattle are misdiagnosed as bovine respiratory disease (BRD) when they are suffering from acidosis. Acidotic cattle get a chance to eat hay or a lower concentrate hospital ration when the up and back system is used.

The two-day hospital system is described as cattle are rotated through the 48-hour hospital pen system before they are reevaluated for additional treatments or returned to their home pen. This system gives cattle a chance to rest and recover before competing with healthy cohorts. They also get a chance for shelter, fresh hay, and a low level of competition with penmates. The negatives are that an animal may miss a ration change and the head counts might not be consistent for the feed crew. Also, staying in the hospital system allows time for nosocomial infections.

The biocontainment system is a new system. Basically, it is an extension of the two-day hospital system. However, if an animal is treated twice, it never goes back to its home pen. New pens of cattle are built with animals that have all been treated more than once for BRD complex. This system is difficult to accomplish if there are multiple owners of cattle in the feeding facility, because of accounting principles. However, it does have some positive attributes when considering biosecurity, along with making groups of like cattle for marketing purposes.

Sick Cattle Nutrition

Sick cattle have decreased feed intakes.[9] Also, cattle with IBR infections have been shown to have decreased nitrogen retention compared with cattle that are healthy. Generally, it is thought that cattle nutrient requirements do not change as a result of stress or sickness; however, they require a more nutrient-dense diet to offset decreased dry matter intake during these times.

Many feedlots have four rations for feeding cattle at their facility. The rations differ in nutrient density and roughage-to-concentrate ratio. The first ration is generally a receiving-type ration that is usually around 60% to 65% concentrate and is more nutrient dense to get newly arrived cattle off to a good start.[10] Cattle are then transitioned from the first ration to the fourth ration, which is the ration that has the most energy for finishing the cattle as efficiently, both economically and biologically, as possible. As one goes from a receiving ration to a finish ration, the rations increase the amount of concentrate feed and decrease the amount of roughage. This allows cattle the ability to change the rumen flora and adapt to diets of little to no roughage to diets (90% concentrate or higher).

No data on the effects of feeding different nutrient densities or roughage levels to sick cattle have been published. Feeding hospital cattle poses logistical problems. The efficiency of the feedyard is dependent on the amount of time that the feed mill is running. Decreasing the number of rations and decreasing the number of cattle that need a special diet (diets other than a finish ration) improve the efficiency of the feed mill and the feed delivery team. Hospital populations are generally small compared with the total number of cattle on feed at a facility. The lack of research on sick cattle nutrition, coupled with the logistic problems of feeding such a small population, leads producers to use one of the four healthy cattle diets in the hospital pen.

Cattle generally get sick with BRD during the first 14 to 28 days on feed. Cattle are transitioned from the first diet after the pen is healthy. Although the pulls are slowing down, there are still cattle from the pen in the hospital system. Cattle are usually on a new diet for 5 to 10 days depending on their intakes before they are transitioned to the next ration. Cattle in the hospital system run the risk of missing a ration step in the home pen depending on the length of stay in the hospital pen. Also, because of the similarity in clinical signs between acidosis and BRD, calves in the hospital pen system may need roughage to help improve rumen health. Considering home pen diet step up, when cattle are pulled to the hospital pen and the possibility of misdiagnosis, using the second ration in a four-ration program makes sense to feed to the hospital pen cattle. It decreases the chance of them missing a step-up ration while still having a large amount of roughage to help stimulate rumen function.

Animal Health Records

Animal health records can be used to improve a manager's or veterinarian's insight as to efficacy of sick cattle management successes or failures. Health records allow management and employees to improve a level of communication and separate bias from fact. Variables such as days on feed, morbidity, treatment success rates, mortality, causes of mortality, railer rates, and necropsy findings are associated with the animals.

Pen morbidity affects most other health parameters. Mortality and railer rates are correlated with morbidity rates.[11] Morbidity patterns in the feedlot setting are not generally a matter of when or why but more of a question of how bad. Morbidity patterns can most easily be explained by looking at the population of the feedyard between high- and low-risk cattle. Second, morbidity patterns can be explained by the number of days on feed that the cattle within each risk group have been in the feedyard. Many other factors such as arrival weight, weather patterns, starter diet, and marketing stress also affect the morbidity of the feedyard. As the morbidity exceeds the human resources in the hospital system, the crews quit doctoring cattle and basically process sick cattle to get through their day.

The case fatality rate (CFR) is also a good method to evaluate both disease identification and treatment regimen. CFR is calculated by dividing the number of cattle treated and died by the number of cattle treated. Typically, the CFR is in the 5% to 10% range depending on the type and risk level of the animals. Case fatality rates can be biased depending on how many high-risk cattle have been recently placed on feed. If there has been a recent increase in morbidity, more cattle are being treated and the mortality resulting from the morbidity has not occurred. An increase in CFR could be due to many reasons including weather patterns, poor pen riding, cattle procurement practices, and not enough hospital employees. Rarely is CFR increased because of which antibiotic veterinarians use for BRD therapy. A low CFR (1%-3%) is usually due to treating too many cattle that are not sick.

The dead-to-pull ratio is calculated by dividing the total number of dead cattle by the total number of cattle pulled to the hospitals during a given period. This ratio should be between 10% and 15%. A dead-to-pull ratio of 20% could mean that personnel are not finding the cattle soon enough, not treating the cattle properly, or that the cattle are dying from something that is not treatable. A high dead-to-pull ratio can be expected during times of the year when mortality resulting from digestive upset is high.

Pull tickets are used to enhance communication between the pen riders and the doctors on why cattle were brought to the hospital. The use of treatment reports from the hospital should be sent back to the pen riders. This information will tell the pen riders what the examination of the cattle revealed and how the cattle were treated. This allows the pen riders to better gauge the sickness rates in the pens that they are riding. The treatment reports also keep both the doctors and pen riders on the same page, which is essential for a seamless cattle health team.

Necropsy is done daily by the hospital crew. The ability to understand why the cattle died and what treatments they received allows management to communicate with the crews to adjust their efforts. Necropsy data can be great teaching tools for crews and management. Likewise,

teaching necropsy to feedlot employees and management can be great teachable moments and a way for practitioners to build credibility with the crews.

SUMMARY

The hospital system in a feedyard takes dedicated employees with compassion for cattle. None of the epidemiology, designs, statistics, and theories can replace good people who know cattle and know how to work. It is hoped that this chapter has shed some light on a subject about which not much has been written. Communication, sanitation, good cattle handling, cattle flow, cattle comfort, bunk management, and many other management issues outweigh any decision on antimicrobials. However, it is difficult to read a four-color advertisement in a trade magazine or get a paid trip to discuss sanitation in the feedyard when no one sells it.

References

1. Hancock DD: Case Study: Salmonella outbreak in the feedyard. Summer Conference, Texas A&M University, College Station, Texas, 1999.
2. Loneragan GH, Thomson DU, Montgomery DL et al: Prevalence, outcome, and animal-health consequences of feedlot cattle persistently infected with bovine viral diarrhea virus, *J Am Vet Med Assoc* 226:595-601, 2005.
3. O'Connor AM, Sorden SD, Apley MD: Association between the existence of calves persistently infected with bovine viral diarrhea virus and commingling on pen morbidity in feedlot cattle, *Am J Vet Res* 66:2130, 2005.
4. Stevens ET, Thomson DU, Lindberg NN: Effects of testing and removal of persistently infected bovine viral diarrhea virus feeder calves on morbidity and mortality of home pen-associated feeder calves, *Proc Am Assoc Bov Pract* 25, 2006.
5. Niskanen R, Lindberg A: Transmission of bovine viral diarrhoea virus by unhygienic vaccination procedures, ambient air, and from contaminated pens, *Vet J* 165:125-130, 2003.
6. Griffin DD: Injection site CD, University of Nebraska-Lincoln, 2003, Great Plains Veterinary Educational Center.
7. Mitlöhner FM, Galyean ML, McGlone JJ: Shade effects on performance, carcass traits, physiology, and behavior of heat-stressed feedlot heifers, *J Anim Sci* 80:2043-2050, 2002.
8. Thomson DU, White BJ: Backgrounding of beef cattle, *Vet Clin North Am Food Anim Pract* 22:373-398, 2006.
9. Hutcheson DP: Nutrient requirements of diseased, stressed cattle, *Vet Clin North Am Food Anim Pract* 4:523-530, 2006.
10. Galyean ML, Perino LJ, Duff GC: Interaction of cattle health/immunity and nutrition, *J Anim Sci* 77:1120-1134, 1999.
11. Renfro DC, Swingle RS, Thomson DU et al: *Effects of castration on arrival on male bovine health and performance in the commercial feedyard*, San Antonio, Texas, 2004, Plains Nutrition Council.

CHAPTER 131

No Loose Parts Necropsy Procedure for the Feedyard

DEE GRIFFIN

It has been said that the most important animal in a feedlot may be the one that dies. Although this seems inappropriate, no doubt valuable management information can be obtained from the thorough examination of each animal that dies in a beef feedlot.

Important Note: If animals are headed for rendering, they must be safe for byproduct consumption. Three classifications of cattle must not be allowed to go to rendering and should be identified so that a renderer does not mistakenly pick them up. These include cattle treated or euthanized with a drug that creates a residue (e.g., heat stable antibiotics, barbiturates), bovine spongiform encephalopathy or rabies suspects, and cattle that die from a chemical toxicosis. Cattle in this category should be buried or composted on the premise.

What is different about the procedure outlined in this chapter and the procedure taught in most veterinary colleges?

This chapter offers four changes that will improve the efficiency of feedlot necropsies. First, the procedure is designed to allow an "assembly line" (or unassembly line) flow. Second, the procedure is designed to minimize hide damage and loose or detached tissues that create a disposal problem for the feedlot. Third, the procedure is designed to make it easy to examine the central nervous system of each animal. Fourth, a necropsy findings check-off form is included to make it easy to record observations and incorporate them into a necropsy database.

EQUIPMENT

Knives. Never leave home without several sharp knives. Although there is considerable individual preference, a stiff-bladed knife 6 inches long is undoubtedly safer than a flexible boning knife for necropsies on cattle weighing more than 600 lb. Stiff boning and sheep-skinning knives are my preferred knife styles. Having several, all sharp, is important. Tips on sharpening knives can be found at http://gpvec.unl.edu/filesdatabase/files/feedlot/sharp1.htm.

Ax. One 32- to 40-oz sharp, single-bit ax is essential for examination of the brain. A 36-oz "boy's" ax is an outstanding choice. Double-bladed axes are unstable and do not provide a blunt side for breaking the cut edges of the skull away from the brain. The blade of a 48-oz ax is too large to make fine cuts along the upper edge of the cranium.

Steels. A ceramic rod, technically not a steel, work wonderfully. Two blade-straightening steels, one fine (smooth) steel, and one medium steel are useful. Steels should be used to straighten the fine edge of a sharp blade.

File. One flat file for sharpening the ax.

Fine emery cloth. A small oiled strip of fine emery cloth for dressing the surface of the steels.

Sterile syringes and needles. Ten-ml syringes and 20-gauge, 1.5-inch needles for collecting needle aspirates and for inoculating agar plates.

Butane lighter. Use a butane lighter for sterilizing the aspiration needle before using a needle to streak the agar plate.

Other standard veterinary necropsy equipment and supplies include leak-proof sterile tissue sample bags, 10% formaldehyde, and personal protection clothing.

SHARP KNIVES

Sharp knives take much of the work out of necropsies. Veterinarians spend more money trying to get and keep sharp knives than any other gross diagnostic item. Keeping a sharp knife is not simple, but it is not hard. The following list should be helpful:

1. Have many sharp knives with you (it is cheaper to buy knives in boxes of six). Knife suppliers include Hantover 800-821-2227 or KOCH 800-456-5624. Select stiff-bladed boning or skinning knives. A sheep skinner is my favorite.
2. Use a sharp ax to make your skin cuts. It will save your knife blade edge. A flat bastard file works great for keeping ax sharp. Get a *Real* sharpening tool such as Flap Wheel Knife Sharpener or a WEN Wet Stone Sharpener for your knives. Flap sanders cost about $250. The WEN sharpener costs about $40. Both will eat knife blades, but they will be sharp. TIP: Keep a thick blade angle ($\approx$15 degrees) and work the final edge to approximately 20 degrees. Another option is to let someone else keep your knives sharp.
3. Use the steel properly. Steels straighten, *not sharpen*, blades.

PROCEDURE

As tissues are collected, they are placed in the foreleg reflection. Do not cut your samples more than a half inch thick. All cultures are collected by aspirate.

Use the ax to pattern the cut for the head. Make two cuts behind the poll, two cuts across the face at the lateral palpebral fissure, and two cuts upper lateral skull connecting the face and poll cuts (Figs. 131-1 and 131-2).

Cut the skin free along the skull cuts. Using the blunt side of the ax blade, break the bones away from the skull. Cut dura and lift the brain out (see Fig. 131-2).

Using the ax, set the skin pattern by cutting the midline from the neck, along the abdomen, and behind the rear leg (Fig. 131-3).

Next, start skinning front to back approximately one third up the side. When you get to the rear leg, cut through the muscles until the hip joint is disarticulated and the leg will remain reflected (Fig. 131-4).

Reflect the foreleg continuing to skin the abdomen (Fig. 131-5).

Cut along the inside of the mouth, exposing the molars to age the animal (age: first [7-12], second [12-18], and third [24-36]). Lift out the larynx and trachea, and examine the esophagus, larynx, and trachea (Fig. 131-6).

Reflect the abdominal musculature.

Using the ax, cut along the distal costal junction. I sometimes use the ax to cut the ribs away from the spine. *Do not remove the first rib.* The first rib will hold the pluck in place, and the reflected ribs will serve as a table for the pluck during examination (see Fig. 131-5).

Cut the pluck free and reflect over the first rib (see Fig. 131-5). Examine the lung, heart, etc.

Next, cut the omentum free and lift the intestines out and fan over the abdominal cavity (see Fig 131-5). Examine the small intestine and associated lymph nodes.

Next, flip the intestines over to examine the large intestine (see Fig. 131-6).

Cut through the surface of the kidney and lift it out but do not remove it. Examine the bladder and rectum.

Examine the gallbladder and bile ducts. Cut the liver free from the diaphragm and reflect back over the rumen. Make 10 to 15 cuts in the liver and closely examine both the surface and cuts in the liver.

Examine the spleen by reaching under the edge of the rumen. Cut a small hole, approximately 12 inches, in the anterior rumen. Pull pillars through the hole and examine.

Examine the hock joint. Cut along the anterior medial aspect of the tibia exposing the fibularis muscle. Cut across the belly and reflect across the cavity of the tarso-crural joint.

FORM

A check-off form improves the efficiency, accuracy, and utility of data collection. You may feel uncomfortable when you first start to use a check-off form, but the advantage gained for data analysis is worth making a check-off form part of your necropsy technique (Box 131-1).

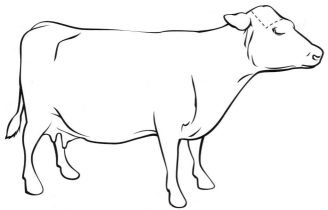

Fig 131-1 Animal with right side up and cranial cuts indicated with dash marks.

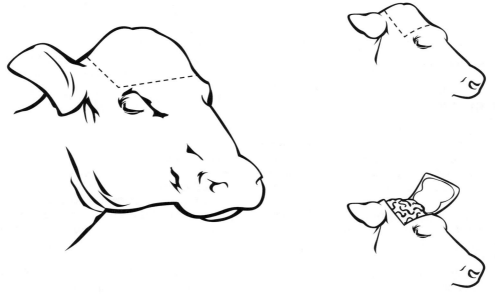

Fig 131-2 Cuts to be made in the cranium for brain removal outlined.

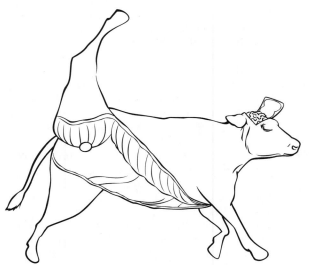

Fig 131-3   Left rear leg dissected and coxofemoral joint opened, with skin open along the midline toward the forelegs. Cranium opened, exposing the brain.

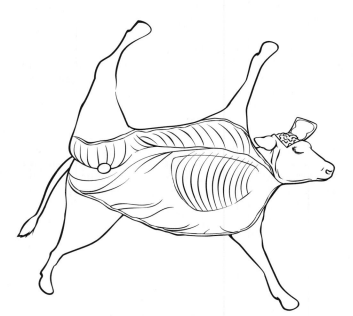

Fig 131-4   Continued dissection to reflect the foreleg.

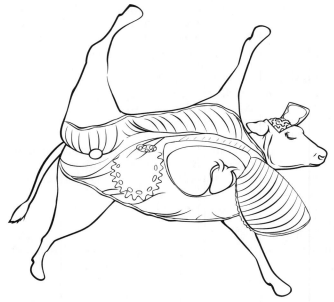

Fig 131-5   Abdominal cavity opened and ribs reflected forward to form a table for holding the lungs and heart after reflecting the pluck.

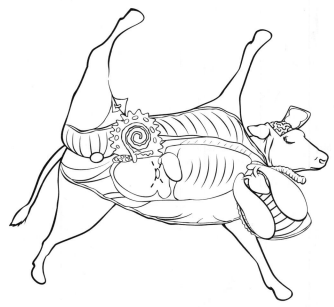

Fig 131-6   Pluck reflected for examination of both right and left sides of the lung lobes. Intestines reflected to expose the small colon.

FIELD MICROBIOLOGY FOR FEEDLOT CATTLE

Bacteriology is not simple and safety precautions must be taken. Starting cultures in the field improves the turn around and can improve the accuracy of diagnosis of some diseases. I take aspirates using a 10-ml syringe and 1.5-inch, 20-gauge needle.

After the necropsy, spray the aspirate on blood agar plates. Next, bend the 1.5-inch needle in a 45-degree angle and flame until sterile. Use the bent needle to streak the agar plate. Tape the edges of the agar plate. Double bag the plate and ship it to a diagnostic laboratory.

A limited number of bacteria would be of routine interest recovered from field feedlot necropsies. These include from the respiratory system *Mannheimia hemolytica*, *Pasteurella multocida*, *Histophilus somni*, and *Mycoplasma bovis*. From the digestive system *Salmonella* spp. and *Escherichia coli* would be of interest. The first three of the respiratory pathogens and the digestive pathogens listed are included in the microbial identification chart listed in Table 131-1. You will need the following identification tests: 3% potassium hydroxide Gram's, oxidase, indole, hydrogen peroxide, and the *Salmonella* Poly O Antiserum. An incubator can be made from an aquarium heater, light socket, thermometer, and ice chest.

Box 131-1

Necropsy Form

Date: _____   Pen/Lot & Animal ID: _____   **Samples taken** (yes or no)

Sex (S-H-B)   **Breed** (Brit-Zebu-Exotic-Dairy)   **Euth or Found dead** (Pen = rcv, hom, hsp, rcv)

Weight: (<4, 4-6, 6-8, 8-10, >10)   **Type stress** (Heat-Cold-Shipping-Weaning-Dust-Rain-Mud)
Previously Sick (N-Y: *<30 or >30 days*)   **H temp:** <30, 30s, 40s, 50s, 60s, 70s, 80s, 90s, >90
Days on last ration: *<7, >7, >30 days*   **L temp:** <0, 0s, 10s, 20s, 30s, 40s, 50s, 60s, 70s
Ration meds: A, O, D, R, T, L, C, M   **DOF:** 0-7, 8-30, 31-60, 61-90, 91-150, >150d

Pull Code _____   **RxAB** (EX, AS, MT, NF, BT, DX, OT, PG) // MM:(Y-N)

General Condition ☐☐
Fat, thin, fresh, stale ☐

Skin ☐
General hair loss ☐
Sinus injury or infection ☐☐
Subcutaneous yellow ☐
Mammary gland infected ☐

Head & Neck ☐
Tongue/Pharynx ☐
Veins distended ☐
Bad IV injection ☐
Dark, blood-filled neck

Esophagus ☐
Ulcers

Trachea ☐
Larynx lesion ☐
Trachea—red or bloody ☐☐
Trachea—yellow membrane ☐
Top thick & bloody
Froth or fluid in lumen ☐

Lung
Fluid around lung ☐☐
Lung collapsed ☐
Lung fluid filled ☐
Lung gas bubbles ☐
Lung dark & infected
Lung abscesses
Lung stuck to ribs ☐
Lung lymph node large & PO
% Affected (<⅓, ⅓-⅔, >⅔)

Heart ☐
Outside infection ☐
Inside infection ☐
Bloody spots on surface ☐

Intestine ☐
Content (white-yellow-red-brown) ☐
Small intestine
Large intestine
Obstructed ☐
Intestine lymph nodes ☐☐

Liver-Pancreas ☐
Rotten, big, yellow spots ☐
General yellow color
Abscess

Gallbladder ☐
Enlarged ☐
Bloody inside surface
Bile ducts-flukes

Adrenal glands ☐
Bloody spots ☐

Muscles ☐
Neck—bloody
Back & side—blood spots ☐
Hind leg—pale
Hind leg—injection site ☐
Muscle injury ☐☐

Reproductive ☐
Infected ☐
pregnant (1-9)

Kidney (Lf/Rt) ☐☐
Pale/dark ☐☐
Rough with scars or streaks
Bloody spots
Swollen ☐
Mushy rotten ☐
Bladder—red spots or infected ☐
Urine—bloody or pusy

Rumen Reticulum ☐
Free gas ☐
Froth ☐
Bloody spots on folds ☐
Ulcers ☐

Abomasum ☐
Thick folds ☐☐
Ulcers ☐
Thick with white spots

Spleen ☐
Swollen and full of blood

Joints & Bones ☐☐
Injury ☐
Infected ☐

Brain
Dark red and watery
Slight pus on the bottom
Small dark rotten areas ☐
Injury ☐

Cancer ... **Location** _____

| **Etiology:** ☐ | C = Circulatory ☐ | G = Genetic ☐ | I = Infectious ☐ | M = Metabolic ☐ |
| N = Neop ☐ | P = Parasitic ☐ | T = Trauma ☐ | Tx = Toxic ☐ | U = Unknown ☐ |

| **System:** ☐ | Gen Body ☐ | Skin/Subcutaneous ☐ | Muscle/Skeletal ☐ | Respiratory ☐ |
| Circ/Hem/Lymph ☐ | Digestive ☐ | Urinary ☐ | Repro ☐ | Nervous ☐ |

General Comments &/or Diagnosis: _____

Table 131-1

Feedlot Necropsy Microbiology Identification Chart

Name	Gram's Reaction	MacConkey	TSI	H₂S	Indole	Oxidase	Catalase	*Salmonella* Poly O
Salmonella	Negative	Colorless +++	K/A H$_2$S	Positive	Negative	Negative	Positive	Positive
Escherichia	Negative	Red/pink +++	A/A	Negative	Positive	Negative	Variable	Negative
Pseudomonas	Negative	Colorless +++	K/NC	Negative	Negative	Positive	Positive	Negative
Mannheimia hemolytica	Negative	Colorless delayed	A/A	Negative	Negative	Positive	Positive	Negative
Histophilus somni	Negative	No growth	No growth	Negative	Negative	Positive	Negative	Negative
Pasteurella multocida	Negative	No growth	A/A	Negative	Positive	Positive	Positive	Negative

Gram's reaction: stringy on 3% KOH = gram (negative); no reaction = gram (positive).
Oxidase and indole: color test (purple/dark blue) on white tissue paper (recheck at 48 hr).
Catalase: bubbles on 0.3% H_2O_2.
Salmonella Poly O Antiserum: agglutination = (+).

A, Acid; *K,* alkaline; *NC,* no change; *TSI,* triple sugar iron; *w,* weak.

Index

Note: Page numbers followed by f indicate illustrations; t, tables; and b, boxed material.